Rapid Reference to the *Exo*

Hints for Using This Formulary,

Table of Contents, p. xvii

Invertebrates, p. 1

Fish, p. 16

Amphibians, p. 53

Reptiles, p. 81

Birds, p. 167

Backyard Poultry and Waterfowl, p. 376

Sugar Gliders, p. 432

Hedgehogs, p. 443

Rodents, p. 459

Rabbits, p. 494

Ferrets, p. 532

Miniature Pigs, p. 558

Primates, p. 575

Wildlife, p. 616

Select Topics for the Exotic Animal Veterinarian, p. 636

Index, p. 665

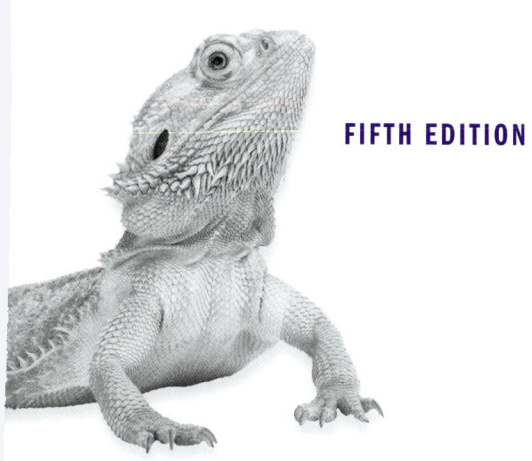

FIFTH EDITION

EXOTIC ANIMAL FORMULARY

Editor

JAMES W. CARPENTER, MS, DVM, DIPLOMATE ACZM
Professor
Zoological Medicine
Department of Clinical Sciences
College of Veterinary Medicine
Kansas State University
Manhattan, Kansas

Assistant Editor

CHRISTOPHER J. MARION, DVM, MPH
Marion Veterinary Consulting
Manhattan, Kansas

ELSEVIER

ELSEVIER

3251 Riverport Lane
St. Louis, Missouri 63043

EXOTIC ANIMAL FORMULARY, FIFTH EDITION   ISBN: 978-0-323-44450-7

Copyright © 2018, Elsevier Inc. All rights reserved.
Previous editions copyrighted 2013, 2005, 2001, and 1996.

No part of this publication may be reproduced or transmitted in any form or by any means, electronic or mechanical, including photocopying, recording, or any information storage and retrieval system, without permission in writing from the publisher. Details on how to seek permission, further information about the Publisher's permissions policies and our arrangements with organizations such as the Copyright Clearance Center and the Copyright Licensing Agency, can be found at our website: www.elsevier.com/permissions.

This book and the individual contributions contained in it are protected under copyright by the Publisher (other than as may be noted herein).

Notices

Knowledge and best practice in this field are constantly changing. As new research and experience broaden our understanding, changes in research methods, professional practices, or medical treatment may become necessary.

Practitioners and researchers must always rely on their own experience and knowledge in evaluating and using any information, methods, compounds, or experiments described herein. In using such information or methods they should be mindful of their own safety and the safety of others, including parties for whom they have a professional responsibility.

With respect to any drug or pharmaceutical products identified, readers are advised to check the most current information provided (i) on procedures featured or (ii) by the manufacturer of each product to be administered, to verify the recommended dose or formula, the method and duration of administration, and contraindications. It is the responsibility of practitioners, relying on their own experience and knowledge of their patients, to make diagnoses, to determine dosages and the best treatment for each individual patient, and to take all appropriate safety precautions.

To the fullest extent of the law, neither the Publisher nor the authors, contributors, or editors, assume any liability for any injury and/or damage to persons or property as a matter of products liability, negligence or otherwise, or from any use or operation of any methods, products, instructions, or ideas contained in the material herein.

Library of Congress Cataloging-in-Publication Data

Names: Carpenter, James W. (James Wyman), editor. | Marion, Christopher J., assistant editor.
Title: Exotic animal formulary / editor, James W. Carpenter, MS, DVM,
   Diplomate ACZM, Professor, Zoological Medicine, Department of Clinical
   Sciences, College of Veterinary Medicine, Kansas State University,
   Manhattan, Kansas; assistant editor, Christopher J. Marion, DVM, MPH,
   Marion Veterinary Consulting, Manhattan, Kansas.
Description: Fifth edition. | St. Louis, Missouri : Elsevier, [2018] | Includes index.
Identifiers: LCCN 2017031268 (print) | LCCN 2017032341 (ebook) | ISBN 9780323498036 (ebook) | ISBN 9780323444507 (pbk. : alk. paper)
Subjects: LCSH: Veterinary drugs. | Veterinary drugs–Dosage. | Exotic animals.
Classification: LCC SF917 (ebook) | LCC SF917 .C27 2018 (print) | DDC 636.089/51–dc23
LC record available at https://lccn.loc.gov/2017031268

Senior Content Strategist: Jennifer Flynn-Briggs
Senior Content Development Manager: Lucia Gunzel
Senior Content Development Specialist: Dee Simpson
Publishing Services Manager: Deepthi Unni
Senior Project Manager: Umarani Natarajan
Design Direction: Brian Salisbury

  Working together to grow libraries in developing countries

www.elsevier.com • www.bookaid.org

Printed in China
Last digit is the print number: 9 8 7 6 5 4 3

DEDICATION

This book is dedicated to the 40 (yes, 40!) interns and residents whom I've had the honor to train from 1991 to 2018, and who have brought great joy to my life and pride to our profession: Dr. Rob Browning (2017-2018), Dr. Louden Wright (2016-2017), Dr. Melissa R. Nau (2015-2016), Dr. Dana M. Lindemann (2014-2015), Dr. Christine Higbee (2013-2014), Dr. Katie Delk (2012-2013), Dr. Daniel V. Fredholm (2011-2012), Dr. Rodney Schnellbacher (2010-2011), Dr. Kristin Phair (2009-2010), Dr. Judilee Marrow (2008-2009), Dr. Kim Wojick (2007-2008), Dr. Julie Swenson (2006-2007), Dr. Gretchen Cole (2005-2006), Dr. Karen Wolf (2004-2005), Dr. Jessica Siegal-Willott (2003-2004), Dr. Jennifer D'Agostino (2002-2003), Dr. Adrian Mutlow (2001-2003), Dr. Nancy Boedeker (2001-2002), Dr. Robert Coke (2000-2001), Dr. Greg Fleming (1999-2000), Dr. Peter Helmer (1999-2000), Dr. Tama Cathers (1998-1999), Dr. Cornelia Ketz (1998-1999), Dr. Geoff Pye (1997-1998), Dr. Nancy Morales (1996-1998), Dr. R. Scott Larsen (1996-1997), Dr. Pilar Hayes (1995-1996), Dr. Cynthia Stadler (1995-1996), Dr. Ray Ball (1994-1996), Dr. Christine Kolmstetter (1994-1995), Dr. James K. Morrisey (1994-1995), Dr. Edward Gentz (1993-1994), Dr. Lisa Harrenstien (1993-1994), Dr. Janette Ackermann (1992-1993), Dr. Ted Y. Mashima (1992-1993), Dr. Sandra C. Wilson (1991-1992; 1992-1995), Dr. Craig A. Harms (1991-1992), Dr. Mel Shaw (1990-1992), and Dr. Mitch Finnegan (1990-1991).

I have always been inspired by them, learned more from them than they realize, and always valued their friendship. I am very proud of all they have accomplished and their contributions to exotic animal, wildlife, and zoo animal medicine.

This formulary is also dedicated to my wife (Terry), son (Michael), daughter (Erin Peterman) and her husband (Steve), and my three grandchildren (Kylie, Hayden, and Asher the Dasher) for their support throughout this project.

James W. Carpenter

DEDICATION

I dedicate this book to my wife, Landa Colvin-Marion, PharmD, and son, Evan, for their support and patience during this project. Landa provided invaluable insight from her area of expertise, veterinary pharmacy. Additionally, I need to thank Dr. James W. Carpenter who has been my mentor during veterinary school, a colleague upon graduation, and most importantly, a great friend throughout my veterinary career. I would not be the individual I am today without their support along the way.

Christopher J. Marion

James K. Morrisey, DVM, Diplomate ABVP (Avian)
Chief, Companion Exotic Animal Medicine Service
Department of Clinical Sciences
College of Veterinary Medicine
Cornell University
Ithaca, New York, USA

Kristie Mozzachio, DVM, CVA, Diplomate ACVP
Mozzachio Mobile Veterinary Services
Hillsborough, North Carolina, USA

Kurt K. Sladky, MS, DVM, Diplomate ACZM, Diplomate ECZM (Herpetology)
Clinical Associate Professor, Zoological Medicine/Special Species Health
Department of Surgical Sciences
School of Veterinary Medicine
University of Wisconsin
Madison, Wisconsin, USA

Julie Swenson, DVM, Diplomate ACZM
Associate Veterinarian
Fossil Rim Wildlife Center
Glen Rose, Texas, USA

Valarie V. Tynes, DVM, Diplomate ACVB
Premier Veterinary Behavior Consulting
Sweetwater, Texas, USA

Brent Whitaker, MS, DVM
Associate Professor
Institute of Marine and Environmental Technology
University of Maryland
Baltimore, Maryland, USA

Roy P.E. Yanong, VMD
Professor and Extension Veterinarian
Tropical Aquaculture Laboratory
Fisheries and Aquaculture Sciences
School of Forest Resources and Conservation
Institute of Food and Agricultural Sciences/University of Florida
Ruskin, Florida, USA

Foreword

The practice of exotic animal medicine is founded on a strong understanding of medical science. With confidence in one's knowledge of medicine, treating many different species is possible. It is absurd to believe that one should know all about every companion exotic animal one treats—so much so that if that were the case, veterinarians would never have even treated the first bird, snake, or rabbit patient when this area of veterinary medicine was in its infancy. As veterinary practitioners who treat exotic animals, we owe much to those who paved the way and revealed the challenging yet rewarding work that has become an accepted veterinary discipline. It was their confidence in their medical knowledge and abilities that allowed early exotic animal practitioners to push veterinary medicine into this new realm. With the information we have available today and the challenges faced by our patients, the question persists: "How did they do it?" There were no books to speak of, no Internet, and no veterinary associations. It was through dedication, collegial interaction, and meeting notes that the dissemination of companion exotic animal medical knowledge first occurred. The need to share and gain information through firsthand knowledge of exotic animal clinical medicine was the genesis of what has quickly grown into the widely recognized area of companion exotic animal medicine. Many influences have contributed to the growth of exotic animal medicine, including the continued consumer demand for veterinary services and an increasing interest over the years among young veterinary students who see both the challenges and rewards of treating these exceptional animals. Also, over the last 35 years, there has been an increase in the availability of published veterinary medical literature, the advent of Internet resources, the formation of veterinary associations, and specialty designations related to companion exotic animals. All of the contributions to the medical knowledge of exotic animal species during the last 3 to 4 decades have allowed many individuals to develop their interest in this area of medicine, who previously may have been reluctant.

Practicing medicine requires treatment of patients who are ill. This is a fact, and so is the fact that proper dosage and duration of medications should be used. As with any medication, there are adverse side effects. Often there are more potential adverse side effects with a medication than therapeutic benefits. Therein lies the basis of many doctors' decision to prescribe medications when the good outweighs the bad. Moreover, that is why there should be knowledge of an appropriate length of treatment. Again, when companion exotic animal medicine began, practitioners used personal communication and published case reports to determine appropriate dose ranges and durations of treatments. Often this information was extrapolated from other species, and possibly the exotic animal patient did not die from the treatment and may have even improved. Of course, all veterinarians knew this had to improve, and there was much to be done to make pharmacologic information more detailed and as verifiable as possible through structured scientific studies. As exotic animal practitioners, we have come a long way but still have a long way to go in this regard. We can extrapolate dosages between species from scientifically determined information, but it is known that this is done at the risk of providing an incorrect treatment dose. It is simply not possible to scientifically determine all of the correct dosages for the approximately 10,000 species of both birds and reptiles, as well as the numerous companion exotic mammals and other species that may be treated by exotic animal veterinarians. Consequently there have been formularies published in exotic animal medical books over the last 35 years that help provide a basis for prescribing medication to a patient. If a veterinarian treats all different groups of companion exotic animals, it is difficult and time consuming to get the most up-to-date information regarding drug dosages for these patients. Dr. James W. Carpenter saw this problem and in the 1990s decided to do something about one of the most important tools used by veterinarians treating exotic animals: the formulary. As editor, he published the first edition of the *Exotic Animal Formulary* (1996) and has subsequently edited three other editions (2001, 2005, 2013), as well as this fifth edition (2018). Since the first edition, the *Exotic Animal Formulary* has arguably become the most important source of information that a veterinarian treating these patients can own. It is quite possible that no other area of veterinary medicine has changed as quickly over time than pharmacology. Drugs are often used by practitioners treating exotic animals long before there is validation of a proper dosage or the effectiveness has been determined. Through the publication of new editions of the *Exotic Animal Formulary*, veterinarians' ability to have within grasp the latest information relating to the treatment of exotic animals has been maintained.

It is an honor for me to be asked to write the foreword for this seminal exotic veterinary text. The *Exotic Animal Formulary* is used on a daily basis in our veterinary hospital and is the "go to" book for students and veterinarians alike when determining a treatment plan for any animal species. The *Exotic Animal Formulary* also allows one to use their veterinary medical knowledge. The extensive drug tables may not provide an exact, scientifically determined dose for the species of animal being treated. One may need to extrapolate from the information provided for another species. There are often wide dosage ranges provided for the drugs listed, and the references may be associated with a single case report. Therefore it is incumbent on the user of this text to assess his or her patient and use the information in the *Exotic Animal Formulary* to determine whether the drug he or she would like to use is advisable and if so, based on the patient's condition, select a proper dose.

Never before has so much valuable information been published in a condensed text covering as many animal groups and species as the fifth edition of the *Exotic Animal Formulary*. In addition to the 295 drug tables that have the most current information and references (over 2400), there are many informative tables and charts at the end of each chapter. The information contained in the tables and charts includes biological information, therapeutic details to treat specific disease conditions, dietary recommendations, common venipuncture sites, and useful websites related to exotic pet practice. All in all the information provided in the fifth edition of the *Exotic Animal Formulary* will elevate the ability of veterinarians to practice exotic animal medicine.

The veterinary medical community, as a whole, owes a debt of gratitude to the 29 authors who contributed to this text and to Dr. James W. Carpenter for his vision and supreme effort to bring this work to fruition. The benefits of their work will be found in veterinary hospitals the world over as patients recover through the use of information provided by the fifth edition of the *Exotic Animal Formulary*.

Thomas N. Tully, Jr., DVM, MS, Dipl ABVP (Avian), Dipl ECZM (Avian)
Louisiana State University—School of Veterinary Medicine
Baton Rouge, Louisiana, USA
August 8, 2017

Preface

Welcome to the fifth edition of the *Exotic Animal Medicine Formulary!* As we know, the medical care of exotic pets has become an integral part of most companion animal practices. The *Exotic Animal Formulary*, fifth edition, therefore, was compiled to accommodate this rapid growth of exotic animal medicine. For this revision, 29 of the most recognized specialists in our field were invited to contribute; their role was to evaluate published drug dosages and related biologic and medical information and references, and to select those that would be most clinically useful and relevant to the practitioner.

Not only is this edition updated and expanded (now containing 295 tables), but we've added a section on "Backyard Poultry and Waterfowl," in addition to sections on invertebrates, fish, amphibians, reptiles, birds, sugar gliders, hedgehogs, rodents, rabbits, ferrets, miniature pigs, primates, and wildlife. The "Selected Topics for the Exotic Animal Veterinarian" has also been expanded and now includes information on compounding resources.

This book is not intended to replace existing medical resources or the use of sound medical judgment, but rather to serve as a guide in providing medical care to exotic animals. This formulary assumes that the reader has a reasonable understanding of veterinary medicine. For example, drug indications are generally listed only in unique situations. Supporting tables have been carefully selected to include those topics of major importance in clinical practice.

As in previous editions of this book, the selection of species, drugs, and other information used in this reference was based on an extensive review of the literature (over 2400 references are cited) and on our collective teaching and clinical experience. The book, therefore, is not intended to be all-inclusive, but rather to serve as a quick reference for the common questions and medical situations we encounter in clinical practice.

Unfortunately, relatively few pharmacokinetic/pharmacodynamic studies in exotic companion pets have been published. Until more pharmacokinetic, efficacy, and safety studies of the drugs that we use are conducted, most dosages used in these species are based on empirical data, observations, and experience.

This book is intended to be a practical, user-friendly, quick reference for veterinary clinicians, students, and technicians working with exotic animals. We hope that you find this formulary and accompanying tables handy to use and that it adds to the quality of the medical care you provide to your exotic animal patients. Because exotic animal practitioners face daily challenges to meet the pharmaceutical and clinical needs of their patients, our hope is that this book will be a valuable tool in helping meet these challenges.

James W. Carpenter MS, DVM, Diplomate ACZM

ACKNOWLEDGMENTS

This book would not have been possible without the invaluable assistance of many dedicated and hard-working people. Certainly, first and foremost, my appreciation goes to Dr. Christopher J. Marion, who, as the Assistant Editor for this edition of the *Exotic Animal Formulary*, provided editorial assistance, technical expertise, and personal encouragement. I am also greatly appreciative of the numerous contributors who unselfishly shared their expertise and gave of their time, and are largely responsible for the success of this book! I am indebted to Megan Cabot, Danielle Windle, Sarah Wilson, and Nichole Arbona for assistance in the preparation of this formulary; to Lea Pearlman and Amanda Wonn for assistance in preparing the Primate chapter; and to Dr. Butch KuKanich for reviewing the appendix on antimicrobial agents.

I also wish to thank all those colleagues, interns and residents, and veterinary students, both national and international, who encouraged me to prepare the *Exotic Animal Formulary*, fifth edition. It let me know that our efforts into preparing this book are appreciated by the veterinary community and provided a powerful incentive for me to continue working on this reference.

In addition, a special thanks to Dr. Bonnie Rush for her many years of strong support and encouragement for me and for our Zoological Medicine Service! And thanks to Dr. Roger Fingland for his role in strengthening KSU's zoo animal medicine program.

I also thank Penny Rudolph (a very special person and strong supporter of this "project"), Jennifer Flynn-Briggs, Umarani Natarajan, Courtney Sprehe, Dee Simpson, and Lucia Gunzel, our publishing team at Elsevier, for their patience and support, and to their commitment to this fifth edition.

James W. Carpenter

DISCLAIMER

The Editor, Assistant Editor, and the Contributors attempted to verify and double-check all references, dosages, and other data contained in this book. However, despite these efforts, errors in the original sources or in the preparation of this book may have occurred. All users of this reference, therefore, should empirically evaluate all dosages to determine that they are reasonable prior to use. The publisher assumes no responsibility for and makes no warranty with respect to results obtained from the uses, procedures, or dosages listed, or for any misstatement or error, negligent or otherwise, contained in this book. In addition, the authors do not necessarily endorse specific products, procedures, or dosages reported in this book. Also, the listing of a drug or commercial product in this book does not indicate approval by the FDA or the manufacturer for use in exotic animals.

About the Editors

ABOUT THE EDITOR

James W. Carpenter, MS, DVM, Diplomate ACZM, is a professor of zoological medicine at the College of Veterinary Medicine, Kansas State University. He has been a clinical and research veterinarian for 42 years in the field of exotic animal, wildlife, and zoo animal medicine, and he has trained 40 interns and residents. He is the author of numerous scientific papers and book chapters; is editor/co-author of the *Exotic Animal Formulary* (1996, 2001, 2005, 2013, 2018) and its Japanese (2002), Spanish (2006), and Portuguese (2010) translations; and was co-editor of *Ferrets, Rabbits, and Rodents: Clinical Medicine and Surgery* (2004, 2012). Dr. Carpenter is also the former editor of the *Journal of Zoo and Wildlife Medicine* (1987-1992), served on the Wildlife Scientific Advisory Board of the Morris Animal Foundation (1998-2001; Chair, 2000-2001), and is the past president of the American Association of Zoo Veterinarians (1998-1999), the Association of Avian Veterinarians (2006-2007), and the American College of Zoological Medicine (2008-2009). He was awarded the Edwin J. Frick Professorship in Veterinary Medicine from the KSU College of Veterinary Medicine in 2002 and the Emil Dolensek Award by the American Association of Zoo Veterinarians in 2004. Dr. Carpenter was named the Exotic DVM of the Year for 2000 and the T.J. Lafeber Avian Practitioner of the Year for 2012. He was also named an Alumni of the Year by the Oklahoma State University College of Veterinary Medicine in 2009. In 2013, the Veterinary Health Center (KSU College of Veterinary Medicine) named the new veterinary facility at Manhattan's Sunset Zoo the "James W. Carpenter Clinic at Sunset Zoo." In 2016, Dr. Carpenter was awarded both the E.R. Frank Award by the KSU College of Veterinary Medicine Alumni Association for "outstanding achievements, humanitarian service, and contributions to the veterinary profession" and the KSU Distinguished Service Award for "outstanding leadership and clinical/diagnostic service to Kansas Veterinary Medical Association members." Dr. Carpenter is currently the editor-in-chief of the *Journal of Avian Medicine and Surgery.*

ABOUT THE ASSISTANT EDITOR

Christopher J. Marion, DVM, MPH, received his doctor of veterinary medicine and master of public health degrees from Kansas State University. He has managed and monitored clinical trials in the clinical research industry for the past 11 years. During this time, he has also consulted with the Association of Avian Veterinarians as an associate to the editor on the quarterly publication of the *Journal of Avian Medicine and Surgery.*

Contents

CHAPTER 1 Invertebrates
Gregory A. Lewbart, MS, VMD, Diplomate ACZM, Diplomate ECZM (Zoo Health Management)

TABLE 1-1	Antimicrobial and Antifungal Agents Used in Invertebrates,	2
TABLE 1-2	Antiparasitic Agents Used in Invertebrates,	5
TABLE 1-3	Chemical Restraint/Anesthetic/Analgesic Agents Used in Invertebrates,	6
TABLE 1-4	Miscellaneous Agents Used in Invertebrates,	9
TABLE 1-5	Common Captive Invertebrate Taxa,	11
REFERENCES	Invertebrates,	12

CHAPTER 2 Fish
Gregory A. Lewbart, MS, VMD, Diplomate ACZM, Diplomate ECZM (Zoo Health Management)
Roy P.E. Yanong, VMD

TABLE 2-1	Antimicrobial and Antifungal Agents Used in Fish,	17
TABLE 2-2	Antiparasitic Agents Used in Fish,	25
TABLE 2-3	Chemical Restraint/Anesthetic/Analgesic Agents Used in Fish,	31
TABLE 2-4	Miscellaneous Agents Used in Fish,	34
TABLE 2-5	Euthanasia Agents Used in Fish,	36
TABLE 2-6	Hematologic and Serum Biochemical Values of Fish,	37
REFERENCES	Fish,	45

CHAPTER 3 Amphibians
Brent R. Whitaker, MS, DVM
Colin T. McDermott, VMD

TABLE 3-1	Antimicrobial Agents Used in Amphibians,	54
TABLE 3-2	Antifungal Agents Used in Amphibians,	56
TABLE 3-3	Antiparasitic Agents Used in Amphibians,	58
TABLE 3-4	Chemical Restraint/Anesthetic/Analgesic Agents Used in Amphibians,	60
TABLE 3-5	Hormones Used in Amphibians,	65
TABLE 3-6	Miscellaneous Agents Used in Amphibians,	65
TABLE 3-7	Physiologic and Hematologic Values of Select Amphibians,	68
TABLE 3-8	Blood Collection Sites in Amphibians,	71
TABLE 3-9	Differential Diagnoses by Predominant Signs in Amphibians,	71
TABLE 3-10	Selected Disinfectants for Equipment and Cage Furniture,	74

TABLE 3-11	Guidelines for Managing Pet Amphibians with Nematode Parasites, 75
TABLE 3-12	Amphibian Quarantine Protocols, 75
REFERENCES	Amphibians, 78

CHAPTER 4 Reptiles

Eric Klaphake, DVM, Diplomate ACZM, Diplomate ABVP (Avian; Reptile/Amphibian)
Paul M. Gibbons, DVM, MS, Diplomate ABVP (Avian; Reptile/Amphibian)
Kurt K. Sladky, MS, DVM, Diplomate ACZM, Diplomate ECZM (Herpetology)
James W. Carpenter, MS, DVM, Diplomate ACZM

TABLE 4-1	Antimicrobial Agents Used in Reptiles, 82
TABLE 4-2	Antiviral Agents Used in Reptiles, 86
TABLE 4-3	Antifungal Agents Used in Reptiles, 87
TABLE 4-4	Antiparasitic Agents Used in Reptiles, 89
TABLE 4-5	Chemical Restraint/Anesthetic Agents Used in Reptiles, 93
TABLE 4-6	Analgesic Agents Used in Reptiles, 104
TABLE 4-7	Hormones and Steroids Used in Reptiles, 106
TABLE 4-8	Nutritional/Mineral/Fluid Support Used in Reptiles, 108
TABLE 4-9	Miscellaneous Agents Used in Reptiles, 113
TABLE 4-10	Hematologic and Serum Biochemical Values of Reptiles, 117
TABLE 4-11	Environmental, Dietary, and Reproductive Characteristics of Reptiles, 137
TABLE 4-12	Urinalysis Values of Chelonians, 139
TABLE 4-13	Selected Products and Guidelines Used in Force-Feeding Anorectic or Debilitated Reptiles, 139
TABLE 4-14	Guidelines for Tracheal/Pulmonary and Colonic Lavage in Reptiles, 141
TABLE 4-15	Venipuncture Sites Commonly Used in Reptiles, 141
TABLE 4-16	Treatment of Dystocia in Reptiles, 142
TABLE 4-17	Treatment of Metabolic Bone Diseases in Reptiles, 144
TABLE 4-18	Selected Sources of Diets and Other Commercial Products for Reptiles, 145
REFERENCES	Reptiles, 149

CHAPTER 5 Birds

Michelle G. Hawkins, VMD, Diplomate ABVP (Avian)
David Sanchez-Migallon Guzman, LV, MS, Diplomate ECZM (Avian; Small Mammal), Diplomate ACZM
Hugues Beaufrère, Dr. med. vet., PhD, Diplomate ACZM, Diplomate ABVP (Avian), Diplomate ECZM (Avian)
Angela M. Lennox, DVM, Diplomate ABVP (Avian; Exotic Companion Mammal), Diplomate ECZM (Small Mammal)
James W. Carpenter, MS, DVM, Diplomate ACZM

TABLE 5-1	Antimicrobial Agents Used in Birds, 168
TABLE 5-2	Antifungal Agents Used in Birds, 189

TABLE 5-3	Antiviral and Immunomodulating Agents Used in Birds,	196
TABLE 5-4	Antiparasitic Agents Used in Birds,	197
TABLE 5-5	Chemical Restraint/Anesthetic/Analgesic Agents Used in Birds,	218
TABLE 5-6	Nonsteroidal Antiinflammatory Agents Used in Birds,	236
TABLE 5-7	Hormones and Steroids Used in Birds,	240
TABLE 5-8	Nebulization Agents Used in Birds,	246
TABLE 5-9	Agents Used in the Treatment of Toxicologic Conditions of Birds,	248
TABLE 5-10	Psychotropic and Antiepileptic Agents Used in Birds,	253
TABLE 5-11	Nutritional/Mineral Support and Supplementation Used in Birds,	258
TABLE 5-12	Ophthalmologic Agents Used in Birds,	263
TABLE 5-13	Oncologic Agents and Radiation Therapy Used in Birds,	267
TABLE 5-14	Antimicrobial-Impregnated Polymethylmethacrylate (PMMA) Agents Used in Birds,	270
TABLE 5-15	Agents Used in the Treatment of Oiled Birds,	272
TABLE 5-16	Agents Used in Bird Emergencies,	272
TABLE 5-17	Euthanasia Agents Used in Birds,	274
TABLE 5-18	Miscellaneous Agents Used in Birds,	275
TABLE 5-19	Hematologic and Biochemical Values of Selected Psittaciformes,	284
TABLE 5-20	Hematologic and Biochemical Values for Juveniles of Selected Psittaciformes,	293
TABLE 5-21	Hematologic and Biochemical Values of Selected Passeriformes,	295
TABLE 5-22	Hematologic and Biochemical Values of Selected Ratites,	296
TABLE 5-23	Hematologic and Biochemical Values of Selected Piciformes and Columbiformes,	297
TABLE 5-24	Hematologic and Biochemical Values of Selected Raptors,	298
TABLE 5-25	Biologic and Physiologic Values of Selected Avian Species,	307
TABLE 5-26	Biologic and Physiologic Values of Selected Raptors,	309
TABLE 5-27	Quick Reference to Abnormalities of the Standard Avian Hematology Profile,	311
TABLE 5-28	Quick Reference to Abnormalities of the Standard Avian Biochemical Profile,	312
TABLE 5-29	Blood Gases of Selected Avian Species,	314
TABLE 5-30	Lipoprotein Panel of Selected Avian Species,	314
TABLE 5-31	T_4 Values of Selected Avian Species,	315
TABLE 5-32	Approximate Resting Respiratory Rates of Selected Avian Species and by Weight,	316
TABLE 5-33	Urinalysis Values Reported in Birds,	316
TABLE 5-34	Values Reported for Selected Ophthalmic Diagnostic Tests in Avian Species,	317
TABLE 5-35	Checklist of Supportive Care Procedures Used in Companion Bird Medicine,	318
TABLE 5-36	Fluid Therapy Recommendations for Birds,	318

TABLE 5-37	Routes of Administration and Maximum Suggested Volumes of Fluids Which Can Be Administered to Psittacines, 319	
TABLE 5-38	Suggested Volumes and Frequency of Gavage Feeding in Anorectic Birds, 319	
TABLE 5-39	Calculation of Enteral Feeding Requirements for Birds, 320	
TABLE 5-40	Doxycycline Recipes Used in Psittacines, 321	
TABLE 5-41	Selected Sources of Formulated and Medicated Diets for Companion and Aviary Birds, 321	
TABLE 5-42	Selected Nutritional Recommendations for Wild Bird Rehabilitation, 322	
TABLE 5-43	Management of Dystocia or Egg Binding in Birds, 323	
TABLE 5-44	Protocols Used in Treating Mycobacteriosis in Birds, 324	
TABLE 5-45	Suggested Chemotherapeutic Protocols Used in Birds, 325	
TABLE 5-46	Drug Dosages and Volumes Suggested for Cardiopulmonary Resuscitation (CPR) and in Critical Birds, 326	
TABLE 5-47	Vaccines Used in Birds (Non-Poultry), 328	
TABLE 5-48	Blood Pressure Values Reported in Birds, 330	
TABLE 5-49	Selected Arrhythmias and Some Documented Causes in Birds, 331	
TABLE 5-50	ECG Measurements Reference Values on Lead II in Selected Avian Species (Amplitude in mV, Interval/Duration in Sec), 332	
TABLE 5-51	Echocardiographic Reference Intervals (mm) in Selected Avian Species Obtained in the Horizontal Four-Chamber View, 333	
TABLE 5-52	Spectral Doppler Echocardiographic Reference Intervals (m/s) in Selected Avian Species Obtained in the Horizontal Four-Chamber View, 333	
TABLE 5-53	Guidelines for Selection of Psychotherapeutic Agents for Birds, 334	
REFERENCES	Birds, 337	

CHAPTER 6 Backyard Poultry and Waterfowl

Cheryl B. Greenacre, DVM, Diplomate ABVP (Avian; Exotic Companion Mammal)
G. Lynne Luna, DVM, MAM, Diplomate ACPV
Teresa Y. Morishita, DVM, MPVM, MS, PhD, Diplomate ACPV

TABLE 6-1	Antimicrobial Agents Used in Backyard Poultry and Waterfowl, 377
TABLE 6-2	Antifungal Agents Used in Backyard Poultry and Waterfowl, 390
TABLE 6-3	Antiviral and Immunomodulating Agents Used in Backyard Poultry and Waterfowl, 391
TABLE 6-4	Antiparasitic Agents Used in Backyard Poultry and Waterfowl, 391
TABLE 6-5	Chemical Restraint/Anesthetic/Analgesic Agents Used in Backyard Poultry and Waterfowl, 399
TABLE 6-6	Nonsteroidal Antiinflammatory Agents Used in Backyard Poultry and Waterfowl, 404
TABLE 6-7	Hormones and Steroids Used in Backyard Poultry and Waterfowl, 406
TABLE 6-8	Nebulization Agents Used in Backyard Poultry and Waterfowl, 406
TABLE 6-9	Agents Used in the Treatment of Toxicologic Conditions of Backyard Poultry and Waterfowl, 407
TABLE 6-10	Nutritional/Mineral Support Used in Backyard Poultry and Waterfowl, 408

TABLE 6-11	Ophthalmologic Agents Used in Backyard Poultry and Waterfowl, 409
TABLE 6-12	Oncologic Agents Used in Backyard Poultry and Waterfowl, 410
TABLE 6-13	Euthanasia Agents Used in Backyard Poultry and Waterfowl, 410
TABLE 6-14	Miscellaneous Agents Used in Backyard Poultry and Waterfowl, 411
TABLE 6-15	Hematologic and Serum Biochemical Values of Selected Galliformes, 412
TABLE 6-16	Hematologic and Serum Biochemical Values of Selected Anseriformes (Waterfowl), 413
TABLE 6-17	Biologic and Physiologic Values of Selected Galliformes, 414
TABLE 6-18	Biologic and Physiologic Values of Selected Anseriformes (Waterfowl) Species, 415
TABLE 6-19	Selected Nutritional Recommendations for Wild Bird Rehabilitation, 416
TABLE 6-20	Veterinary Feed Directive (VFD) Order Information, 416
TABLE 6-21	Partial List of Antimicrobials Transitioning From Over-the-Counter (OTC) to Veterinary Feed Directive (VFD) Status (as of January 2016), 416
TABLE 6-22	Serologic Tests for Poultry, 417
TABLE 6-23	Definitions of the Various Designations of Drugs in Food-Producing Animals According to the U.S. Food and Drug Administration (FDA) as They Pertain to Poultry, 419
TABLE 6-24	Water and Feed Consumption Rates for Backyard Poultry, 420
TABLE 6-25	Sources of Information on Meat and Egg Withdrawal for Backyard Poultry and Waterfowl, 420
TABLE 6-26	Values Reported for Selected Ophthalmic Diagnostic Tests in Avian Species, 420
TABLE 6-27	Selected Vaccines Used in Backyard Poultry, 421
REFERENCES	Backyard Poultry and Waterfowl, 422

CHAPTER 7 Sugar Gliders

David M. Brust, DVM

Christoph Mans, Dr. med. vet., Diplomate ACZM, Diplomate ECZM (Zoo Health Management)

TABLE 7-1	Antimicrobial and Antifungal Agents Used in Sugar Gliders, 433
TABLE 7-2	Antiparasitic Agents Used in Sugar Gliders, 433
TABLE 7-3	Chemical Restraint/Anesthetic Agents Used in Sugar Gliders, 434
TABLE 7-4	Analgesic Agents Used in Sugar Gliders, 435
TABLE 7-5	Miscellaneous Agents Used in Sugar Gliders, 436
TABLE 7-6	Hematologic and Serum Biochemical Values of Sugar Gliders, 437
TABLE 7-7	Biologic and Physiologic Values of Sugar Gliders, 438
TABLE 7-8	Urinalysis Values of Sugar Gliders, 438
TABLE 7-9	Growth and Development of Sugar Gliders, 439
TABLE 7-10	Dietary Components for Sugar Gliders in Captivity, 439
TABLE 7-11	Suggested Sugar Glider Diets, 440
TABLE 7-12	Feed Estimates for Hand-Rearing Sugar Gliders, 441
REFERENCES	Sugar Gliders, 441

CHAPTER 8 Hedgehogs
Peter J. Helmer, DVM, Diplomate ABVP (Avian)
James W. Carpenter, MS, DVM, Diplomate ACZM

TABLE 8-1	Antimicrobial Agents Used in Hedgehogs,	444
TABLE 8-2	Antifungal Agents Used in Hedgehogs,	445
TABLE 8-3	Antiparasitic Agents Used in Hedgehogs,	446
TABLE 8-4	Chemical Restraint/Anesthetic Agents Used in Hedgehogs,	447
TABLE 8-5	Analgesic Agents Used in Hedgehogs,	448
TABLE 8-6	Miscellaneous Agents Used in Hedgehogs,	449
TABLE 8-7	Hematologic and Serum Biochemical Values of Hedgehogs,	451
TABLE 8-8	Biological and Physiological Values of Hedgehogs,	452
TABLE 8-9	Suggested Diets for Hedgehogs,	452
TABLE 8-10	Hand-Rearing Orphaned Hedgehogs,	453
TABLE 8-11	Common Injection and Venipuncture Sites in Hedgehogs,	453
TABLE 8-12	Preventive Medicine in Hedgehogs,	454
TABLE 8-13	Common Differential Diagnoses Based on Physical Examination Findings,	454
TABLE 8-14	Confirmed Zoonotic Diseases Carried by Hedgehogs,	454
TABLE 8-15	Common Vocalizations in Hedgehogs,	454
TABLE 8-16	Cardiac Measurements in Hedgehogs,	455
REFERENCES	Hedgehogs,	456

CHAPTER 9 Rodents
Jörg Mayer, Dr. med. vet., MSc, Diplomate ACZM, Diplomate ECZM (Small Mammal), Diplomate ABVP (Exotic Companion Mammal)
Christoph Mans, Dr. med. vet., Diplomate ACZM, Diplomate ECZM (Zoo Health Management)

TABLE 9-1	Antimicrobial and Antifungal Agents Used in Rodents,	460
TABLE 9-2	Antiparasitic Agents Used in Rodents,	464
TABLE 9-3	Chemical Restraint/Anesthetic Agents Used in Rodents,	467
TABLE 9-4	Analgesic Agents Used in Rodents,	470
TABLE 9-5	Cardiovascular Agents Used in Rodents,	473
TABLE 9-6	Emergency Drugs Used in Rodents,	474
TABLE 9-7	Miscellaneous Agents Used in Rodents,	476
TABLE 9-8	Common and Scientific Names of Pet Rodents,	480
TABLE 9-9	Hematologic and Serum Biochemical Values of Rodents,	481
TABLE 9-10	Biologic and Physiologic Data of Rodents,	482
TABLE 9-11	Blood Volumes of Rodents with Safe-Bleeding Volume Recommendations,	483
TABLE 9-12	Urinalysis Reference Values of Rodents,	483
TABLE 9-13	Reproductive Data for Rodents,	484

CONTENTS xxiii

TABLE 9-14	Determining the Sex of Mature Rodents, 485
TABLE 9-15	Nutritional Data for Rodents, 485
TABLE 9-16	Zoonotic Diseases in Rodents, 485
TABLE 9-17	Disease Testing in Rodents, 486
TABLE 9-18	Endocrine Values in Rodents, 487
TABLE 9-19	Echocardiographic Measurements in Rodents, 488
TABLE 9-20	Electrocardiographic Measurements in Rodents, 488
REFERENCES	Rodents, 488

CHAPTER 10 Rabbits

Peter Fisher, DVM, Diplomate ABVP (Exotic Companion Mammal)
Jennifer Graham, DVM, Diplomate ABVP (Avian; Exotic Companion Mammal), Diplomate ACZM

TABLE 10-1	Antimicrobial Agents Used in Rabbits, 495
TABLE 10-2	Antifungal Agents Used in Rabbits, 498
TABLE 10-3	Antiparasitic Agents Used in Rabbits, 500
TABLE 10-4	Chemical Restraint/Sedative/Anesthetic/Analgesic Agents Used in Rabbits, 503
TABLE 10-5	Constant Rate Infusion (CRI) Protocols Used in Rabbits, 511
TABLE 10-6	Ophthalmologic Agents Used in Rabbits, 511
TABLE 10-7	Miscellaneous Agents Used in Rabbits, 513
TABLE 10-8	Hematologic and Serum Biochemical Values of Rabbits, 517
TABLE 10-9	Rabbit Blood Glucose and Sodium Levels as Prognostic Indicators, 518
TABLE 10-10	Biologic and Physiologic Data of Rabbits, 519
TABLE 10-11	Urinalysis Values in Rabbits, 519
TABLE 10-12	Cerebrospinal Fluid Values in Rabbits, 520
TABLE 10-13	Electrocardiographic (ECG) and Echocardiographic Values in Rabbits, 520
TABLE 10-14	Determining the Sex of Mature Rabbits, 521
TABLE 10-15	Drugs Reported to Be Toxic in Rabbits, 521
TABLE 10-16	Treatments Used in the Management of Rabbit Gastrointestinal Syndrome (RGIS), 522
TABLE 10-17	Bronchoalveolar Lavage (BAL) in Rabbits, 523
TABLE 10-18	Clinical Signs and Behavioral Changes Used in the Assessment of Pain in Rabbits, 523
TABLE 10-19	Percentage of Antibiotic Susceptibility Results for the Most Common Bacteria Isolated from Nasal Cultures of 121 Rabbits with Signs of Upper Respiratory Disease, 524
TABLE 10-20	Sensitivity and Specificity Calculators for IgM and IgG Titers and CRP Levels Relative to the Diagnosis of Suspected *Encephalitozoon cuniculi* Infections in Pet Rabbits, 524
REFERENCES	Rabbits, 525

CHAPTER 11 Ferrets
James K. Morrisey, DVM, Diplomate ABVP (Avian)
Matthew S. Johnston, VMD, Diplomate ABVP (Avian)

- TABLE 11-1 Antimicrobial and Antifungal Agents Used in Ferrets, 533
- TABLE 11-2 Antiparasitic Agents Used in Ferrets, 535
- TABLE 11-3 Chemical Restraint/Anesthetic Agents Used in Ferrets, 536
- TABLE 11-4 Analgesic Agents Used in Ferrets, 539
- TABLE 11-5 Cardiopulmonary Agents Used in Ferrets, 540
- TABLE 11-6 Adrenal Gland Disease Agents Used in Ferrets, 542
- TABLE 11-7 Miscellaneous Agents Used in Ferrets, 543
- TABLE 11-8 Hematologic and Biochemical Values of Ferrets, 549
- TABLE 11-9 Protein Electrophoresis Values for Ferrets, 550
- TABLE 11-10 Biologic and Physiologic Data of Ferrets, 550
- TABLE 11-11 Urinalysis Values of Ferrets, 551
- TABLE 11-12 Proposed Schedule of Vaccinations and Routine Prophylactic Care for Ferrets, 552
- TABLE 11-13 Chemotherapy Protocols for Lymphoma in Ferrets, 552
- TABLE 11-14 Conversion of Body Weight (kg) to Body Surface Area (m^2), 554
- REFERENCES Ferrets, 555

CHAPTER 12 Miniature Pigs
Valarie V. Tynes, DVM, Diplomate ACVB
Kristie Mozzachio, DVM, CVA, Diplomate ACVP

- TABLE 12-1 Antimicrobial Agents Used in Miniature Pigs, 559
- TABLE 12-2 Antiparasitic Agents Used in Miniature Pigs, 561
- TABLE 12-3 Chemical Restraint/Anesthetic Agents Used in Miniature Pigs, 561
- TABLE 12-4 Analgesic Agents Used in Miniature Pigs, 566
- TABLE 12-5 Miscellaneous Agents Used in Miniature Pigs, 568
- TABLE 12-6 Hematologic and Serum Biochemical Values of Miniature Pigs, 569
- TABLE 12-7 Urinalysis Reference Values for Miniature Pigs, 570
- TABLE 12-8 Biological and Physiologic Data of Miniature Pigs, 570
- TABLE 12-9 Preventive Medicine Recommendations for Miniature Pigs, 571
- TABLE 12-10 Blood Collection Sites in Miniature Pigs, 572
- TABLE 12-11 Recommendations for Feeding Miniature Pigs, 572
- TABLE 12-12 Tips for Oral Dosing of Miniature Pigs, 573
- REFERENCES Miniature Pigs, 573

CHAPTER 13 Primates
Kathryn C. Gamble, DVM, MS, Diplomate ACZM, Diplomate ECZM (Zoo Health Management)

- TABLE 13-1 Antimicrobial and Antifungal Agents Used in Primates, 576

CONTENTS xxv

TABLE 13-2	Antiparasitic Agents Used in Primates,	580
TABLE 13-3	Chemical Restraint/Anesthetic/Analgesic Agents Used in Primates,	586
TABLE 13-4	Miscellaneous Agents Used in Primates,	594
TABLE 13-5	Hematologic and Serum Biochemical Values of Primates,	602
TABLE 13-6	Biologic and Physiologic Data of Primates,	604
TABLE 13-7	Identifying Characteristics of Small Nonhuman Primates by their Taxonomic Classification,	605
TABLE 13-8	ECG Intervals and Durations,	605
TABLE 13-9	Preventive Medicine Recommendations for Primates,	606
TABLE 13-10	Immunization Recommendations for Primates,	607
TABLE 13-11	Nonhuman Primate Laboratories,	609
REFERENCES	Primates,	611

CHAPTER 14 Wildlife
David L. McRuer, MSc, DVM, Diplomate ACVPM
Heather Barron, DVM, Diplomate ABVP (Avian)

TABLE 14-1	Checklist for the Care of Sick, Injured, or Orphaned Wildlife,	617
TABLE 14-2	Considerations for Developing a Wildlife Policy in Private Practice,	619
TABLE 14-3	Recommendations for Safe Restraint of Native Wildlife,	620
TABLE 14-4	Recommendations for Venipuncture Sites in Native Wildlife,	622
TABLE 14-5	Recommendations for Meat Withdrawal Times in Game Species for Select Medications,	623
TABLE 14-6	Antimicrobial Agents Used in Wild Mammals,	623
TABLE 14-7	Antiparasitic Agents Used in Wild Mammals,	625
TABLE 14-8	Antifungal Agents Used in Wild Mammals,	626
TABLE 14-9	Chemical Restraint/Anesthetic Agents Used in Wild Mammals,	627
TABLE 14-10	Analgesic and Nonsteroidal Antiinflammatory Agents Used in Wild Mammals,	628
TABLE 14-11	Agents Used in Wild Mammal Emergencies,	629
TABLE 14-12	Miscellaneous Agents Used in Wild Mammals,	631
REFERENCES	Wildlife,	632

CHAPTER 15 Select Topics for the Exotic Animal Veterinarian
Julie Swenson, DVM, Diplomate ACZM
James W. Carpenter, MS, DVM, Diplomate ACZM

TABLE 15-1	Classification of Select Antimicrobials Used in Exotic Animal Medicine,	637
TABLE 15-2	General Efficacy of Select Antimicrobial Agents Used in Exotic Animals,	639
TABLE 15-3	Antimicrobial Therapy Used in Exotic Animals According to Site of Infection,	641
TABLE 15-4	Antimicrobial Combination Therapies Commonly Used in Exotic Animals,	643
TABLE 15-5	Select Laboratories Conducting Exotic Animal Diagnostic Procedures,	643

TABLE 15-6	Professional Associations for Veterinarians Interested in Exotics,	648
TABLE 15-7	Exotic Animal Online Resources for Practitioners,	648
TABLE 15-8	Captive Husbandry Web Sites for Owners of Exotic Animals,	650
TABLE 15-9	Emergency Drug Doses (in mL) Commonly Used in Exotic Animals,	654
TABLE 15-10	Fluid Solutions Used in Exotic Animal Medicine,	656
TABLE 15-11	Common Abbreviations Used in Prescription Writing,	657
TABLE 15-12	Common Weight, Liquid Measure, Length, Percentage, and Milliequivalent Conversions,	658
TABLE 15-13	Equivalents of Celsius (Centigrade) and Fahrenheit Temperature Scales,	659
TABLE 15-14	System of International (SI) Units Conversion Factors of Hematology Commonly Used in Exotic Animal Medicine,	659
TABLE 15-15	System of International (SI) Units Conversion Factors of Clinical Chemistries Commonly Used in Exotic Animal Medicine,	660
TABLE 15-16	Select Compounding Pharmacies,	661
TABLE 15-17	Additional Compounding Resources,	663

INDEX 665

Chapter 1 Invertebrates

Gregory A. Lewbart

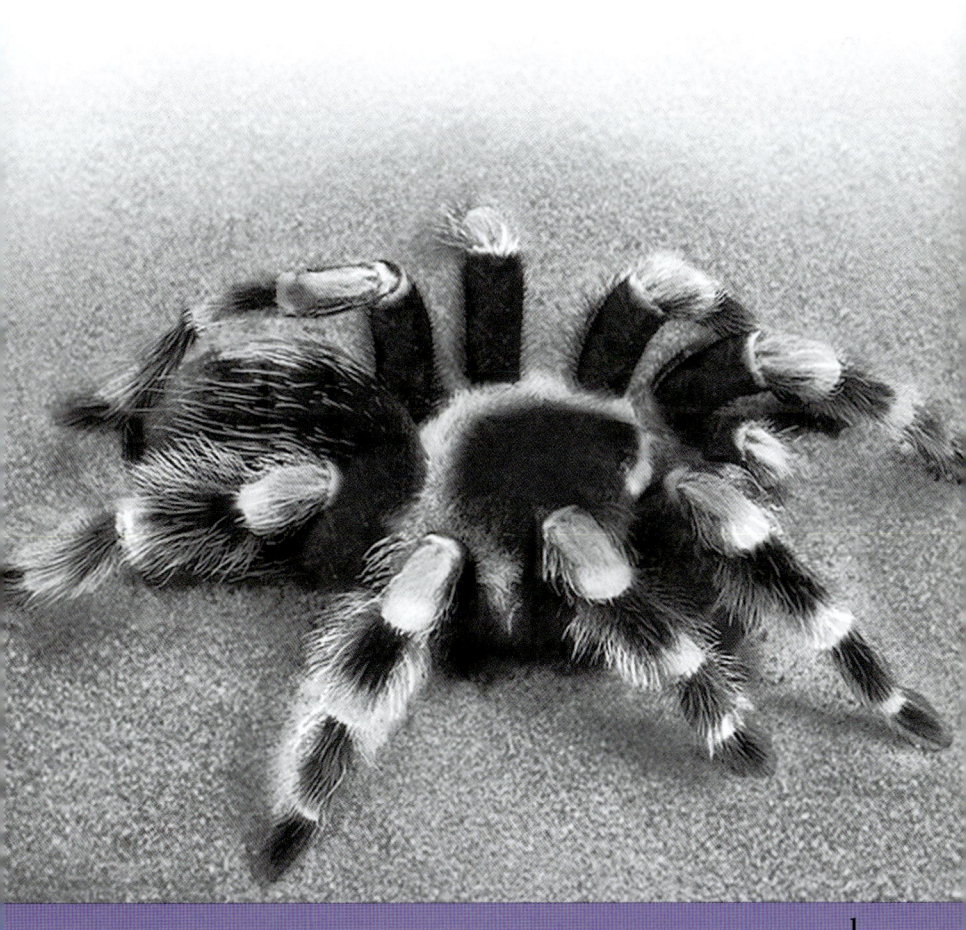

TABLE 1-1 Antimicrobial and Antifungal Agents Used in Invertebrates.[a-e]

Agent	Dosage	Comments
Ampicillin	100 mg/L q12h × 7 days[69]	Control of white band disease (WBD) in *Acropora* sp.
Benzalkonium chloride	0.5 mg/L long-term[71] 10 mg/L for 10 min[60]	Quaternary amine with broad disinfection properties, not for use on live animals
Ceftazidime (Fortaz, Pfizer)	20 mg/kg intracardiac q72h × 3 wk[60]	Spiders/cephalosporin with good activity against Gram-negative bacteria (e.g., *Pseudomonas*); although this regimen appears safe, efficacy has not been determined
Chloramphenicol	75 mg/kg PO, IM q12h × 6 days[63]	Cephalopods
	10-50 mg/L as an immersion treatment for several days[10,66,68] (prepare fresh solution with 100% water change q24h)	Corals/reduce lighting for treated animals if possible (slows metabolic rate and may reduce stress and improve drug tolerance); rinse animals well with fresh seawater before return to primary habitat; properly treat any effluent before discharge; florfenicol may be a better alternative (risk to humans from chloramphenicol)
Enrofloxacin	5 mg/kg IM, IV[33,63]	Cuttlefish (PD) and possibly other cephalopods
	5 mg/kg IV[60]	Spiders
	5 mg/kg ICe[62]	Purple sea stars (*Pisaster ochraceus*)/PD
	10 mg/kg PO[33,63]	Cuttlefish (PD) and possibly other cephalopods
	10 mg/kg ICe[59]	Green sea urchins (*Strongylocentrotus droebachiensis*)/PD
	10-20 mg/kg IM[70]	Chinese mitten crabs/PD
	10-20 mg/kg PO q24h[60]	Spiders
	2.5 mg/L × 5 hr immersion q12-24 h[33,63]	Cuttlefish (PD) and possibly other cephalopods
	5 mg/L × 24 hr immersion[14]	Manila clams (*Ruditapes philippinarum*)/PD; decreasing temperature and/or salinity slowed elimination
	5 mg/L immersion for 6 hr[62]	Purple sea stars (*Pisaster ochraceus*)/PD
	10 mg/L immersion for 6 hr[59]	Green sea urchins (*Strongylocentrotus droebachiensis*)/PD
Fluconazole	3 mg/kg intracardiac q4d × 6 treatments[64]	Horseshoe crabs

TABLE 1-1 Antimicrobial and Antifungal Agents Used in Invertebrates. (cont'd)

Agent	Dosage	Comments
Formalin	1-1.5 ppm immersion for 4 hr[42]	Horseshoe crabs/ectocommensals; can also be administered indefinitely (i.e., until diluted out)
Furazolidone	50 mg/L q12h for 10 min immersion[63]	Cephalopods
Iodine, Lugol's 5% solution	5-10 drops/L of seawater; use as an immersion for 10-20 min[68]	Corals/antiseptic; cauterize wounds; strong oxidizing agent; some corals are sensitive, including pulse corals (*Xenia* sp.), *Anthelia* spp., and star polyps (*Pachyclavularia* spp.); remove corals at first signs of stress (polyp expulsion)
	Topically at full strength (5%) for 20-30 sec[68]	
Itraconazole (Sporanox, Janssen)	10 mg/kg IV q24h[2]	Horseshoe crabs/PD
Nitrofurazone	1.5 mg/L for 72 hr[67] immersion	Cephalopods/nitrofuran; carcinogenic; drug inactivated in bright light; water soluble formulations preferred
	25 mg/L q12h for 1 hr[67] immersion	
Oxolinic acid	10 mg/kg intrasinus[72]	Kuruma shrimp/PD; quinolone; Gram-negative bacteria; decreased uptake in hard water; better uptake pH <6.9
	50 mg/kg PO[72]	Kuruma shrimp/PD
Oxytetracycline	10 mg/kg intrasinus[72,73]	Tiger shrimp/PD; cooking reduced muscle levels by 30%-60% and shell levels by 20%
	25 mg/kg intrasinus[72]	Kuruma shrimp/PD
	25-50 mg/kg IV[56]	Horseshoe crabs/PD
	50 mg/kg PO[72,73]	Kuruma shrimp/PD; tiger shrimp/PD; cooking reduced muscle levels by 30%-60% and shell levels by 20%
	100 mg/kg PO[61]	White shrimp/PD
	200 mg/colony PO q4-5d × 3 treatments[75,76]	Honeybees/for treating American and European foulbrood; withdrawal time of 6 wk; should not be used on hives where honey will be consumed by humans
	10-15 mg/L q48-72 h × 3-5 treatments[38]	Chocolate chip sea stars/cutaneous ulcerations; may be applicable to other echinoderms with bacterial lesions
	1 g/lb of feed[55]	American lobsters/gaffkemia; approved for use in food animals by the FDA
Paromomycin	100 mg/L q12h immersion with a 25% water change × 6 days[69]	Control of white band disease (WBD) in *Acropora* sp.

Continued

TABLE 1-1 Antimicrobial and Antifungal Agents Used in Invertebrates. (cont'd)

Agent	Dosage	Comments
Silver sulfadiazine cream (Silvadene, Marion Merrill Dow)	Apply topically to lesions	Proceed with caution (biotest if possible) as treatments are empirical
Sulfadimethoxine	50-100 mg/kg in feed × 14 days[55]	Penaeid shrimp
Sulfadimethoxine/ ormetoprim (Romet-30, Alpharma)	42 mg/kg intrapericardial[7]	American lobster/PD; although no frequency is given, it appears that q3-5d may be reasonable based on the long half-life
Sulfamethoxazole/ trimethoprim	Bioencapsulated in brine shrimp PO q12h[13,45,53,54]	White shrimp/PD; combine 20%-40% trimethoprim sulfamethoxazole with a lipid emulsion (Selco, INVE Aquaculture) at a concentration of 1:5
Tetracycline	10 mg/kg PO q24h[63]	Cephalopods
	10 mg/L bath[41,68]	Corals/efficacy questionable in saltwater; anecdotal evidence of successful treatment for bacterial infections
Trifluralin	0.01-0.1 ppm as an immersion[55]	Penaeid shrimp/larval oomycetosis
Tris EDTA and neomycin (Tricide-Neo, Molecular Therapeutics)	100 mL/L for 45 min q24h × 7 days as an immersion[38]	Cushion sea stars/cutaneous ulcers; may be applicable to other echinoderms
Tylosin (Tylan, Elanco)	200 mg/colony q7d × 3 treatments[75,76]	Honeybees/antibiotic applied topically to the brood chamber for control of American foulbrood (*Paenibacillus larvae*); approved by the FDA; should not be used in hives where the honey will be consumed by humans
Winter savory extract (*Satureja montana*)	0.01% in microcrystalline sugar[16]	Honeybees/chalkbrood fungal disease (*Ascosphaera apis*); a number of plant aromatic oils have been tested, some with more promise than others, on various diseases of honeybees[22,75,76]

[a]Not to be used with invertebrates intended for human consumption unless government approved.
[b]Preferable to treat a single animal of a species (biotest) to determine toxicity.
[c]Tank treatment: when treating the invertebrates' resident aquarium, disconnect activated carbon filtration to prevent drug removal. Many drugs adversely affect the nitrifying bacteria, so water quality should be monitored closely (especially ammonia and nitrite concentrations). Keep water well aerated when appropriate and monitor patient(s) closely. Perform water changes and reconnect filtration to remove residual drug following treatment. Discard carbon following drug removal.
[d]Bath (immersion) treatment: remove invertebrates from resident aquarium and place in container with known volume of water and concentration of therapeutic agent. Watch closely for signs of toxicity.
[e]Invertebrate species, temperature, and water quality parameters can influence the pharmacodynamics of many drugs, especially antimicrobials.

TABLE 1-2 Antiparasitic Agents Used in Invertebrates.[a-e]

Agent	Dosage	Comments
Acetic acid, glacial	3%-5% solution for 1 hr[12]	Horseshoe crabs
Amitraz (Apivar, Véto-pharma)	Use as directed[75,76]	Honeybees/acariasis; commercial packaging should be consulted prior to use
Diflubenzuron	0.03 mg/L for 7 days[21]	Control of amphipods in *Chrysaora* jellyfish
Formalin	50-100 µL/L for 4 hr or 25 µL/L indefinitely[55]	Shrimp/protozoal ectoparasites; approved for use by the FDA in food animals
Formic acid	Use as directed[75,76]	Honeybees/acariasis; commercial packaging should be consulted prior to use; an empty super must be used on hive during treatment
Freshwater	1-3 min dip[68]	Stony corals, some soft corals/flatworms, and other ectoparasites; buffer to pH 8.2 and use clean, dechlorinated water; do not use on small polyp corals or xenids; biotest first, if possible, especially when attempting with a new species
Fumagillin	Use as directed[75,76]	Honeybees/nosemosis (caused by microsporidian parasites); commercial packaging should be consulted prior to use
Ivermectin	Stock solution of 1:1 (1% ivermectin and propylene glycol); dilute 1:50 with distilled water prior to topical use[60]	Spiders/for the treatment of individual parasitic mites; apply carefully to mites with fine paintbrush or similar implement
Levamisole (Levasole, Schering Plough)	8 mg/L immersion for 24 hr[68]	Corals/metazoan parasites; well tolerated by *Acropora* spp., *Montipora digitata*, *M. capricornis*, *Seriatopora histrix*, *Stylophora pistillata*
Menthol	Use as directed[75]	Honeybees/acariasis; commercial packaging should be consulted prior to use
Metronidazole	50 mg/kg intracardiac × 1 treatment[60]	Spiders/appears safe, but efficacy is unknown
	100 mg/L immersion for 16 hr[63]	Cephalopods/antiprotozoal
Milbemycin oxime (Interceptor, Novartis)	0.625 mg/L as an immersion[26,37,43]	Stony corals (*Acropora*)/ "red bug" (*Tegastes acroporanus*)
	0.16 mg/L as an immersion q6-7d × 2 treatments[9]	For amphipod parasites of jellyfish; use with caution on hydrozoans
Potassium permanganate	25-30 ppm for 30-60 min[55]	Penaeid shrimp/external parasiticide
Povidone iodine	0.75% solution for topical treatment[60]	Spiders/fungal infections; use water-based solution

Continued

TABLE 1-2 Antiparasitic Agents Used in Invertebrates. (cont'd)

Agent	Dosage	Comments
Thymol	Use as directed[75,76]	Honeybees/acariasis; commercial packaging should be consulted prior to use

[a]Not to be used with invertebrates intended for human consumption unless government approved.
[b]Preferable to treat a single animal of a species (biotest) to determine toxicity.
[c]Tank treatment: when treating the invertebrates' resident aquarium, disconnect activated carbon filtration to prevent drug removal. Many drugs adversely affect the nitrifying bacteria, so water quality should be monitored closely (especially ammonia and nitrite concentrations). Keep water well aerated when appropriate and monitor patient(s) closely. Perform water changes and reconnect filtration to remove residual drug following treatment. Discard carbon following drug removal.
[d]Bath (immersion) treatment: remove invertebrates from resident aquarium and place in container with known volume of water and concentration of therapeutic agent. Watch closely for signs of toxicity.
[e]Invertebrate species, temperature, and water quality parameters can influence the pharmacodynamics of many drugs.

TABLE 1-3 Chemical Restraint/Anesthetic/Analgesic Agents Used in Invertebrates.

Agent	Dosage	Comments
Alfaxalone	200 mg/kg intracardiac[31]	Used as a general anesthetic for tarantulas (*Grammostola roseae*)
Benzocaine	100 mg/L[4,35] bath	Abalone/anesthesia; not sold as anesthetic in United States; available from chemical supply companies; do not use topical anesthetic products marketed for mammals; prepare stock solution in ethanol (benzocaine is poorly soluble in water); store in dark bottle at room temperature
	400 mg/L[20]	Leeches/this could be applied, with caution, to other aquatic annelids
	1 g/L[29]	Prepare as 1:4 w/v added to 95°C water to dissolve the benzocaine; for use in apple snails (*Pomacea paludosa*)
	2.5-3 g/L[63] bath	Cephalopods/euthanasia
Butorphanol	Fish, amphibian, and reptile dosages can be employed with care	Analgesia; use with caution as dosing regimens are empirical; biotest when possible
Carbon dioxide	3%-5%[36]	Terrestrial arthropods/euthanasia; isoflurane and sevoflurane may be preferable with regard to recovery; an anesthetic chamber has been developed/described for use in the fruit fly[71]
Clove oil (eugenol)	0.125 mL/L (approx. 125 mg/L) as an immersion[28]	Crustaceans/stock solution: 100 mg/mL of eugenol by diluting 1 part clove oil with 9 parts 95% ethanol (eugenol is poorly soluble in water); over-the-counter preparation (pure) available at most pharmacies contains approximately 1 g eugenol per mL clove oil
	0.35 g/L[29]	Apple snails (*Pomacea paludosa*)

TABLE 1-3 Chemical Restraint/Anesthetic/Analgesic Agents Used in Invertebrates. (cont'd)

Agent	Dosage	Comments
Ethanol	1.5%-3% solution[39]	Cuttlefish/anesthesia may not be effective for cold water cephalopods[35]
	3% solution[35]	Abalone/anesthesia
	5% solution[27,36]	Aquatic gastropods/anesthesia
	5% solution[18,46]	Oligochaetes/adequate anesthesia for terrestrial earthworms such as *Lumbricus terrestris*
	5% solution[32]	Octopuses for general anesthesia
	10% solution[63]	Cephalopods/euthanasia
Ethanol/menthol (Listerine, McNeil-PPC)	10% in saline[79]	Aquatic gastropods/anesthesia
Isoflurane	Can be used with an anesthetic chamber	Terrestrial gastropods,[30] arachnids[18,24,47,50,60,80]/anesthesia; fast induction with a possible excitatory period; anesthetic depth may not be appropriate for invasive surgery;[27] usually applied at a 5% concentration for arachnids
	5% with 1 L/min oxygen[25]	Tarantulas (*Grammostola roseae*)/ sedation and anesthesia (depending on the amount of time in the anesthetic chamber
	2 mL on a cotton ball[5]	Place cotton ball in a 500 mL beaker with the tarantula; cotton ball should be placed/protected to avoid direct contact
Ketamine	40-90 mcg/g IM[11]	Crayfish/induction time of less than 1 min and anesthetic duration of 10 min at low dose and 2 hr at high dose
	0.025-1 mg/kg[28]	Australian giant crabs/fast induction (less than 30 sec) with an excitatory phase; dose dependent anesthetic duration of 8-40 min
	20 mg/kg intracardiac with 200 mg/kg alfaxalone[31]	Tarantulas/results in deep plane of anesthesia
Lidocaine	0.4-1 mg/g IM[11]	Crayfish/induction time of less than 2 min and duration of anesthesia of 5-30 min when injected into the tail
Magnesium chloride	Intracoelomic, 25-50% bodyweight with a 1000 milliosmolar solution[15,49a]	Sea hares/short induction time (2-5 min) and good muscle relaxation
	6.8 g/L[33,35]	Cephalopods/induction time of 6-12 min in cuttlefish
	30-50 g/L[40]	Scallops/fast induction and recovery
	1:1 mixture of 7.5% with seawater[38,49]	Echinoderms/concentration adjustments may be required for prolonged anesthesia

Continued

TABLE 1-3 Chemical Restraint/Anesthetic/Analgesic Agents Used in Invertebrates. (cont'd)

Agent	Dosage	Comments
Magnesium chloride (cont'd)	7.5% immersion[45,52]	Polychaetes
	10% solution prn[63]	Cephalopods/euthanasia
	30 g/L for 20 min[1]	Queen conch (*Strombus gigas*)
	32.5 g/L for 20 min[32]	Octopuses
Magnesium sulfate	4-22 g/100 mL[78]	Abalone/fast induction and good recovery
Morphine	5 mg/kg intracardiac with 200 mg/kg alfaxalone[31]	Tarantulas
MS-222 (Finquel, Argent)	—	See tricaine methanesulfonate
2-phenoxyethanol	0.5-3 mL/L[78]	Abalone/quick induction and short recovery
	1-2 mL/L[35]	Quick induction and short recovery
Potassium chloride	1 g/kg (330 mg/mL solution) IV[8]	Lobsters/euthanasia; inject at base of second walking leg
Procaine	25 mg/kg IV[58]	Crabs/very short induction time (less than 30 sec) and prolonged anesthesia (2-3 hr)
Propylene phenoxetol	1-3 mL/L of a 1% solution[35,51,57]	Oysters/anesthesia; this concentration should produce anesthesia in less than 15 min; recovery time is short (under 30 min); higher doses can be used but induce a deeper level of anesthesia; can also be used for giant clams[51]
	2 mL/L[35,74]	Echinoderms
Sevoflurane	Can be used with an anesthetic chamber at a 5% concentration[35,81]	Terrestrial arthropods/see isoflurane for details of administration; use with a 1 L/min oxygen flow in tarantulas[81]
Sodium bicarbonate tablets (Alka-Seltzer, Bayer)	2-4 tablets/L bath[34]	Euthanasia; generates CO_2; use when other agents unavailable; keep aquatic invertebrate in solution >10 min after respiration stops; dosage based on piscine literature
Sodium pentobarbital	400 mg/L[48]	Aquatic gastropods/anesthesia; very slow onset but apparently safe; controlled drug
	1 mL/L[4]	Abalone

TABLE 1-3 Chemical Restraint/Anesthetic/Analgesic Agents Used in Invertebrates. (cont'd)

Agent	Dosage	Comments
Tricaine methanesulfonate (MS-222; Finquel, Argent)	Dosages and efficacy vary widely depending on species and application; consult taxon-specific literature[35,36]	Anesthesia; stock solution: 10 g/L, buffer the acidity by adding sodium bicarbonate at 10 g/L or to saturation; store stock in dark container; shelf-life of stock extended by refrigeration or freezing; stock that develops an oily film should be discarded; aerate water to prevent hypoxemia; euthanasia: keep animal in solution >20 min after respiration stops
	0.4-0.8 g/L immersion[3]	Purple sea urchin (*Arbacia punctulata*)/safe and effective
Xylazine	16-22 mg/kg IV[28]	Giant crabs/fast induction (3-5 min) and approximately 30 min of anesthesia (dose dependent)
	20 mg/kg intracardiac with 200 mg/kg alfaxalone[31]	Tarantulas/results in a deep plane of anesthesia

TABLE 1-4 Miscellaneous Agents Used in Invertebrates.

Agent	Dosage	Comments
Barium sulfate	4 mL/15 g food[23]	Tarantulas, scorpions, millipedes, hissing cockroaches/contrast radiography; inject into a strawberry and feed to millipedes; inject into crickets and/or other prey for carnivorous invertebrates
Benzocaine topical (Orabase, Colgate-Palmolive)	Topically[68]	Corals and, potentially, other aquatic invertebrates/used as a water-resistant paste; chemotherapeutics can be combined for topical therapy
Carbon, activated	75 g/40 L tank water[55]	Removal of medications and other organics from water; usually added to filter system; discard after 2 wk; 75 g ≈ 250 cc dry volume
Chlorine/chloramine neutralizer	Use as directed	See sodium thiosulfate
Diatrizoate meglumine and diatrizoate sodium (Hypaque-76, Amersham Health)	4 mL/15 g food[23]	Tarantulas, scorpions, millipedes, hissing cockroaches/contrast radiography; combine with/inject into the food item and feed 1-3 hr prior to radiography
Hydrogen peroxide (3%)	0.25 mL/L water[54]	Acute environmental hypoxia; dose from the piscine literature
Iohexol	12 mL/kg IV[65]	Horseshoe crabs/contrast radiography
	15 mL PO[65]	

Continued

TABLE 1-4 Miscellaneous Agents Used in Invertebrates. (cont'd)

Agent	Dosage	Comments
Methylmethacrylate	Apply topically as needed[19,60]	Arthropods (spiders, scorpions, insects)/repair fractured exoskeleton; there are numerous references for the application of surgical adhesives, so consult the appropriate taxon-based literature
Mineral oil	1 mL/kg PO	Insects/laxative[19]
Nitrifying bacteria	Use as directed for commercial products	Seed or improve development of biological filtration to detoxify ammonia, nitrite, and nitrate; numerous commercial preparations; do not expose products to extreme temperatures; use before expiration date
	Add material (e.g., floss, gravel) from a tank with an active biological filter and healthy fish to new tank[54]	Must evaluate risk of disease transmission with this technique
Oxygen (100%)	Fill plastic bag with O_2 containing ⅓ vol of water[34]	Acute environmental hypoxia common with transportation; close bag tightly with rubber band; keep animals in bag until normal swimming and respiratory behavior
Sodium thiosulfate	Use as directed for chlorine/chloramine neutralizers	Active ingredient in numerous chlorine/chloramine neutralizers; chlorine and chloramine are common additions to municipal water supplies and are toxic to many aquatic invertebrates; ammonia released by detoxification of chloramine is removed by functioning biological filter (see nitrifying bacteria) or chemical means (see zeolite)
	10 mg/L tank water[44]	
	10 g neutralizes chlorine (up to 2 mg/L) in 1000 L water[44]	
	100 mg/L tank water[67]	Chlorine exposure
Zeolite (i.e., clinoptilite) (Ammonex, Argent)	Use as directed	Ion-exchange resin that exchanges ammonia for sodium ions; clinoptilite is an active form of zeolite; used to reduce or prevent ammonia toxicity
	20 g/L tank water[54]	

CHAPTER 1 Invertebrates

TABLE 1-5 Common Captive Invertebrate Taxa.[a]

Arthropods

Chelicerates: This group includes the spiders, scorpions, and horseshoe crabs. Some common species are listed here.[60,64]
Chilean rosehair tarantula (*Grammostola spatulata*)
Mexican fireleg tarantula (*Brachypelma boehmei*)
Mexican redknee tarantula (*Brachypelma smithi*)
Emperor scorpion (*Pandinus imperator*)
American horseshoe crab (*Limulus polyphemus*)
Myriapods (centipedes, millipedes):[24]
African banded millipedes (*Isulus* spp.)
Desert millipede (*Orthoporus* sp.)
Giant desert centipede (*Scolopendra heros*)
Giant train millipedes (*Spirostreptida* spp.)
Madagascar fire millipedes (*Aphistogoniulus* spp.)
Crustaceans: Decapods are a diverse group of readily recognized species including the crabs, lobsters, and shrimp. Some common examples include the banded shrimps, crayfish (numerous species), marine hermit crabs, and terrestrial hermit crabs (*Coenobita* sp.).[55]
Sea monkeys (*Artemia* sp.).[55]
Insects: Insects, sometimes referred to as the phylum Hexapoda, are an immense group of over a million described species. Some common captive insects include the beetles (Order Coleoptera), butterflies and moths (Order Lepidoptera), crickets (grey crickets [*Acheta domestica*]; black prairie cricket [*Gryllus* sp.]), honeybee (*Apis mellifera*), Madagascar hissing cockroach (*Gromphadorhina portentosa*), and the silkworm (*Bombyx mori*).[19,24,60,75,76]

Coelenterates

Scyphozoans (jellyfishes): Although not common as pets, some individuals, and many public institutions and establishments, maintain jellyfish aquaria. Some popular species include fried egg jellies (*Phacellophora camtschatica*), moon jellies (*Aurelia aurita*), and the sea nettles (*Chrysaora* sp.).[68]
Anthozoans (anemones and corals): Numerous species of sea anemones and corals (hard and soft) are commonly maintained in reef aquaria. Frequently maintained soft coral groups include members of the families Alcyoniidae, Nephtheidae, and Xeniidae.[43] Commonly maintained scleractinian (hard coral) genera include *Acropora*, *Montipora*, and *Porites*.[43]

Echinoderms

This entirely marine phylum includes five major classes:[38]
Asteroidea: sea stars
Crinoidea: feather stars, sea lilies
Echinoidea: sand dollars, sea biscuits, sea urchins
Holothuroidea: sea cucumbers
Ophiuroidea: basket stars, brittle stars

Mollusks

Gastropods (nudibranchs, sea hares, slugs, and snails): This group includes a diverse array of terrestrial, freshwater, and marine species.[15,30,43]
Cephalopods (cuttlefish, nautilus, octopuses, squid): This group includes a diverse group of marine species. Some species of octopus, and the chambered nautilus (*Nautilus pompilius*), are occasionally found in home aquaria.[63]
Bivalves (clams, mussels, oysters): This group includes a diverse group of freshwater and marine species. One of the most common reef genera is the giant clam (*Tridacna* sp.).[43,51,57]

[a]This is not a comprehensive list of taxa. The reader should be aware that taxonomy is a dynamic science and taxonomists frequently assign different taxonomic levels to the same groups depending on the anatomical, genetic, and other criteria being considered.

REFERENCES

1. Acosta-Salmón H, Davis M. Inducing relaxation in the queen conch *Strombus gigas* (L.) for cultured pearl production. *Aquaculture* 2007;262:73-77.
2. Allender MC, Schumacher J, Milam J, et al. Pharmacokinetics of intravascular itraconazole in the American horseshoe crab (*Limulus polyphemus*). *J Vet Pharmacol Therap* 2007;31:83-86.
3. Applegate JR, Dombrowski D, Christian LS, et al. Tricaine methanesulfonate (MS-222) sedation and anesthesia in the purple-spined sea urchin (*Arbacia punctulata*). *J Zoo Wildl Med* 2016;47:1025-1033.
4. Aquilina B, Roberts R. A method for inducing muscle relaxation in the abalone, *Haliotis iris*. *Aquaculture* 2000;190:403-408.
5. Archibald KE, Minter LJ, Lewbart GA, Bailey CS. Semen collection and characterization in the Chilean rose tarantula (*Grammostola rosea*). *Am J Vet Res* 2014;75:929-936.
6. Avery L, Horvitz HR. Effects of starvation and neuroactive drugs on feeding in *Caenorhabditis elegans*. *J Exp Zool* 2000;253:263-270.
7. Barron MG, Gedutis C, James MO. Pharmacokinetics of sulphadimethoxine in the lobster, *Homarus americanus*, following intrapericardial administration. *Xenobiotica* 1988;18:269-276.
8. Battison A, MacMillans R, MacKenzie A, et al. Use of injectable potassium chloride for euthanasia of American lobsters (*Homarus americanus*). *Comp Med* 2000;50:545-550.
9. Boonstra JL, Koneval ME, Clark JD, et al. Milbemycin oxime (Interceptor) treatment of amphipod parasites (Hyperiidae) from several host jellyfish species. *J Zoo Wildl Med* 2015;46:158-160.
10. Borneman EH. *Aquarium Corals: Selection, Husbandry, and Natural History*. Neptune City, NJ: TFH; 2001.
11. Brown PB, White MR, Chaille J, et al. Evaluation of three anesthetic agents for crayfish (*Orconectes virilis*). *J Shellfish Res* 1996;15:433-435.
12. Bullis RA. Care and maintenance of horseshoe crabs for use in biomedical research. In: Stolen JS, Fletcher TC, Rowley AF, et al, eds. *Techniques in Fish Immunology*. Vol 3. Fair Haven, NJ: SOS Publications; 1994:A9-A10.
13. Chair M, Nelis HJ, Leger P, et al. Accumulation of trimethoprim, sulfamethoxazole, and N-acetylsulfamethoxazole in fish and shrimp fed medicated *Artemia franciscana*. *Antimicrob Agents Chemother* 1996;40:1649-1652.
14. Chang Z-Q, Gao A-X, Li J, Liu P. The effect of temperature and salinity on the elimination of enrofloxacin in the Manila clam *Ruditapes philippinarum*. *J Aquat Anim Health* 2012;24:17-21.
15. Clark TR, Nossov PC, Apland JP, et al. Anesthetic agents for use in the invertebrate sea snail, *Aplysia californica*. *Contemp Top Lab Anim Sci* 1996;35:75-79.
16. Colin ME, Duclos J, Larribau E, et al. Activité des huiles essentielles de Labiés sur *Ascosphaera apis* et traitement d'un rucher. *Apidologie* 1989;20:221-228.
17. Cooper EL. Transplantation immunity in annelids. *Transplantation* 1968;6:322-337.
18. Cooper JE. Invertebrate anesthesia. *Vet Clin North Am Exot Anim Pract* 2001;4:57-67.
19. Cooper JE. Insects. In: Lewbart GA, ed. *Invertebrate Medicine*. 2nd ed. Ames: Wiley-Blackwell Publishing; 2012:267-283.
20. Cooper JE, Mahaffey P, Applebee K. Anaesthesia of the medicinal leech (*Hirudo medicinalis*). *Vet Rec* 1986;118:589-590.
21. Crossley SMG, George AL, Keller CJ. A method for eradicating amphipod parasites (Hyperiidae) from host jellyfish, *Chrysaora fuscescens* (Brandt, 1835), in a closed recirculating system. *J Zoo Wild Med* 2009;40:174-180.
22. Davis C, Ward W. Control of chalkbrood disease with natural products. A report for the Rural Industries Research and Development Corporation. RIRDC Publication No 03/107 RIRDC Project No DAQ-269A; 2003:1-23.
23. Davis MR, Gamble KC, Matheson JS. Diagnostic imaging in terrestrial invertebrates: Madagascar hissing cockroach (*Gromphadorhina portentosa*), desert millipede (*Orthoporus* sp.), emperor scorpion (*Pandinus imperator*), Chilean rosehair tarantula (*Grammostola spatulata*), Mexican fireleg tarantula (*Brachypelma boehmei*) and Mexican redknee tarantula (*Brachypelma smithi*). *Zoo Biol* 2008;27:109-125.

24. Dombrowski D, De Voe R. Emergency care of invertebrates. *Vet Clin North Am Exot Anim Pract* 2007;10:621-645.
25. Dombrowski D, De Voe R, Lewbart GA. Comparison of isoflurane and carbon dioxide anesthesia in rose-haired tarantulas (*Grammostola rosea*). *J Zoo Biol* 2012; http://dx.doi.org/10.1002/zoo21026.
26. Dorton D. The "cure" for red acro bugs. Available at: http://www.reefs.org/forums/viewtopic .php?p=439155. Accessed November 14, 2016.
27. Flores DV, Salas PJI, Vedra JPS. Electroretinography and ultrastructural study of the regenerated eye of the snail, *Cryptomphallus aspera*. *J Neurobiol* 1983;14:167-176.
28. Gardner C. Options for immobilization and killing crabs. *J Shellfish Res* 1997;16:219-224.
29. Garr AL, Posch H, McQuillan M, Davis M. Development of a captive breeding program for the Florida apple snail, *Pomacea paludosa*: relaxation and sex ratio recommendations. *Aquaculture* 2012;370-371:166-171.
30. Girdlestone D, Cruickshank SGH, Winlow W. The actions of three volatile anaesthetics on withdrawal responses of the pond-snail, *Lymnaea stagnalis* (L). *Comp Biochem Physiol C* 1989;92:39-43.
31. Gjeltema J, Posner LP, Stoskopf MK. The use of injectable alphaxalone as a single agent and in combination with ketamine, xylazine, and morphine in the Chilean rose tarantula, *Grammostola rosea*. *J Zoo Wildl Med* 2014;45:792-801.
32. Gleadall IG. The effects of prospective anaesthetic substances on cephalopods: summary of original data and a brief review of studies over the last two decades. *J Exp Mar Biol and Ecol* 2013;447:23-30.
33. Gore SR, Harms CA, Kukanich B, et al. Enrofloxacin pharmacokinetics in the European cuttlefish, *Sepia officinalis*, after a single i.v. injection and bath administration. *J Vet Pharm Therap* 2005;28:433-439.
34. Gratzek JB, ed. *Aquariology: The Science of Fish Health Management: Master Volume (Aquariology Series)*. Morris Plains, NJ: Tetra Press; 1994.
35. Gunkel C, Lewbart GA. Invertebrates. In: West G, Heard D, Caulkett N, eds. *Zoo Animal and Wildlife Immobilization and Anesthesia*. Ames: Blackwell Publishing; 2007:147-158.
36. Gunkel C, Lewbart GA. Anesthesia and analgesia of invertebrates. In: Fish R, Danneman P, Brown M, et al. *Anesthesia and Analgesia in Laboratory Animals*. 2nd ed. St. Louis: Elsevier; 2008:535-546.
37. Hadfield CA, Clayton LA, O'Neill KL. Milbemycin treatment of parasitic copepods on *Acropora* corals. *Proc 33rd Eastern Fish Health Workshop* 2008;76.
38. Harms CA. Echinoderms. In: Lewbart GA, ed. *Invertebrate Medicine*. 2nd ed. Ames: Wiley-Blackwell Publishing; 2012:365-379.
39. Harms CA, Lewbart GA, McAlarney R, et al. Surgical excision of mycotic (*Cladosporium* sp.) granulomas from the mantle of a cuttlefish (*Sepia officinalis*). *J Zoo Wildl Med* 2006;37:524-530.
40. Heasman MP, O'Connor WA, Frazer AWJ. Induction of anaesthesia in the commercial scallop, *Pecten fumatus* Reeve. *Aquaculture* 1995;131:231-238.
41. Hodgson G. Tetracycline reduces sedimentation damage to corals. *Mar Biol* 1990;104:493-496.
42. Landy RB, Leibovitz L. A preliminary study of the toxicity and therapeutic efficacy of formalin in the treatment of triclad turbellarid worm infestations in *Limulus polyphemus*. *Proc Annu Meet Soc Invert Pathol* 1983.
43. Lehmann DW. Reef systems. In: Lewbart GA, ed. *Invertebrate Medicine*. 2nd ed. Ames: Wiley-Blackwell Publishing; 2012:57-75.
44. Lewbart GA. Emergency and critical care of fish. *Vet Clin North Am Exot Anim Pract* 1998;1:233-249.
45. Lewbart G, Riser NW. Nuchal organs of the polychaete *Parapionosyllis manca* (Syllidae). *Invert Biol* 1996;115:286-298.
46. Marks DH, Cooper EL. *Aeromonas hydrophila* in the coelomic cavity of the earthworms *Lumbricus terrestris* and *Eisenia foetida*. *J Invert Pathol* 1977;29:382-383.

47. Marnell C. Tarantula and hermit crab emergency care. *Vet Clin Exot Anim Med* 2016;19:627-646.
48. Martins-Sousa RL, Negrao-Correa D, Bezerra FSM, et al. Anesthesia of *Biomphalaria* spp. (Mollusca, Gastropoda): sodium pentobarbital is the drug of choice. *Mem Inst Oswaldo Cruz* 2001;96:391-392.
49. McCurley RS, Kier WM. The functional morphology of starfish tube feet: the role of a crossed-fiber helical array in movement. *Biol Bull* 1995;188:197-209.
49a. McManus JM, Lu H, Chiel HJ. An in vitro preparation for eliciting and recording feeding motor programs with physiological movements in Aplysia californica. *J Vis Exp* 2012; http://dx.doi.org/10.3791/4320.
50. Melidone R, Mayer J. How to build an invertebrate surgery chamber. *Exot DVM* 2005;7.5:8-10.
51. Mills D, Tlili A, Norton J. Large-scale anesthesia of the silver-lip pearl oyster, *Pinctada maxima* Jameson. *J Shellfish Res* 1997;16:573-574.
52. Müller MCM, Berenzen A, Westheide W. Regeneration experiments in *Eurythoe complanata* ("Polychaeta," Amphinomidae): reconfiguration of the nervous system and its function for regeneration. *Zoomorphology* 2003;122:95-103.
53. Nelis HJ, Léger F, Sorgeloos P, et al. Liquid chromatographic determination of efficacy of incorporation of trimethoprim and sulfamethoxazole in brine shrimp (*Artemia* spp.) used for prophylactic chemotherapy of fish. *Antimicrob Agents Chemother* 1991;35:2486-2489.
54. Noga EJ. *Fish Disease: Diagnosis and Treatment*. 2nd ed. Ames: Wiley-Blackwell; 2010.
55. Noga EJ, Hancock A, Bullis R. Crustaceans. In: Lewbart GA, ed. *Invertebrate Medicine*. 2nd ed. Ames: Wiley-Blackwell Publishing; 2012:235-254.
56. Nolan MW, Smith SA, Jones D. Pharmacokinetics of oxytetracycline in the American horseshoe crab, *Limulus polyphemus*. *J Vet Pharmacol Therap* 2007;30:451-455.
57. Norton JH, Dashorst M, Lansky TM, et al. An evaluation of some relaxants for use with pearl oysters. *Aquaculture* 1996;144:39-52.
58. Oswald RL. Immobilization of decapod crustaceans for experimental purposes. *J Mar Biol Assoc UK* 1977;57:715-721.
59. Phillips B, Harms CA, Lewbart GA, et al. Population pharmacokinetics of enrofloxacin and its metabolite ciprofloxacin in the green sea urchin (*Strongylocentrotus droebachiensis*) following intracoelomic and immersion administration. *J Zoo Wild Med* 2016;47:175-186.
60. Pizzi R. Spiders. In: Lewbart GA, ed. *Invertebrate Medicine*. 2nd ed. Ames: Wiley-Blackwell Publishing; 2012:187-221.
61. Reed LA, Siewicki TC, Shah C. The biopharmaceutics and oral bioavailability of two forms of oxytetracycline to the white shrimp, *Litopenaeus setiferus*. *Aquaculture* 2006;258:42-54.
62. Rosenberg J, Haulena M, Phillips B, et al. Population pharmacokinetics of enrofloxacin in purple sea stars (*Pisaster ochraceus*) following an intracoelomic injection or extended immersion. *Am J Vet Res* 2016;77:1266-1275.
63. Scimeca J. Cephalopods. In: Lewbart GA, ed. *Invertebrate Medicine*. 2nd ed. Ames: Wiley-Blackwell Publishing; 2012:113-125.
64. Smith S. Horseshoe crabs. In: Lewbart GA, ed. *Invertebrate Medicine*. 2nd ed. Ames: Wiley-Blackwell Publishing; 2012:173-185.
65. Spotswood T, Smith SA. Cardiovascular and gastrointestinal radiographic contrast studies in the horseshoe crab (*Limulus polyphemus*). *Vet Rad Ultrasound* 2007;48:14-20.
66. Sprung J, Delbeek JC. *The Reef Aquarium: A Comprehensive Guide to the Identification and Care of Tropical Marine Invertebrates*. Vol 2. Coconut Grove, FL: Ricordea; 1997.
67. Stoskopf MK. Appendix V: Chemotherapeutics. In: Stoskopf MK, ed. *Fish Medicine*. 2nd ed. Philadelphia: WB Saunders Co; 1993:832-839.
68. Stoskopf MK. Coelenterates. In: Lewbart GA, ed. *Invertebrate Medicine*. 2nd ed. Ames: Wiley-Blackwell Publishing; 2012:21-56.
69. Sweet MJ, Croquer A, Bythell JC. Experimental antibiotic treatment identifies potential pathogens of white band disease in the endangered Caribbean coral *Acropora cervicornis*. *Proc R Soc B* 2014;281:20140294.

70. Tang J, Yang X, Zheng Z, et al. Pharmacokinetics and the active metabolite of enrofloxacin in Chinese mitten-handed crab (*Eriocheir sinensis*). *Aquaculture* 2006;260:69-76.
71. Treves-Brown KM. *Applied Fish Pharmacology*. Dodrecht, The Netherlands: Kluwer Academic Publishers; 2000.
72. Uno K. Pharmacokinetics of oxolinic acid and oxytetracycline in kuruma shrimp, *Penaeus japonicus*. *Aquaculture* 2004;230:1-11.
73. Uno K, Aoki T, Kleechaya W, et al. Pharmacokinetics of oxytetracycline in black tiger shrimp, *Penaeus monodon*, and the effect of cooking on the residues. *Aquaculture* 2006;254:24-31.
74. Van den Spiegel D, Jangoux M. Cuvierian tubules of the holothuroid *Holothuria forskali* (Echinodermata): a morphofunctional study. *Mar Biol* 1987;96:263-275.
75. Vidal-Naquet N. Honeybees. In: Lewbart GA, ed. *Invertebrate Medicine*. 2nd ed. Ames: Wiley-Blackwell Publishing; 2012:285-321.
76. Vidal-Naquet N. *Honeybee Veterinary Medicine: Apis mellifera L*. Sheffield, UK: 5M Publishing; 2016:288.
77. Walcourt A, Ide D. A system for the delivery of general anesthetics and other volatile agents to the fruit fly *Drosophila melanogaster*. *J Neurosci Meth* 1998;84:115-119.
78. White HI, Hecht T, Potgieter B. The effect of four anaesthetics on *Haliotis midae* and their suitability for application in commercial abalone culture. *Aquaculture* 1996;140:145-151.
79. Woodall AJ, Naruo H, Prince DJ, et al. Anesthetic treatment blocks synaptogenesis but not neuronal regeneration of cultured Lymnaea neurons. *J Neurophysiol* 2003;90:2232-2239.
80. Zachariah TT, Mitchell MA, Guichard CM, Singh RS. Isoflurane anesthesia of wild-caught goliath birdeater spiders (*Theraphosa blondi*) and Chilean rose spiders (*Grammostola rosea*). *J Zoo Wildl Med* 2009;40:347-349.
81. Zachariah TT, Mitchell MA, Watson MK, et al. Effects of sevoflurane anesthesia on righting reflex and hemolymph gas analysis variables for Chilean rose tarantulas (*Grammostola rosea*). *Am J Vet Res* 2014;75:521-526.

Chapter 2 **Fish**

Gregory A. Lewbart | *Roy P.E. Yanong*

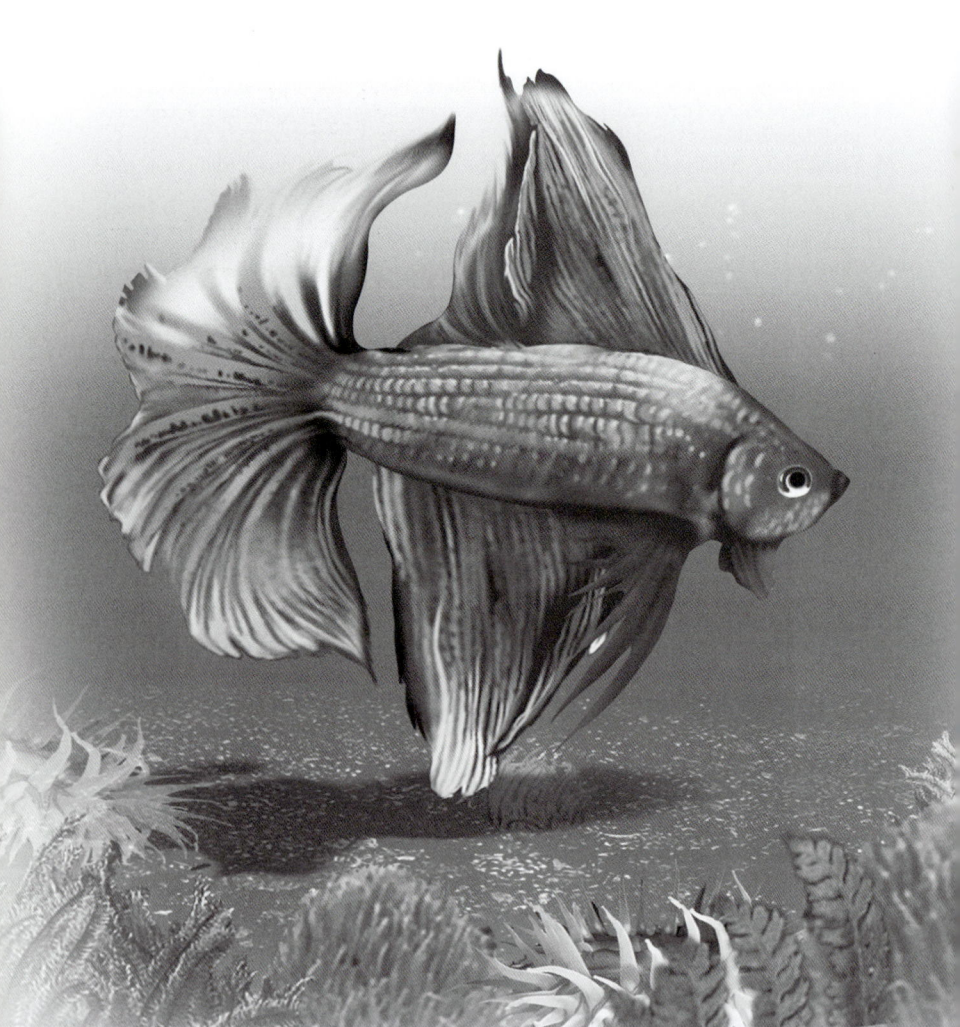

TABLE 2-1 Antimicrobial and Antifungal Agents Used in Fish.[a-f]

Agent	Dosage	Comments
Acriflavine	4 mg/L × 4h[118]	Rainbow trout/organic dye and antifungal agent
	10 mg/L × 4h[111]	Channel catfish/PK
Amikacin	5 mg/kg IM q12h[152]	
	5 mg/kg IM q72h × 3 treatments[152]	
	5 mg/kg ICe q24h × 3 days, then q48h × 2 treatments[77]	Koi/PK
Amoxicillin	—	Infrequently indicated in ornamental fish because few pathogens are Gram-positive
	12.5 mg/kg IM[16]	Atlantic salmon/PK
	25 mg/kg PO q12h[142]	
	40 mg/kg IV q24h[32]	Seabream/PK
	80 mg/kg PO q24h × 10 days[32]	Seabream/PK
	40-80 mg/kg/day in feed × 10 days[100]	
	110 mg/kg/day in feed[8]	Channel catfish/PK
Ampicillin	—	Infrequently indicated in ornamental fish because few pathogens are Gram-positive
	10 mg/kg q24h IM[16,149]	
	10 mg/kg q24h IV[110]	Striped bass
	50-80 mg/kg/day in feed × 10 days[100]	
Azithromycin (Zithromax, Zoetis)	30 mg/kg q24h × 14 days[39]	Chinook salmon/PK
	40 mg/kg ICe[40]	Chinook salmon/PK
Aztreonam (Azactam, Bristol-Myers Squibb)	100 mg/kg IM, ICe q48h × 7 treatments[120]	Koi/*Aeromonas salmonicida*; used by hobbyists
Benzalkonium chloride	0.5 mg/L long-term[149]	Quaternary amine with broad disinfection properties
	10 mg/L for 10 min[149]	
Bronopol (Pyceze, Novartis)	15-50 mg/L × 30-60 min bath[114,152]	For mycotic infections (eggs and fish); eggs may require the higher dose
Cefovecin (Convenia, Zoetis)	—	Some intraspecies variability; rapidly eliminated in white bamboo sharks (not recommended)[138]
	16 mg/kg SC[133]	Adult copper rockfish/plasma levels of >1 µg/mL persisted for 7 days
Ceftazidime (Fortaz, Zoetis)	22 mg/kg IM, ICe q72-96h × 3-5 treatments[120]	Cephalosporin with good activity against Gram-negative bacteria (e.g., *Pseudomonas*)

Continued

TABLE 2-1 Antimicrobial and Antifungal Agents Used in Fish. (cont'd)

Agent	Dosage	Comments
Chloramine-T	2.5-20 mg/L as immersion treatment[29,149] for 60 min/day up to 3 days[3]	Disinfectant; used to control bacterial gill disease and some ectoparasites; dosage and duration varies widely with species and water quality
	20 mg/L as immersion × 4 hr[95]	Rainbow trout, striped bass, yellow perch/PK
Chloramphenicol	—	Florfenicol may be a better alternative than chloramphenicol (risk to humans)
	40-182 mg/kg q24h ICe[84]	Carp/PK
	50 mg/kg PO, IM once, then 25 mg/kg q24h[143]	
	50 mg/kg PO q24h[27]	Rainbow trout/PK
Ciprofloxacin	15 mg/kg IM, IV[102]	Carp, African catfish, rainbow trout/PK
Difloxacin	10 mg/kg PO q24h[37]	Atlantic salmon/PK; plasma levels were higher in marine fish compared with freshwater fish
	10 mg/kg PO q24h[144]	Olive flounder/PK
	20 mg/kg PO q24h × 3 days[34]	Goldfish/PK
Diquat dibromide (Reward, Syngenta)	2-18 mg/L for 1-4 hr × 1-4 treatments q24-48h; 19-28 mg/L for 30-60 min × 1-3 treatments q48h[1]	For control of columnaris disease in freshwater fish
Doxycycline	20 mg/kg PO q24h[158]	Tilapia/PK; possible intrahepatic cycling; dosing intervals not established
	20 mg/kg PO, IV[158]	
Enrofloxacin (Baytril, Bayer)	—	For a review of quinolones used in fishes, see Samuelsen, 2006[126]
	2.5 mg/kg IV q24h[31]	Seabream/PK; no ciprofloxacin detected
	5 mg/kg PO, IM, ICe q24h[142]	Red pacu/PK[89]
	5-10 mg/kg PO q24h[149]	
	5-10 mg/kg IM, ICe q48h[92] × 7 treatments	
	10 mg/kg PO q24h × 10 days[108]	Pacu (Piaractus mesopotamicus)/ withdrawal period (non-USA) 23 days at 27°C; ciprofloxacin detected
	10 mg/kg PO q24h[31,126]	Atlantic salmon, seabream/PK; no ciprofloxacin detected
	10 mg/kg PO, IV[81]	Korean catfish/PK; ciprofloxacin detected
	10 mg/kg ICe q96h × 4 treatments[90]	Koi/PK (21°C, 70°F)

TABLE 2-1 Antimicrobial and Antifungal Agents Used in Fish. (cont'd)

Agent	Dosage	Comments
Enrofloxacin (Baytril, Bayer) (cont'd)	30 mg/kg PO q24h[156]	Grass carp (*Ctenopharyngodon idella*)/prevention of resistance mutation for *Aeromonas hydrophila* strain AH10
	10 mg/kg of feed q24h[88,100,139]	Atlantic salmon/PK
	0.1% feed × 10-14 days[88]	Oral or injectable form can be used; equivalent to 10 mg/kg of feed
	2.5-5 mg/L × 5 hr bath q24h × 5-7 days[92]	Red pacu/PK; change 50%-75% of water between treatments
Erythromycin	—	Commonly sold as tank treatment for aquarium fish; not generally recommended because of toxicity to nitrifying bacteria[100]
	10-25 mg/kg IM, ICe;[38] 10-25 mg/kg IM, ICe 1-3 × q3wk[38]	For treatment of bacterial kidney disease; second dose is for control of vertical transmission of bacterial kidney disease
	75 mg/kg PO q24h × 7 days[28]	Barramundi/successful treatment of *Streptococcus iniae*
	75 mg/kg PO q24h × 10 days[35]	For control of *Streptococcus iniae* in seabream/PD
	100 mg/kg PO, IM q24h × 7-21 days[142,149]	
	100-200 mg/kg PO q24h × 21 days[97]	Salmonids/to control *Renibacterium salmoninarum*
Florfenicol (Nuflor, Merck Animal Health; Aquaflor [Veterinary Feed Directive-medicated feed], Merck Animal Health)	5-20 mg/kg PO q24h[72]	Atlantic salmon/PK
	10 mg/kg IM q24h[160,161]	Koi/PK (for MICs [minimum inhibitory concentration] of 1-6 µg/mL)
	10-15 mg/kg PO q24h[10]	Catfish/PK
	10-20 mg/kg PO q24h[127,130] × 10 days	Cod/PK
	10, 25, or 50 mg/kg PO q24h[160,161]	Koi/PK, for MIC of 1, 3, and 6 µg/mL, respectively
	10, 25, or 50 mg/kg PO q12h[160,161]	Gourami/PK; for MICs of 1, 3, and 6 µg/mL, respectively
	10 or 100 mg/kg IM q12h[160,161]	Gourami/PK; for MICs of 1 µg/mL or 6 µg/mL
	40 mg/kg IM[162]	White-spotted bamboo shark/PK
	40-50 mg/kg PO, IM, ICe q12-24h[91,142]	Red pacu/PK[91]
Flumequine (Apoquin aqualtes, Sigma-Aldrich)	—	Quinolone; Gram-negative bacteria; freshwater fish at pH 6.8-7.2; decreased uptake in hard water; increase dose for marine fish
	10 mg/kg PO q48h[54]	Cod, goldsinny wrasse/PK
	12-25 mg/kg PO, ICe, IV q24h[128]	Atlantic halibut/PK
	25 mg/kg ICe q24h[129]	Corkwing wrasse/PK

Continued

TABLE 2-1 Antimicrobial and Antifungal Agents Used in Fish. (cont'd)

Agent	Dosage	Comments
Flumequine (Apoquin aqualtes, Sigma-Aldrich) (cont'd)	25-50 mg/kg PO q24h[122]	Atlantic salmon
	30 mg/kg IM, ICe[100]	High antibiotic levels for several days when given IM
	50-100 mg/L × 3 hr bath[100]	
	10 mg/kg q24h in feed × 10 days[100]	
Formalin	All doses based on volumes of 100% formalin (=37% formaldehyde solution)	Mycotic infections on eggs; do not treat within 24 hr of hatching; caution: carcinogenic; do not use if highly toxic white precipitates of paraformaldehyde are present; some fish are very sensitive; test on small number first, monitor fish for respiratory distress and pale color; increased toxicity in soft, acidic water and at high temperature; treat with vigorous aeration because of oxygen depletion; toxic to plants
	0.23 mL/L bath up to 60 min[100]	
	1 mL/38 L as 12-24 hr bath followed by 30%-70% water change, may be repeated[48]	
		Degradation in saltwater recirculating aquaculture systems occurred rapidly by day 3 presumptively due to microbial digestion (biotic) or abiotic factors; for intended multiple day treatments, testing and variable additions may be required to achieve target dose above 15 mg/L[83]
	1-2 mL/L bath, up to 15 min[100]	For eggs only
	25 mg/L (9.3 mg formaldehyde/L) bath for 144 hr[155]	Striped bass
Furazolidone	—	Nitrofuran; caution: carcinogenic; toxic to scaleless fish; absorbed from water; drug inactivated in bright light
	1 mg/kg PO, IV q24h[112]	Channel catfish
	30 mg/kg PO[157]	Nile tilapia
	67.5 mg/kg PO q12h × 10 days[85]	Rainbow trout/PK; at 14°C (57°F), half-life ≈ 30 days and residue present at 40 days post 10-day treatment
	25-35 mg/kg q24h in feed for 20 days[63]	Some salmonids/not approved for fish intended for human consumption in the United States
	50-100 mg/kg q24h in feed × 10-15 days[100]	
	1-10 mg/L tank water for ≥ 24 hr[100]	

TABLE 2-1	Antimicrobial and Antifungal Agents Used in Fish. (cont'd)	
Agent	Dosage	Comments
Gentamicin	1 mg/kg IM, ICe q24h[134]	Channel catfish/PK
	2 mg/kg IM, then 1 mg/kg IM at 8 and 72 hr[143]	Brown shark/PK
	2.5 mg/kg IM q72h[88]	Nephrotoxic; substantial risk in species for which dosages have not been determined[117]
	3.5 mg/kg IM q24h[78]	Goldfish, toadfish/PK
Hydrogen peroxide (HP) (3%)	0.1 mL/L × 1 hr[123]	For treatment of external bacteria in swordtails
Hydrogen peroxide (HP) (35% PEROX-AID, Eka Chemicals)	—	Each mL of 35% PEROX-AID contains 350 mg HP
	50 mg/L × 1 hr[109]	For control of columnaris disease in channel catfish fry
	50-75 mg/L × 1 hr[109]	For control of columnaris disease in channel catfish fingerlings and adults
Iodine, potentiated (Betadine, Purdue Frederick)	Topical to wound, rinse immediately[100]	Do not use solutions combined with detergent (e.g., Betadine scrub)
	20-100 mg/L for 10 min[149]	For disinfecting eggs (available iodine)
Itraconazole	1-5 mg/kg q24h in feed q1-7d[142]	Systemic mycoses
Kanamycin sulfate (Kantrex, Apothecon)	20 mg/kg ICe q3d × 5 treatments[100]	Toxic to some fish
	50 mg/kg q24h in feed[100]	
	40-640 mg/L × 2 hr bath[46]	Channel catfish
	50-100 mg/L q72h × 3 treatments[100]	Change 50%-75% of water between treatments; absorbed from water
Ketoconazole	2.5-10 mg/kg PO, IM, ICe[142]	Systemic mycoses
Malachite green (zinc-free)	—	Freshwater fish/mycotic infections; caution: mutagenic, teratogenic; toxic to some fish species and to fry; increased toxicity at higher temperatures and lower pH; stains objects, especially plastic; toxic to plants; not approved for use on fish intended for human consumption
	0.1 mg/L tank water q3d × 3 treatments[100]	Remove residual chemical with activated carbon after final treatment
	0.25 mg/L × 15 min q24h[153]	Fungal control on fish eggs
	0.5 mg/L × 1 hr bath[100]	Freshwater fish eggs
	1 mg/L × 30-60 min bath[100]	Use 2 mg/L if pH is high
	1 mg/L × 1 hr[149]	Fungal control on fish eggs
	2 mg/L × 15 min q24h[149]	Fungal control on fish eggs
	10 mg/L × 10-30 min bath[100]	Freshwater fish eggs
	50-60 mg/L × 10-30 sec bath[100]	
	100 mg/L topical to skin lesions[100]	

Continued

TABLE 2-1 Antimicrobial and Antifungal Agents Used in Fish. (cont'd)

Agent	Dosage	Comments
Methylene blue	2 mg/L tank water q48h, up to 3 treatments[100]	Preventing infections of freshwater eggs; toxic to nitrifying bacteria and to plants; stains many objects
Miconazole (Monistat, McNeil-PPC)	10-20 mg/kg PO, IM, ICe[142]	Systemic mycoses
Nalidixic acid (NegGram, Sanofi-Aventis)	5 mg/kg PO, IM q24h[142]	Quinolone; Gram-negative bacteria
	5 mg/kg PO, IV q24h[76]	Rainbow trout/PK
	20 mg/kg PO q24h[149]	
	13 mg/L × 1-4 hr bath, repeat prn[100]	
Neomycin	66 mg/L tank water q3d, up to 3 treatments[100]	Commonly sold as tank treatment for aquarium fish; toxic to nitrifying bacteria; keep fish densities low
Nifurpirinol	—	Nitrofuran; caution: carcinogenic; toxic to scaleless fish; absorbed from water; drug inactivated in bright light
	0.45-0.9 mg/kg PO q24h × 5 days[100]	
	4-10 mg/kg in feed q12h × 5 days[100]	
	0.1 mg/L tank water q24h × 3-5 days[100]	
	1-2 mg/L × 5 min-6 hr bath[100]	
Nitrofurazone	—	Nitrofuran; caution: carcinogenic; toxic to scaleless fish; absorbed from water; drug inactivated in bright light; water soluble formulations preferred; change 50%-75% of water between treatments
	2-5 mg/L tank water q24h × 5-10 days[152]	
	50 mg/L × 3 hr[23]	Seabream/no residues were found in muscle following treatment
	100 mg/L × 30 min bath[100]	
	100 mg/L × 6 hr[23]	Tilapia/no residues were found in muscle following treatment
Oxolinic acid	—	Quinolone; Gram-negative bacteria
	5-25 mg/kg PO q24h[142]	
	10 mg/kg q24h PO[149]	Freshwater species/PK in many species
	25 mg/kg ICe q24h[129]	Corkwing wrasse/PK
	25-50 mg/kg q24h PO[149]	Marine species
	50 mg/kg q24h × 5 days PO[24,25]	Rainbow trout/PK

TABLE 2-1 Antimicrobial and Antifungal Agents Used in Fish. (cont'd)

Agent	Dosage	Comments
Oxolinic acid (cont'd)	10 mg/kg q24h in feed × 10 days[100]	
	3-10 mg/L tank water × 24 hr[100]	
	25 mg/L × 15 min bath q12h × 3 days[100]	Decreased uptake in hard water; better uptake in pH <6.9
Oxytetracycline	3 mg/kg IV q24h[36]	Red pacu/PK
	7 mg/kg IM q24h[36]	Red pacu/PK
	10 mg/kg IM q24h[142]	Produces high levels for several days when given IM
	20 mg/kg ICe[149]	Some salmonids
	20 mg/kg PO q8h[142]	
	25-50 mg/kg IM, ICe[100]	
	60 mg/kg IM q7d[50]	Carp/PK
	70 mg/kg PO q24h × 10-14 days[151]	
	82.8 mg/kg PO × 10 days[21]	Walleye pike, tilapia, hybrid striped bass, summer flounder/PK
	100 mg/kg IM q24h[119]	Tench/PK
	10-100 mg/L tank water[100]	Higher doses in hard water; if fish still sick, retreat on day 3 after 50% water change; light sensitive, so keep tank covered to prevent photo-inactivation; drug turns dark brown when decomposing: change 50% of water immediately; change 50%-75% of water between treatments
	7 mg/g feed q24h × 10 days[151]	
	55-83 mg/kg q24h in feed × 10 days[100]	
	75 mg/kg PO q24h in feed × 10 days[149]	
	10-50 mg/L × 1 hr bath[100]	Surface bacterial infections; yellow-brown foam may develop in treatment water
Potassium permanganate	2 mg/L as an indefinite bath[152]	Heavily organic systems may require a higher dose; test efficacy by adding the appropriate amount of $KMnO_4$ to a small amount of system water (without fish); red color should remain for at least 4 hr (if not, then $KMnO_4$ should be added until the 4-hr test is completed); however, in systems with lower organic loading (e.g., moderate to lower intensity recirculating aquaculture systems), and for sensitive species, treatment durations may need to be shortened to 1-2 hr

Continued

TABLE 2-1 Antimicrobial and Antifungal Agents Used in Fish. (cont'd)

Agent	Dosage	Comments
Potassium permanganate (cont'd)	5 mg/L × 30-60 min bath[100] 1000 mg/L × 10-40 sec bath[100]	Freshwater fish/skin and gill bacterial infections; toxic in water with high pH; do not mix with formalin; can be toxic in goldfish[140]
Sarafloxacin (Sarafloxacin hydrochloride, Enzo Life Sciences)	10-14 mg/kg PO q24h × 10 days[142] 10 mg/kg PO q24h[149] 10 mg/kg PO q24h × 5 days[47]	Fluoroquinolone Marine Atlantic salmon Channel catfish
Silver sulfadiazine cream (Silvadene, Pfizer)	Topical q12h[88]	External bacterial infection; keep lesion out of water 30-60 sec after application; keep gills submerged
Sulfadimethoxine/ormetoprim (Romet, Zoetis)	50 mg/kg/day in feed × 5 days[100] Medicated brine shrimp[100]	Available as a powder to add to feed and as medicated feed Place brine shrimp nauplii (larvae) in 3 mg/L seawater for 4 hr, rinse in seawater with brine shrimp net, then feed immediately to fish; may also work with adult brine shrimp and other live feeds
Thiamphenicol	15 and 30 mg/kg PO[73]	Sea bass/PK; drug was not detected in plasma or tissues at either dose on day 7; recommended withdrawal times of 5 and 6 days, respectively
Tobramycin	2.5 mg/kg IM, then 1 mg/kg IM q4d[143]	Brown shark/PK
Trimethoprim/sulfamethoxazole	30 mg/kg PO q24h × 10-14 days[100] 20 mg/L × 5-12 hr bath q24h × 5-7 days[100] 0.2% feed × 10-14 days[100]	Change 50%-75% of water between treatments
Triple antibiotic ointment (polymyxin B sulfate/bacitracin/neomycin sulfate)	Topical q12h[88]	External bacterial infection; keep lesion out of water 30-60 sec following application; keep gills submerged

[a]Not to be used in fish for human consumption.
[b]Preferable to treat a single fish of a species (biotest) to determine toxicitxy.
[c]Tank treatment: When treating the fishes' resident aquarium, disconnect activated carbon filtration to prevent drug removal. Many drugs adversely affect the nitrifying bacteria, so water quality should be monitored closely (especially ammonia and nitrite concentrations). Always keep water well aerated and monitor fish closely. Perform water changes and reconnect filtration to remove residual drug following treatment. Discard carbon following drug removal.[89]
[d]Bath (immersion) treatment: Remove fish from resident aquarium and place in container with known volume of water and concentration of therapeutic agent. Watch closely for signs of toxicity (e.g., listing and dyspnea). Always keep water well aerated.
[e]Species of fish, temperature, and water quality parameters can influence the pharmacodynamics of many drugs, especially antimicrobials.
[f]For more information, refer to the Web site by Reimschuessel et al.[118] This is a comprehensive and informative resource for many drugs and other compounds used with aquatic animals.

TABLE 2-2 Antiparasitic Agents Used in Fish.[a-d]

Agent	Dosage	Comments
Acetic acid, glacial	1-2 mL/L × 30-45 sec bath[100,152]	Monogeneans, crustacean ectoparasites; safe for goldfish; may be toxic to smaller tropical fish
Albendazole	5 mg/kg PO once[99]	Atlantic salmon/PK
	10 mg/kg PO once[135]	Atlantic salmon, rainbow trout, tilapia/PK
	10-50 mg/L × 2-6 hr[132]	Sticklebacks/treating *Glugea anomala* infection
Chloramine-T	—	See Table 2-1
Chloroquine diphosphate	50 mg/kg PO once[93]	Red drum
	10 mg/L tank water, once[100]	*Amyloodinium ocellatum*; monitor for 21 days, repeat prn; use activated carbon to remove drug if no relapse
Closantel (50 mg/mL)/mebendazole (75 mg/mL) (Supaverm, Janssen-Cilag)	1 mL/400 L once; may repeat in 3-7 days following a water change if necessary[152]	Koi/very safe and effective for external monogeneans; reported to be highly toxic to goldfish and medaka; used in the United Kingdom to kill digenean trematodes of sheep
Copper sulfate	—	Marine fish/protozoan, monogenean ectoparasites; copper levels must be assessed with a commercial kit, and adjusted as needed; blue copper sulfate is copper sulfate (II) pentahydrate ($= CuSO_4 \cdot 5H_2O$); when calculating free copper 2^+ ion levels, copper sulfate pentahydrate is approximately 25% free copper; in marine systems, concentration should be increased gradually to target concentration over the course of 3-4 days; toxic to gill tissue; immunosuppressive; extremely toxic to invertebrates and many plants; copper removed by activated carbon
	Total alkalinity (TA) (mg/L)/100 = mg/L ($CuSO_4 \cdot 5H_2O$)	General dose recommendation for use in freshwater systems (FS), for 50 < total alkalinity (TA) < 250 mg/L; not recommended for use in freshwater systems with TA < 50 mg/L; chelation may be required for TA > 250 mg/L[100]
	0.012 and 0.094 mg/L bath for 28 days[51]	European eel
	0.02 mg/L bath × 65 or 72 hr[52,53]	Rainbow trout
	0.1-0.2 mg/L[149]	Use higher dose in hard water
	Maintain free ion levels at 0.15-0.2 mg/L tank water, until therapeutic effect[100]	
	Maintain copper levels at 0.2 mg/L tank water × 14-21 days[151]	Citrated copper sulfate; prepare stock solution of 1 mg/mL (3 g $CuSO_4 \cdot 5H_2O$ and 2 g citric acid monohydrate in 750 mL distilled water)

Continued

TABLE 2-2 Antiparasitic Agents Used in Fish. (cont'd)

Agent	Dosage	Comments
Copper sulfate (cont'd)	Maintain free ion levels at 0.25-1 mg/L × 24-48 hr bath[57]	
	100 mg/L × 1-5 min bath[20]	Prepare stock solution of 1 mg/mL (1 g $CuSO_4 \cdot 5H_2O$ in 250 mL distilled water)
Diflubenzuron (Dimilin 25W, Chemtura)	0.01 mg/L tank water × 48 hr q6d × 3 treatments[140]	Crustacean ectoparasites; inhibits chitin synthesis; drug persists in water long-term; marketed for control of terrestrial insects; may need EPA restricted use pesticide license for use in the United States
Dimethyl phosphonate	—	See trichlorfon
Dimetridazole	28 mg/kg in feed q24h × 10 days[116]	Rainbow trout/*Ichthyophthirius multifiliis*; available through compounding veterinary pharmacies
	80 mg/L × 3 days (minimum)	Experimental evidence suggests some control of *Cryptobia iubilans* and/or associated mortalities[159]
Doramectin	200 µg/kg PO once	Carp (*Labeo fimbriatus* and *Catla catla*)/*Lernaea*
	750 µg/kg PO[64]	Carp (rohu, *Labeo rohita*)/*Argulus*
	1 mg/kg PO q24h × 10 days[65]	Carp (fringed-lipped peninsula carp, [*Labeo fimbriatus*] and major/Indian carp [*Catla catla*])/*Lernacea*
Emamectin (SLICE, Merck Animal Health)	5 µg/kg PO q24h × 7 days[56]	Koi/*Argulus*
	50 µg/kg PO q24h × 7 days[131]	Atlantic salmon/PK; an avermectin compound used to control sea lice (*Lepeophtheirus salmonis, Caligus elongatus, C. teres,* and *C. rogercressyi*)
	50 µg/kg PO q24h × 7 days[56]	Goldfish/*Argulus*
Fenbendazole	1 mg/kg IV[30]	Channel catfish
	5 mg/kg PO × 1 dose[82]	Channel catfish
	6 mg/kg q24h PO[75]	Rainbow trout
	50 mg/kg PO q24h × 2 days, repeat in 14 days[151]	
	0.2% in feed × 3 days, repeat in 14-21 days[88]	
	40 mg/kg in feed q4d × 2 treatments[149]	Carp/*Bothriocephalus acheilognathi*
	1.5 mg/L × 12-hr bath[75]	Rainbow trout
	2 mg/L tank water q7d × 3 treatments[100]	Nonencysted gastrointestinal nematodes
	2.5 mg/g feed × 2-3 days, repeat in 14 days[151]	
	Bioencapsulation of brine shrimp[7]	Place 1 tablespoon of strained adult brine shrimp and 4 g fenbendazole per 500 mL volume for 30 min to achieve 15.3 µg fenbendazole per shrimp

TABLE 2-2 Antiparasitic Agents Used in Fish. (cont'd)

Agent	Dosage	Comments
Formalin	—	Formalin combination follows
	All doses based on volumes of 100% formalin (=37% formaldehyde)	Protozoan, monogenean, crustacean ectoparasites; caution: carcinogenic; do not use if highly toxic white precipitates are present; some fish are very sensitive: test on small number first, monitor for piping and pale color; increased toxicity in soft, acidic water and at high temperature; treat with vigorous aeration because of oxygen depletion; toxic to plants
	0.015-0.025 mL/L tank water[100]	For *Ichthyophthirius*, use 0.025 mL/L tank water q48h × 3 treatments; change up to 50% of water on alternate days
	0.125-0.25 mL/L, up to 60 min bath, repeat q24h × 2-3 days prn[100]	When using maximum dose, treat q3d
	0.4 mL/L up to 1 hr bath q3d, up to 3 treatments[140]	Soft water
	0.5 mL/L up to 1 hr bath q3d, up to 3 treatments[140]	Hard water
Formalin (F)/malachite green (M)	(F) 0.025 mL/L + (M) 0.1 mg/L tank water q48h × 3 treatments[100]	Combination synergistic for *Ichthyophthirius*; change up to 50% water on alternate days; several premixed commercial products available; malachite green should never be used on fish intended for human consumption
Freshwater	3-15 min bath, repeat q7d prn[100]	Marine fish/ectoparasites; aerate well; match pH with seawater pH; monitor closely; some small fish are sensitive
	4-5 min bath[87]	
Hydrogen peroxide (HP) (3%; 30 mg/mL)	—	Not recommended for use in blue gourami or suckermouth catfish (*Pterygoplichthys* spp.)[124]
	0.22 mL/L × 1 bath[123]	Swordtails/*Ichthyobodo*
	1-1.5 mL/L × 20 min bath[147]	Atlantic salmon/sea lice
	5 mg/L × 24 hr or 10 mg/L × 1 hr[123]	Tiger barb
	5.4 mg/L × 24 hr or 20.2 mg/L × 1 hr[123]	Swordtail
	5.6 mg/L × 24 hr or 7 mg/L × 1 hr[123]	Serpae tetra
	17.5 mL/L × 4-10 min bath, once[57]	Ectoparasites; monitor closely; may be harmful to smaller fish
Hydrogen peroxide (HP) (PEROX-AID 35%, Eka Chemicals)	—	These are unlabeled experimental treatments
	170-560 mg/L (static bath) × 30 min[115]	Rainbow trout/*Ambiphrya* and *Gyrodactylus*[115]
	75 mg/L × 30 min[98]	Pacific threadfin (*Polydactylus sexfilis*) juveniles/*Amyloodinium*
	300 mg/L × 10 min[94]	Kingfish/monogenean *Zeuxapta seriolae*

Continued

TABLE 2-2 Antiparasitic Agents Used in Fish. (cont'd)

Agent	Dosage	Comments
Ivermectin	—	Do not use; neurologic signs and death at therapeutic doses;[57,149] toxic to many environmental invertebrates[149]
Levamisole	0.5 mg/kg ICe[79]	Rainbow trout/immunostimulant
	10 mg/kg PO q7d × 3 treatments[57]	
	11 mg/kg IM q7d × 2 treatments[57]	
	1 mg/L × 24 hr bath[145]	Eels/swimbladder nematodes
	1-2 mg/L × 24 hr bath[57]	Internal nematodes, especially larval
	50 mg/L × 2 hr bath[57]	
	4 g/kg feed q7d × 3 treatments[57]	External monogeneans
Lufenuron (Program, Novartis)	0.13 mg/L prn[120,152]	Control of crustacean ectoparasites
Malachite green	—	See formalin for combination
	0.1 mg/L tank water q3d × 3 treatments[100]	
	1 mg/L × 30-60 min bath[100]	Use 2 mg/L if pH high
	50-60 mg/L × 10-30 sec bath[100]	
	100 mg/L topical to skin lesions[100]	Freshwater fish/protozoan ectoparasites; prepare stock solution of 3.7 mg/mL (1.4 g malachite green in 380 mL water); caution: mutagenic; teratogenic; toxic to some fish species (e.g., tetras) and fry; increased toxicity at higher temperatures and lower pH; toxic to plants; stains objects, especially plastic; remove residual chemical with activated carbon after last tank treatment; not to be used on fish intended for human consumption
Mebendazole	20 mg/kg PO q7d × 3 treatments[142]	Gastrointestinal nematodes; do not administer to brood fish: embryotoxic and teratogenic
	1 mg/L × 24 hr bath[57,74]	Monogeneans
	1 mg/L × 72 hr bath[17]	European eels/branchial monogeneans (*Pseudodactylogyrus bini* and *P. anguillae*)
	10-50 mg/L for 2-6 hr immersion[132]	Sticklebacks/*Glugea anomala*
	100 mg/L × 10 min-2 hr bath[57]	Monogeneans
Methylene blue	1-3 mg/L tank water[100]	Freshwater fish/ectoparasites; not recommended because of poor efficacy; toxic to nitrifying bacteria; stains objects; toxic to plants

TABLE 2-2 Antiparasitic Agents Used in Fish. (cont'd)

Agent	Dosage	Comments
Metronidazole	25 mg/kg q24h in feed × 5-10 days[100]	Equivalent to 0.25% in feed (250 mg/100 g food) at 1% BW/day
	50 mg/kg PO q24h × 5 days[57]	
	100 mg/kg q24h in feed × 3 days[100]	Equivalent to 1% in feed (1 g/100 g food) at 1% BW/day
	6.6 mg/L tank water q24h × 3 days[100]	*Spironucleus* (*Hexamita*) and other internal flagellates; some external flagellates; poorly soluble in water: dissolve before adding to water or feed; change water between tank treatments
	25 mg/L tank water q48h × 3 treatments[100]	
	6.25-18 mg/g feed × 5 days[151]	
	Brine shrimp encapsulation of metronidazole[6]	One Tbs of live strained adult brine shrimp is approximately 16 g wet weight (≈262 shrimp/g); 5 g metronidazole plus 1 Tbs brine shrimp in 500 mL water for 0.25 hr will yield 9.32 μg metronidazole per shrimp (2500 μg per g of shrimp)
Niclosamide	0.055 mg/L × 24 hr bath[71]	Rainbow trout/lampricide
Piperazine	10 mg/kg q24h in feed × 3 days[100]	Nonencysted gastrointestinal nematodes; equivalent to 0.1% in feed at 1% BW/day
Potassium permanganate	5 mg/L × 30-60 min bath[100]	Freshwater fish/protozoan, crustacean ectoparasites; toxic in water with high pH; do not mix with formalin; can be toxic in goldfish[140]
	100 mg/L × 5-10 min bath[100]	
	1 g/L × 10-40 sec bath[100]	
Praziquantel	5 mg/kg PO q24h × 3 treatments[149]	
	5 mg/kg PO in feed q7d, up to 3 treatments[142]	
	5 mg/kg PO, ICe, repeat in 14-21 days[87]	Cestodes, some internal digenean trematodes; could be administered in feed
	50 mg/kg PO once[100]	Adult cestodes; gavage or give 0.5% in feed at 1% BW/day
	2 mg/L × 2-4 hr[113]	Metacercaria
	2-10 mg/L up to 4 hr bath[151]	Monitor closely for lethargy, incoordination, loss of equilibrium
	5-10 mg/L × 3-6 hr bath, repeat in 7 days[87]	Monogenean ectoparasites, cestodes; aerate water well; some marine fish sensitive; may be toxic to *Corydoras* catfish
	5-12 mg/kg feed × 3 days[151]	
	Bioencapsulation of praziquantel in brine shrimp[5]	Place 1 Tbs of strained adult brine shrimp and 2.5 g praziquantel per 500 mL volume for 30 min to achieve 8.6 μg praziquantel per shrimp

Continued

TABLE 2-2 Antiparasitic Agents Used in Fish. (cont'd)

Agent	Dosage	Comments
Pyrantel pamoate	10 mg/kg in feed, once[142]	Gastric nematodes
Salt (as sodium chloride, seawater, or artificial sea salts)	—	Freshwater fish/protozoan, monogenean ectoparasites; seawater or artificial sea salts preferred; seawater is normally 30-35 g/L; use non-iodized table/rock salts; some anticaking agents in solar salts are highly toxic; species sensitivity is highly variable (some catfish sensitive); may be toxic to plants
	1-5 g/L tank water, indefinitely[100]	Prophylaxis or treatment of ectoparasites
	3 g/L[149]	Supportive care
	10-30 g/L up to 30 min bath[100]	With salt-sensitive or weak fish, use lower dosage and repeat in 24 hr
	30 g/L for 10 min[149]	Fish >100 g only
	30-35 g/L × 4-5 min bath[87]	Safe for goldfish and koi in most cases
Thiabendazole	10-25 mg/kg in feed, repeat in 10 days[142]	Gastric nematodes; anorexia may be seen (more severe at higher doses), generally resolves within 2-4 days
	66 mg/kg PO, once[142]	
Trichlorfon (dimethyl phosphonate)	—	Caution: organophosphate, neurotoxic, avoid inhalation and skin contact; aerate water well; especially toxic to larval fish, some characins (i.e., pacu, piranha, and silver dollars); other species sensitivities; liquid form marketed for cattle is convenient to dispense
	0.25 mg/L tank water;[100] 96 hr bath at this concentration in channel catfish[118]	Freshwater fish/use 0.5 mg/L tank water if >27°C (80°F); treat q3d × 2 treatments for Dactylogyrus and other oviparous monogeneans; treat q7d × 4 treatments for anchor worms (Lernaea) and fish louse (Argulus); single treatment will usually suffice for other copepods, other monogeneans, leeches
	0.5 mg/L tank water q10d × 3 treatments[87]	Crustacean ectoparasites; change 20%-30% of water 24-48 hr following each treatment
	0.5-1 mg/L tank water[100]	Marine fish/treat q3d × 2 treatments for oviparous monogeneans; use 1 mg/L q48h × 3 treatments for turbellarians; single treatment will usually suffice for copepods (except sea lice), other monogeneans, leeches

[a]Not to be used in fish for human consumption.
[b]Preferable to treat single fish of a species to determine toxicity.
[c]Tank treatment: when treating the fishes' resident aquarium, disconnect activated carbon filtration to prevent drug removal; many drugs adversely affect the nitrifying bacteria, so water quality should be monitored closely (especially ammonia and nitrite concentrations); always keep water well aerated and monitor fish closely; perform water changes and reconnect filtration to remove residual drug following treatment; discard carbon following drug removal.[89]
[d]Bath (immersion) treatment: remove fish from resident aquarium and place in container with known volume of water and concentration of therapeutic agent; watch closely for signs of toxicity, e.g., listing and dyspnea; always keep water well aerated.

TABLE 2-3 Chemical Restraint/Anesthetic/Analgesic Agents Used in Fish.[a-d]

Agent	Dosage	Comments
Alfaxalone (Alfaxan, Jurox)	5 mg/L induction[18]	Oscar (cichlid)/sedation and anesthesia
	10 mg/L induction; 1-2.5 mg/L maintenance[96]	Koi/sedation and anesthesia; not recommended as an injectable agent for koi carp;[13] may have opercular cessation at 2.5 mg/L
Atipamezole (Antisedan, Zoetis)	0.2 mg/kg IM[43]	Reversal agent (α_2 antagonist) for medetomidine
Benzocaine	—	Not sold as fish anesthetic in United States; available from chemical supply companies; do not use topical anesthetic products marketed for mammals; prepare stock solution in ethanol (benzocaine is poorly soluble in water); store in dark bottle at room temperature
	15-40 mg/L bath[100]	Transport sedation
	50-500 mg/L bath[100]	Anesthesia
	70 mg/L for 5 min then 35 mg/L for 30 min[118]	Channel catfish
	1 g/L spray[100]	Large fish/anesthesia; spray onto gills with an aerosol pump sprayer
Butorphanol	0.05-0.1 mg/kg IM[142]	Postoperative analgesia
	0.4 mg/kg IM[59,60]	Koi/postoperative analgesia
	10 mg/kg IM[14]	Koi/postoperative analgesia; respiratory depression at this dose; lower dosage might be warranted
Carbon dioxide	—	Euthanasia; bubble gas through water until respiration stops >10 min; other agents preferred[100]
Clove oil (also see Eugenol)	—	Clove oil consists of a mixture of eugenol, methyleugenol, isoeugenol, and other compounds and in this generic form is not approved by the FDA for use in fish intended for human consumption
	40-120 mg/L bath[87]	Stock solution: 100 mg/mL of clove oil by diluting 1 part clove oil with 9 parts 95% ethanol (eugenol is poorly soluble in water); over-the-counter preparation (pure) available at most pharmacies contains approximately 1 g eugenol per mL of clove oil; recovery may be prolonged; use lower end of this range to start; many bony fishes readily anesthetized with 25-50 mg/L
Dexmedetomidine[d]	—	See medetomidine for comments
Ethanol	1%-1.5% bath[58]	Anesthetic levels difficult to control, resulting in overdose; not recommended
	>3% bath[58]	Euthanasia; other agents preferred
Etomidate	1-4 mg/L[149]	Lower doses should be used with striped bass and related species[149]

Continued

TABLE 2-3 Chemical Restraint/Anesthetic/Analgesic Agents Used in Fish. (cont'd)

Agent	Dosage	Comments
Eugenol (a purified derivative of clove oil; also see clove oil)	10-100 mg/L bath for sedation to handleable[2] 17-25 mg/L bath[149]	Aqui-SE contains 50% eugenol and Aqui-S20E, 10% eugenol, a compound mixture of eugenol and polysorbate 80 (for solubility); lower doses (6 mg/L) will produce sedation without general anesthesia[2,149]
Isoflurane	0.5-2 mL/L bath or vaporize then bubble in water[58]	Anesthetic levels difficult to control, resulting in overdose; not recommended
Ketamine	— 66-88 mg/kg IM[142]	Ketamine combination follows Immobilization for short procedures; complete recovery can take >1 hr
Ketamine (K)/medetomidine (M)[d]	(K) 1-2 mg/kg + (M) 0.05-0.1 mg/kg IM[58]	Immobilization; reverse (M) with atipamezole (0.2 mg/kg IM); see medetomidine
Ketoprofen (Ketofen, Zoetis)	2 mg/kg IM[60]	As a postoperative analgesic in koi
Lidocaine	—	Local anesthetic; use cautiously in small fish; do not exceed 1-2 mg/kg total dose[59]
Medetomidine[d]	0.03-0.07 mg/kg IV[4]	See ketamine for combination; medetomidine is off-market, but is available through selected compounding services
Metomidate (Aquacalm, Syndel USA)	—	Gouramis may be sensitive; contraindicated in cichlids in water of pH <5
	0.06-0.2 mg/L water[141]	Transport sedation
	0.1-1 mg/L[9]	
	1 mg/L[80]	Convict cichlids/for 24 hr transport sedation
	0.5-1 mg/L water[58]	Light sedation
	1-10 mg/L bath induction; 0.1-1 mg/L maintenance[141]	Freshwater fish/anesthesia
	2.5-5 mg/L water[58]	Heavy sedation
	2.5-5 mg/L bath induction; 0.2-0.3 mg/L maintenance[141]	Marine fish/anesthesia
	3 mg/kg IV[55]	Atlantic halibut, turbot/PK
	5-10 mg/L bath[58]	Anesthesia; some species require 10-30 mg/L bath
	7 mg/kg PO[55]	Turbot/PK
	9 mg/L bath for 5 min[55]	Atlantic halibut, turbot/PK
Morphine	5 mg/kg IM[14]	Koi/analgesia
MS-222 (Tricaine-S, Syndel USA)	—	See tricaine methanesulfonate
Pentobarbital	60 mg/kg ICe[100]	Euthanasia
2-Phenoxyethanol	0.1-0.5 mL/L bath[149] 0.6 mL/L bath[149]	 Carp/surgery

TABLE 2-3 Chemical Restraint/Anesthetic/Analgesic Agents Used in Fish. (cont'd)

Agent	Dosage	Comments
Propofol	3.5-7.5 mg/kg IV[43]	Gulf of Mexico sturgeon
	7 mg/L bath[45]	Goldfish/anesthesia; induction time, 7.4 min; recovery, 8.5 min
Quinaldine sulfate	25 mg/L bath[149]	Channel catfish, salmonids/do not use with largemouth bass; not recommended for long surgical procedures
	50-100 mg/L bath induction; 15-60 mg/L maintenance[58]	Anesthesia; not sold as fish anesthetic in United States; stock solution: 10 g/L, buffer the acidity by adding sodium bicarbonate to saturation; store stock in dark container; shelf-life of stock extended by refrigeration or freezing; aerate water to prevent hypoxemia; drug not metabolized, excreted unchanged; euthanasia: keep in solution >10 min after respiration stops
Sodium bicarbonate	30 g/L bath[100]	Euthanasia; generates CO_2; use when other agents unavailable; keep fish in solution >10 min after respiration stops; generally not recommended; not an AVMA-approved method of euthanasia
Sodium bicarbonate tablets (Alka-Seltzer, Bayer)	2-4 tablets/L bath[48]	Euthanasia; generates CO_2; use when other agents unavailable; keep fish in solution >10 min after respiration stops; generally not recommended; not an AVMA-approved method of euthanasia
Tricaine methanesulfonate (MS-222; Tricaine-S, Syndel USA)	15-50 mg/L water[58]	Sedation
	50-100 mg/L bath induction; 50-60 mg/L maintenance[141]	Anesthesia; stock solution: 10 g/L, buffer the acidity by adding sodium bicarbonate at 10 g/L or to saturation (unbuffered solution may cause some ectoparasites to leave fish)[20] store stock in dark container; shelf-life of stock extended by refrigeration or freezing; stock that develops an oily film should be discarded; aerate water to prevent hypoxemia; narrower margin of safety in young fish, and soft, warm water; euthanasia: keep fish in solution >20 min after respiration stops
	100-200 mg/L bath induction; 50-100 mg/L maintenance[58]	
	1 g/L spray[100]	Large fish/anesthesia; spray onto gills with an aerosol pump sprayer

[a]Not to be used in fish for human consumption.
[b]Preferable to treat single fish of a species to determine toxicity.
[c]Aerate water during anesthetic procedures; dissolved oxygen concentrations should be maintained between 6 and 10 mg/L (ppm).
[d]Medetomidine is no longer commercially available although it can be obtained from select compounding services; a dosage is listed here as a guide for possible use with dexmedetomidine, an α_2 agonist that is the active optical enantiomer of racemic compound medetomidine; in other species, dexmedetomidine is used at {1/2} the dose of medetomidine but the same volume due to a higher concentration. However, the effects of the v/v use of the two drugs may not be equivalent, so the dose of dexmedetomidine may need to be adjusted based on clinical response.

TABLE 2-4 Miscellaneous Agents Used in Fish.[a-c]

Agent	Dosage	Comments
Atropine	0.1 mg/kg IM, IV, ICe[140]	Organophosphate, chlorinated hydrocarbon toxicity
Becaplermin (Regranex, Smith & Nephew)	Topically as a thin layer for 3 min[42]	Ocean surgeonfish/light debridement of the head and lateral line erosion (HLLE) lesions is recommended prior to treatment; multiple treatments are not warranted, but fish should be returned to a habitat without predisposing factors to HLLE
Carbon, activated	75 g/40 L tank water[100]	Removal of medications and other organics from water; usually added to filter system; discard after 2 wk; 75 g ≈ 250 cc dry volume
Carp pituitary extract	0.75 mg/kg IM[149]	Female fish (<2 kg)
	1-1.5 mg/kg IM[149]	Male fish
	1.5 mg/kg IM[149]	Female fish (2-5 kg)
	2.5-3 mg/kg IM[149]	Female fish (>5 kg)
	5 mg/kg IM, repeat in 6 hr[142]	Dose when combined with human chorionic gonadotropin (20 U/kg); hormone to stimulate release of eggs (may be given in 2 doses, 24 hr apart; the first "preparatory" dose ≤10% of the total dose); does not cause eggs to mature; do not administer unless eggs are mature
Chlorine/chloramine neutralizer	Use as directed	See sodium thiosulfate
Dexamethasone	1-2 mg/kg IM, ICe[142]	Adjunct to treatment of shock, trauma, chronic stress syndromes
	2 mg/kg IV, ICe q12h[87]	Chlorine toxicity; may improve prognosis
Doxapram	5 mg/kg IV, ICe[140]	Respiratory depression
Epinephrine (1:1000)	0.2-0.5 mL IM, IV, ICe, intracardiac[140]	Cardiac arrest
Furosemide	2-5 mg/kg IM q12-72 h[142]	Diuretic; ascites, generalized edema; of questionable value since fish lack a loop of Henle
Glucans (MacroGard, Orffa)	2-10 mg/kg ICe[121,149]	Polysaccharides; immunostimulant
	1 g/kg in feed × 24 days fed at 3% BW[124]	Red-tailed black sharks/significant decrease in mortalities from Streptococcus iniae
	2 g/kg in feed × 7 days[136]	Rainbow trout/tested with positive results
sGnRHa (salmon gonadotropin-releasing hormone analogue) + domperidone (Ovaprim, Syndel USA)	0.5 mL/kg (0.5 μL/g) IM, ICe[66,106]	For use as a spawning aid in fish; enhances/triggers ovulation and spermiation; for ovulation of eggs
Haloperidol	0.5 mg/kg IM[142]	Dopamine blocking agent; use with luteinizing releasing hormone analog (LRH-A) to stimulate release of eggs

TABLE 2-4 Miscellaneous Agents Used in Fish. (cont'd)

Agent	Dosage	Comments
Human chorionic gonadotropin (hCG) (Chorulon, Merck Animal Health)	20 U/kg IM, repeat in 6 hr[142]	Dose when combined with carp pituitary extract (5 mg/kg)
	30 U/kg (22.7-232 U/kg for males; 30.5-828 U/kg for females) IM, repeat in 6 hr[142] × 1-3 injections[22]	Indicated for use as an aid in improving spawning function in male and female broodfish; hormone to stimulate release of eggs (ovulation) and sperm (spermiation); does not cause eggs to mature: do not administer unless eggs are mature
	800-1000 U/kg IM q8h[154]	Carp
Hydrocortisone	1-4 mg/kg IM, ICe[142]	Adjunct to treatment of shock, trauma, chronic stress syndromes
Hydrogen peroxide (3%)	0.25 mL/L water[100]	Acute environmental hypoxia; see oxygen
Luteinizing releasing hormone analog (LRH-A)	2 µg/kg IM, then 8 µg/kg 6 hr later[142]	Synthetic luteinizing releasing hormone analog; stimulates release of eggs; does not cause eggs to mature: do not administer unless eggs are mature; in species that do not respond to LRH-A alone, administer with haloperidol or reserpine with the first injection of LRH-A
Methyltestosterone	30 mg/kg PO q24h × 2 or 4 days[118]	Rainbow trout/PD; functional masculinization of genetic females
Nitrifying bacteria	Use as directed for commercial products	Seed or improve development of biological filtration to detoxify ammonia and nitrite; numerous commercial preparations; do not expose products to extreme temperatures; use before expiration date
	Add material (e.g., floss, gravel) from a tank with an active biological filter and healthy fish to new tank[100]	Must evaluate risk of disease transmission with this technique
Nucleotide (Aquagen, Novartis)	2 g/kg feed at 3% BW × 24 days[124]	Red-tailed black sharks/reduced mortalities from *Streptococcus iniae*; product may be difficult to find as commercial production has been discontinued.
Oxygen (100%)	Fill plastic bag with O_2 containing ⅓ vol of water[87]	Acute environmental hypoxia common with transportation; close bag tightly with rubber band; keep fish in bag until normal swimming and respiratory behavior
Reserpine	50 mg/kg IM[142]	Dopamine blocking agent; use with LRH-A to stimulate release of eggs
Salt (sodium chloride)	1-3 g/L tank water[86] 3-5 g/L tank water[100]	Freshwater fish/prevention of stress-induced mortality; seawater or artificial sea salts preferred; use non-iodized table/rock salts; some anticaking agents in solar salts are highly toxic; highly variable species sensitivity to salt (some catfish sensitive); may be toxic to plants
	Add chloride to produce at least a 6:1 ratio (w/w) of Cl: NO_2 ions[100]	Treatment of nitrite toxicity; table/rock salt = 60% Cl, artificial sea salts = 55% Cl

Continued

TABLE 2-4 Miscellaneous Agents Used in Fish. (cont'd)

Agent	Dosage	Comments
Sodium thiosulfate	Use as directed for chlorine/chloramine neutralizers 10 mg/L tank water[87]	Active ingredient in numerous chlorine/chloramine neutralizers; chlorine and chloramine are common additions to municipal water supplies and are toxic to fish; ammonia released by detoxification of chloramine is removed by functioning biological filter (see nitrifying bacteria) or chemical means (see zeolite)
	100 mg/L tank water[140]	Chlorine exposure
	10 g neutralizes chlorine (up to 2 mg/L) from 1000 L water[87]	
Zeolite (i.e., clinoptilolite)	Use as directed 20 g/L tank water[100]	Ion-exchange resin that exchanges ammonia for sodium ions; clinoptilolite is an active form of zeolite; used to reduce or prevent ammonia toxicity; more effective for removal of some compounds (e.g., sulfonamides, enrofloxacin) than activated carbon[15,67,104]

[a]Not to be used in fish for human consumption.
[b]Preferable to treat single fish of a species to determine toxicity.
[c]Bath treatment: remove fish from resident aquarium and place in container with known volume of water and concentration of therapeutic agent; watch closely for signs of toxicity, e.g., listing and dyspnea; always keep water well aerated.

TABLE 2-5 Euthanasia Agents Used in Fish.[a]

Agent	Dosage	Comments
Benzocaine	≥250 mg/L immersion for at least 10 min[12]	Solution should be buffered; once the fish loses consciousness, a secondary method (double pithing, decapitation, injectable pentobarbital) should be used
Carbon dioxide	Immersion to effect[12]	Fish may become hyperactive before losing consciousness; use in a well ventilated area
Ethanol	10-30 mL 95%/L as an immersion to effect[12]	
Eugenol (a purified derivative of clove oil; also see clove oil)	≥17 mg/L as an immersion to effect[12]	Concentrations up to 5 times this amount can be used; once the fish loses consciousness, a secondary method (double pithing, decapitation, injectable pentobarbital) should be used
Isoflurane/sevoflurane	5-20 mL/L as an immersion to effect[12]	Due to the volatility of these comppounds and risk to humans, ventilation precautions should be taken
Ketamine	66-88 mg/kg IM[12]	Follow with a lethal pentobarbital injection
Ketamine (K)/dexmedetomidine (D)	(K) 1-2 mg/kg + (D) 0.05-0.1 mg/kg IM[12]	Follow with a lethal pentobarbital injection

TABLE 2-5	Euthanasia Agents Used in Fish. (cont'd)	
Agent	**Dosage**	**Comments**
2-phenoxyethanol	≥0.5-0.6 mL/L or 0.3-0.4 mg/L as an immersion to effect[12]	
Propofol	1.5-2.5 mg/L IM[12]	Follow with a lethal pentobarbital injection
	5-10 mg/L as an immersion to effect[103]	Once the fish loses consciousness, a secondary method (double pithing, decapitation, injectable intracardiac pentobarbital) should be used
Quinaldine sulfate	≥100 mg/L as an immersion to effect[12]	Buffering may be required in some cases
Tricaine methanesulfonate (MS-222) (Tricaine-S, Syndel USA)	250-500 mg/L as an immersion for at least 10 min after cessation of respiration[12]	Buffering is required and a secondary method (double pithing, decapitation, injectable intracardiac pentobarbital) should be used

[a]Not to be used in fish for human consumption; CO_2 euthanasia is the exception.

TABLE 2-6	Hematologic and Serum Biochemical Values of Fish.[a]	
Measurement	**Goldfish (*Carassius auratus*)[49]**	**Koi (*Cyprinus carpio*)[49,107,150]**
Hematology		
PCV (%)	31 ± 7.3	35 (24-43)
RBC ($10^6/\mu L$)	1.5 ± 0.1	1.61-1.91
Hgb (g/dL)	9.1 ± 0.4	6.32-7.55
MCV (fL)	—	166.3-190
MCH (pg)	—	37.7-42.7
MCHC (g/dL)	—	20.4-22.9
WBC ($10^3/\mu L$)	—	19.8-28.1
Heterophils (%)	29 ± 3	7.96-13.89
Lymphocytes (%)	70 ± 5	74.5-83.7
Monocytes (%)	1 ± 0.1	2.3-3.4
Basophils (%)	—	3.5-5.6
Chemistries		
ALP (U/L)	—	12 (4-56)
ALT (U/L)	106 (97-115)	31 (9-98)
Anion gap	—	17 (14-23)
AST (U/L)	220 (111-433)	121 (40-381)
Bicarbonate (mmol/L)	—	6 (3-8)
Bile acids (μmol/L)	—	1 (0-6)
BUN (mg/dL)	28	2 (0.2-5)
Calcium (mg/dL)	9.1 (4.3-13.5)	8.7 (7.8-11.4)
Chloride (mEq/L)	—	114 (108-119)
Cholesterol (mg/dL)	—	149 (94-282)

Continued

TABLE 2-6 Hematologic and Serum Biochemical Values of Fish. (cont'd)

Measurement	Goldfish (*Carassius auratus*)	Koi (*Cyprinus carpio*)
Chemistries (cont'd)		
Creatine kinase (U/L)	4515 (0-10,000)	4123 (80-9014)
Creatinine (mg/dL)	—	—
Glucose (mg/dL)	35.7 (15-93)	37 (22-65)
GGT (U/L)	—	1 (0-6)
LDH (U/L)	—	359 (41-1675)
Phosphorus (mg/dL)	8.83 (3.1-16.3)	6.1 (3.5-7.7)
Potassium (mEq/L)	2.16 (0.1-5.6)	1.4 (0-2.9)
Protein, total (g/dL)	2.03 (0.1-4.02)	3.4 (2.7-4.3)
Albumin (g/dL)	1.9 (0.3-3.2)	2 (1.4-2.7)
Globulin (g/dL)	0.69 (0.3-1.2)	0.9 (0.6-1.1)
A:G (ratio)	2.75	1.1 (0.8-1.6)
Sodium (mEq/L)	139 (126-176)	133 (110-143)
Total bilirubin (mg/dL)	—	0.5 (0.2-2)
Uric acid (mg/dL)	0.08 (0-0.2)	0.1 (0-0.5)

Measurement	Striped bass (*Morone saxatilis*)[62,101]	Palmetto bass (*Morone saxatilis* × *M. chrysops*)[69,70,101]
Hematology		
PCV (%)	42 (34-28)	20-34
RBC ($10^6/\mu L$)	—	2.42-4.96
Hgb (g/dL)	—	4.2-8.4
MCV (fL)	—	65-117
MCH (pg)	—	16.2-24.8
MCHC (g/dL)	—	19-26
WBC ($10^3/\mu L$)	—	32.6-118.2
Neutrophils ($10^3/\mu L$)	—	0-6.8
Lymphocytes (small and large) ($10^3/\mu L$)	—	23.7-125.1
Monocytes ($10^3/\mu L$)	—	0-3.2
Eosinophils (%)	—	0-2.7
Chemistries		
ALP (U/L)	—	72
Anion gap	29 ± 5	24 ± 1
AST (U/L)	23 ± 6	45 ± 21
Calcium (mg/dL)	10.6 ± 0.1	11.1 ± 0.2
Chloride (mEq/L)	143 ± 2	144 ± 2
Cholesterol (mg/dL)	—	164
Creatinine (mg/dL)	0.5 ± 0	0.3 ± 0
Glucose (mg/dL)	100 ± 28	118 ± 10
LDH (U/L)	221 ± 92	164 ± 54

TABLE 2-6	Hematologic and Serum Biochemical Values of Fish. (cont'd)	
Measurement	Striped bass (*Morone saxatilis*)	Palmetto bass (*Morone saxatilis* × *M. chrysops*)
Chemistries (cont'd)		
Osmolality (mOsm/kg)	348 ± 2	356 ± 2
Phosphorus (mg/dL)	10 ± 0.3	9.8 ± 0.2
Potassium (mEq/L)	3.9 ± 0.1	3.3 ± 0.2
Protein, total (g/dL)	3.8 ± 0.1	3.0
Albumin (g/dL)	1.1 ± 0	1.3
Globulin (g/dL)	—	1.7
A:G (ratio)	0.4 ± 0	0.76
Sodium (mEq/L)	181 ± 4	151
Chloride (mEq/L)	150	
Total CO_2 (mmol/L)	9.5 ± 1	10.7 ± 0.9

Measurement	[a]Red pacu (*Piaractus brachypomum*)[125,148]	Rainbow trout (*Oncorhynchus mykiss*)[33,68a,137]
Hematology		
PCV (%)	26 (22-32)	34.8-56.9
RBC ($10^6/\mu L$)	1.7 (1.2-2.9)	1.4-1.8
Hgb (g/dL)	—	6.4-9.5
MCH (pg)	—	35.3-62.4
MCHC (g/dL)	—	14.2-18.9
WBC ($10^3/\mu L$)	33.5 (13.6-52.3)	9.9 ± 1.3
Heterophils (%)	5.2 (0.3-36.7)	—
Lymphocytes (%)	84 (53-96)	—
Monocytes (%)	4 (0.8-11.2)	—
Eosinophils (%)	0.3 (0.3-0.7)	—
Chemistries		
Anion gap	6.9 (1.2-12.5)	—
AST (U/L)	49 (0-125)	102
BUN (mg/dL)	—	—
Calcium (mg/dL)	10.8 (9.5-12.5)	2.3
Chloride (mEq/L)	139 (146-159)	137
Creatine kinase (U/L)	—	—
Creatinine (mg/dL)	0.3 (0.2-0.4)	0.4
Glucose (mg/dL)	—	103
Lactate (mmol/L)	—	—
LDH (U/L)	238 (65-692)	—
Osmolality (mOsm/kg)	—	—
Phosphorus (mg/dL)	7.3 (4.1-8.9)	
Potassium (mEq/L)	3.9 (2.7-5)	

Continued

TABLE 2-6 Hematologic and Serum Biochemical Values of Fish. (cont'd)

Measurement	Red pacu (*Piaractus brachypomum*)	Rainbow trout (*Oncorhynchus mykiss*)
Chemistries (cont'd)		
Protein, total (g/dL)	—	—
Albumin (g/dL)	0.9 (0.5-1)	—
Sodium (mEq/L)	150 (146-159)	—
Total CO_2 (mmol/L)	7.5 (6-10)	—
Uric acid (mg/dL)	—	—

Measurement	[a]Mbuna cichlid (*Metriaclima greshakei*)[137a]	[a]*Cichlasoma dimerus* (a South American cichlid)[150a]
Hematology		
>PCV (%)	25.3 (21-29.5)	31.3 (22.5-39.1)
RBC (10^6/μL)	2.3 (1.7-2.7)	3.1 (1.7-4.3)
Hgb (g/L)	75 (63-91.3)	68.2 (52.3-83.3)
MCV (fL)	113.8 (95.3-132.4)	110.3 (70.1-198)
MCH (pg)	33.6 (26.9-40.3)	24.5 (14.5-40.6)
MCHC (g/dL)	3.0 (2.7-3.2)	22.3 (17.4-30.3)
WBC (10^3/μL)	33.2 (22.9-55.2)	12.2 (6.6-18.6)
Granulocytes (10^3/μL)	1.48 (0.3-2.4)	3.4 (1.9-5.2) (heterophils)
Lymphocytes (10^3/μL)	30.9 (21.2-52.4)	4.7 (2.5-7.1)
Monocytes (10^3/μL)	—	2.2 (1.2-3.3)
Eosinophils (%)	—	1.9 (1-2.8)
Chemistries		
ALP (U/L)	44.5 (30.1-61.9)	—
ALT (U/L)	59.8 (34.7-236.1)	—
AST (U/L)	12.5 (3.5-46.3)	—
Calcium (mmol/L)	2.6 (2.5-2.7)	—
Chloride (mEq/L)	147 (143-150)	—
Cholesterol (mmol/L)	10.6 (6.8-13.9)	—
Creatinine (μmol/dL)	512 (265-941)	—
Glucose (mmol/L)	2.4 (2.1-2.7)	—
Phosphorus (mmol/L)	1.5 (1.3-1.6)	—
Potassium (mmol/L)	3.1 (2.4-3.6)	—
Protein, total (g/L)	39 (34.6-46.2)	—
Albumin (g/L)	9.5 (8.1-10.5)	—
Globulin (g/L)	29 (25.8-37)	—
A:G (ratio)	0.33	—
Sodium (mmol/L)	161 (156.3-163.4)	—
Chloride (mmol/L)	147 (143-150)	—

TABLE 2-6　Hematologic and Serum Biochemical Values of Fish. (cont'd)

Measurement	[a]Tilapia (*Orechromis* hybrid)[68]	[a]Channel catfish (*Ictalurus punctatus*)[146]
Hematology		
PCV (%)	33 (27-37)	31 (27-54)
RBC (10^6/μL)	6.1 (4.8-7.8)	3 (15-41)
Hgb (g/dL)	8.2 (7.0-9.8)	7 (4.4-10.9)
MCV (fL)	135.7 (115-183)	108 (88.6-186.7)
MCH (pg)	34.9 (28.3-42.3)	—
MCHC (g/dL)	25.7 (22-29)	22 (15.7-28.7)
WBC (10^3/μL)	7.6	—
Heterophils (%)	1.8 (0.56-9.9) (neutrophils)	—
Lymphocytes (small) (%)	61 (6.8-136)	—
Lymphocytes (large) %	10.7 (2.9-31)	—
Monocytes (%)	1.5 (0.4-4.3)	—
Eosinophils (%)	0.3 (0.03-1.6)	—
Thromobocytes (10^3/μL)	52.8 (25-85)	—
Thromobocyte-like cells (10^3/μL)	1 (0.03-4.3)	—
Chemistries		
ALP (U/L)	26 (16-38)	—
ALT (U/L)		—
AST (U/L)	18 (5-124)	—
Calcium (mmol/L)	2.9 (2.6-4.7)	2.7 (2.3-3.3)
Chloride (mEq/L)	141 (136-147)	108 (80-147)
Cholesterol (mg/dL)	156 (64-299)	—
Creatinine (mg/dL)	0.2-1.1	—
Glucose (mg/dL)	52 (39-96)	35.1 (17-86.5)
Magnesium (mEq/L)	2.5 (2.3-2.8)	1.2 (1.0-2.0)
Phosphorus (mg/dL)	4.6 (3.5-7.2)	—
Potassium (mEq/L)	3.9 (3.2-4.3)	3 (2.1-4.8)
Protein, total (g/dL)	2.9 (2.3-3.6)	4.2 (2.6-6.6)
Albumin (g/dL)	1.2 (1.0-1.6)	—
Globulin (g/dL)	1.6 (1.3-2.1)	—
A:G (ratio)	0.75	—
Sodium (mEq/L)	150 (140-156)	141 (132-155)
Total bilirubin (mg/dL)	0 (0-0.1)	—
Measurement	Rainbow trout (*Oncorhynchus mykiss*)[33,68a,137]	
Hematology		
PCV (%)	34.8-56.9	
RBC (10^6/μL)	1.4-1.8	
Hgb (g/dL)	6.4-9.5	
MCV (fL)	192-393	
MCH (pg)	35.3-62.4	

Continued

TABLE 2-6 Hematologic and Serum Biochemical Values of Fish. (cont'd)

Measurement	Rainbow trout (*Oncorhynchus mykiss*)
Hematology (cont'd)	
MCHC (g/dL)	14.2-18.9
WBC ($10^3/\mu L$)	9.9 ± 1.3
Chemistries	
ALP (U/L)	31
AST (U/L)	102
Calcium (mmol/L)	2.3
Chloride (mEq/L)	137
Cholesterol (mg/dL)	144
Creatinine (mg/dL)	0.4
Glucose (mg/dL)	103
Magnesium (mg/dL)	2.3
Phosphorus (mg/dL)	10.5
Potassium (mEq/L)	2.3
Protein, total (g/dL)	2.7
Albumin (g/dL)	1.2
Globulin (g/dL)	1.5
A:G (ratio)	0.8
Sodium (mEq/L)	152
Total bilirubin (mg/dL)	0.1

Measurement	[a]Bonnethead shark (*Sphyrna tiburo*)[61]	[a]Sandbar shark (*Carcharhinus plumbeus*)[11]
Hematology		
PCV (%)	24 (17-28)	17.5-23
Hgb (g/dL)	—	7.6-10.1
WBC ($10^3/\mu L$)	—	—
Heterophils (%)	—	40-58 (total granulocytes)
Lymphocytes (%)	—	40-55
Monocytes (%)	—	2-6
Chemistries		
Anion gap	−5.8 (−15.7-7.5)	—
AST (U/L)	42 (15-132)	—
Bicarbonate (mmol/L)	3 (0-5)	—
BUN (mg/dL)	2812 (2644-2992)	—
Calcium (mg/dL)	16.8 (15.8-18.2)	—
Chloride (mEq/L)	290 (277-304)	—
Cholesterol (mg/dL)	—	—
Creatine kinase (U/L)	82 (18-725)	—
Creatinine (mg/dL)	—	—
Glucose (mg/dL)	184 (155-218)	—
Lactate (mmol/L)	—	—

TABLE 2-6 Hematologic and Serum Biochemical Values of Fish. (cont'd)

Measurement	Bonnethead shark (*Sphyrna tiburo*)	Sandbar shark (*Carcharhinus plumbeus*)
Chemistries (cont'd)		
LDH (U/L)	<5 (<5-11)	—
Osmolality (mOsm/kg)	1094 (1056-1139)	—
Phosphorus (mg/dL)	8.8 (5.9-12.7)	—
Potassium (mEq/L)	7.3 (5.7-9.2)	—
Protein, total (g/dL)	2.9 (2.2-4.3)	—
Albumin (g/dL)	0.4 (0.3-0.5)	—
Globulin (g/dL)	2.6 (1.9-3.8)	—
A:G (ratio)	0.1 (0.1-0.2)	—
Sodium (mEq/L)	282 (273-292)	—

Measurement	Sand tiger shark (*Carcharias taurus*)[105]	Cownose ray (*Rhinoptera bonasus*)[41]
Hematology		
PCV (%)	31 (24-38)	—
RBC ($10^6/\mu L$)	—	5.11 (2.6-7.15)
WBC ($10^3/\mu L$)	—	0.55 (0.16-1.98)
Fine segmented eosinophilic granulocytes (%)	—	4 (0-13)
Fine nonsegmented eosinophilic granulocytes (%)	—	2 (0-10)
Lymphocytes (%)	—	86 (72-95)
Monocytes (%)	—	1 (0-3)
Coarse segmented eosinophilic granulocytes (%)	—	4 (0-14)
Coarse nonsegmented granulocytes (%)	—	3 (0-15)
Chemistries		
ALP (U/L)	8-31	33 (22-46)
ALT (U/L)	3	—
AST (U/L)	13-45	39 (15-78)
Bilirubin, total (μmol/L)	1.5	—
BUN (mg/dL)	—	1,154 (1010-1270)
Calcium (mmol/L)	3.3-4.4	4.2 (3.75-4.85)
Chloride (mEq/L)	227-257	255 (192-290)
Cholesterol (mg/dL)	0.9-2.1	166 (118-321)
Creatine kinase (U/L)	5-79	—
Creatinine (μmol/L)	32	8.84
Glucose (mmol/L)	2.2-3.2	2.78 (1.94-4.0)
Magnesium (mmol/L)	1.6-2.2	
Phosphorus (mmol/L)	1.7-2	5.8 (4.4-7.1)

Continued

TABLE 2-6 Hematologic and Serum Biochemical Values of Fish. (cont'd)

Measurement	Sand tiger shark (*Carcharias taurus*)	Cownose ray (*Rhinoptera bonasus*)
Chemistries (cont'd)		
Potassium (mmol/L)	4.3-5.7	1.5 (1-2.4)
Protein, total (g/L)	24-36	2.9 (1.9-4.2)
Albumin (g/dL)	—	0.6 (0.5-0.8)
Globulin (g/dL)	—	2.2 (1.4-3.6)
A:G (ratio)	—	0.29 (0.17-0.38)
Sodium (mEq/L)	249-267	276 (208-312)
Total bilirubin (mg/dL)	—	0.17 (0.1-0.3)
Triglyceride (mmol/L)	0.5-0.6	9.16 (3.16-22.8)

Measurement	Southern stingray (*Dasyatis americana*)[19]
Hematology	
PCV (%)	22 (15-25)
RBC ($10^6/\mu L$)	—
WBC ($10^3/\mu L$)	22.1-42.2
Heterophils (%)	—
Lymphocytes (%)	—
Monocytes (%)	—
Eosinophils (%)	—
Chemistries	
Anion gap	—
AST (U/L)	14.5 (3.6-61.2)
BUN (mg/dL)	1243 (1185-1293)
Calcium (mg/dL)	16.5 (12.06-19.3)
Chloride (mEq/L)	342 (301-362)
Creatine kinase (U/L)	80.5 (11.7-296.5)
Creatinine (mg/dL)	0.3 (0.2-0.4)
Glucose (mg/dL)	30.5 (16.9-42.4)
Lactate (mmol/L)	3.1 (<2-6.2)
LDH (U/L)	—
Osmolality (mOsm/kg)	1065 (1007-1144)
Phosphorus (mg/dL)	4.7 (3-6.4)
Potassium (mEq/L)	5 (3.2-6.4)
Protein, total (g/dL)	—
Albumin (g/dL)	—
Sodium (mEq/L)	315 (301-362)
Total CO_2 (mmol/L)	—
Uric acid (mg/dL)	—

[a]Values listed are means except where indicated with an [a], which are medians. In some cases the data are not based on a large sample size. These values are only meant to be guidelines. Age of fish, time of year, and water temperature may all affect "normal" clinical pathological data.

REFERENCES

1. AADAP/FDA. Web site: www.fws.gov/fisheries/aadap/inads-available/immersion/diquat/. Accessed December 20, 2016.
2. AADAP-FWS FDA INAD. Web site: www.fws.gov/fisheries/aadap/inads-available/index.html. Accessed December 20, 2016.
3. AADAP-FWS FDA INAD. Web site: www.fws.gov/fisheries/aadap/inads-available/immersion/chloramine-t/index.html. Accessed December 20, 2016.
4. Adamovicz L, Trosclair M, Lewbart GA. Biochemistry panel reference intervals for juvenile goldfish (*Carassius auratus*). *J Zoo Wildl Med*. In press.
5. Allender MC, Kastura M, George R, et al. Bioencapsulation of praziquantel in adult *Artemia*. *J Bioanal Biomed* 2010;2:96-99.
6. Allender MC, Kastura M, George R, et al. Bioencapsulation of metronidazole in adult brine shrimp (*Artemia* sp.). *J Zoo Wildl Med* 2011;42:241-246.
7. Allender MC, Kastura M, George R, et al. Bioencapsulation of fenbendazole in adult *Artemia*. *J Exot Pet Med* 2012;21:207-212.
8. Ang CY, Liu FF, Lay JO Jr, et al. Liquid chromatographic analysis of incurred amoxicillin residues in catfish muscle following oral administration of the drug. *J Agric Food Chem* 2000;48:1673-1677.
9. Aquacalm (metomidate hydrochloride) package insert. Syndel USA, Ferndale, WA, USA.
10. Aquaflor (florfenicol) product label. Merck Animal Health, Summit, NJ, USA.
11. Arnold J. Hematology of the sandbar shark (*Carcharhinus plumbeus*). *Vet Clin Path* 2005;34:115-123.
12. American Veterinary Medical Association. Guidelines for the euthanasia of animals. *J Am Vet Med Assoc* 2013. 102 pp.
13. Bailey KM, Minter LJ, Lewbart GA, et al. Alfaxalone as an intramuscular injectable anesthetic in koi carp (*Cyprinus carpio*). *J Zoo Wildl Med* 2014;45:852-858.
14. Baker TR, Baker BB, Johnson SM, Sladky KK. Comparative analgesic efficacy of morphine sulfate and butorphanol tartrate in koi (*Cyprinus carpio*) undergoing unilateral gonadectomy. *J Am Vet Med Assoc* 2013;243:882-890.
15. Braschi I, Blasioli S, Gigli L, et al. Removal of sulfonamide antibiotics from water: evidence of adsorption into an organophilic zeolite Y by its structural modifications. *J Hazard Mater* 2010;178:218-225.
16. Brown AG, Grant AN. Use of amoxycillin by injection in Atlantic salmon broodstock. *Vet Rec* 1992;131:237.
17. Buchmann K, Bjerregaard J. Mebendazole treatment of pseudodactylogyrosis in an intensive eel-culture system. *Aquaculture* 1990;86:139-153.
18. Bugman AM, Langer PT, Hadzima E, et al. Evaluation of the anesthetic efficacy of alfaxalone in oscar fish (*Astronotus ocellatus*). *Am J Vet Res* 2016;77:239-244.
19. Cain DK, Harms CA, Segars A. Plasma biochemistry reference values of wild-caught southern stingrays (*Dasyatis americana*). *J Zoo Wildl Med* 2004;35:471-476.
20. Callahan HA, Noga EJ. Tricaine dramatically reduces the ability to diagnose protozoan ectoparasite (*Ichthyobodo necator*) infections. *J Fish Dis* 2002;25:433-437.
21. Chen CY, Getchel RG, Wooster GA, et al. Oxytetracycline residues in four species of fish after 10-day oral dosing in feed. *J Aquat Anim Health* 2004;16:208-219.
22. Chorulon (human chorionic gonadotropin; hCG) product label. Merck Animal Health, Summit, NJ, USA.
23. Colorni A, Paperna I. Evaluation of nitrofurazone baths in the treatment of bacterial infections of *Sparus aurata* and *Oreochromis mossambicus*. *Aquaculture* 1983;25:181-186.
24. Coyne R, Bergh O, Smith P, et al. A question of temperature related differences in plasma oxolinic acid concentrations achieved in rainbow trout (*Oncorhynchus mykiss*) under laboratory conditions following multiple oral dosing. *Aquaculture* 2004;245:13-17.

25. Coyne R, Samuelsen O, Kongshaug H, et al. A comparison of oxolinic acid concentrations in farmed and laboratory held rainbow trout (*Oncorhynchus mykiss*) following oral therapy. *Aquaculture* 2004;239:1-13.
26. Cravedi JP, Boudry G, Baradat M, et al. Metabolic fate of 2,4-dichloroaniline, prochloraz and nonylphenol diethoxylate in rainbow trout: a comparative in vivo/in vitro approach. *Aquat Toxicol* 2001;53:159-172.
27. Cravedi JP, Heuillet G, Peleran JC, et al. Disposition and metabolism of chloramphenicol in trout. *Xenobiotica* 1985;15:115-121.
28. Creeper JH, Buller NB. An outbreak of *Streptococcus iniae* in barramundi (*Lates calcarifera*) in freshwater cage culture. *Aust Vet J* 2006;84:408-411.
29. Cross DG, Hursey PA. Chloramine-T for the control of *Ichthyophthirius multifiliis* (Fouquet). *J Fish Dis* 1973;10:789-798.
30. Davis LE, Davis CA, Koritz GD, et al. Comparative studies of pharmacokinetics of fenbendazole in food-producing animals. *Vet Hum Toxicol* 1988;30(Suppl 1):9-11.
31. della Rocca G, Di Salvo A, Malvisi J, et al. The disposition of enrofloxacin in seabream (*Sparus aurata* L.) after single intravenous injection or from medicated feed administration. *Aquaculture* 2004;232:53-62.
32. della Rocca G, Zaghini A, Zanoni R, et al. Seabream (*Sparus aurata* L.): disposition of amoxicillin after single intravenous or oral administration and multiple dose depletion studies. *Aquaculture* 2004;232:1-10.
33. Denton JE, Yousef MK. Seasonal changes in hematology of rainbow trout, *Salmo gairdneri*. *Comp Biochem Physiol* 1975;51A:151-153.
34. Ding F, Cao J, Ma L, et al. Pharmacokinetics and tissue residues of difloxacin in crucian carp (*Carassius auratus*) after oral administration. *Aquaculture* 2006;256:121-128.
35. Di Salvo A, Pellegrino RM, Cagnardi P, della Rocca G. Pharmacokinetics and residue depletion of erythromycin in gilthead seabream *Sparus aurata* L. after oral administration. *J Fish Dis* 2014;37:797-803.
36. Doi A, Stoskopf MK, Lewbart GA. Pharmacokinetics of oxytetracycline in the red pacu (*Colossoma brachypomum*) following different routes of administration. *J Vet Pharmacol Therap* 1998;21:364-368.
37. Elston RA, Drum AS, Schweitzer MG, et al. Comparative update of orally administered difloxacin in Atlantic salmon in freshwater and seawater. *J Aquat Anim Health* 1994;6:341-348.
38. Erythromycin FWS-FDA INAD. Web site: www.fws.gov/fisheries/aadap/inads-available/injectable/Erythromycin/index.html. Accessed December 20, 2016.
39. Fairgrieve WT, Masada CL, McAuley WC, et al. Accumulation and clearance of orally administered erythromycin and its derivative, azithromycin, in juvenile fall Chinook salmon *Oncorhynchus tshawytscha*. *Dis Aquat Organ* 2005;64:99-106.
40. Fairgrieve WT, Masada CL, Peterson ME, et al. Concentrations of erythromycin and azithromycin in mature Chinook salmon *Oncorhynchus tshawytscha* after intraperitoneal injection, and in their progeny. *Dis Aquat Organ* 2006;68:227-234.
41. Ferreira CM, Field CL, Tuttle AD. Hematological and plasma biochemical parameters of aquarium-maintained cownose rays. *J Aquat Anim Health* 2010;22:123-128.
42. Fleming GJ, Corwin A, McCoy AJ, et al. Treatment factors influencing the use of recombinant platelet-derived growth factor (Regranex®) for head and lateral line erosion syndrome in ocean surgeonfish (*Acanthurus bahianus*). *J Zoo Wildl Med* 2008;39:155-160.
43. Fleming GJ, Heard DJ, Francis-Floyd R, et al. Evaluation of propofol and medetomidine-ketamine for short-term immobilization of Gulf of Mexico sturgeon (*Acipenser oxyrinchus de soti*). *J Zoo Wildl Med* 2003;34:153-158.
44. FWS. The Aquatic Animal Drug Approval Partnership Program. Web site: www.fws.gov/fisheries/aadap/home.htm. Accessed December 20, 2016.
45. GholipourKanani H, Ahadizadeh S. Use of propofol as an anesthetic and its efficacy on some hematological values of ornamental fish *Carassius auratus*. *SpringerPlus* 2013;2:76.

46. Gilmartin WG, Camp BJ, Lewis DH. Bath treatment of channel catfish with three broad-spectrum antibiotics. *J Wildl Dis* 1976;12:555-559.
47. Gingerich WH, Meinertrz JR, Dawson VK, et al. Distribution and elimination of [14C]sarafloxacin hydrochloride from tissues of juvenile channel catfish (*Ictalurus punctatus*). *Aquaculture* 1995;131:23-36.
48. Gratzek JB, Shotts EB, Dawe DL. Infectious diseases and parasites of freshwater ornamental fish. In: Gratzek JB, Matthews FR, eds. *Aquariology: The Science of Fish Health Management*. Morris Plains, NJ: Tetra Press; 1992:227-274.
49. Groff JM, Zinkl JG. Hematology and clinical chemistry of cyprinid fish. *Vet Clin North Am Exot Anim Pract* 1999;2:741-776.
50. Grondel JL, Nouws JFM, De Jong M, et al. Pharmacokinetics and tissue distribution of oxytetracycline in carp, *Cyprinus carpio* L., following different routes of administration. *J Fish Dis* 1987;10:153-163.
51. Grosell MH, Hansen HJM, Rosenkilde P. Cu update, metabolism and elimination in fed and starved European eels (*Anguilla anguilla*) during adaptation to water-borne Cu exposure. *Comp Biochem Physiol C* 1998;120:295-305.
52. Grosell MH, Hogstrand C, Wood CM. Cu update and turnover in both Cu-acclimated and non-acclimated rainbow trout (*Oncorhynchus mykiss*). *Aquat Toxicol* 1997;38:257-276.
53. Grosell MH, Hogstrand C, Wood CM. Renal Cu and Na excretion and hepatic Cu metabolism in both Cu acclimated and non acclimated rainbow trout (*Oncorhynchus mykiss*). *Aquat Toxicol* 1998;40:275-291.
54. Hansen MK, Horsberg TE. Single-dose pharmacokinetics of flumequine in cod (*Gadus morhua*) and goldsinny wrasse (*Ctenolabrus rupestris*). *J Vet Pharmacol Ther* 2000;23:163-168.
55. Hansen MK, Nymoen U, Horsberg TE. Pharmacokinetic and pharmacodynamic properties of metomidate in turbot (*Scophthalmus maximus*) and halibut (*Hippoglossus hippoglossus*). *J Vet Pharmacol Ther* 2003;26:95-103.
56. Hanson SK, Hill JE, Watson CA, et al. Evaluation of emamectin benzoate for the control of experimentally induced infestations of *Argulus* sp. in goldfish and koi carp. *J Aquat Anim Health* 2011;23:30-34.
57. Harms CA. Treatments for parasitic diseases of aquarium and ornamental fish. *Semin Avian Exot Pet Med* 1996;5:54-63.
58. Harms CA. Anesthesia in fish. In: Fowler ME, Miller RE, eds. *Zoo and Wild Animal Medicine: Current Therapy 4*. Philadelphia: WB Saunders Co; 1999:158-163.
59. Harms CA, Lewbart GA. Surgery in fish. *Vet Clin North Am Exot Anim Pract* 2000;3:759-774.
60. Harms CA, Lewbart GA, Swanson CR, et al. Behavioral and clinical pathology changes in koi carp (*Cyprinus carpio*) subjected to anesthesia and surgery with and without intra-operative analgesics. *Comp Med* 2005;55:221-226.
61. Harms CA, Ross T, Segars A. Plasma biochemistry reference values of wild bonnethead sharks, *Sphyrna tiburo*. *Vet Clin Pathol* 2002;31:111-115.
62. Harms CA, Sullivan CV, Hodson RG, et al. Clinical pathology and histopathology characteristics of net-stressed striped bass with "red tail." *J Aquat Anim Health* 1996;8:82-86.
63. Heaton LH, Post G. Tissue residues and oral safety of furazolidone in four species of trout. *Prog Fish-Cult* 1968;30:208-215.
64. Hemaprasanth KP, Kar B, Garnayak SK, et al. Efficacy of two avermectins, doramectin and ivermectin against *Argulus siamensis* infestation in Indian major carp, *Labeo rohita*. *Vet Parasitol* 2012;190:297-304.
65. Hemaprasanth KP, Raghavendra A, Singh R, et al. Efficacy of doramectin against natural and experimental infections of *Lernaea cyprinacea* in carps. *Vet Parasitol* 2008;156:261-269.
66. Hill JE, Kilgore KH, Pouder DB, et al. Survey of Ovaprim use as a spawning aid in ornamental fishes in the United States as administered through the University of Florida Tropical Aquaculture Laboratory. *North Am J Aquacult* 2009;71:206-209.
67. Homem V, Santos L. Degradation and removal methods of antibiotics from aqueous matrices – a review. *J Environ Manag* 2011;92:2304-2347.

68. Hrubec TC, Cardinale JL, Smith SA. Hematology and plasma chemistry reference intervals for cultured tilapia (*Oreochromis hybrid*). *Vet Clin Path* 2000;29:7-12.
68a. Hrubec TC, Smith SA. Differences between plasma and serum samples for the evaluation of blood chemistry values in rainbow trout, channel catfish, hybrid tilapias, and hybrid striped bass. *J Aquat Anim Health* 1999;11:116-122.
69. Hrubec TC, Smith SA, Robertson JL. Age-related changes in hematology and plasma chemistry values of hybrid striped bass (*Morone chrysops* × *Morone saxatilis*). *Vet Clin Path* 2001;30:8-15.
70. Hrubec TC, Smith SA, Robertson JL, et al. Blood biochemical reference intervals for sunshine bass (*Morone chrysops* × *Morone saxatilis*) in three culture systems. *Am J Vet Res* 1996;57:624-627.
71. Hubert TD, Bernardy JA, Vue C, et al. Residues of the lampricides 3-trifluoromethyl-4-nitrophenol and niclosamide in muscle tissue of rainbow trout. *J Agric Food Chem* 2005;53:5342-5346.
72. Inglis V, Richards RH, Varma KJ, et al. Florfenicol in Atlantic salmon, *Salmo salar* L., parr: tolerance and assessment of efficacy against furunculosis. *J Fish Dis* 1991;14:343-351.
73. Intorre L, Castells G, Cristofol C, et al. Residue depletion of thiamphenicol in the sea-bass. *J Vet Pharmacol Ther* 2002;25:59-63.
74. Iosifidou EG, Haagsma N, Olling M, et al. Residue study of mebendazole and its metabolites hydroxymebendazole and amino-mebendazole in eel (*Anguilla anguilla*) after bath treatment. *Drug Metab Dispos* 1997;25:317-320.
75. Iosifidou EG, Haagsma N, Tanck MWT, et al. Depletion study of fenbendazole in rainbow trout (*Oncorhynchus mykiss*) after oral and bath treatment. *Aquaculture* 1997;154:191-199.
76. Jarboe H, Toth BR, Shoemaker KE, et al. Pharmacokinetics, bioavailability, plasma protein binding and disposition of nalidixic acid in rainbow trout (*Oncorhynchus mykiss*). *Xenobiotica* 1993;23:961-972.
77. Johnson EL. *Koi Health and Disease*. Athens: Reade Printers; 2006.
78. Jones J, Kinnel M, Christenson R, et al. Gentamicin concentrations in toadfish and goldfish serum. *J Aquat Anim Health* 1997;9:211-215.
79. Kajita Y, Sakai M, Atsuta S, et al. The immunomodulatory effects of levamisole on rainbow trout, *Oncorhynchus mykiss*. *Fish Pathol* 1990;25:93-98.
80. Kilgore KH, Hill JE, Powell JF, et al. Investigational use of metomidate hydrochloride as a shipping additive for two ornamental fishes. *J Aquat Anim Health* 2009;21:133-139.
81. Kim MS, Lim JH, Park BK, et al. Pharmacokinetics of enrofloxacin in Korean catfish (*Silurus asotus*). *J Vet Pharmacol Ther* 2006;29:397-402.
82. Kitzman JV, Holley JH, Huber WG, et al. Pharmacokinetics and metabolism of fenbendazole in channel catfish. *Vet Res Com* 1990;14:217-226.
83. Knight SJ, Boles L, Stamper MA. Response of recirculating saltwater aquariums to long-term formalin treatment. *J Zoo Aquar Res* 2016;4:77-84.
84. Kozlowski F. Chloromycetin levels in the blood and some tissues of carps in the prophylactic treatment of dropsy. *Bull Vet Instit Pulway* 1964;8:188-195.
85. Law FCP. Total metabolic depletion and residue profile of selected drugs in trout: furazolidone. Final FDA Report (Contract 223-90-7016); 1994.
86. Lewbart GA. Emergency pet fish medicine. In: Bonagura JD, ed. *Kirk's Current Veterinary Therapy XII: Small Animal Practice*. Philadelphia: WB Saunders Co; 1995:1369-1374.
87. Lewbart GA. Emergency and critical care of fish. *Vet Clin North Am Exot Anim Pract* 1998;1:233-249.
88. Lewbart GA. Koi medicine and management. *Suppl Comp Contin Educ Pract Vet* 1998;20:5-12.
89. Lewbart GA. Fish supplement. In: Johnson-Delaney C, ed. *Exotic Companion Medicine Handbook*. West Palm Beach, FL: Zoological Medicine Network; 2006:1-58.

90. Lewbart GA, Butkus DA, Papich M, et al. A simple catheterization method for systemic administration of drugs to fish. *J Am Vet Med Assoc* 2005;226:784-788.
91. Lewbart GA, Papich MG, Whitt-Smith D. Pharmacokinetics of florfenicol in the red pacu (*Piaractus brachypomus*) after single dose intramuscular administration. *J Vet Pharmacol Ther* 2005;28:317-319.
92. Lewbart GA, Vaden S, Deen J, et al. Pharmacokinetics of enrofloxacin in the red pacu (*Colossoma brachypomum*) after intramuscular, oral and bath administration. *J Vet Pharmacol Ther* 1997;20:124-128.
93. Lewis DH, Wenxing W, Ayers A, et al. Preliminary studies on the use of chloroquine as a systemic chemotherapeutic agent for amyloodinosis in red drum (*Sciaenops ocellatus*). *Marine Sci Suppl* 1988;30:183-189.
94. Mansell B, Powell MD, Ernst I, Nowak BF. Effects of the gill monogenean *Zeuxapta seriolae* (Meserve, 1938) and treatment with hydrogen peroxide on pathophysiology of kingfish, *Seriola lalandi* Valenciennes, 1833. *J Fish Dis* 2005;28:253-262.
95. Meinertz JR, Stehly GR, Greseth SL, et al. Depletion of the chloramine-T marker residue, paratoluenesulfonamide, from skin-on fillet tissue of hybrid striped bass, rainbow trout, and yellow perch. *Aquaculture* 2004;232:1-10.
96. Minter LJ, Bailey KM, Harms CA, et al. The efficacy of alfaxalone for immersion anesthesia in koi carp (*Cyprinus carpio*). *Vet Anesth Analg* 2014;41:398-405.
97. Moffitt CM. Survival of juvenile Chinook salmon challenged with *Renibacterium salmoninarum* and administered oral doses of erythromycin thiocyanate for different durations. *J Aquat Anim Health* 1992;4:119-125.
98. Montgomery-Brock D, Sato VT, Brock JA, Tamaru CS. The application of hydrogen peroxide as a treatment for the ectoparasite *Amyloodinium ocellatum* on the Pacific threadfin *Polydactylus sexfilis*. *J World Aquacult Soc* 2001;32:250-254.
99. Nafstad I, Ingebrigsten K, Langseth W, et al. Benzimidazoles for antiparasite therapy in salmon. *Acta Vet Scand Suppl* 1991;87:302-304.
100. Noga EJ. *Fish Disease: Diagnosis and Treatment.* 2nd ed. Ames: Wiley-Blackwell; 2010.
101. Noga EJ, Wang C, Grindem CB, et al. Comparative clinicopathological responses of striped bass and palmetto bass to acute stress. *Trans Am Fish Soc* 1999;128:680-686.
102. Nouws JFM, Grondel JL, Schutte AR, et al. Pharmacokinetics of ciprofloxacin in carp, African catfish and rainbow trout. *Vet Quart* 1988;10:211-216.
103. Oda A, Bailey KM, Lewbart GA, et al. Physiologic and biochemical assessments of koi carp, *Cyprinus carpio*, following immersion in propofol. *J Am Vet Med Assoc* 2014;245:1286-1291.
104. Ötker HM, Akmehmet-Balcıoğlu I. Adsorption and degradation of enrofloxacin, a veterinary antibiotic on natural zeolite. *J Hazard Mat* 2005;122:251-258.
105. Otway NM. Serum biochemical reference intervals for free-living sand tiger sharks (*Carcharias taurus*) from east Australian waters. *Vet Clin Path* 2015;44:262-274.
106. Ovaprim (salmon gonadotropin releasing hormone analog 20 µg/mL plus dormperidone 10 mg/mL) product label. Syndel USA, Ferndale, WA, USA.
107. Palmeiro BS, Rosenthal KL, Lewbart GA, et al. Plasma biochemical reference intervals for koi. *J Am Vet Med Assoc* 2007;230:708-712.
108. Paschoal JAR, Quesada SP, Goncalves LU, et al. Depletion study and estimation of the withdrawal period for enrofloxacin in pacu (*Piaractus mesopotamicus*). *J Vet Pharmacol Therap* 2013;36:594-602.
109. PEROX-AID (33% hydrogen peroxide) product label. Syndel USA, Ferndale, WA, USA.
110. Plakas SM, DePaola A, Moxey MB. *Bacillus stearothermophilis* disk assay for determining ampicillin residues in fish muscle. *J Assoc Off Anal Chem Internat* 1991;74:910-912.
111. Plakas SM, El Said KR, Bencsath FA, et al. Pharmacokinetics, tissue distribution and metabolism of acriflavine and proflavine in the channel catfish (*Ictalurus punctatus*). *Xenobiotica* 1998;28:605-616.

112. Plakas SM, El Said KR, Stehly GR. Furazolidone disposition after intravascular and oral dosing in the channel catfish. *Xenobiotica* 1994;24:1095-1105.
113. Plumb JA, Rogers WA. Effect of Droncit (praziquantel) on yellow grubs *Clinostomum marginatum* and eye flukes *Diplostomum spathaceum* in channel catfish. *J Aquat Anim Health* 1990;2:204-206.
114. Pottinger TG, Day JG. A *Saprolegnia parasitica* challenge system for rainbow trout: assessment of Pyceze as an anti-fungal agent for both fish and ova. *Dis Aquatic Org* 1999;36:129-141.
115. Rach JJ, Gaikowski MP, Ramsay RT. Efficacy of hydrogen peroxide to control parasitic infestations on hatchery-reared fish. *J Aquat Anim Health* 2000;12:267-273.
116. Rapp J. Treatment of rainbow trout (*Oncorhynchus mykiss* Walb.) fry infected with *Ichthyophthirius multifiliis* by oral administration of dimetridazole. *Bull Euro Assoc Fish Pathol* 1995;15:67-69.
117. Reimschuessel R, Chamie SJ, Kinnel M. Evaluation of gentamicin-induced nephrotoxicosis in toadfish. *J Am Vet Med Assoc* 1996;209:137-139.
118. Reimschuessel R, Stewart L, Squibb E, et al. Fish Drug Analysis—Phish-Pharm: A Searchable Database of Pharmacokinetics Data in Fish. www.fda.gov/AnimalVeterinary/ScienceResearch/ToolsResource/Phish-Pharm/default.htm. Accessed December 20, 2016.
119. Reja A, Moreno L, Serrano JM, et al. Concentration-time profiles of oxytetracycline in blood, kidney and liver of tench (*Tinca tinca* L.) after intramuscular administration. *Vet Hum Toxicol* 1996;38:344-347.
120. Roberts HE, Palmeiro B, Weber ES III. Bacterial and parasitic diseases of pet fish. *Vet Clin North Am Exot Anim Pract* 2009;12:609-638.
121. Robertson B, Rorstad G, Engstad R, et al. Enhancement of non-specific disease resistance in Atlantic salmon, *Salmo salar* L., by a glucan from *Saccharomyces cerevisiae* cell walls. *J Fish Dis* 1990;13:391-400.
122. Rogstad A, Ellingsen OF, Syvertsen C. Pharmacokinetics and bioavailability of flumequine and oxolinic acid after various routes of administration to Atlantic salmon in seawater. *Aquaculture* 1993;110:207-220.
123. Russo R, Curtis EW, Yanong RPE. Preliminary investigations of hydrogen peroxide treatment of selected ornamental fishes and efficacy against external bacteria and parasites in green swordtails. *J Aquat Anim Health* 2007;19:121-127.
124. Russo R, Yanong RPE, Mitchell H. Dietary beta-glucans and nucleotides enhance resistance of redtail black shark (*Epalzeorhynchos* bicolor, fam. Cyprinidae) to *Streptococcus iniae* infection. *J World Aquacult Soc* 2006;37:298-306.
125. Sakamoto K, Lewbart GA, Smith TM II. Blood chemistry values of juvenile red pacu (*Piaractus brachypomus*). *Vet Clin Path* 2001;30:50-52.
126. Samuelsen OB. Pharmacokinetics of quinolones in fish: a review. *Aquaculture* 2006; 255:55-75.
127. Samuelsen OB, Bergh O. Efficacy of orally administered florfenicol and oxolinic acid for the treatment of vibriosis in cod (*Gadus morhua*). *Aquaculture* 2004;235:27-35.
128. Samuelsen OB, Ervik A. Single dose pharmacokinetic study of flumequine after intravenous, intraperitoneal and oral administration to Atlantic halibut (*Hippoglossus hippoglossus*) held in seawater at 9°C. *Aquaculture* 1997;158:215-227.
129. Samuelsen OB, Ervik A. Absorption, tissue distribution, and excretion of flumequine and oxolinic acid in corkwing wrasse (*Symphodus melops*) following a single intraperitoneal injection or bath treatment. *J Vet Pharmacol Ther* 2001;24:111-116.
130. Samuelsen OB, Bergh O, Ervik A. Pharmacokinetics of florfenicol in cod (*Gadus morhua*) and in vitro antibacterial activity against *Vibrio anguillarum*. *Dis Aquat Organ* 2003;56:127-133.
131. Schering Plough (later became Merck Animal Health, Summit, NJ, USA). Emamectin benzoate (SLICE). http://aqua.merck-animal-health.com/products/slice/information.aspx. Accessed June 1, 2017.
132. Schmahl G, Benini J. Treatment of fish parasites 11. Effects of different benzimadazole derivatives (albendazole, mebendazole, fenbendazole) on *Glugea anomala*, Moniez, 1887 (Microsporidia): Ultrastructural aspects and efficacy studies. *Parasitol Res* 1998;60:41-49.

133. Seeley KE, Wolf KN, Bishop MA, et al. Pharmacokinetics of long-acting cefovecin in copper rockfish (*Sebastes caurinus*). *Am J Vet Res* 2016;77:260-264.
134. Setser MD. Pharmacokinetics of gentamicin in channel catfish (*Ictalurus punctatus*). *Am J Vet Res* 1985;46:2558-2561.
135. Shaikh B, Rummel N, Gieseker C, et al. Metabolism and residue depletion of albendazole in rainbow trout, tilapia, and Atlantic salmon after oral administration. *J Vet Pharmacol Ther* 2003;26:421-428.
136. Siwicki AK, Anderson DP, Rumsey GL. Dietary intake of immunostimulants by rainbow trout affects non-specific immunity and protection against furunculosis. *Vet Immunol Immunopathol* 1994;41:125-139.
137. Smith CJ, Shaw BJ, Handy RD. Toxicity of single walled carbon nanotubes to rainbow trout (*Oncorhynchus mykiss*): respiratory toxicity, organ pathologies, and other physiological effects. *Aquat Tox* 2007;82:94-109.
137a. Snellgrove DL, Alexander LG. Haematology and plasma chemistry of the red top ice blue mbuna cichlid (*Metriaclima greshakei*). *Br J Nutr* 2011;106:S154-S157.
138. Steeil JC, Schumacher J, George RH, et al. Pharmacokinetics of cefovecin (Convenia®) in white bamboo sharks (*Chiloscyllium plagiosum*) and Atlantic horseshoe crabs (*Limulus polyphemus*). *J Zoo Wildl Med* 2014;45:389-392.
139. Stoffregen DA, Chako AJ, Backman S, et al. Successful therapy of furunculosis in Atlantic salmon *Salmo salar* L. using the fluoroquinolone antimicrobial agent enrofloxacin. *J Fish Dis* 1993;16:219-227.
140. Stoskopf MK. Appendix V: chemotherapeutics. In: Stoskopf MK, ed. *Fish Medicine*. Philadelphia: WB Saunders Co; 1993:832-839.
141. Stoskopf MK. Anesthesia of pet fishes. In: Bonagura JD, ed. *Kirk's Current Veterinary Therapy XII: Small Animal Practice*. Philadelphia: WB Saunders Co; 1995:1365-1369.
142. Stoskopf MK. Fish pharmacotherapeutics. In: Fowler ME, Miller RE, eds. *Zoo and Wild Animal Medicine: Current Therapy 4*. Philadelphia: WB Saunders Co; 1999:182-189.
143. Stoskopf MK, Kennedy-Stoskopf S, Arnold J, et al. Therapeutic aminoglycoside antibiotic levels in brown shark, *Carcharhinus plumbeus* (Nardo). *J Fish Dis* 1986;9:303-311.
144. Sun M, Li J, Gai CL, et al. Pharmacokinetics of difloxacin in olive flounder *Paralichthys olivaceus* at two water temperatures. *J Vet Pharm Therap* 2013;37:186-191.
145. Tarascheewski H, Renner C, Melhorn H. Treatment of fish parasites 3. Effects of levamisole HCl, metrifonate, fenbendazole, mebendazole, and ivermectin in *Anguillicola crassus* (nematodes) pathogenic in the air bladder of eels. *Parasitol Res* 1988;74:281-289.
146. Tavares-Dias M, Moraes FR. Haematological and biochemical reference intervals for farmed channel catfish. *J Fish Biol* 2007;71:383-388.
147. Thomasen JM. Hydrogen peroxide as a delousing agent for Atlantic salmon. In: Boxshall GA, Defaye D, eds. *Pathogens of Wild and Farmed Fish: Sea Lice*. Chichester, England: Ellis Horwood; 1993:290-295.
148. Tocidlowski ME, Lewbart GA, Stoskopf MK. Hematologic study of red pacu (*Colossoma brachypomum*). *Vet Clin Path* 1997;26:119-125.
149. Treves-Brown KM. *Applied Fish Pharmacology*. Dodrecht, The Netherlands: Kluwer Academic Publishers; 2000.
150. Tripathi NK, Latimer KS, Brunley VV. Hematologic reference intervals for koi (*Cyprinus carpio*), including blood cell morphology, cytochemistry, and ultrastructure. *Vet Clin Pathol* 2004;33:74-83.
150a. Vázquez GR, Guerrero GA. Characterization of blood cells and hematological parameters in *Cichlasoma dimerus* (Teleostei, Perciformes). *Tissue Cell* 2007;39:151-160.
151. Whitaker BR. Preventive medicine programs for fish. In: Fowler ME, Miller RE, eds. *Zoo and Wild Animal Medicine: Current Therapy 4*. Philadelphia: WB Saunders Co; 1999:163-181.
152. Wildgoose WH, Lewbart GA. Therapeutics. In: Wildgoose WH, ed. *Manual of Ornamental Fish*. 2nd ed. Gloucester, England: British Small Animal Veterinary Association; 2001:237-258.

153. Willoughby LG, Roberts RJ. Towards strategic use of fungicides against *Saprolegnia parasitica* in salmonid fish hatcheries. *J Fish Dis* 1992;15:1-13.
154. Woynarovich E, Horvath L. The Artificial Propagation of Warm-Water Finfishes—A Manual for Extension Fisheries. Technical Paper 201, FAO, Rome, 1980.
155. Xu D, Rogers WA. Formaldehyde residue in striped bass muscle. *J Aquat Anim Health* 1993;5:306-312.
156. Xu L, Wang H, Yang X, Lu L. Integrated pharmacokinetics/pharmacodynamics parameters-based dosing guidelines of enrofloxacin in grass carp *Ctenopharyngodon idella* to minimize selection of drug resistance. *BMC Vet Res* 2013;9:126.
157. Xu W, Zhu X, Wang X, et al. Residues of enrofloxacin, furazolidone and their metabolites in Nile tilapia (*Oreochromis niloticus*). *Aquaculture* 2006;254:1-8.
158. Yang F, Li ZL, Shan Q, Zeng ZL. Pharmacokinetics of doxycycline in tilapia (*Oreochromis aureus* × *Oreochromis niloticus*) after intravenous and oral administration. *J Vet Pharmacol Therap* 2014;37:388-393.
159. Yanong RP, Curtis E, Russo R, et al. *Cryptobia iubilans* infection in juvenile discus. *J Am Vet Med Assoc* 2004;224:1644-1650.
160. Yanong RPE. Personal observation. 2016.
161. Yanong RPE, Curtis EW, Simmons R, et al. Pharmacokinetic studies of florfenicol in koi carp and threespot gourami *Trichogaster trichopterus* after oral and intramuscular treatment. *J Aquat Anim Health* 2005;17:129-137.
162. Zimmerman DM, Armstrong DL, Curro TG, et al. Pharmacokinetics of florfenicol after a single intramuscular dose in white-spotted bamboo sharks (*Chiloscyllium plagiosum*). *J Zoo Wildl Med* 2006;37:165-173.

Chapter 3 **Amphibians**

Brent R. Whitaker | *Colin T. McDermott*

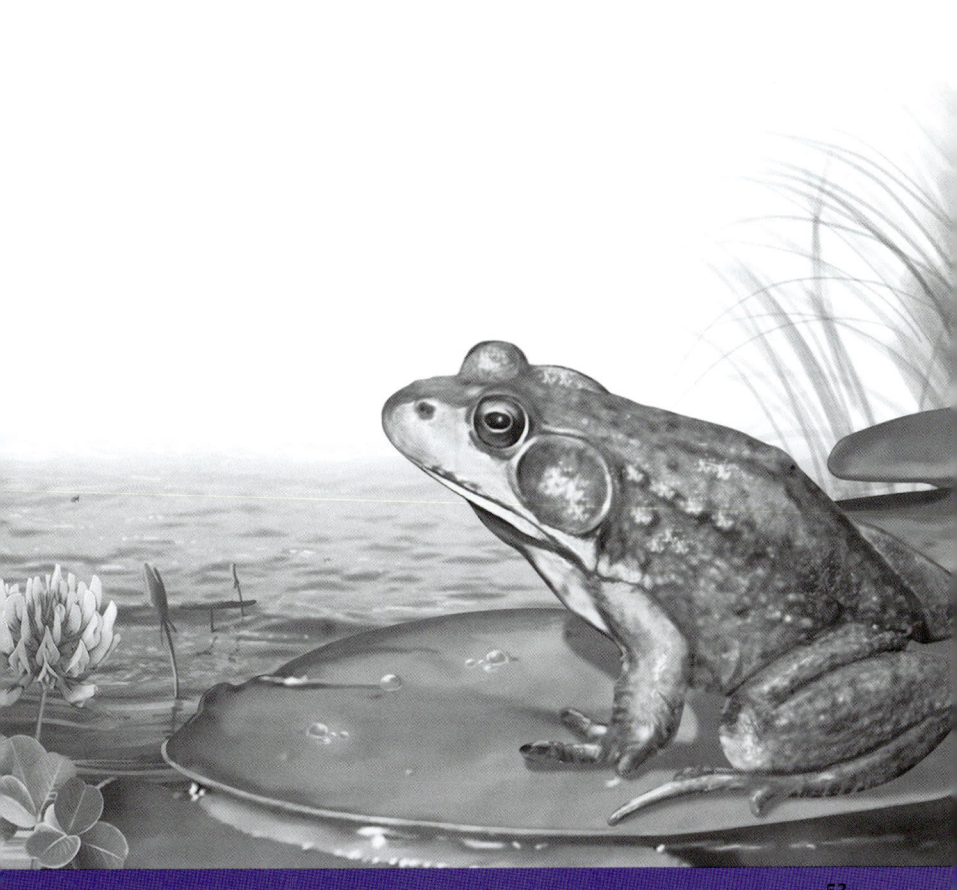

TABLE 3-1 Antimicrobial Agents Used in Amphibians.[a,b]

Agent	Dosage	Species/Comments
Amikacin	5 mg/kg IM q36h[59]	Bullfrogs/PK
	5-10 mg/kg SC, IM, ICe q24-48 h[58]	Most species; may be used in combination with piperacillin
Carbenicillin	100 mg/kg SC, IM q72h[59]	
	200 mg/kg SC, IM, ICe q24h[59]	
Ceftazidime	20 mg/kg SC, IM q48-72h[59]	
Chloramphenicol	50 mg/kg SC, IM, ICe q12-24h[59]	Caution: even miniscule exposure carries risk of aplastic anemia in susceptible individuals; wear disposable gloves when handling; aplastic anemia-like findings in *Bufo regularis* exposed to 125 mg/kg PO q24h × 12 wk[14]
	20 mg/L bath[a] changed daily[59]	
Ciprofloxacin	10 mg/kg PO,[59] ICe[58] q24h	
	500-750 mg/75 L as 6-8 hr bath[a] q24h[59]	May be used for large numbers of animals
Doxycycline (Psittavet, Vetafarm)	50 mg/kg IM q7d[59]	Broad-spectrum antibiotic, part of 4-quadrant therapy; may have antiinflammatory effect; chlamydiosis
Doxycycline (Vibramycin, Zoetis)	5-10 mg/kg PO q24h[59]	Chlamydiosis
	10-50 mg/kg PO q24h[59]	African clawed frogs/chlamydiosis
Doxycycline 1% topical gel, compounded	Apply topically q8-12h not to exceed 10 mg/kg per day[59]	Useful for localized lesions; may have antiinflammatory effect
Enrofloxacin	5-10 mg/kg PO, SC, IM q24h[59]	Most species/PK (bullfrogs);[59] ICe and topical routes also used but with limited PK data[59]
	10 mg/kg SC, IM[15]	African clawed frogs/PK; high kidney concentrations of enrofloxacin and ciprofloxacin;[15] no significant difference between routes[23]
	10 mg/kg topically[52]	Coqui frogs/detectable tissue concentration for >24 hr, no correlation to plasma concentration
	500 mg/L × 6-8 hr bath[a] q24h[59]	
Enrofloxacin and silver sulfadiazine solution (Baytril Otic, Bayer)	Apply topically to lesions q12h[59]	May have some antifungal effect, but does not appear effective against chytrid
Gentamicin	2-4 mg/kg IM q72h × 4 treatments[59]	
	2.5 mg/kg IM q72h[50]	Coldwater salamanders (i.e., *Necturus*)/PD; more frequent dosing may be needed if temperature >4°C (39.2°F)
	3 mg/kg IM q24h at 22.2°C (72°F)[59]	Leopard frogs/PD; at higher temperatures, serum concentrations will be lower

TABLE 3-1　Antimicrobial Agents Used in Amphibians. (cont'd)

Agent	Dosage	Species/Comments
Gentamicin (cont'd)	Topical to eyes[59]	All species/ocular infections; dilute to 2 mg/mL
	Intracameral injection once; not to exceed 4 mg/kg[59]	Panophthalmitis
Metronidazole	10 mg/kg PO q24h × 5-10 days[42]	For chronic diarrhea
	10 mg/kg IV q24h × 2 days[59]	Anaerobic infections
	12 mg/kg topically q24h × 5-10 days[59]	For chronic diarrhea
	20 mg/kg PO q48h × 20 days[59]	Anaerobic infections
	50 mg/kg PO q24h × 3 days[59]	Anaerobic infections
	60 mg/kg topically q24h × 3 days[59]	Anaerobic infections
	50 mg/L × 24 hr bath[a,59]	Anaerobic infections
Ofloxacin 0.3% ophthalmic solution	1 drop q2-4h × 10 days[58]	Keratitis; may also be applied topically to wounds
Oxytetracycline	25 mg/kg SC, IM q24h[59]	Most species
	50 mg/kg PO q12-24h[59]	Most species
	50-100 mg/kg IM q48h[59]	Bullfrogs/PK; especially useful in cases of chlamydiosis (use up to 30 days)[59]
	100 mg/L × 1hr bath[a,59]	Most species
	1 g/kg feed × 7 days[59]	Most useful with axolotls and *Xenopus* fed compounded pelleted diet[59]
Piperacillin	100 mg/kg SC, IM q24h[59]	Anaerobes; may be used in combination with amikacin
Silver sulfadiazine (Silvadine Cream 1%, Marion)	Topical q24 h[59]	Antibiotic cream
Sulfadiazine	132 mg/kg PO q24h[59]	
Sulfamethazine	1 g/L bath[a] to effect[59]	Change daily
Tetracycline	50 mg/kg PO q12h[59]	
	150 mg/kg PO q24h × 5-7 days[59]	
	167 mg/kg (5 mg/30 g) PO q12h × 7 days[59]	
Trimethoprim/sulfa	3 mg/kg PO, SC, IM q24h[59]	Unspecified sulfa
Trimethoprim/ sulfadiazine	15-20 mg/kg IM q48h[59]	Chronic diarrhea[59]
Trimethoprim/ sulfamethoxazole	15 mg/kg PO q24h[59]	Chronic diarrhea

[a]Water baths containing antibiotics or topical applications may not provide as consistent distribution as parenteral administration.
[b]SC can be administered in the dorsal lymph sac of anurans.[59]

TABLE 3-2 Antifungal Agents Used in Amphibians.

Agent	Dosage	Species/Comments
Amphotericin B	1 mg/kg ICe q24h[59]	Internal mycoses; acutely toxic to *Alytes muletensis* tadpoles at 8 µg/mL bath[33]
Benzalkonium chloride	0.25 mg/L × 72 hr bath[59] 2 mg/L × 1 hr bath q24h[59]	Saprolegniasis
Chloramphenicol	20 mg/kg topically (applied as Chlorsig 1% ointment [Sigma] which also contains paraffin and wool fat)[5] 10-30 mg/L (10-30 ppm) as continuous bath replaced fresh daily for up to 30 days[59]	Chytridiomycosis; safe for larvae, recent metamorphs, and adults; confirm negative result by real-time PCR;[5,59] caution: even miniscule exposure carries risk of aplastic anemia in susceptible individuals; wear disposable gloves when handling; aplastic anemia-like findings in *Bufo regularis* exposed to 125 mg/kg PO q24h × 12 wk[14]
	20 mg/L by continuous shallow immersion × 14 days, changed daily[61]	Australian green frog (*Litoria caerulea*); severely ill frogs treated with combination of chloramphenicol, SC fluids q8-12h × 6 days, and temperature increased to 28°C × 14 days[61]
Florfenicol	10 µg/mL topical spray q24h × 14 days[39]	Experimentally infected *Alytes muletensis* adults/reduced zoosporangia numbers but did not eliminate infection; GI and renal toxicity to tadpoles at 100 µg/mL[39]
	30 ppm as continuous bath replaced fresh daily for up to 30 days[59]	Chytridiomycosis; safe for larvae, recent metamorphs, and adults; confirm negative result by real-time PCR[59]
Fluconazole	60 mg/kg PO q24h[59]	
Itraconazole	10 mg/kg PO q24h[59] 0.01% in 0.6% salt solution × 5 min bath q24h × 11 days[59]	Topical route best choice to treat chytridiomycosis; caution with tadpoles[17,59]
	0.01% in buffered solution × 5 min bath q24h × 11-14 days[18]	Multiple species/cleared chytridiomycosis by PCR 14 days post-treatment; 6-15 mo post-treatment follow-up yielded positive PCR in some individuals
	0.5-1.5 mg/L × 5 min bath q24h × 7 days[17]	*Alytes muletensis* tadpoles/safe at varying concentrations and duration of 7-28 days; confirmed negative PCR post-treatment; varying levels of depigmentation observed in all individuals[17]
	50 mg/L × 5 min bath q24h × 10 days[25]	Multiple species/cleared chytridiomycosis in subclinical animals; confirmed with PCR

TABLE 3-2 Antifungal Agents Used in Amphibians. (cont'd)

Agent	Dosage	Species/Comments
Itraconazole (cont'd)	0.0025% × 5 min bath q24h × 6 days[8]	Australian green tree frog (*Litoria caerulea*), coastal plains toad (*Incillus nebulifer*)/cleared PCR positive juveniles with no clinically apparent side effects
Ketoconazole	10-20 mg/kg PO q24h[59] Topical cream[59]	
Methylene blue	2-4 mg/L bath to effect[59]	Tadpoles/may reduce mortality in newly hatched tadpoles
	4 mg/L × 1 hr bath q24h[59]	Saprolegniasis
Miconazole	5 mg/kg ICe q24h × 14-28 days[59]	Systemic mycoses
	Topical cream or solution[59]	Topical route best choice for chytridiomycosis; solutions containing alcohol may cause irritation; do not use with larvae[59]
Neomycin, polymixin B, bacitracin (Neosporin, Pfizer)	Apply topically to wound q24h[20]	Microsporidian infections; not recommended for bacterial infections, appears to inhibit re-epithelialization[59]
Nystatin 1% cream	Topical[59]	Cutaneous mycoses
Potassium permanganate	1:5000 water × 5 min bath q24h[59]	Cutaneous mycoses
Sodium chlorite (NaOCl$_2$)	20 mg/L × 6-8 hr bath[59]	Cutaneous mycoses
Temperature elevation	30°C (86°F) × 10 days[11]	*Rana catesbeiana, Acris crepitans*/ confirm negative result by real-time PCR[11]
	37°C (98.6°F) for 16 hr[56]	Chytridiomycosis, caution with temperature elevation in sensitive species
Terbinafine hydrochloride (Lamisil AT, Novartis)	0.005%-0.01% in distilled water × 5 min bath q24h × 5 days, or q48h × 6 treatments[7]	Various species/no adverse clinical effects noted with treatment; pH 7.0; confirm negative result by real-time PCR[7]
Voriconazole	1.25 μg/mL q24h topically via spray × 7 days[33]	Poison dart frogs, Iberian midwife toad (*Alytes cisternasii*)/cleared chytridiomycosis in naturally infected individuals in vivo; performed poorly with in vitro assays[33]
Voriconazole (V) + polymixin E (P) + elevated temperature (T)	(V) 12.5 μg/mL q24h topically via spray + (P) 2000 IU/mL × 10 min bath q12h + (T) 20°C (68°F) continuous × 10 days[6]	Fire salamanders/treatment of *Batrachochytrium salamandrivorans*; no effect of medications at 15°C (59°F)[6]

TABLE 3-3 Antiparasitic Agents Used in Amphibians.[a]

Agent	Dosage	Species/Comments
Acriflavin	0.025% bath × 5 days[59]	Protozoa
	500 mg/L × 30 min bath[59]	Protozoa
Benzalkonium chloride	2 mg/L × 1 hr bath q24h to effect[59]	Protozoa
Distilled water	3 hr bath[59]	Protozoa
Febantel (in combination with pyrantel pamoate and praziquantel; Drontal Plus, Bayer)	0.01 mL/1 g (10 mL/kg) PO q2-3wk[40]	Nematodes, cestodes, possibly trematodes
Fenbendazole	—	Fenbendazole combinations follow
	30-50 mg/kg PO[59]	Gastrointestinal nematodes
	50 mg/kg PO q24h × 3-5 days, repeat in 14-21 days[59]	Gastrointestinal nematodes
	50-100 mg/kg PO[42] repeat in 2-3 wk prn	Most species/gastrointestinal nematodes
	100 mg/kg PO,[59] repeat in 14 days	Gastrointestinal nematodes
Fenbendazole (F)/ ivermectin (I)	(F) 100 mg/kg PO on day 1, then (I) 0.2 mg/kg PO on days 2,11[59]	Gastrointestinal nematodes
Fenbendazole (F)/ metronidazole (M)	(F) 100 mg/kg PO, repeat in 10-14 days + (M) 10 mg/kg PO q24h for 5 days[59]	Concurrent gastrointestinal nematodes and protozoa
Formalin (10%)	—	Do not use if skin is ulcerated; may be toxic to some species
	1.5 mL/L × 10 min bath q48h to effect[59]	Protozoans; may be toxic in some species
	0.5% × 10 min bath once[59]	Monogenic trematodes; may be toxic to some species
Ivermectin	—	See fenbendazole for combination; caution: may cause flaccid paralysis with overdosage; caffeine or physostigmine may ameliorate effects[59]
	0.2-0.4 mg/kg PO, SC, repeat q14d as needed[59]	Nematodes, including lungworms; mites
	2 mg/kg topically, repeat in 2-3 wk[30]	Especially useful for small specimens[59] and *Rana* spp.[30]
	10 mg/L × 60 min bath, repeat q14d prn[59]	Mites
Levamisole	—	May cause paralysis in some species at suggested dosages;[59] caffeine or physostigmine may ameliorate effects[59]
	6.5-13.5 mg/kg topically to pelvic patch, repeat in 10 days[4]	*Anaxyrus houstonensis*/reduced nematode egg counts
	10 mg/kg IM, ICe, topically,[59] repeat in 2 wk	Nematodes, including lungworms
	12 mg/L bath × 4 days[24]	African clawed frogs/cutaneous nematodes; use ≥4.2 L of tank water/frog

TABLE 3-3 Antiparasitic Agents Used in Amphibians. (cont'd)

Agent	Dosage	Species/Comments
Levamisole (cont'd)	100 mg/L × ≥72 hr bath[59]	Resistant nematodes
	100-300 mg/L × 24 hr bath, repeat in 1-2 wk[59]	Nematodes, including subcutaneous nematodes in aquatic amphibians; water soluble form is available through aquaculture supply companies
Metronidazole	—	See fenbendazole for combination; toxicity possible at high doses
	10 mg/kg PO q24h × 5-10 days[59]	Protozoa; for unfamiliar or sensitive species
	50 mg/kg PO q24h × 3-5 days[59]	Confirmed cases of amoebiasis and flagellate overload
	100 mg/kg PO q3d[59]	Protozoa
	100-150 mg/kg PO, repeat in 2-3 wk or prn[59]	Protozoa (i.e., *Entamoeba, Hexamita, Opalina*)
	50 mg/L × 24 hr bath[59]	Aquatic amphibians/protozoa
	500 mg/100 g feed × 3-4 treatments[59]	Ciliates
Moxidectin	200 μg/kg SC q4mo[44]	Nematodes
Oxfendazole	5 mg/kg PO[59]	Gastrointestinal nematodes
Oxytetracycline	25 mg/kg SC, IM q24h[59]	Protozoa
	50 mg/kg PO q12h[59]	Protozoa
	1 g/kg feed × 7 days[59]	Protozoa
Paromomycin	50-75 mg/kg PO q24h[59]	Gastrointestinal protozoa
Piperazine	50 mg/kg PO, repeat in 2 wk[59]	Gastrointestinal nematodes
Ponazuril	30 mg/kg PO q12h × 3 days, repeat in 3 wk; often more effective at 30 mg/kg PO q24h × 30 days; may work with less frequent treatments[59]	Coccidia but not *Cryptosporidium*; may have some effect on unidentified protozoan cysts
Potassium permanganate	7 mg/L × 5 min bath q24h to effect[59]	Ectoparasitic protozoa
Praziquantel	8-24 mg/kg PO, SC, ICe, topically,[59] repeat q14d	Trematodes, cestodes
	10 mg/L × 3 hr bath,[59] repeat q7-21d	Trematodes, cestodes
Pyrantel pamoate	5 mg/kg PO q14d[40]	Nematodes
Ronidazole	10 mg/kg PO q24h × 10 days[59]	Flagellated protozoa, amoebas
Salt (sodium chloride)	4-6 g/L continuous bath[59]	Ectoparasitic protozoa
	5 g/L bath up to 12h, 10 g/L bath up to 1h[32]	Axolotls, immediate negative clinical effects in baths >20 g/L[32]
	6 g/L × 5-10 min bath q24h × 3-5 days[59]	Ectoparasitic protozoa
	25 g/L × ≤10 min bath[59]	Ectoparasitic protozoa
Selamectin (Revolution, Zoetis)	6 mg/kg topically[12]	Bullfrogs/PK

Continued

TABLE 3-3 Antiparasitic Agents Used in Amphibians. (cont'd)

Agent	Dosage	Species/Comments
Sulfadiazine	132 mg/kg PO q24h[59]	Coccidiosis
Sulfamethazine	1 g/L bath[59]	Coccidiosis; change daily to effect
Tetracycline	50 mg/kg PO q12h[59]	Protozoa
Thiabendazole	50-100 mg/kg PO,[59] repeat in 2 wk prn	Gastrointestinal nematodes
	100 mg/L bath, repeat in 2 wk[59]	Verminous dermatitis
Trimethoprim/sulfa	3 mg/kg PO, SC, IM q24h[59]	Coccidiosis; unspecified sulfa

[a]SC can be administered in the dorsal lymph sac of anurans.[59]

TABLE 3-4 Chemical Restraint/Anesthetic/Analgesic Agents Used in Amphibians.[a]

Agent	Dosage	Species/Comments
Alfaxalone	5-25 mg/kg IM[28]	Most species/recommend starting at lower dose (5-10 mg/kg) and titrating up
	10-17.5 mg/kg IM[41]	Bullfrogs/immobilization, respiratory depression, still responsive to noxious stimuli; dose dependent time to recumbency and time to recovery; no effect by immersion at 2 g/L for 30 min[41]
	18 mg/kg IM, IV, ICe[22]	African clawed frogs/deep sedation for 1-3 hr (IM, IV), 10-60 min ICe; no effect via immersion at 18 mg/L[22]
	20-30 mg/kg IM[46]	Australian tree frogs/initial effect within 10 min, respiratory depression; insufficient anesthesia as sole agent for painful procedures
	5 mg/L in fresh water bath[35]	Axolotls/single individual; induction of anesthesia, maintained continuous irrigation of gills and skin with additional 0.03 mL drops of alfaxalone for maintenance of anesthesia during surgery[35]
	200 mg/L in fresh water bath[2]	Fire-bellied toads/buffer with sodium bicarbonate to pH 7.2; anesthetic induction in 14 ± 4 min, variable duration of anesthesia up to 30 min; not sufficient for painful procedures
Alfaxalone (A)/ morphine (M)	(A) 3 mg/100 mL + (M) 5 mg/100 mL as bath[1]	Fire-bellied toads/provided anesthetic induction and antinociception
Atipamezole (Antisedan, Zoetis)	Titrate to effect IM, IV	Antagonist for dexmedetomidine[31]

TABLE 3-4 Chemical Restraint/Anesthetic/Analgesic Agents Used in Amphibians. (cont'd)

Agent	Dosage	Species/Comments
Benzocaine (Sigma Chemical)	—	Anesthesia; not sold as fish anesthetic in United States; available from chemical supply companies; do not use topical anesthetic products marketed for mammals; prepare stock solution in ethanol (poorly soluble in water); store in dark bottle at room temperature
	50 mg/L bath to effect[59]	Larvae/dissolve in ethanol first
	200-300 mg/L bath to effect[59]	Frogs, salamanders/dissolve in ethanol first
	200-500 mg/L bath[59]	Dissolve in acetone first
Buprenorphine	38 mg/kg SC[31]	Analgesia >4 hr; ED_{50}^b in leopard frogs[31]
	50 mg/kg ICe q24h[26]	Eastern red spotted newts/return to normal behavior following limb amputation; may take >1 hr for onset of clinical effects; postsurgical bath in 0.1% sulfamerazine (w/v; Sigma Chemical Company)[26]
Butorphanol	0.2-0.4 mg/kg IM[59]	Analgesia; efficacy uncertain[59]
	0.5 mg/L continuous immersion for 3 days[26]	Eastern red spotted newts/return to normal behavior following limb amputation; may take >4 hr for onset of clinical effects; postsurgical bath in 0.1% sulfamerazine (w/v; Sigma Chemical Company)[26]
Clove oil (eugenol)	0.3 mL/L (~310-318 mg/L)[59]	Anesthesia; deep anesthesia after 15 min bath; caused reversible gastric prolapse in 50% of leopard frogs
	0.35 mL in 1 L purified water[19]	African clawed frogs/anesthetic plane for frogs <10 g after 5 min immersion, for frogs ~30 g after 10 min immersion
	0.45 mL/L (~473 mg/L)[38]	Anesthesia; deep anesthesia induced in 80% of tiger salamanders
Codeine	53 mg/kg SC[31]	Analgesia >4 hr; ED_{50}^b in leopard frogs
Dexmedetomidine	40-120 mg/kg SC[31]	Analgesia >4 hr; ED_{50}^b in leopard frogs
Diazepam	—	See ketamine for combination
Fentanyl	0.5 mg/kg SC[31]	Analgesia >4 hr; ED_{50}^b in leopard frogs
Flunixin meglumine	25 mg/kg intralymphatic[10]	African clawed frogs
Isoeugenol (Aqui-S; 0.54 μg/mL isoeugenol)	20-50 μL/L[47]	*Litoria ewingii* tadpoles/higher doses resulted in faster induction and longer recovery

Continued

TABLE 3-4 Chemical Restraint/Anesthetic/Analgesic Agents Used in Amphibians. (cont'd)

Agent	Dosage	Species/Comments
Isoflurane	—	Anesthesia; induction chamber
	3%-5% induction, 1%-2% maintenance[59]	Terrestrial species
	5%[59]	Terrestrial species/euthanasia; induction chamber
	Topical application of liquid isoflurane[59]	*Bufo* spp. (0.015 mL/g BW), African clawed frogs (0.007 mL/g BW)/induce in closed container; once induced, remove excess from animal
	Topical mixture of isoflurane (3 mL), KY jelly (3.5 mL), and water (1.5 mL)[59]	*Bufo* spp. (0.035 mL/g BW), African clawed frogs (0.025 mL/g BW)/induce in closed container; once induced, remove excess from animal
	Topical mixture of 1.5 parts distilled water, 3.5 parts nonspermicidal jelly, and 1.8 parts isoflurane[63]	American tree frogs/induced in closed container; once induced remove excess from animal; erythematous lesions and signs of systemic illness noted following application[63]
	0.28 mL/100 mL bath[59]	Induce in closed container
	Bubbled into water to effect[59]	Aquatic species
Ketamine	—	May have long induction and recovery times; does not provide good analgesia so may not be suited for major surgical procedures; other agents preferred; ketamine combination follows; see lidocaine
	50-150 mg/kg SC, IM[59]	Most species
Ketamine (K)/diazepam (D)	(K) 20-40 mg/kg + (D) 0.2-0.4 mg/kg IM[59]	Variable results
Lidocaine 1%-2%	Local infiltration[59]	All/local anesthesia; with or without epinephrine; 2% lidocaine in combination with ketamine has been used for minor surgeries;[59] use with caution
Meloxicam	0.1 mg/kg[37]	American bullfrogs/decreased circulating prostaglandin E2 (PGE2) levels measured 24 hr post muscle biopsy[37]
	0.4-1 mg/kg PO, SC, ICe q24h[59]	Analgesia
Metomidate hydrochloride	30 mg/L bath[13]	*Rana pipiens*/immersion for 60 min then transferred to amphibian Ringer's solution; clinical sedation in 11/11 frogs; surgical anesthesia in 3/11; prolonged recovery; not recommended as sole anesthetic agent
Morphine	38-42 mg/kg SC[31]	Analgesia >4 hr
Nalorphine	122 mg/kg SC[31]	Analgesia >4 hr

TABLE 3-4 Chemical Restraint/Anesthetic/Analgesic Agents Used in Amphibians. (cont'd)

Agent	Dosage	Species/Comments
Naloxone	10 mg/kg SC;[31] titrate to effect	Antagonist for buprenorphine, butorphanol, codeine, fentanyl, morphine
Naltrexone	1 mg/kg SC;[31] titrate to effect	Antagonist for buprenorphine, butorphanol, codeine, fentanyl, morphine
Pentobarbital sodium	60 mg/kg IV, ICe[59]	Euthanasia; can also be administered in lymph sacs in anurans
Pentobarbital sodium + sodium phenytoin	1100 mg/kg + 141 mg/kg ICe[51]	African clawed frogs/complete cardiac arrest within 3 hr
Propofol	10-30 mg/kg ICe[59]	White's tree frogs/pilot study; use the lower dosage for sedation or light anesthesia; induction within 30 min; recovery in 24 hr
	35 mg/kg ICe[38]	Deep anesthesia in 83% of tiger salamanders[38]
	35 mg/kg ICe[57]	Sonoran desert toads/sedation only; did not achieve surgical plane of anesthesia
	60-100 mg/kg ICe[59]	Euthanasia
	88 mg/L by immersion[21]	African clawed frogs/induced for 15 min, then rinsed; respiratory depression, darkened skin color; death at doses over 175 mg/L
	100-140 mg/kg topically[59]	Maroon-eyed tree frogs (*Agalychnis litodryas*)/unpublished data; 15-20 min to max effect at 100 mg/kg dose; 10-15 min to max effect at 140 mg/kg;[59] sedation to deep anesthesia; remove and rinse when desired level achieved; recommended only for animals <50 g
Sevoflurane	Topical application	Rapid recovery unless constant reapplication
	Topical mixture of 1.5 parts distilled water, 3.5 parts nonspermicidal jelly, and 3 parts sevoflurane[48,63]	American tree frogs/induced in closed container with 2 mL of sevoflurane jelly per individual; once induced, remove excess from animal; recovery 4.5 times faster than topical isoflurane jelly;[63] in cane toads, reliable loss of righting reflex when 37.5 µg/g sevoflurane in jelly was applied to dorsum[48]
Tiletamine/zolazepam (Telazol, Fort Dodge)	10-20 mg/kg IM[59]	Results variable between species; rapid recovery; not suitable as single anesthetic agent for anurans[29]

Continued

TABLE 3-4 Chemical Restraint/Anesthetic/Analgesic Agents Used in Amphibians. (cont'd)

Agent	Dosage	Species/Comments
Tricaine methanesulfonate (MS-222) (Finquel, Argent)	—	Anesthesia; buffer the acidity by adding sodium bicarbonate to buffer the solution to a pH of 7.0-7.1; aerate water to prevent hypoxemia; remove from bath on induction or overdosing can readily occur; following bath, place terrestrial amphibians on moist towel or in very shallow water to recovery; some species can be induced at much lower concentrations than listed here; in some cases, anesthesia can be maintained by dripping a dilute solution of this drug (100-200 mg/L) over the skin or by covering animal with a paper towel moistened with the anesthetic[59]
	50-200 mg/kg SC, IM, ICe[59]	Most species/may be irritating administered SC, IM (neutral solution is preferred)[59]
	100-200 mg/kg ICe[49]	Leopard frogs
	100-400 mg/kg ICe[49]	Bullfrogs
	100-200 mg/L bath to effect[59]	Larvae/induction
	200-500 mg/L bath to effect[59]	Tadpoles, newts/induction in 15-30 min
	0.5-2 g/L bath to effect[59]	Frogs, salamanders/induction in 15-30 min
	1 g/L bath to effect[59]	Most gill-less adult species (unless very large)/induction
	1 g/L by immersion, buffered with 1 g/L sodium bicarbonate[57]	Sonoran desert toads/surgical plane of anesthesia
	1-2 g/L by immersion[27]	African clawed frogs/buffered to pH of 7.0 ± 0.4; 20 min induction then rinsed; respiratory depression; longer duration of surgical anesthesia with higher dosing
	2-3 g/L bath to effect[59]	Toads/induction in 15-30 min
	5 g/L immersion[51]	African clawed frogs/immersion for 1 hr; death within 3 hr
	10 g/L bath[59]	Euthanasia; can be administered ICe or in lymph sacs

[a]SC can be administered in dorsal lymph sac in anurans.[59]
[b]ED_{50}, effective dose for 50% of the population.

TABLE 3-5 Hormones Used in Amphibians.[a]

Agent	Dosage	Species/Comments
Gonadotropin-releasing hormone (GnRH)	10 μg SC to female followed by additional 20 μg after 18 hr; 5 μg SC to male[54]	Tomato frogs (*Dyscophus guineti*)/ovulation and spermiation
	0.1 mg/kg SC, IM, repeat prn[59]	Induction of ovulation in those non-responsive to pregnant mare serum gonadotropin (PMSG) or human chorionic gonadotropin (hCG); administer to females 8-12 hr before males
Human chorionic gonadotropin (hCG)	50-300 U[59] SC, IM	For mating or release of sperm in males; follow with GnRH in 8-24 hr
	250-400 U SC, IM[59]	African clawed frogs, axolotls/induction of ovulation; may be used with PMSG and/or progesterone
Luteinizing hormone–releasing hormone (LHRH)	5 μg ICe per animal[53]	Salamanders (*Desmognathus ochrophaeus*)/induced oviposition in 94% of animals
	10 μg in 0.05 mL of 40% DMSO applied to ventral drink patch[43]	*Bufo americanus, B. valliceps*/induced spermiation in 70% of males
Pregnant mare serum gonadotropin (PMSG)	50-200 U SC, IM[59]	African clawed frogs, axolotls/induction of ovulation; administer 600 U hCG SC, IM 72 hr later[59]
Progesterone	1-5 mg SC, IM[59]	African clawed frogs, axolotls/use in addition to PMSG or hCG for induction of ovulation

[a]SC can be administered into the dorsal lymph sac of anurans.[59]

TABLE 3-6 Miscellaneous Agents Used in Amphibians.[a]

Agent	Dosage	Species/Comments
Amphibian Ringer's solution (ARS)	6.6 g NaCl, 0.15 g KCl, 0.15 g $CaCl_2$, and 0.2 g $NaHCO_3$ in 1 L water[59]	For treating hydrocoelom and subcutaneous edema; place animal in shallow ARS bath until stabilized ($\approx$24 hr or more); replace with fresh solution daily; may need to wean animal off ARS by placing it in gradually more dilute solutions; hypertonic solution created by using 800-950 mL water instead of 1 L and may be more effective for some cases of hydrocoelom; up to 10 g of glucose may be added per L, but then solution must be made fresh daily[59]
Atropine	0.1 mg/animal SC, IM prn[59]	Organophosphate toxicosis
Caffeine	Use caffeinated tea bag; steep (soak) until solution is "weak tea"; place amphibian in shallow bath, replace q6h[59]	Stimulant; may help reverse ivermectin or levamisole toxicosis, or excessively deep anesthesia[59]
Calcium glubionate (Calcionate, 1.8 g/5 mL, Rugby Laboratories)	1 mL/kg PO q24h[59]	Nutritional secondary hyperparathyroidism

Continued

TABLE 3-6 Miscellaneous Agents Used in Amphibians. (cont'd)

Agent	Dosage	Species/Comments
Calcium gluconate	100-200 mg/kg SC[59]	Hypocalcemic tetany
	2.3% continuous bath (with 2-3 U/mL vitamin D_3)[59]	Nutritional secondary hyperparathyroidism
Critical care diets	—	Dosages are approximate; may be more appropriate to offer larger volume less frequently for easily stressed animals
• Carnivore Critical Care (Oxbow)	3% bodyweight PO q24-72h[59]	
• Emeraid for Carnivores (Lafeber)	3% body weight PO q24-48h[59]	
• Feline Clinical Care Liquid (Pet-Ag)	1-2 mL/50 g PO q24h[59] 3-6 mL/50 g PO q72h[59]	
• Hill's Feline a/d (Hill's Pet Nutrition)	PO[59]	Nutritional support; mix 1:1 with water; generally gavaged
Cyanoacrylate surgical adhesive (Vet Bond, 3M)	Topical on wounds[59]	Produces a seal for aquatic and semiaquatic species
Dexamethasone	1.5 mg/kg SC, IM[59]	Vascularizing keratitis
	1.5 mg/kg IM, IV[59]	Shock
Dextrose 5% solution	Bath[59]	For treating hydrocoelom and subcutaneous edema;[59] place animal in shallow bath until stabilized ($\approx$24 hr or more); replace with fresh solution daily; may need to wean animal off dextrose by placing it in gradually more dilute solutions; 7.5%-10% solutions may be more effective for some cases of hydrocoelom
	Topically to affected tissues[34]	Small amount can be applied to edematous/inflamed tissue in cases of cloacal prolapse to aid in prolapse reduction
Doxycycline	1.25-2.5 mg/kg PO, SC, ICe q24h[59]	Antiinflammatory
	1% gel topically q12h[59]	Antiinflammatory
Hetastarch (6% in 0.9% saline)	Bath not to exceed 1 hr without reassessment[59]	May help with initial treatment of hydrocoelom
Hypertonic saline, 5% ophthalmic solution	Topically to affected tissues[34]	Small amount can be applied to edematous/inflamed tissue in cases of cloacal prolapse to aid in prolapse reduction
Laxative (Laxatone, Evsco)	PO[59]	Laxative, especially for intestinal foreign bodies
Meloxicam	0.4-1 mg/kg PO, SC, ICe q24h[58]	Antiinflammatory; presumptive analgesia; adjunct therapy for septicemia
	0.5% gel topically q24h; do not exceed 0.4 mg/kg[59]	Antiinflammatory for localized wounds
Methylene blue	2 mg/mL bath to effect[59]	Nitrite and nitrate toxicoses

TABLE 3-6 Miscellaneous Agents Used in Amphibians. (cont'd)

Agent	Dosage	Species/Comments
Oxygen	100% for up to 24 hr[59]	Adjunct treatment for septicemia, toxicoses
Physostigmine (ophthalmic drops)	1 drop/50 g topically q1-2h to effect[59]	May ameliorate flaccid paralysis from ivermectin or levamisole toxicosis
Prednisolone sodium succinate	5-10 mg/kg IM, IV[59]	Shock
Sodium thiosulfate	1% solution as continuous bath to effect[59]	Halogen toxicoses
Vitamin A (Aquasol A, 50,000 U/mL, Mayne Pharma)	Dilute 1:9 with sterile water; make fresh weekly; apply 1 drop from a tuberculin syringe with 27 g needle to amphibians under 5 g; 1 drop from tuberculin syringe w/out needle is about 200 U and useful for 15-30 g BW; >30 g, try 1 drop per 10 g BW; topically q24h × 14 days, then q4-7d[59]	Hypovitaminosis A; given the plethora of organ systems that hypovitaminosis A may affect, it is reasonable to institute vitamin A supplementation of any clinically ill amphibian, particularly ones with signs similar to "short tongue syndrome," swollen eyelids, evidence of infectious dermatitis, hydrocoelom, or simply "failing to thrive";[59] the use of mixed dietary carotenoids may also be effective in some species[9]
	Dilute 1:10 in sterile water; applied as one drop from 18g needle; estimated as 50 U/frog q48h to q7d[45]	African foam-nesting frogs/weight range, 2-7 g; dosing q48h and once weekly significantly increased whole body vitamin A levels over control group and group treated with vitamin A fortified supplement dusted over crickets[45]
	1 U/g PO daily × 14 days[59]	
Vitamin A gel caps (10,000 U/cap)	Dilute 1:9 with corn oil to yield 1000 U/mL; give 1 U/g PO q24h × 14 days, then q7d[59]	Hypovitaminosis A; given the plethora of organ systems that hypovitaminosis A may affect, it is reasonable to institute vitamin A supplementation of any clinically ill amphibian, particularly ones with signs similar to "short tongue syndrome," swollen eyelids, evidence of infectious dermatitis, hydrocoelom, or simply "failing to thrive;"[59] the use of mixed dietary carotenoids may also be effective in some species[9]
Vitamin B$_1$	25 mg/kg PO[59]	Deficiency resulting from thiaminase-containing fish
	25-100 mg/kg IM, ICe[60]	
Vitamin D$_3$	2-3 U/mL continuous bath (with 2.3% calcium gluconate)[59]	Nutritional secondary hyperparathyroidism
	100-400 U/kg PO q24h[59]	
Vitamin E (alpha-tocopherol)	1 mg/kg PO, IM q7d[59]	
	200 U/kg feed[59]	Steatitis

[a]SC can be administered into the dorsal lymph sac of anurans.[59]

TABLE 3-7 Physiologic and Hematologic Values of Select Amphibians.[59]

Measurement	African clawed frog (Xenopus laevis)[55,59]	American bullfrog (Rana catesbeiana)[59]	Australian common green tree frog (Litoria caerulea)[62]	Australian white-lipped tree frog (Litoria infrafrenata)[62]	Cuban tree frog (Hyla septentrionalis)[59]	Leopard frog (Rana pipiens)[59] ♂	Leopard frog (Rana pipiens)[59] ♀	Tiger salamander (Ambystoma tigrinum)[59]
BW (g)	—	—	—	—	28-35	25-42	25-46	35
Blood volume (mL/100 g BW)	—	3.1-3.6	—	—	7.2-7.8	—	—	—
Hematology[a]								
PCV (%)	23.3-47.0	39-42	34-40.8	26.0-34.0	20-24	19-52	16-51	40
RBC (10^6/μL)	0.80-1.48	0.45	0.62-0.82	0.63-0.82	—	0.23-0.77	0.17-0.70	1.66
Hgb (g/dL)	6.06-15.19	9.3-9.7	8.0-10.6	6.1-8.2	5.6-6.8	3.8-14.6	2.7-14	9.4
MCV (fL)	31.6-62.8	—	461-602	374-486	—	722-916	730-916	—
MCH (pg)	6.9-22.1	—	111-148	84-115	—	182-221	182-238	—
MCHC (g/dL)	19.3-32.3	21.1-25.9	236-268	210-250	25-31	22.7-26.8	19.9-27.7	4.6
WBC[b] (10^3/μL)	0.64-9.56	—	12.4-22.1	14.2-29.1	—	3.1-22.2	2.8-25.9	—
Early stages[b] (%)	—	—	—	—	—	—	—	—
Neutrophils[b] (%)	8±1.1	—	14-27	15.0-32.0	—	—	—	—
Lymphocytes[b] (%)	65.3±2.7	—	—	57.0-78.3	—	—	—	—
Monocytes[b] (%)	0.5	—	5.0-10.0	4.0-8.0	—	—	—	—
Eosinophils[b] (%)	—	—	1.0-5.0	0-1.3	—	—	—	—
Basophils[b] (%)	8.5±1.4	—	0	0-1.0	—	—	—	—
Plasmocytes[b] (%)	0.2	—	—	—	—	—	—	—
Thrombocytes (10^3/μL)	17.1	—	23.2-33.5	25.8-38.8	—	—	—	—

Chemistry

ALP (U/L)	59-282	—	—	—	—
ALT (U/L)	10-39	—	—	—	—
AST (U/L)	27-1774	—	66-122	41-119	—
Bilirubin, total (mg/dL)	0.01-0.26	—	—	—	—
BUN (mg/dL)	2-10	—	—	—	—
Calcium (mg/dL)	5.2-12.3	—	10.6-13.1	8.6-11.3	—
Chloride (mEq/L)	72.7-92.7	—	—	—	—
Cholesterol (mg/dL)	56-563	—	—	—	—
Creatine kinase (U/L)	10-5400	—	347-705	233-722	—
Creatinine (mg/dL)	0.1-1.1	—	—	—	—
GGT (U/L)	1-19	—	—	—	—
Glucose (mg/dL)	18-111	—	55-78	45-81	—
LDH (U/L)	21-240	—	—	—	—
Phosphorus (mg/dL)	3.5-11.6	—	3.3-5.0	3.2-4.9	—
Potassium (mEq/L)	2.3-7.3	—	4.9-7.7	3.2-4.7	—
Protein, total (g/dL)	2.0-4.6	—	5.5-6.8	3.0-4.1	—
Albumin (g/dL)	0.1-2.3	—	—	—	—
Globulin (g/dL)	1.1-4.1	—	—	—	—

Continued

TABLE 3-7 Physiologic and Hematologic Values of Select Amphibians. (cont'd)

Measurement	African clawed frog (*Xenopus laevis*)	American bullfrog (*Rana catesbeiana*)	Australian common green tree frog (*Litoria caerulea*)	Australian white-lipped tree frog (*Litoria infrafrenata*)	Cuban tree frog (*Hyla septentrionalis*)	Leopard frog (*Rana pipiens*) ♂	Leopard frog (*Rana pipiens*) ♀	Tiger salamander (*Ambystoma tigrinum*)
Sodium (mEq/L)	111-134	—	107-114	104-108	—	—	—	—
Triglyceride (mg/dL)	57-555	—	—	—	—	—	—	—
Uric acid (mg/dL)	0.1-0.4	—	0.2-0.7	0.1-0.2	—	—	—	—

[a]Hematology is presently of limited diagnostic value because of the lack of normal data and the wide variation in hematologic and biochemical values according to sex, season, and state of hydration.
[b]For leukocyte totals and percentages for various species, refer to The Wildlife Leukocytes Web site at wildlifehematology.uga.edu.

TABLE 3-8 Blood Collection Sites in Amphibians[3,a]

Collection Site	Species Reported	Notes
Ventral abdominal vein	Anurans	Vessel present on midline along the ventral coelom, between sternum and pelvis; risk of hitting coelomic organs; visualization may be confirmed via transillumination of coelom in some species
Lingual plexus	Anurans	With mouth open, depress tongue to expose buccal surface of the oral cavity; lingual plexus can be visualized as superficial vessels; sedation may be needed in some species; safely used in frogs as small as 25 g, possible salivary contamination
Femoral vein	Anurans	Superficial vessel present along the medial aspect of the femur; runs parallel with femoral nerve; sedation may be needed
Heart	Multiple	Sedation recommended; aim needle at ventricle, allow heart to passively fill syringe to avoid collapsing ventricle; visualization may be assisted with ultrasound
Ventral tail vein	Urodelans	Similar to reptiles; caudal vein runs along the ventral caudal vertebrate and can be accessed via ventral or lateral approach; tail autotomy possible in some species
Facial vein/musculo-cutaneous vein[16]	Anurans (Ranidae)	Facial vein forms at the middle of the orbit and courses caudally to the angle of the jaw, turning into the musculo-cutaneous vein as it passes the caudal half of the tympanum; blood may be collected just rostral or just caudal to the tympanum; insert needle in rostrocaudal direction at 30° angle to the skin[16]

[a]Blood volume has been reported to vary by species or genus. In general, it is safe to collect 10% of the blood volume from healthy animals (approx. 1% of body weight). Clinical judgment should be used in collecting blood from sick or debilitated animals.

TABLE 3-9 Differential Diagnoses by Predominant Signs in Amphibians.[a]

Sign	Common Causes	Suggested Diagnostics[b]
Changes in skin color	Infectious agents: virus, bacteria, mycobacteria nodules, saprolegniasis, chromoblastomycosis, other mycoses, protozoa, myxosporeans, microsporidia, helminths (*Capillaroides xenopi*), leeches, fly larvae, other arthropods, fish lice, mollusks	Biology review of species in question; husbandry review (diet, water quality tests, soil pH, temperature); skin scrapes (wet mount and stained); PCR tests for ranavirus and chytrid; skin and blood cultures; fecal parasite exams; plasma cholesterol and triglycerides; radiograph for skeletal density; plasma calcium and phosphorus; CBC and other plasma biochemistries
	Noninfectious causes: toxicosis, hypothermia, hyperthermia, dehydration, desiccation, burn, frostbite, trauma, neoplasia, nutritional secondary hyperparathyroidism, xanthomatosis/hyperlipidosis, drug reaction	
Changes in skin texture	Infectious agents: virus, bacteria, mycobacteria, mycoses, protozoa, myxosporeans, microsporidia, helminths, fly larvae, leeches, mites, ticks, fish lice, other arthropods, mollusks	Biology review of species in question; husbandry review (diet, water quality tests, soil pH, temperature); skin scrapes (wet mount and stained); PCR tests for ranavirus and chytrid; skin and blood cultures; fecal parasite exams; CBC and plasma biochemistries
	Noninfectious causes: toxicosis, hypothermia, hyperthermia, dehydration, desiccation, stress, trauma (especially rostral abrasion), neoplasia, normal (e.g., dorsal crests in European newts, egg brood patch of Surinam toad, nuptial pads in male anurans)	

Continued

TABLE 3-9 Differential Diagnoses by Predominant Signs in Amphibians. (cont'd)

Sign	Common Causes	Suggested Diagnostics
Excess mucus production	Infectious agents: virus, bacteria, mycoses, protozoa, helminths, arthropods, mollusks Noninfectious causes: toxicosis (ammonia, nitrite, chlorine, chloramine, salt, nicotine), poor water quality (pH, hardness, supersaturation), stress (cagemate, escape behavior, inappropriate soil pH or composition), hyperthermia, trauma	Husbandry review (diet, water quality tests, soil pH, temperature); skin scrapes (wet mount and stained); PCR tests for ranavirus and chytrid; skin and blood culture; fecal parasite exams; CBC and plasma biochemistries
Fluctuant mass	Infectious agents: bacterial abscess, mycobacteria (rare), mycoses (rare), protozoal cyst, myxosporeans, helminths (e.g., immature trematodes and cestodes), subcutaneous leeches, fly larvae, mites, pentastomes Noninfectious causes: lymphatic blockage (e.g., gout), xanthomatosis, toxicosis, trauma, fluid overload, thermal injury, hypocalcemia, neoplasia, normal (e.g., active marsupium of *Gastrotheca* spp. females, water sacs of *Cycloderma rana*, distended lymphatic sacs of *Ceratophrys* spp.)	Biology review of species in question; husbandry review (diet, water quality tests, soil pH, temperature); aspirate (wet mount, stained, culture); fecal parasite exams; plasma uric acid, cholesterol, and triglycerides; radiograph for skeletal density; plasma calcium and phosphorus; skin and blood cultures; CBC and other plasma chemistries
Corneal opacity	Infectious agents: bacteria, mycoses, nematodes Noninfectious causes: scar, corneal lipidosis/xanthomatosis, trauma, chemical irritation, toxicosis, neoplasia	Husbandry review; slit lamp ophthalmic exam; culture and sensitivity; plasma cholesterol and triglycerides
Sudden death	Infectious agents: iridovirus, bacteria, chamydiosis, chytridiomycosis Noninfectious causes: toxicosis (ammonia, household pesticides, chlorine), electrocution, hypothermia, hyperthermia, trauma, gastric overload/impaction, stress, drowning, neoplasia	Biology review of species in question; husbandry review (diet, water quality tests, soil pH, temperature); PCR tests for ranavirus and chytrid; necropsy; physical exam of cagemates (include CBC, plasma biochemistries, blood culture, fecal parasite exams); consider euthanasia and necropsy of one or more cagemates
Weight loss	Infectious agents: bacteria, virus, chromomycosis, other mycoses, mycobacteria, coccidiosis, flagellate or ciliate overgrowth, helminths Noninfectious causes: heavy metal toxicosis (e.g., copper), chemical irritation (e.g., ammonia, chlorine, salt, pH), stress from inappropriate husbandry (e.g., environmental temperature too high, cagemate aggression), ocular disease with vision impairment, xanthomatosis	Biology review of species in question; husbandry review (diet, water quality tests, soil pH, temperature); skin scrapes (wet mount and stained); fecal parasite exams; PCR tests for ranavirus and chytrid; CBC; skin and blood cultures; plasma calcium, phosphorus, cholesterol, and triglycerides; radiograph for skeletal density; other plasma biochemistries

CHAPTER 3 Amphibians

TABLE 3-9 **Differential Diagnoses by Predominant Signs in Amphibians. (cont'd)**

Sign	Common Causes	Suggested Diagnostics
Anorexia, inappetence	Infectious agents: iridovirus, Lucke's herpesvirus, other virus, bacteria, mycobacteria, chytridiomycosis, chromoblastomycosis, mucormycosis, protozoa, myxosporean, microsporidial, helminth, fly larvae, pentastomes, mites, ticks Noninfectious causes: inappropriate environment (e.g., substrate, temperature, illumination, photoperiod, humidity, lack of furnishings and hiding spots, inappropriate cagemates, too many cagemates or visible specimens in adjacent cages, activity in room), inappropriate feeding practices (e.g., wrong kind of food/prey, wrong size of food/prey, feeding at wrong times, too many prey items offered at one time), frequent handling or cage servicing, nutritional secondary hyperparathyroidism, hypocalcemia, toxicosis (e.g., copper, ammonia, chlorine), xanthomatosis, ocular disease with vision impairment, neoplasia, geriatric/senescence, normal (i.e., estivation or hibernation cues)	Biology review of species in question; husbandry review (diet, water quality tests, soil pH, temperature); skin scrapes (wet mount and stained); PCR tests for ranavirus and chytrid; skin and blood cultures; fecal parasite exams; plasma cholesterol and triglycerides; radiograph for skeletal density; plasma calcium and phosphorus; CBC and other plasma biochemistries
Bloating	Infectious agents: virus, bacteria, mycoses, mycobacteria, gastrointestinal nematodes Noninfectious causes: hypocalcemia (especially in hylid frogs), toxicosis, hypothermia, decomposition of ingesta (e.g., gastric overload, low or high temperatures), pneumocoelom (i.e., ruptured lung or trachea), gas supersaturation	Biology review of species in question; husbandry review (diet, water quality tests, soil pH, temperature); fecal parasite exams; PCR tests for ranavirus and chytrid; plasma calcium and phosphorus; radiograph; aspirate (wet mount, stained, culture); plasma biochemical analysis; ultrasonography; radiograph; skin and blood cultures; CBC
Hydrocoelom	Infectious agents: virus, bacteria, mycoses, mycobacteria, verminous granulomata, filarids, other helminths Noninfectious causes: toxicosis (e.g., heavy metal, chlorine, ammonia, insecticide, distilled or reverse osmosis water), hepatic failure, renal failure, hypocalcemia, xanthomatosis, gout, neoplasia (especially ovarian, hepatic, or renal), failure to oviposit, normal (e.g., ovulation)	Biology review of species in question; husbandry review (diet, water quality tests, soil pH, temperature); aspirate (wet mount, stained, culture); fecal parasite exams; PCR tests for ranavirus and chytrid; plasma biochemical analysis; ultrasonography; radiograph; skin and blood cultures; CBC
Cloacal prolapse	Infectious agents: helminths, protozoa, colitis/cloacitis (bacterial, fungal) Non-infectious causes: mechanical ileus, dehydration, gastric overload, intussusception, hypocalcemia, nutritional secondary hyperparathyroidism, constipation, physiologic behavior, iatrogenic (handling, sedation), straining with oviposition (females), neoplasia	Biology review of species in question; husbandry review (diet, water quality tests, soil pH, temperature); fecal parasite exams/ impression smear of prolapsed tissue; radiograph; ultrasonography; plasma biochemical analysis; CBC

Continued

TABLE 3-9 Differential Diagnoses by Predominant Signs in Amphibians. (cont'd)

Sign	Common Causes	Suggested Diagnostics
Lameness	Infectious agents: virus, bacteria, mycobacteria, mycoses, protozoa, myxosporeans, microsporidia, helminths, fly larvae, pentastomes, mites Noninfectious causes: nutritional secondary hyperparathyroidism, trauma, malnutrition (e.g., hypovitaminosis B), thiaminosis, hypervitaminosis D, gout, xanthomatosis/hyperlipidosis, toxicosis (especially insecticides), neoplasia, drug reaction	Husbandry review (diet, water quality tests, soil pH, temperature); radiograph; plasma calcium and phosphorus; plasma cholesterol and triglycerides; fecal parasite exams; CBC and other plasma chemistries
Spindly leg	Infectious agents: iridovirus, larval cestodes or trematodes, subcutaneous nematodes Noninfectious causes: nutritional secondary hyperparathyroidism, malnutrition (e.g., hypovitaminosis B, protein deficiency, iodine deficiency, trace mineral deficiency, diet of parents, outdated food or vitamin supplements), toxicosis (ammonia, chlorine, nitrites), water quality (pH, hardness, temperature), crowding, poor illumination, trauma, genetic, hybridization	Biology review of species in question; husbandry review (water quality tests, temperature); diet (inspect actual food items and supplements in original containers); PCR tests for ranavirus and chytrid; necropsy; physical exam of cagemates and parents; consider euthanasia and complete necropsy of one or more cagemates

[a]This is based on the previous author's (Dr. Kevin M. Wright) clinical impressions of the most common underlying etiologies for gross symptomology; a patient's differential list should be a comprehensive review of all potential etiologies regardless of likelihood. Edited by current authors.
[b]Suggested diagnostics are presented in prioritized order.

TABLE 3-10 Selected Disinfectants for Equipment and Cage Furniture.[40,a]

Batrachochytrium dendrobatidis

- Sodium hypochlorite (household bleach) 1% for 1 min contact time
- Ethanol 70% for 1 min exposure time
- Benzalkonium chloride 1 mg/mL for 1 min contact time
- Desiccation and exposure to 50-60°C (122-140°F) heat for 30 min
- Exposure to 1:1000 quaternary ammonium compound Quat-128 (Waxie Sanitary Supply, San Diego, CA; 800-995-4466; www.waxie.com) for 30 sec; this contains 6.8% didecyl dimethyl ammonium chloride (DDAC) as the active ingredient

Ranavirus

- Nolvasan (chlorhexidine) 0.75% for 1 min contact time
- Sodium hypochlorite (household bleach) 3% for 1 min contact time
- Virkon S 1.0% for 1 min contact time
- Desiccation and exposure to 60°C (140°F) heat for 15-30 min

[a]In order to increase efficacy of disinfectants, rinse all organic material and debris from the surface before applying disinfectants.

TABLE 3-11 Guidelines for Managing Pet Amphibians with Nematode Parasites.[59]

- Determine purpose of captive amphibian
  - Pet amphibians are often kept for different purposes than captive assurance colonies
  - Plan must be with owner's informed consent
- Assess current health and body condition score (BCS)
  - If unthrifty
    - Consider any nematode ova, larvae, or adults significant. Treat for nematodes appropriately in light of other clinical findings
  - If well-fleshed, score the fecal parasite exam
    - If diarrhea, blood, mucus, or visible nematodes are present at any stage of the fecal parasite examination, treat
    - If stool appears grossly normal
      - and there are ≤5 RBC/HPF or <1 WBC/HPF, parasites may not be significant
      - and there are >5-10 RBC/HPF or >1-5 WBC/HPF, parasites are likely significant, treatment may be indicated
      - or there are >5 strongyle larvae/HPF on direct or float, treat
- Treatment of amphibians that are apparently healthy, eating well, and maintaining or gaining weight, should be done with caution despite the presence of a few nematode ova or larvae per high-power field on direct or flotation fecal parasite exams
- If any amphibians in the collection appear unthrifty, there are mortalities with nematodes implicated, or there are otherwise unexplained mortalities, treat for nematodes
- Monitor with regular direct fecal parasite exams to evaluate a shift in cytology and fluctuations in nematode ova and larvae; while there is often no correlation between reduction in nematode ova or larvae in feces and actual reduction in nematode numbers, improvements in BCS and weight often happen when the ova or larvae counts go down and the feces has ≤5 RBC/HPF and <1 WBC/HPF
- Success is measured by an amphibian having a normal weight and BCS, producing normal-appearing feces, and exhibiting normal behaviors
- With problematic pets, routine randomly collected feces should be assessed for parasites

TABLE 3-12 Amphibian Quarantine Protocols.[59]

Because of worldwide amphibian population declines and local extinctions, assurance colonies are being brought into captivity in hopes of preserving species for the future. The importance of these assurance colonies, and the possibility of future reintroduction efforts, makes proper quarantine and infectious disease testing paramount. In most cases, amphibians destined for use in reintroduction programs should remain in permanent quarantine to prevent introduction of novel pathogens. A 30-day quarantine is the minimum suggested time for quarantine of low risk amphibians, and moderate to high-risk animals should be quarantined for 60-90 days. Release from quarantine is predicated on interpretation of morbidity and mortality, appropriate testing to detect important diseases, and a healthy body condition score and normal physical examination prior to release. Any quarantine plan must have the owner's informed consent before implementation.

Husbandry

- Facilities and equipment
  - Ideally, each quarantine area is spatially separated from areas containing other animals. In addition, separate air-handling systems should exist for individual areas. Tools should be designated for use only in quarantine areas. Some facilities may employ shower-in/shower-out protocols, but at the very least boots, smocks/coveralls should be worn when servicing quarantine animal areas.
  - Enclosures

Continued

TABLE 3-12   Amphibian Quarantine Protocols. (cont'd)

- Enclosures should be escape-proof and made of non-abrasive, non-toxic material that is easy to clean and disinfect. Enclosures with spartan furnishings are easiest to monitor and maintain in quarantine situations; however, many animals will not thrive in such conditions. Critical husbandry requirements should always take precedence over other needs.
- Food
- Transmission of infectious disease through food animals is possible. In cases where this is of significant concern, it may be prudent to establish on-site breeding colonies of prey items and occasionally screen for various pathogens.

Quarantine Examination

- Physical examination can be facilitated via manual restraint, restraint in a clear container, or via anesthesia.
- To control the spread of *Batrachochytrium dendrobatidis*, new gloves should be changed after handling each patient. Nitrile gloves are preferred for their ability to kill zoospores on contact. Bare hands are preferred over rinsing the same pair of gloves between patients.[36]
- It is important to individually identify animals maintained in groups. Microchips and subcutaneous polymers can be placed; however, retention can be a problem. Charting of characteristic colors/patterns can be useful in some species (maintaining a database of digital photographs can be helpful in this regard). Toe-clipping has been used as a last resort, but is not recommended in zoological or private collections for humane and health reasons.
- Body weight and body condition scores should be assessed on arrival, periodically throughout quarantine, and immediately prior to release.

Diagnostic Testing

- Fecal flotation and direct examination
  - Quality samples can be obtained by placing the animal in a small container lined with damp, plain paper toweling overnight following a meal. It is best to assume wild amphibians are parasitized even though fecal exams can often be negative for the presence of parasites or ova.
- Complete blood count and chemistry panel
  - A large percentage of amphibians are too small to safely take routine blood samples. Even larger specimens can present venipuncture challenges. See Table 3.8 for venipuncture sites in amphibians. Normal ranges for bloodwork parameters are not available for the vast majority of species which creates interpretive challenges.
- Specific infectious disease testing
  - It is paramount that all amphibians entering quarantine (whether wild caught or captive bred) be screened for chytridiomycosis and ranavirus infection. Polymerase chain reaction tests are available for both pathogens, although chytrid fungus may also be detected via cytology of skin scrapings. Other specific pathogen testing will depend on individual circumstances.

Prophylactic Treatment

- Fluid therapy
  - Newly captured or shipped amphibians can be stressed and dehydrated. Amphibian Ringer's solution (see Table 3.6) can be used as a bath to help hydrate the animal and replenish solutes.
- Deworming
  - It is impractical to impossible to completely clear most amphibians of parasites. Treatment is aimed at reducing overall parasite burden. Treatment should address the results of diagnostic testing, otherwise empirical therapy with broad-spectrum anthelminthics is recommended.
- Treatment for chytridiomycosis
  - Animals brought into captivity from areas suffering local declines due to chytridiomycosis should always be prophylactically treated. In other situations, it is recommended to avoid treatment unless an infection is diagnosed to avoid development of resistance to available drugs.

TABLE 3-12 Amphibian Quarantine Protocols. (cont'd)

Maintenance and Hygiene

- A variety of disinfectants are available for use in amphibian applications. Care should be taken to choose a product that meets the disinfection needs but is not unsafe for the amphibians.
- Heat, desiccation, and ultraviolet light can be used, in some cases, to disinfect equipment and materials without the hazards associated with chemical use.
- Proper disposal of solid waste/water is paramount to avoid exposure of native amphibians in the area to novel pathogens. At the least, wastewater should only be discarded into a sanitary sewer and solid waste be deeply buried or transferred to a landfill. Best practices involve treating all waste that comes in contact with quarantined amphibians as potential biohazardous waste and disposing of accordingly. Wastewater and other materials should never be discarded into the environment in a manner where exposure to native amphibians is likely.

Infectious Disease Screening

There are a number of laboratories that will perform various tests to document exposure to or presence of chytrid fungus or ranavirus particles via PCR. It is up to the clinician to evaluate the tests run by the various laboratories and interpret the results accordingly. The following are contact information for laboratories that perform ranavirus and/or chytrid testing. This list is by no means conclusive, and contact information was verified as of September 16, 2016.

Amphibian Disease Laboratory
San Diego Zoo Institute for Conservation Research
15600 San Pasqual Valley Rd.
Escondido, CA 92027, USA
760-291-5472 or 760-291-5470
http://institute.sandiegozoo.org/resources/amphibian-disease-laboratory
Chytridiomycosis and ranavirus

Pisces Molecular
1600 Range St., Suite 201
Boulder, CO 80301, USA
303-546-9300
www.pisces-molecular.com
Chytridiomycosis

Research Associates Laboratory
14556 Midway Rd.
Dallas, TX 75244, USA
972-960-2221
www.vetdna.com
Chytridiomycosis

Zoologix
9811 Owensmouth Ave., Suite 4
Chatsworth, CA 91311, USA
818-717-8880
www.zoologix.com
Chytridiomycosis, ranavirus, and various *Mycobacterium* species

A more complete list of laboratories for *Batrachochytrium dendrobatidis* testing can be found at: http://www.amphibianark.org/the-crisis/chytrid-fungus/
A more complete list of laboratories in various countries for ranavirus testing can be found through the Global Ranavirus Consortium at: http://www.ranavirus.org/resources/testing-labs/

REFERENCES[a]

1. Adami C, d'Ovidio D, Casoni D. Alfaxalone-butorphanol versus alfaxalone-morphine combination for immersion anaesthesia in oriental fire-bellied toads (*Bombina orientalis*). *Lab Anim* 2016;50:204-211.
2. Adami C, Spadavecchia C, Angeli G, d'Ovidio D. Alfaxalone anesthesia by immersion in oriental fire-bellied toads (*Bombina orientalis*). *Vet Anaesth Analg* 2015;42:547-551.
3. Allender MC, Fry MM. Amphibian hematology. *Vet Clin North Am Exot Anim Pract* 2008;11:463-480.
4. Bianchi CM, Johnson CB, Howard LL, Crump P. Efficacy of fenbendazole and levamisole treatments in captive Houston toads (*Bufo [Anaxyrus] houstonensis*). *J Zoo Wildl Med* 2014;45:564-568.
5. Bishop PJ, Spear R, Poulet R, et al. Elimination of the amphibian chytrid fungus *Batrachochytrium dendrobatidis* by Archey's frog *Leiopelma archeyi*. *Dis Aquat Org* 2009;84:9-15.
6. Blooi M, Pasmans F, Rouffaer L, et al. Successful treatment of *Batrachochytrium salamandrivorans* infections in salamanders requires synergy between voriconazole, polymixin E and temperature. *Sci Rep* 2015;5:11788. http://dx.doi.org/10.1038/srep11788.
7. Bowerman J, Rombough C, Weinstock SR, et al. Terbinafine hydrochloride in ethanol effectively clears *Batrachochytrium dendrobatidis* in amphibians. *J Herp Med Surg* 2010;20:24-28.
8. Brannelly LA, Richards-Zawacki CL, Pessier AP. Clinical trials with itraconazole as a treatment for chytrid fungal infections in amphibians. *Dis Aquat Organ* 2012;101:95-104.
9. Brenes-Soto A, Dierenfeld ES. Effect of dietary carotenoids on vitamin A status and skin pigmentation in false tomato frogs (*Dyscophus guineti*). *Zoo Biol* 2014;33:544-552.
10. Coble DJ, Taylor DK, Mook DM. Analgesic effects of meloxicam, morphine sulfate, flunixin megulumine, and xylazine hydrochloride in African-clawed frogs (*Xenopus laevis*). *J Am Assoc Lab Anim Sci* 2011;50:355-360.
11. Chatfield MWH, Richards-Zawacki CL. Elevated temperature as a treatment for *Batrachochytrium dendrobatidis* infection in captive frogs. *Dis Aquat Organ* 2011;94:235-238.
12. D'Agostino JJ, West G, Boothe DM, et al. Plasma pharmacokinetics of selamectin after a single topical administration in the American bullfrog (*Rana catesbeiana*). *J Zoo Wildl Med* 2007;38:51-54.
13. Doss GA, Nevarez JG, Fowlkes N, et al. Evaluation of metomidate hydrochloride as an anesthetic in leopard frogs (*Rana pipiens*). *J Zoo Wildl Med* 2014;45:53-59.
14. El-Mofty MM, Abdelmeguid NE, Sadek IA, et al. Induction of leukaemia in chloramphenicol-treated toads. *E Mediter Health J* 2000;6:1026-1034.
15. Felt S, Papich MG, Howard A, et al. Tissue distribution of enrofloxacin in African clawed frogs (*Xenopus laevis*) after intramuscular and subcutaneous administration. *J Am Assoc Lab Anim Sci* 2013;52:186-188.
16. Forzan MJ, Vanderstichel RV, Ogbuah CT, et al. Blood collection from the facial (maxillary)/musculo-cutaneous vein in true frogs (family Ranidae). *J Wildl Dis* 2012;48:176-180.
17. Garner TWJ, Garcia G, Carroll B, et al. Using itraconazole to clear *Batrachochytrium dendrobatidis* infection, and subsequent depigmentation of *Alytes muletensis* tadpoles. *Dis Aquat Organ* 2009;83:257-260.
18. Georoff TA, Moore RP, Rodriguez C, et al. Efficacy of treatment and long-term follow-up of *Bactrachochytrium dendrobatidis* PCR-positive anurans following itraconazole bath treatment. *J Zoo Wildl Med* 2013;44:395-403.
19. Goulet F, Hélie P, Vachon P. Eugenol anesthesia in African clawed frogs (*Xenopus laevis*) of different body weights. *J Am Assoc Lab Anim Sci* 2010;49:460-463.

---

[a]Note: Pessier AP, Mendelson JR[40] remains an important and convenient source of information on amphibian medicine and is available free online.

20. Graczyk TK, Cranfield MR, Bichnese EJ, et al. Progressive ulcerative dermatitis in a captive wild-caught South American giant treefrog (*Phyllomedusa bicolor*) with microsporidial septicemia. *J Zoo Wildl Med* 1996;27:522-527.
21. Guenette SA, Beaudry F, Vachon P. Anesthetic properties of propofol in African clawed frogs (*Xenopus laevis*). *J Am Assoc Lab Anim Sci* 2008;47:35-38.
22. Hadzima E, Mitchell MA, Knotek Z, et al. Alfaxalone use in *Xenopus laevis*: comparison of IV, IM, IP, and water immersion of alfaxalone with doses of 18 mg/kg and 18 mg/L. *Proc Annu Conf Assoc Rept Amph Vet* 2013;60–64.
23. Howard AW, Papich MG, Felt SA, et al. Pharmacokinetics of enrofloxacin in adult African clawed frogs (*Xenopus laevis*). *J Am Assoc Lab Anim Sci* 2010;49:800-804.
24. Iglauer F, Willmann F, Hilken G, et al. Anthelmintic treatment to eradicate cutaneous capillariasis in a colony of South African clawed frogs (*Xenopus laevis*). *Lab Anim Sci* 1997;47:477-482.
25. Jones MEB, Paddock D, Bender L, et al. Treatment of chytridiomycosis with reduced-dose itraconazole. *Dis Aquat Organ* 2012;99:243-249.
26. Koeller CA. Comparison of buprenorphine and butorphanol analgesia in the eastern red spotted newt (*Notophthalmus viridescens*). *J Am Assoc Lab Anim Sci* 2009;48:171-175.
27. Lalonde-Robert V, Beaudry F, Vachon P. Pharmacologic parameters of MS222 and physiologic changes in frogs (*Xenopus laevis*) after immersion at anesthetic doses. *J Am Assoc Lab Anim Sci* 2012;51:464-468.
28. Lennox AM. Sedation with alfaxalone and local analgesia as an alternative to general anesthesia in reptile and amphibians. *Proc Annu Conf Assoc Rept Amph Vet* 2013;66–68.
29. Letcher J. Evaluation of use of tiletamine/zolazepam for anesthesia of bullfrogs and leopard frogs. *J Am Vet Med Assoc* 1995;207:80-82.
30. Letcher J, Glade M. Efficacy of ivermectin as an anthelmintic in leopard frogs. *J Am Vet Med Assoc* 1992;200:537-538.
31. Machin KL. Amphibian pain and analgesia. *J Zoo Wildl Med* 1999;30:2-10.
32. Marcec R, Mitchell MA, Kirshenbaum J, et al. Clinical and physiologic effects of sodium chloride baths in axolotls, *Ambystomma mexicanum*. *Proc Annu Conf Assoc Rept Amph Vet* 2011;1.
33. Martel A, Van Rooij P, Vercauteren G, et al. Developing a safe antifungal treatment protocol to eliminate *Batrachochytrium dendrobatidis* from amphibians. *Med Mycol* 2011;49:143-149.
34. McDermott C, Hadfield K, Clayton L, Nelson J. Cloacal prolapses in anurans: a ten-year retrospective review. *Proc Annu Conf Assoc Rept Amph Vet* 2015;477.
35. McMillan MW, Leece EA. Immersion and branchial/transcutaneous irrigation anaesthesia with alfaxalone in a Mexican axolotl. *Vet Anaesth Analg* 2011;38:619-623.
36. Mendez D, Webb R, Berger L, Speare R. Survival of the amphibian chytrid fungus *Batrachochytrium dendrobatidis* on bare hands and gloves: hygiene implications for amphibian handling. *Dis Aquat Organ* 2008;82:97-104.
37. Minter LJ, Clarke EO, Gjeltema JL, et al. Effects of intramuscular meloxicam administration on prostaglandin E2 synthesis in the North American bullfrog (*Rana catesbeiana*). *J Zoo Wildl Med* 2011;42:680-685.
38. Mitchell MA, Riggs SM, Singleton CB, et al. Evaluating the clinical and cardiopulmonary effects of clove oil and propofol in tiger salamanders (*Ambystoma tigrinum*). *J Exot Pet Med* 2009;18:50-56.
39. Muijsers M, Martel A, Van Rooij P, et al. Antibacterial therapeutics for the treatment of chytrid infection in amphibians: Columbus's egg? *BMC Vet Res* 2012;8:175.
40. Pessier AP, Mendelson JR, eds. *A Manual for Control of Infectious Diseases in Amphibian Survival Assurance Colonies and Reintroduction Programs*. Apple Valley, MN: IUCN/SSC Conservation Breeding Specialist Group. Available at: http://amphibianark.org/pdf/Amphibian_Disease_Manual.pdf. Accessed September 16, 2016.
41. Posner LP, Bailey KM, Richardson EY, et al. Alfaxalone anesthesia in bullfrogs (*Lithobates catesbeiana*) by injection or immersion. *J Zoo Wildl Med* 2013;44:965-971.
42. Poynton SL, Whitaker BR. Protozoa in poison dart frogs (Dentrobatidae): clinical assessment and identification. *J Zoo Wildl Med* 1994;25:29-39.

43. Rowson AD, Obringer AR, Roth TL. Non-invasive treatments of luteinizing hormone-releasing hormone for inducing spermiation in American (*Bufo americanus*) and Gulf Coast (*Bufo valliceps*) toads. *Zoo Biol* 2001;20:63-74.
44. Shilton CM, Smith DA, Crawshaw GJ, et al. Corneal lipid deposition in Cuban tree frogs (*Osteopilus septentrionalis*) and its relationship to serum lipids: an experimental study. *J Zoo Wildl Med* 2001;32:305-319.
45. Sim RR, Sullivan KE, Valdes EV, et al. A comparison of oral and topical vitamin A supplementation in African foam-nesting frogs (*Chiromantis xerampelina*). *J Zoo Wildl Med* 2010;41:456-460.
46. Sladakovic I, Johnson RS, Vogelnest L. Evaluation of intramuscular alfaxalone in three Australian frog species (*Litoria caerulea, Litoria aurea, Litorea booroolongensis*). *J Herp Med Surg* 2014;24:36-42.
47. Speare R, Speare B, Muller R, et al. Anesthesia of tadpoles of the southern brown tree frog (*Litoria ewingii*) with isoeugenol (Aqui-S). *J Zoo Wildl Med* 2014;45:492-496.
48. Stone SM, Clarke-Price SC, Boesch JM, Mitchell MA. Evaluation of righting reflex in cane toads (*Bufo marinus*) after topical application of sevoflurane jelly. *Am J Vet Res* 2013;74:823-827.
49. Stoskopf MK. Pain and analgesia in birds, reptiles, amphibians, and fish. *Invest Ophthalmol Visual Sci* 1994;35:775-780.
50. Stoskopf MK, Arnold J, Mason M. Aminoglycoside antibiotic levels in the aquatic salamander (*Necturus necturus*). *J Zoo Anim Med* 1987;18:81-85.
51. Torreilles SL, McClure DE, Green SL. Evaluation and refinement of euthanasia methods for *Xenopus laevis*. *J Am Assoc Lab Anim Sci* 2009;48:512-516.
52. Valitutto MT, Raphael BL, Calle PP, et al. Tissue concentrations of enrofloxacin and its metabolite ciprofloxacin after a single topical dose in the coqui frog (*Eleutherodactylus coqui*). *J Herp Med Surg* 2013;23:69-73.
53. Verrel PA. Hormonal induction of ovulation and oviposition in the salamander *Desmognathus ochrophaeus* (Plethodontidae). *Herp Rev* 1989;20:42-43.
54. Whitaker BR. Reproduction. In: Wright KM, Whitaker BR, eds. *Amphibian Medicine and Captive Husbandry*. Malabar, FL: Krieger Publishing Co; 2001:285-299.
55. Wilson S, Felt S, Torreilles S, et al. Serum clinical biochemical and hematological reference ranges of laboratory-reared and wild-caught *Xenopus laevis*. *J Am Assoc Lab Anim Sci* 2011;50:635-640.
56. Woodhams DC, Alford RA, Marantelli G. Emerging disease of amphibians cured by elevated body temperature. *Dis Aquat Org* 2003;55:65-67.
57. Wojick KB, Langan JN, Mitchell MA. Evaluation of MS-222 (tricaine methanosulfonate) and propofol as anesthetic agents in Sonoran desert toads (*Bufo alvarius*). *J Herp Med Surg* 2010;20:79-83.
58. Wright KM, Carpenter JW, DeVoe RS. Abridged formulary for amphibians. In: Mader DR, Divers SJ, eds. *Current Therapy in Reptile Medicine and Surgery*. St. Louis, MO: Elsevier; 2014:411-416.
59. Wright KM, DeVoe RS. Amphibians. In: Carpenter JW, ed. *Exotic Animal Formulary*. 4th ed. St. Louis: Saunders/Elsevier; 2013:53-82.
60. Wright KM, Whitaker BR. Nutritional disorders. In: Wright KM, Whitaker BR, eds. *Amphibian Medicine and Captive Husbandry*. Malabar, FL: Krieger Publishing Co; 2001:73-87.
61. Young S, Speare R, Berger L, Skerratt LF. Chloramphenicol with fluid and electrolyte therapy cures terminally ill green tree frogs (*Litoria caerulea*) with chytridiomycosis. *J Zoo Wildl Med* 2012;43:330-337.
62. Young S, Warner J, Speare R, et al. Hematologic and plasma biochemical reference intervals for health monitoring of wild Australian tree frogs. *Vet Clin Pathol* 2012;41:478-492.
63. Zec S, Clark-Price S, Mitchell M. Loss of return of righting reflex in American green tree frogs (*Hyla cinerea*) after topical application of compounded sevoflurane or isoflurane jelly: a pilot study. *J Herp Med Surg* 2014;24:72-76.

Chapter 4 **Reptiles**

Eric Klaphake | Paul M. Gibbons | Kurt K. Sladky | James W. Carpenter

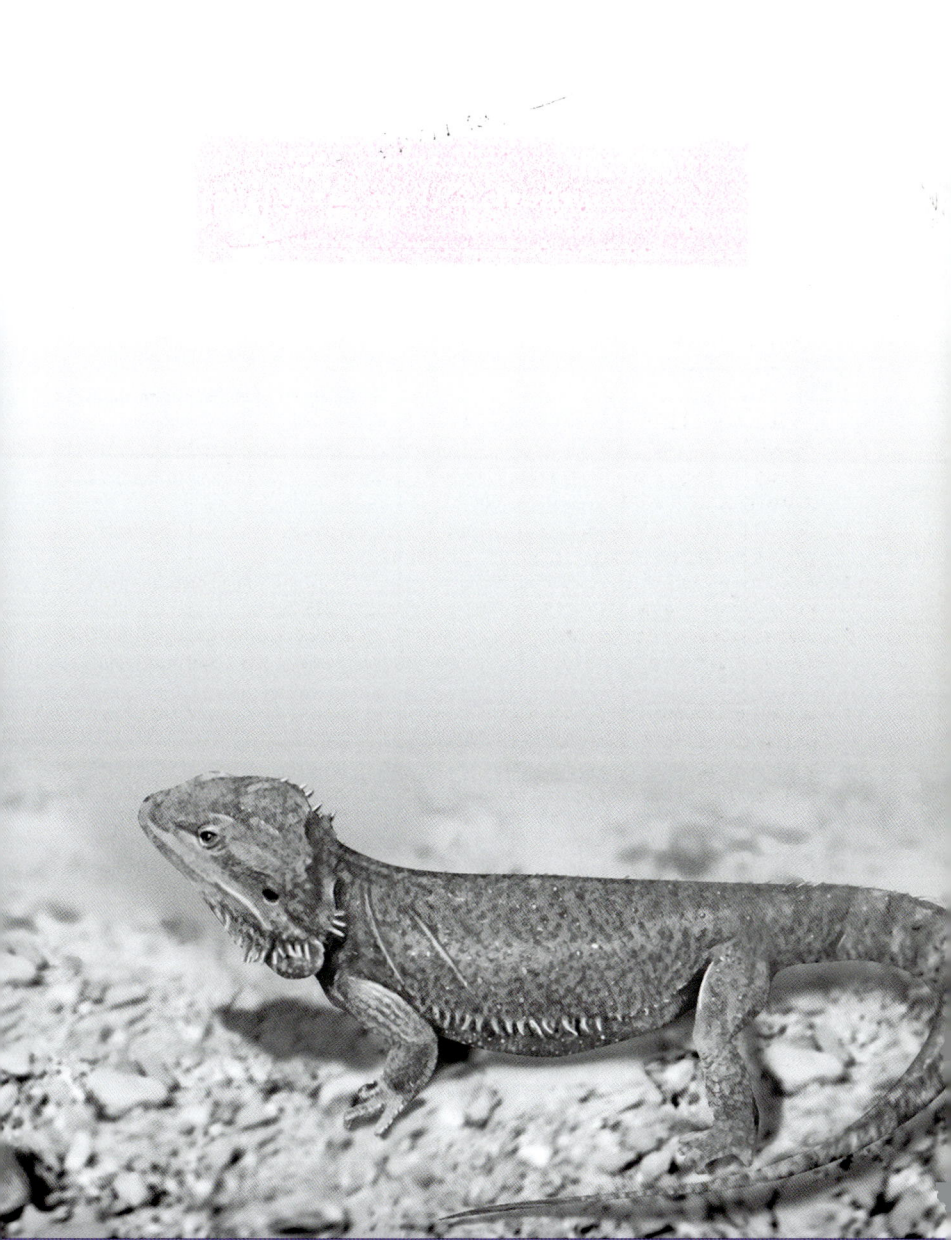

TABLE 4-1 Antimicrobial Agents Used in Reptiles.[a,b]

Agent	Dosage	Species/Comments
Amikacin	—	Potentially nephrotoxic; maintain hydration; frequently used with a penicillin or cephalosporin
	26 µg/kg/hr via osmotic infusion pump implant[55,374]	Snakes/PD; consider loading dose at time of implant
	3.48 mg/kg IM once[182]	Pythons/PK (ball pythons)
	5 mg/kg IM, then 2.5 mg/kg q72h[233]	Gopher snakes/PD; house at high end of optimum temperature range during treatment
	5 mg/kg IM, then 2.5 mg/kg q72h[16,363]	Lizards
	5 mg/kg IM q48h[44]	Gopher tortoises/PK; 30°C (86°F)
	2.25 mg/kg IM q72h[172]	Alligators/PD
	50 mg/10 mL saline × 30 min nebulization q12h[117]	Most species/pneumonia; aminophylline at 25 mg/9 mL of sterile saline in nebulizer before antibiotics for bronchodilation[316]
Amoxicillin	22 mg/kg PO q12-24h[79,103]	Most species/use with an aminoglycoside
Ampicillin	—	May use with an aminoglycoside
	10-20 mg/kg SC, IM q12h[174]	Most species, including chameleons
	50 mg/kg SC, IM q12h[343]	Chelonians
	20 mg/kg IM q24h[117]	Tortoises
	50 mg/kg IM q12h[357]	Tortoises/PD
Azithromycin	10 mg/kg PO q2-7d[59]	Ball pythons/PK; single dose study; may cause nonregenerative anemia; *Mycoplasma*, *Cryptosporidium*, *Giardia*, and other susceptible organisms; location dictates dosage frequency: skin, q3d; respiratory tract, q5d; liver/kidneys, q7d
Carbenicillin	—	Discontinued; more stable than ampicillin; extended G-spectrum
	200 mg/kg IM q24h[158]	Carpet pythons/PK
	400 mg/kg IM q24h[215]	Snakes/PD; 30°C (86°F)
	400 mg/kg IM q48h[214]	Chelonians/PD (*Testudo* spp.)
Cefazolin	22 mg/kg IM q24h[307]	Chelonians
Cefoperazone (Cefobid, Pfizer)	100 mg/kg IM q96h[106]	Snakes/PD (false water cobras; 24°C [75°F])
	125 mg/kg IM q24h[106]	Lizards/PD (tegus; 24°C [75°F])
Cefotaxime	20-40 mg/kg IM q24h[117]	Most species/may use with an aminoglycoside
	100 mg/10 mL saline × 30 min nebulization q24h[278]	Most species/pneumonia
Cefovecin	—	Short dosing interval is likely for most reptile species[281,378]
	10 mg/kg SC q12h[281]	Green iguanas/PD (25°C [77°F])

TABLE 4-1	Antimicrobial Agents Used in Reptiles. (cont'd)	
Agent	Dosage	Species/Comments
Ceftazidime	20-40 mg/kg SC, IM, q48-72h[106,363,391]	Most species/chameleons use q24h
	20 mg/kg SC, IM, IV q72h[16,213]	Snakes/PD; 30°C (86°F); often effective against Gram-negative aerobes (i.e., *Pseudomonas*)
	22 mg/kg IM, IV q72h[165,366]	Sea turtles
Ceftiofur	2.2 mg/kg IM q48h[79]	Snakes/ceftiofur sodium
	15 mg/kg IM q24-120h[1]	Snakes/PK; ceftiofur crystalline-free acid; ball pythons; 26.1°C (79°F); dosing interval based on MIC
	5 mg/kg SC, IM q24h[26]	Lizards/PK; ceftiofur sodium; (green iguanas)
	30 mg/kg IM, SC[54]	Lizards/PK; ceftiofur crystalline-free acid; bearded dragons 30°C (86°F); interval may be q10-12d
	2.2 mg/kg IM q24h[79]	Turtles/ceftiofur sodium
	4 mg/kg IM q24h[79]	Tortoises/ceftiofur sodium; upper respiratory infection
Cefuroxime	100 mg/kg IM q24h[79]	Most species/30°C (86°F)
Cephalexin	20-40 mg/kg PO q12h[106]	Most species/unknown absorption
Cephalothin	20-40 mg/kg IM q12h[106]	Most species
Chloramphenicol	—	Most species/public health concern; reserve for meningitis or encephalitis caused by susceptible organisms
	40 mg/kg PO, SC, IM q24h, or 20 mg/kg PO, SC, IM q12h[106]	Most species/20 mg/kg may be given q24h in larger crocodilians
	40 mg/kg SC q24h[42]	Snakes/PD (gopher snakes, 29°C [84°F])
	50 mg/kg SC q12-72h[56]	Snakes/PD; q12h in indigo, rat, king snakes; q24h in boids, moccasin snakes; q48h in rattlesnakes; q72h in red-bellied water snakes
Chlorhexidine (Nolvasan 2%, Fort Dodge)	Topical 0.05% aqueous solution q24h[264]	All species/topical disinfection; dermatitis; infectious stomatitis; periodontal disease in lizards q24h
	Topical 0.07% (1:30 [solution:water])[35,277]	Most species/topical disinfection; infectious stomatitis; abscess lavage; middle ear infection flush in box turtles
Chlortetracycline	200 mg/kg PO q24h[106]	Most species
Ciprofloxacin	10 mg/kg PO q48h[79]	Most species
	11 mg/kg PO q48-72h[198]	Pythons/PD (reticulated pythons)
Ciprofloxacin ophthalmic ointment or drops (Ciloxan, Alcon)	Topical[117]	All species/infectious stomatitis; gingivitis
Clarithromycin	15 mg/kg PO q84h[397]	Tortoises/PD (desert tortoises); upper respiratory tract disease (mycoplasmosis)

Continued

TABLE 4-1 Antimicrobial Agents Used in Reptiles. (cont'd)

Agent	Dosage	Species/Comments
Clindamycin	10 mg/kg PO, IM, IV q12h[135]	Loggerhead sea turtles/PK; 29.1-30.3°C (84.4-86.5°F) insufficient to be effective
Danofloxacin	6 mg/kg SC, IM[247]	Loggerhead sea turtles
	6 mg/kg SC q48h × 30 days[117]	Tortoises/upper respiratory tract disease
Dihydrostreptomycin	5 mg/kg IM q12-24h[103,117]	Most species/maintain hydration
Doxycycline (Vibramycin, Pfizer)	5-10 mg/kg PO q24h × 10-45 days[117]	Most species/respiratory infection (i.e., mycoplasmosis)
	50 mg/kg IM, then 25 mg/kg q72h[38,357]	Tortoises/Hermann's tortoise; 27°C (81°F)
Enrofloxacin	5-10 mg/kg q24h PO, SC, IM, ICe[117]	Most species/IM administration is painful and may result in tissue necrosis and sterile abscesses; may cause skin discoloration or tissue necrosis if given SC; to administer SC, dilute with sterile NaCl
	6.6 mg/kg IM q24h, or 11 mg/kg IM q48h[198]	Pythons/PD (reticulated pythons); *Pseudomonas*
	10 mg/kg IM q48h[391,392,407]	Snakes/PK (Burmese pythons, rattlesnakes, pit vipers)
	5 mg/kg PO, IM q24h[255]	Lizards/PD (green iguanas); marked pharmacokinetic variability with PO administration may make IM more suitable in critically ill animals
	10 mg/kg IM q5d[160]	Monitors/PK (savannah monitors); preliminary data
	5 mg/kg IM q24-48h[310]	Chelonians and most other reptiles/PD (gopher tortoises); hyperexcitation, incoordination, diarrhea reported in a Galapagos tortoise[49]
	5 mg/kg IM q12-24h[320]	Chelonians/PK (Indian star tortoises); q12h for *Pseudomonas* and *Citrobacter*; q24h for other bacteria
	5 mg/kg IV, IM q48h[210]	Sea turtles/PK (loggerhead sea turtles)
	10 mg/kg ICe q48h[123,332]	Chelonians/PD (Hermann's tortoises; yellow-bellied sliders) dilute with saline to 10 mg/mL
	10 mg/kg IM q24h[357]	Chelonians/PD (Hermann's tortoises)
	5 mg/kg IV q36-72h[146,250]	Crocodilians/PK; PO pharmacokinetics not fully determined; mycoplasmosis
	Nasal flush 50 mg/250 mL sterile water; 1-3 mL/naris q24-48h[117]	Tortoises/URT syndrome; use until no more discharge (5-10 days); may use concurrently with parenteral antibiotics
Gentamicin	—	Nephrotoxicity has been reported,[275] especially in snakes; maintain hydration; use with a penicillin or cephalosporin
	2.5 mg/kg IM q72h[42,43]	Snakes/PD (gopher snakes)
	2.5-3 mg/kg IM, then 1.5 mg/kg q96h[154]	Snakes/PK (blood pythons)

TABLE 4-1 Antimicrobial Agents Used in Reptiles. (cont'd)

Agent	Dosage	Species/Comments
Gentamicin (cont'd)	3 mg/kg IM q > 96h[18]	Turtles/PD (eastern box turtles; 29°C [84°F]); lower dose may be more appropriate
	6 mg/kg IM q72-96h[318]	Turtles/PD (red-eared sliders; 24°C, [75°F])
	1.75-2.25 mg/kg IM q72-96h[172]	Crocodilians/PK (alligators); respiratory infection
Gentamicin ophthalmic ointment or drops	Topical[103]	Most species/superficial ocular infection; lesions in oral cavity
Gentamicin/betamethasone ophthalmic drops (Gentocin Durafilm, Merck)	1-2 drops to eye q12-24h[178]	Tortoises/upper respiratory infections; may also be given as a reverse nasal flush q48-72h, or intranasal q12-24h
Kanamycin	10-15 mg/kg IM, IV q24h (or divided doses)[79,103]	Most species/24°C (75°F); give with fluid therapy; avoid in cases of dehydration or renal or hepatic dysfunction
Lincomycin	5 mg/kg IM q12-24h[79]	Most species/wound infection; potentially nephrotoxic; maintain hydration
	10 mg/kg PO q24h[79]	Most species
Marbofloxacin	10 mg/kg PO q48h[60]	Ball pythons/PD
Metronidazole	20 mg/kg PO q48h × ≥7 days[107]	Most species/anaerobes
	50 mg/kg PO q24h × 7-14 days[198]	Most species/may be administered concurrently with amikacin for broader spectrum; because of potential side effects at this dose, a lower dose may be prudent
	20 mg/kg PO q48h[32,206]	Snakes/PK (corn and rat snakes)
	20 mg/kg PO q24-48h[207]	Iguanas/PK; use q24h for resistant anaerobes
Oxytetracycline	6-10 mg/kg PO, IM, IV q24h[79,103]	Most species/may produce local inflammation at injection site
	10 mg/kg IM, IV q5d[145]	Crocodilians/PK (alligators; 27°C [81°F]); mycoplasmosis
Penicillin, benzathine	10,000-20,000 U/kg IM q48-96h[106]	Most species/may use with an aminoglycoside
Penicillin G	10,000-20,000 U/kg SC, IM, IV, ICe q8-12h[103]	Most species/infrequently used
Piperacillin	50-100 mg/kg IM q24h[79,103]	Most species/broad-spectrum bactericidal agent; maintain hydration; may use with an aminoglycoside
	50 mg/kg IM, then 25 mg/kg q24h[79,117]	Snakes
	100 mg/kg IM q48h[155]	Snakes/PK (blood pythons)
	100-200 mg/kg SC, IM q24-48h[174]	Chameleons
	100 mg/10 mL saline × 30 min nebulization q12h[278]	Most species/pneumonia
Polymyxin B sulfate, neomycin sulfate, bacitracin zinc ointment	Topical[117]	All species/rostral abrasions, dermal wounds

Continued

TABLE 4-1	Antimicrobial Agents Used in Reptiles. (cont'd)	
Agent	**Dosage**	**Species/Comments**
Povidone-iodine solution (0.05%) or ointment	Topical/lavage[103,300]	All species/fungal dermatitis; dermatophilosis; contaminated wound; can soak in 0.005% aqueous solution ≤1 hr q12-24h
Silver sulfadiazine cream (Silvadene, Marion)	Topical q24-72h[231]	All species/broad-spectrum antibacterial for skin (i.e., wounds, burns) or oral cavity; dressing is generally not necessary
Streptomycin	10 mg/kg IM q12-24h[103]	Most species/potentially nephrotoxic; maintain hydration; avoid in cases of dehydration or renal or hepatic dysfunction
Sulfadiazine	25 mg/kg PO q24h[117]	Most species/maintain hydration
Sulfadimethoxine	90 mg/kg IM, then 45 mg/kg q24h[103]	Most species/potentially nephrotoxic; maintain hydration
Ticarcillin (Ticar, SmithKline-Beecham)	50-100 mg/kg IM q24h[103]	Most species/maintain hydration
	50-100 mg/kg IM, IV q24-48h[237]	Loggerhead sea turtles/PK
Tobramycin	—	Potentially nephrotoxic; maintain hydration; potentiated by β-lactams
	2.5 mg/kg IM q24-72h[79]	Most species
	10 mg/kg IM q24-48h[79]	Chelonians/can be given q48h in tortoises; fluid therapy recommended
Trimethoprim/sulfadiazine or sulfamethoxazole	—	Maintain hydration; parenteral form must be compounded
	10-30 mg/kg PO q24h[117]	Most species/maintain hydration
	30 mg/kg IM q24h × 2 days, then q48h[357]	Tortoises/PD
Tylosin	5 mg/kg IM q24h × 10-60 days[79]	Most species/mycoplasmosis

[a]Because reptiles are ectothermic, pharmacokinetics of drugs are influenced by ambient temperature. Antimicrobial therapy should be conducted at the upper end of the patient's preferred (selected) optimum temperature zone.
[b]See Table 15-4 for antimicrobial combination therapies, some of which are commonly used in reptiles.

TABLE 4-2	Antiviral Agents Used in Reptiles.	
Agent	**Dosage**	**Species/Comments**
Acyclovir	40-80 mg/kg PO[5]	Box turtles/PK, low maximum plasma concentrations; uncertain efficacy
	≥80 mg/kg PO q24h[108]	Tortoises/PK; herpesvirus; poor oral absorption
	80 mg/kg PO q8h, or 240 mg/kg PO q24h[258]	Tortoises/herpesvirus; uncertain efficacy; unlikely to eliminate infection; combine with supportive care
	80 mg/kg PO q24h[299]	Mediterranean tortoises/decreased mortality in those infected with TeHV-3
	80 mg/kg PO q24h[63]	Australian Krefft's river turtles/herpesvirus; uncertain efficacy
	Topical (5% ointment) q12h[103]	All species/antiviral (i.e., herpesvirus-associated dermatitis)

CHAPTER 4 Reptiles 87

TABLE 4-2 Antiviral Agents Used in Reptiles. (cont'd)

Agent	Dosage	Species/Comments
Chlorhexidine solution	0.5% dilution, topical on oral lesions q24h[191]	Tortoises/herpesvirus
Famcyclovir	10-30 mg/kg PO q24h using allometric scaling[348]	Eastern box turtles/treated during outbreak of concurrent terHV-1 and ranavirus (FV-3); uncertain efficacy
Valacyclovir	40 mg/kg PO q24h[5]	Box turtles/PK, effective plasma concentrations compared to humans; uncertain efficacy or toxicity

TABLE 4-3 Antifungal Agents Used in Reptiles.

Agent	Dosage	Species/Comments
Amphotericin B	0.5 mg/kg IV q48-72h[104]	Most species/nephrotoxic; can use in combination with ketoconazole; administer slowly
	0.5-1 mg/kg IV, ICe q24-72h × 14-28 days[79]	Most species/aspergillosis
	1 mg/kg IT q24h × 14-28 days[173]	Most species/respiratory infection; dilute with water or saline
	0.1 mg/kg intrapulmonary q24h × 28 days[147]	Greek tortoises/pneumonia
	1 mg/kg q24h ICe × 2-4 wk[218]	Crocodilians
	5 mg/150 mL saline × 1 hr nebulization q12h × 7 days[169]	Most species/pneumonia
Chlorhexidine (Nolvasan 2%, Fort Dodge)	20 mL/g water bath[398]	Lizards/dermatophytosis
Clotrimazole (Veltrim, Haver-Lockhart; Otomax, with gentamicin and betamethasone, Schering-Plough)	Topical[328]	Most species/dermatitis; may bathe q12h with dilute organic iodine prior to use
F10 super concentrate disinfectant (Health and Hygiene, Roodeport, S Africa)	1:250 nasal flush, 0.1 mL each nare q24h[52]	Terrestrial chelonians/ benzalkonium chloride/ polyhexamethylene biguanide HCl
Fluconazole	5 mg/kg PO q24h[398]	Lizards/dermatophytosis
	21 mg/kg SC once, then 10 mg/kg SC 5 days later[136,235]	Loggerhead sea turtles/PK
Griseofulvin	15 mg/kg PO q72h[175-177]	Most species
	20-40 mg/kg PO q72h × 5 treatments[328]	Most species/dermatitis; limited success
Itraconazole	5 mg/kg PO q24h[249]	Most species/some hepatotoxicity noted when used for *Chrysosporium* anamorph of *Nannizziopsis vriesii*; can cause anorexia in bearded dragons without evidence of hepatotoxicity[114]
	10 mg/kg PO q24h[271]	Snakes

Continued

TABLE 4-3 Antifungal Agents Used in Reptiles. (cont'd)

Agent	Dosage	Species/Comments
Itraconazole (cont'd)	5 mg/kg PO q24h[142]	Panther chameleons
	10 mg/kg PO q48h × 60 days[29]	Chameleons (Parson's)/osteomyelitis
	23.5 mg/kg PO q24h[110]	Lizards/PD (spiny lizards); following a 3-day treatment, a therapeutic plasma concentration persists for 6 days beyond peak concentration; treatment interval was not determined
	5 mg/kg PO q24h, or 15 mg/kg PO q72h[238]	Kemp's ridley sea turtles
Ketoconazole	—	May use antibiotics concomitantly to prevent bacterial overgrowth; may use concurrently with thiabendazole
	15 mg/kg q72h PO[175-177]	Most species
	25 mg/kg PO q24h × 21 days[170]	Snakes, turtles
	15-30 mg/kg PO q24h × 14-28 days[254,304]	Chelonians/PK (gopher tortoises); systemic infection
	50 mg/kg PO q24h × 14-28 days[117]	Crocodilians
Malachite green	0.15 mg/L water × 1 hr bath × 14 days[79]	Dermatitis
Miconazole (Monistat-Derm, Ortho)	Topical[328]	Most species/dermatitis; may bathe q12h with dilute organic iodine before use
Nystatin	100,000 U/kg PO q24h × 10 days[169]	Most species/enteric yeast infections; limited success
Terbinafine	3.4 mg/kg PO q24h × 15 mo[369]	Aldabra tortoises/severe phaeohyphomycosis of carapace; non-responsive to itraconazole
	Topical[186]	Use in conjunction with oral azoles for *Chrysosporium* anamorph of *Nannizziopsis vriesii*; expect long treatment calendar
Tolnaftate 1% cream (Tinactin, Schering-Plough)	Topical q12h prn[4]	Most species/dermatitis; may bathe q12h with dilute organic iodine before use
Voriconazole	10 mg/kg per cloacal 3 ×/wk × 4 wk[261]	Rattlesnakes/*Ophidiomyces ophiodiicola*; crushed in suspension (Ora-Plus, Paddock Laboratories)
	10 mg/kg PO × 47 days[347,383]	Bearded dragons for *Chrysosporium* anamorph of *Nannizziopsis vriesii*; possible hepatocellular injury
	5 mg/kg SC[162]	Red-eared sliders/exceeded MIC only until 4 hr postinjection; 26°C (78°F)

TABLE 4-3 Antifungal Agents Used in Reptiles. (cont'd)

Agent	Dosage	Species/Comments
Voriconazole (cont'd)	10 mg/kg SC q12h × 7 days[167]	Red-eared sliders/resulted in trough concentrations considered subtherapeutic in humans but may reach MIC for some reptile fungal isolates; possible side effects seen
Voriconazole (V)/F10 super concentrate disinfectant (F10, Health and Hygiene, Roodeport, S Africa)	(V) 10 mg/kg PO q24h × 60 days + (F10) 1:250 dilution for 20 min bath q24h × 60 days[335]	Luthega skinks/systemic *Lecanicillium* sp. infection; nonresponsive to oral voriconazole and terbinafine ointment

TABLE 4-4 Antiparasitic Agents Used in Reptiles.

Agent	Dosage	Species/Comments
Albendazole	50 mg/kg PO[117]	Most species/ascarids; most toxic of the benzimidazoles
Carbaryl powder (5%)	Lightly dust animal and environment; rinse after 1 hr; repeat in 7 days[92,106]	Lizards, snakes/mites
Chloroquine	125 mg/kg PO q48h × 3 treatments[117]	Tortoises/hemoprotozoa
Dichlorvos (Vapona No-Pest Strip; United Industries)	6 mm strip/10 ft^3 in cage × 3 hr q48h × 2-4 wk[103,400]	Most species/mites; toxicity occurs;[106] prevent contact with animals (e.g., place strip above cage or inside perforated container); avoid in cases of renal or hepatic dysfunction; remove water container; use is discouraged
Dimetridazole (Emtryl, Rhône-Poulenc)	—	Not available in the United States
	100 mg/kg PO once, repeat in 2 wk[117]	Most species/amoebae
	40 mg/kg PO q24h × 5-8 days[169]	Snakes (except milk and indigo)/amoebae, flagellates
	40 mg/kg PO, repeat in 14 days[117]	Milk and indigo snakes/amoebae; flagellates
Emodepside (1.98%) + praziquantel (7.94%) (Profender, Bayer)	1.12 mL/kg[265,337]	Many species/PD; nematodes; cestodes; aquatic turtles must be kept dry for 48 hr after application; appears to be safe, but need more safety and efficacy data
Fenbendazole	—	Drug of choice for nematodes; least toxic of the benzimidazoles; may have an antiprotozoan effect; overdose may cause leukopenia, avoid in septicemic patients[285]
	25-100 mg/kg PO q14d for up to 4 treatments[38,169,196]	All species/nematodes
	100 mg/kg once[113]	Tortoises/nematodes; shedding of ova continues for 30 days
Fipronil (0.29%; Frontline Spray, Merial)	Wipe on then wash off in 5 min q7-10d prn[88,92]	Most species/mites, ticks; beware of reactions to alcohol carrier; needs safety evaluation[117]

Continued

TABLE 4-4	Antiparasitic Agents Used in Reptiles. (cont'd)	
Agent	Dosage	Species/Comments
Imidocloprid and moxidectin (Advantage multi/Advocate, Bayer)	0.2 mg/kg topical q14d × 3 treatments[130]	Lizards/eliminated hookworms and pinworms; needs safety and pharmacokinetic evaluation
Ivermectin	—	Do not use in chelonians,[377] crocodilians, indigo snakes, or skinks[38,117,199]
	0.2 mg/kg PO, SC, IM, repeat in 14 days[93,117]	Snakes (except indigos), lizards (except skinks)[38]/nematodes (including lungworms),[223] mites; can dilute with propylene glycol for oral use; colored animals may have skin discoloration at injection site; rare adverse effects reported in chameleons, possibly associated with breakdown of parasites;[16] do not use within 10 days of diazepam or tiletamine/zolazepam; rare death and occasional nervous system signs, lethargy, or inappetence have been reported;[199] used for pentastomids in monitor lizards (with dexamethasone 0.2 mg/kg q2d)[93]
	5-10 mg/L water topical spray q3-5d up to 28 days[199]	Snakes (except indigos), lizards (except skinks)/mites; less effective than fipronil; spray on skin and in newly cleaned cage, then allow to dry before replacing water dish
Levamisole (Levasole 13.65%, Mallinckrodt)	5-10 mg/kg SC, ICe, repeat in 14 days[16,117,169]	Most species/lungworms; 5 mg/kg in chelonians; 10 mg/kg in lizards, snakes; very narrow range of safety; main advantage is that it can be administered parenterally; avoid concurrent use with chloramphenicol; avoid use in debilitated animals; low dose may stimulate depressed immune system; can be used IM, but less effective
Mebendazole	20-25 mg/kg PO, repeat in 14 days prn[169]	Most species/strongyles, ascarids, effective dosage of 400 mg/kg;[208] may be toxic
Metronidazole	—	Protozoan (i.e., flagellates, amoebae) overgrowth; may stimulate appetite; may cause severe neurologic signs at doses >200 mg/kg;[272] death occurred in indigo and mountain king snakes at 100 mg/kg;[169] injectable form can be administered PO; oral suspension is not available in the United States, but can be compounded
	40-100 mg/kg PO, repeat in 10-14 days[103]	Most species/flagellate overgrowth
	20 mg/kg PO q48h[32]	Corn snakes/PK; 28°C (82°F); protozoa
	40 mg/kg PO, repeat in 14 days[106,169]	Uracoan rattler, milk, tricolor king, and indigo snakes/flagellates

TABLE 4-4 Antiparasitic Agents Used in Reptiles. (cont'd)

Agent	Dosage	Species/Comments
Metronidazole (cont'd)	40-60 mg/kg PO q7d × 2-3 doses[364]	Chameleons/flagellates; amoebae
	40-200 mg/kg PO, repeat in 14 days[268]	Geckos/ocular lesions (40 mg/kg) and subcutaneous lesions (200 mg/kg) caused by *Trichomonas*
	20 mg/kg ICe q48h[161]	Red-eared sliders/PK; ICe administration not recommended; needs further safety evaluation
	25 mg/kg PO q24h × 5 days[117]	Chelonians/amoebiasis
Milbemycin	0.25-0.5 mg/kg SC prn[31]	Chelonians/nematodes; parenteral form is not commercially available in United States; fenbendazole preferred
Nitrofurazone	25.5 mg/kg PO[393]	Most species/coccidia; seldom used
Olive oil	Coat skin q7d[16,92]	Most species, especially small, delicate lizards/mites; wash animal with mild soap (and rinse well) the next day; messy to use; environment must be treated with acaricide
Oxfendazole (Benzelmin, Fort Dodge)	66 mg/kg PO once[113]	Most species/nematodes; may be repeated after 28 days prn
Paromomycin (Humatin, Parke Davis)	35-100 mg/kg PO q24h × ≤28 days[103,169]	Most species/amoebae
	100 mg/kg PO q24h × 7 days, then 2×/wk × 3 mo[64]	Snakes/cryptosporidia; reduced clinical signs and oocyte shedding; does not eliminate the organism
	300-360 mg/kg PO q48h × 14 days[305]	Lizards (gila monsters)/cryptosporidia
	300-800 mg/kg PO q24h prn[58]	Geckos/cryptosporidia; reduced clinical signs; does not eliminate the organism
	360 mg/kg PO q48h × 10 days[129]	Bearded dragons/intestinal cryptosporidia
Permethrin (Provent-a-Mite, Pro Products)	Environmental treatment, 1 sec of spray/ft^2; wait until dry before returning animal to enclosure[92]	Lizards, snakes/mites; ticks; FDA approved; safe and effective; wash immediately if accidentally applied to skin
	Topical[92]	Tortoises/ticks
Piperazine	40-60 mg/kg PO, repeat in 14 days[208]	Most species/strongyles, ascarids; poor efficacy at <400 mg/kg[208]
	100-200 mg/kg PO[159]	Crocodilians
Ponazuril	30 mg/kg PO q48h × 2 treatments[33,273]	Bearded dragons/coccidiosis
Praziquantel	—	See also emodepside
	8 mg/kg PO, SC, IM, repeat in 14 days[16,117,174]	Most species/cestodes, trematodes; higher dosages have been administered[106]
	25-50 mg/kg PO q3h × 3 treatments[2,171]	Sea turtles (green, loggerhead)/PD; spirorchidiasis

Continued

TABLE 4-4 Antiparasitic Agents Used in Reptiles. (cont'd)

Agent	Dosage	Species/Comments
Pyrantel pamoate	5 mg/kg PO, repeat in 14 days[199]	Most species/nematodes
	25 mg/kg PO q24h × 3 days; repeat in 3 wk[106]	Most species/ascarids, hookworms, pinworms
Pyrethrin spray (0.09%)	Topical q7d × 2-3 treatments[92]	Most species/use water-based sprays labeled for kittens and puppies; apply with cloth; can also spray cage, wash out after 30 min; use sparingly and with caution; pyrethroids are safer (see permethrin, resmethrin)
Quinacrine (Atabrine, Winthrop)	19-100 mg/kg PO q48h × 14-21 days[393]	Most species/some hematozoa
Quinine sulfate	75 mg/kg PO q48h × 14-28 days[393]	Most species/some hematozoa; toxic at >100 mg/kg q24h; ineffective against exoerythrocytic forms
Spiramycin (Spirasol, May and Baker)	160 mg/kg PO q24h × 10 days, then 2×/wk × 3 mo[64]	Snakes/cryptosporidia; may reduce clinical signs and oocyte shedding; does not eliminate the organism
Sulfadiazine, sulfamerazine	—	Most species/coccidia; avoid sulfa drugs in cases of dehydration, urinary calculi, or renal dysfunction[272]
	75 mg/kg PO, then 45 mg/kg q24h × 5 days[103,393]	Most species/coccidia
	25 mg/kg PO q24h × 21 days[16,393]	Snakes, lizards/coccidia
Sulfadimethoxine	50 mg/kg PO q24h × 3-5 days, then q48h prn[199]	Most species/coccidia; ensure adequate hydration and renal function
	90 mg/kg PO, IM, IV, then 45 mg/kg q24h × 5-7 days[103,169,393]	Most species/coccidia
	50 mg/kg PO q24h × 21 days[384]	Bearded dragons/coccidia
Sulfadimidine (33% solution)	0.3-0.6 mL/kg PO q24h × 10 days[393]	Most species/coccidia; alternatively, 0.3-0.6 mL/kg, then 0.15-0.3 mL/kg q24h × 10 days
	1 oz/gal drinking water × 10 days[393]	Most species/coccidia
Sulfamethazine	25 mg/kg PO, IM q24h × 21 days[393]	Most species/coccidia
	50 mg/kg PO q24h × 3 days, off 3 days, on 3 days[117]	Most species/coccidia
	75 mg/kg PO, IM, IV, then 40 mg/kg q24h × 5-7 days[169]	Most species/coccidia; ensure adequate hydration and renal function
Sulfaquinoxaline	75 mg/kg PO, then 40 mg/kg q24h × 5-7 days[169]	Most species/coccidia
Thiabendazole	50-100 mg/kg PO, repeat in 14 days[104,169]	Most species/nematodes; fenbendazole preferred
Toltrazuril 5% (Baycox, Bayer)	5-15 mg/kg q24h × 3 days[83]	Bearded dragons/coccidiosis
	15 mg/kg q48h × 30 days[118]	Tortoises/coccidiosis; needs safety, efficacy, and pharmacokinetic study
Trimethoprim/sulfa	—	Most species/coccidia; avoid potentiated sulfa drugs in cases of dehydration or renal dysfunction[272]

CHAPTER 4 Reptiles   93

TABLE 4-4 Antiparasitic Agents Used in Reptiles. (cont'd)

Agent	Dosage	Species/Comments
Trimethoprim/sulfa (cont'd)	30 mg/kg PO q24h × 2 days, then q48h × 21 days[16,393]	Most species/coccidia
	30 mg/kg IM q24h × 2 days, then 15 mg/kg IM q48h × 10-28 days[393]	Most species/coccidia
	30 mg/kg PO q24h × 14 days, then 1-3 ×/wk × 3-6 mo[64]	Most species/cryptosporidia; can reduce shedding but does not clear infection
Water	Bath × 30 min[92,228]	Snakes, lizards/mites; use lukewarm (29°C [85°F]) water; monitor to avoid drowning; not 100% effective; does not kill mites on head; must treat environment with acaricide

TABLE 4-5 Chemical Restraint/Anesthetic Agents Used in Reptiles.

Agent	Dosage	Species/Comments
Acepromazine	0.05-0.25 mg/kg IM[117]	Most species/can be used as a preanesthetic with ketamine
	0.1-0.5 mg/kg IM[269,303]	Most species/preanesthetic; reduce by 50% if used with barbiturates
Acepromazine (A)/ propofol (P)	(A) 0.5 mg/kg IM + (P) 5 mg/kg IV; (A) 0.5 mg/kg IM + (P) 10 mg/kg IV[6]	Giant Amazon pond turtles/sedation with both protocols, longer duration with higher propofol dosage
Alphaxalone (Alfaxan, Jurox)	6-9 mg/kg IV, or 9-15 mg/kg IM[216]	Most species/good muscle relaxation; variable results; drug requires more evaluation; may have violent recovery;[19] don't use within 10 days of DMSO treatment
	6-15 mg/kg IM, IV[344]	Most species
	9 mg/kg IV[336]	Snakes,lizards/induction; not effective for blotched blue-tongued skinks
	15 mg/kg IM[269]	Lizards, chelonians/induction, 35-40 min; duration, 15-35 min; good muscle relaxation; variable results
	24 mg/kg ICe[131]	Chelonians (red-eared sliders)/ surgical anesthesia with good relaxation
	5 mg/kg IV[201]	Turtles, tortoises/induction
	10-20 mg/kg IM[133,193,346]	Horsfield's tortoises (males only)/ light to moderate sedation with no to minimal analgesia; red-eared slider turtles/light sedation of short duration; PD turtles administered 10 mg/kg at low temperature more relaxed than warm and turtles administered 20 mg/kg at warm temperature were most relaxed

Continued

TABLE 4-5 Chemical Restraint/Anesthetic Agents Used in Reptiles. (cont'd)

Agent	Dosage	Species/Comments
Alphaxalone (Alfaxan, Jurox) (cont'd)	20 mg/kg IM[166]	Red-eared slider turtles, Eastern painted turtles, yellow-spotted Amazon river turtles, other undocumented turtle species/anesthetic induction
	3 mg/kg IV[296]	Crocodilians/induction, but unpredictable results
Alfaxalone (Al)/medetomidine (Me)	(Al) 10 mg/kg + (Me) 0.10 mg/kg IM; (Al) 20 mg/kg + (Me) 0.05 mg/kg IM[133]	Horsfield's tortoises (males only)/deeper sedation than alfaxalone alone with analgesia
Atipamezole (Antisedan, Zoetis)	Give same volume SC, IV, IP as medetomidine, or dexmedetomidine (5× medetomidine, or 10× dexmedetomidine dose in mg)[a,95,355]	Most species/medetomidine and dexmedetomidine reversal; causes severe hypotension in gopher tortoises when given IV[69]
	0.2-0.5 mg/kg IM[94]	Chelonians/shell repair 5-10 min before finished
	0.5-0.75 mg/kg IM,[319] 0.75 mg/kg SC[244]	Chelonians
Atropine	0.01-0.04 mg/kg SC, IM,[34] IV,[104] ICe[341]	Most species/preanesthetic; bradycardia; rarely indicated; generally use only in profound or prolonged bradycardia;[341] may help prevent intracardiac shunting;[175] ineffective at this dose in green iguanas[302]
	0.5 mg/kg IM, IV, IT, IO[272]	Most species/bradycardia, decrease secretions, CPR
Bupivicaine (0.5%)	1 mg/kg intrathecal[240]	Turtles and tortoises/spinal anesthesia
	0.1 mL/10 cm carapace[17]	Green sea turtles/spinal anesthesia
Butorphanol	—	Butorphanol combinations follow; see ketamine for combinations; inadequate for analgesia
	0.4-1 mg/kg SC, IM[341]	Most species/sedation; preanesthetic
	0.5-2 mg/kg IM, or 0.2-0.5 mg/kg IV, IO[24]	Most species/preanesthetic
	1-1.5 mg/kg SC, IM[341]	Lizards/administer 30 min prior to isoflurane for smoother, shorter induction
	0.2 mg/kg IM[139,319]	Chelonians/minimal sedation
Butorphanol (B)/medetomidine (Me)[a]	(B) 0.4 mg/kg + (Me) 0.08 mg/kg IM[112]	Green tree monitors/sedation
Butorphanol (B)/midazolam (Mi)	(B) 0.4 mg/kg + (Mi) 2 mg/kg IM[23]	Most species/preanesthetic; administer 20 min before induction
Dexmedetomidine[a] (Dexdomitor, Zoetis)	—	Dexmedetomidine combinations follow; α₂ agonist that has replaced medetomidine;[a] reverse with atipamezole
Dexmedetomidine (De)/ketamine (K)	(De) 0.03 mg/kg + (K) 6 mg/kg IV[137]	Hatchling leatherback sea turtles/anesthesia; reversal with atipamezole (0.3 mg/kg IM, IV)

TABLE 4-5　Chemical Restraint/Anesthetic Agents Used in Reptiles. (cont'd)

Agent	Dosage	Species/Comments
Dexmedetomidine (De)/midazolam (Mi)/ ketamine (K)	(De) 0.1 mg/kg + (Mi) 1 mg/kg + (K) 2 mg/kg SC[245]	Red-eared slider turtles/deep sedation
Dexmedetomidine (De)/ketamine (K)/morphine (Mo)	(De) 0.075 mg/kg + (K) 8 mg/kg + (Mo) 1 mg/kg IM[263]	Gopher tortoises/anesthesia, reversed with atipamezole
Dextroketamine (DK)	10 mg/kg IV, ICe[156]	Spectacled caiman/mild sedation ICe; PK
Dextroketamine (DK)/midazolam (Mi)	(Mi) 0.5 mg/kg + (DK) 10 mg/kg IV, ICe[156]	Spectacled caiman/deep sedation IV; PK; no analgesia
Diazepam	—	Diazepam has been replaced by the use of midazolam in many cases; see ketamine for combinations; muscle relaxation; give 20 min prior to anesthesia; potentially reversible with flumazenil; drug interaction with ivermectin
	0.5 mg/kg IM, IV[272]	All species/seizures
	2.5 mg/kg IM, IV[329]	Most species/seizures
	0.2-0.8 mg/kg IM[341]	Snakes/use in conjunction with ketamine for anesthesia with muscle relaxation
	0.2-2 mg/kg IM, IV[344]	Snakes, lizards
	2.5 mg/kg PO[341]	Iguanas/reduce anxiety which often leads to aggression
	0.2-1 mg/kg IM[341,344]	Chelonians/use in conjunction with ketamine for anesthesia with muscle relaxation
Disoprofol	5-15 mg/kg IV to effect[37]	All species/anesthesia; similar characteristics to propofol; not available in United States
Doxapram	4-12 mg/kg IM, IV[341]	Most species/respiratory stimulant
	5 mg/kg IM, IV[23] q10min prn	Most species/respiratory stimulant; reduces recovery time; reported to partially "reverse" effects of dissociatives[217]
	20 mg/kg IM, IV, IO[272]	Most species/respiratory stimulant
	5-10 mg/kg IV[349]	American alligators/immediate dose-dependent increase in breathing frequency
Epinephrine (1:1000)	0.5-1 mg/kg IV, IO, IT[272]	Most species/CPR, cardiac arrest
	0.1 mg/kg IM[125]	Snapping turtles/reduction in time to spontaneous respiration after isoflurane anesthesia
Etorphine (M-99, Wildlife Pharmaceuticals)	0.3-0.5 mg/kg IM[269] 0.3-2.75 mg/kg IM[216]	Crocodilians, chelonians/very potent narcotic; crocodilians: induction, 5-30 min; duration, 30-180 min; chelonians: induction, 10-20 min; duration, 40-120 min; not very effective in reptiles other than

Continued

TABLE 4-5   Chemical Restraint/Anesthetic Agents Used in Reptiles. (cont'd)

Agent	Dosage	Species/Comments
Etorphine (M-99, Wildlife Pharmaceuticals) (cont'd)		alligators;[303] poor relaxation; adequate for immobilization and minor procedures; requires an antagonist; limited use because of expense and legal restrictions
Flumazenil (Romazicon, Hoffman-LaRoche)	—	All species/reversal of benzodiazepines, including diazepam and midazolam; seldom indicated
	0.05 mg/kg IM, SC, IV[241]	All species/reversal of midazolam; extrapolated from mammals and birds
	1 mg/20 mg of zolazepam[220] IM, IV[319]	Crocodilians, chelonians/reversal of zolazepam
Fospropofol	25-50 mg/kg ICe[340]	Red-eared slider turtles/muscle relaxation and immobility especially at higher dosage, but prolonged recovery, and profound respiratory depression with resuscitation in 2/8 subjects; use with caution
Gallamine (Flaxedil, American Cyanamid)	0.4-1.25 mg/kg IM[20] 0.6-4 mg/kg IM[221] 0.7 mg/kg IM[276] 1.2-2 mg/kg IM[95]	Crocodiles/results in flaccid paralysis, but no analgesia; larger animals require lower dosage; reverse with neostigmine;[221] use in alligators questionable; unsafe in alligators at $\geq$1 mg/kg,[303] deaths reported in American alligators and false gharials[218]
	0.5-2 mg/kg IM[211]	Crocodilians
Glycopyrrolate	0.01 mg/kg SC,[34] IM, IV[23]	Most species/preanesthetic; for excess oral or respiratory mucus; rarely indicated; generally use only in profound or prolonged bradycardia; may be preferable to atropine;[104] does not work at this dose in green iguanas[302]
Haloperidol	0.5-10 mg/kg IM q7-14d[367]	Boids/aggression management
Hyaluronidase (Wydase, Wyeth)	25 U/dose SC[220]	Crocodilians/combine with premedication, anesthetic, or reversal drugs to accelerate SC absorption
Isoflurane	3%-5% induction,[173] 1%-3% maintenance[38]	Most species/inhalation anesthetic of choice in reptiles; induction, 6-20 min; recovery, 30-60 min; not as smooth in reptiles compared to other animals; intubation and intermittent positive pressure ventilation advisable; may preanesthetize with low dose propofol, ketamine, etc.
	3% in 100% O_2 and 21% O_2[292]	Bearded dragons/trend toward shorter induction and recovery with 21% O_2 group compared to use of 100% O_2

TABLE 4-5 Chemical Restraint/Anesthetic Agents Used in Reptiles. (cont'd)

Agent	Dosage	Species/Comments
Isoflurane (cont'd)	5% via chamber in 5 L/min O_2[153]	Green iguanas/15-35 min loss of righting reflex; mean MAC, 1.62%; pH 7.49
Ketamine	—	Ketamine combinations follow; muscle relaxation and analgesia may be marginal; prolonged recovery with higher doses; larger reptiles require lower dose; painful at injection site; safety is questionable in debilitated patients; avoid use in cases with renal dysfunction; snakes may be permanently aggressive after ketamine anesthesia;[19] generally recommend use only as a preanesthetic prior to isoflurane for surgical anesthesia
	10 mg/kg SC, IM q30min[34]	Most species/maintenance of anesthesia; recovery, 3-4 hr
	20-60 mg/kg IM, or 5-15 mg/kg IV[117]	Most species/muscle relaxation improved with midazolam or diazepam
	22-44 mg/kg SC, IM[19,20]	Most species/sedation
	55-88 mg/kg SC, IM[20]	Most species/surgical anesthesia; induction, 10-30 min; recovery, 24-96 hr
	10-20 mg/kg IM[271,272]	Snakes, chelonians/sedation
	20-60 mg/kg SC, IM[34,180]	Snakes/sedation; induction, 30 min; recovery, 2-48 hr
	60-80 mg/kg IM[38]	Snakes/light anesthesia; intermittent positive pressure ventilation may be needed at higher doses
	5-10 mg/kg[271,341]	Lizards, snakes/decreases the incidence of breath-holding during chamber induction
	20-30 mg/kg IM[90]	Iguanas/sedation (i.e., facilitates endotracheal intubation); preanesthetic; requires lower dose than other reptiles
	30-50 mg/kg SC, IM[34,180]	Lizards/sedation; variable results
	20-60 mg/kg IM[157,180,303]	Chelonians/sedation; induction, 30 min; recovery, ≥24 hr; potentially dangerous in dehydrated and debilitated tortoises
	25 mg/kg IM, IV[117]	Sea turtles/sedation; used at higher doses (50-70 mg/kg); recovery times may be excessively long and unpredictable; combination of ketamine and acepromazine gives a more rapid induction and recovery
	38-71 mg/kg ICe[399]	Green sea turtles/anesthesia; induction, 2-10 min; duration, 2-10 min; recovery, <30 min

Continued

TABLE 4-5 Chemical Restraint/Anesthetic Agents Used in Reptiles. (cont'd)

Agent	Dosage	Species/Comments
Ketamine (cont'd)	60-90 mg/kg IM[180,269]	Chelonians/light anesthesia; induction, <30 min; recovery, hours to days; requires higher doses than most other reptiles
	20-40 mg/kg SC, IM, ICe (sedation), to 40-80 mg/kg (anesthesia)[220]	Crocodilians/induction, <30-60 min; recovery, hours to days; in larger animals, 12-15 mg/kg may permit tracheal intubation;[341] not recommended alone in Nile crocodiles[211]
	20-100 mg/kg IM[218]	Crocodilians/lower dose for sedation, higher for anesthesia (requires intermittent positive pressure ventilation for hours)
Ketamine (K)/ butorphanol (B)	See (K) dosages + (B) ≤1.5 mg/kg IM[341]	Snakes/anesthesia with improved muscle relaxation
	(K) 10-30 mg/kg + (B) 0.5-1.5 mg/kg IM[341]	Chelonians/minor surgical procedures (i.e., shell repair)
Ketamine (K)/ dexmedetomidine (De)	(K) 5-7 mg/kg + (De) 0.025-0.07 mg/kg IV[166]	Red-eared slider turtles, Eastern painted turtles, yellow-spotted Amazon river turtles, other undocumented turtle species/anesthetic induction
	(K) 10 mg/kg + (De) 0.05 mg/kg IM, IV[311,312]	Desert tortoises/premedication
Ketamine (K)/ diazepam (D)	See (K) dosages + (D) 0.2-0.8 mg/kg IM[341]	Snakes/anesthesia with improved muscle relaxation
	(K) 60-80 mg/kg[269] + (D) 0.2-1 mg/kg IM[341]	Chelonians/anesthesia; muscle relaxation
Ketamine (K)/ medetomidine (M)[a]	—	Medetomidine is no longer commercially available, but can be compounded;[a] reverse medetomidine with atipamezole
	(K) 10 mg/kg + (M) 0.1-0.3 mg/kg IM[80]	Most species
	(K) 5-10 mg/kg + (M) 0.1-0.15 mg/kg IM, IV[141]	Lizards (iguanas)
	(K) 3-8 mg/kg + (M) 0.025-0.08 mg/kg IV[222]	Giant tortoises (Aldabra)
	(K) 4 mg/kg + (M) 0.04 mg/kg IM[144]	Green sea turtles
	(K) 4-10 mg/kg + (M) 0.04-0.14 mg/kg IM[94]	Chelonians/sedation and muscle relaxation for shell repair
	(K) 5 mg/kg + (M) 0.05 mg/kg IV[51]	Loggerhead sea turtles/induction of anesthesia for intubation
	(K) 5 mg/kg + (M) 0.05 mg/kg IM[291]	Tortoises (gopher)/light anesthesia; tracheal intubation; inconsistent results
	(K) 5-10 mg/kg IM + (M) 0.1-0.15 mg/kg IM, IV[141]	Tortoises (small-medium)
	(K) 7.5 mg/kg + (M) 0.075 mg/kg IM[291]	Tortoises (gopher)/anesthesia; tracheal intubation

TABLE 4-5 Chemical Restraint/Anesthetic Agents Used in Reptiles. (cont'd)

Agent	Dosage	Species/Comments
Ketamine (K)/ medetomidine (M)[a] (cont'd)	(K) 10 mg/kg + (M) 0.1 mg/kg IM[200]	Hybrid Galapagos tortoises/sedation
	(K) 10-20 mg/kg IM + (M) 0.15-0.3 mg/kg IM, IV[141]	Turtles (fresh water)
	(K) 5-10 mg/kg + (M) 0.1-0.15 mg/kg IM[143]	Alligators/adults
	(K) 10-15 mg/kg + (M) 0.15-0.25 mg/kg IM[143]	Alligators/juveniles
Ketamine (K)/medetomidine (Me)/midazolam (Mi)	(K) 5 mg/kg + (Me) 0.15 mg/kg + (Mi) 1 mg/kg SC[243]	Leopard tortoises/deep sedation
Ketamine (K)/medetomidine (Me)/morphine (Mo)	(K) 2.5 mg/kg + (Me) 0.15 mg/kg + (Mo) 1 mg/kg SC[244]	African spurred tortoises/deep sedation and analgesia
Ketamine (K)/midazolam (Mi)	(K) 20 mg/kg + (Mi) 2 mg/kg IM, (K) 60 mg/kg + (Mi) 2 mg/kg IM[7]	Giant Amazon river turtles/sedation with both combinations; more rapid and prolonged sedation with higher K dosage
	(K) 20-40 mg/kg + (Mi) ≤2 mg/kg IM[30]	Chelonians/sedation; muscle relaxation
	(K) 60-80 mg/kg[269] + (Mi) ≤2 mg/kg IM[341]	Chelonians/anesthesia; muscle relaxation
Ketamine (K)/propofol (P)	(K) 25-30 mg/kg IM[269] + (P) 7 mg/kg IV[313]	Chelonians/administer propofol ≈ 70-80 min post-ketamine; see propofol
Ketamine (K)/xylazine (X)	(K) 30 mg/kg + (X) 1 mg/kg IM[47]	Broad-snouted caiman juveniles/provided mild sedation after either forelimb or hind limb administration
Lidocaine (0.5%-2%)	Local or topical[341]	Most species/local analgesia; infiltrate to effect (e.g., 0.01 mL 2% lidocaine used for local block for IO catheter placement in iguanas);[21] often used in conjunction with chemical immobilization
	0.158 mg/cm intrathecal (combined with epinephrine hemitartrate)[333]	Green iguana/spinal anesthesia
	2 mg/kg intrathecal (IT)[240]	Turtles and toroises/surgical analgesia/anesthesia of caudal body
	0.038 mL/kg (1 mL/20-25 kg)[324]	Hybrid Galapagos tortoises/surgical analgesia/anesthesia for phallectomy
Medetomidine[a]	—	Medetomidine is no longer commercially available, but can be compounded;[a] reverse with atipamezole; produces poor immobilization alone; see ketamine and butorphanol for combinations
	0.1-0.15 mg/kg IM[23]	Most species
	0.06-0.15 mg/kg[342]	Lizards
	0.15 mg/kg IM[354,355]	Desert tortoises, crocodilians/sedation; incomplete immobilization; generally produces bradycardia and bradypnea

Continued

TABLE 4-5 Chemical Restraint/Anesthetic Agents Used in Reptiles. (cont'd)

Agent	Dosage	Species/Comments
Medetomidine[a] (cont'd)	0.04-0.15 mg/kg IM[218]	Crocodilians/need to reverse
	0.13-0.17 mg/kg IM[294,295]	Crocodilians/moderate sedation/atipamezole (0.1 mg/kg IM) for reversal
	0.5-0.75 mg/kg IM[294,295]	Crocodilians/sedation only when administered in thoracic limb (versus pelvic limb and tail), with atipamezole (2.5 mg/kg) reversal
Meperidine (Mp)/Midazolam (Mi)	(Mp) 1 mg/kg + (Mi) 1 mg/kg IM[17]	Green sea turtles/premedication
Methohexital (Brevital, Lilly)	—	Recovery time of red-sided garter snakes at 21°C (70°F), 125 min; 26°C (79°F), 86 min; 31°C (88°F), 64 min; thinner snakes had longer recovery times; if within 5 wk of parturition, mean recovery time 2× as long as nongravid; time postfeeding had no effect at 1, 3, 10 days[309]
	5-20 mg/kg SC,[20] IV[104]	Most species/induction, 5-30 min; recovery, 1-5 hr; use at 0.125%-0.5% concentration; much species variability; decrease dose 20%-30% for young animals; avoid use in debilitated animals
	9-10 mg/kg SC,[287] ICe	Colubrids/induction, ≥22 min; recovery, 2-5 hr; does not produce soft-tissue irritation seen with other barbiturates; may need to adjust dosage in obese snakes
Metomidate	10 mg/kg IM[80,334]	Snakes/profound sedation; not available in the United States
Midazolam	—	See butorphanol, ketamine for combinations; can be reversed by flumazenil
	0.1-1 mg/kg[12]	Multiple species/mild to moderate sedation
	2 mg/kg IM[19,20]	Most species/preanesthetic; increases the efficacy of ketamine; effective in snapping turtles, not in painted turtles[20]
	0.5-2 mg/kg[342]	Lizards
	1.5 mg/kg IM[298]	Turtles (red-eared sliders)/sedation; onset, 5.5 min; duration, 82 min; recovery, 40 min; much individual variability
	2-3 mg/kg IV[137]	Hatchling leatherback sea turtles/sedation
Naloxone	0.04-2 mg/kg SC[350,353]	Corn snakes, bearded dragons, red-eared sliders/μ-opioid agonist reversal
	4 mg/kg IM[112]	Green tree monitors/reversal of butorphanol

TABLE 4-5 Chemical Restraint/Anesthetic Agents Used in Reptiles. (cont'd)

Agent	Dosage	Species/Comments
Neostigmine	0.03-0.25 mg/kg IM[221] 0.063 mg/kg IV[221] 0.07-0.14 mg/kg IM[276]	Crocodiles/gallamine reversal; may cause emesis and lacrimation; fast 24-48 hr before use; effects enhanced if combined with 75 mg hyaluronidase per dose when administered SC, IM[221]
Pentobarbital	—	Rarely used as an anesthetic agent in reptiles
	15-30 mg/kg ICe[269]	Snakes/induction, 30-60 min; duration, ≥ 2 hr; prolonged recovery (risk of occasional fatalities); venomous snakes require twice as much as nonvenomous snakes;[19] avoid use in lizards
	10-18 mg/kg ICe[269]	Chelonians
	7.5-15 mg/kg ICe, or 8 mg/kg IM[19,269]	Crocodilians
Propofol	—	If administered in supravertebral sinus, be aware for potential submeningeal delivery;[314] see ketamine for combination; anesthesia; rapid, smooth induction; may give 15-25 min anesthesia and restraint in most species; rapid, excitement-free recovery; must be administered IV (slowly; no inflammation if goes perivascularly); may be administered IO; dosages may be reduced by as much as 50% in premedicated (e.g., ketamine) animals; may cause apnea and bradycardia; intubation and assisted ventilation generally required; considered by many to be parenteral agent of choice for inducing anesthesia
	0.3-0.5 mg/kg/min IV, IO constant rate infusion, or 0.5-1 mg/kg IV, IO periodic bolus[344]	Most species/maintenance anesthesia; must provide respiratory and thermal support
	5-10 mg/kg IV, intracardiac[10,334]	Snakes
	10 mg/kg intracardiac[262]	Ball pythons/anesthetic induction for isoflurane maintenance, but prolonged recovery; mild, resolving cardiac lesions
	15 mg/kg IV[28]	South American rattlesnakes/anesthetic induction
	3-5 mg/kg IV, IO[140,141]	Lizards (iguanas)/intubation and minor diagnostic procedures; may need to give an additional dose in 3-5 min; less cardiopulmonary depression than with higher doses
	5-10 mg/kg IV, IO[25]	Iguanas/higher dose is recommended for induction for short-duration procedures or intubation

Continued

TABLE 4-5 Chemical Restraint/Anesthetic Agents Used in Reptiles. (cont'd)

Agent	Dosage	Species/Comments
Propofol (cont'd)	10 mg/kg IV, IO[25,80,282]	Lizards, snakes/0.25 mg/kg/min may be given for maintenance;[117] green iguanas/anesthetic induction[282]
	2 mg/kg IV[23]	Giant tortoises
	3-5 mg/kg IV supravertebral sinus[94]	Chelonians/sedation (i.e., shell repair)
	5 mg/kg IV[125]	Snapping turtles/anesthetic induction
	10 mg/kg IV (supravertebral sinus)[406]	Red-eared sliders/40-85 min anesthesia
	12-15 mg/kg IV[77,365]	Chelonians/lower dosages (5-10 mg/kg IV[341]) may be used; 1 mg/kg/min may be given for maintenance[341]
	20 mg/kg IV (supravertebral sinus)[406]	Red-eared sliders/60-120 min anesthesia
	10-15 mg/kg IV[220]	Crocodilians/duration, 0.5-1.5 hr; maintain on gas anesthetics; experimental IM with hyaluronidase
Rocuronium (Zemuron, Organon)	0.25-0.5 mg/kg IM[185]	Box turtles/neuromuscular blocking agent; no analgesia; for intubation only and small, nonpainful procedures
Sevoflurane	To effect[16,326]	Most species/anesthesia; rapid induction and recovery when intubated
Succinylcholine	—	No analgesia; narrow margin of safety; generally not recommended, but included for completeness; intermittent positive pressure ventilation generally required; paralysis occurs in 5-30 min; avoid if exposed to organophosphate parasiticides within last 30 days; administer minimal amount required to perform procedure
	0.25-1 mg/kg IM[173]	Most species
	0.75-1 mg/kg IM[34]	Large lizards
	0.25-1.5 mg/kg IM[303]	Chelonians/induction, 15-30 min; recovery, 45-90 min; facilitates intubation
	0.5-1 mg/kg IM[35]	Box turtles/induction, 20-30 min
	0.25 mg/kg IM[211]	Crocodilians
	0.4-1 mg/kg IM[303]	Alligators/rapid onset; 3-5 mg/kg in smaller animals have been used
	0.5-5 mg/kg IM[20,218]	Crocodilians/variable induction and recovery periods
Thiopental	19-31 mg/kg IV[399]	Green sea turtles/anesthesia; induction, 5-10 min; recovery, <6 hr; erratic anesthesia
Tiletamine/ zolazepam (Telazol, Fort Dodge)	—	Sedation, anesthesia; severe respiratory depression possible (may need to ventilate);[38] variable results; may have prolonged recovery; use lower end of dose range in heavier species; good for muscle relaxation prior to intubation;[96,319] other anesthetic agents may be preferable

TABLE 4-5 Chemical Restraint/Anesthetic Agents Used in Reptiles. (cont'd)

Agent	Dosage	Species/Comments
Tiletamine/ zolazepam (Telazol, Fort Dodge) (cont'd)	4-5 mg/kg SC, IM[20]	Most species/sedation; induction, 9-15 min; recovery, 1-12 h; adequate for most noninvasive procedures
	5-10 mg/kg IM[23]	Most species
	3 mg/kg IM[141]	Snakes/facilitates handling and intubation of large snakes; induction, 30-45 min; prolongs recovery
	3-5 mg/kg IM[272]	Snakes, lizards/sedation
	10-30 mg/kg IM[269] to 20-40 mg/kg IM[173,339]	Snakes, lizards/induction, 8-20 min; recovery, 2-10 hr; variable results; longer sedation and recovery times at 22°C (72°F) than at 30°C (86°F);[368] good sedation in boa constrictors at 25 mg/kg IM;[368] generally need to supplement with inhalation agents for surgical anesthesia; some snakes died at 55 mg/kg
	3.5-14 mg/kg IM[269] (generally 4-8 mg/kg)	Chelonians/sedation; induction, 8-20 min; does not produce satisfactory anesthesia even at 88 mg/kg[303]
	5-10 mg/kg IM, IV[341]	Large tortoises/facilitates intubation; if light, mask with isoflurane rather than redosing
	1-2 mg/kg IM[218]	Crocodilians/recovery takes several hours
	2-10 mg/kg IM[341]	Large crocodilians/may permit intubation
	5-10 mg/kg SC, IM, ICe (sedation), 10-40 mg/kg (anesthesia)[220]	Crocodilians
	15 mg/kg IM[57]	Alligators/induction, >20 min; adequate for minor procedures
Xylazine	—	Infrequently used; variable effects; potentially reversible with yohimbine; preanesthetic for ketamine; see ketamine for combination
	0.1-1.25 mg/kg IM, IV[104]	Most species
	0.1-1 mg/kg IM[218]	Crocodilians/atipamezole better reversal than yohimbine
	1-2 mg/kg IM[220,303]	Nile crocodiles
Yohimbine (Yobine, Lloyd)	—	Xylazine reversal; rarely indicated; atipameazole commonly used to reverse all α_2 agonists

[a]Medetomidine is no longer commercially available although it can be obtained from select compounding services; dosages are listed here as a guide for possible use with dexmedetomidine, an α_2 agonist that is the active optical enantiomer of racemic compound medetomidine; dexmedetomidine is generally used at ½ the dose of medetomidine but the same volume due to higher concentration; both compounds tend to have similar effects.

TABLE 4-6 Analgesic Agents Used in Reptiles.

Agent	Dosage	Species/Comments
Bupivacaine	1-2 mg/kg local q4-12h prn[344]	Most species/local anesthesia; 4 mg/kg maximum dose
	1 mg/kg intrathecal[240]	Turtles, tortoises/regional analgesia/anesthesia
Buprenorphine	0.2 mg/kg SC[246]	No evidence of analgesic efficacy in red-eared slider turtles or other reptile species
Butorphanol	—	Recent studies call into question use of particular doses or of this drug in general in providing analgesia in reptiles, including red-eared sliders, ball pythons, corn snakes, bearded dragons, and green iguanas; respiratory depression is a common side effect[338,351,353]
	0.4-1 mg/kg SC, IM[341]	Most species; sedation; preanesthetic; 0.2 mg/kg IM used experimentally in tortoises[115]
	1 mg/kg IM[97]	Green iguanas/ineffective for analgesia; presence of observer may affect iguana response
	20 mg/kg SC[190]	Red-eared slider turtles/ineffective for surgical analgesia
Carprofen	1-4 mg/kg PO, SC, IM, IV q24h,[217] follow with half the dose q24-72h[259]	Most species/nonsteroidal antiinflammatory; no efficacy data in any reptile species
Etodolac	5 mg/kg PO q72h × 30 days[301]	Komodo dragons
Fentanyl	12.5 µg/hr transdermal patch to cranial epaxial muscles[188]	Ball pythons/high plasma concentrations (above analgesic threshold in mammals); analgesic efficacy not proven in any snake species, but anecdotal evidence from certain snake clinical cases demonstrated improved condition after application of patch
	12.5 µg/hr transdermal patch to caudodorsal lumbar region[109]	Prehensile-tailed skinks/no side effects reported after 24 hr when skink blood levels reached human therapeutic levels; environmental temperature can significantly affect absorption
Flunixin meglumine	0.1-0.5 mg/kg IM q12-24h[217]	Most species/nonsteroidal antiinflammatory; use for maximum of 3 days; no evidence of efficacy
	0.5-2 mg/kg IM q12-24h[344]	Most species/nonsteroidal antiinflammatory; no evidence of efficacy
	1-2 mg/kg IM q24h × 2 treatments[37,360]	Lizards/postsurgical nonsteroidal antiinflammatory; no evidence of efficacy
Hydromorphone	0.5-1 mg/kg SC[246]	Red-eared sliders/analgesic efficacy
Ketoprofen	—	Nonsteroidal antiinflammatory
	2 mg/kg PO, SC, IM q24-48h[225,381]	Most species/green iguanas/PK study;[381] loggerhead sea turtles/frequently used due to historical evidence of safety;[225] no efficacy data
Lidocaine (0.5%-2%)	2-5 mg/kg local[344]	Most species/10 mg/kg maximum dosage
	Local or topical[341]	Most species/local analgesia; infiltrate to effect (e.g., 0.01 mL 2% lidocaine used for local block for IO catheter placement in iguanas);[21] often used in conjunction with chemical immobilization
	4 mg/kg intrathecal[240]	Turtles, tortoises/regional analgesia

TABLE 4-6   Analgesic Agents Used in Reptiles. (cont'd)

Agent	Dosage	Species/Comments
Lidocaine (L)/ morphine (Mo)	2 mg/kg (L) + 0.1 mg/kg (Mo) intrathecal[312]	Desert tortoises/orchiectomy analgesia
Meloxicam	0.1-0.5 mg/kg PO, SC q24-48h[175-177]	Most species
	0.3 mg/kg IM[293]	Ball pythons/physiologic changes not consistent with analgesia
	0.2 mg/kg PO, IV q24h[82]	Green iguanas/PD; no evidence of efficacy
	0.1 mg/kg IM, IV[209]	Loggerhead sea turtles/PK; plasma concentrations not consistent with analgesia
	0.1-0.2 mg/kg PO, IM q24h × 4-10 days[94]	Chelonians; no evidence of efficacy
	0.2 mg/kg IM, IV;[382] SC[311,312]	Red-eared slider turtles/PK; plasma concentrations consistent with therapeutic efficacy for 48 hr by IM and IV administration routes;[382] Mojave desert tortoises, postsurgical nonsteroidal antiinflammatory[311,312]
	0.2-0.4 mg/kg IM[166]	Red-eared slider turtles, Eastern painted turtles, yellow-spotted Amazon river turtles, other undocumented turtle species/nonsteroidal antiinflammatory; no evidence of efficacy
	0.5 mg/kg PO, IM, or 0.22 mg/kg IV[325]	Red-eared sliders/PK; found better absorption IM vs PO;[325] after IV administration, plasma levels decreased rapidly and the elimination half-life was 7.57 hr
Meperidine	5-10 mg/kg IM q12-24h[139]	Most species/analgesia; no noticeable effect in snakes even at 200 mg/kg
	20 mg/kg IM q12-24h[217]	Most species/analgesia
	2-4 mg/kg ICe q6-8h[175]	Lizards
	1-5 mg/kg IM[184,351,386]	Turtles, crocodiles/analgesic efficacy of short duration
	2-4 mg/kg ICe[4]	Nile crocodiles/analgesia
Methadone	3-5 mg/kg SC, IM[63,351]	Aquatic turtles/analgesia
Morphine	—	No effective dose for analgesia documented in corn snakes[353]
	10 mg/kg IM[353,394]	Bearded dragons/analgesia; ball pythons/no analgesia
	1.5-6.5 mg/kg SC, IM[90,350,351,353]	Red-eared sliders (long lasting respiratory depression), freshwater crocodiles, Anolis lizards/ may be effective thermal analgesia
	0.1-0.2 mg/kg intrathecal[240]	Turtles, tortoises/thermal analgesia for 48 hr; regional analgesia caudal body
	2 mg/kg SC[190]	Red-eared slider turtles/surgical analgesia
	1 mg/kg IM[166]	Red-eared slider turtles, Eastern painted turtle, yellow-spotted Amazon river turtle, other undocumented turtle species/analgesia
	0.5-4 mg/kg ICe[355]	Crocodilians/analgesia

Continued

TABLE 4-6 Analgesic Agents Used in Reptiles. (cont'd)

Agent	Dosage	Species/Comments
Naloxone	0.04-2 mg/kg SC[350a,350,353]	Red-eared sliders, bearded dragons, corn snakes/ μ-opioid agonist reversal
Oxymorphone	0.025-0.1 mg/kg IV[104] 0.05-0.2 mg/kg SC, IM q12-48h[139] 0.5-1.5 mg/kg IM[104]	Anecdotal evidence of analgesia in some lizard and turtle species; no efficacy or PK/PD studies; avoid in cases with hepatic or renal dysfunction; no observable effects in snakes even at 1.5 mg/kg
Pethidine	—	See meperidine
Prednisolone	2-5 mg/kg PO, IM[217]	Most species/antiinflammatory
Proparacaine (0.5%)	Topical to eye[126,229,331,345]	Iguanas/desensitizes surface of eye; ineffective in animals with spectacles; bearded dragons/IOP by rebound tonometry;[345] Kemp's ridley sea turtles/ one drop provided 45 min duration of action;[126] do not exceed toxic dose 2 mg/kg;[117] Yacare caiman/ IOP by applanation tonometry[331]
Tapentadol	10 mg/kg IM[121,122]	Red-eared and yellow-bellied slider turtles/ analgesia
Tramadol	11 mg/kg PO[128]	Bearded dragons
	5-10 mg/kg PO, SC[14]	Red-eared slider turtles, sea turtles/thermal analgesia, higher doses may affect ventilation
	5-10 mg/kg PO[289]	Loggerhead sea turtles/PK; plasma concentrations consistent with efficacy for 48 hr (5 mg/kg PO) or 72 hr (10 mg/kg PO)
	10 mg/kg PO[356]	Turtles, tortoises/analgesia
	10 mg/kg IM[124]	Yellow-bellied slider turtles/PK/PD comparing forelimb and hind limb administration; analgesia; plasma concentrations consistent with analgesia in both forelimb and hind limb

TABLE 4-7 Hormones and Steroids Used in Reptiles.

Agent	Dosage	Species/Comments
Arginine vasotocin (AVT) (Sigma Chemical)	0.01-1 μg/kg IV (preferred), ICe[219] q12-24h × several treatments	Most species/dystocias; administer 30-60 min after Ca lactate/Ca glycerophosphate; more effective in reptiles than oxytocin but not commercially available for use in animals; higher doses have been reported; 0.5 μg/kg commonly recommended
Calcitonin	1.5 U/kg SC q8h × 14-21 days prn[104] 50 U/kg IM, repeat in 14 days[22,117]	Most species (e.g., iguanas)/severe nutritional secondary hyperparathyroidism; administer after Ca supplementation; do not give if hypocalcemic
	50 U/kg q7d × 2-3 doses[226,230]	Green iguanas/salmon calcitonin; do not give if hypocalcemic

TABLE 4-7　Hormones and Steroids Used in Reptiles. (cont'd)

Agent	Dosage	Species/Comments
Deslorelin acetate	—	No success with use in female reptile reproductive issues
	4.75 mg implant SC[330]	Bearded dragons/abnormal aggression in juveniles; decreased serum testosterone, behavior ceased
Dexamethasone	0.2 mg/kg IM, IV[343]	Most species/laryngeal or pharyngeal edema and inflammation
	0.6-1.25 mg/kg IM, IV[104]	Most species/shock (septic/traumatic)
	0.3-1.5 mg/kg IM, IV, IO[177]	Chelonians/hyperthermia
Dexamethasone sodium phosphate	0.1-0.25 mg/kg SC, IM, IV[117]	Most species/shock (septic/traumatic)
Insulin	1-5 U/kg IM, ICe q24-72h[362]	Snakes, chelonians/doses are empirical and must be adjusted based on response to therapy and serial blood glucose; doses administered ICe may take 24-48 hr before a response is noted
	5-10 U/kg IM, ICe q24-72h[362]	Lizards, crocodilians/see above
Leuprolide acetate (Lupron Depot 1.875 mg/mL, Abbott)	0.4 mg/kg IM[192]	Iguanas/did not suppress testosterone levels in males
Levothyroxine	0.02 mg/kg PO q48h[132]	Geckos/post-thyroidectomy, lifetime management
	0.02 mg/kg PO q48h[290]	Tortoises/hypothyroidism; stimulates feeding in debilitated tortoises
	0.025 mg/kg q24h in AM[101]	Tortoises/monitor T_4 levels
Methylprednisolone	1 mg/kg IV q24h[177]	Chelonians/ivermectin toxicity
Nandrolone (Deca-Durabolin, Orgamon)	0.5-5 mg/kg IM q7-28d[149]	Most species/hepatic lipidosis
	1 mg/kg IM q7-28d[78]	Lizards/anabolic steroid; reduces protein catabolism; may stimulate erythropoiesis
Oxytocin	—	Dystocias; results are variable; works well in chelonians, less so in snakes and lizards; generally administer 1 hr after Ca administration; use multiple doses with caution
	1-10 U/kg IM[90,117]	Most species/higher end of the range is commonly used; may be repeated up to 3 treatments at 90 min intervals with increasing dosage[164]
	2 U/kg IM q4-6h × 1-3 treatments[11]	Most species
	1-5 U/kg IM,[76] repeat in 1 hr	Lizards/alternatively, 5 U/kg by slow IV or IO over 4-8 hr[76]
	1-2,[36] 2-20,[254] or 10-20[35] U/kg IM	Chelonians
	1-20 U/kg IM q90min × 3 treatments at increased doses, or 50%-100% first dose 1-12 hr later, or IO drip[373]	Chelonians
	2 U/kg IV q2h[74]	Red-eared sliders/faster onset vs IM; fewer animals required second or third doses vs IM route

Continued

TABLE 4-7 Hormones and Steroids Used in Reptiles. (cont'd)

Agent	Dosage	Species/Comments
Prednisolone	2-5 mg/kg PO, IM[217]	Most species/analgesia (chronic pain)
	0.5 mg/kg q24h × 14 days, then q48h until PCV stable[175]	Lizards/autoimmune hemolytic anemia
Prednisolone Na succinate (Solu-Delta Cortef, Pharmacia and Upjohn)	5-10 mg/kg IM, IV,[95] IO[78]	Most species/shock; brain swelling from hyperthermia; may help reduce nephrocalcinosis
Prednisone	0.5-1 mg/kg PO, SC, IM, IV[253]	Most species/lymphoma, leukemia, myeloproliferative disease
	0.8 mg/kg q48h[112]	Most species/chronic T-lymphocytic leukemia; may combine with chlorambucil, but need to monitor uric acid levels
Stanozolol (Winstrol-V, Winthrop)	5 mg/kg IM q7d prn[117]	Most species/anabolic steroid; management of catabolic disease states

TABLE 4-8 Nutritional/Mineral/Fluid Support Used in Reptiles.[a]

Agent	Dosage	Species/Comments
Calcium	PO prn[84]	Most species/dietary sources include crushed cuttlebone, oyster shell, egg shell, tablets of Ca salts, or other commercially available products
Calcium carbonate (Rep-Cal, Rep-Cal Labs; Repti Calcium, Zoo Med; Fluker's powdered or liquid forms of calcium)	PO prn[84]	Omnivores, herbivores, insectivores/dietary Ca supplement
Calcium glubionate (Neo-Calglucon, Sandoz; Calciquid, Breckenridge Pharmaceuticals; Calcionate, Rugby)	10 mg/kg PO q12-24h prn[107]	All species/nutritional secondary hyperparathyroidism
	25-50 mg/kg PO q24h prn[242]	All species/nutritional secondary hyperparathyroidism
	360 mg/kg (1 mL/kg) PO q12-24h prn[22,38]	Most species/nutritional secondary hyperparathyroidism; hypocalcemia; dystocia; ensure adequate UVB exposure and proper nutrition
Calcium gluconate	50-100 mg/kg SC, IM, IV[242]	Most species/hypocalcemia (low ionized Ca); hypocalcemic muscle tremors, seizures, dystocia, or flaccid paresis in lizards; when patient is stable, switch to oral Ca; should be diluted in fluids

TABLE 4-8 Nutritional/Mineral/Fluid Support Used in Reptiles. (cont'd)

Agent	Dosage	Species/Comments
Calcium gluconate (cont'd)	100 mg/kg SC, IM, ICe[234,259] q6-24h[22,38]	Most species/hypocalcemia (low ionized Ca); hypocalcemic muscle tremors, seizures, dystocia, or flaccid paresis in lizards; when patient is stable, switch to oral Ca
Calcium gluconate/ borogluconate	10-50 mg/kg SC, IM[107]	Most species/hypocalcemia; hypocalcemic dystocia
Calcium glycerophosphate/ calcium lactate (Calphosan, Glenwood)	1-5 mg/kg SC, IM[107]	Most species/hypocalcemia; hypocalcemic dystocia
	10 mg/kg SC, IM, ICe q24h × 1-7 days[16,22]	Lizards (iguanas)/hypocalcemia
Carnivore Care (Oxbow Animal Health)	10-20 mL/kg PO or via gavage/ esophagostomy q24-48h[115]	Carnivores/short-term nutritional support; anorexia; prepare according to directions; begin after rehydration and stable condition; more dilute in first feeding after anorexia, gradually increase concentration over 3-5 days
	30 mL/kg (3% of body weight) PO or via gavage/esophagostomy q24h;[71] range of 2%-10% body weight PO or via gavage/ esophagostomy q24h[242]	Carnivores
Clinicare—feline and canine (Abbott Animal Health)	Gavage prn[401]	Most species/post-omphalectomy; use canine formula for herbivores and omnivores, and feline formula for carnivores; initially dilute 1:1 with water and gradually increase to full strength over 48 hr; generally precede nutritional supplementation with 48-96 hr of water or electrolyte solution PO
Critical Care for Herbivores (Oxbow Animal Health)	10-20 mL/kg PO or via gavage/ esophagostomy q24-48h[115]	Herbivores/long-term nutritional support; prepare according to directions; begin after rehydration and stable condition
	30 mL/kg (3% of body weight) PO or via gavage/esophagostomy q24h;[71] range of 2%-10% body weight PO or via gavage/ esophagostomy q24h[242]	Herbivores
Dextrose in water (2.5%, 5%)	PO, SC, IV, IO, ICe, EpiCe, prn[191]	All species/hyperkalemia;[191] can mix with electrolye solutions
	Calculated water deficit IV, IO[232]	Most species/for intracellular rehydration when mentation is altered and plasma Na >160 mEq/L; for acute Na toxicosis replace deficit in 12-24 hr; for chronic dehydration slowly replace deficit over 48-72 hr

Continued

TABLE 4-8 Nutritional/Mineral/Fluid Support Used in Reptiles. (cont'd)

Agent	Dosage	Species/Comments
Electrolyte solutions (Pedialyte, Abbott; Gatorade, S-VC, Inc.)	Voluntary drinking (whole body soak)[115]	All species/oral fluid therapy; early treatment of anorexia; dilute 1:1 with water; caution against drowning
	10-20 mL/kg via gavage or esophagostomy tube q24h[115]	All species/rehydration; when stable; first stage in supplemental nutrition
Emeraid Exotic Carnivore (Lafeber)	5-30 mL/kg gavage or esophagostomy tube q24-72h[117]	Carnivores/nutritional support, severely debilitated, cachectic patients; prepare according to directions; use when hydrated and stable condition; greater dilution in first few feedings
	3% body weight PO or via gavage/esophagostomy q24h;[71] range of 2%-10% body weight PO or via gavage/esophagostomy q24h[242]	Carnivores
Emeraid Herbivore (Lafeber)	5-20 mL/kg gavage or esophagostomy tube q12-48h[117]	Herbivores/nutritional support, severely debilitated, cachectic patients; prepare according to directions; use when hydrated and stable condition; greater dilution in first few feedings
	3% body weight PO or via gavage/esophagostomy q24h;[71] range of 2%-10% body weight PO or via gavage/esophagostomy q24h[242]	Herbivores
Emeraid Omnivore (Lafeber)	5-20 mL/kg gavage or esophagostomy tube q12-48h[115]	Most species/nutritional support, severely debilitated, cachectic patients; prepare according to directions; use when hydrated and stable condition; greater dilution in first few feedings
	3% body weight PO or via gavage/esophagostomy q24h;[71] range of 2%-10% body weight PO or via gavage/esophagostomy q24h[242]	Omnivores
Hydroxyethyl starch (Hetastarch, HES)	3-5 mL/kg slow IV or IO bolus prn[115,232]	All species/hypoalbuminemia; hypovolemic perfusion deficits; increased capillary permeability; use with crystalloids; reduce crystalloid volume 40%-60%; max volume 20 mL/kg[390]
Iodine	2-4 mg/kg PO q24h × 14-21 days, then q7d[117]	Herbivores/iodine deficiency (i.e., goiter); use in species fed a goitrogenic diet; can use a multivitamin-mineral mixture or iodized salt; suggested daily dietary iodine 0.03 mg/kg BW[84]

TABLE 4-8 Nutritional/Mineral/Fluid Support Used in Reptiles. (cont'd)

Agent	Dosage	Species/Comments
Iron dextran	12 mg/kg IM 1-2×/wk ×45 days[371]	Crocodilians/iron deficiency; in other species for anemia[117]
Lactated Ringer's solution (LRS)	15-40 mL/kg SC, IV, IO prn[232]	Land turtles/fluid replacement; use extracoelomically after warming the patient; avoid lactate if hepatic insufficiency
LRS + 0.9% saline (1:1 solution)	20 mL/kg/day ICe[46]	Loggerhead sea turtles/highest percentage of acid-base recovery and electrolyte balance compared to LRS, saline, or 5% dextrose in saline (1:1)
Maintenance crystalloid solution: ½-strength LRS and 2.5% dextrose	SC, IV, IO, ICe, EpiCe, prn[232]	All species/maintenance fluid therapy after losses have been replaced
Metronidazole	12.5-50 mg/kg PO[103]	Most species/appetite stimulant (anecdotal; presumably associated with antiprotozoal activity)
	50-100 mg/kg PO[174]	Chameleons/appetite stimulant (anecdotal; presumably associated with antiprotozoal activity)
Multivitamin Products (ReptiVite, Zoo Med; Herptivite, RepCal; Repta-Vitamin, Fluker's; Exo-Terra; Nekton)	Dust on vegetables, fruits, or insects q84-168h[358]	Herbivores, omnivores, insectivores/preformed vitamin A; minerals; multivitamin
Polymerized bovine hemoglobin (Oxyglobin, OPK Biotech)	3-5 mL/kg slow IV or IO bolus prn[115,232]	All species/hemoglobin polymer; hypoalbuminemia; hemorrhage; severe anemia; hypovolemic perfusion deficits; increased capillary permeability; use with crystalloids; reduce crystalloid volume 40%-60%; max volume 20 mL/kg;[390] currently under FDA testing by a new manufacturer and unavailable
Replacement crystalloid solutions (Normosol-R, Ceva; Plasma-Lyte, Baxter)	15-25 mL/kg/d PO, SC, IV, IO, ICe, EpiCe prn[37]	All species/replacement fluid therapy; warm to 29°C (84°F)[232]
	10-30 mL/kg q24h, or divided into 2-3 boluses several hours apart[191]	All species/ongoing regurgitation or severe diarrhea
Ringer's solution for reptiles: 1 part Normosol-R + 2 parts 2.5% dextrose in 0.45% saline[141] or, 1 part Normosol-R + 1 part 5% dextrose + 1 part 0.9% saline	10-20 mL/kg q24h[117]	All species/hypertonic dehydration or to prevent nephrotoxicity due to aminoglycosides
	15 (large reptiles) to 25 (small reptiles) mL/kg q24h, or divided into 2 doses per day[37]	All species/hypertonic dehydration; warm fluids to 28°C (82°F)
	20 mL/kg q12h[38]	Chelonians/severe dehydration
Selenium	0.028 mg/kg IM[16]	Lizards/deficiency; myopathy
Sodium chloride (0.45%)	PO, SC, IV, IO, ICe, EpiCe, prn[191]	All species/hypertonic dehydration; correct deficits over 3 days

Continued

TABLE 4-8 Nutritional/Mineral/Fluid Support Used in Reptiles. (cont'd)

Agent	Dosage	Species/Comments
Sodium chloride (0.9%)	SC, IV, IO, ICe, EpiCe, prn[191,232]	All species/hyperkalemia, hypercalcemia, hypochloremic metabolic alkalosis;[232] can mix with other crystalloid solutions, particularly 5% dextrose; use SC, ICe, EpiCe routes after patient is warm
Vitamin A	—	Overdose causes epidermal sloughing; greater risk with aqueous parenteral formulation; for less severe cases, commercial formulated diets or reptile multivitamin supplements may suffice;[84,270,358] may help infectious stomatitis
	2000 U/kg PO, SC, IM q7-14d × 2-4 treatments[35,38]	Most species/hypovitaminosis A
	2000 U/30 g BW PO once, repeat in 7 days[134,358]	Chameleons/eye swelling, respiratory disease, hemipenile plugs, dysecdysis
	200-300 U/kg[84] SC, IM	Turtles/hypovitaminosis A; give in conjunction with PO vitamin A (2-8 U/g feed DM)
Vitamins A, D_3, E (Vital E + A + D, Stuart Products)	0.15 mL/kg IM, repeat in 21 days[117]	Most species/hypovitaminosis A, D_3, or E; product contains alcohol and may sting when administered; a product without alcohol can be compounded commercially
	0.3 mL/kg PO, then 0.06 mL/kg q7d × 3-4 treatments[35]	Box turtles/hypovitaminosis A; parenteral use may result in hypervitaminosis A and D; given PO may enhance Ca uptake
Vitamin B complex	0.3 mL/kg SC, IM q24h[117]	Most species/anorexia; hypovitaminosis B; use with caution as B_6 toxicity may occur
	25 mg thiamine/kg PO q24h × 3-7 days[11]	Most species/appetite stimulant; hypovitaminosis B
Vitamin B_1 (thiamine)	50-100 mg/kg PO, SC, IM q24h[45]	Piscivores/thiamine deficiency from thawed fish
	30 g/kg feed fish PO[117]	Crocodilians/treat or prevent deficiency
Vitamin B_{12} (cyanocobalamin)	0.05 mg/kg SC, IM[117]	Snakes, lizards/appetite stimulant
Vitamin C	10-20 mg/kg SC, IM q24h[102,264]	All species/empirical for hypovitaminosis C; stomatitis; skin slough in snakes; supportive therapy for bacterial infections

TABLE 4-8 Nutritional/Mineral/Fluid Support Used in Reptiles. (cont'd)

Agent	Dosage	Species/Comments
Vitamin D_3	—	Nutritional secondary hyperparathyroidism; hypocalcemia; deficiency and excess may result in soft-tissue calcification
	1000 U/kg IM, repeat in 1 wk[38]	Most species/deficiency; use with oral calcium glubionate and carbonate, general dietary management, and UVB irradiation
	200 U/kg PO, IM q7d[16,22]	Lizards/PO may be safer than IM, but absorption is poor in some species[27,297]
	400 U/kg IM q7d × 3 treatments[230]	Green iguanas/nutritional secondary hyperparathyroidism; use with calcitonin after normocalcemic; also supplement oral calcium
Vitamin E/selenium (L-Se, Schering)	1 U vitamin E/kg[84] IM	Piscivores/hypovitaminosis E; myopathy, anorexia, swollen subcutaneous nodule
	50 U vitamin E/kg + 0.025 mg selenium/kg IM[89]	Lizards/hypovitaminosis E (vitamin E/selenium)
Vitamin K_1	0.25-0.5 mg/kg IM[117]	Most species/hypovitaminosis K_1; coagulopathies

[a]Also see Table 4-13.

TABLE 4-9 Miscellaneous Agents Used in Reptiles.

Agent	Dosage	Species/Comments
Activated charcoal-kaolin suspension (ToxiBan, Vet-a-Mix)	5-10 mL/kg PO q24h × 1-3 days[236]	Sea turtles/reduce exposure to brevitoxin
Allopurinol	—	Careful when giving with urine acidifiers and uricosuric drugs (probenecid)[66]
	10-20 mg/kg PO q24h[78,254,315]	Most species/gout; decreases production of uric acid;[227] long-term therapy; tortoises may respond best
	25 mg/kg PO q24h[151]	Green iguanas
	50 mg/kg PO q24h × 30 days, then q72h[204]	Chelonians/hyperuricemia
Aluminum hydroxide (Amphogel, Wyeth-Ayerst)	100 mg/kg PO q12-24h[227]	Most species/hyperphosphatemia (associated with renal disease); decreases intestinal absorption of P; use cautiously in patients with gastric outlet obstruction

Continued

TABLE 4-9 Miscellaneous Agents Used in Reptiles. (cont'd)

Agent	Dosage	Species/Comments
Amidotrizoate (Gastrografin, Squibb)	5-7.7 mL/kg PO[239]	Gastrointestinal contrast agent; reported faster transit vs barium; no risk if regurgitation
	7.5 mL/kg PO[267]	Tortoises/gastrointestinal contrast agent; give via gavage; mean transit times: 2.6 hr at 87°F (30.6°C); 6.6 hr at 71°F (21.5°C)
Aminophylline	2-4 mg/kg IM[104]	Most species/bronchodilator
Atropine	0.01-0.04 mg/kg IM, IV q8-24h[266]	Most species/dries up excess mucous secretions with infectious stomatitis
	0.1-0.2 mg/kg IM prn[117]	Most species/organophosphate toxicity
	0.2 mg/kg SC, IM[329]	Most species/respiratory distress associated with excessive secretions
Barium sulfate	5-20 mL/kg PO[48]	Most species/gastrointestinal contrast studies
	25 mL/kg PO, 35% wt:vol concentration[15]	Ball pythons/best gastrointestinal image quality
Bleomycin with high voltage electrical pulses	1 U/cm^3 intralesional, repeat in 33 days[39]	Green sea turtles/fibropapillomas electrochemotherapy; use concurrent local anesthesia
	3.65 mg/kg (1 mg/mL) intralesional, repeat in 2 wk[212]	Yellow-bellied slider turtles/squamous cell carcinoma, post-partial surgical excision
Calcium EDTA	10-40 mg/kg IM q12h[288]	Most species/heavy metal chelation; ensure hydration
Carboplatin	2.5-5 mg/kg IV, intracardiac[253]	Most species/carcinoma, osteosarcoma, mesothelioma, carcinomatosis
Carboplatin 4.6 mg implantable bead (compounded, Wedgewood Pharmacy)	≤10 mg/kg total q3wk intralesional or surgical excision sites[179]	Chameleons/squamous cell carcinoma, carcinoma; cut bead into smaller pieces to avoid overdose
Chlorambucil (Leukeran, Glaxo SmithKline)	0.1-0.2 mg/kg PO[253]	Most species/lymphoma, leukemia, myeloproliferative tumors
CHOP Therapy (Modified)	See original paper for full protocol details[100]	Green iguanas/successful management of lymphoma post-radiation therapy
Cimetidine	4 mg/kg PO, IM q8-12h[117]	Most species/gastric and duodenal ulceration; esophagitis; gastroesophageal reflux; may use in renal failure to increase phosphate secretion
Cisapride (Propulsid, Janssen)	0.5-2 mg/kg PO q24h[117]	Most species/motility modifier; gastrointestinal stasis; not commercially available in the United States; may be compounded; ineffective in desert tortoises at 1 mg/kg[379]
	1-4 mg/kg PO q24h until defecates[387]	Bearded dragons/constipation

TABLE 4-9 Miscellaneous Agents Used in Reptiles. (cont'd)

Agent	Dosage	Species/Comments
Cisplatin	0.5-1 mg/kg IV (prehydrate), intracardiac, intralesional (in oil)[253]	Most species/carcinoma, osteosarcoma, infiltrative sarcoma (intralesional), mesothelioma, carcinomatosis
Cyclophosphamide	10 mg/kg SC, IM, IV, intracardiac[253]	Most species/lymphoma, leukemia, myeloproliferative tumors
Dioctyl Na sulfosuccinate	1-5 mg/kg PO[119]	Most species/constipation; use 1:20 dilution
Diphenhydramine	2 mg/kg IM q24h[236]	Sea turtles/brevitoxicosis; rapidly reduced conjunctival edema, prevented corneal ulceration
Doxorubicin	1 mg/kg IV q7d × 2 treatments, then q14d × 2 treatments, then q21d × 2 treatments[327]	Snakes/chemotherapy for sarcoma (also lymphoma, carcinoma, etc.); treatment periods variable
Famotidine	0.5 mg/kg SC q3d[395]	Kemp's ridley sea turtles
Furosemide	2-5 mg/kg PO, IM, IV q12-24h[175-177]	Most species/diuretic for edema and pulmonary congestion; while lacking loop of Henle, may effect via other mechanisms
	5 mg/kg IM q24h × 1-3 days[236]	Sea turtles/intentional dehydration with brevitoxicosis, no concurrent fluids given
Hydrochlorothiazide	1 mg/kg q24-72h[78]	Lizards/promotes diuresis; monitor hydration status
Iodine compound (Conray 280, Mallinckrodt)	500 mg/kg IV, IO[78]	Lizards/IV urography; take radiographs 0, 5, 15, 30, and 60 min postinjection
Iohexol (240 mg I/mL; Omnipaque, Sanofi Winthrop)	5-20 mL/kg PO[117]	Most species/gastrointestinal contrast studies; nonionic, organic iodine solution; good alternative to barium;[37] faster transit time than barium; can be diluted 1:1 with water
	75 mg/kg IV[187]	Kemp's ridley turtles (juveniles)/GFR assessment
K-Y jelly (Johnson & Johnson)	1-3 mL of 50% K-Y jelly and 50% warm water/100 g[9]	Most species/enema
Lactulose	0.5 mL/kg PO q24h[175,177,361]	Lizards, chelonians/hepatic lipidosis
L-asparaginase (Elspar, Merck)	400 U/kg SC, IM, intracardiac[253]	Most species/lymphoma, leukemia, myeloproliferative tumors
Maropitant citrate (Cerenia, Zoetis)	1 mg/kg PO, SC q24h[195]	Antiemetic; antinausea; no adverse effects seen; Substance P conserved across classes
Melphalan (Alkeran, Celegene)	0.05-0.1 mg/kg PO[253]	Most species/lymphoma, leukemia, myeloproliferative tumors
Methimazole	2 mg/kg q24h × 30 days[134]	Snakes/excessive shedding from hyperthyroidism; limited effectiveness

Continued

TABLE 4-9 Miscellaneous Agents Used in Reptiles. (cont'd)

Agent	Dosage	Species/Comments
Methotrexate	0.25 mg/kg PO, SC, IV[253]	Most species/lymphoma, leukemia, myeloproliferative tumors
Metoclopramide	0.06 mg/kg PO q24h × 7 days[75,117]	Most species/stimulates gastric motility
	0.05 mg/kg PO q24h × 7 days[236]	Sea turtles/intestinal motility stimulant
	0.5 mg/kg IM q24h[87]	Sea turtles/supportive care
	1-10 mg/kg PO q24h[402]	Tortoises/stimulates gastric motility; ineffective in desert tortoises at 1 mg/kg[379]
Milk thistle (*Silybum marianum*)	4-15 mg/kg PO q8-12h[175,177]	Lizards, chelonians/hepatoprotectant
Pentobarbital	60-100 mg/kg IV, ICe[8,41]	Euthanasia
Pimobendan	0.2 mg/kg PO q24h[175]	Lizards
Potassium chloride	2 mEq/kg IV, ICe[22]	Most species/euthanasia; cardioplegic; administer following a euthanasia solution
Probenecid	250 mg/kg PO q12h[308]	Most species/gout; increases uric acid excretion; can be increased prn
S-adenosylmethionine (Denosyl, Nutramax)	30 mg/kg PO q24h[280]	Savannah monitors/liver disease
Sodium bicarbonate	0.5-1 mg/kg IV[117]	Most species/hypoxic acidosis postanesthesia
Sucralfate	500-1000 mg/kg PO q6-8h[104]	Most species/oral, esophageal, gastric, and duodenal ulcers
	200 mg/kg PO q24h[396]	Green iguanas/post-duodenoileal anastomosis
Tamoxifen 60-day time-release pellets (Innovative Research of America)	Pellets containing 5 mg tamoxifen implants ICe[68]	Leopard geckos/inhibition of follicular development for 60 days if implanted before vitellogenesis
Terbutaline	0.01-0.02 mg/kg IM[306]	Reduce bronchospasm
	Nebulization, 15-45 min/session q4-12h × 3+ days[306]	Lower respiratory tract particle size should be ≤0.5 μm, 2-10 μm for trachea; oxygen flow rates <10 kg 1-2 L/min, 5 L/min for larger reptiles; use bubble humidifier; possible adverse cardiovascular effects
Tricaine methanesulfonate (MS-222)	250-500 mg/kg ICe 1% solution followed by 0.1-1 mL 50% solution ICe or intracardiac[13,61]	Fence lizards, desert iguanas, garter snakes, house geckos, anole species/ euthanasia
Vincristine	0.025 mg/kg IV[253]	Most species/lymphoma, leukemia, myeloproliferative tumors

TABLE 4-10 Hematologic and Serum Biochemical Values of Reptiles.[a]

Measurement	Boa constrictor (Boa constrictor)[50,117,224,376]	Emerald tree boa (Corallus caninus)[117,376]	Rainbow boa (Epicrates cenchria)[117,376]
Hematology			
PCV (%)	29 (12-40)	26 (7-44)	29 (15-44)
RBC (10^6/µL)	0.71 (0.16-1.4)	2.16 (0.54-5.05)	0.87 (0.23-1.74)
Hgb (g/dL)	8.2 (3.1-13.2)	8.2 (6.1-11.4)	10.6 (8-13.1)
MCV (fL)	395 (122-669)	237 (37-360)	314 (45-619)
MCH (pg)	117 (51-184)	120 (113-128)	160
MCHC (g/dL)	31 (21-40)	34 (30-36)	36 (33-40)
WBC (10^3/µL)	7.37 (1.47-19.6)	4.87 (0.48-11.1)	7.64 (1-21.23)
Heterophils (10^3/µL)	1.93 (0.20-6.50)	1.25 (0.18-3.64)	1.07 (0.03-3.67)
Lymphocytes (10^3/µL)	2.89 (0.34-11.9)	1.92 (0.14-5.68)	4.71 (0.1-14.1)
Monocytes (10^3/µL)	0.27 (0.03-2.38)	0.17 (0.02-1.11)	0.9 (0.03-3.06)
Azurophils (10^3/µL)	0.84 (0-4.74)	0.23 (0-3.22)	0.60 (0-2.47)
Eosinophils (10^3/µL)	0.13 (0-0.60)	0.07 (0.06-0.08)	0.11 (0.04-0.22)
Basophils (10^3/µL)	0.21 (0.03-1.01)	0.06 (0.03-0.21)	0.1 (0.02-0.27)
Chemistries			
ALP (U/L)	189 (46-652)	87 (0-236)	27 (14-37)
ALT (U/L)	11 (0-30)	7 (0-27)	4 (1-6)
Amylase (U/L)	14 (0-76)	371 (61-847)	—
AST (U/L)	15 (2-64)	23 (2-61)	18 (3-54)
Bilirubin, total (mg/dL)	0.2 (0-0.6)	0.2 (0.2-0.3)	0.4 (0-0.8)
BUN (mg/dL)	2 (0-8)	2 (1-4)	2 (1-3)
Calcium (mg/dL)	15.3 (10-20)	12.8 (8.1-17.5)	13.8 (10.2-17.5)
Chloride (mEq/L)	125 (108-138)	131 (112-149)	129 (94-158)
Cholesterol (mg/dL)	120 (46-289)	304 (77-614)	206 (140-314)
Creatine kinase (U/L)	489 (57-2099)	454 (41-1445)	95 (0-347)
Creatinine (mg/dL)	0.2 (0-0.5)	0.6 (0.4-0.9)	0.4 (0.1-0.7)
GGT (U/L)	4 (0-23)	2 (1-2)	5
Glucose (mg/dL)	34 (7-74)	27 (5-64)	36 (2-80)
Iron (µg/dL)	113 (103-122)	—	—
LDH (U/L)	149 (0-452)	128 (14-754)	401 (141-661)
Lipase (U/L)	2730	—	—
Magnesium (mEq/L)	2.95 (2.9-3)	—	—
Osmolarity (mOsm/L)	306	—	—
Phosphorus (mg/dL)	4.3 (2.4-8.6)	4.1 (1.8-8)	4.3 (1.6-7.1)
Potassium (mEq/L)	4.7 (3.1-7.3)	5 (3-8.7)	4.8 (2.4-6.7)
Protein, total (g/dL)	7.0 (4.0-10.3)	4.5 (2.6-7.2)	6.8 (4.7-8.9)
Albumin (g/dL)[b]	2.9 (1.6-4.3)	2.6 (2-3.6)	2.4 (1.1-3.6)
Globulin (g/dL)[b]	3.9 (2.0-6.8)	2.8 (1.8-3.6)	4.2 (1.9-6.5)
Sodium (mEq/L)	159 (143-173)	157 (148-167)	162 (142-181)
Triglyceride (mg/dL)	103 (3-457)	24 (10-49)	72 (64-90)
Uric acid (mg/dL)	4.0 (0.3-15.0)	4.7 (1.4-19.2)	3.6 (1.1-9.7)

Continued

TABLE 4-10 Hematologic and Serum Biochemical Values of Reptiles. (cont'd)

Measurement	Rosy boa (Lichanura trivirgata)[376]	Ball python (Python regius)[181,376]	Blood python (Python curtus)[117]
Hematology			
PCV (%)	37 (20-54)	24 (10-33)	25 (15-49)
RBC ($10^6/\mu L$)	—	0.74 (0.31-1.16)	0.65
Hgb (g/dL)	—	7.8 (4.5-11.1)	—
MCV (fL)	—	328 (131-524)	340
MCH (pg)	—	102 (28-175)	—
MCHC (g/dL)	—	32 (24-40)	—
WBC ($10^3/\mu L$)	4.65 (0.57-8.73)	7.46 (2.22-21.6)	11.7 (1.13-42.5)
Heterophils ($10^3/\mu L$)	1.67 (0.39-4.13)	1.78 (0.32-6.17)	1.82 (0.31-3.99)
Lymphocytes ($10^3/\mu L$)	1.74 (0.18-4.92)	3.21 (0.35-13.8)	6.71 (0.34-33.6)
Monocytes ($10^3/\mu L$)	0.10 (0.03-0.65)	0.73 (0.01-3.26)	0.62 (0.13-2.12)
Azurophils ($10^3/\mu L$)	0.40 (0-1.68)	0.65 (0.01-4.12)	2.82 (0.27-6.8)
Eosinophils ($10^3/\mu L$)	—	0.10 (0.02-0.53)	0.08
Basophils ($10^3/\mu L$)	—	0.22 (0.04-1.08)	0.93 (0.32-1.83)
Chemistries			
ALP (U/L)	—	37 (11-98)	44 (8-56)
ALT (U/L)	—	9 (1-25)	10 (3-17)
Amylase (U/L)	—	1647 (383-2911)	—
AST (U/L)	20 (1-107)	25 (4-97)	56 (6-209)
Bilirubin, total (mg/dL)	—	0.1 (0-0.2)	0.3 (0.2-0.5)
BUN (mg/dL)	—	2 (0-7)	1 (0-2)
Calcium (mg/dL)	13.1 (9.4-17.4)	14.7 (10.4-19.3)	14.7 (13.5-16.2)
Chloride (mEq/L)	—	121 (107-134)	131 (123-138)
Cholesterol (mg/dL)	—	111 (15-232)	214 (76-445)
Creatine kinase (U/L)	—	526 (55-2136)	668 (327-1009)
Creatinine (mg/dL)	—	0.2 (0-0.7)	0.9 (0.5-1.3)
GGT (U/L)	—	—	8 (0-16)
Glucose (mg/dL)	37 (3-73)	25 (8-53)	30 (13-74)
LDH (U/L)	—	122 (4-376)	207 (49-364)
Phosphorus (mg/dL)	2.9 (0.8-6.1)	3.0 (1.4-7.3)	3.7 (3.1-4.5)
Potassium (mEq/L)	5.9 (3.7-10.3)	5.5 (2.4-10.0)	6.3 (3.3-11.2)
Protein, total (g/dL)	5.8 (3.7-8.3)	6.8 (3.6-9.0)	6.2 (3.6-8.1)
Albumin (g/dL)[b]	2.1 (1.2-2.9)	2.1 (1.1-3.6)	2.3 (1.6-2.8)
Globulin (g/dL)[b]	3.7 (2.3-4.8)	4.5 (2.1-6.5)	4.1 (3.1-4.9)
Sodium (mEq/L)	155 (115-174)	153 (137-171)	160 (155-164)
Triglyceride (mg/dL)	—	—	16 (13-22)
Uric acid (mg/dL)	6.4 (1.9-19.0)	3.0 (0.8-8.3)	4.3 (2.1-7.1)

TABLE 4-10 Hematologic and Serum Biochemical Values of Reptiles. (cont'd)

Measurement	Burmese python (Python bivittatus)[117,376]	Reticulated python (Python reticulatus)[117,376]	Green tree python (Morelia viridis)[117,376]
Hematology			
PCV (%)	28 (13-38)	26 (13-39)	25.3 (13-38)
RBC (10^6/μL)	0.83 (0.13-1.54)	0.72 (0.41-1.25)	0.85 (0.4-1.3)
Hgb (g/dL)	9.0 (4-11)	10.7 (5.2-30)	5.9 (4-7)
MCV (fL)	319 (84-554)	343 (176-429)	229 (208-250)
MCH (pg)	98 (32-143)	138 (60-186)	100
MCHC (g/dL)	32 (18-44)	37 (29-45)	36 (33-40)
WBC (10^3/μL)	7.6 (2.19-24.2)	7.48 (1.32-15.8)	7.28 (1.2-18.7)
Heterophils (10^3/μL)	2.25 (0.31-5.76)	1.92 (0.08-4.83)	1.59 (0.24-3.49)
Lymphocytes (10^3/μL)	3.73 (0.46-17.4)	2.24 (0.12-7.47)	3.46 (0.07-11.8)
Monocytes (10^3/μL)	0.17 (0.02-2.13)	1.22 (0.02-5.50)	0.61 (0.02-2.86)
Azurophils (10^3/μL)	0.27 (0.01-5.89)	0.10 (0.01-4.30)	0.72 (0.00-3.17)
Eosinophils (10^3/μL)	0.45 (0.10-1.4)	0.68 (0.04-1.95)	0.16 (0.1-0.22)
Basophils (10^3/μL)	0.12 (0.03-0.33)	0.06 (0.06-0.7)	0.17 (0.04-0.70)
Chemistries			
ALP (U/L)	58 (4-230)	61 (4-211)	177 (43-425)
ALT (U/L)	7 (0-26)	16 (0-51)	18 (0-52)
Amylase (U/L)	3255	1690 (416-2963)	902 (564-1240)
AST (U/L)	14 (3-65)	12 (2-34)	18 (1-63)
Bilirubin, total (mg/dL)	0.6 (0-2)	0.3	0.2
BUN (mg/dL)	2 (1-5)	2 (1-7)	2 (0-2)
Calcium (mg/dL)	16.1 (7.2-25.0)	16.3 (10.9-26.6)	13.8 (9.8-17.9)
Chloride (mEq/L)	118 (104-132)	118 (92-141)	124 (90-153)
Cholesterol (mg/dL)	264 (120-479)	285 (81-531)	251 (72-561)
Creatine kinase (U/L)	381 (39-1577)	351 (24-2338)	606 (21-1843)
Creatinine (mg/dL)	0.3 (0-1.6)	0.2 (0.1-0.4)	0.2 (0.2-0.5)
GGT (U/L)	25 (4-51)	22	—
Glucose (mg/dL)	24 (1-83)	31 (1-77)	37 (1-76)
LDH (U/L)	144 (12-807)	313 (43-1048)	206
Phosphorus (mg/dL)	4.4 (2.3-9.2)	5.6 (2.4-13.0)	5.1 (2.3-10.2)
Potassium (mEq/L)	4.8 (2.6-7.0)	5.0 (3.4-8.1)	5.5 (3.6-7.9)
Protein, total (g/dL)	7.2 (4.4-11.1)	7.8 (4.8-10.7)	7.2 (3.6-10.9)
Albumin (g/dL)[b]	2.3 (1.2-3.4)	2.1 (0.8-3.9)	2.0 (0.4-3.7)
Globulin (g/dL)[b]	4.9 (1.9-7.8)	5.0 (0.8-9.0)	4.9 (3.2-8.1)
Sodium (mEq/L)	158 (145-172)	160 (142-178)	161 (142-179)
Triglyceride (mg/dL)	114 (16-532)	45	—
Uric acid (mg/dL)	4.3 (0.4-10.1)	7.8 (3.5-17.4)	3.6 (0-11.0)

Continued

TABLE 4-10   Hematologic and Serum Biochemical Values of Reptiles. (cont'd)

Measurement	Carpet python (Morelia spilota ssp)[40,117,376]	Gopher snake (Pituophis catenifer)[117,234,376]	Indigo snake (Drymarchon corais)[85,117,376]
Hematology			
PCV (%)	24 (16-32)	35 (13-49)	26 (10-41)
RBC ($10^6/\mu L$)	0.89 (0.32-1.45)	0.67 (0.14-1.4)	0.62 (0.43-0.76)
Hgb (g/dL)	7.9 (4.9-9.7)	9.7 (4.3-12.3)	9.2 (7.3-11.1)
MCV (fL)	327 (260-386)	578 (246-1571)	369 (221-558)
MCH (pg)	111 (86-170)	111 (81-132)	258
MCHC (g/dL)	34 (29-39)	33 (27.5-36)	40 (33-46)
WBC ($10^3/\mu L$)	13.4 (2.7-24.8)	7.31 (1.66-24.0)	8.4 (1.5-21.6)
Heterophils ($10^3/\mu L$)	7.13 (1.79-16.8)	1.58 (0.33-5.99)	1.64 (0.14-3.94)
Lymphocytes ($10^3/\mu L$)	2.59 (0.60-6.91)	4.06 (0.21-13.2)	3.89 (0.24-14.5)
Monocytes ($10^3/\mu L$)	0.67 (0.03-2.67)	0.14 (0.01-0.86)	0.24 (0.04-2.50)
Azurophils ($10^3/\mu L$)	1.09 (0.01-5.72)	0.58 (0.01-3.23)	0.47 (0-3.51)
Basophils ($10^3/\mu L$)	0.16 (0-1.01)	0.14 (0.01-0.44)	0.35 (0.03-1.09)
Chemistries			
ALP (U/L)	36 (10-81)	61 (15-128)	123 (6-547)
ALT (U/L)	17 (6-78)	15 (1-70)	10 (3-16)
Amylase (U/L)	—	711 (107-1315)	—
AST (U/L)	17 (2-45)	20 (5-103)	15 (2-61)
Bilirubin, total (mg/dL)	0.5	0.4 (0.3-0.6)	2.1 (0.6-3.5)
BUN (mg/dL)	3 (2-3)	2.2 (1-5)	7 (0-22)
Calcium (mg/dL)	14.3 (10.9-20.5)	15.5 (11.0-20.0)	39 (12-97)[c]
Chloride (mEq/L)	118 (102-131)	120 (103-138)	121 (104-138)
Cholesterol (mg/dL)	318 (126-630)	368 (118-630)	93 (17-272)
Creatine kinase (U/L)	349 (3-1230)	330 (34-1702)	15
Creatinine (mg/dL)	1.3 (0.3-3.7)	0.3 (0.1-0.6)	644 (68-1923)
GGT (U/L)	32 (9-55)	10 (0-34)	0.3 (0.2-0.3)
Glucose (mg/dL)	30 (3-57)	57 (23-99)	57 (16-103)
LDH (U/L)	201 (11-728)	112 (1-405)	46 (28-89)
Magnesium (mEq/L)	330 (48-547)	76 (20-191)	313 (13-1055)
Phosphorus (mg/dL)	4.1 (0.8-7.9)	3.6 (1.7-7.9)	10.1 (0.1-39.6)[c]
Potassium (mEq/L)	4.9 (3.0-7.1)	4.8 (2.2-7.4)	4.7 (2.1-7.3)
Protein, total (g/dL)	7.2 (5.4-10.3)	6.0 (3.7-8.8)	8.1 (4.2-13.1)
Albumin (g/dL)[b]	2.1 (1.6-2.9)	2.0 (1.1-3.0)	2.4 (1.0-4.3)
Globulin (g/dL)[b]	5.1 (3.7-7.6)	4.0 (1.7-6.3)	5.1 (0.7-9.2)
Sodium (mEq/L)	156 (140-172)	163 (146-180)	162 (149-175)
Triglyceride (mg/dL)	30	27 (16-37)	92 (76-118)
Uric acid (mg/dL)	4.1 (0-9.3)	4.6 (1.9-12.6)	3.8 (0-9.1)

TABLE 4-10 Hematologic and Serum Biochemical Values of Reptiles. (cont'd)

Measurement	Corn snake (Pantherophis guttata)[117,376]	Common kingsnake (Lampropeltis getula)[117,376]	Rat snake (Elaphe obsoleta)[117,317,376]
Hematology			
PCV (%)	30 (13-50)	31 (9-47)	30 (12-46)
RBC (10^6/μL)	0.88 (0.40-1.60)	0.77 (0.10-1.88)	0.83 (0.23-1.43)
Hgb (g/dL)	11.5 (9.7-13.5)	—	9.8 (2.8-16.2)
MCV (fL)	307 (67-546)	311 (28-618)	354 (73-636)
MCH (pg)	127 (110-143)	—	121 (90-175)
MCHC (g/dL)	35 (32-40)	—	31 (18-45)
WBC (10^3/μL)	5.93 (1.12-16.9)	7.45 (1.55-27.7)	7.83 (1.02-25.2)
Heterophils (10^3/μL)	1.24 (0.23-5.08)	1.01 (0.16-5.50)	1.20 (0.10-3.89)
Lymphocytes (10^3/μL)	2.92 (0.29-11.8)	3.92 (0.35-20.9)	3.89 (0.41-16.1)
Monocytes (10^3/μL)	0.31 (0.03-1.78)	1.98 (0.05-5.83)	0.48 (0.02-2.52)
Azurophils (10^3/μL)	0.42 (0.01-3.29)	0.24 (0-4.77)	0.41 (0-3.50)
Eosinophils (10^3/μL)	0.09 (0.03-0.48)	0.08 (0.02-0.37)	0.11 (0.01-0.55)
Basophils (10^3/μL)	0.19 (0.04-1.04)	0.27 (0.04-1.08)	0.18 (0.01-0.72)
Chemistries			
ALP (U/L)	35 (0-85)	41 (13-102)	70 (11-212)
ALT (U/L)	19 (1-57)	11 (0-50)	10 (0-32)
Amylase (U/L)	540 (255-2225)	1268 (371-2671)	1337 (630-2626)
AST (U/L)	25 (4-149)	20 (4-107)	19 (3-75)
Bilirubin, total (mg/dL)	0.3 (0-1.0)	0.4 (0.1-0.7)	0.2 (0-0.8)
BUN (mg/dL)	3 (1-6)	2 (1-10)	2 (1-12)
Calcium (mg/dL)	15.6 (11.9-19.9)	14.9 (9.1-22.2)	15.3 (10.6-21.0)
Chloride (mEq/L)	122 (105-139)	119 (97-141)	121 (96-146)
Cholesterol (mg/dL)	473 (267-678)	294 (75-513)	340 (92-588)
Creatine kinase (U/L)	270 (31-967)	406 (59-1909)	228 (41-1049)
Creatinine (mg/dL)	0.6 (0.2-2)	9	0.3 (0-0.8)
GGT (U/L)	9 (0-25)	0.6 (0-1.6)	9 (1-35)
Glucose (mg/dL)	49 (17-92)	38 (8-92)	62 (11-121)
Iron (μg/dL)	—	190 (30-488)	—
LDH (U/L)	178 (10-585)	126 (15-417)	175 (4-452)
Lipase (U/L)	—	—	4 (3-4)
Magnesium (mg/dL)	—	—	2.5
Phosphorus (mg/dL)	3.7 (1.8-8.0)	3.8 (1.7-11.3)	3.8 (1.5-9.3)
Potassium (mEq/L)	4.9 (1.8-9.1)	4.6 (2.3-9.2)	5.0 (1.2-8.7)
Protein, total (g/dL)	7.0 (3.3-10.7)	6.4 (3.8-10.3)	6.3 (3.8-10.7)
Albumin (g/dL)[b]	2.1 (1.0-3.4)	1.8 (0.8-2.9)	2.3 (1.4-3.6)
Globulin (g/dL)[b]	4.7 (2.6-7.4)	4.4 (2.1-7.2)	4.0 (1.5-6.6)
Sodium (mEq/L)	162 (149-181)	161 (140-180)	164 (148-180)
Triglyceride (mg/dL)	331 (47-1118)	—	195 (21-1017)
Uric acid (mg/dL)	4.4 (1.0-13.6)	4.6 (1.4-16.0)	4.1 (0.9-14.0)

Continued

TABLE 4-10 Hematologic and Serum Biochemical Values of Reptiles. (cont'd)

Measurement	Milk snake (*Lampropeltis triangulum*)[117,376]	Prehensile-tailed skink (*Corucia zebrata*)[376,403]	Blue-tongued skink (*Tiliqua scincoides*)[117,376]
Hematology			
PCV (%)	30 (10-43)	32 (21-43)	28 (16-39)
RBC (10^6/μL)	0.88 (0.36-1.45)	1.59 (0.91-2.28)	0.89 (0.30-2.00)
Hgb (g/dL)	10.4 (6.9-11.9)	9.3 (5.7-12.0)	10.4 (6-13)
MCV (fL)	354 (135-615)	213 (126-311)	297 (34-441)
MCH (pg)	119 (89-164)	61 (35-91)	98 (44-173)
MCHC (g/dL)	34 (29-45)	28 (19-35)	33 (16-57)
WBC (10^3/μL)	7.33 (1.66-23.8)	11.5 (3.4-31.2)	5.93 (2.00-17.7)
Heterophils (10^3/μL)	1.29 (0.09-5.32)	3.66 (0.70-10.6)	2.24 (0.43-6.64)
Lymphocytes (10^3/μL)	3.55 (0.61-10.33)	3.87 (0.50-16.2)	1.93 (0.31-7.31)
Monocytes (10^3/μL)	0.12 (0.03-1.19)	0.68 (0.07-4.55)	0.16 (0.03-1.03)
Azurophils (10^3/μL)	0.76 (0.02-6.13)	0.11 (0.02-4.28)	0.16 (0.01-1.93)
Eosinophils (10^3/μL)	—	0.45 (0.05-1.48)	0.37 (0.02-1.50)
Basophils (10^3/μL)	0.24 (0.02-0.67)	1.26 (0.10-5.30)	0.67 (0.03-2.27)
Chemistries			
ALP (U/L)	115 (27-338)	118 (33-344)	80 (25-159)
ALT (U/L)	8 (3-17)	6 (1-20)	20 (5-34)
Amylase (U/L)	665	792 (255-1971)	—
AST (U/L)	19 (1-74)	14 (3-54)	20 (5-80)
Bilirubin, total (mg/dL)	0.4 (0.1-0.9)	0.2 (0-0.5)	—
BUN (mg/dL)	2 (1-14)	1 (0-4)	2 (1-27)
Calcium (mg/dL)	14.9 (11.0-18.9)	11.8 (8.9-15.2)	12.7 (10.0-15.9)
Chloride (mEq/L)	122 (106-137)	124 (107-138)	116 (100-132)
Cholesterol (mg/dL)	446 (51-631)	97 (39-265)	207 (49-601)
Creatine kinase (U/L)	157 (7-566)	234 (26-1319)	629 (59-5570)
Creatinine (mg/dL)	0.5 (0.3-1.1)	0.3 (0-0.6)	0.3 (0.1-0.6)
GGT (U/L)	8 (3-13)	2 (0-11)	8
Glucose (mg/dL)	52 (12-128)	107 (35-171)	127 (72-202)
LDH (U/L)	816 (18-2807)	183 (28-625)	735 (364-1106)
Lipase (U/L)	—	25 (8-63)	364
Phosphorus (mg/dL)	3.5 (1.0-7.3)	4.3 (2.3-9.8)	4.4 (2.3-10.8)
Potassium (mEq/L)	4.6 (2.2-8.1)	5.0 (2.9-8.1)	5.1 (3.3-7.9)
Protein, total (g/dL)	6.5 (3.9-10.0)	5.8 (4.1-8.3)	6.1 (3.7-8.5)
Albumin (g/dL)[b]	2.0 (0.8-3.2)	2.3 (1.4-3.4)	2.1 (1.1-3.1)
Globulin (g/dL)[b]	4.6 (2.4-6.8)	3.5 (2.3-5.0)	3.9 (2.4-5.8)
Sodium (mEq/L)	164 (148-180)	160 (145-177)	151 (139-175)
Triglyceride (mg/dL)	428 (68-1620)	48 (12-309)	—
Uric acid (mg/dL)	4.9 (1.3-15.0)	1.8 (0.3-5.0)	2.7 (0.6-9.5)

TABLE 4-10 Hematologic and Serum Biochemical Values of Reptiles. (cont'd)

Measurement	Panther chameleon (*Furcifur pardalis*)[117,376]	Veiled chameleon (*Chameleo calyptratus*)[376]	Spiny-tailed lizard (*Uromastyx* spp.)[117,279]
Hematology			
PCV (%)	31 (17-46)	24 (12-37)	29 (4.9-44.5)
RBC (10^6/μL)	0.83 (0.42-1.6)	—	0.78 (0.33-4.1)
Hgb (g/dL)	—	—	9.9 (3.3-17.4)
MCV (fL)	330 (200-418)	—	415 (119-614)
MCH (pg)	—	—	133 (1.2-203)
MCHC (g/dL)	—	—	33 (22-41)
Thrombocytes (10^3/μL)	—	—	958 (290-2290)
WBC (10^3/μL)	9.92 (0.47-25.1)	6.30 (1.20-21.0)	3.1 (1-8.1)
Heterophils (10^3/μL)	2.68 (0.09-6.64)	2.35 (0.50-8.32)	2 (0.59-5.36)
Lymphocytes (10^3/μL)	5.98 (0.21-16.8)	2.18 (0.07-10.8)	0.99 (0.27-4.05)
Monocytes (10^3/μL)	—	—	0.04 (0-0.5)
Azurophils (10^3/μL)	0.46 (0-2.29)	0.50 (0-2.75)	—
Eosinophils (10^3/μL)	—	—	0.04 (0-0.2)
Basophils (10^3/μL)	0.13 (0.03-0.92)	—	0.03 (0-0.33)
Chemistries			
ALP (U/L)	32 (1-109)	—	31 (5.9-139)
ALT (U/L)	—	—	11 (2.4-35)
Amylase (U/L)	—	—	134
AST (U/L)	23 (2-70)	397 (93-967)	73 (29-172)
Bilirubin, total (mg/dL)	—	—	0.3 (0.1-0.7)
BUN (mg/dL)	—	—	0.56 (0-3)
Calcium (mg/dL)	10.9 (7.1-14.6)	11.9 (8.7-14.5)	9.9 (7.2-13.2)
Chloride (mEq/L)	—	—	126 (111-135)
Cholesterol (mg/dL)	—	—	161 (64-295)
Creatine kinase (U/L)	367 (47-1474)	1873 (5-8905)	1778 (141-10 k)
Creatinine (mg/dL)	—	—	0.4 (0.1-3)
GGT (U/L)	—	—	0.8 (0-5.0)
Glucose (mg/dL)	319 (174-465)	270 (125-444)	200 (68-356)
LDH (U/L)	—	—	209 (22-899)
Magnesium (mg/dL)	—	—	3.48 (2.1-10.2)
Phosphorus (mg/dL)	9.8 (2.1-17.5)	8.4 (4.4-16.1)	4.5 (1.3-10)
Potassium (mEq/L)	5.5 (1.1-10.0)	6.5 (3.5-12.0)	3.7 (3-4.6)
Protein, total (g/dL)	5.9 (3.3-8.5)	6.4 (4.4-10.9)	4 (2.6-7.4)
Albumin (g/dL)[b]	2.6 (1.2-4.1)	3.1 (1.4-4.2)	2 (1.2-3.1)
Globulin (g/dL)[b]	3.2 (2.0-4.4)	3.3 (2.0-5.9)	2.9 (2.2-4.6)
Sodium (mEq/L)	143 (127-159)	144 (132-169)	173 ± 4
Triglyceride (mg/dL)	—	—	175 (111-238)
Uric acid (mg/dL)	5.1 (0-12.9)	5.6 (0-21.9)	2.94 (0.3-7.3)

Continued

TABLE 4-10 Hematologic and Serum Biochemical Values of Reptiles. (cont'd)

Measurement	Bearded dragon (*Pogona vitticeps*)[86,117]	Gila monster (*Heloderma suspectum*)[62]	Green iguana (*Iguana iguana*)[70,81,150,260,286,376]
Hematology			
PCV (%)	30 (17-45)	37 (22-50)	25-38
RBC ($10^6/\mu L$)	1 (0.40-1.60)	0.50 (0.22-0.67)	1-1.9
Hgb (g/dL)	9.3 (4.7-14)	7.4 (6.0-9.5)	8-12
MCV (fL)	292 (77-506)	812 (415-1773)	165-305
MCH (pg)	90 (16-163)	—	65-105
MCHC (g/dL)	32 (19-46)	21 (14-36)	20-38
WBC ($10^3/\mu L$)	6.21 (1.45-19.0)	4.72 (3.30-6.40)	3-10
Heterophils ($10^3/\mu L$)	2.09 (0.24-7.77)	2.17 (1.35-3.31)	0.35-5.2
Lymphocytes ($10^3/\mu L$)	2.77 (0.29-11.3)	1.54 (0.58-3.39)	0.5-5.5
Monocytes ($10^3/\mu L$)	0.25 (0.03-1.39)	0.07 (0-0.19)	0-0.1
Azurophils ($10^3/\mu L$)	0.11 (0.01-1.98)	0.38 (0-1.14)	0-1.7
Eosinophils ($10^3/\mu L$)	0.12 (0.01-0.37)	—	0-1
Basophils ($10^3/\mu L$)	0.26 (0.04-1.28)	0.57 (0.23-1.05)	0-0.5
Fibrinogen (mg/dL)	180 (0-300)	—	0-300
Chemistries			
ALP (U/L)	133 (21-569)	—	40 (4-170)
ALT (U/L)	9 (0-33)	—	21 (0-97)
Amylase (U/L)	1670 (497-3430)	—	1815 (996-2988)
AST (U/L)	20 (2-90)	42 (20-66)	52 (2-100)
Bile acids (rest; μmol/L)	—	16.2 (2.6-55.1)	7.5 (2.6-30.3)
Bile acids (7.5 h; μmol/L)	—	—	32.5 (15.2-44.1)
Bilirubin, total (mg/dL)	0.4 (0-1.4)	—	0.3 (0-4.9)
BUN (mg/dL)	2 (1-5)	15 (6-30)	2 (0-10)
Calcium (mg/dL)	11.9 (8.6-18)	12.2 (10.2-13.4)	12 (6-18)[d]
Ionized Ca^{++} (mmol/L)	—	1.26 (1.09-1.50)	1.01-1.62
Chloride (mEq/L)	120 (94-149)	—	117 (102-130)
Cholesterol (mg/dL)	271 (79-606)	—	104-333[d]
Creatine kinase (U/L)	563 (33-4042)	600 (144-1812)	1876 (174-8768)[d]
Creatinine (mg/dL)	0.2 (0-0.7)	—	0.5 (0.2-1.3)
GGT (U/L)	1 (0-21)	—	3 (0-10)
Glucose (mg/dL)	202 (108-333)	48 (4-109)	169-288
Iron (μg/dL)	—	—	88-133
LDH (U/L)	347 (25-1906)	—	617 (36-7424)[d]
Lipase (U/L)	—	—	21 (17-24)
Magnesium (mEq/L)	—	—	2.4-4
Phosphorus (mg/dL)	4.4 (2.1-10.6)	3.4 (1.1-8.6)	5 (2.5-21)[d]
Potassium (mEq/L)	4.0 (1.5-7.1)	3.9 (2.8-4.6)	1.3-3
Protein, total (g/dL)	5.0 (3.0-8.1)	6.3 (5.4-6.9)	5.4 (4.1-7.4)[d]

TABLE 4-10 Hematologic and Serum Biochemical Values of Reptiles. (cont'd)

Measurement	Bearded dragon (*Pogona vitticeps*)	Gila monster (*Heloderma suspectum*)	Green iguana (*Iguana iguana*)
Albumin (g/dL)[b]	2.5 (1.2-4.0)	—	2.1-2.8
Albumin (PEP; g/dL)[b]	—	2.61 (2.14-3.23)	1.8 (1.4-3.1)
Globulin (g/dL)[b]	2.5 (1.1-4.5)	—	2.5-4.3[d]
α-1 (PEP; g/dL)[b]	—	2.09 (1.48-2.60)	0.9 (0.4-1.2)
α-2 (PEP; g/dL)[b]	—	0.59 (0.44-0.76)	—
β (PEP; g/dL)[b]	—	0.58 (0.41-0.77)	2.2 (1.6-3.8)[d]
γ (PEP; g/dL)[b]	—	0.33 (0.18-0.68)	0.3 (0.1-0.4)
A/G ratio	—	—	0.5 (0.41-0.78)
Sodium (mEq/L)	157 (140-179)	144 (140-151)	158-183
Triglyceride (mg/dL)	261 (93-437)	—	383 (7-1323)[d]
Uric acid (mg/dL)	3.1 (0.5-9.8)	16.8 (9.8-24.7)	2.6 (0-8.2)[d]
Vitamin D_3 (25-OH; nmol/L)	—	—	51-393[d]

Measurement	Green iguana (*Iguana iguana*) male[e,138,183]	Green iguana (*Iguana iguana*) female[e,138,183]	Green iguana (*Iguana iguana*) juvenile[e,138]
Hematology			
PCV (%)	34 (29-39)	38 (33-44)	38 (30-47)
RBC (10^6/µL)	1.3 (1-1.7)	1.4 (1.2-1.8)	1.4 (1.3-1.6)
Hgb (g/dL)	8.6 (6.7-10.2)	10.6 (9.1-12.2)	9.6 (9.2-10.1)
MCV (fL)	266 (228-303)	270 (235-331)	—
MCHC (g/dL)	25 (23-28)	28 (25-31)	—
WBC (10^3/µL)	15 (11-25)	15 (8-25)	16 (8-22)
Heterophils (10^3/µL)	3.6 (1-5.4)	3.2 (0.6-6.4)	2.2 (1-3.8)
Lymphocytes (10^3/µL)	9.7 (5-16.5)	9.9 (5.2-14.4)	12.9 (6.2-17.2)
Monocytes (10^3/µL)	1.3 (0.2-2.7)	1.2 (0.4-2.3)	0.4 (0.3-0.6)
Eosinophils (10^3/µL)	0.1 (0-0.3)	0.1 (0-0.2)	0.3 (0-0.4)
Basophils (10^3/µL)	0.4 (0.1-1)	0.5 (0.2-1.2)	0.5 (0.1-0.7)
Fibrinogen (mg/dL)	100 (100-200)	100 (100-300)	100 (100-300)
Chemistries			
ALP (U/L)	39 (14-65)	59 (22-90)	—
ALT (U/L)	32 (4-76)	45 (5-96)	—
Anion gap (mEq/L)	22 (12-30)	29 (19-41)	—
AST (U/L)	33 (19-65)	40 (7-102)	41 (13-72)
Bilirubin, total (mg/dL)	0.8 (0.1-1.4)	1.5 (0.3-3.1)	—
Calcium (mg/dL)	11.3 (8.6-14.1)	12.5 (10.8-14)	14.3 (12.1-23.2)
Chloride (mEq/L)	119 (115-124)	121 (113-129)	—
Cholesterol (mg/dL)	161 (82–214)	255 (204-347)	—

Continued

TABLE 4-10 Hematologic and Serum Biochemical Values of Reptiles. (cont'd)

Measurement	Green iguana (Iguana iguana) male	Green iguana (Iguana iguana) female	Green iguana (Iguana iguana) juvenile
CO_2 (mEq/L)	19.9 (15.2-24.7)	19 (16-23)	—
Estradiol (pg/mL)	79 (36-162)	270 (81-512)	—
Glucose (mg/dL)	166 (70-244)	170 (105-258)	273 (131-335)
Phosphorus (mg/dL)	5.3 (3.2-7.6)	6.3 (2.8-9.3)	7.7 (4.3-9)
Potassium (mEq/L)	4 (2.8-6.1)	3.6 (2-5.8)	—
Protein, total (g/dL)	5.4 (4.4-6.5)	6.1 (4.9-7.6)	5 (4.2-6.1)
Albumin (g/dL)[b]	2 (1.3-3)	2.4 (1.5-3)	2.3 (2-2.8)
Globulin (g/dL)[b]	3.5 (2.5-4.4)	3.8 (2.8-5.2)	2.7 (2.2-3)
A:G (ratio)	0.6 (0.4-0.9)	0.7 (0.3-1)	0.8 (0.7-0.9)
Sodium (mEq/L)	157 (152-162)	163 (156-172)	—
Testosterone (ng/mL)	10.2 (2.2-15.7)	0.26 (0.07-0.35)	—
Uric acid (mg/dL)	2.7 (1.5-5.8)	3.6 (0.9-6.7)	3.3 (0.7-5.7)

Measurement	Chinese (Asian) water dragon (Physignathus cocincinus)[256]	Crested gecko (Rhacodactylus ciliatus) male[257]	Crested gecko (Rhacodactylus ciliatus) female[257]
Hematology			
PCV (%)	35 (32-40)	36 (23-45)	31 (24-43)
WBC (10^3/μL)	13.5 (11.7-18.2)	15.4 (3.5-38.9)	15.4 (3.5-38.9)
Heterophils (10^3/μL)	5.1 (3.9-6.9)	1.5 (0.6-4.2)	1.5 (0.6-4.2)
Lymphocytes (10^3/μL)	7.2 (5.6-9.5)	10.7 (2.2-24.9)	10.7 (2.2-24.9)
Monocytes (10^3/μL)	1.1 (0.4-1.9)	1.9 (0.8-5.1)	1.9 (0.8-5.1)
Azurophils (10^3/μL)	0 (0-0.6)	—	—
Eosinophils (10^3/μL)	0.2 (0.1-0.3)	0 (0-0.2)	0 (0-0.2)
Basophils (10^3/μL)	0.5 (0.2-0.8)	0.3 (0-0.8)	0.3 (0-0.8)
Chemistries			
AST (U/L)	16.5 (8-52)	30 (12-84)	30 (12-84)
Bile acids (μmol/L)	—	43 (<35-89)	43 (<35-89)
Calcium (mg/dL)	12.4 (11.6-13.3)	12.5 (11.8-13.9)	>20 (15.6-20.0)
Creatine kinase (U/L)	1747 (19-6630)	489 (89-2104)	489 (89-2104)
Glucose (mg/dL)	157 (112-243)	107 (56-180)	107 (56-180)
Phosphorus (mg/dL)	5.7 (3.4-8.2)	4.0 (2.6-6.2)	9.6 (3.8-18.8)
Potassium (mEq/L)	4.2 (3.8-4.5)	2.6 (1.5-4.5)	2.6 (1.5-4.5)
Protein, total (g/dL)	7 (6.6-7.5)	6.0 (4.9-7.7)	6.6 (5.2-8.0)
Albumin (g/dL)[b]	2.2 (2.1-2.3)	2.7 (2.3-3.2)	2.9 (2.4-3.4)
Globulin (g/dL)[b]	4.7 (4.5-5.3)	3.5 (2.6-5.2)	3.5 (2.6-5.2)
Sodium (mEq/L)	150 (147-153)	143 (136-148)	143 (136-148)
Uric acid (mg/dL)	2.3 (1.9-2.7)	2.6 (0.9-6.0)	2.6 (0.9-6.0)

TABLE 4-10 Hematologic and Serum Biochemical Values of Reptiles. (cont'd)

Measurement	Savannah monitor (*Varanus exanthematicus*)[117,376]	Water monitor (*Varanus salvator*)[117,376]	Tegu lizard (*Tupinambus* spp.)[f,117,380]
Hematology			
PCV (%)	34 (16-51)	34 (20-47)	25 ± 2.6
RBC ($10^6/\mu L$)	1.23 (0.63-1.58)	0.98 (0.42-1.42)	0.96 ± 0.14
Hgb (g/dL)	10.5 (6.2-13.2)	10.5 (9.8-11.5)	11.4 ± 1.6
MCV (fL)	284 (229-382)	335 (227-595)	261 ± 23
MCH (pg)	94 (89-99)	140 (104-177)	119 ± 12.5
MCHC (g/dL)	32 (26-38)	33 (30-40)	45.6 ± 3.4
WBC ($10^3/\mu L$)	4.67 (0.10-10.9)	9.49 (2.9-18.8)	16.8 ± 2.5
Heterophils ($10^3/\mu L$)	1.58 (0.03-4.55)	4.30 (0.16-8.44)	2.2 ± 0.45
Lymphocytes ($10^3/\mu L$)	1.87 (0.06-4.88)	2.84 (0.3-7.98)	7.5 ± 0.58
Monocytes ($10^3/\mu L$)	0.42 (0.01-2.32)	0.81 (0.06-3.38)	1 ± 0.41
Azurophils ($10^3/\mu L$)	0.02 (0-0.69)	0.75 (0.01-3.72)	1.8 ± 0.56
Eosinophils ($10^3/\mu L$)	—	—	4.1 ± 0.11
Basophils ($10^3/\mu L$)	0.15 (0.07-0.28)	0.11 (0.06-0.14)	0.4 ± 0.01
Fibrinogen (mg/dL)	156 (100-300)	500 (200-700)	133 (0-200)
Chemistries			
ALP (U/L)	20 (4-101)	176 (14-405)	160 ± 85
ALT (U/L)	70 (7-374)	19 (1-93)	33 ± 24
Amylase (U/L)	—	1021 (265-1868)	—
AST (U/L)	26 (5-80)	24 (2-58)	18 ± 14
Bilirubin, total (mg/dL)	0.1 (0-0.3)	0.1 (0-0.3)	0.3 ± 0.2
BUN (mg/dL)	1 (0-5)	2 (1-5)	1 ± 1
Calcium (mg/dL)	13.6 (10.8-16.5)	14.0 (9.8-18.2)	12.2 ± 0.8
Chloride (mEq/L)	115 (93-133)	111 (97-124)	121 ± 7
Cholesterol (mg/dL)	116 (49-231)	78 (22-126)	206 ± 67
Creatine kinase (U/L)	1529 (7-6624)	772 (176-1818)	641 ± 568
Creatinine (mg/dL)	8.7 (0-67)	0.5 (0-1)	0.3 ± 0.1
GGT (U/L)	7 (1-11)	24 (7-48)	7
Glucose (mg/dL)	108 (54-163)	98 (29-170)	128 ± 30
Iron (μg/dL)	—	242 (111-429)	—
LDH (U/L)	427 (29-3699)	157 (34-1288)	540 ± 537
Magnesium (mEq/L)	3.1	2.5 (2.2-2.7)	—
Osmolarity (mOsm/L)	332 (319-345)	—	—
Phosphorus (mg/dL)	4.2 (0.8-7.7)	5.2 (2.9-8.9)	5.6 ± 2.1
Potassium (mEq/L)	4.9 (3.0-6.9)	4.6 (3.5-6.1)	2.4 ± 1.4
Protein, total (g/dL)	6.6 (3.4-9.8)	7.0 (5.1-9.8)	6.6 ± 1.3
Albumin (g/dL)[b]	2.0 (0.6-3.3)	2.4 (1.4-3.4)	3.6 ± 0.7
Albumin (PEP; g/dL)[b]	3.2 (3.1-3.3)	3.1 (3-3.2)	—

Continued

TABLE 4-10   Hematologic and Serum Biochemical Values of Reptiles. (cont'd)

Measurement	Savannah monitor (*Varanus exanthematicus*)	Water monitor (*Varanus salvator*)	Tegu lizard (*Tupinambus* spp.)
Globulin (g/dL)[b]	4.6 (1.4-7.9)	4.7 (2.0-7.3)	2.9 ± 1.2
α-1 (PEP; g/dL)[b]	—	0.1	—
α-2 (PEP; g/dL)[b]	—	0.9 (0.8-1)	—
β (PEP; g/dL)[b]	—	0.9	—
γ (PEP; g/dL)[b]	—	4.7 (2.6-6.8)	—
Sodium (mEq/L)	156 (142-169)	156 (143-170)	159 ± 4
Triglyceride (mg/dL)	135 (17-476)	35 (6-78)	31
Uric acid (mg/dL)	6.5 (2.0-14.6)	4.7 (1-12.2)	3.2 ± 2

Measurement	American alligator (*Alligator mississippiensis*)[117,376]	Dwarf caiman (*Paleosuchus palpebrosus*)[117,376]	Aldabra tortoise (*Aldabrachelys gigantea*)[376]
Hematology			
PCV (%)	24 (9-39)	22 (12-35)	22 (11-34)
RBC ($10^6/\mu L$)	0.57 (0.21-1.3)	0.66 (0.43-0.89)	0.45 (0.13-0.77)
Hgb (g/dL)	7.8 (4.0-12.2)	7.7 (6.2-8.8)	7.1 (3.8-10.5)
MCV (fL)	430 (122-786)	362 (180-535)	469 (195-742)
MCH (pg)	135 (37-246)	98	154 (63-244)
MCHC (g/dL)	32 (18-45)	33 (23-38)	32 (21-42)
WBC ($10^3/\mu L$)	6.39 (2.03-21.3)	6 (2.1-14.7)	5.45 (1.54-17.5)
Heterophils ($10^3/\mu L$)	2.51 (0.50-8.19)	2.95 (0.51-7.73)	3.17 (0.69-8.79)
Lymphocytes ($10^3/\mu L$)	2.21 (0.29-12.1)	2.10 (0.28-9.66)	1.52 (0.11-5.53)
Monocytes ($10^3/\mu L$)	0.31 (0.04-2.04)	0.10 (0.02-0.44)	0.14 (0.02-0.79)
Azurophils ($10^3/\mu L$)	0.05 (0.01-1.25)	0.04 (0.01-0.73)	0.04 (0-0.68)
Eosinophils ($10^3/\mu L$)	0.22 (0.03-1.02)	0.12 (0.03-0.43)	0.13 (0.01-0.44)
Basophils ($10^3/\mu L$)	0.71 (0.04-3.23)	0.15 (0.04-0.46)	0.11 (0.02-0.40)
Fibrinogen (mg/dL)	267 ± 115	100 (0-200)	100 (0-200)
Chemistries			
ALP (U/L)	34 (12-105)	13 (2-26)	64 (15-142)
ALT (U/L)	37 (8-92)	37 (5-74)	3 (0-22)
Amylase (U/L)	58 (25-1067)	47 (25-234)	947 (144-3266)
AST (U/L)	246 (111-539)	88 (36-218)	59 (19-155)
Bilirubin, total (mg/dL)	0.2 (0-0.8)	0.2 (0-0.6)	0.4 (0.1-1.2)
BUN (mg/dL)	2 (1-18)	2 (0-4)	18 (4-43)
Calcium (mg/dL)	11.2 (8.1-15.1)	10.4 (8.1-13.8)	11.7 (8.5-42.7)
Chloride (mEq/L)	112 (94-123)	121 (99-144)	93 (86-104)
Cholesterol (mg/dL)	108 (32-291)	115 (29-241)	229 (69-564)
Creatine kinase (U/L)	911 (145-7408)	1926 (89-9228)	59 (11-380)

TABLE 4-10 Hematologic and Serum Biochemical Values of Reptiles. (cont'd)

Measurement	American alligator (*Alligator mississippiensis*)	Dwarf caiman (*Paleosuchus palpebrosus*)	Aldabra tortoise (*Aldabrachelys gigantea*)
Creatinine (mg/dL)	0.3 (0-0.7)	0.3 (0-0.6)	0.2 (0-0.4)
Glucose (mg/dL)	88 (34-177)	64 (13-146)	43 (12-85)
LDH (U/L)	346 (13-1726)	1269 (62-4058)	473 (131-1077)
Osmolarity (mOsm/L)	—	303 (301-304)	—
Phosphorus (mg/dL)	4.3 (1.6-9.9)	4.4 (2.0-9.7)	3.9 (1.9-13)
Potassium (mEq/L)	3.8 (2.4-5.3)	4.3 (3.0-6.3)	5.5 (3.8-8.1)
Protein, total (g/dL)	5.1 (2.6-7.8)	5.4 (2.6-7.8)	5.3 (2.5-7.7)
Albumin (g/dL)[b]	1.5 (0.4-2.6)	1.4 (0.6-2.7)	1.6 (0.7-3.0)
Albumin (PEP; g/dL)[b]	—	2.2 (1.8-2.5)	—
Globulin (g/dL)[b]	3.3 (0.7-5.5)	4.0 (1.8-6.2)	3.7 (1.0-5.5)
Sodium (mEq/L)	147 (134-160)	151 (134-167)	128 (119-141)
Triglyceride (mg/dL)	83 (7-505)	92 (9-174)	425 (17-1010)
Uric acid (mg/dL)	1.3 (0.2-4.0)	2.1 (0.4-5.6)	1.5 (0.2-3.4)

Measurement	Radiated tortoise (*Astrochelys radiata*)[248,376,405]	Red-footed tortoise (*Chelonoidis carbonaria*)[117,376]	Indian star tortoise (*Geochelone elegans*)[117,376]
Hematology			
PCV (%)	10-51	25 (6-38)	23 (14-38)
RBC (10⁶/μL)	0.3-1.1	0.46 (0.14-0.19)	0.37 (0.24-0.55)
Hgb (g/dL)	5.6 (4-8)	7.5 (7-7.9)	7.9 (6.9-8.5)
MCV (fL)	454 (319-571)	482 (22-940)	—
MCH (pg)	108 (82-133)	136 (123-149)	—
MCHC (g/dL)	28 (26-33)	31 (29-32)	27 (26-28)
WBC (10^3/μL)	2.5-14	6.51 (1.15-20.0)	6.71 (1.35-27.9)
Heterophils (10^3/μL)	0.7-8	1.67 (0.16-7.26)	2.56 (0.24-10.9)
Lymphocytes (10^3/μL)	0.4-5.8	1.89 (0.12-9.10)	2.83 (0.20-15.4)
Monocytes (10^3/μL)	0.02-0.5	0.16 (0.02-0.58)	0.20 (0.02-0.75)
Azurophils (10^3/μL)	0-0.82	0.05 (0-0.87)	0.05 (0.01-0.87)
Eosinophils (10^3/μL)	0.03-0.82	0.17 (0.02-0.80)	0.26 (0.03-1.51)
Basophils (10^3/μL)	0.1-2.5	0.92 (0.03-3.48)	0.49 (0.09-1.79)
Fibrinogen (mg/dL)	117 (100-200)	—	—
Chemistries			
ALP (U/L)	72-392	60 (6-145)	72 (20-164)
ALT (U/L)	0-17	7 (0-18)	4 (0-14)
Amylase (U/L)	—	—	1235
AST (U/L)	25-348	130 (20-406)	54 (14-152)
Bile acids (μmol/L)	0.3-31.3	—	—
Bilirubin, total (mg/dL)	0-0.5	0.5 (0.1-1.1)	0.2 (0-0.5)

Continued

TABLE 4-10 Hematologic and Serum Biochemical Values of Reptiles. (cont'd)

Measurement	Radiated tortoise (*Astrochelys radiata*)	Red-footed tortoise (*Chelonoidis carbonaria*)	Indian star tortoise (*Geochelone elegans*)
BUN (mg/dL)	2-34	14 (1-34)	3 (0-9)
Calcium (mg/dL)	8.6-18	12.2 (7.1-24.1)	11.7 (7.6-21.2)
Chloride (mEq/L)	91-112	99 (81-111)	100 (88-112)
Cholesterol (mg/dL)	56-154	121 (10-257)	115 (15-255)
Creatine kinase (U/L)	33-5666	695 (54-3593)	374 (22-2644)
Creatinine (mg/dL)	0.1-0.5	0.4 (0.2-1.3)	0.3 (0.2-0.5)
GGT (U/L)	5 (0-11)	28 (7-130)	4 (0-5)
Glucose (mg/dL)	21-93	67 (13-154)	76 (37-186)
Iron (µg/dL)	60	107	—
LDH (U/L)	213-6444	638 (118-1644)	438 (12-863)
Lipase (U/L)	5-50	—	5
Phosphorus (mg/dL)	2.5-7	3.5 (1.0-8.3)	3.6 (1.4-9.4)
Potassium (mEq/L)	3.1-5.8	5.5 (2.8-9.4)	4.8 (2.0-7.7)
Protein, total (g/dL)	3-6.6	4.7 (1.9-7.4)	4.7 (2.2-7.6)
Albumin (g/dL)[b]	0.6-2.4	1.6 (0-3.0)	1.7 (0.4-3.0)
Albumin (PEP; g/dL)[b]	0.9-2.4	—	—
Globulin (g/dL)[b]	1.4-3.2	3.1 (0.2-4.8)	2.9 (1.3-4.6)
α-1 Glob (PEP; g/dL)[b]	0.1-0.5	—	—
α-2 Glob (PEP; g/dL)[b]	0.6-1.9	—	—
β Glob (PEP; g/dL)[b]	0.6-1.5	—	—
γ Glob (PEP; g/dL)[b]	0.4-0.9	—	—
Sodium (mEq/L)	121-146	130 (117-143)	127 (117-137)
Triglyceride (mg/dL)	26-303	246 (28-480)	60 (27-110)
Uric acid (mg/dL)	0.3 (0-0.6)	0.6 (0.1-2.1)	3.3 (0.2-7.9)

Measurement	Desert tortoise (*Gopherus agassizii*)[3,53,72,127]	Gopher tortoise (*Gopherus polyphemus*)[375]	Russian tortoise (*Testudo horsfieldii*)[202,252]
Hematology			
PCV (%)	15-39	23 (15-30)	23 (22-34)
RBC (10⁶/µL)	0.28-1.34	0.54 (0.24-0.91)	—
Hgb (g/dL)	3.6-10.3	6.4 (4.2-8.6)	—
MCV (fL)	197-688	—	—
MCH (pg)	39-189	—	—
MCHC (g/dL)	19-35	—	—
WBC (10³/µL)	0.97-10.9	15.7 (10-22)	8.5 (5-12.5)
Heterophils (10³/µL)	0.49-7.3	4.7 (1-12.5)[g]	3.7 (1.3-4.6)
Lymphocytes (10³/µL)	0-3.8	—	4.7 (3.6-7.6)
Monocytes (10³/µL)	0-0.57	8.9 (3.2-17.4)[g]	0.01 (0-0.02)

TABLE 4-10 | Hematologic and Serum Biochemical Values of Reptiles. (cont'd)

Measurement	Desert tortoise (*Gopherus agassizii*)	Gopher tortoise (*Gopherus polyphemus*)	Russian tortoise (*Testudo horsfieldii*)
Azurophils ($10^3/\mu L$)	0-0.9	1.1 (0.3-2.9)[g]	0.05 (0.03-0.12)
Eosinophils ($10^3/\mu L$)	0-0.95	—	0.05 (0.02-0.06)
Basophils ($10^3/\mu L$)	0-4.3	0.94 (0.2-2.4)[g]	0.05 (0.02-0.08)
Chemistries			
ALP (U/L)	43-176	39 (11-71)	498 (181-1188)
ALT (U/L)	21 (0-66)	15 (2-57)	1 (0-2)
AST (U/L)	41-106	136 (57-392)	20 (12-32)
Bile acids (μmol/L)	0-5.4	—	—
Bilirubin, total (mg/dL)	0-0.9	0.02 (0-0.1)	0.015 (0-0.09)
BUN (mg/dL)	0-4	30 (1-130)	12 (4-17)
Calcium (total; mg/dL)	9.3-14.7	12 (10-14)	13.2 (9.9-19.5)
Ionized calcium (mmol/L)	—	—	1.28 (1-1.6)
Chloride (mEq/L)	94-112	102 (35-128)	—
Cholesterol (mg/dL)	56-233	76 (19-150)	109 (25-210)
Creatine kinase (U/L)	2262 (944-3880)	160 (32-628)	123 (6-344)
Creatinine (mg/dL)	0.11-0.37	0.3 (0.1-0.4)	—
GLDH (U/L)	—	—	1 (0.6-1.5)
Glucose (mg/dL)	92-165	75 (55-128)	59 (40-86)
LDH (U/L)	25-250	273 (18-909)	—
Magnesium (mEq/L)	2.1 (1.8-2.4)	4.1 (3.3-4.8)	—
Phosphorus (mg/dL)	1-6.3	2.1 (1-3.1)	2.6 (1.3-3.9)
Potassium (mEq/L)	3.5-4.7	5 (2.9-7)	5.3 (1.9-7.2)
Protein, total (g/dL)	3-4.6	3.1 (1.3-4.6)	3 (2.5-4.6)
Albumin (g/dL)[b]	1.2-2.2	1.5 (0.5-2.6)	1.6 (1.2-2.3)
Albumin (PEP; g/dL)[b]	—	—	—
Globulin (g/dL)[b]	1.2-2.6	—	1.4 (1.3-2.3)
α-1 Glob (PEP; g/dL)[b]	1	—	—
α-2 Glob (PEP; g/dL)[b]	1	—	—
β Glob (PEP; g/dL)[b]	0.6	—	—
γ Glob (PEP; g/dL)[b]	—	—	—
Sodium (mEq/L)	122-139	138 (127-148)	138 (131-149)
Triglyceride (mg/dL)	0-425	—	—
Uric acid (mg/dL)	2.7-7.2	3.5 (0.9-8.5)	1.2 (0.8-3.9)
Vitamin A (μg/mL)	0.2-0.6	—	—
Zinc (ppm)	0.4-3.7	—	—

Continued

TABLE 4-10 Hematologic and Serum Biochemical Values of Reptiles. (cont'd)

Measurement	African spurred tortoise (Centrochelys sulcata)[117,376]	Leopard tortoise (Stigmochelys pardalis)[117,376]	Galapagos tortoise (Chelonoidis nigra)[376]
Hematology			
PCV (%)	28 (9-43)	23 (8-37)	18 (7-29)
RBC ($10^6/\mu L$)	0.61 (0.08-1.15)	0.52 (0.15-1.06)	0.40 (0.16-0.63)
Hgb (g/dL)	7.7 (2.4-13.1)	16.1 (8.8-28)	5.5 (3.3-8.9)
MCV (fL)	418 (156-678)	488 (179-833)	535 (266-769)
MCH (pg)	116 (2.1-193)	83	160 (100-239)
MCHC (g/dL)	30 (20-40)	44 (42-46)	31 (24-38)
WBC ($10^3/\mu L$)	4.41 (0.87-13.23)	4.24 (0.6-10.0)	4.57 (0.71-17.5)
Heterophils ($10^3/\mu L$)	1.92 (0.23-7.43)	1.92 (0.11-4.87)	1.57 (0.10-6.76)
Lymphocytes ($10^3/\mu L$)	1.41 (0.17-6.06)	1.61 (0.05-4.74)	1.45 (0.04-6.56)
Monocytes ($10^3/\mu L$)	0.01 (0.01-0.37)	0.08 (0.02-0.62)	0.08 (0.02-0.33)
Azurophils ($10^3/\mu L$)	0.04 (0-0.84)	0.02 (0-0.51)	0.03 (0-0.52)
Eosinophils ($10^3/\mu L$)	0.10 (0.01-0.43)	0.15 (0.02-0.37)	0.09 (0.02-0.40)
Basophils ($10^3/\mu L$)	0.12 (0.01-0.36)	0.11 (0.01-0.34)	0.34 (0.03-1.38)
Chemistries			
ALP (U/L)	36 (10-70)	107 (21-278)	77 (27-235)
ALT (U/L)	9 (0-33)	8	3 (0-18)
Amylase (U/L)	1359 (399-2240)	—	22 (3-41)
AST (U/L)	108 (34-401)	54 (5-119)	40 (16-122)
Bilirubin, total (mg/dL)	0.1 (0-0.7)	0.1	0.3 (0-0.8)
BUN (mg/dL)	3 (1-6)	12 (1-36)	12 (3-35)
Calcium (mg/dL)	11.4 (7.8-21.2)	11.8 (6.5-18.3)	10.4 (6.6-17.8)
Chloride (mEq/L)	109 (93-124)	104 (90-119)	98 (83-112)
Cholesterol (mg/dL)	129 (36-283)	111 (9-239)	172 (42-450)
Creatine kinase (U/L)	407 (31-2088)	359 (223-704)	592 (35-2378)
Creatinine (mg/dL)	0.3 (0.1-0.4)	0.6	0.2 (0-0.4)
GGT (U/L)	14 (3-19)	—	4 (0-11)
Glucose (mg/dL)	107 (55-220)	75 (10-152)	98 (35-312)
Iron (μg/dL)	81 (80-82)	—	73 (8-593)
LDH (U/L)	977 (140-3264)	446 (346-546)	469 (71-1212)
Phosphorus (mg/dL)	3.8 (1.5-6.5)	2.7 (1.1-5.2)	3.7 (2.0-8.0)
Potassium (mEq/L)	6.1 (3.3-11.9)	5.4 (2.3-8.8)	4.8 (3.4-7.2)
Protein, total (g/dL)	3.8 (1.2-6.3)	3.3 (1.9-6.2)	4.7 (1.8-7.9)
Albumin (g/dL)[b]	1.5 (0-2.3)	1.6 (0.3-2.9)	1.6 (0.4-2.7)
Globulin (g/dL)[b]	2.3 (0.4-3.8)	2.6 (0.6-4.6)	3.1 (1.1-5.5)
Sodium (mEq/L)	139 (125-154)	132 (115-148)	130 (119-140)
α-tocopherol (μg/dL)	—	—	2 (1,2)
Triglyceride (mg/dL)	163 (53-388)	—	271 (29-1345)
Free T_3	—	—	29
Uric acid (mg/dL)	4.6 (0.6-10.4)	2.5 (0.5-6.6)	1.7 (0.1-4.0)

TABLE 4-10	Hematologic and Serum Biochemical Values of Reptiles. (cont'd)		
Measurement	Eastern box turtle (*Terrapene carolina*)[73,99,103,189,376]	Ornate box turtle (*Terrapene ornata*)[117,376]	Wood turtle (*Glyptemys insculpta*)[376]
Hematology			
PCV (%)	24 (8-37)	23 (10-37)	25 (9-41)
RBC (10^6/µL)	0.56 (0.08-1.03)	0.62 (0.46-0.8)	—
Hgb (g/dL)	6.8 (2.6-11.0)	7.2 (6-9)	—
MCV (fL)	396 (117-750)	408 (350-463)	—
MCH (pg)	110 (30-207)	122 (108-136)	—
MCHC (g/dL)	29 (14-43)	33 (31-33)	—
WBC (10^3/µL)	5.48 (1.34-15.9)	5.76 (1.2-13.4)	5.20 (0.8-20.0)
Heterophils (10^3/µL)	1.61 (0.15-6.4)	2.01 (0.10-5.9)	—
Lymphocytes (10^3/µL)	1.61 (0.15-9.82)	2.19 (0.10-7.60)	3.15 (0.59-13.0)
Monocytes (10^3/µL)	0.19 (0.18-0.80)	0.13 (0.02-0.74)	—
Azurophils (10^3/µL)	0.03 (0-0.80)	0.03 (0-0.13)	0.08 (0-1.11)
Eosinophils (10^3/µL)	0.47 (0.42-3.01)	0.23 (0.03-1.32)	—
Basophils (10^3/µL)	0.55 (0.4-2.14)	0.25 (0.02-0.92)	—
Chemistries			
ALP (U/L)	77 (20-225)	61 (14-139)	71 (21-268)
ALT (U/L)	6 (0-20)	30 (25-33)	—
Amylase (U/L)	1033 (87-2526)	691 (2-1893)	—
AST (U/L)	64 (14-191)	61 (11-141)	79 (14-212)
Bilirubin, total (mg/dL)	0.1 (0.1-0.4)	0.3 (0.1-0.4)	—
BUN (mg/dL)	52 (6-121)	60 (4-154)	—
Calcium (mg/dL)	10.5 (6.8-23.2)[d]	10.3 (6.2-17.5)	11.8 (6.3-29.4)
Chloride (mEq/L)	106 (89-121)	108 (93-124)	—
Cholesterol (mg/dL)	205 (42-483)	201 (20-469)	—
Creatine kinase (U/L)	153 (23-747)	196 (0-777)	—
Creatinine (mg/dL)	0.2 (0-0.5)	1 (0.2-2.4)	—
Glucose (mg/dL)	48 (23-114)	67 (13-120)	53 (13-108)
LDH (U/L)	307 (20-1032)	362 (300-424)	—
Phosphorus (mg/dL)	3.5 (1.7-7.5)	3.3 (1.9-5.8)	3.2 (1.6-10)
Potassium (mEq/L)	4.7 (3.1-9.4)	4.7 (2.4-8.2)	—
Protein, total (g/dL)	3.20 (3.10-3.90)	4.0 (1.4-6.6)	4.7 (1.5-6.5)

Continued

TABLE 4-10 Hematologic and Serum Biochemical Values of Reptiles. (cont'd)

Measurement	Eastern box turtle (*Terrapenecarolina*)	Ornate box turtle (*Terrapene ornata*)	Wood turtle (*Glyptemys insculpta*)
Protein, total (male; g/dL)	3.00 (1.80-5.20)	—	—
Protein, total (female; g/dL)	4.00 (2.20-6.20)	—	—
Haptoglobin	0.25 (0.27-0.38)	—	—
Albumin (g/dL)[b]	2.2 (1.2-3.2)	1.5 (0.2-2.8)	—
Pre-alb (PEP; g/dL)[b]	0 (0-0.002)	—	—
Albumin (PEP; g/dL)[b]	0.71-0.85	—	—
Globulin (g/dL)[b]	3.4 (2.5-4.7)	2.4 (0.6-4.3)	—
α-1 Glob (PEP; g/dL)[b]	0.25 (0.25-0.30)	—	—
α-2 Glob (PEP; g/dL)[b]	0.80 (0.76-0.92)	—	—
β Glob (PEP; g/dL)[b]	1.27 (1.27-1.55)	—	—
γ Glob (PEP; g/dL)[b]	0.26 (0.27-0.32)	—	—
A:G ratio	0.27-0.31	—	—
Sodium (mEq/L)	139 (120-155)	141 (129-154)	—
Uric acid (mg/dL)	0.7 (0.1-2.9)	0.6 (0-1.9)	1.0 (0-4.1)

Measurement	Pacific pond turtle (*Actinemys marmorata*)[376]	Sliders (*Trachemys scripta* spp.)[65,111,117,168,376]	Painted turtle (*Chrysemys picta*)[111,168,376]
Hematology			
PCV (%)	24 (7-42)	26 (8-44)	25 (6-43)
RBC (10^6/μL)	0.69 (0.24-1.20)	0.84 (0.33-2.21)	0.57 (0.41-0.68)
Hgb (g/dL)	7.6 (3.0-12.6)	11.1 (10-12.2)	11.2 (10.7-11.7)
MCV (fL)	377 (200-634)	409 (179-697)	271 (183-365)
MCH (pg)	107 (19-186)	108	—
MCHC (g/dL)	27 (18-42)	30	—
WBC (10^3/μL)	5.94 (1.02-17.0)	6.73 (1.0-19.4)	9.49 (0.40-23.2)
Heterophils (10^3/μL)	1.83 (0.14-5.52)	2.33 (0.18-5.86)	2.30 (0.17-8.39)
Lymphocytes (10^3/μL)	2.46 (0.22-8.48)	2.28 (0.03-6.90)	2.60 (0.01-7.07)
Monocytes (10^3/μL)	—	0.18 (0.04-0.65)	—
Azurophils (10^3/μL)	0.04 (0-0.43)	0.05 (0-0.48)	0.05 (0-0.26)
Eosinophils (10^3/μL)	0.37 (0.02-1.81)	0.52 (0.01-3.06)	—
Basophils (10^3/μL)	0.62 (0.05-2.09)	1.07 (0.01-3.56)	1.95 (0.04-5.91)
Chemistries			
ALP (U/L)	—	113 (30-372)	208
ALT (U/L)	—	14 (1-66)	—
Amylase (U/L)	—	493 (411-535)	—
AST (U/L)	105 (26-228)	141 (44-358)	132 (45-284)

TABLE 4-10 Hematologic and Serum Biochemical Values of Reptiles. (cont'd)

Measurement	Pacific pond turtle (*Actinemys marmorata*)	Sliders (*Trachemys scripta* spp.)	Painted turtle (*Chrysemys picta*)
Bilirubin, total (mg/dL)	—	0.2 (0.1-0.5)	0.1
BUN (mg/dL)	—	23 (2-64)	37
Calcium (mg/dL)	10.0 (7.0-14.5)	12.6 (6.5-22.6)	11.7 (5.5-19.1)
Chloride (mEq/L)	—	98 (88-112)	96 (73-109)
Cholesterol (mg/dL)	—	162 (106-227)	—
Creatine kinase (U/L)	242 (63-747)	516 (108-2125)	352 (35-1608)
Creatinine (mg/dL)	—	0.3 (0.2-0.5)	—
GGT (U/L)	—	7 (0-21)	—
Glucose (mg/dL)	53 (4-113)	54 (21-143)	63 (10-133)
Iron (μg/dL)	—	—	—
LDH (U/L)	—	1713 (371-5763)	412
Lipase (U/L)	—	6 (1-15)	—
Magnesium (mEq/L)	—	2.2	4.8
Phosphorus (mg/dL)	3.6 (1.9-6.6)	4.0 (1.8-8.8)	3.6 (1.7-7.2)
Potassium (mEq/L)	4.3 (2.3-7.1)	3.8 (2.4-7.5)	3.6 (2.2-11.6)
Protein, total (g/dL)	4.4 (1.8-7.0)	4.8 (1.1-8.8)	4.4 (1.8-7.7)
Albumin (g/dL)[b]	1.7 (0.7-2.7)	1.8 (0.6-3.3)	1.3 (0-2.7)
Globulin (g/dL)[b]	2.8 (1.0-4.6)	3.2 (1.1-5.9)	3.0 (0.1-5.9)
Sodium (mEq/L)	135 (123-147)	134 (123-147)	137 (119-146)
Triglyceride (mg/dL)	—	304 (30-664)	—
Uric acid (mg/dL)	0.9 (0-3.1)	0.8 (0.1-1.9)	0.7 (0.1-1.8)

Measurement	Loggerhead sea turtle (*Caretta caretta*)[67,376]	Green sea turtle (*Chelonia mydas*)[98,370,376]	Hawksbill sea turtle (*Eretmochelys imbricata*)[h,376,392]
Hematology			
PCV (%)	32 (18-40)	33 (23-45)	13-41
RBC (10^6/μL)	0.52 (0.22-1.22)	0.52 (0.21-0.97)	—
Hgb (g/dL)	10.7	10.7	—
MCV (fL)	416 (82-1027)	717 (320-1429)	—
MCH (pg)	55	55	—
MCHC (g/dL)	36	36	—
WBC (10^3/μL)	9.00 (5.00-12.50)	9.98 (3.76-21.7)	—
Heterophils (10^3/μL)	3.67 (0.35-7.16)	6.69 (1.57-15.7)	—
Lymphocytes (10^3/μL)	2.72 (0.30-4.83)	2.14 (0.94-4.34)	—
Monocytes (10^3/μL)	0.96 (0.22-1.84)	0.91 (0.23-1.81)	—
Azurophils (10^3/μL)	—	—	—
Eosinophils (10^3/μL)	1.15 (0.45-2.10)	0.12 (0-0.48)	—
Basophils (10^3/μL)	—	0.13 (0-1.94)	—

Continued

TABLE 4-10 Hematologic and Serum Biochemical Values of Reptiles. (cont'd)

Measurement	Loggerhead sea turtle (*Caretta caretta*)	Green sea turtle (*Chelonia mydas*)	Hawksbill sea turtle (*Eretmochelys imbricata*)
Chemistries			
ALP (U/L)	64 (11-254)	6-67	7-80
ALT (U/L)	—	32 (3-241)	1-23
Amylase (U/L)	—	534	—
AST (U/L)	154 (10-480)	74-245	74-245
Bilirubin, total (mg/dL)	—	0.03-0.2	0-10
BUN (mg/dL)	105 (19-162)	64 (13.9-173)	7-34
Calcium (mg/dL)	6.9 (2.2-11.5)	8-8.8	2.6-11.6
Chloride (mEq/L)	118 (103-137)	101-121	106-134
Cholesterol (mg/dL)	—	221 (142-354)	—
Creatine kinase (U/L)	899 (258-3586)	326-2729	14-6008
Creatinine (mg/dL)	—	0.25 (0.1-1.6)	—
GGT (U/L)	—	6 (0-21)	—
Glucose (mg/dL)	120 (66-177)	67-178	79-162
Iron (μg/dL)	—	362 (117-600)	6-67
LDH (U/L)	—	75-477	—
Lipase (U/L)	—	—	—
Magnesium (mEq/L)	—	4.8-12.2	3.4-7.1
Phosphorus (mg/dL)	9.3 (3.7-14.0)	4.9-11.1	1.9-8.7
Potassium (mEq/L)	3.9 (2.7-5.1)	3-7.1	3.0-5.3
Protein, total (g/dL)	3.3 (1.2-6.9)	2.1-6.2	1.3-5.1
Albumin (g/dL)[b]	1.5 (0.7-2.6)	0.7-1.8	0.3-1.4
Globulin (g/dL)[b]	2.2 (0.2-4.9)	1.5-4.7	0.8-4.8
Sodium (mEq/L)	153 (142-164)	139-158	146-159
Triglyceride (mg/dL)	—	492 (124-932)	—
Uric acid (mg/dL)	0.5 (0-1.2)	1.1 (0-2.7)	0.6 (0-1.8)

[a]Listed values are median followed by either min-max or a confidence interval in parentheses depending on reported methods and the authors' judgment from the available evidence, unless a single value indicating n=1, or a range that is not enclosed in parentheses indicating a reported reference interval.
[b]Albumin is measured by colorimetry (e.g., bromocresol green) and globulin value is calculated unless otherwise indicated (PEP = protein electrophoresis).
[c]Remarkably high reference ranges for Ca (mean, 159 mg/dL; range, 30-337 mg/dL) and P (mean, 35 mg/dL; range, 8-69) have also been reported.[85]
[d]Can be elevated in gravid females[189,286]
[e]These data were obtained from iguanas housed outdoors with unfiltered sunlight.
[f]Adults.
[g]Calculated from data.
[h]Juveniles.

TABLE 4-11 Environmental, Dietary, and Reproductive Characteristics of Reptiles.[117,284,322]

Species	Environmental Preference		Diet[d]	Method of Reproduction[e]	Gestation/Incubation Period (days)[f]
	Temperature[a-c]	RH (%)			
Snakes					
Ball (Royal) python (*Python regius*)	25-30°C (77-86°F)	70-80 (use humidity box)[g]	C	Ov	90
Boa constrictor (*Boa constrictor*)	28-34°C (82-93°F)	50-70 (use humidity box)[g]	C	V	120-240
Garter snake (*Thamnophis sirtalis*)	22-30°C (72-86°F)	60-80 (use humidity box)[g]	C	V	90-110
King snake (*Lampropeltis getulus*)	23-30°C (73-86°F)	50-70 (use humidity box)[g]	Op/c	Ov	50-60
Sand boa (*Eryx sp.*)	25-30°C (77-86°F)	20-30	C	V	120-180
Lizards					
Bearded dragon (*Pogona vitticeps*)	21-35°C (70-95°F)	— (use humidity box)[g]	I—young H–adult	Ov	65-90
Crested gecko (*Correlophus ciliatus*)	25-28°C (77-82°F)	50-70 (use humidity box)[g]	F/i	Ov	60-150
Leopard gecko (*Eublepharis macularius*)	25-30°C (77-86°F)	20-30 (use humidity box)[g]	I	Ov	55-60
Uromastyx/ spiny-tailed lizard (*Uromastyx sp.*)	26-49°C (80-120°F) Large cage for gradient	— (use humidity box)[g]	H/seeds	Ov	60-80
Veiled chameleon (*Chameleo calyptratus*)	20-30°C (75-95°F)	50-70 Need good ventilation	I	Ov	200
Water dragon (*Physignathus cocincinus*)	25-34°C (77-93°F)	80-90 Need water with filter[h]	I/om	Ov	90
Chelonians					
Common box turtle (*Terrapene carolina*)	24-29°C (75-84°F)	60-80 (use humidity box)[g]	C/f	Ov	50-90

Continued

TABLE 4-11 Environmental, Dietary, and Reproductive Characteristics of Reptiles. (cont'd)

Species	Environmental Preference		Diet	Method of Reproduction	Gestation/ Incubation Period (days)
	Temperature	RH (%)			
Desert tortoise (*Gopherus agassizii*)	25-30°C (77-86°F)	— (use humidity box)[g]	H	Ov	84-120
Greek tortoise (*Testudo graeca*)	20-27°C (68-81°F)	30-50 (use humidity box)[g]	H/om	Ov	60
Painted turtle (*Chrysemys picta*)	23-28°C (73-82°F)	80-90 Need water with filter[h]	H/I/o	Ov	47-99
Red-eared slider (*Trachemys scripta elegans*)	22-30°C (72-86°F)	80-90 Need water with filter[h]	C	Ov	59-93
Russian tortoise (*Agrionemys horsfieldii*)	21-32°C (70-90°F)	— (use humidity box)[g]	H	Ov	56-84
Crocodilian					
American alligator (*Alligator mississippiensis*)	30-35°C (86-95°F)	80-90 Need water with filter[h]	C/p	Ov	62-65

C, carnivorous; *F*, frugivorous; *H*, herbivorous; *I*, insectivorous; *O*, molluscavorous; *Om*, omnivorous; *Op*, ophiophagus; *P*, piscivorous; *RH*, relative humidity; *V*, viviparous; *Ov*, oviparous.

[a]Temperatures shown are ideal ambient daytime temperature gradients. These should be allowed to fall by approximately 5°C (9°F) during the night. "Hot-spot" temperatures should generally be 5°C (9°F) greater than the highest temperature shown.

[b]Preferred daytime temperature range for other commonly housed captive snakes are: rosy boa (*Lichanura trivirgata*) = 27-29.5°C (81-85°F); green tree python (*Morelia viridis*): 24-28°C (75-82°F); carpet python (*Morelia spilota*): 27-29.5°C (81-85°F); corn snake (*Pantherophis guttata*): 25-30°C (77-86°F); yellow rat snake (*Elaphe obsoleta*): 25-29°C (77-84°F); gopher/bullsnake (*Pituophis melanoleucus*): 25-29°C (77-84°F).

[c]Preferred daytime temperature range for other commonly housed captive lizards are: day gecko (*Phelsuma* sp.): 29.5°C (85°F); chameleons (montane) (*Chamaeleo* spp.): 21-27°C (70-81°F); chameleons (lowland) (*Chamaeleo* spp.): 27-29°C (81-84°F); bearded dragon (*Pogona vitticeps*): 26.7-29.5°C (80-85°F); blue-tongued skink (*Tiliqua* sp.): 27-29.5°C (81-85°F); monitor lizards (*Varanus* spp.): 29-31°C (84-88°F); tegus (*Tupinambis* spp.): 27-30°C (81-86°F).

[d]Uppercase letters denote principal dietary requirements; lowercase denotes secondary preference.

[e]Temperature-dependent.

[f]Can have long hatch times dependent on incubation parameters.

[g]This simulates humid underground burrow. Use dark colored plastic container with cut entrance, moistened paper towels or sphagnum moss.

[h]Need to set up water component like fish tank with proper filter (use one for koi or turtles), pump, water quality testing, dechlorinator.

TABLE 4-12 Urinalysis Values of Chelonians.[116,163,203,205]

Measurement	Normal Values	Abnormal Values
Specific gravity	1.003-1.014 (mean, 1.008)	Up to 1.034
pH	Herbivores: alkaline Omnivores: 5-8	Acidic[a]
Color	Colorless to pale yellow with white urates	Dark yellow, yellow-brown, yellow-green
Turbidity	Clear	Cloudy
Protein	Trace proteinuria	Increased proteinuria
Glucose	Glucosuria up to 30 mg/dL	Glucosuria can be higher than 50 mg/dL with anorexia
Renal casts	None	Various types present
Calcium, phosphorus, ammonia, urea, creatinine	Detectable in urine	Significantly increased in urine of *Testudo* spp. with renal disease
AST, CK, LDH	Detectable in urine	Significantly increased in urine of *Testudo* spp. with renal disease
Crystals	Amorphous urates/ammonium biurates	Many other crystals found in renal failure; uric acid crystals in gout; bilirubin and tyrosine crystals in liver disease

[a]May be associated with hibernation, anorexia, and improper diet.

TABLE 4-13 Selected Products and Guidelines Used in Force-Feeding Anorectic or Debilitated Reptiles.[a,b]

Agent	Guidelines	Species/Comments
Alfalfa pellets (e.g., iguana or rabbit pellets) or powder (Alfalfa Powder, NOW Foods)	Blend (1:4) with electrolyte solution or water; 20-30 mL/kg PO q48h (lizards) to q84h (chelonians)[36,359]	Herbivorous reptiles/administer via gavage or esophagostomy tube; may clog feeding tube; for iguanas, may gavage equal volume of water on alternate days until patient is stable and eating;[359] soaked pellets can also be hand-fed (especially by owner)
Baby foods	Vegetable; blend in with other food sources	Herbivorous reptiles/administer via gavage; for some species, some fruit baby food can be added
	Meat (small amount); blend in with other food sources	Omnivorous species/administer by gavage
Commercial dry or moist diets, which are Genera specific (e.g., Fluker's, Zilla, Tetra, Zoo Med, etc.)	Blend (1:4) with electrolyte solution or water; 20-30 mL/kg or 3% body weight PO q48h (lizards) to q72h (chelonians)	Herbivorous, omnivorous, insectivorous reptiles/administer via gavage or esophagostomy tube; may clog feeding tube; for iguanas, may gavage equal volume of water on alternate days until patient is stable and eating; soaked pellets can also be hand-fed (especially by owner)

Continued

TABLE 4-13 Selected Products and Guidelines Used in Force-Feeding Anorectic or Debilitated Reptiles. (cont'd)

Agent	Guidelines	Species/Comments
Dog/cat food, canned (a/d, Hill's; Maximum-Calorie, Iams; Nutritional Recovery Formula, Eukanuba)	30 mL/kg POq7-14d[117,197]	Carnivorous species/administer via gavage; although low protein (8.5%), some concern over high purine and vitamin A levels (probably OK unless concurrent renal disease); in dehydrated animals, dilute 1:1 with physiologic solution, pediatric oral human electrolyte solution (Pedialyte, Ross), or Gatorade (Gatorade); once stabilized, small whole animals (lubricated with egg white) can be force-fed
Electrolyte solutions (Pedialyte, Ross; Gatorade, Gatorade)	15-25 mL/kg PO q24h	Most species; no data with respect to costs/benefits
Emeraid Omnivore, Herbivore, Carnivore, and Piscivore Critical Care Powder Formulas	Mix as labeled, generally to pancake batter consistency, feed small amount to start (see bag suggestion) once daily	Herbivorous, omnivorous, insectivorous, carnivorous, piscivorous reptiles/administer via gavage or esophagostomy tube; may clog feeding tube; typically follow the general feeding sequence: first feed 1% body weight, second feed 2% body weight, third feed 3% body weight
High protein powders (Carnivore Care, Oxbow Pet Products; Emeraid Carnivore, Lafeber)	Mix as labeled, generally to pancake batter consistency, feed small amount to start (see bag suggestion) once daily	Insectivorous and carnivorous species/once reconstituted, can be mixed 1:1 with an alfalfa or timothy product for true omnivorous reptiles; administer via gavage
Vetark Professional Critical Care Formula (CCF) Powder	Mix as labeled	Herbivorous, omnivorous reptiles/administer via gavage or esophagostomy tube; may clog feeding tube

[a]General guidelines for force-feeding: generally provide nutrition following rehydration of patient; needs may vary with specific disease (e.g., low protein with renal disease); force-feeding volumes are frequently started at a low/modest level and gradually brought up to the desired level (for patients with severe disease/cachexia, transition should be very gradual); concurrent to force-feeding and hydrating a patient, highly palatable food items should be provided for voluntary food intake.

[b]Dietary fiber supplements (alfalfa pellets or powder; barley powder; purified cellulose) should be an integral part of enteral therapy for herbivorous reptiles.

TABLE 4-14 Guidelines for Tracheal/Pulmonary and Colonic Lavage in Reptiles.[19,251,278]

Snakes

Tracheal/pulmonary lavage	Anesthesia often not necessary in debilitated animals; pass red rubber catheter through glottis to premeasured distance; infuse with 5-10 mL/kg of tepid (29°C, 85°F), sterile 0.9% saline; massage and rock the snake's body to loosen debris; aspirate
Colonic lavage	Pass lubricated soft red rubber catheter into cloaca; infuse with 10-20 mL/kg of tepid (29°C, 85°F), sterile saline; massage coelomic cavity and gently aspirate

Lizards

Tracheal/pulmonary lavage	General anesthesia is typically necessary; if possible, intubate with sterile endotracheal tube; pass sterile catheter inside lumen (premeasure distance to sample site); infuse 5-10 mL/kg of tepid (29°C, 85°F), sterile 0.9% saline and aspirate several times; not all fluid will be recovered
Colonic lavage	Pass lubricated soft red rubber catheter into cloaca without excessive force; infuse 10 mL/kg of tepid (29°C, 85°F), sterile saline and gently aspirate several times

Chelonians

Tracheal/pulmonary lavage	Sedation or anesthesia usually necessary; intubate with sterile endotracheal tube if possible; pass radiomarked catheter into affected lung lobe; may be helpful to bend it in the direction of the lobe prior to insertion, though location cannot be assured without orthogonal radiographic evidence of placement; infuse with tepid (29°C, 85°F), sterile saline at 5-10 mL/kg; gently aspirate
Colonic lavage	Pass lubricated red rubber catheter into cloaca; infuse with tepid (29°C, 85°F), sterile saline at no more than 10 mL/kg; gently aspirate; repeat several times

TABLE 4-15 Venipuncture Sites Commonly Used in Reptiles.[a,148,152,321,372,385]

Snakes

Ventral caudal vein	Ventral aspect of tail caudal to cloaca under central scute; avoid hemipenes and anal sacs, can be difficult to collect from in boas, pythons, anacondas; may in rare cases lead to tail necrosis/paresis
Heart	Dorsal recumbency; insertion of needle under central abdominal scale at 45° angle caudal to heart; pericardial fluid contamination can occur

Lizards

Ventral caudal vein	Ventral aspect of vertebral body under center of middle scale; avoid hemipenes and anal sacs; this vein can also be approached laterally by inserting needle under lateral process of vertebral body aiming toward midline; ventral approach may in rare cases lead to tail necrosis/paresis
Ventral abdominal vein	Vein is located on caudal to middle midline within inner surface of abdominal wall; insert 25-g needle (bent at 45° angle) cranially, at acute angle to skin and in midline of abdomen, just caudal to umbilicus; avoid urinary bladder in species that have one
Jugular vein	Veins are lateral and deep; insert needle caudal to tympanum; best tried in larger animals

Continued

TABLE 4-15 Venipuncture Sites Commonly Used in Reptiles. (cont'd)

Chelonians

Jugular vein	Lymphatic contamination can be a concern with most locations of phlebotomy in chelonians, however, jugular considered less likely
	Right vein often larger than left; runs level with tympanum to base of neck with head extended; may require sedation
Subcarapacial vein and plexus	The sinus accessed with patient's head either extended or retracted; depending on conformation of carapace, needle may be bent up to 60° and positioned in midline just caudal to skin insertion of dorsal aspect of neck and ventral aspect of cranial rim of carapace; needle is advanced in caudodorsal direction, with slight negative pressure; can cause significant internal hemorrhage or paresis in some cases
Dorsal caudal vein	Close to carapace, dorsal to dorsal aspect of vertebral body; lymph dilution common
Brachial vein/plexus	Near triceps tendon at lateral aspect of radiohumeral joint (elbow), foreleg grasped/extended, triceps tendon palpated near caudal aspect of elbow joint, needle inserted ventral to tendon with syringe perpendicular to forearm
Interdigital vessels of rear flippers	Adult leatherback sea turtles, about 2.5 cm deep, near phalangeal junctions, best at P1-P2; along side of phalanx, 20°-30° angle to flipper surface

Crocodilians

Ventral caudal vein	Ventral aspect of vertebral body under center of middle scale; avoid hemipenes and anal sacs; this vein can also be approached laterally by inserting needle under lateral process of vertebral body aiming toward midline; ventral approach may in rare cases lead to tail necrosis/paresis
Supravertebral vein	Position needle in dorsal midline, just caudal to occiput and perpendicular to skin surface, slowly advance needle with slight negative pressure; excessive penetration can cause spinal trauma

[a]Generally recommended to collect only 0.7% body weight in healthy reptiles, less in debilitated animals, so 0.7 mL total in 100 g animal.

TABLE 4-16 Treatment of Dystocia in Reptiles.[a,16,37,74,91,283,373]

Etiologies

- Poor environmental conditions (improper thermal environment, lack of suitable nesting substrate, shallow nesting substrate; underground obstructions [e.g., roots or buried rocks], disturbance, lack of visual security, etc.)
- Social factors (e.g., competition, fighting, recent introduction of male)
- Dietary imbalances (e.g., calcium deficiency, hypovitaminosis A), malnutrition
- Endocrine imbalances
- Nutritional secondary hyperparathyroidism
- Uterine inertia
- Dehydration
- Renal disease
- Egg yolk coelomitis
- Cystic or cloacal calculi
- Infections (e.g., uterus)
- Anatomic anomalies of the reproductive tract, eggs, pelvis, or shell of chelonians
- Other (substrate ingestion, overfeeding, other illness, inadequate exercise)

TABLE 4-16 Treatment of Dystocia in Reptiles. (cont'd)

Diagnosis

- History and clinical signs (prolonged anorexia, lethargy, posterior paresis, straining/tenesmus, increased pacing/seeking, excavating nests without oviposition, straining to pass eggs, passage of a few eggs but not a full clutch, fluid discharge from cloaca)
- Knowledge of normal egg retention time or usual season for laying
- Physical examination (gentle palpation of inguinal or prefemoral fossa or caudal coelom; eggs may not be palpable)
- CBC (anemia, elevated or decreased WBCs)
- Plasma biochemical analysis (hyperproteinemia, elevated ALP activity, hypercalcemia [total calcium elevated], hypocalcemia [ionized Ca <1 mmol/L])
- Coelomic effusion aspirate and cytology—carefully avoid aspirating from the urinary bladder, oviducts, or eggs when collecting coelomic fluid samples
- Radiography (tortoise eggs have a calcified outer shell and appear radiographically similar to avian eggs; turtles, lizards, and snakes generally have soft-shelled eggs with soft-tissue density on radiographs)
- Ultrasound
- Coelioscopy—particularly to confirm coelomitis, salpingitis, or oviduct rupture; determine whether early surgical management is appropriate

Treatment

- If patient is stable, provide proper environmental conditions (appropriate thermal environment, humidity, nesting site, substrate material, substrate depth, and substrate moisture; minimal stimulus; isolation)
- Handle gently and infrequently
- Tepid ($\sim$29°C; $\sim$85°F) water soak, 30-60 min q24h
- Rehydration—fluid therapy prn; do not administer fluids intracoelomically
- Alert, strong, stable, responsive females that are eating well will often oviposit without further therapy if given sufficient time
- Dextrose (SC, IV) may be of value in some cases
- Calcium (see Table 4-8; only if hypocalcemic; low Ca^{++} not generally a problem in snakes)
  - Ca glycerophosphate/Ca lactate (Calphosan, Glenwood) (5 mg each/mL): 5 mg/kg SC, IM
  - Ca gluconate: 100-200 mg/kg SC, IM
- Oxytocin[b] (see Table 4-7)
  - Generally administer 1 hr after Ca^{++} injection
  - 1-10 U/kg IM, ICe in lizards and snakes (results are variable); 1-20 U/kg IM, IV, ICe for chelonians
  - Repeat dose q1h; response is more rapid after IV administration in turtles
- Arginine vasotocin[c] (Sigma Chemical) (alternative to oxytocin) (see Table 4-7)
  - 0.01-1 µg/kg IV (preferred), ICe
- Dinoprostone gel (Prepidil, Upjohn) 0.9 mg/kg intracloacally followed 20 min later by prostaglandin $F_{2\alpha}$ (Lutalyse, Zoetis) 0.6 mg/kg IM
- Propranolol 1 mg/kg followed by prostaglandin $F_{2\alpha}$ 0.025 mg/kg[d]
- Prostaglandin $F_{2\alpha}$ (Lutalyse, 5 mg/mL)
  - 1.5 mg/kg SC in turtles
  - Efficacy may improve if given 20 min after an α_2 agonist (dexmedetomidine 0.035 mg/kg or xylazine 8 mg/kg)
- Lubricate cloaca with water soluble gel
- Manual massage may be useful in some situations—avoid causing oviduct rupture or prolapse
- Salpingotomy may be required if declining clinical condition (i.e., anorexia, dehydration, lethargy)

[a]Although most reptiles are oviparous, some, including garter snakes, water snakes, boas (not pythons), vipers, Jackson's chameleons, horned lizards, and Solomon Island prehensile-tailed skinks are viviparous.
[b]Use only if *no* evidence of obstructive dystocia or broken eggs.
[c]Appears to be more effective than oxytocin in many reptiles, but it is not commercially available for use in animals.
[d]Effective in healthy *Sceloporus* sp., did not induce oviposition in iguanas; may be effective in chelonians.

TABLE 4-17 Treatment of Metabolic Bone Diseases in Reptiles.[194]

Etiology

- Improper Ca:P ratio; lack of dietary Ca
- Lack of vitamin D_3
- Lack of UVA and UVB light spectrum
- Renal disease
- Other: low ambient temperature, protein deficiency, small intestinal disease, parathyroid disease, etc.

Clinical Signs

- Lethargy, reluctance to move
- Poor appetite or anorexia
- Weight loss or poor weight gain
- Softening of the mandible; shortened/rounded mandible and maxilla; symmetrical swelling of the mandible (fibrous osteodystrophy)
- Fibrous osteodystrophy of the long bones of the legs
- Difficulty in lifting body off ground when walking
- Pathologic fractures
- Ataxia, paresis, or paralysis of the rear legs due to collapsed vertebrae or vertebral luxation
- Osteoporosis
- Hypocalcemic muscle fasciculations and seizures
- Soft shell in chelonians
- Constipation
- Inability to evert/replace hemipenes

Diagnosis

- Dietary and environmental history
- Clinical signs
- Physical examination
- Radiography
- Serum Ca:P ratio; usually inverse (1:2+) with renal etiology
- Uric acid levels
- Ionized calcium levels
- Calcidiol (25-hydroxyvitamin D) levels (Michigan State University)
- UV meter readings of enclosure
- Dual energy x-ray absorptiometry (DEXA) scan
- Determination of glomerular filtration rate
- Renal nuclear medicine
- Renal biopsy

Treatment

- Provide species-correct environmental temperature ranges for day and night
- Correct diet as needed; usually changing to improve calcium:phosphorus ratio
- Use species-appropriate UVA/UVB lighting arrangement
    - Use fluorescent or mercury vapor bulbs, or light emitting plasma lamps
    - Provide areas to hide, as corneal and skin burns can occur
    - In general:
        - Desert-dwelling diurnal lizards/chelonians, high UVB levels (10% or full unfiltered sun, 6 hr)
        - Diurnal arboreal lizards/semiaquatic basking chelonians, moderate levels of UVB (5%, 4 hr)
        - Diurnal terrestrial lizards/chelonians from forested environment, low levels of UVB (5%, 2 hr)
        - Nocturnal lizards, low levels of UVB (2%, 2 hr)—focus more on oral vitamin D_3
        - Snakes seem to get adequate levels of calcium/cholecalciferol from ingestion of whole vertebrate prey (or earthworms); exceptions are diamond and green tree pythons, indigo snakes, some aquatic species, rough/smooth green snakes, other arboreal, diurnal snakes
        - Albino (amelanistic), hypomelanistic, snow, blizzard, pastel, tangerine, lavender, yellow, pied, anerythristic, leucistic, xanthochromistic, or any other genetic mutant with less than normal levels of melanin are more susceptible to UV light burns of the eyes and dorsal skin, so lower levels of UV supplementation (if any) should be provided, oral vitamin D_3 may need to be considered

TABLE 4-17 Treatment of Metabolic Bone Diseases in Reptiles. (cont'd)

- Force-feeding (following rehydration) (see Table 4-13)
    - Use species-appropriate diet, especially useful for immature animals as maintenance until improving and closer to adult size, esophageal feeding tube usually needed for chelonians to avoid beak fractures
- Ca supplementation options (see Table 4-8)—best to use human products
    - Calcium carbonate (400 mg calcium/g product)
    - Calcium citrate (210 mg calcium/g product)
    - Calcium phosphate
- Maintain hydration
    - Fluid therapy, as needed
    - Soak in warm water (shallow) for 10-20 min q12-24 h to encourage drinking and defecation (caution: head may need to be supported; do not leave unattended)
- Vitamin D_3 (see Table 4-8)
    - Best source is UVA/UVB exposure from sun or appropriate lamp
    - Some species may benefit from judicious oral supplementation
- Calcitonin to prevent further transfer of Ca from bone to blood (hormone therapies should always be performed cautiously)
    - 50 U/kg IM q7d × 2 treatments
    - Ca supplementation should be given prior to and during calcitonin therapy
    - Serum Ca should be within normal limits prior to calcitonin therapy; if Ca levels cannot be determined, administer calcium 7 days prior to calcitonin
- Gut-load invertebrates (crickets, mealworms, superworms, cockroaches) on high calcium diet (high calcium leafy greens, Mazuri Hi-Ca Cricket Diet) for several days before feeding to insectivores
- Feed high-calcium invertebrates such as phoenix worms, snails, and earthworms when appropriate for diet in insectivores
- Dusting invertebrates may be beneficial; but they often remove dust quickly, can make unpalatable, and be careful with dusts containing vitamins; avoid those with phosphorus
- Feed only leafy greens and other high calcium plants for herbivores, minimizing thicker vegetables and avoiding most fruits
- In mammals, condition considered painful, appropriate analgesics may be warranted
- Both short-term and long-term prognosis is often guarded at best
- Other
    - Handle gently
    - Remove climbing branches to prevent injuries

TABLE 4-18 Selected Sources of Diets and Other Commercial Products for Reptiles.[a,b]

Foods and Supplements

Fluker Farms	800-735-8537	www.flukerfarms.com
Drs Foster and Smith	800-443-1160	www.drsfostersmith.com
JurassiPet	706-343-6060	www.jurassipet.com
Mazuri	800-227-8941	www.mazuri.com
National Geographic/Petsmart	888-839-9638	www.petsmart.com/featured-shops/reptile/cat-36-catid-800506
Oxbow Animal Health	800-249-0366	www.oxbowanimalhealth.com

Continued

TABLE 4-18	Selected Sources of Diets and Other Commercial Products for Reptiles. (cont'd)			
Pretty Pets	800-356-5020	www.prettybird.com		
Reliable Protein Products	480-361-3940	www.zoofood.com		
Repashy Superfoods	855-737-2749	www.store.repashy.com		
Rep-Cal	800-406-6446	www.repcal.com		
San Francisco Bay Brand	510-792-7200	http://sfbb.com		
Sticky Tongue Farms	951-244-3434	www.stickytonguefarms.com		
Tetra Fauna	800-423-6458	www.tetra-fish.com		
T-Rex Products	800-991-8739	www.t-rexproducts.com		
Wombaroo	(08)83911713 (Aust)	www.wombaroo.com.au/reptiles		
Zilla	888-255-4527	www.zilla-rules.com		
Zoo Med Laboratories	888-496-6633	www.zoomed.com		
Live/Frozen Foods for Carnivores				
American Rodent Supply	317-899-1599	www.americanrodent.com	Frozen mice, rats	
Backwater Reptiles	Unpublished	www.backwaterreptiles.com	Frozen mice, rats	
Big Apple Herp	561-923-9510	www.bigappleherp.com	Frozen mine, rats, chicks, quail, rabbits	
Big Cheese Rodents	800-887-0921	www.bigcheeserodents.com	Frozen mice, rats, chicks	
The Gourmet Rodent	352-472-9189	www.gourmetrodent.com	Frozen mice, rats, rabbits, and chicks	
Hoosier Mouse Supply	317-831-1219	www.hoosiermousesupply.com	Live (local) and frozen mice, rats	
Layne Laboratories, Inc	Unpublished	www.laynelabs.com	Frozen mice, rats	
Mack Natural Reptile Food	888-372-9570	www.macksnaturalreptilefood.com	Frozen mice, rats	
Perfect Pets Inc	800-366-8794	www.perfectpet.net	Frozen mice, rats, hamsters, gerbils, guinea pigs, rabbits, chicks	
Rodent Pro	812-867-7598	www.rodentpro.com	Frozen mice, rats, rabbits, guinea pigs, chicks, quail	
T-Rex Products	800-991-8739	www.t-rexproducts.com	Frozen pinkies, fuzzies, small mice	

TABLE 4-18 Selected Sources of Diets and Other Commercial Products for Reptiles. (cont'd)

Live Foods for Insectivores

Arbico Organics	800-827-2847	www.arbico-organics.com	Live Tiny Wigglers, Tiny Wasp, Cocoon Capers, many other insects
Backwater Reptiles	Unpublished	www.Backwaterreptiles.com	Crickets, roaches, hornworms, mealworms, superworms, silkworms
Bassett's Cricket Ranch	800-634-2445	www.bcrcricket.com	Crickets, mealworms
Big Apple Herp	561-923-9510	www.bigappleherp.com	Butterworms, mealworms, waxworms, nightcrawlers
Fluker Farms	800-735-8537	www.flukerfarms.com	Crickets, mealworms, superworms, cockroaches, fruit flies, soldier worms
Ghann's Cricket Farm	800-476-2248	www.ghann.com	Crickets, soldier fly larvae, mealworms, superworms, wax worms
Grubco	800-222-3563	www.grubco.com	Crickets, superworms, mealworms, fly larvae, wax worms
Josh's Frogs	800-691-8178	www.joshsfrogs.com	Fruit flies, mealworms, hornworms, soldier fly larvae, roaches, rice flour beetles
Knutson's	800-248-9318	www.knutsonlivebait.com	Night crawlers, crickets, mealworms, wax worms
Millbrook Cricket Farm	800-654-3506	www.millbrookcrickets.com	Crickets, superworms
Mulberry Farms	760-731-6088	www.mulberryfarms.com	Silkworm larvae, soldier fly larvae, mealworms, superworms, waxworms, roaches
The Phoenix Worm Store		www.phoenixworm.com	Soldier fly larvae
Rainbow Mealworms	800-777-9676	www.rainbowmealworms.net	Crickets, mealworms, cockroaches
Reptile Food	Unpublished	www.reptilefood.com	Mealworms, giant mealworms, zophobas worms, waxworms, nightcrawlers, red worms, fruit flies, crickets
Russell's Cricket Farm	234-738-3663	www.livecrickets.com	Crickets, mealworms, superworms, roaches
Timberline Fresh	800-423-2248	http://timberlinefresh.com	Crickets, superworms, hornworms, waxworms, mealworms
Top Hat Cricket Farm	800-638-2555	www.tophatcrickets.com	Crickets, mealworms, superworms, hornworms, waxworms

Lights

Exo Terra	800-724-2436	www.exo-terra.com	Ultraviolet, visible, infrared/heat
Fluker Farms	800-735-8537	www.flukerfarms.com	Incandescent, heat
General Electric	800-435-4448	www.gelighting.com	Incandescent, heat

Continued

TABLE 4-18 Selected Sources of Diets and Other Commercial Products for Reptiles. (cont'd)

Mac Industries, Inc	252-241-4584	www.reptileuv.com	Brightrite halogen, self-ballasted lamps, heat projector lamps, reptileUV
Philips	800-555-0050	www.lighting.philips.com	Incandescent, heat
Sylvania	978-777-1900	www.sylvania.com	350BL blacklights
T-Rex Products	800-991-8739	www.t-rexproducts.com	Mercury vapor UVB, incandescent, heat
Zilla	888-255-4527	www.zilla-rules.com	Incandescent, heat, UVB fluorescent, halogen
Zoo Med Laboratories	888-496-6633	www.zoomed.com	Incandescent, heat, mercury vapor UVB, fluorescent UVB

Heating Devices

Avitec	800-646-2473	www.avitec.com	Ceramic heat elements, infrared heat panels, fluorescent
The Bean Farm	877-708-5882	www.beanfarm.com	Heat tape, heat pads, cords, ceramic heaters
Big Apple Pet Supply	800-922-7753	www.bigappleherp.com	Ceramic bulbs, heat mats, heat tape, incandescent bulbs
Fluker Farms	800-735-8537	www.flukerfarms.com	Under-cage heat pads
Helix Controls	760-726-4464	www.helixcontrols.com	Thermostats, heat tape, heat panels
LLL Reptile	888-547-3784	http://lllreptile.com	Pearlco conical ceramic heat emitters
National Geographic/ Petsmart	888-839-9638	www.petsmart.com/featured-shops/reptile/cat-36-catid-800506	Heat lamps
Zilla	800-255-4527	www.zilla-rules.com	Conical ceramic heat emitters, thermostats, heat mats
Zoo Med Laboratories	888-496-6633	www.zoomed.com	Thermostats, rheostats, heat pads, tape, cables, cermaic heat emitter, rock heater, under tank heater

Humidity Devices

Exo Terra (Hagen)	800-724-2436	www.exo-terra.com	Ultrasonic fogger, Monsoon rainfall
Humidifirst	561-752-1936	www.humidifirst.com	Mist Pac ultrasonic humidifiers
Zoo Med Laboratories	888-496-6633	www.zoomed.com	Ultrasonic fogger, Repti fogger, Habba mist, Hygro-Therm humidity controller

Environmental Sensing and Monitoring Devices

The Bean Farm	877-708-5882	www.beanfarm.com	Thermostats
Exo Terra (Hagen)	800-724-2436	www.exo-terra.com	Remote digital thermometers, hygrometers
Onset Computer Corp	800-564-4377	www.onsetcomp.com	Relative humidity, temperature

TABLE 4-18	Selected Sources of Diets and Other Commercial Products for Reptiles. (cont'd)			
Raytek	800-227-8074	www.raytek.com	Digital infrared thermometer	
Solartech	800-798-3311	www.solarmeter.com	Solarmeter 6.2 UVB meter	
Zilla	800-255-4527	www.zilla-rules.com	Digital infrared thermometer	
Zoo Med Laboratories	888-496-6633	www.zoomed.com	Hygro-Therm humidity/heat monitor and controller, ReptiTemp rheostat, many thermometer and humidity gauges	

[a]Many pet stores sell live and frozen food for reptiles, and many of the products listed.
[b]Numerous sources of information were used to compile this table, particularly Internet sources.

REFERENCES

1. Adkesson MJ, Fernandez-Varon E, Cox S, et al. Pharmacokinetics of a long-acting ceftiofur formulation (ceftiofur crystalline free acid) in the ball python (*Python regius*). *J Zoo Wildl Med* 2011;42:444-450.
2. Adnyana W, Ladds PW, Blair D. Efficacy of praziquantel in the treatment of green sea turtles with spontaneous infection of cardiovascular flukes. *Aust Vet J* 1997;75:405-407.
3. Alleman AR, Jacobson ER, Raskin RE. Morphologic and cytochemical characteristics of blood cells from the desert tortoise (*Gopherus agassizii*). *Proc Annu Conf Assoc Rept Amph Vet* 1996;51-55.
4. Allen DG, Pringle JK, Smith D. *Handbook of Veterinary Drugs*. Philadelphia: JB Lippincott Co; 1993;534-567.
5. Allender MC, Mitchell MA, Yarborough J, et al. Pharmacokinetics of a single oral dose of acyclovir and valacyclovir in North American box turtles (*Terrapene* sp.). *J Vet Pharmacol Therap* 2012;36:205-208.
6. Alves-Junior JRF, Bosso ACS, Andrade MB, et al. Association of acepromazine with propofol in giant Amazon river turtles *Podocnemis expansa* breed in captivity. *Acta Cir Bras* 2012;27:552-556.
7. Alves-Junior JRF, Bosso ACS, Andrade MB, et al. Association of midazolam with ketamine in giant Amazon river turtles *Podocnemis expansa* reared in captivity. *Acta Cir Bras* 2012;27:144-147.
8. American Veterinary Medical Association. AVMA guidelines on euthanasia. Available at: www.avma.org/issues/animal_welfare/euthanasia.pdf. Accessed May 6, 2011.
9. Anderson NL, Wack RF. Basic husbandry and medicine of pet reptiles. In: Birchard SJ, Sherding RG, eds. *Saunders Manual of Small Animal Practice*. 2nd ed. Philadelphia: WB Saunders Co; 2000:1539-1567.
10. Anderson NL, Wack RF, Calloway L. Cardiopulmonary effects and efficacy of propofol as an anesthetic agent in brown tree snakes, *Boiga irregularis*. *Bull Assoc Rept Amph Vet* 1999;9:9-15.
11. Antinoff N, Bauck L, Boyer TH, et al. *Exotic Animal Formulary*. 2nd ed. Lakewood, CO: AAHA Press; 1999.
12. Arnett-Chinn ER, Hadfield CA, Clayton LA. Review of intramuscular midazolam for sedation in reptiles at the National Aquarium, Baltimore. *J Herp Med Surg* 2016;26:59-63.
13. Ascher JM, Bates W, Ng J, et al. Assessment of xylazine for euthanasia of anoles (*Anolis carolinensis* and *Anolis distichus*). *J Am Assoc Lab Anim Sci* 2012;51:83-87.
14. Baker BB, Sladky KK, Johnson SM. Evaluation of the analgesic effects of oral and subcutaneous tramadol administration in red-eared slider turtles. *J Am Vet Med Assoc* 2011;238:220-227.
15. Banzato T, Russo E, Finotti L, Zotti A. Development of a technique for contrast radiographic examination of the gastrointestinal tract in ball pythons (*Python regius*). *Am J Vet Res* 2012;73:996-1001.

16. Barten SL. The medical care of iguanas and other common pet lizards. *Vet Clin North Am Small Anim Pract* 1993;23:1213-1249.
17. Baruffaldi LC, da Silva A, Sellera FP, et al. Spinal anesthesia in a green turtle (*Chelonia mydas*) for surgical removal of cutaneous fibropapillomatosis. *J Agri Vet Sci* 2016;9:83-86.
18. Beck K, Loomis M, Lewbart G, et al. Preliminary comparison of plasma concentrations of gentamicin injected into the cranial and caudal limb musculature of the eastern box turtle (*Terrapene carolina carolina*). *J Zoo Wildl Med* 1995;26:265-268.
19. Bennett RA. A review of anesthesia and chemical restraint in reptiles. *J Zoo Wildl Med* 1991;22:282-303.
20. Bennett RA. Anesthesia. In: Mader DR, ed. *Reptile Medicine and Surgery.* Philadelphia: WB Saunders Co; 1996:241-247.
21. Bennett RA. Clinical, diagnostic, and therapeutic techniques. *Proc Annu Conf Assoc Rept Amph Vet* 1998;35-40.
22. Bennett RA. Management of common reptile emergencies. *Proc Annu Conf Assoc Rept Amph Vet* 1998;67-72.
23. Bennett RA. Reptile anesthesia. *Semin Avian Exot Pet Med* 1998;7:30-40.
24. Bennett RA, Divers SJ, Schumacher J, et al. Roundtable: anesthesia. *Bull Assoc Rept Amph Vet* 1999;9:20-27.
25. Bennett RA, Schumacher J, Hedjazi-Haring K, et al. Cardiopulmonary and anesthetic effects of propofol administered intraosseously to green iguanas. *J Am Vet Med Assoc* 1998;212: 93-98.
26. Benson KG, Tell LA, Young LA, et al. Pharmacokinetics of ceftiofur sodium after intramuscular or subcutaneous administration in green iguanas (*Iguana iguana*). *Am J Vet Res* 2003;64:1278-1282.
27. Bernard JB, Oftedal OT, Citino SB, et al. The response of vitamin D-deficient green iguanas (*Iguana iguana*) to artificial ultraviolet light. *Proc Annu Conf Am Assoc Zoo Vet* 1991; 147-150.
28. Bertelsen MF, Buchanan R, Jensen HM, et al. Assessing the influence of mechanical ventilation on blood gases and blood pressure in rattlesnakes. *Vet Anaesth Analg* 2015;42:386-393.
29. Bicknese E, Pessier A, Boedeker N. Successful treatment of fungal osteomyelitis in a Parson's chameleon (*Calumma parsonii*) using surgical and anti-fungal treatments. *Proc Annu Conf Assoc Rept Amph Vet* 2008;86.
30. Bienzle D, Boyd CJ. Sedative effects of ketamine and midazolam in snapping turtles. *J Zoo Wildl Med* 1992;23:201-204.
31. Bodri MS, Hruba SJ. Safety of milbemycin (A_3-A_4 oxime) in chelonians. *Proc Joint Conf Am Assoc Zoo Vet/Am Assoc Wildl Vet* 1992;156-157.
32. Bodri MS, Rambo TM, Wagner RA, et al. Pharmacokinetics of metronidazole administered as a single oral bolus to red rat snakes, *Elaphe guttata. J Herpetol Med Surg* 2006;16:15-19.
33. Bogoslavsky B. The use of ponazuril to treat coccidiosis in eight inland bearded dragons (*Pogona vitticeps*). *Proc Annu Conf Assoc Rept Amph Vet* 2007;8-9.
34. Boyer TH. Clinical anesthesia of reptiles. *Bull Assoc Rept Amph Vet* 1992;2:10-13.
35. Boyer TH. Common problems of box turtles (*Terrapene* spp.) in captivity. *Bull Assoc Rept Amph Vet* 1992;2:9-14.
36. Boyer TH. Emergency care of reptiles. *Semin Avian Exot Pet Med* 1994;3:210-216.
37. Boyer TH. Emergency care of reptiles. *Vet Clin North Am Exot Anim Pract* 1998;1:191-206.
38. Boyer TH. *Essentials of Reptiles: A Guide for Practitioners.* Lakewood, CO: AAHA Press; 1998:1-253.
39. Brunner CHM, Dutra G, Silva CB, et al. Electrochemotherapy for the treatment of fibropapillomas in *Chelonia mydas. J Zoo Wild Med* 2014;45:213-218.
40. Bryant GL, Fleming PA, Twomey L, Warren K. Factors affecting hematology and plasma biochemistry in the southwest carpet python (*Morelia spilota imbricata*). *J Wildl Dis* 2012; 48:282-294.

41. Burns RB, McMahan W. Euthanasia methods for ectothermic vertebrates. In: Bonagura JD, ed. *Kirk's Current Veterinary Therapy XII: Small Animal Practice*. Philadelphia: WB Saunders Co; 1995:1379-1381.
42. Bush M, Smeller JM, Charache PN, et al. Preliminary study of antibiotics in snakes. *Proc Annu Conf Am Assoc Zoo Vet* 1976;50-54.
43. Bush M, Smeller JM, Charache P, et al. Biological half-life of gentamicin in gopher snakes. *Am J Vet Res* 1978;39:171-173.
44. Caligiuri R, Kollias GV, Jacobson E, et al. The effects of ambient temperature on amikacin pharmacokinetics in gopher tortoises. *J Vet Pharm Therapeut* 1990;13:287-291.
45. Calvert I. Nutritional problems. In: Girling SJ, Raiti P, eds. *BSAVA Manual of Reptiles*. 2nd ed. Quedgeley, Gloucester: British Small Animal Veterinary Association; 2004:289-308.
46. Camacho M, del Pino Quintana M, Calabuig P, et al. Acid-base and plasma biochemical changes using crystalloid fluids in stranded juvenile loggerhead sea turtles (*Caretta caretta*). *Plos One* 2015;10:1371-1381.
47. Campagnol D, Lemos FR, Silva ELF, et al. Comparacao da contencao farmacologica com cetamina e xilazina, administradas pela via intramuscular no membro toracico ou pelvico, em jacares-do-papo-amarelo juvenis. *Pesq Vet Bras* 2014;34:675-681.
48. Carpenter JW. Radiographic imaging of reptiles. *Proc North Am Vet Conf* 1998;873-875.
49. Casares M, Enders F. Enrofloxacin side effects in a Galapagos tortoise (*Geochelone elephantopus nigra*). *Proc Annu Conf Am Assoc Zoo Vet* 1996;446-448.
50. Chiodini RJ, Sundberg JP. Blood chemical values of the common boa constrictor (*Constrictor constrictor*). *Am J Vet Res* 1982;43:1701-1702.
51. Chittick EJ, Stamper MA, Beasley JF, et al. Medetomidine, ketamine, and sevoflurane for anesthesia of injured loggerhead sea turtles: 13 cases (1996-2000). *J Am Vet Med Assoc* 2002;221:1019-1025.
52. Chitty JR. Use of a novel disinfectant agent in reptile respiratory disease. *Proc Annu Conf Assoc Rept Amph Vet* 2003;65-67.
53. Christopher MM, Berry KH, Wallis IR, et al. Reference intervals and physiologic alterations in hematologic and biochemical values of free-ranging desert tortoises in the Mojave Desert. *J Wildl Dis* 1999;35:212-238.
54. Churgin SM, Musgrave KE, Cox SK, et al. Pharmacokinetics of subcutaneous versus intramuscular administration of ceftiofur crystalline-free acid to bearded dragons (*Pogona vitticeps*). *Am J Vet Res* 2014;75:453-459.
55. Clancy MM, Newton AL, Sykes JM. Management of osteomyelitis caused by *Salmonella enteritica* subsp. *houtenae* in a Taylor's cantil (*Agkistrodon bilineatus taylori*) using amikacin delivered via osmotic pump. *J Zoo Wildl Med* 2016;47:691-694.
56. Clark CH, Rogers ED, Milton JL. Plasma concentrations of chloramphenicol in snakes. *Am J Vet Res* 1985;46:2654-2657.
57. Clyde VL, Cardeilhac PT, Jacobson ER. Chemical restraint of American alligators (*Alligator mississippiensis*) with atracurium or tiletamine-zolazepam. *J Zoo Wildl Med* 1994;25:525-530.
58. Coke RL, Tristan TE. *Cryptosporidium* infection in a colony of leopard geckos, *Eublepharis macularius*. *Proc Annu Conf Assoc Rept Amph Vet* 1998;157-163.
59. Coke RL, Hunter RP, Isaza R, et al. Pharmacokinetics and tissue concentrations of azithromycin in ball pythons (*Python regius*). *Am J Vet Res* 2003;64:225-228.
60. Coke RL, Isaza R, Koch DE, et al. Preliminary single-dose pharmacokinetics of marbofloxacin in ball pythons (*Python regius*). *J Zoo Wildl Med* 2006;37:6-10.
61. Conroy CJ, Papenfuss T, Parker J, et al. Use of tricaine methanesulfonate (MS222) for euthanasia of reptiles. *J Am Assoc Lab Anim Sci* 2009;48:28-32.
62. Cooper-Bailey K, Smith SA, Zimmerman K, et al. Hematology, leukocyte cytochemical analysis, plasma biochemistry, and plasma electrophoresis of wild-caught and captive bred Gila monsters (*Heloderma suspectum*). *Vet Clin Pathol* 2011;40:316-323.
63. Cowan ML, Raidal SR, Peters A. Herpesvirus in a captive Australian Krefft's river turtle (*Emydura macquarii krefftii*). *Aust Vet J* 2015;93:46-49.

64. Cranfield MR, Graczyk TK. Cryptosporidiosis. In: Mader DR, ed. *Reptile Medicine and Surgery*. 2nd ed. St. Louis: Saunders/Elsevier; 2006:756-762.
65. Crawshaw GJ, Holz P. Comparison of plasma biochemical values in blood and blood-lymph mixtures from red-eared sliders, *Trachemys scripta elegans*. *Bull Assoc Rept Amph Vet* 1996;6:7-9.
66. Dallwig R. Allopurinol. *J Exot Pet Med* 2010;19:255-257.
67. Deem SL, Norton TM, Mitchell M, et al. Comparison of blood values in foraging, nesting, and stranded loggerhead turtles (*Caretta caretta*) along the coast of Georgia, USA. *J Wildl Dis* 2009;45:41-56.
68. DeNardo DF, Helminski G. Birth control in lizards? Therapeutic inhibition of reproduction. *Proc Annu Conf Assoc Rept Amph Vet* 2000;65-66.
69. Dennis PM, Heard DJ. Cardiopulmonary effects of a medetomidine-ketamine combination administered intravenously in gopher tortoises. *J Am Vet Med Assoc* 2002;220:1516-1519.
70. Dennis PM, Bennett RA, Harr KE, et al. Plasma concentration of ionized calcium in healthy iguanas. *J Am Vet Med Assoc* 2001;219:326-328.
71. DeVoe R. Nutritional support of reptile patients. *Vet Clin Exot Anim* 2014;17:249-261.
72. Dickinson VM, Jarchow JL, Trueblood MH. Hematology and plasma biochemistry reference range values for free-ranging desert tortoises in Arizona. *J Wildl Dis* 2002;38:143-153.
73. Diethelm G, Stein G. Hematologic and blood chemistry values in reptiles. In: Mader DR, ed. *Reptile Medicine and Surgery*. 2nd ed. St. Louis: Saunders/Elsevier; 2006:1103-1118.
74. Di Ianni F, Parmigiani E, Pelizzone I, et al. Comparison between intramuscular and intravenous administration of oxytocin in captive-bred red-eared sliders (*Trachemys scripta elegans*) with nonobstructive egg retention. *J Exot Pet Med* 2014;23:79-84.
75. Divers SJ. Constipation in snakes with particular reference to surgical correction in a Burmese python (*Python molurus bivittatus*). *Proc Annu Conf Assoc Rept Amph Vet* 1996;67-69.
76. Divers SJ. Medical and surgical treatment of pre-ovulatory ova stasis and post-ovulatory egg stasis in oviparous lizards. *Proc Annu Conf Assoc Rept Amph Vet* 1996;119-123.
77. Divers SJ. The use of propofol in reptile anesthesia. *Proc Annu Conf Assoc Rept Amph Vet* 1996;57-59.
78. Divers SJ. Clinician's approach to renal disease in lizards. *Proc Annu Conf Assoc Rept Amph Vet* 1997;5-11.
79. Divers SJ. Empirical doses of antimicrobial drugs commonly used in reptiles. *Exot DVM* 1998;1:23.
80. Divers SJ. Anesthetics in reptiles. *Exot DVM* 1999;1(3):7-8.
81. Divers SJ, Redmayne G, Aves EK. Haematological and biochemical values of 10 green iguanas (*Iguana iguana*). *Vet Rec* 1996;138:203-205.
82. Divers SJ, Papich MG, McBride M, et al. Pharmacokinetics of meloxicam following intravenous and oral administration in green iguanas (*Iguana iguana*). *Am J Vet Res* 2010;71:1277-1283.
83. Doneley B. Caring for the bearded dragon. *Proc North Am Vet Conf* 2006;1607-1611.
84. Donoghue S. Nutrition. In: Mader DR, ed. *Reptile Medicine and Surgery*. 2nd ed. St. Louis: Saunders/Elsevier; 2006:251-298.
85. Drew ML. Hypercalcemia and hyperphosphatemia in indigo snakes (*Drymarchon corais*) and serum biochemical reference values. *J Zoo Wildl Med* 1994;25:48-52.
86. Ellman MM. Hematology and plasma chemistry of the inland bearded dragon, *Pogona vitticeps*. *Bull Assoc Rept Amph Vet* 1997;7:10-12.
87. Erlacher-Reid CD, Norton TM, Harms CA, et al. Intestinal and cloacal strictures in free-ranging and aquarium-maintained green sea turtles (*Chelonia mydas*). *J Zoo Wildl Med* 2013;44:408-429.
88. Farmaki R, Simou C, Papadopoulos E, et al. Effectiveness of a single application of 0.25% fipronil solution for the treatment of hirstiellosis in captive green iguanas (*Iguana iguana*): an open label study. *Parasitol* 2013;140:1144-1148.
89. Farnsworth RJ, Brannian RE, Fletcher KC, et al. A vitamin E-selenium responsive condition in a green iguana. *J Zoo Anim Med* 1986;17:42-43.

90. Faulkner JE, Archambault A. Anesthesia and surgery in the green iguana. *Semin Avian Exot Pet Med* 1993;2:103-108.
91. Feldman M, Feldman E. New methods to induce egg laying in turtles. *Proc 14th Annu Symp Cons Biol Tortoises Freshwater Turtles* 2016;26.
92. Fitzgerald KT, Vera R. Acariasis. In: Mader DR, ed. *Reptile Medicine and Surgery*. 2nd ed. St. Louis: Saunders/Elsevier; 2006:720-738.
93. Flach EJ, Riley J, Mutlow AG, et al. Pentastomiasis in Bosc's monitor lizards (*Varanus exanthematicus*) caused by an undescribed *Sambonia* species. *J Zoo Wildl Med* 2000;31:91-95.
94. Fleming G. Clinical technique: chelonian shell repair. *J Exot Pet Med* 2008;17:246-258.
95. Fleming GJ. Capture and chemical immobilization of the Nile crocodile (*Crocodylus niloticus*) in South Africa. *Proc Annu Conf Assoc Rept Amph Vet* 1996;63-66.
96. Fleming GJ. Crocodilian anesthesia. *Vet Clin North Am Exot Anim Pract* 2001;4:119-145.
97. Fleming GJ, Robertson SA. Assessments of thermal antinociceptive effects of butorphanol and human observer effect on quantitative evaluation of analgesia in green iguanas (*Iguana iguana*). *Am J Vet Res* 2012;73:1507-1511.
98. Flint M, Morton JM, Limpus CJ, et al. Development and application of biochemical and haematological reference intervals to identify unhealthy green sea turtles (*Chelonia mydas*). *Vet J* 2010;185:299-304.
99. Flower JE, Byrd J, Cray C, Allender MC. Plasma electrophoretic profiles and hemoglobin binding protein reference intervals in the Eastern box turtle (*Terrapene carolina carolina*) and influences of age, sex, season, and location. *J Zoo Wildl Med* 2014;45:836-842.
100. Folland DW, Johnston MS, Thamm DH, Reavill D. Diagnosis and management of lymphoma in a green iguana (*Iguana iguana*). *J Am Vet Med Assoc* 2011;239:985-991.
101. Franco KH, Hoover JP. Levothyroxine as a treatment for presumed hypothyroidism in an adult male African spurred tortoise (*Centrochelys* (formerly *Geochelone*) *sulcata*). *J Herpetol Med Surg* 2009;19:42-44.
102. Fraser MA, Girling SJ. Dermatology. In: Girling SJ, Raiti P, eds. *BSAVA Manual of Reptiles*. 2nd ed. Quedgeley, Gloucester: British Small Animal Veterinary Association; 2004:184-198.
103. Frye FL. *Reptile Care: An Atlas of Diseases and Treatments*. Neptune City, NJ: TFH Publications, Inc; 1991:1-637.
104. Frye FL. *Reptile Clinician's Handbook*. Malabar, FL: Krieger Publishing; 1994.
105. Fudge AM. Laboratory reference ranges for selected avian, mammalian, and reptilian species. In: Fudge AM, ed. *Laboratory Medicine: Avian and Exotic Pets*. Philadelphia: WB Saunders Co; 2000:375-400.
106. Funk RS. A formulary for lizards, snakes, and crocodilians. *Vet Clin North Am Exot Anim Pract* 2000;3:333-358.
107. Funk RS, Diethelm G. Reptile formulary. In: Mader DR, ed. *Reptile Medicine and Surgery*. 2nd ed. St. Louis: Saunders/Elsevier; 2006:1119-1139.
108. Gaio C, Rossi T, Villa R, et al. Pharmacokinetics of acyclovir after a single oral administration in marginated tortoises, *Testudo marginata*. *J Herpetol Med Surg* 2007;17:8-11.
109. Gamble KC. Plasma fentanyl concentrations achieved after transdermal fentanyl patch application in prehensile-tailed skinks, *Corucia zebrata*. *J Herpetol Med Surg* 2008;18:81-85.
110. Gamble KC, Alvarado TP, Bennett CL. Itraconazole plasma and tissue concentrations in the spiny lizard (*Sceloporus* sp.) following once-daily dosing. *J Zoo Wildl Med* 1997;28:89-93.
111. Gaumer A, Goodnight CJ. Some aspects of the hematology of turtles as related to their activity. *Am Midland Nat* 1957;58:332-340.
112. Georoff TA, Stacy NI, Newton AN, et al. Diagnosis and treatment of chronic T-lymphocytic leukemia in a green tree monitor (*Varanus prasinus*). *J Herpetol Med Surg* 2009;19:106-114.
113. Giannetto S, Brianti E, Poglayen G, et al. Efficacy of oxfendazole and fenbendazole against tortoise (*Testudo hermanni*) oxyurids. *Parasitol Res* 2007;100:1069-1073.
114. Gibbons P. Advances in reptile clinical therapeutics. *J Exot Pet Med* 2014;23:21-38.

115. Gibbons PM. Critical care nutrition and fluid therapy in reptiles. In: *Proc 15th Annu Intl Vet Emerg Crit Care Symp*; 2009:91-94.
116. Gibbons PM, Horton SJ, Brandl SR. Urinalysis in box turtles, *Terrapene* spp. *Proc Annu Conf Assoc Rept Amph Vet* 2000;161-168.
117. Gibbons PM, Klaphake E, Carpenter JW. Reptiles. In: Carpenter JW, ed. *Exotic Animal Formulary*. 4th ed. St. Louis: Elsevier; 2013:83-182.
118. Gibbons PM, Steffes ZJ. Emerging infectious diseases of chelonians. *Vet Clin North Am Exot Anim Pract* 2013;16:303-317.
119. Gillespie D. Reptiles. In: Birchard SJ, Sherding RG, eds. *Saunders Manual of Small Animal Practice*. Philadelphia: WB Saunders Co; 1994:1390-1411.
120. Gimenez M, Saco Y, Pato R, et al. Plasma protein electrophoresis of *Trachemys scripta* and *Iguana iguana*. *Vet Clin Pathol* 2010;39:227-235.
121. Giorgi M, De Vito V, Owen H, et al. PK/PD evaluations of the novel atypical opioid tapentadol in red-eared slider turtles. *Med Weter* 2014;70:530-535.
122. Giorgi M, Lee H-K, Rota S, et al. Pharmacokinetic and pharmacodynamics assessments of tapentadol in yellow-bellied slider turtles (*Trachemys scripta scripta*) after a single intramuscular injection. *J Exot Pet Med* 2015;24:317-325.
123. Giorgi M, Rota S, Giorgi T, et al. Blood concentrations of enrofloxacin and the metabolite ciprofloxacin in yellow-bellied slider turtles (*Trachemys scripta scripta*) after a single intracoelomic injection of enrofloxacin. *J Exot Pet Med* 2013;22:192-199.
124. Giorgi M, Salvadori M, De Vito V, et al. Pharmacokinetic/pharmacodynamics assessments of 10 mg/kg tramadol intramuscular injection in yellow-bellied slider turtles (*Trachemys scripta scripta*). *J Vet Pharmacol Therap* 2015;38:488-496.
125. Goe A, Shmalberg J, Gatson B, et al. Epinephrine or GV-26 electrical stimulation reduces inhalant anesthetic recovery time in common snapping turtles (*Chelydra serpentina*). *J Zoo Wildl Med* 2016;47:501-507.
126. Gornik KR, Pirie CG, Marrion RM, et al. Baseline corneal sensitivity and duration of action of proparacaine in rehabilitated juvenile Kemp's ridley sea turtles (*Lepidochelys kempii*). *J Herp Med Surg* 2015;25:116-121.
127. Gottdenker NL, Jacobson ER. Effect of venipuncture sites on hematologic and clinical biochemical values in desert tortoises (*Gopherus agassizii*). *Am J Vet Res* 1995;56:19-21.
128. Greenacre CB, Massi K, Schumacher JP, et al. Comparative antinociception of various opioids and non-steroidal anti-inflammatory medications versus saline in the bearded dragon (*Pogona vitticeps*) using electrostimulation. *Proc Annu Conf Rept Amph Vet* 2008;87.
129. Grosset C, Villeneuve A, Brieger A, Lair S. Cryptosporidiosis in juvenile bearded dragons (*Pogona vitticeps*): effects of treatment with paromomycin. *J Herpetol Med Surg* 2011;21:10-15.
130. Groza A, Mederle N, Darabus G. Advocate-therapeutical solution in parasitical infestation in frillneck lizard (*Chlamydosaurus kingii*) and bearded dragon (*Pogona vitticeps*). *Lucrari Stiintifice - Universitatea Stiinte Agricole Banatului Timisoara, Med Vet* 2009;42:105-108.
131. Hackenbroich C, Failing K, Axt-Findt U, et al. Alphaxalone-alphadolone anesthesia in *Trachemys scripta elegans* and its influence on respiration, circulation and metabolism. *Proc 2nd Conf Euro Assoc Zoo Wildl Vet* 1998;431-436.
132. Hadfield CA, Clayton LA, Clancy MM. Proliferative thyroid lesions in three diplodactylid geckos: *Nephrurus amyae*, *Nephrurus levis*, and *Oedura marmorata*. *J Zoo Wildl Med* 2012;43:131-140.
133. Hansen LL, Bertelsen MF. Assessment of the effects of intramuscular administration of alfaxalone with and without medetomidine in Horsfield's tortoises (*Agrionemys horsfieldii*). *Vet Anaesth Analg* 2013;40:68-75.
134. Harkewicz KA. Dermatologic problems of reptiles. *Semin Avian Exot Pet Med* 2002;11:151-161.
135. Harms CA, Cranston EA, Papich MG, et al. Pharmacokinetics of clindamycin in loggerhead sea turtles (*Caretta caretta*) after a single intravenous, intramuscular, or oral dose. *J Herpetol Med Surg* 2011;21:113-119.

136. Harms CA, Lewbart GA, Beasley J. Medical management of mixed nocardial and unidentified fungal osteomyelitis in a Kemp's ridley sea turtle, *Lepidochelys kempii*. *J Herpetol Med Surg* 2002;12:21-26.
137. Harms CA, Piniak WED, Eckert SA, et al. Sedation and anesthesia of hatchling leatherback sea turtles (*Dermochelys coriacea*) for auditory evoked potential measurement in air and in water. *J Zoo Wildl Med* 2014;45:86-92.
138. Harr KE, Alleman AR, Dennis PM, et al. Morphologic and cytochemical characteristics of blood cells and hematologic and plasma biochemical reference ranges in green iguanas. *J Am Vet Med Assoc* 2001;218:915-921.
139. Heard DJ. Principles and techniques of anesthesia and analgesia for exotic practice. *Vet Clin North Am Small Anim Pract* 1993;23:1301-1327.
140. Heard DJ. Advances in reptile anesthesia and medicine. *Proc Annu Conf Assoc Avian Vet/Avian Speciality Advanced Prog/Small Mam Rept Prog* 1998;113-119.
141. Heard DJ. Advances in reptile anesthesia. *Proc North Am Vet Conf* 1999;770.
142. Heatley J, Mitchell M, Williams J, et al. Fungal periodontal osteomyelitis in a chameleon, *Furcifer pardalis*. *J Herpetol Med Surg* 2001;11:7-12.
143. Heaton-Jones TG, Ko J, Heaton-Jones DL. Evaluation of medetomidine-ketamine anesthesia with atipamezole reversal in American alligators (*Alligator mississippiensis*). *J Zoo Wildl Med* 2002;33:36-44.
144. Helmick KE, Bennett RA, Ginn P, et al. Intestinal volvulus and stricture associated with a leiomyoma in a green turtle (*Chelonia mydas*). *J Zoo Wildl Med* 2000;31:221-227.
145. Helmick KE, Papich MG, Vliet KA, et al. Pharmacokinetic disposition of a long-acting oxytetracycline formulation after single-dose intravenous and intramuscular administrations in the American alligator (*Alligator mississippiensis*). *J Zoo Wildl Med* 2004;35:341-346.
146. Helmick KE, Papich MG, Vliet KA, et al. Pharmacokinetics of enrofloxacin after single-dose oral and intravenous administration in the American alligator (*Alligator mississippiensis*). *J Zoo Wildl Med* 2004;35:333-340.
147. Hernandez-Divers SJ. Pulmonary candidiasis caused by *Candida albicans* in a Greek tortoise (*Testudo graeca*) and treatment with intrapulmonary amphotericin B. *J Zoo Wildl Med* 2001;32:352-359.
148. Hernandez-Divers SJ. Diagnostic techniques. In: Mader DR, ed. *Reptile Medicine and Surgery*. 2nd ed. St. Louis: Saunders/Elsevier; 2006:490-532.
149. Hernandez-Divers SJ, Cooper JE. Hepatic lipidosis. In: Mader DR, ed. *Reptile Medicine and Surgery*. 2nd ed. St. Louis: Saunders/Elsevier; 2006:806-813.
150. Hernandez-Divers SJ, Knott CD, MacDonald J. Diagnosis and surgical treatment of thyroid adenoma-induced hyperthyroidism in a green iguana (*Iguana iguana*). *J Zoo Wildl Med* 2001;32:465-475.
151. Hernandez-Divers SJ, Martinez-Jimenez D, Bush S, et al. Effects of allopurinol on plasma uric acid levels in normouricaemic and hyperuricaemic green iguanas (*Iguana iguana*). *Vet Rec* 2008;162:112-115.
152. Hernandez-Divers SM. Reptile critical care. *Exot DVM* 2003;5(3):81-87.
153. Hess JC, Benson J, Grimm KA, et al. Minimum alveolar concentration of isoflurane and arterial blood gas values in anesthetized green iguanas, *Iguana iguana*. *J Herpetol Med Surg* 2008;17:118-124.
154. Hilf M, Swanson D, Wagner R, et al. A new dosing schedule for gentamicin in blood pythons (*Python curtus*): a pharmacokinetic study. *Res Vet Sci* 1991;50:127-130.
155. Hilf M, Swanson D, Wagner R, et al. Pharmacokinetics of piperacillin in blood pythons (*Python curtus*) and in vitro evaluation of efficacy against aerobic gram-negative bacteria. *J Zoo Wildl Med* 1991;22:199-203.
156. Hirano LQL. Contenção química e perfil farmacocinético da dextrocetamina, isolada em associação ao midazolam em jacaré-tinga *Caiman crocodilus Linnaeus* (1758) (Crocodylia: Alligatoridae) [Master's dissertation]. http://repositorio.bc.ufg.br/tede/handle/tede/46944,2015.

157. Holz P, Holz RM. Evaluation of ketamine, ketamine/xylazine, and ketamine/midazolam anesthesia in red-eared sliders (*Trachemys scripta elegans*). *J Zoo Wildl Med* 1994;25:531-537.
158. Holz PH, Burger JP, Baker R, et al. Effect of injection site on carbenicillin pharmacokinetics in the carpet python, *Morelia spilota*. *J Herpetol Med Surg* 2002;12:12-16.
159. Huchzermeyer FW. *Crocodiles: Biology, Husbandry and Diseases*. Cambridge, MA: CABI Publishing; 20031-337.
160. Hungerford C, Spelman L, Papich M. Pharmacokinetics of enrofloxacin after oral and intramuscular administration in savannah monitors (*Varanus exanthematicus*). *Proc Annu Conf Am Assoc Zoo Vet* 1997;89-92.
161. Innis C, Papich M, Young D. Pharmacokinetics of metronidazole in the red-eared slider turtle (*Trachemys scripta elegans*) after single intracoelomic injection. *J Vet Pharm Therapeut* 2007;30:168-171.
162. Innis C, Young D, Wetzlich S, et al. Plasma voriconazole concentrations in four red-eared slider turtles (*Trachemys scripta elegans*) after a single subcutaneous injection. *Proc Annu Conf Assoc Rept Amph Vet* 2008;72.
163. Innis CJ. Observations on urinalysis of clinically normal captive tortoises. *Proc Annu Conf Assoc Rept Amph Vet* 1997;109-112.
164. Innis CJ, Boyer TH. Chelonian reproductive disorders. *Vet Clin North Am Exot Anim Pract* 2002;5:555-578.
165. Innis CJ, Ceresia ML, Merigo C, et al. Single-dose pharmacokinetics of ceftazidime and fluconazole during concurrent clinical use in cold-stunned Kemp's ridley turtles (*Lepidochelys kempii*). *J Vet Pharmacol Therap* 2012;35:82-89.
166. Innis CJ, Feinsod R, Hanlon J, et al. Coelioscopic orchiectomy can be effectively and safely accomplished in chelonians. *Vet Rec* 2013;172:526-531.
167. Innis CJ, Young D, Wetzlich S, et al. Plasma concentrations and safety assessment of voriconazole in red-eared slider turtles (*Trachemys scripta elegans*) after single and multiple subcutaneous injections. *J Herp Med Surg* 2014;24:28-35.
168. Jacobson ER. Evaluation of the reptile patient. In: Jacobson ER, Kollias Jr GV, eds. *Exotic Animals*. New York: Churchill Livingstone; 1988:1-18.
169. Jacobson ER. Use of chemotherapeutics in reptile medicine. In: Jacobson ER, Kollias Jr GV, eds. *Exotic Animals*. New York: Churchill Livingstone; 1988:35-48.
170. Jacobson ER. Antimicrobial drug use in reptiles. In: Prescott JF, Baggot JD, eds. *Antimicrobial Therapy in Veterinary Medicine*. Ames: Iowa State University Press; 1993:543-552.
171. Jacobson E, Harman G, Laille E, et al. Plasma concentrations of praziquantel in loggerhead sea turtles (*Caretta caretta*) following oral administration of single and multiple doses. *Proc Annu Conf Assoc Rept Amph Vet* 2002;37-39.
172. Jacobson ER, Brown MP, Chung M, et al. Serum concentration and disposition kinetics of gentamicin and amikacin in juvenile American alligators. *J Zoo Anim Med* 1988;19:188-194.
173. Jenkins JR. A formulary for reptile and amphibian medicine. In: *Proc 4th Annu Avian/Exot Anim Med Symp*, Davis: University of California; 1991:24-27.
174. Jenkins JR. Husbandry and diseases of Old World chameleons. *J Small Exot Anim Med* 1992;1:166-171.
175. Jepson L. Lizards. *Exotic Animal Medicine: A Quick Reference Guide*. Philadelphia: Saunders/Elsevier; 2009268-314.
176. Jepson L. Snakes. *Exotic Animal Medicine: A Quick Reference Guide*. Philadelphia: Saunders/Elsevier; 2009315-357.
177. Jepson L. Turtles and tortoises. *Exotic Animal Medicine: A Quick Reference Guide*. Philadelphia: Saunders/Elsevier; 2009358-411.
178. Johnson JD, Mangone B, Jarchow JL. A review of mycoplasmosis infections in tortoises and options for treatment. *Proc Annu Conf Assoc Rept Amph Vet* 1998;89-92.
179. Johnson JG, Naples LM, Chu C, et al. Cutaneous squamous cell carcinoma in a panther chameleon (*Furcifer pardalis*) and treatment with carboplatin implantable beads. *J Zoo Wildl Med* 2016;47:931-934.

180. Johnson JH. Anesthesia, analgesia, and euthanasia of reptiles and amphibians. *Proc Annu Conf Am Assoc Zoo Vet* 1991;132-138.
181. Johnson JH, Benson PA. Laboratory reference values for a group of captive ball pythons (*Python regius*). *Am J Vet Res* 1996;57:1304-1307.
182. Johnson JH, Jensen JM, Brumbaugh GW, et al. Amikacin pharmacokinetics and the effects of ambient temperature on the dosage regimen in ball pythons (*Python regius*). *J Zoo Wildl Med* 1997;28:80-88.
183. Judd HL, Laughlin GA, Bacon JP, et al. Circulating androgen and estrogen concentrations in lizards (*Iguana iguana*). *Gen Comp Endocrinol* 1976;30:391-395.
184. Kanui TI, Hole K. Morphine and pethidine antinociception in the crocodile. *J Vet Pharmacol Ther* 1992;15:101-103.
185. Kaufman GE, Seymour RE, Bonner BB, et al. Use of rocuronium for endotracheal intubation of North American Gulf Coast box turtles. *J Am Vet Med Assoc* 2003;222:1111-1115.
186. Keller K. Terbinafine. *J Exot Pet Med* 2012;2:181-185.
187. Kennedy A, Innis C, Rumbeiha W. Determination of glomerular filtration rate in juvenile Kemp's ridley turtles (*Lepidochelys kempii*) using iohexol clearance, with preliminary comparison of clinically healthy turtles vs. those with renal disease. *J Herp Med Surg* 2012;22:25-29.
188. Kharbush R, Gutwillig A, Hartzler K, et al. Transdermal fentanyl in ball pythons (Python regius) does not provide antinociception and decreases breathing frequency despite high plasma fentanyl levels and brain mu-opioid receptor expression similar to opioid-responsive turtles. *Am J Vet Res*. In press.
189. Kimble SJA, Williams RN. Temporal variance in hematologic and plasma biochemical reference intervals for free ranging Eastern box turtles (*Terrapene carolina carolina*). *J Wildl Dis* 2012;799-802.
190. Kinney ME, Johnson SM, Sladky KK. Behavioral evaluation of red-eared slider turtles (*Trachemys scripta elegans*) administered either morphine or butorphanol following unilateral gonadectomy. *J Herp Med Surg* 2011;21:54-62.
191. Kirchgessner M, Mitchell MA. Chelonians. In: Mitchell MA, Tully Jr TN, eds. *Manual of Exotic Pet Practice*. St. Louis: Saunders/Elsevier; 2009:207-249.
192. Kirchgessner M, Mitchell M, Domenzain L, et al. Evaluating the effect of leuprolide acetate on testosterone levels in captive male green iguanas (*Iguana iguana*). *J Herpetol Med Surg* 2009;19:128-131.
193. Kischinovsky M, Duse A, Wang T, et al. Intramuscular administration of alfaxalone in red-eared slider turtles (*Trachemys scripta elegans*) – effects of dose and body temperature. *Vet Anaesth Analg* 2013;40:13-20.
194. Klaphake E. A fresh look at metabolic bone diseases in reptiles and amphibians. *Vet Clin North Am Exot Anim Pract* 2010;13:375-392.
195. Klaphake E. *Personal observation;* 2016.
196. Klingenberg RJ. A comparison of fenbendazole and ivermectin for the treatment of nematode parasites in ball pythons, *Python regius. Bull Assoc Rept Amph Vet* 1992;2:5-6.
197. Klingenberg RJ. Management of the anorectic ball python. *Proc North Am Vet Conf* 1996;830.
198. Klingenberg RJ. Therapeutics. In: Mader DR, ed. *Reptile Medicine and Surgery*. Philadelphia: WB Saunders Co; 1996:299-321.
199. Klingenberg RJ. *Understanding Reptile Parasites*. Irvine, CA: Advanced Vivarium Systems; 20071-200.
200. Knafo SE, Divers SJ, Rivera S, et al. Sterilisation of hybrid Galapagos tortoises (*Geochelone nigra*) for island restoration. Part 1: endoscopic oophorectomy of females under ketamine-medetomidine anaesthesia. *Vet Rec* 2011;168:78-82.
201. Knotek Z. Alfaxalone as an induction agent for anaesthesia in terrapins and tortoises. *Vet Rec* 2014;175:327-329.
202. Knotkova Z, Doubek J, Knotek Z, et al. Blood cell morphology and plasma biochemistry in Russian tortoises (*Agrionemys horsfieldi*). *Acta Vet Brno* 2002;71:191-198.

203. Koelle P. Urinalysis in tortoises. *Proc Annu Conf Assoc Rept Amph Vet* 2000;111-113.
204. Koelle P. Efficacy of allopurinol in European tortoises with hyperuricemia. *Proc Annu Conf Assoc Rept Amph Vet* 2001;185-186.
205. Koelle P, Hoffmann R. Urinalysis in European tortoises - part II. *Proc Annu Conf Assoc Rept Amph Vet* 2002;117.
206. Kolmstetter CM, Cox S, Ramsay EC. Pharmacokinetics of metronidazole in the yellow rat snake, *Elaphe obsoleta quadrivitatta*. *J Herpetol Med Surg* 2001;11:4-8.
207. Kolmstetter CM, Frazier D, Cox S, et al. Pharmacokinetics of metronidazole in the green iguana, *Iguana iguana*. *Bull Assoc Rept Amph Vet* 1998;8:4-7.
208. Konda ME. The therapeutic effects of mebendazole and piperazine on certain helminth parasites of the garden lizard, *Calotes versicolor*. *Int J Parasitol* 1992;22:843-845.
209. Lai OR, Di Bello A, Soloperto S, et al. Pharmacokinetic behavior of meloxicam in loggerhead sea turtles (*Caretta caretta*) after intramuscular and intravenous administration. *J Wildl Dis* 2015;51:509-512.
210. Lai OR, Marín P, Laricchiuta P, et al. Pharmacokinetics of marbofloxacin in loggerhead sea turtles (*Caretta caretta*) after single intravenous and intramuscular doses. *J Zoo Wildl Med* 2009;40:501-507.
211. Lane T. Crocodilians. In: Mader DR, ed. *Reptile Medicine and Surgery*. 2nd ed. St. Louis: Saunders Elsevier; 2006:100-117.
212. Lanza A, Baldi A, Spugnini EP. Surgery and electrochemotherapy for the treatment of cutaneous squamous cell carcinoma in a yellow-bellied slider (*Trachemys scripta scripta*). *J Am Vet Med Assoc* 2015;246:455-457.
213. Lawrence K, Muggleton PW, Needham JR. Preliminary study on the use of ceftazidime, a broad spectrum cephalosporin antibiotic, in snakes. *Res Vet Sci* 1984;36:16-20.
214. Lawrence K, Palmer GH, Needham JR. Use of carbenicillin in 2 species of tortoise (*Testudo graeca* and *Testudo hermanni*). *Res Vet Sci* 1986;40:413-415.
215. Lawrence K, Needham JR, Palmer GH, et al. A preliminary study on the use of carbenicillin in snakes. *J Vet Pharmacol Therapeut* 1984;7:119-124.
216. Lawton MPC. Anaesthesia. In: Benyon PH, Lawton MPC, Cooper JE, eds. *Manual of Reptiles*. Ames: Iowa State University Press; 1992:170-183.
217. Lawton MPC. Pain management after surgery. *Proc North Am Vet Conf* 1999;782.
218. Lloyd M. Crocodilia. In: Fowler ME, Miller RE, eds. *Zoo and Wild Animal Medicine*. 5th ed. Philadelphia: Elsevier Saunders; 2003:59-70.
219. Lloyd ML. Reptilian dystocias review – causes, prevention, management, and comments on the synthetic hormone vasotocin. *Proc Annu Conf Am Assoc Zoo Vet* 1990;290-296.
220. Lloyd ML. Crocodilian anesthesia. In: Fowler ME, Miller RE, eds. *Zoo & Wild Animal Medicine: Current Therapy 4*. Philadelphia: WB Saunders Co; 1999:205-216.
221. Lloyd ML, Reichard T, Odum RA. Gallamine reversal in Cuban crocodiles (*Crocodilus rhombifer*) using neostigmine alone vs. neostigmine with hyaluronidase. *Proc Annu Conf Assoc Rept Amph Vet* 1994;117-120.
222. Lock BA, Heard DJ, Dennis P. Preliminary evaluation of medetomidine/ketamine combinations for immobilization and reversal with atipamezole in three tortoise species. *Bull Assoc Rept Amph Vet* 1998;8:6-9.
223. Luppi M, Costa M, Malta M, et al. Treatment of *Rhabdias labiata* with levamisole and ivermectin in boa constrictor (*Boa constrictor amarali*). *Veterinaria Noticias* 2007;13:61-65.
224. Machado CC, Silva LFN, Ramos PRR, et al. Seasonal influence on hematologic values and hemoglobin electrophoresis in Brazilian *Boa constrictor amarali*. *J Zoo Wildl Med* 2006;37:487-491.
225. MacLean RA, Harms CA, Braun-McNeill J. Propofol anaesthesia in loggerhead (*Caretta caretta*) sea turtles. *J Wildl Dis* 2008;44:143-150.
226. Mader DR. IME – Use of calcitonin in green iguanas, *Iguana iguana*, with metabolic bone disease. *Bull Assoc Rept Amph Vet* 1993;3:5.

227. Mader DR. Gout. In: Mader DR, ed. *Reptile Medicine and Surgery*. Philadelphia: WB Saunders Co; 1996:374-379.
228. Mader DR. Specific diseases and conditions. In: Mader DR, ed. *Reptile Medicine and Surgery*. Philadelphia: WB Saunders Co; 1996:341-346.
229. Mader DR. Understanding local analgesics: practical use in the green iguana, *Iguana iguana*. *Proc Annu Conf Assoc Rept Amph Vet* 1998;143-147.
230. Mader DR. Metabolic bone diseases. In: Mader DR, ed. *Reptile Medicine and Surgery*. 2nd ed. St. Louis: Saunders/Elsevier; 2006:841-851.
231. Mader DR. Thermal burns. In: Mader DR, ed. *Reptile Medicine and Surgery*. 2nd ed. St. Louis: Saunders/Elsevier; 2006:916-923.
232. Mader DR, Rudloff E. Emergency and critical care. In: Mader DR, ed. *Reptile Medicine and Surgery*. 2nd ed. St. Louis: Saunders/Elsevier; 2006:533-548.
233. Mader DR, Conzelman GM, Baggot JD. Effects of ambient temperature on half life and dosage regimen of amikacin in the gopher snake. *J Am Vet Med Assoc* 1985;187:1134-1136.
234. Mader DR, Horvath CC, Paul-Murphy J. The hematocrit and serum profile of the gopher snake (*Pituophis melanoleucas catenifer*). *J Zoo Anim Med* 1985;16:139-140.
235. Mallo KM, Harms CA, Lewbart GA, et al. Pharmacokinetics of fluconazole in loggerhead sea turtles (*Caretta caretta*) after single intravenous and subcutaneous injections, and multiple subcutaneous injections. *J Zoo Wildl Med* 2002;33:29-35.
236. Manire CA, Anderson ET, Byrd L, Fauquier DA. Dehydration as an effective treatment for brevetoxicosis in loggerhead sea turtles (*Caretta caretta*). *J Zoo Wildl Med* 2013;44:447-452.
237. Manire CA, Hunter RP, Koch DE, et al. Pharmacokinetics of ticarcillin in the loggerhead sea turtle (*Caretta caretta*) after single intravenous and intramuscular injections. *J Zoo Wildl Med* 2005;36:44-53.
238. Manire CA, Rhinehart HL, Pennick GJ, et al. Steady-state plasma concentrations of itraconazole after oral administration in Kemp's ridley sea turtles, *Lepidochelys kempi*. *J Zoo Wildl Med* 2003;34:171-178.
239. Mans C. Clinical update on diagnosis and management of disorders of the digestive system of reptiles. *J Exot Pet Med* 2013;22:141-162.
240. Mans C. Clinical technique: intrathecal drug administration in turtles and tortoises. *J Exot Pet Med* 2014;23:67-70.
241. Mans C. Sedation of pet birds. *J Exot Pet Med* 2014;23:152-157.
242. Mans C, Braun J. Update on common nutritional disorders of captive reptiles. *Vet Clin North Am Exot Anim Pract* 2014;17:369-395.
243. Mans C, Foster JD. Endoscopy-guided ectopic egg removal from the urinary bladder in a leopard tortoise (*Stigmochelys pardalis*). *Can Vet J* 2014;58:569-572.
244. Mans C, Sladky KK. Endoscopically guided removal of cloacal calculi in three African spurred tortoises (*Geochelone sulcate*). *J Am Vet Med Assoc* 2012;240:869-875.
245. Mans C, Drees R, Sladky KK, et al. Effects of body position and extension of the neck and extremities on lung volume measured via computed tomography in red-eared slider turtles (*Trachemys scripta elegans*). *J Am Vet Med Assoc* 2013;243:1190-1196.
246. Mans C, Lahner LL, Baker BB, et al. Antinociceptive efficacy of buprenorphine and hydromorphone in red-eared slider turtles (*Trachemys scripta elegans*). *J Zoo Wildl Med* 2012;43:662-665.
247. Marin P, Bayon A, Fernandez-Varon E, et al. Pharmacokinetics of danofloxacin after single dose intravenous, intramuscular, and subcutaneous administration to loggerhead turtles *Caretta caretta*. *Dis Aquat Organ* 2008;82:231-236.
248. Marks SK, Citino SB. Hematology and serum chemistry of the radiated tortoise (*Testudo radiata*). *J Zoo Wildl Med* 1990;21:342-344.
249. Martel A, Hellebuyck T, Van Waeyenberghe L. Treatment of infections with *Nannizziopsis vriesii*, an emergent reptilian dermatophytea. *Proc Annu Conf Assoc Rept Amph Vet* 2009;69-70.

250. Martelli P, Lai OR, Krishnasamy K, et al. Pharmacokinetic behavior of enrofloxacin in estuarine crocodile (*Crocodylus porosus*) after single intravenous, intramuscular, and oral doses. *J Zoo Wildl Med* 2009;40:696-704.
251. Martinez-Jimenez D, Hernandez-Divers SJ. Emergency care of reptiles. *Vet Clin North Am Exot Anim Pract* 2007;10:557-585.
252. Mathes KA, Holz A, Fehr M. Blood reference values of terrestrial tortoises (*Testudo* spp.) kept in Germany. *Tierarztl Prax Ausg K Klientiere Heimtiere* 2006;34:268-274.
253. Mauldin GN, Done LB. Oncology. In: Mader DR, ed. *Reptile Medicine and Surgery*. 2nd ed. St. Louis: Saunders/Elsevier; 2006:299-322.
254. Mautino M, Page CD. Biology and medicine of turtles and tortoises. *Vet Clin North Am Small Anim Pract* 1993;23:1251-1270.
255. Maxwell LK, Jacobson ER. Preliminary single-dose pharmacokinetics of enrofloxacin after oral and intramuscular administration in green iguanas (*Iguana iguana*). *Proc Annu Conf Am Assoc Zoo Vet* 1997;25.
256. Mayer J. Characterizing the hematologic and plasma chemistry profiles of captive Chinese water dragons, *Physignathus cocincinus*. *J Herpetol Med Surg* 2005;15:45-52.
257. Mayer J, Knoll J, Wrubel KM, Mitchell MA. Characterizing the hematologic and plasma chemistry profiles of captive crested geckos (*Rhacodactylus ciliatus*). *J Herpetol Med Surg* 2011;21:68-75.
258. McArthur S. Problem solving approach to common diseases of terrestrial and semi-aquatic chelonians. In: McArthur S, Wilkinson R, Meyer J, eds. *Medicine and Surgery of Tortoises and Turtles*. Oxford, UK: Blackwell Publishing Ltd; 2004:309-377.
259. McArthur SDJ, Wilkinson RJ, Barrows MG. Tortoises and turtles. In: Meredith A, Redrobe S, eds. *BSAVA Manual of Exotic Pets*. 4th ed. Gloucestershire, GB: British Small Animal Veterinary Association; 2002:208-222.
260. McBride M, Hernandez-Divers SJ, Koch T, et al. Preliminary evaluation of pre- and postprandial 3[alpha]-hydroxy bile acids in the green iguana, *Iguana iguana*. *J Herpetol Med Surg* 2006;16:129-134.
261. McBride MP, Wojick KB, Georoff TA, et al. *Ophidiomyces ophiodiicola* dermatitis in eight free-ranging timber rattlesnakes (*Crotalus horridus*) from Massachusetts. *J Zoo Wildl Med* 2015;46:86-94.
262. McFadden MS, Bennett RA, Reavill DR, et al. Clinical and histologic effects of intracardiac administration of propofol for induction of anesthesia in ball pythons (*Python regius*). *J Am Assoc Vet Med* 2011;239:803-807.
263. McGuire JL, Hernandez SM, Smith LL, et al. Safety and utility of an anesthetic protocol for the collection of biological samples from gopher tortoises. *Wildl Soc Bull* 2014;38:43-50.
264. Mehler SJ, Bennett RA. Upper alimentary tract disease. In: Mader DR, ed. *Reptile Medicine and Surgery*. 2nd ed. St. Louis: Saunders/Elsevier; 2006:924-930.
265. Mehlhorn H, Schmahl G, Frese M, et al. Effects of a combinations of emodepside and praziquantel on parasites of reptiles and rodents. *Parasitol Res* 2005;97(Suppl 1):S65-S69.
266. Messonnier S. Formulary for exotic pets. *Vet Forum* 1996;Aug:46-49.
267. Meyer J. Gastrographin as a gastrointestinal contrast agent in the Greek tortoise (*Testudo hermanni*). *J Zoo Wildl Med* 1998;29:183-189.
268. Miller HA, Brandt PJ, Frye FL, et al. *Trichomonas* associated with ocular and subcutaneous lesions in geckos. *Proc Annu Conf Assoc Rept Amph Vet* 1994;102-107.
269. Millichamp NJ. Surgical techniques in reptiles. In: Jacobson ER, Kollias Jr GV, eds. *Exotic Animals*. New York: Churchill Livingstone; 1988:49-74.
270. Millichamp NJ. Ophthalmology. In: Girling SJ, Raiti P, eds. *BSAVA Manual of Reptiles*. 2nd ed. Quedgeley, Gloucester: British Small Animal Veterinary Association; 2004:199-209.
271. Mitchell M. Ophidia. In: Fowler ME, Miller RE, eds. *Zoo and Wild Animal Medicine*. 5th ed. Philadelphia: Saunders/Elsevier; 2003:82-91.
272. Mitchell MA. Therapeutics. In: Mader DR, ed. *Reptile Medicine and Surgery*. 2nd ed. St. Louis: Saunders/Elsevier; 2006:631-664.

273. Mitchell MA. Ponazuril. *J Exot Pet Med* 2008;17:228-229.
274. Mitchell MA. Managing the reptile patient in the veterinary hospital: establishing a standards of care model for nontraditional species. *J Exot Pet Med* 2010;19:56-72.
275. Montali RJ, Bush M, Smeller JM. Pathology of nephrotoxicity of gentamicin in snakes – model for reptilian gout. *Vet Pathol* 1979;16:108-115.
276. Morgan-Davies AM. Immobilization of the Nile crocodile (*Crocodilus niloticus*) with gallamine triethiodide. *J Zoo Anim Med* 1980;11:85-87.
277. Murray MJ. Aural abscesses. In: Mader DR, ed. *Reptile Medicine and Surgery*. 2nd ed. St. Louis: Saunders/Elsevier; 2006:742-746.
278. Murray MJ. Pneumonia and lower respiratory tract disease. In: Mader DR, ed. *Reptile Medicine and Surgery*. 2nd ed. St. Louis: Saunders/Elsevier; 2006:865-877.
279. Naldo JL, Libanan NL, Samour JH. Health assessment of a spiny-tailed lizard (*Uromastyx* spp.) population in Abu Dhabi, United Arab Emirates. *J Zoo Wildl Med* 2009;40:445-452.
280. Naples LM, Langan JN, Mylniczenko ND, et al. Islet cell tumor in a Savannah monitor (*Varanus exanthematicus*). *J Herpetol Med Surg* 2009;19:97-105.
281. Nardini G, Barbarossa A, Dall'Occo A, et al. Pharmacokinetics of cefovecin sodium after subcutaneous administration to Hermann's tortoises (*Testudo hermanni*). *Am J Vet Res* 2014;75:918-923.
282. Nardini G, Di Girolamo N, Leopardi S, et al. Evaluation of liver parenchyma and perfusion using dynamic contrast-enhanced computed tomography and contrast-enhanced ultrasonography in captive green iguanas (*Iguana iguana*) under general anesthesia. *BMC Vet Res* 2014;10:112-120.
283. Nathan R. Treatment with ovicentesis, prostaglandin E_2 then prostaglandin $F_{2\alpha}$ to aid oviposition in a spotted python, Antaresia maculosa. *Bull Assoc Rept Amph Vet* 1996;6:4.
284. Necas P. *Chameleons, Nature's Hidden Jewels*. Malabar, FL: Krieger Publishing; 1999113-119.
285. Neiffer DL, Lydick D, Burks K, et al. Hematologic and plasma biochemical changes associated with fenbendazole administration in Hermann's tortoises (*Testudo hermanni*). *J Zoo Wildl Med* 2005;36:661-672.
286. Nevarez JG, Mitchell MA, Le Blanc C, et al. Determination of plasma biochemistries, ionized calcium, vitamin D_3, and hematocrit values in captive green iguanas (*Iguana iguana*) from El Salvador. *Proc Annu Conf Assoc Rept Amph Vet* 2002;87-91.
287. Nichols DK, Lamirande EW. Use of methohexital sodium as an anesthetic in two species of colubrid snakes. *Proc Joint Conf Am Assoc Zoo Vet/Assoc Rept Amph Vet* 1994;161-162.
288. Norton TM. Chelonian emergency and critical care. *Semin Avian Exot Pet Med* 2005;14:106-130.
289. Norton TM, Cox S, Nelson SE, et al. Pharmacokinetics of tramadol and O-desmethyltramadol in loggerhead sea turtles (*Caretta caretta*). *J Zoo Wildl Med* 2015;46:262-265.
290. Norton TM, Jacobson ER, Caligiuri R, et al. Medical management of a Galapagos tortoise (*Geochelone elephantopus*) with hypothyroidism. *J Zoo Wildl Med* 1989;20:212-216.
291. Norton TM, Spratt J, Behler J, et al. Medetomidine and ketamine anesthesia with atipamezole reversal in free-ranging gopher tortoises, *Gopherus polyphemus*. *Proc Annu Conf Assoc Rept Amph Vet* 1998;25-27.
292. O O, Churgin SM, Sladky KK, Smith LJ. Anesthetic induction and recovery parameters in bearded dragons (*Pogona vitticeps*): comparison of isoflurane delivered in 100% oxygen versus 21% oxygen. *J Zoo Wildl Med* 2015;46:534-539. http://dx.doi.org/10.1638/2014-0193.1.
293. Olesen MG, Bertelsen MF, Perry SF, et al. Effects of preoperative administration of butorphanol or meloxicam on physiologic responses to surgery in ball pythons. *J Am Vet Med Assoc* 2008;233:1883-1888.
294. Olsson A, Phalen D. Medetomidine immobilization and atipamazole reversal in large estuarine crocodiles (*Crocodylus porosus*) using metabolically scaled dosages. *Aust Vet J* 2012;90:240-244.
295. Olsson A, Phalen D. Preliminary studies of chemical immobilization of captive juvenile estuarine (*Crocodylus porosus*) and Australian freshwater crocodiles (*Crocodylus johnstoni*) with medetomidine and reversal with atipamazole. *Vet Anaesth Analg* 2012;39:345-356.

296. Olsson A, Phalen D, Dart C. Preliminary studies of alfaxalone for intravenous immobilization of juvenile captive estuarine crocodiles (*Crocodylus porosus*) and Australian freshwater crocodiles (*Crocodylus johnstoni*) at optimal and selected suboptimal thermal zones. *Vet Anaesth Analg* 2013;40:494-502.
297. Oonincx DGAB, Stevens Y, van den Borne JJGC, et al. Effects of vitamin D-3 supplementation and UVB exposure on the growth and plasma concentration of vitamin D-3 metabolites in juvenile bearded dragons (*Pogona vitticeps*). *Comp Biochem Physiol B Biochem Mol Biol* 2010;156:122-128.
298. Oppenheim YC, Moon PF. Sedative effects of midazolam in red-eared sliders (*Trachemys scripta elegans*). *J Zoo Wildl Med* 1995;26:409-413.
299. Origgi FC. Testudinid herpesviruses: a review. *J Herp Med Surg* 2012;22:42-54.
300. Origgi F, Roccabianca P, Gelmetti D. Dermatophilosis in *Furcifer* (*Chamaleo*) *pardalis*. *Bull Assoc Rept Amph Vet* 1999;9:9-11.
301. O'Shea R, Ball RL. Use of bovine tendon collagen for wound repair in *Varanus komodoensis*. *Proc Annu Conf Assoc Rept Amph Vet* 2010;66-69.
302. Pace L, Mader DR. Atropine and glycopyrrolate, route of administration and response in the green iguana (*Iguana iguana*). *Proc Annu Conf Assoc Rept Amph Vet* 2002;79.
303. Page CD. Current reptilian anesthesia procedures. In: Fowler ME, ed. *Zoo & Wild Animal Medicine: Current Therapy 3*. Philadelphia: WB Saunders Co; 1993:140-143.
304. Page CD, Mautino M, Derendorf H, et al. Multiple dose pharmacokinetics of ketoconazole administered orally to gopher tortoises (*Gopherus polyphemus*). *J Zoo Wildl Med* 1991;22:191-198.
305. Paré JA, Crawshaw GJ, Barta JR. Treatment of cryptosporidiosis in Gila monsters (*Heloderma suspectum*) with paromomycin. *Proc Annu Conf Assoc Rept Amph Vet* 1997;23.
306. Petersen NT. Terbutaline. *J Exot Pet Med* 2012;21:260-263.
307. Plumb DC. Cefazolin. In: *Plumb's Veterinary Drug Handbook*. 8th ed Ames: Wiley-Blackwell; 2015:230-232.
308. Plumb DC. Probenecid. In: *Plumb's Veterinary Drug Handbook*. 8th ed Ames: Wiley-Blackwell; 2015:1214-1216.
309. Preston DL, Mosley CAE, Mason RT. Sources of variability in recovery time from methohexital sodium anesthesia in snakes. *Copeia* 2010;3:496-501.
310. Prezant RM, Isaza R, Jacobson ER. Plasma concentrations and disposition kinetics of enrofloxacin in gopher tortoises (*Gopherus polyphemus*). *J Zoo Wildl Med* 1994;25:82-87.
311. Proneca LM, Fowler S, Kleine S, et al. Coelioscopic-assisted sterilization of female Mojave desert tortoises (*Gopherus agassizii*). *J Herp Med Surg* 2014;24:95-100.
312. Proneca LM, Fowler S, Kleine S, et al. Single surgeon coelioscopic orchiectomy of desert tortoises (*Gopherus agassizii*) for population management. *Vet Rec* 2014;175:404-409.
313. Pye GW, Carpenter JW. Ketamine sedation followed by propofol anesthesia in a slider, *Trachemys scripta*, to facilitate removal of an esophageal foreign body. *Bull Assoc Rept Amph Vet* 1998;8:16-17.
314. Quesada RJ, Aitken-Palmer C, Conley K, et al. Accidental submeningeal injection of propofol in gopher tortoises (*Gopherus polyphemus*). *Vet Rec* 2010;167:494-495.
315. Raiti P. Veterinary care of the common kingsnake, *Lampropeltis getula*. *Bull Assoc Rept Amph Vet* 1995;5:11-18.
316. Raiti P. Administration of aerosolized antibiotics in reptiles. *Exot DVM* 2002;4(3):87-90.
317. Ramsay EC, Dotson TK. Tissue and serum enzyme activities in the yellow rat snake (*Elaphe obsoleta quadrivitatta*). *Am J Vet Res* 1995;56:423-428.
318. Raphael B, Clark CH, Hudson Jr R. Plasma concentration of gentamicin in turtles. *J Zoo Anim Med* 1985;16:136-139.
319. Raphael BL. Chelonians. In: Fowler ME, Miller RE, eds. *Zoo and Wild Animal Medicine*. 5th ed. Philadelphia: Saunders/Elsevier; 2003:48-58.
320. Raphael BL, Papich M, Cook RA. Pharmacokinetics of enrofloxacin after a single intramuscular injection in Indian star tortoises (*Geochelone elegans*). *J Zoo Wildl Med* 1994;25:88-94.

321. Redrobe S, MacDonald J. Sample collection and clinical pathology of reptiles. *Vet Clin North Am Exot Anim Pract* 1999;2:709-730.
322. *Reptiles Magazine*. www.reptilesmagazine.com. Accessed December 11, 2016.
323. Rivera S. Health assessment of the reptilian reproductive tract. *J Exot Pet Med* 2008;17: 259-266.
324. Rivera S, Divers SJ, Knafo SE, et al. Sterilisation of hybrid Galapagos tortoises (*Geochelone nigra*) for island restoration. Part 2: phallectomy of males under intrathecal anaesthesia with lidocaine. *Vet Rec* 2011;168:78-81.
325. Rojo-Solís C, Ros-Rodriguez JM, Valls M. Pharmakokinetics of meloxicam (Metacam) after intravenous, intramuscular, and oral administration in red-eared slider turtles (*Trachemys scripta elegans*). *Proc Joint Conf Am Assoc Zoo Vet/Am Assoc Wildl Vet* 2009;228.
326. Rooney MB, Levine G, Gaynor J, et al. Sevoflurane anesthesia in desert tortoises (*Gopherus agassizii*). *J Zoo Wildl Med* 1999;30:64-69.
327. Rosenthal K. Chemotherapeutic treatment of a sarcoma in a corn snake. *Proc Joint Conf Am Assoc Zoo Vet/Assoc Rept Amph Vet* 1994;46.
328. Rossi J. Practical reptile dermatology. *Proc North Am Vet Conf* 1995;648-649.
329. Rossi JV. Emergency medicine of reptiles. *Proc North Am Vet Conf* 1998;799-801.
330. Rowland MN. Use of a deslorelin implant to control aggression in a male bearded dragon (*Pogona vitticeps*). *Vet Rec* 2011;169:127.
331. Ruiz T, Campos WNS, Peres TPS, et al. Intraocular pressure, ultrasonographic and echobiometric findings of juvenile Yacare caiman (*Caiman yacare*) eye. *Vet Ophthalmol* 2015;18: 40-45.
332. Salvadori M, DeVito V, Owen H, et al. Pharmacokinetics of enrofloxacin and its metabolite ciprofloxacin after intracoelomic administration in tortoises (*Testudo hermanni*). *Israel J Vet Med* 2015;70:45-48.
333. Sanches L. Anestesia espinhal no lagarto Iguana iguana (Linnaeus, 1758). [Master's dissertation]. Available at: https://repositorio.unesp.br/handle/11449/115707. Accessed April 25, 2017.
334. Schaeffer DO. Anesthesia and analgesia in nontraditional laboratory animal species. In: Kohn DF, Wixson SK, White WJ, et al. *Anesthesia and Analgesia in Laboratory Animals*. New York: Academic Press; 1997:338-378.
335. Scheelings F, Dobson E, Hooper C, Eden P. Cutaneous and systemic mycoses from infection with *Lecanicillium* spp. in captive Guthega skinks (*Liopholis guthega*). *Aust Vet J* 2015;93: 248-251.
336. Scheelings TF, Holz P, Haynes L, et al. A preliminary study of the chemical restraint of selected squamate reptiles with alfaxalone. *Proc Annu Conf Assoc Rept Amph Vet* 2010;114-115.
337. Schilliger L, Betremieux O, Rochet J, et al. Absorption and efficacy of a spot-on combination containing emodepside plus praziquantel in reptiles. *Rev Med Vet (Toulouse)* 2009;160: 557-561.
338. Schnellbacher R. Butorphanol. *J Exot Pet Med* 2010;19:192-195.
339. Schobert E. Telazol use in wild and exotic animals. *Vet Med* 1987;82:1080-1088.
340. Schroeder CA, Johnson RA. The efficacy of intracoelomic fospropofol in red-eared sliders (*Trachemys scripta elegans*). *J Zoo Wildl Med* 2013;44:941-950.
341. Schumacher J. Reptiles and amphibians. In: Thurman JC, Tranquilli WJ, Benson GJ, eds. *Lumb and Jones' Veterinary Anesthesia*. 3rd ed. Baltimore, MD: Williams & Wilkins; 1996:670-685.
342. Schumacher J. Lacertilia. In: Fowler ME, Miller RE, eds. *Zoo and Wild Animal Medicine*. 5th ed. Philadelphia: Saunders/Elsevier; 2003:73-81.
343. Schumacher J. Respiratory medicine of reptiles. *Vet Clin North Am Exot Anim Pract* 2011;14:207-224.
344. Schumacher J, Yelen T. Anesthesia and analgesia. In: Mader DR, ed. *Reptile Medicine and Surgery*. 2nd ed. St. Louis: Saunders/Elsevier; 2006:442-452.
345. Schuster EJ, Strueve J, Fehr MJ, et al. Measurement of intraocular pressure in healthy unanesthetized inland bearded dragons (*Pogona vitticeps*). *Am J Vet Res* 2015;76:494-499.

346. Shepard MK, Divers S, Braun C, et al. Pharmacodynamics of alfaxalone after single-dose intramuscular administration in red-eared sliders (*Trachemys scripta elegans*): a comparison of two different doses at two different ambient temperatures. *Vet Anaesth Analg* 2013;40: 590-598.
347. Sim R. Voriconazole. *J Exot Pet Med* 2016;25:342-347.
348. Sim RR, Allender MC, Crawford LK, et al. Ranavirus epizootic in captive Eastern box turtles (*Terrapene carolina carolina*) with concurrent herpesvirus and *Mycoplasma* infection: management and monitoring. *J Zoo Wildl Med* 2016;47:256-270.
349. Skovgaard N, Crossley DA, Wang T. Low cost of pulmonary ventilation in American alligators (*Alligator mississippiensis*) stimulated with doxapram. *J Exp Biol* 2016;219:933-936.
350. Sladky KK, Kinney ME, Johnson SM. Analgesic efficacy of butorphanol and morphine in bearded dragons and corn snakes. *J Am Vet Med Assoc* 2008;233:267-273.
350a. Sladky KK. *Unpublished data;* 2017.
351. Sladky KK, Kinney ME, Johnson SM. Effects of opioid receptor activation on thermal antinociception in red-eared slider turtles (*Trachemys scripta*). *Am J Vet Res* 2009;70:1072-1078.
352. Sladky KK, Mans C. Clinical analgesia in reptiles. *J Exot Pet Med* 2012;21:17-32.
353. Sladky KK, Miletic V, Paul-Murphy J, et al. Analgesic efficacy and respiratory effects of butorphanol and morphine in turtles. *J Am Vet Med Assoc* 2007;230:1356-1362.
354. Sleeman JM, Gaynor J. Sedative and cardiopulmonary effects of medetomidine and reversal with atipamezole in desert tortoises (*Gopherus agassizii*). *J Zoo Wildl Med* 2000;31:28-35.
355. Smith JA, McGuire NC, Mitchell MA. Cardiopulmonary physiology and anesthesia in crocodilians. *Proc Annu Conf Assoc Rept Amph Vet* 1998;17-21.
356. Spadola F, Morici M, Knotek Z. Combination of lidocaine/prilocaine with tramadol for short time anaesthesia-analgesia in chelonians: 18 cases. *Acta Vet Brno* 2015;84:71-75.
357. Spörle H, Gobel T, Schildger B. Blood levels of some anti-infectives in the spur-thighed tortoise (*Testudo hermanni*). *Proc 4th Intl Colloq Path Med Rept Amph* 1991;120-128.
358. Stahl SJ. Captive management, breeding, and common medical problems of the veiled chameleon (*Chamaeleo calyptratus*). *Proc Annu Conf Assoc Rept Amph Vet* 1997;29-40.
359. Stahl SJ. Common diseases of the green iguana. *Proc North Am Vet Conf* 1998;806-809.
360. Stahl SJ. Reproductive disorders of the green iguana. *Proc North Am Vet Conf* 1998;810-813.
361. Stahl SJ. Medical management of bearded dragons. *Proc North Am Vet Conf* 1999;789-792.
362. Stahl SJ. Diseases of the reptile pancreas. *Vet Clin North Am Exot Anim Pract* 2003;6:191-212.
363. Stahl SJ. Pet lizard conditions and syndromes. *Semin Avian Exot Pet Med* 2003;12:162-182.
364. Stahl SJ. Clinician's approach to the chameleon patient. *Proc North Am Vet Conf* 2006;1667-1670.
365. Stahl S, Donoghue S. Pharyngostomy tube placement, management and use for nutritional support in chelonian patients. *Proc Annu Conf Assoc Rept Amph Vet* 1997;93-97.
366. Stamper MA, Papich MG, Lewbart GA, et al. Pharmacokinetics of ceftazidime in loggerhead sea turtles (*Caretta caretta*) after single intravenous and intramuscular injections. *J Zoo Wildl Med* 1999;30:32-35.
367. Stegman N, Heatley JJ. The use of haloperidol in mitigation of human-directed aggression in boid snakes. *Proc Annu Conf Assoc Rept Amph Vet* 2010;113.
368. Stirl R, Krug P, Bonath KH. Tiletamine/zolazepam sedation in boa constrictors and its influence on respiration, circulation, and metabolism. *Proc Conf Euro Assoc Zoo Wildl Vet* 1996;115-119.
369. Stringer EM, Garner MM, Proudfoot JS, et al. Phaeohyphomycosis of the carapace in an Aldabra tortoise (*Geochelone gigantea*). *J Zoo Wildl Med* 2009;40:160-167.
370. Suarez-Yana T, Montes D, Zuniga R, et al. Hematologic, morphometric, and biochemical analytes of clinically healthy green sea turtles (*Chelonia mydas*) in Peru. *Chelonian Conserv Biol* 2016;15:153-157.
371. Suedmeyer WK. Iron deficiency in a group of American alligators: diagnosis and treatment. *J Small Exot Anim Med* 1991;1:69-72.
372. Sykes JM. Updates and practical approaches to reproductive disorders in reptiles. *Vet Clin North Am Exot Anim Pract* 2010;13:349-373.

373. Sykes JM, Klaphake E. Reptile hematology. *Vet Clin North Am Exot Anim Pract* 2015;18:63-82.
374. Sykes JM, Ramsay EC, Schumacher J, et al. Evaluation of an implanted osmotic pump for delivery of amikacin to corn snakes (*Elaphe guttata guttata*). *J Zoo Wildl Med* 2006;37: 373-380.
375. Taylor Jr RW, Jacobson ER. Hematology and serum chemistry of the gopher tortoise, *Gopherus polyphemus*. *Comp Biochem Physiol A* 1982;72:425-428.
376. Teare JA, ed. Species360 physiological reference intervals for captive wildlife. Species360, Bloomington, MN. 2013. Available at: https://zims.species360.org/Main.aspx. Accessed November 5, 2016.
377. Teare JA, Bush M. Toxicity and efficacy of ivermectin in chelonians. *J Am Vet Med Assoc* 1983;183:1195-1197.
378. Theusen LR, Bertelsen MF, Brimer L, et al. Selected pharmokinetic parameters for cefovecin in hens and green iguanas. *J Vet Pharmacol Therap* 2009;32:613-617.
379. Tothill A, Johnson J, Branvold H, et al. Effect of cisapride, erythromycin, and metoclopramide on gastrointestinal transit time in the desert tortoise, *Gopherus agassizii*. *J Herpetol Med Surg* 2000;10:16-20.
380. Troiano J, Gould E, Gould I. Hematological reference intervals in Argentine lizard *Tupinambis merianae*. *Comp Clin Path* 2008;17:169-174.
381. Tuttle AD, Papich M, Lewbart GA, et al. Pharmacokinetics of ketoprofen in the green iguana (*Iguana iguana*) following single intravenous and intramuscular injections. *J Zoo Wildl Med* 2006;37:567-570.
382. Uney K, Altan F, Aboubakr M, et al. Pharmacokinetics of meloxicam in red-eared slider turtles (*Trachemys scripta scripta*) after single intravenous and intramuscular injections. *Am J Vet Res* 2016;77:439-444.
383. Van Waeyenberghe L, Baert K, Pasmans F, et al. Voriconazole, a safe alternative for treating infections caused by the *Chrysosporium* anamorph of *Nannizziopsis vriesii* in bearded dragons (*Pogona vitticeps*). *Med Mycol* 2010;48:880-885.
384. Walden M, Mitchell M. Evaluation of three treatment modalities against *Isospora amphiboluri* in inland bearded dragons (*Pogona vitticeps*). *J Exot Pet Med* 2012;21:213-218.
385. Wallace BP, George RH. Alternative techniques for obtaining blood samples from leatherback turtles. *Chelonian Conser Biol* 2007;6:147-149.
386. Wambugu SN, Towett PK, Kiama SG, et al. Effects of opioids in the formalin test in the Speke's hinged tortoise (*Kinixy's spekii*). *J Vet Pharmacol Ther* 2010;33:347-351.
387. Wangen K. Cisapride. *J Exot Pet Med* 2013;22:301-304.
388. Waxman S, Prados AP, de Lucas JJ, et al. Pharmacokinetic behavior of enrofloxacin and its metabolite ciprofloxacin in Urutu pit vipers (*Bothrops alternatus*) after intramuscular administration. *J Zoo Wildl Med* 2014;45:78-85.
389. Waxman S, Prados AP, de Lucas JJ, et al. Pharmacokinetics of enrofloxacin and its metabolite ciprofloxacin after single intramuscular administration in South American rattlesnake (*Crotalus durissus terrificus*). *Pakistan Vet J* 2015;35:494-498.
390. Wellehan JFX, Gunkel CI. Emergent diseases in reptiles. *Semin Avian Exot Pet Med* 2004;13:160-174.
391. White SD, Bourdeau P, Bruet V, et al. Reptiles with dermatological lesions: a retrospective study of 301 cases at two university veterinary teaching hospitals (1992-2008). *Vet Dermatol* 2010;22:150-161.
392. Whiting SD, Guinea ML, Fomiatti K, et al. Plasma biochemical and PCV ranges for healthy, wild, immature hawksbill sea turtles (*Eretmochelys imbricata*). *Vet Rec* 2014;174:608.
393. Willette-Frahm M, Wright KM, Thode BC. Select protozoal diseases in amphibians and reptiles. *Bull Assoc Rept Amph Vet* 1995;5:19-29.
394. Williams CJ, James LE, Bertelsen MF, et al. Tachycardia in response to remote capsaicin injections as a model for nociception in the ball python (*Python regius*). *Vet Anaesth Analg* 2015;43:429-434.

395. Williams SR, Sims MA, Roth-Johnson L, Wickes B. Surgical removal of an abscess associated with *Fusarium solani* from a Kemp's ridley sea turtle (*Lepidochelys kempii*). *J Zoo Wildl Med* 2012;43:402-406.
396. Wills S, Beaufrère H, Watrous G, et al. Proximal duodenoileal anastomosis for treatment of small intestinal obstruction and volvulus in a green iguana (*Iguana iguana*). *J Am Vet Med Assoc* 2016;249:1061-1066.
397. Wimsatt J, Tothill A, Offermann CF, et al. Long-term and per-rectum disposition of clarithromycin in the desert tortoise (*Gopherus agassizii*). *J Am Assoc Lab Anim Sci* 2008;41-45.
398. Wissman MA, Parsons B. Dermatophytosis of green iguanas (*Iguana iguana*). *J Small Exot Anim Med* 1993;2:133-136.
399. Wood FE, Critchley KH, Wood JR. Anesthesia in green the sea turtle Chelonia mydas. *Am J Vet Res* 1982;43:1882.
400. Wozniak EJ, DeNardo DF. The biology, clinical significance and control of the common snake mite, *Ophionyssus natricis*, in captive reptiles. *J Herpetol Med Surg* 2000;10:4-10.
401. Wright K. Omphalectomy of reptiles. *Exot DVM* 2001;3(1):11-15.
402. Wright KM. Common medical problems of tortoises. *Proc North Am Vet Conf* 1997;769-771.
403. Wright KM, Skeba S. Hematology and plasma chemistries of captive prehensile-tailed skinks (*Corucia zebrata*). *J Zoo Wildl Med* 1992;23:429-432.
404. Young LA, Schumacher J, Papich MG, et al. Disposition of enrofloxacin and its metabolite ciprofloxacin after intravascular injection in juvenile Burmese pythons (*Python molurus bivittatus*). *J Zoo Wildl Med* 1997;28:71-79.
405. Zaias J, Norton T, Fickel A, et al. Biochemical and hematologic values for 18 clinically healthy radiated tortoises (*Geochelone radiata*) on St Catherines Island, Georgia. *Vet Clin Pathol* 2006;35:321-325.
406. Ziolo M, Bertelsen M. Effects of propofol administered via the supravertebral sinus in red-eared sliders. *J Am Vet Med Assoc* 2009;234:390-393.

Chapter 5 **Birds**

Michelle G. Hawkins | David Sanchez-Migallon Guzman | Hugues Beaufrère | Angela M. Lennox | James W. Carpenter

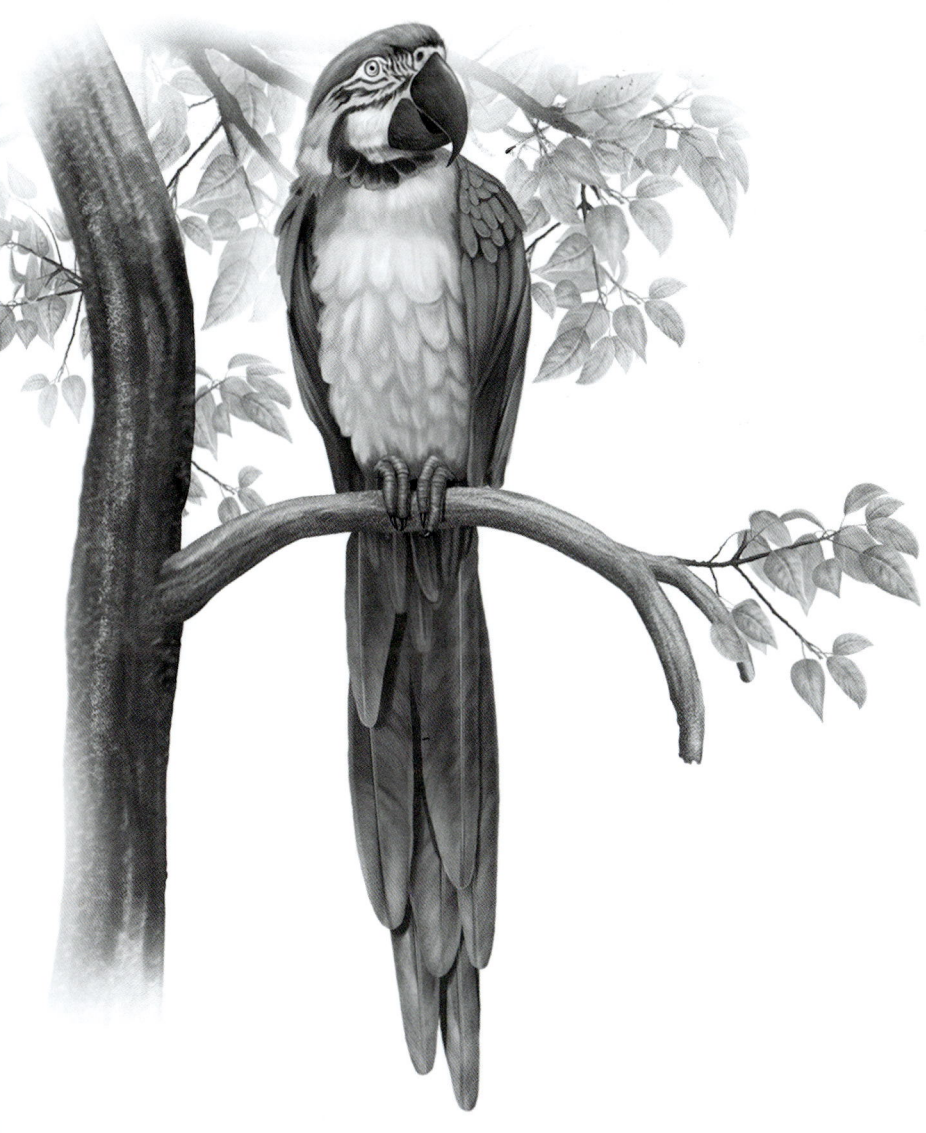

Exotic Animal Formulary

TABLE 5-1 Antimicrobial Agents Used in Birds.

Agent	Dosage	Species/Comments
Amikacin	—	Extended spectrum aminoglycoside; least nephrotoxic of the aminoglycosides; maintain hydration and avoid concurrent use of other nephroactive drugs[90]
	7 mg/kg IV q24h[342]	Emus/PD; mean serum levels declined below a target trough of 4 µg/mL at 24 hr
	7.6 mg/kg IM q8h[374]	Ostriches/PD; causes myositis; painful injection
	10 mg/kg IM q12h[566]	Cranes
	10-15 mg/kg IM q24h[333]	Raptors
	10-15 mg/kg IM q12h[473]	Amazon parrots, cockatiels, cockatoos/PD
	10-15 mg/kg IM, IV q8-12h[333]	Most species, including psittacines
	10-20 mg/kg IM, IV q8-12h[298]	African grey parrots/PD
	15 mg/kg IM q12h, IV q8h[721]	Blue-fronted Amazon parrots/PD
	15-20 mg/kg/day divided q8-24h[86]	Red-tailed hawks/PD; use low end of dose range for smaller hawks
	15-20 mg/kg SC, IM, IV q8-12h[203]	Passerines, pigeons/5 days maximum[686]
	15-20 mg/kg IM q8-12h[637]	Cockatiels/PD
	15-30 mg/kg IM q12-24h[203,822]	Most species, including passerines/use in combination with other agents for *Mycobacterium*; see Table 5-44
	528 mg/L drinking water[806]	Ratites/egg dip
	3 g/40 packet bone cement[810]	PMMA bead formation (1:14 ratio); same dose for all aminoglycoside beads
Amoxicillin/clavulanate (Clavamox, Zoetis)	—	β-lactamase inhibitor[90]
	7-14 mg/kg IM q24h[112]	Ostriches
	10-15 mg/kg PO q12h[806]	Ratites
	60-120 mg/kg IM q8-12h[204]	Collared doves/PD
	125 mg/kg PO q12h[255,607]	Most species, including pigeons, psittacines, raptors
	125 mg/kg PO q8h[575]	Blue-fronted Amazon parrots/PD
	125 mg/kg PO q6h[148]	Psittacines
	125-250 mg/kg PO q8-12h[204]	Collared doves/PD
Amoxicillin sodium	—	Broad-spectrum β-lacatamase-sensitive penicillin[90]
	50 mg/kg IM q12-24h[198,202]	Pigeons/PD; Gram-positive bacteria
	100 mg/kg IM, IV q4-8h[697]	Bustards/PD; administer q4h IM or q8h IV to maintain blood levels >2 mg/mL
	150 mg/kg IM q8h[689]	Passerines, soft bills
	250 mg/kg IM q12-24h[198,202]	Pigeons/PD; Gram-positive and Gram-negative bacteria

TABLE 5-1	Antimicrobial Agents Used in Birds. (cont'd)	
Agent	Dosage	Species/Comments
Amoxicillin trihydrate	—	Broad-spectrum β-lacatamase-sensitive penicillin;[90] may have minimal activity for common Gram-negative infections of birds; higher doses are needed in birds to achieve the same peak levels as in mammals[206]
	15-22 mg/kg PO q8h[806]	Ratites
	20 mg/kg PO q12-24h[200]	Pigeons/PD; mean half-life 66 min
	30 mg/kg IM q12h × 5 days[112]	Pigeons
	40-80 mg/kg PO q12h × 5 days[112]	Pigeons
	55-110 mg/kg PO q12h[318]	Pigeons
	100 mg/kg PO q12-24h[207]	Pigeons/PD
	100 mg/kg PO q8h[51]	Most species, including raptors
	100-150 mg/kg PO q12h[149a]	Raptors
	100-200 mg/kg PO, IM q4-8h[207]	Pigeons
	150 mg/kg SC, IM q24h × 5 days (administer q48h with long-acting preparation)[697]	Pigeons
	150 mg/kg PO, IV[753]	Pigeons/PD; *Streptococcus bovis*
	150-175 mg/kg PO q12h[148]	Passerines (towhees), psittacines
	150-175 mg/kg PO q4-8h[689,808]	Pigeons, psittacines
	65 mg/L drinking water[806]	Ratites
	200-400 mg/L drinking water[311]	Canaries/aviary use
	500-800 mg/L drinking water[318]	Pigeons
	1500 mg/L drinking water × 5 days[753]	Pigeons/*Streptococcus bovis*
	1500-4500 mg/L drinking water[148]	Psittacines
	300-500 mg/kg soft feed[311]	Canaries/aviary use
	600 mg/kg soft feed[148]	Psittacines
Ampicillin sodium	—	Broad-spectrum β-lactamase-sensitive penicillin[90]
	50 mg/kg IM q6-8h[217]	Amazon parrots/PD; localized infections
	100 mg/kg IM q4h[217]	Amazon parrots/PD
	150 mg/kg IM q12-24h[198,202]	Pigeons/PD
	150 mg/kg IM q12-24h[201]	Passerines, soft bills
	150-200 mg/kg PO q8-12h[217]	Amazon parrots/PD; therapeutic levels not achieved in blue-naped Amazons at this dosage

Continued

TABLE 5-1   Antimicrobial Agents Used in Birds. (cont'd)

Agent	Dosage	Species/Comments
Ampicillin sodium (cont'd)	174 mg/kg PO q24h[175]	Pigeons/PD; *Streptococcus bovis*
	528 mg/L drinking water[175]	Pigeons/PD; *Streptococcus bovis*
Ampicillin trihydrate	—	Broad-spectrum β-lactamase-sensitive penicillin; minimal activity for common Gram-negative infections of birds; poor gastrointestinal absorption; may be useful for treating sensitive gastrointestinal infections[697]
	4-7 mg/kg SC, IM q8h[806]	Ratites (excluding emus)
	11-15 mg/kg PO q8h[806]	Ratites
	15 mg/kg IM q12h[111]	Raptors/PD
	15-20 mg/kg SC, IM q12h[111]	Emus, cranes (PD)
	25 mg/kg PO q12-24h[198,202]	Pigeons/PD
	100 mg/kg PO q12-24h[198,202]	Pigeons/PD
	100 mg/kg IM q12h[566]	Cranes
	100 mg/kg IM q4h[333]	Most species, including psittacines
	100-200 mg/kg PO q6-8h[333]	Psittacines
	155 mg/kg IM q12-24h[207]	Pigeons/PD; amoxicillin preferred over ampicillin for IM use in pigeons
	500 mg powder/L drinking water[333]	Psittacines/*Pseudomonas*
	1000-2000 mg/L drinking water[311]	Canaries/aviary use
	2000-3000 mg/kg soft feed[311]	Canaries/aviary use
Azithromycin (Zithromax, Pfizer)	—	Macrolide antibiotic; effective against most aerobic and anaerobic Gram-positive bacteria, may be effective against Gram-negative organisms; active against *Mycobacterium* (including atypical species), *Chlamydia*, and *Mycoplasma*[90]
	10-20 mg/kg PO q48h × 5 treatments[124]	Blue and gold macaws/PD; nonintracellular infections
	40 mg/kg PO q48h × 21 days[305]	Cockatiels/PD; Chlamydia
	40 mg/kg PO q24h × 30 days[124]	Blue and gold macaws/PD; intracellular infections (i.e., *Chlamydia*)
	43-45 mg/kg PO q24h[333]	Most species including psittacines, passerines/intracellular infections including mycobacterial sp.; used with ethambutol and rifabutin (see Table 5-44)
	50-80 mg/kg PO q24h × 3 days on, off 4 days, repeat up to 3 wk[667]	Most species/mycobacterial sp.; do not use if hepatic or renal disease; can mix with lactulose (stable refrigerated for 3-4 wk)

TABLE 5-1 Antimicrobial Agents Used in Birds. (cont'd)

Agent	Dosage	Species/Comments
Bacitracin methylene disalicylate (Solutracin 200, A.L. Laboratories; BMD Soluble, Alpharma)	50-400 mg/L drinking water[333] 100-500 mg/kg feed[112]	Ratites/*Clostridium perfringens*; prepare daily Ostriches <3 mo of age
Carbenicillin (Geocillin, Roerig)	—	Broad-spectrum β-lactamase-sensitive penicillin with extended spectra including *Pseudomonas*, *Proteus*, and others[90]
	11-15 mg/kg IV q8h[806]	Ratites
	100 mg/kg PO q12h[508]	Most species
	100 mg/kg IM q8h[49]	Most species
	100 mg/kg intratracheal q24h[139]	Most species/*Pseudomonas* respiratory infections
	100-200 mg/kg IM, IV q6-12h[333]	Most species, including psittacines, passerines, soft bills, pigeons, cranes, raptors
	250 mg/kg IM q12h[647]	Raptors
	1058 mg/L drinking water[508]	Most species
Cefadroxil	—	First-generation cephalosporin; limited activity against Gram-negative pathogens[90]
	20 mg/kg PO q12h[843]	Ratites
	100 mg/kg PO q12h × 7 days[318,685]	Most psittacines, pigeons/14-21 day therapy may be indicated for severe or deep pyodermas
Cefazolin	—	First-generation cephalosporin; limited activity against Gram-negative pathogens[90]
	25-30 mg/kg IM, IV q8h[118]	Cranes
	25-50 mg/kg IM, IV q12h[667]	Most species
	50-75 mg/kg IM q12h[685]	Most species
	50-100 mg/kg PO, IM q12h[619]	Raptors
Cefotaxime	—	Third-generation cephalosporin with broad-spectrum activity for many Gram-positive and Gram-negative pathogens; may penetrate cerebrospinal fluid in some species[90]
	25 mg/kg IM q8h[809]	Ratites/young birds
	50-100 mg/kg IM q8-12h[566]	Cranes
	75-100 mg/kg IM q12h[358]	Raptors
	75-100 mg/kg IM, IV q4-8h[333]	Most species, including soft bills, psittacines, passerines
	100 mg/kg IM q8-12h[318]	Pigeons
Cefovecin (Convenia, Zoetis)	10 mg/kg SC, IM, IV q1h[715]	Pigeons/PD; third-generation cephalosporin;[90] not recommended for use in birds due to short half-life; cannot be used q14d as in dogs and cats

Continued

TABLE 5-1 Antimicrobial Agents Used in Birds. (cont'd)

Agent	Dosage	Species/Comments
Cefoxitin	—	Second-generation cephalosporin with a wide range of activity against many Gram-positive and Gram-negative bacteria[90]
	50-75 mg/kg IM, IV q6-8h[333]	Most species, including soft bills
	50-100 mg/kg IM, IV q6-12h[333]	Psittacines
Ceftazidime	—	Third-generation cephalosporin; extensive activity against Gram-negative bacteria; may penetrate central nervous system[90]
	50-100 mg/kg IM, IV q4-8h[333]	Most species
Ceftiofur (Naxcel, Zoetis)	—	Third-generation cephalosporin with activity against *Pasteurella*[90]
	10 mg/kg IM q8-12h[795]	Orange-winged Amazon parrots/PD
	10 mg/kg IM q4h[795]	Cockatiels/PD; higher doses may be required for resistant infections
	10-20 mg/kg IM q12h[333]	Ratites
	50 mg/kg IM q12h[333]	Ostrich chicks
	50-100 mg/kg q4-8h[333]	Most species, including psittacines and passerines
Ceftiofur extended release formulation (Excede, Zoetis)	10 mg/kg IM[693]	Red-tailed hawks/PK; 10 mg/kg may allow targeted plasma levels for 36-45 hr
	10 mg/kg IM[403a]	Flamingos/PK; 10 mg/kg reached levels above MIC through 96 hr in 9/11 birds
	20 mg/kg IM[693]	Red-tailed hawks/PK; may provide target plasma levels for 96 hr
Ceftriaxone	—	Third-generation cephalosporin; effective against Gram-positive and Gram-negative bacteria including some activity against *Pseudomonas*[90]
	75-100 mg/kg IM q4-8h[333]	Most species
Cephalexin	—	First-generation cephalosporin; active against many Gram-positive and some Gram-negative bacteria[90]
	15-22 mg/kg PO q8h[806]	Ratites (excluding emus)
	35-50 mg/kg PO, IM q6-8h[110]	Pigeons, emus, cranes, raptors, psittacines >500 g/dose psittacines q6h
	35-50 mg/kg IM q2-3h[110]	Psittacines <500 g
	40-100 mg/kg PO, IM q6-8h[333]	Most species, including raptors, psittacines, passerines
	50 mg/kg PO q6h × 3-5 days[333]	Raptors, pigeons

TABLE 5-1 Antimicrobial Agents Used in Birds. (cont'd)

Agent	Dosage	Species/Comments
Cephalexin (cont'd)	100 mg/kg PO q8-12h[318]	Pigeons/14-21 day therapy may be indicated for severe or deep pyodermas
	100 mg/kg PO q4-6h[110]	Pigeons, emus, cranes/PD
Cephalothin	—	First-generation cephalosporin; active against many Gram-positive and some Gram-negative bacteria[90]
	30-40 mg/kg IM, IV q6h[806]	Ratites (excluding emus)
	100 mg/kg IM q8-12h[358]	Raptors
	100 mg/kg IM, IV q6-8h[333]	Most species, including psittacines, ratites
	100 mg/kg IM q6h[110]	Pigeons, emus, cranes/PD
	100 mg/kg IM, IV q2-6h[203]	Passerines
Cephradine	—	First-generation cephalosporin; active against many Gram-positive and some Gram-negative bacteria[90]
	35-50 mg/kg PO q4-6h[666]	Most species/14-21 day therapy may be indicated for severe or deep pyodermas
	100 mg/kg PO q4-6h[666]	Pigeons, emus, cranes
Chloramphenicol palmitate (oral suspension)	—	Phenicol; broad spectrum, including anaerobes, but causes blood dyscrasias in humans;[90] because large differences in pharmacokinetics exist between birds and mammals, and even between avian species, extrapolation between species is not recommended;[206] not commercially available in the United States, but can be compounded
	25 mg/kg PO q8h × 5 days[112]	Pigeons
	30-50 mg/kg PO q6-8h[333]	Psittacines, including budgerigars
	35-50 mg/kg PO q8h × 3 days[806]	Ratites
	50 mg/kg PO q6-12h[333]	Raptors
	50-100 mg/kg PO q6-12h[333]	Most species, including passerines
	250 mg/kg PO q6h[318]	Pigeons
	100-200 mg/L drinking water[667]	Canaries
Chloramphenicol succinate	30 mg/kg IM q8h × 3-5 days[255]	Raptors
	35-50 mg/kg SC, IM, IV q8h × 3 days[806]	Ratites
	50 mg/kg IM q24h[136]	Eagles (PD)
	50 mg/kg IM q8-12h[203]	Passerines
	50 mg/kg IM, IV q6-12h[136,333]	Most species, including budgerigars, passerines, pigeons, raptors

Continued

TABLE 5-1 Antimicrobial Agents Used in Birds. (cont'd)

Agent	Dosage	Species/Comments
Chloramphenicol succinate (cont'd)	50 mg/kg IM q6h[136]	Macaws, conures (PD)
	50-80 mg/kg IM q12-24h[203]	Passerines
	60-100 mg/kg IM q8h[320]	Pigeons
	100 mg/kg SC q8h[566]	Cranes
	100 mg/kg IM q6h[203]	Passerines
	200 mg/kg IM q12h × 5 days[364]	Budgerigars/PD
Chlorhexidine	—	Biguanides; antiseptic activity against most Gram-positive and some Gram-negative bacteria; not bacterial spores[850]
	2.6-7.9 mL of 2% solution/L drinking water[668]	Most species/bacterial infection; topical application may be fatal to nun and parrot finches[667]
	7.9 mL/L water[806]	Ratites/egg disinfectant spray at 104-108°F (40-42°C)
Chlorine (Na hypochlorite)	5 mg/L drinking water[685]	Water disinfectant; 0.1 mL of 5.25% bleach/L approximates this concentration
Chlortetracycline (Aureomycin Soluble Powder, Cyanamid)	—	Broad-spectrum tetracycline with activity against a wide range of Gram-positive and Gram-negative bacteria including *Chlamydia* and *Mycoplasma*[90]
	6-10 mg/kg IM q24h[340]	Raptors
	15-20 mg/kg PO q8h[806]	Ratites
	40-50 mg/kg PO q8h (w/grit), or q12h (w/o grit)[333]	Pigeons/PD
	100 mg/kg PO q6h[148]	Psittacines
	250 mg/kg PO q24h[340]	Raptors
	130-400 mg/L drinking water[318,697,804]	Pigeons
	500 mg/L drinking water or nectar[333]	Most species/prepare fresh q8-12h
	1000-1500 mg/L drinking water[333]	Canaries, psittacines/prophylaxis against *Chlamydia*
	5000 mg/L drinking water × 45 days[148]	Psittacines/*Chlamydia*
	100 mg/kg feed[804]	Pigeons/*Salmonella*
	500 mg/kg feed[202]	Budgerigars/*Chlamydia*
	1000-2000 mg/kg soft mixed feed × 45 days[77,200,201]	Most psittacines, canaries
	5000 mg/kg soft feed × 45 days[148]	Psittacines/*Chlamydia*
	0.5% pellets × 30-45 days[199]	Small psittacines/reduce calcium content of diet to 0.7%
	1% pellets × 30-45 days[199]	Large psittacines/reduce calcium content of diet to 0.7%

TABLE 5-1 Antimicrobial Agents Used in Birds. (cont'd)

Agent	Dosage	Species/Comments
Ciprofloxacin	—	Fluoroquinolone with wide spectrum against Gram-negative and some Gram-positive bacteria; activity against *Chlamydia* and *Mycoplasma*[90]
	3-6 mg/kg PO q12h[806]	Ratites
	5-20 mg/kg PO q12h × 5-7 days[686]	Pigeons
	10 mg/kg PO q12h × 7 days[2]	Ostrich chicks
	10-20 mg/kg PO q12h[257]	Raptors
	15-20 mg/kg PO, IM q12h[203,333,807]	Most species, including psittacines, passerines
	20-40 mg/kg PO, IV q12h[333]	Most species, including psittacines, canaries, raptors
	50 mg/kg PO q12h[363]	Raptors/PD
	80 mg/kg PO q24h[822]	Most species/*Mycobacterium*; use in combination with other agents (see Table 5-44)
	250 mg/L drinking water × 5-10 days[686]	Pigeons
Clarithromycin	—	Macrolide; effective against most aerobic and anaerobic Gram-positive bacteria, may be effective against Gram-negative organisms; active against *Mycobacterium* (including atypical species), *Chlamydia*, and *Mycoplasma*;[90] see Table 5-44
	10 mg/kg PO q24h[547]	Penguins
	60 mg/kg q24h[446]	Psittacines
	85 mg/kg PO q24h[688]	Most species/mycobacterial sp.; allometrically scaled
Clindamycin	—	Lincosamide; broad spectrum against anaerobic bacteria, limited against aerobic pathogens; widely distributed to tissues including bone[90]
	5.5 mg/kg PO q8h[525]	Ostriches
	12.5 mg/kg PO q12h[312]	Great horned owls/skin grafts; given in combination with enrofloxacin
	25 mg/kg PO q8h[240]	Psittacines, raptors
	50 mg/kg PO q8-12h[242]	Most species/7-10 day course recommended for raptors with osteomyelitis[76]
	100 mg/kg PO q24h × 3-5 days[333]	Most species, including psittacines, passerines, raptors, pigeons/*Clostridium*
	100 mg/kg PO q12h × 7 days[607]	Psittacines
	150 mg/kg PO q24h[296]	Pigeons, raptors/osteomyelitis
	200 mg/L drinking water[158]	Pigeons

Continued

TABLE 5-1   Antimicrobial Agents Used in Birds. (cont'd)

Agent	Dosage	Species/Comments
Clofazimine	—	Antimycobacterial agent
(Lamprene, Novartis)	1-5 mg/kg PO q24h × 3-12 mo[333]	Psittacines, raptors/*Mycobacterium*; use in combination with other agents (see Table 5-44)
	6-12 mg/kg PO q12h[333]	Most species/*Mycobacterium*; use in combination with other agents (see Table 5-44)
Cloxacillin	—	Narrow-spectrum β-lactamase-resistant penicillin inactive against many Gram-positive organisms[90]
	100-250 mg/kg PO, IM q24h[333]	Most species
	250 mg/kg PO q12h × 7-10 days[76]	Raptors
Cycloserine (Seromycin, Lilly)	5 mg/kg PO q12-24h × 3-12 mo[333]	Raptors/*Mycobacterium*; use in combination with other agents (see Table 5-44)
Danofloxacin mesylate (A180, Zoetis)	—	Fluoroquinolone with wide spectrum against Gram-negative and some Gram-positive bacteria; activity against *Chlamydia* and *Mycoplasma*[90]
	5 mg/kg PO, IM, IV[512]	Hyacinth macaws
Doxycycline	—	Broad-spectrum tetracycline with activity against a wide range of Gram-positive and Gram-negative bacteria; drug of choice for *Chlamydia* and *Mycoplasma*; products or foods containing Al, Ca, Mg, and Fe reduce or alter absorption; readily penetrates blood-brain barrier;[90] 12.5-25 mg/kg PO q12-24h resulted in elevations in AST and serum bile acids as well as hepatocellular damage in lorikeets[876]
	2-3.5 mg/kg PO q12h[806]	Ratites
	7.5-8 mg/kg PO q12-24h[198,667]	Passerines, nectar feeders, pigeons/PD; administer without grit[200]
	10-20 mg/kg PO q24h × 3-5 days[112]	Pigeons
	25 mg/kg (w/grit) PO q12h[877]	Pigeons/PD
	25 mg/kg PO q12h[384]	Psittacines, raptors/some Gram-negative bacterial infections and possibly *Leucocytozoon*
	25-50 mg/kg PO q12-24h[333]	Most species, including parrots (African grey parrots, Amazon parrots, cockatoos, macaws) and pigeons/may cause regurgitation; use low end of dose range for macaws and cockatoos
	35 mg/kg PO q24h × 21 days[305]	Cockatiels/PD; *Chlamydia*

TABLE 5-1 Antimicrobial Agents Used in Birds. (cont'd)

Agent	Dosage	Species/Comments
Doxycycline (cont'd)	40 mg/kg PO q24h[175]	Pigeons/PD; *Streptococcus bovis*
	130 mg/L drinking water[148]	Psittacines
	200 mg/L drinking water[221]	Pigeons
	250 mg/L drinking water[200]	Canaries
	280 mg/L drinking water[621]	Cockatiels/see Table 5-40 for recipe
	400 mg/L drinking water[224]	Cockatiels/PD; spiral bacteria
	500 mg/L drinking water[148,175]	Psittacines, pigeons/*Streptococcus bovis* in pigeons
	500 mg/L drinking water[577]	Fruit doves/PD; erratic drug concentrations (while most birds reached or exceeded therapeutic drug levels, some birds did not)
	800 mg/L drinking water (mix the contents of 16 × 100 mg capsules with 2 L water)[247]	African grey parrots, Goffin's cockatoos/PD; protect solution from exposure to light; make fresh daily
	250-300 mg/kg seed[76,239]	Budgerigars
	500 mg/kg wet weight seeds[621]	Cockatiels/PD; see Table 5-40 for recipe
	1000 mg/kg feed[333,626]	Large psittacines on dehulled seed (PD), macaws on corn (PD), canaries, large psittacines on soft feed (10 mg/mL syrup mixed into 29% kidney beans, 29% canned corn, 29% cooked rice, 13% dry oatmeal cereal)
Doxycycline (Vibravenös, Pfizer)	—	Broad-spectrum tetracycline with activity against a wide range of Gram-positive and Gram-negative bacteria;[90] drug of choice for *Chlamydia* and *Mycoplasma*; not available in the United States
	25-50 mg/kg IM q5-7d × 5-7 treatments[333]	Psittacines
	60-100 mg/kg SC, IM q5-7d[200]	Psittacines, pigeons
	75 mg/kg IM q7d × 4-6 wk[51]	Macaws
	75-100 mg/kg IM q5-7d × 4-6 wk[333]	Psittacines, including macaws, budgerigars
	100 mg/kg SC, IM q5-7d × 7 doses[293]	Houbara bustards/PD; *Chlamydia*
Doxycycline (Pharmacist-compounded micronized doxycycline hyclate)	75-100 mg/kg IM q7d[689]	Cockatoos/anecdotal reports of sudden death with compounded product; inadequate drug levels achieved in cockatiels at 100 mg/kg IM q10d;[621] adequate drug levels achieved with 100 mg/kg given IM in cockatoos, Amazon parrots and SC in African grey parrots, but severe soft-tissue reactions seen[244]

Continued

TABLE 5-1 Antimicrobial Agents Used in Birds. (cont'd)

Agent	Dosage	Species/Comments
Doxycycline hyclate (injection)	—	Cardiovascular collapse associated with the propylene glycol carrier can occur after rapid IV injection[265]
	25-50 mg/kg slow bolus IV q24h × 3 days[689]	Psittacines
	75-100 mg/kg SC, IM q5-7d[198]	Pigeons/PD
Doxycyline hyclate capsule	300 mg doxycycline mixed in soybean oil/kg low fat psittacine pellets[251]	Cockatiels/*Chlamydia* and spiral bacterial infections; feed as sole diet for 47 days
Doxycycline (Doxirobe gel, Zoetis)	Topical[761]	Most species/apply to beak or pododermatitis lesions; use in conjuction with debridement; antibiotic is released for 28 days
Enrofloxacin	—	Fluoroquinolone with wide spectrum against Gram-negative and some Gram-positive bacteria; activity against *Chlamydia* and *Mycoplasma*;[90] administration may be associated with emesis;[697] given PO, the IM formulation produces therapeutic plasma concentration;[358] labeled for single IM use only; multiple IM dosages not recommended; best to avoid IV use in raptors;[324] some fluoroquinolones have been used in PMMA beads with success;[213] joint deformities reported in squab chondrocytes with 200-800 mg/L drinking water;[425] however enrofloxacin has been commonly used at the recommended dosages without reports of adverse effects;[248,667] no detected effect on cartilage in day-old poultry chicks[601]
	1.5-2.5 mg/kg PO, SC q12h[806]	Ratites
	2.2 mg/kg IV q12h[343]	Emus/PD
	5 mg/kg SC, IM q12h[807]	Cockatiels
	5 mg/kg PO, IM q12-24h[807]	African grey parrots
	5 mg/kg IM q12h × 2 days[806]	Ratites
	5-10 mg/kg SC, IM q24h[200,202]	African grey parrots
	5-10 mg/kg PO q8h[333]	Passerines, pigeons (PD)
	5-15 mg/kg PO, SC, IM q12h[333]	Raptors, psittacines, pigeons/drug of choice for *Salmonella typhimurium*
	5-20 mg/kg PO q12-24h × 5-10 days[333]	Pigeons
	10 mg/kg PO q12h[113]	Cockatiels
	10 mg/kg PO, IV q24h[431]	Emus/PK
	10-15 mg/kg PO, IM q12h × 5-7 days[333]	Raptors

TABLE 5-1 Antimicrobial Agents Used in Birds. (cont'd)

Agent	Dosage	Species/Comments
Enrofloxacin (cont'd)	10-20 mg/kg PO q24h[200,203]	Passerines, psittacines, pigeons (PD)
	15 mg/kg PO q24h[607]	Psittacines
	15 mg/kg PO q12h[469]	Ostrich chicks, pigeons (administration to adult birds led to therapeutic levels in crop milk)
	15 mg/kg PO, IM, IV q12h[234]	Raptors/PD; IV administration in owls may result in weakness, tachycardia, vasoconstriction
	15 mg/kg PO, SC q12h[242]	Most species
	15-30 mg/kg PO, IM q12h[246]	African grey parrots/PD
	20 mg/kg PO, SC, IM q12h[333]	Pigeons/administer parenterally, followed by oral treatment
	20-30 mg/kg PO q12-24h[221]	Pigeons
	30 mg/kg PO, IM q24h[808]	Psittacines
	45 mg/kg PO q24h[320]	Pigeons
	25-50 mg/L drinking water[98]	Cranes (sandhill)/did not provide sufficient plasma levels
	100-200 mg/L drinking water[194,686,697]	Psittacines, pigeons/PD; may need up to 300 mg/L to prevent recurrence of infection in pigeons[697]
	190-750 mg/L drinking water[248]	African grey parrots/PD
	200 mg/L drinking water[245]	Psittacines/PD; maintains plasma concentrations adequate only for highly susceptible bacteria
	200 mg/L drinking water[201]	Canaries
	500 mg/L drinking water[458]	Psittacines
	200 mg/kg soft feed[201]	Canaries
	250 mg/kg feed[200]	Budgerigars/PD
	250-1000 mg/kg feed q24h[333]	Psittacines, passerines
	500 mg/kg feed[458]	Psittacines, including Patagonian conures/PD; mix into steamed corn diet
	1000 mg/kg feed[458]	Senegal parrots/PD; mix into steamed corn diet
	0.2 mg/mL saline, flush q24h × 10 days[76]	Raptors/nasal flush
Erythromycin	—	Macrolides antibiotic; effective against most aerobic and anaerobic Gram-positive bacteria, may be effective against Gram-negative organisms; active against *Mycobacterium* (including atypical species), *Chlamydia*, and *Mycoplasma*;[90] IM injection may cause severe muscle necrosis[331]
	5-10 mg/kg PO q8h[806]	Ratites

Continued

TABLE 5-1 Antimicrobial Agents Used in Birds. (cont'd)

Agent	Dosage	Species/Comments
Erythromycin (cont'd)	10-20 mg/kg IM q24h[202]	Passerines
	10-20 mg/kg PO q12h[697]	Psittacines
	50-100 mg/kg PO q8-12h[202]	Passerines
	60 mg/kg PO q12h[347]	Most species
	71 mg/kg PO q24h[175]	Pigeons/PD; *Streptococcus bovis*
	100 mg/kg PO[823]	Pigeons/PD; low plasma levels, but higher lung and trachea levels
	125 mg/kg PO q8h[318]	Pigeons
	125 mg/L drinking water[201]	Canaries
	132 mg/L drinking water (10 days on, 5 days off, 10 days on)[333]	Most species, including canaries
	250-500 mg/L drinking water × 3-5 days[148]	Psittacines
	525-800 mg/L drinking water[318]	Psittacines
	1000 mg/L drinking water[175,823]	Pigeons/PD; *Streptococcus bovis*; plasma levels low; one study reported that lung and trachea levels were sub-therapeutic
	1500 mg/L drinking water[697]	Most species
	200 mg/kg soft feed[201]	Canaries, psittacines
Ethambutol	—	Anti-mycobacterial agent; use in combination with other agents (see Table 5-44)
	10 mg/kg PO q12h[51]	Most species
	15-20 mg/kg PO q12h × 3-12 mo[333]	Psittacines, raptors/*Mycobacterium*
	15-30 mg/kg PO q12-24h[203]	Passerines/*Mycobacterium*
	30 mg/kg PO q24h[688]	Most species/*Mycobacterium*
Flumequine (Biocik, Amacol)	—	Fluoroquinolone antibiotic with wide spectrum against Gram-negative and some Gram-positive bacteria; activity against *Chlamydia* and *Mycoplasma*;[90] not available in the United States
	30 mg/kg PO, IM q8-12h[198]	Passerines, pigeons (PD)
Furazolidone (NF180, Hess and Clark)	—	Nitrofuran antibiotic, wide spectrum but potency is relatively low[90] in birds linked with cardiomyopathy; therapeutic action is confined to the gastrointestinal tract
	15-20 mg/kg PO q24h[203]	Passerines
	100-200 mg/L drinking water[667]	Canaries
	200 mg/kg soft food[667]	Canaries
	908 mg/kg feed[804]	Pigeons/*Salmonella*

TABLE 5-1 Antimicrobial Agents Used in Birds. (cont'd)

Agent	Dosage	Species/Comments
Gentamicin	—	Extended spectrum aminoglycoside; potentially nephrotoxic; maintain hydration and avoid concurrent use of other nephroactive drugs;[81,82,90] avoid doses higher than 2.5-5 mg/kg q8-12h[82,250]
	1-2 mg/kg IM q8h[806]	Ratites (excluding emus)/use only as last resort
	2.5 mg/kg IM q8h[82]	Raptors/PD
	3-10 mg/kg IM q6-12h[203]	Passerines
	5 mg/kg IM q8h[109,164,375]	Emus/PD; cranes/PD[164]
	5-10 mg/kg IM q8-12h[637]	Cockatiels/PD
	5-10 mg/kg IM q4h[109,691]	Pigeons/PD;[691] Salmonella
	7 mg/kg q8h[374]	Ostriches/PD; use with caution
	40 mg/kg PO q8-24h[203]	Passerines/15-25 g
	2-3 drops ophthalmic solution intranasal q8h[807]	Most species
Isoniazid	—	Antimycobacterial agent; should be used in combination with other drugs (see Table 5-44)
	5-15 mg/kg PO q12h[333]	Most species, including passerines
	30 mg/kg PO q24h[822]	Most species
Kanamycin	—	Extended spectrum aminoglycoside; potentially nephrotoxic, maintain hydration and avoid concurrent use of other nephroactive drugs[90]
	10-20 mg/kg IM q12h[333]	Most species, including passerines/ enteric infections
	13-65 mg/L drinking water × 3-5 days[333]	Most species/make fresh daily
Lincomycin	—	Lincosamide antibiotic; broad spectrum against anaerobic bacteria; limited activity against aerobic organisms; wide distribution, including bone[90]
	0.25-0.5 mL intraarticular q24h × 7-10 days[697]	Raptors
	25-50 mg/kg PO q12h[315]	Raptors/musculoskeletal surgical repair
	35-50 mg/kg PO q12-24h[203]	Passerines
	35-50 mg/pigeon PO q24h × 7-14 days[499]	Pigeons
	50-75 mg/kg PO, IM q12h × 7-10 days[333]	Psittacines, raptors/pododermatitis, osteomyelitis
	100 mg/kg PO q24h[666]	Raptors
	100 mg/kg IM q12h[77]	Psittacines

Continued

TABLE 5-1 Antimicrobial Agents Used in Birds. (cont'd)

Agent	Dosage	Species/Comments
Lincomycin (cont'd)	100-200 mg/L drinking water[201]	Canaries
	Topical[315]	Raptors/mixture of 50 mg/mL lincomycin and 10 mg/mL tobramycin was used to flush the flexor tendon sheath
Lincomycin/spectinomycin (LS-50 Water Soluble, Zoetis; Linco-Spectin 100 Soluble Powder, Zoetis)	—	Lincosamide in combination with an aminoglycoside; combination is effective against *Mycoplasma*[90]
	50 mg/kg PO q24h[333]	Most species
	¼-½ tsp/L drinking water × 10-14 days[139]	Most species/using soluble powder 16.7 g lincomycin and 33.3 g spectinomycin per 2.55 oz packet of powder
Marbofloxacin (Zeniquin, Zoetis)	—	Fluoroquinolone with wide-spectrum against Gram-negative and some Gram-positive bacteria; activity against *Chlamydia* and *Mycoplasma*[90]
	2-3 mg/kg IV, IO q24h[278,279]	Raptors (buzzards, vultures)/PD
	2.5-5 mg/kg PO q24h[123]	Blue and gold macaws/PD
	5 mg/kg IM, IV[176]	Ostriches/PD
	10-15 mg/kg PO, IM q12-24h[76,149a,277,697]	Raptors, bustards (PO dosage is PD)[277]
Meropenem	—	Broad-spectrum β-lactamase-sensitive penicillin with extended spectra including *Pseudomonas*, and many anaerobes[90]
	175 mg/kg IM q24h[722]	Pigeons/PD
Metronidazole	—	Nitroimidazole antibiotic and antiprotozoal agent active against most anaerobes; penetrates blood-brain barrier;[90] see Table 5-4
	10 mg/kg IM q24h × 2 days[333]	Psittacines
	10-30 mg/kg PO q12h × 10 days[808]	Psittacines
	50 mg/kg PO q24h × 5-7 days[333]	Most species, including raptors, psittacines/anaerobes
	50 mg/kg PO q12h × 30 days[685]	Amazon parrots, cockatoos/anaerobic and hemorrhagic enteritis
Minocycline	—	Broad-spectrum tetracycline with activity against a wide range of Gram-positive and Gram-negative bacteria; drug of choice for *Chlamydia* and *Mycoplasma*; readily penetrates blood-brain barrier[90]
	10 mg/kg PO q12h[547]	Penguins
	15 mg/kg PO q12h[643]	Raptors
	5000 mg/kg feed[13]	Parakeets/use as antibiotic impregnated millet

TABLE 5-1 Antimicrobial Agents Used in Birds. (cont'd)

Agent	Dosage	Species/Comments
Neomycin	—	Aminoglycoside antibiotic; poorly absorbed from gastrointestinal tract; potentially nephrotoxic and ototoxic[90]
	5-10 mg/kg IM q12h[340]	Raptors/toxic if overdosed
	10 mg/kg PO q24h[203]	Passerines
	10 mg/kg PO q8-12h[108]	Most species
	80-100 mg/L drinking water[667]	Canaries
	Topical q6-12h[667]	Most species/superficial wounds; cover with bandage; may be absorbed systemically and may cause ototoxicity and nephrotoxicity
Nitrofurazone	—	Nitrofuran antibiotic; wide spectrum but potency is relatively low;[90] may be hepatotoxic; do not use in finches or pigeons[686]
	0.3 mg/L drinking water × 7 days[666]	Lories, mynahs/do not put in lory nectar
	0.6 mg/L drinking water × 7-10 days[508]	Most species
Norfloxacin	—	Fluoroquinolone with wide spectrum against Gram-negative and some Gram-positive bacteria; activity against *Chlamydia* and *Mycoplasma*[90]
	3-5 mg/kg PO q12h[806]	Ratites
Oleandomycin	—	Macrolide antibiotic; not available in the United States
	25 mg/kg IM q24h[203]	Passerines
	50 mg/kg PO q24h[203]	Passerines
Ormetoprim-sulfadimethoxine (Primor, Zoetis)	—	Potentiated sulfonamide combination antibiotic; broad spectrum[90]
	60 mg/kg PO q12h[320]	Pigeons
	475-951 mg/L drinking water × 7-10 days[320]	Pigeons
Oxytetracycline	—	Broad-spectrum tetracycline with activity against a wide range of Gram-positive and Gram-negative bacteria; drug of choice for *Chlamydia* and *Mycoplasma*; IM administration may cause muscle irritation or necrosis[90]
	2 mg/mL nebulization q4-6h[211]	Parakeets/requires ultrasonic nebulizer; therapeutic concentrations of antibiotic were present in lung and trachea; not effective in treating systemic infections outside the respiratory tract
	5 mg/kg IM q12h[843]	Ratites
	10 mg/kg IM q3d[806]	Ratites
	16 mg/kg IM q24h[794]	Great horned owls/PD

Continued

TABLE 5-1 Antimicrobial Agents Used in Birds. (cont'd)

Agent	Dosage	Species/Comments
Oxytetracycline (cont'd)	25-50 mg/kg PO, IM q8h × 5-7 days[76]	Raptors
	48 mg/kg IM q48h[358]	Owls
	50 mg/kg IM q24h × 5-7 days[697]	Psittacines
	50 mg/kg PO q6-8h[318]	Pigeons
	50-75 mg/kg SC[240]	Goffin's cockatoos, blue and gold macaws
	50-100 mg/kg SC, IM q2-3d[203,249]	Cockatoos (PD), passerines
	50-200 mg/kg IM q3-5d[697]	Raptors
	58 mg/kg IM q24h[794]	Amazon parrots/PD
	80 mg/kg IM q48h[697]	Pigeons <400 g
	200 mg/kg IM q24h[51,76]	Most species, including waterfowl/ *Pasteurella*
	130-400 mg/L drinking water[85,318]	Pigeons
	650-2000 mg/L drinking water × 5-14 days[148]	Psittacines
	300 mg/kg soft feed × 5-14 days[148]	Psittacines
	8 g/40 g packet bone cement[810]	PMMA beads (ratio 1:5)
Penicillin benzathine/ procaine	—	Anecdotal reports suggest procaine penicillin should not be used in birds <1 kg BW because of possible toxic effects[807]
	200 mg/kg IM q24h[51]	Most species
Penicillin G	6 mg/kg IV[137]	Ostriches, emus/PD; rapidly eliminated; small volume of distribution
Penicillin procaine	—	Anecdotal reports suggest procaine penicillin should not be used in birds <1 kg BW; adverse reactions (possible toxic effects) described in finches, canaries, budgerigars, cockatiels[237,807]
Piperacillin	—	Broad-spectrum β-lactamase-sensitive penicillin with extended spectra including *Pseudomonas*, *Proteus*, and others;[90] see piperacillin/tazobactam
	25 mg/kg IM[807]	Ratites (chicks <6 mo of age)
	75-100 mg/kg IM q4-6h[807,808]	Amazon parrots
	100 mg/kg IM q12h[200]	Psittacines/PD
	100 mg/kg IM q12h[1]	Ostrich chicks/administer concurrent with amikacin (20 mg/kg IM q12h)
	100 mg/kg IM, IV q8-12h[566,643,697]	Pigeons, raptors, cranes

TABLE 5-1 Antimicrobial Agents Used in Birds. (cont'd)

Agent	Dosage	Species/Comments
Piperacillin (cont'd)	100 mg/kg IM q4-6h[674]	Red-tailed hawks, great horned owls/PD
	100-200 mg/kg IM, IV q6-12h[689,697]	Most species, including psittacines
	200 mg/kg IM q8h[660]	Budgerigars (PD), raptors
	200 mg/kg IM, IV q4-8h[242,689,807]	Most species, including passerines
	0.02 mL (4 mg) in macaw eggs; 0.01 mL (2 mg) in small eggs[507]	Eggs/inject 200 mg/mL solution into air cell on days 14, 18, and 22
Piperacillin/tazobactam	—	β-lactamase-protected penicillin combination; synergistic effect allows activity against organisms resistant to piperacillin alone;[90] broad-spectrum activity
	100 mg/kg IM q3-4h[125]	Hispaniolan Amazon parrots/PK; to control infections attributed to susceptible bacteria with an MIC of ≤4 µg/mL
	100 mg/kg IM, IV q8-12h[553]	Most species, including psittacines/reports of good clinical response; recommended at 100 mg/kg IV q6h for severe polymicrobic bacteremia
Polymyxin B	—	Polypeptide antibiotic; toxicity limits use to topical preparations or PO for gastrointestinal infections; narrow spectrum against some Gram-negative bacteria[90]
	10-15 mg/kg IM q24h[340]	Raptors/not absorbed if given PO
	50,000 U/L drinking water[377]	Canaries
	50,000 U/kg soft feed[377]	Canaries
Povidone-iodine	Topical to lesions, then wash off[76]	Raptors/wound cleansing; antibacterial, antifungal activity
Rifabutin (Mycobutin, Pfizer)	15-45 mg/kg PO q24h[333]	Antimycobacterial agent; use in combination with other agents (see Table 5-44)
Rifampicin	—	See rifampin
Rifampin	—	Most species/*Mycobacterium*; use with other agents (see Table 5-44); may cause/be associated with hepatitis, CNS signs, depression, and vomiting; yellow-orange urates observed in bustards[697]
	10-20 mg/kg PO q12-24h[203,697,807]	Most species, including passerines, psittacines/*Mycobacterium*
	45 mg/kg PO q24h[752,822]	Most species, including Amazon parrots, cranes
Silver sulfadiazine	Topical q12-24h[226,667]	Most species/topical sulfonamide, specifically for burn wounds;[90] ulcers; Amazon foot necrosis; bandage application preferred

Continued

TABLE 5-1 Antimicrobial Agents Used in Birds. (cont'd)

Agent	Dosage	Species/Comments
Spectinomycin		Aminoglycoside antibiotic[90]
	10-30 mg/kg IM q8-12h[77]	Psittacines
	25-35 mg/kg IM q8-12h[319]	Pigeons
	165-275 mg/L drinking water[320]	Pigeons
	200-400 mg/L drinking water[201]	Canaries
	400 mg/kg soft feed[201]	Canaries
Spiramycin	—	Macrolide antibiotic; effective against most aerobic and anaerobic Gram-positive bacteria; may be effective against Gram-negative organisms; active against *Mycobacterium* (including atypical species), *Chlamydia*, and *Mycoplasma*;[90] not available in the United States
	20 mg/kg IM q24h[340]	Raptors
	250 mg/kg PO q24h[500]	Most species, including raptors/poorly absorbed
	200-400 mg/L drinking water[201]	Canaries
	400 mg/kg soft feed[201]	Canaries
Streptomycin	—	Narrow-spectrum aminoglycoside; activity against Gram-negative aerobic bacteria[90] and *Mycobacterium*; use in combination with other agents (see Table 5-44)
	30 mg/kg IM q12h[51]	Most species
Sulfachlorpyridazine	—	Potentiated sulfonamide combination antibiotic and antiprotozoal; broad spectrum[90]
	150-300 mg/L drinking water[667]	Canaries
	400 mg/L drinking water × 7-10 days[684]	Pigeons
Sulfadimethoxine	—	Potentiated sulfonamide combination antibiotic, broad spectrum; antiprotozoal[90]
	25-55 mg/kg PO q24h × 3-7 days[382,659]	Raptors/loading dose at higher end × 1 day
	50 mg/kg PO q24h[119]	Cranes
	190-250 mg/L drinking water[500]	Pigeons/loading dose 375 mg/L drinking water
	330-400 mg/L drinking water on day 1 followed by 200-265 mg/L × 4 days[320]	Pigeons

TABLE 5-1 Antimicrobial Agents Used in Birds. (cont'd)

Agent	Dosage	Species/Comments
Tetracycline	—	Broad-spectrum tetracycline with activity against a wide range of Gram-positive and Gram-negative bacteria; drug of choice for *Chlamydia* and *Mycoplasma*[90]
	50 mg/kg PO q8h[203,667]	Most species, including passerines
	200-250 mg/kg PO q12-24h[666]	Most species/gavage
	40-200 mg/L drinking water[333]	Most species, including game birds
	100 mg/L drinking water[639]	Rheas
	200 mg/L drinking water[685]	Pigeons
	666 mg/L drinking water[697]	Pigeons
Tiamulin (Denagard; Elanco)	—	Tiamulin fumarate antibiotic; activity against Gram-positive organisms including anaerobes[90]
	25-50 mg/kg PO q24h[180]	Most species
Ticarcillin (Ticar, SmithKline Beecham)	—	Broad-spectrum β-lactamase-sensitive penicillin with extended spectra including *Pseudomonas* and many anaerobes[90]
	75-100 mg/kg IM q4-6h[689]	Amazon parrots
	150-200 mg/kg IV q2-4h[203]	Passerines, soft bills
	200 mg/kg IM, IV q6-12h[333]	Most species, including pigeons, raptors/*Pseudomonas*[240]
	200 mg/kg IM q2-4h[721]	Blue-fronted Amazon parrots/PD
Ticarcillin/clavulanate (Timentin, Glaxo SmithKline)	100 mg/kg IM, IV[147]	Most species/frequency not reported
	200 mg/kg IM, IV q12h[685]	Most species
Tilmicosin (Micotil 300 Injection, Provitil-powder and Pulmotil AC-liquid, Elanco)	—	Macrolide antibiotic; effective against most aerobic and anaerobic Gram-positive bacteria; may be effective against Gram-negative organisms; active against *Mycobacterium* (including atypical species), *Chlamydia*, and *Mycoplasma*;[90] handle with caution; potentially fatal to humans;[614] see Table 6-1 for poultry dosages
Tobramycin	—	Extended spectrum; potentially nephrotoxic; maintain hydration and avoid concurrent use of other nephroactive drugs[90]
	0.25-0.5 mL intraarticular flush q24h × 7-10 days[76]	Raptors/septic arthritis
	2.5-5 mg/kg IM, IV q8-12h[148]	Psittacine, passerines, raptors
	10 mg/kg IM q12h × 5-7 days[333]	Raptors
	Topical	A mixture of lincomycin (50 mg/mL) and tobramycin (10 mg/mL) was used to flush the flexor tendon sheath[315]

Continued

TABLE 5-1 Antimicrobial Agents Used in Birds. (cont'd)

Agent	Dosage	Species/Comments
Trimethoprim	—	Bacteriostatic activity against some Gram-positive and Gram-negative bacteria
	10-20 mg/kg PO q8h[198,202,500]	Psittacines, passerines, pigeons (PD)
Trimethoprim/sulfadiazine	—	Potentiated sulfonamide combination antibiotic; broad spectrum[90]
	8 mg/kg SC, IM q12h[566]	Cranes
	12-60 mg/kg PO q12h × 5-7 days[76]	Raptors/useful for sensitive infections in neonates
	16-24 mg/kg PO q8-12h[566]	Cranes
	20 mg/kg SC, IM q12h[148]	Psittacines
	30 mg/kg PO q8h[341]	Psittacines/combine with pyrimethamine for treatment of sarcocystosis
	30 mg/kg PO, IM, IV q12h[314]	Ostriches/PD
	60 mg/kg PO q12h[320]	Pigeons
	107 mg/L drinking water[85]	Galliformes
	475-950 mg/L drinking water × 7-10 days[320]	Pigeons
Trimethoprim/sulfatroxazole	—	Potentiated sulfonamide combination antibiotic; broad spectrum[90]
	10-50 mg/kg PO q12h[203]	Passerines
Trimethoprim/sulfamethoxazole	—	Potentiated sulfonamide combination antibiotic; broad spectrum[90]
	8 mg/kg IM q12h[697]	Psittacines
	10-50 mg/kg PO q24h[203]	Passerines
	20 mg/kg PO q8-12h[697]	Psittacines
	21 mg/kg PO q12h[1]	Ostriches
	40-50 mg/kg PO q12h[242]	Psittacines
	48 mg/kg PO, IM q12h[384]	Raptors
	60 mg/kg PO q24h[198]	Pigeons/PD
	60-72 mg/kg PO q12h[118]	Cranes
	75 mg/kg IM q12h[51]	Most species/reduce dose if regurgitation occurs[240]
	100 mg/kg PO q12h[51]	Most species, including psittacines
	144 mg/kg PO q8-12h[689]	Most species
	360-400 mg/L drinking water × 10-14 days[684]	Most species, including pigeons
Tylosin	—	Macrolide antibiotic; effective against most aerobic and anaerobic Gram-positive bacteria, may be effective against Gram-negative organisms; active against *Mycobacterium* (including atypical species), *Chlamydia*, and *Mycoplasma*; potentially irritating to muscles when administered IM[90]

TABLE 5-1 Antimicrobial Agents Used in Birds. (cont'd)

Agent	Dosage	Species/Comments
Tylosin (cont'd)	3-5 mg/kg IM, IV q12h[806]	Ratites
	5-10 mg/kg PO q8h[806]	Ratites
	15 mg/kg IM q8h[461]	Cranes/PD
	15-30 mg/kg IM q12h × 3 day[333]	Raptors
	17 mg/kg IM q24h × 7 days[520]	Emus/*Mycoplasma*
	20-40 mg/kg IM q8h[697]	Psittacines
	25 mg/kg IM q8h[461]	Emus/PD
	25 mg/kg IM q6h[461]	Pigeons, quail/PD
	30 mg/kg IM q12h[76]	Most species/*Mycoplasma*
	50 mg/kg PO q24h[333]	Passerines, pigeons
	50 mg/L drinking water[685]	Most species
	250-400 mg/L drinking water[201]	Canaries
	300 mg/L drinking water × 6 wk[558]	House finches/*Mycoplasma*
	500 mg/L drinking water × 3-28 days[333]	Pigeons, emus/*Mycoplasma*
	800 mg/L drinking water[320]	Pigeons
	1000 mg/L drinking water × 21 days[501]	House finches/*Mycoplasma*; give in conjunction with ophthalmic ciprofloxacin
	2000 mg/L drinking water[333]	Pigeons/*Mycoplasma, Haemophilus*

^aMost drug doses used in birds should be considered experimental. Patients should be monitored for adverse effects and treatment failure.[240]

TABLE 5-2 Antifungal Agents Used in Birds.

Agent	Dosage	Species/Comments
Acetic acid (vinegar)	16 mL/L drinking water[377]	Most species/gastrointestinal yeast infections
Amphotericin B	—	Polyene macrolide antifungal agent; broad activity against various types of fungi, but susceptibility varies as to species; ineffective against dermatophytes; primary use is for systemic fungal infections[91]
	1.5 mg/kg IV q8h × 3-7 days[333,644]	Most species
	1 mg/kg intratracheal q8-12h, dilute to 1 mL with sterile water[644,667]	Psittacines, raptors/aspergillosis
	1 mg/kg intratracheal q12h × 12 days, then q48h × 5 wk[76]	Raptors/syringeal aspergilloma

Continued

TABLE 5-2 Antifungal Agents Used in Birds. (cont'd)

Agent	Dosage	Species/Comments
Amphotericin B (cont'd)	100-109 mg/kg PO by gavage q12h × 10-30 days[526]	Budgerigars/*Macrorhabdus*; compound in simple syrup; resistance reported in budgerigars in Australia[607]
	0.05 mg/mL sterile water[52]	Most species/nasal flush
	0.2 mL PO q12h × 10 days[148]	Budgerigars/*Macrorhabdus*; use IV formulation (5 mg/mL)
	0.25-1 mL PO q24h × 4-5 days[76]	Raptor neonates/candidiasis
	1000 mg/L drinking water × 10 days[229]	Budgerigars/*Macrorhabdus*
	Topical[148]	Apply 10% solution to oropharynx
	1.35 mg/kg topical q24h of a liposomally encapsulated formulation in a sterile, water-soluble lubricating gel[87]	Herons
	7 mg/mL saline q12h[810]	Most species/nebulization × 15 min
	1 mg/kg intralesionally[625]	Conures/pulmonary lesions; administered endoscopically with injection needle along with systemic therapy
Amphotericin B (3% cream)	Topical to affected area q12h[667]	Most species/mycoses
Clotrimazole	—	Imidazole antifungal agent; variable sensitivity between yeasts and fungi; superficial mycoses and candidiasis[91]
	2 mg/kg intratracheal q24h × 5 days[685]	Psittacines/syringeal aspergilloma; apply with catheter directly into syrinx during anesthesia
	Inject 10 mg/kg into air sacs[685]	Psittacines/dilute in propylene glycol to 2.5 mg/mL; divide total dose between the 4 most accessible air sacs; toxic and may result in death in African grey parrots and other birds if injected into the viscera or IM[685]
	10 mg/mL saline flush[607]	Most species/effective against *Aspergillus* at sites that can be flushed; nasal flush using 1% solution
	1% solution[810]	Nebulization × 30-60 min
Enilconazole emulsion	—	Imidazole antifungal agent; variable sensitivity between yeasts and fungi; superficial mycoses and candidiasis;[91] used topically and for nasal flush
	6 mg/kg PO q12h[13]	Eclectus parrots/glossal candidiasis; an elevation of AST was seen after 7 days of treatment
	1 mg (0.5 mL)/kg intratracheal of a 1:10 dilution q24h × 7-14 days[697]	Falcons/aspergillosis
	200 mg/L drinking water[13]	Canaries/cutaneous dermatophytosis

TABLE 5-2 Antifungal Agents Used in Birds. (cont'd)

Agent	Dosage	Species/Comments
Enilconazole emulsion (cont'd)	Topical 1:10 dilution q12h × 21-28 days[76]	Raptors/cutaneous aspergillosis, candidiasis
	Topical or intratracheal 1:10-1:100 dilution[77]	Psittacines/aspergillosis, candidiasis
	3 topical soakings q3d[644]	Raptors, ostriches/dermatophytosis
	0.1 mL/kg in 5 mL sterile water, nebulize × 30 min, 5 days on, 2 off, up to 3 mo[338]	Raptors/aspergillosis
Fluconazole	—	Imidazole antifungal agent; variable sensitivity between yeasts and fungi; systemic mycoses and candidiasis; realtively good penetration into CSF;[91] death observed in budgerigars at 10 mg/kg PO q12h (this dose was also ineffective against avian gastric yeast)[607]
	2-5 mg/kg PO q24h × 7-10 days[76,583]	Most species, including raptors/gastrointestinal, systemic candidiasis; CNS, ocular mycoses
	4-6 mg/kg PO q12h[238]	Juvenile psittacines/candidiasis
	5 mg/kg PO q24h[641]	Cockatiels/candidiasis
	10 mg/kg PO q48h[641]	
	5-10 mg/kg PO q24h[50]	Gouldian finches/candidiasis
	8 mg/kg PO q24h × 30 days[808]	Psittacines/cryptococcosis
	10-20 mg/kg PO × 30 days[377]	Red-tailed hawks, gyrfalcons/aspergillosis
	15 mg/kg PO q12h × ≥28 days[687]	Pigeons/aspergillosis
	15 mg/kg PO q12h × 30 days following cessation of clinical signs[10]	Psittacines/chronic nasal aspergillosis
	20 mg/kg PO q48h[238]	Psittacines/PD; mucosal, systemic yeast infections; 2-3 treatments for resistant candidiasis
	25 mg/L nectar[329]	Hummingbirds/aspergillosis
	50 mg/L drinking water × 14-60 days[685]	Most species/systemic mycoses; candidiasis
	100 mg/L drinking water × 8 days[641]	Cockatiels/candidiasis
	150 mg/L drinking water[50]	Gouldian finches/candidiasis
	100 mg/kg soft food[50]	Gouldian finches/candidiasis
Flucytosine	—	Fluorinated pyrimidine antifungal agent; as resistance develops rapidly, not used as sole antifungal agent; effective against *Cryptococcus*, *Candida*, and *Aspergillus*; excellent CSF, aqueous humor penetration;[91] use prophylactically in raptors (especially falcons) to prevent aspergillosis[a]
	20-30 mg/kg PO q6h × 20-90 days[358]	Raptors/aspergillosis

Continued

TABLE 5-2 Antifungal Agents Used in Birds. (cont'd)

Agent	Dosage	Species/Comments
Flucytosine (cont'd)	20-75 mg/kg PO q12h × 21 days[697]	Psittacines/generalized yeast or fungal infections
	50 mg/kg PO q12h × 14-28 days[148,572]	Psittacines, passerines, raptors
	50-75 mg/kg PO q8h[644] 75 mg/kg q12h × 5-7 days, then q24h × 14 days[644]	Raptors/aspergillosis prophylaxis; consider treatment 1 wk prior to and 2 wk after move; used routinely for domestically raised gyrfalcons and gyrfalcon hybrids from age 45 days
	75-120 mg/kg PO q6h[572]	Most species
	80-100 mg/kg PO q12h[806]	Ratites
	100-250 mg/kg PO q12h[386]	Psittacine neonates
	250 mg/kg PO q12h × 14-17 days[782]	Finches/endoventricular mycoses; can use with chlorhexidine in drinking water
	50-250 mg/kg feed[667]	Psittacines, mynah birds
Griseofulvin	—	Systemic antifungal agent; effective against common dermatophytes[91]
	10 mg/kg PO q12h × 21 days[697]	Pigeons/dermatophytosis; gavage
	30-50 mg/kg in drinking water q24h[806]	Ostriches/mycotic dermatitis
Iodine, 1% solution	Topical[644]	Most species/oral or cutaneous candidiasis
Itraconazole	—	Imidazole antifungal agent; variable sensitivity between yeasts and fungi; systemic mycoses and candidiasis; relatively good penetration into CSF;[91] commercially available suspension is recommended as a first choice; use caution using compounded formulations because bulk drug may not be bioavailable or stable[107,170]
	5-10 mg/kg PO q24h[574]	Blue-fronted Amazon parrots/PD; aspergillosis; 10 mg/kg is required to achieve therapeutic concentrations in poorly perfused tissues; anorexia, depression, and toxicity reported at higher doses in African grey parrots[239,607]
	5-10 mg/kg PO q12-24h × 10-14 days, then q48h[358]	Raptors/aspergillosis prophylaxis[a]
	5-10 mg/kg PO q12h × 5 days, followed by q24h for a total of 14 days[644]	Raptors/suggested for Class I aspergillosis (mild, vague signs with inconclusive diagnostics or without histologic confirmation)
	5-10 mg/kg PO q12h × 5 days, followed by q24h × 60-90 days[644]	Raptors/Class II-IV aspergillosis
	5-10 mg/kg PO q12h[394,666]	Passerines (towhees), penguins/aspergillosis prophylaxis in passerines; aspergillosis, candidiasis, and cryptococcosis in others

TABLE 5-2 Antifungal Agents Used in Birds. (cont'd)

Agent	Dosage	Species/Comments
Itraconazole (cont'd)	6 mg/kg PO q12h[475]	Pigeons/PD; dosage will achieve fungicidal plasma concentrations
	6-8 mg/kg PO q12h × 5-7 days then q24h × 14 days[644]	Raptors/prevention of aspergillosis; consider treating for 1 wk prior and 2 wk after move, and routinely for domestically raised gyrfalcons and gyrfalcon hybrids from age 45 days
	6-10 mg/kg PO[375]	Ratites
	10 mg/kg PO q24h[333,383]	Red-tailed hawks (PD), gentoo penguins
	10 mg/kg PO q24h × 14-90 days with food[572,573,607]	Psittacines/use in combination with non-azoles
	10 mg/kg PO q12h × 21-60 days[148,782]	Finches/endoventricular mycoses; can use with chlorhexidine in drinking water
	15 mg/kg PO q12h up to 4-6 wk[358]	Raptors/aspergillosis
	20 mg/kg PO q24h[107]	Penguins/PD
	26 mg/kg PO q12h[475]	Pigeons/PD; fungicidal levels achieved in respiratory tissue; further toxicologic studies are required
	200 mg/kg feed up to 100 days[657]	Gouldian finches/PD; dermatomycoses; beads from capsules were mixed with small amount of oil and seed
Ketoconazole	—	Imidazole antifungal agent; fungistatic; variable sensitivity between yeasts and fungi; systemic fungal infections[91]
	5-10 mg/kg PO q24h[806]	Ratites
	8 mg/kg PO q12h × 30 days[85]	Ostriches
	10-20 mg/kg PO q24h[85]	Ostriches
	15 mg/kg PO q12h[384]	Raptors/candidiasis
	20 mg/kg PO q8h × 7-14 days[607]	Psittacines/refractory candidiasis
	20 mg/kg PO q24h × 14 days[148]	Psittacines, passerines, raptors
	20-30 mg/kg PO q8h[326]	Cockatoos
	20-40 mg/kg PO q12h × 15-60 days[686]	Pigeons
	25 mg/kg PO q12h × 14 days[697]	Ratites, raptors/aspergillosis
	30 mg/kg PO q12h × 7-14 days[415]	Amazon parrots/PD
	50 mg/kg/day PO[150]	Toucans
	60 mg/kg PO q12h[837]	Raptors, common buzzards (PD)/aspergillosis
	200 mg/L drinking water, nectar, or soft feed × 7-14 days[50,201,329]	Canaries, hummingbirds, Gouldian finches/dissolve crushed tablet in ½-1 tsp vinegar

Continued

TABLE 5-2 Antifungal Agents Used in Birds. (cont'd)

Agent	Dosage	Species/Comments
Miconazole	—	Imidazole antifungal agent, topical preparations for local dermatophytosis;[91] injectable product not available in the United States
	5 mg/kg intratracheal q12h × 5 days[333]	Psittacines/10 mg/mL solution diluted with saline; syringeal mycoses; use with flucytosine; clotrimazole may be an alternative
	10 mg/kg IM q24h × 6-12 days[697]	Raptors/generalized aspergillosis
	20 mg/kg IV q8h[697]	Psittacines/candidiasis, cryptococcosis
	Topical to affected areas q12h[644]	Most species/cutaneous fungal infections; used in conjunction with oral itraconazole; dermatophytosis
Nystatin	—	Polyene macrolide antifungal agent; used topically or orally to treat GI candidiasis; can be effective against other yeast and fungi; poorly absorbed from the GI tract[91]
	5000 U/bird PO q12h × 10 days[229,230]	Goldfinches/*Macrorhabdus*; ineffective in budgerigars
	20,000-100,000 U/bird PO q24h × 7 days[85,697]	Pigeons/candidiasis
	100,000 U/kg PO q12h[319,384]	Pigeons, raptors
	250,000-430,000 U/kg PO q12h[148]	Hummingbirds
	250,000-500,000 U/kg PO q12h[806]	Ratites
	300,000 U/kg PO q12h × 7-14 days[76,236]	Most species
	300,000-600,000 U/kg PO q8-12h × 7-14 days[148]	Psittacines
	500,000 U/kg PO q8h × 5 days[159]	Toucannettes (safron)/candidiasis
	Topical q6h[362]	Hummingbirds/candidiasis; direct application using a cotton swab
	25,000 U/L nectar[362]	Hummingbirds
	100,000 U/L drinking water[50,201]	Canaries, finches
	200,000 U/kg soft feed[50,76]	Canaries, finches
Povidone-iodine	Topical to lesions, then rinse[76]	Raptors/wound cleansing; antibacterial, antifungal activity
Sodium benzoate	1 tsp/L water × 5 wk[354]	Budgerigars/cleared infection in nonbreeding birds; 0.5 tsp/L resulted in neurologic signs and death in breeding birds, likely due to increased water intake[354]
Silver sulfadiazine	Topical to affected areas q12-24h[226,667]	Most species/bandage application preferred

TABLE 5-2 Antifungal Agents Used in Birds. (cont'd)

Agent	Dosage	Species/Comments
STA solution (salicyclic acid 3 g, tannic acid 3 g, ethyl alcohol to 100 mL)	Topical[697]	Fungal dermatitis
Terbinafine	—	Allylamine antifungal used topically for dermatophtyes; fungicidal; data are emerging to potentially support its use for systemic fungal infections;[90] questionable therapeutic potential for the treatment of aspergillosis in avian species; higher dose or use in combination with itraconazole may be more effective[243]
	10-15 mg/kg PO q12-24h[169]	Most species
	15 mg/kg PO q24h[68]	Penguins/PD
	15-30 mg/kg PO q12h[243]	Most species
	22 mg/kg PO q24h[69]	Raptors/PD
	1 mg/mL solution via nebulization[216]	Hispaniolan Amazon parrots/raw powder maintained MIC concentrations for 4 hr vs. 1 hr for crushed tablets
Voriconazole	—	Imidazole antifungal agent; indicated for aspergillosis infections in humans;[91] used in avian species for the treatment of aspergillosis, but there are limited PK studies; some strains in pigeons found to be resistant;[73] difficult to extrapolate drug doses between species; safety unproven in birds; increased anecdotal reporting of voriconazole toxicity in penguins;[359b] PO and IV solutions available; may need to adjust dose for long-term treatment to maintain therapeutic concentrations;[243] compounded suspensions stable up to 30 days at room temperature[556]
	10 mg/kg PO q12h or 20 mg/kg q24h[71-73]	Pigeons/PD
	10 mg/kg PO q8h[725]	Red-tailed hawks/PD
	12-18 mg/kg PO q12h[252]	African grey parrots/PD
	12.5 mg/kg PO q12h[720]	Falcons/PD; red-tailed hawks
	18 mg/kg PO q8h[306]	Amazon parrots/PD
	20 mg/kg PO q24h × 21 days[584]	Many species

[a]Prophylatic use of antifungal agents may be indicated in newly captured or admitted birds of susceptible species, and in birds undergoing change of management or transfer of enclosure.[644]

TABLE 5-3 Antiviral and Immunomodulating Agents Used in Birds.

Agent	Dosage	Species/Comments
Acyclovir	—	Antiviral agent; useful against DNA viral infections, particularly herpesvirus; available in topical and parenteral formulations; IM injection of the water-soluble sodium salt (IV formulation) may cause severe muscle necrosis; phlebitis and neurologic signs may occur with IV administration; most effective when administered before clinical signs begin; birds should be treated for a minimum of 7 days; the reconstituted solution is unstable and should be divided into aliquots and frozen[333]
	20-40 mg/kg IM q12h[681]	Psittacines/psittacine herpesvirus
	29 mg/bird PO q8h × 7 days[76]	Pigeons/herpesvirus
	80 mg/kg PO q8h × 7 days[561]	Quaker parakeets/PD; psittacine herpesvirus prophylaxis or treatment
	330 mg/kg PO q12h × 4-7 days[387]	Psittacine neonates/psittacine herpesvirus
	330 mg/kg PO q12h × 7-14 days[358]	Raptors/falcon and owl herpesvirus; may cause vomiting
	1000 mg/L drinking water[157,665]	Quaker parakeets/herpesvirus; gavage
	≤400 mg/kg feed[157]	Quaker parakeets/herpesvirus
Amantadine	—	Antiviral agent; inhibits replication of influenza A viruses
	1 mg/kg PO q24h × 3 wk[289]	African grey parrots/no effect on avian bornavirus infection[289]
Cyclosporine	10 mg/kg PO q12h[273,412]	Psittacines/immunosuppressant agent; palliative treatment of proventricular dilatation disease (3/6 cockatiels treated survived)[412,273]
Echinacea (Echinacea solution, Biobotania)	0.5 mL/kg per L drinking water q24h × 5 days[697]	Psittacines/herbal immunostimulant
	1 mL/L drinking water[666]	Psittacines/use alcohol-free formulation
Imiquimod cream	—	Immune response inhibitor used to inhibit viral-induced tumor formation; has no direct antiviral activity
	Apply topically 3×/wk several hr before the morning feeding[445]	Psittacines/cloacal papillomatosis; thought to boost host cell-mediated immunity; masses decreased in size in one report, but not in another;[443] complete remission did not occur in either
Interferon α_2	—	Antiviral cytokine glycoprotein with immunomodulating and antiproliferative capabilities as well as antiviral activity
	60-240 U/kg SC, IM q12h[731] or 300-1200 U/kg PO q12h[685]	Most species/stock solution: mix 1 mL (3,000,000 U/mL) with 100 mL sterile water (30,000 U/mL); can freeze as 2 mL vials up to 1 yr; mix 2 mL of stock into 1 L LRS (=60 U/mL); refrigerate up to 3 mo

TABLE 5-3	Antiviral and Immunomodulating Agents Used in Birds. (cont'd)	
Agent	Dosage	Species/Comments
Interferon α_2 (cont'd)	1500 U/kg PO q24h[13]	Psittacines
	1,000,000 U IM q2-7d × 3 treatments[762]	African grey parrots/circovirus; birds treated with poultry origin gamma interferon survived, those treated with α feline origin did not
	1000 U/L drinking water × 14-28 days[684]	Pigeons/circovirus
Propionibacterium Acnes, (ImmunoRegulin, Neogen)	0.13 mg/kg (up to 0.08 mg [0.2 mL] max) SC, IM days 1, 3, 7, 14, 28, 42, then q30d[40]	Psittacines/immunomodulatory drug; used to manage FIV infection in cats; anecdotally reported as an alternative therapy for chronic feather destructive disease[40]
Silymarin (milk thistle)	100-150 mg/kg PO divided q8-12h[10]	Most species/hepatic antioxidant; used in patients with liver disease and as ancillary to chemotherapy; use an alcohol-free liquid formulation
Vaccines	—	See Table 5-47 (Vaccines Used in Birds)

TABLE 5-4	Antiparasitic Agents Used in Birds.	
Agent	Dosage	Species/Comments
Albendazole (11.36%) (Valbazen, Zoetis)	—	Broad-spectrum anthelmintic; may be toxic in keas, some columbiformes and other spp. at 50-100 mg/kg[356,760]
	5.2 mg/kg PO q12h × 3 days, repeat in 14 days[806]	Ratites/flagellates, cestodes
	6 mg/kg PO once[178]	Ostriches/100% effective against *Libyostrongylus dentatus* and *L. douglassii*
	15-20 mg/kg PO once[333]	Toucans
	20 mg/kg PO, repeat in 7 days[482]	Cranes/effective against some trematodes
	25 mg/kg PO q24h × 90 days, then repeat × 120 days when signs returned[610]	Cockatoos/*Encephalitozoon hellem* keratoconjunctivitis
	25-50 mg/kg PO q24h × 3-4 days[760]	Doves, rock partridges/*Capillaria*; toxicity occurred in some birds, use with caution
	50 mg/kg PO q24h × 5 days[115]	Amazon parrots/microsporidian keratoconjunctivitis
	113-116 mg/23 kg q12h × 3 days, repeat in 14 days[38]	Ratites/protozoal infections

Continued

TABLE 5-4 Antiparasitic Agents Used in Birds. (cont'd)

Agent	Dosage	Species/Comments
Amprolium	—	Pyridimine derivative coccidiostat; although rarely encountered, efficacy can be reduced by high doses of thiamine;[759] resistance common; some coccidial organisms of mynahs, toucans have shown resistance[38]
	2.2 mg/kg PO[122]	Sandhill cranes/ineffective in preventing experimentally induced disseminated visceral coccidiosis
	15-30 mg/kg PO q24h × 1-5 days[194]	Most species/treatment should be repeated after 5 days due to coccidial prepatent period[194]
	30 mg/kg PO q24h[432b]	Merlins/thiamine deficiency
	30 mg/kg PO q24h × 5 days[38,432b]	Raptors
	5-100 mg/L drinking water × 5-7 days[38,747]	Most species/flock treatment
	50-100 mg/L drinking water × 5-7 days[171,194,333]	Most species, including passerines, parakeets
	60 mg/L drinking water[333]	Cranes
	200 mg/L drinking water[321]	Pigeons/flock treatment
	250 mg/L drinking water × 7 days[333]	Psittacines (keas)/*Sarcocystis;* use in combination with pyrimethamine and primaquine
	¼ tsp/L drinking water × 3-5 days[333]	Pigeons/20% soluble powder
	0.0125 mg/kg feed[482]	Cranes/coccidiosis prophylaxis
	0.025 mg/kg feed × 14 days[482]	Cranes/coccidiosis treatment
	115-235 mg/kg feed[333]	Poultry/coccidia; *Sarcocystis;* lower dose is prophylactic; higher dose is therapeutic
Cambendazole (Equiben, Merial)	60-100 mg/kg PO q24h × 3-7 days[194,333]	Most species
	75 mg/kg PO q24h × 2 day[38,323]	Pigeons
Carbaryl 5% (Sevin Dust, Garden Tech)	Topical; light dusting of plumage or nest box litter (1-2 tsp)[38,482]	Most species/ants, ectoparasites; remove treated litter after 24 hr
Carnidazole (Spartrix, Wildlife Pharmaceuticals)	—	Treatment for *Trichomonas, Hexamita, Histomonas*[38]
	5 mg/bird PO[333]	Doves (adults), pigeons (squabs)
	10 mg/bird PO[788a]	Pink pigeons (adults)/*Trichomonas;* squabs ≤18 days old administer 5 mg
	12.5-25 mg/kg PO once[38,135]	Pigeons, raptors/*Trichomonas,* use lower dose with juvenile birds; combine with dimetridazole to treat flock
	20 mg/kg PO once[333]	Pigeons

TABLE 5-4 Antiparasitic Agents Used in Birds. (cont'd)

Agent	Dosage	Species/Comments
Carnidazole (Spartrix, Wildlife Pharmaceuticals) (cont'd)	20 mg/kg q24h PO × 2 days[333]	Raptors
	20-25 mg/kg PO once[38,194,432b]	Raptors/single dose not always effective in falcons, bustards with advanced infections; use lower dose for juveniles
	20-30 mg/kg PO q24h × 1-2 days[38,135]	Most species, including pigeons, psittacines
	20-30 mg/kg PO q24h × 5 days[20,747]	Passerines/*Trichomonas*; house finches reliably cleared *Trichomonas gallinae* if caught prior to clinical signs
	30 mg/kg PO once[256]	Raptors/*Trichomonas*
	30 mg/kg PO q12-24h × 3 days[382,654]	Raptors/*Trichomonas*
	30-50 mg/kg PO, repeat in 10-14 days[667]	Cockatiels/*Giardia*
	33 mg/kg PO, repeat in 14 and 28 days[50]	Society finches, Gouldian finches/flagellates; 0.5 mg/adult (based on 15 g); 0.25 mg/nestling (based on 7.5 g)
	50 mg/kg PO once[358]	Raptors
	120 mg/kg PO as single dose or divided over 2-5 days[811]	American kestrels, screech owls/*Trichomonas* infections resistant to treatment with lower doses
Chloroquine phosphate[a]	—	Generally used with primaquine for *Plasmodium, Haemoproteus,* and *Leucocytozoon*; overdose can result in death[38]
	10 mg/kg PO q7d [333]	Most species/preventive treatment for *Plasmodium* once bird is stable; use with primaquine (1 mg/kg PO q7d)
	10 mg/kg PO, then 5 mg/kg at 6, 12, 18 hr, then q24h × 10 days[38,826]	Magellanic penguins/upon diagnosis of *Plasmodium*; if still positive on blood smear after this regime, continue with sulfadiazine-trimethoprim 40 mg/kg PO × 10 days
	10 mg/kg PO, then 5 mg/kg at 6, 24, 48 hr[120]	Raptors/use with 0.3 mg/kg primaquine (at 24 hr following the initial chloroquine dose) q24h × 7 days
	10-15 mg/kg PO q12h × 2 doses, then q24h[432b]	Raptors/*Plasmodium*; use with primaquine
	10-25 mg/kg PO, then 5-15 mg/kg at 6, 18, 24 hr[194]	Use in conjunction with primaquine
	20 mg/kg PO or IV, then 10 mg/kg at 6, 18, 24 hr; repeat q7d × 3-5 treatments[333]	Raptors/*Plasmodium*; IV is recommended for initial dose in acute cases; use with 1 mg/kg primaquine q24h × 2 days

Continued

TABLE 5-4 Antiparasitic Agents Used in Birds. (cont'd)

Agent	Dosage	Species/Comments
Chloroquine phosphate[a] (cont'd)	25 mg/kg PO, then 15 mg/kg PO at 12, 24, 48 hr [38,333,714a]	Most species, including raptors/use with 0.75-1.3 mg/kg primaquine at 0 hr
	60 mg/kg PO q24h × 7 days[333]	Raptors/*Haemoproteus*; use in conjunction with mefloquine and primaquine
	2000 mg/L drinking water q24h × 14 days[135]	Passerines/juice covers bitter taste of drug
Chlorsulon (Curatrem, Merial)	—	Benzenesulfonamide anthelmintic and flukicide
	20 mg/kg PO q2wk × 3 treatments[432b]	Raptors
Clazuril (Appertex, Janssen)	—	Benzene-acetonitrile anticoccidial
	2.5 mg/bird PO once; can repeat monthly[827a]	Pigeons/oocyst shedding commences 20 days post-treatment
	5 mg/kg PO once[135]	Pigeons
	5-10 mg/kg PO q24h × 2 days[340,432b]	Raptors
	5-10 mg/kg PO q72h × 3 treatments[38,149a,432b]	Raptors
	6.25 mg/kg PO once[38]	Pigeons
	7 mg/kg PO × 3 days, off 2 days, on 3 days[38,194]	Most species
	30 mg/kg PO once[135]	Raptors
	1.1 or 5.5 mg/kg feed[122]	Sandhill cranes/ineffective in preventing experimentally induced disseminated visceral coccidiosis
Coumaphos (Powder containing 3% w/v coumaphos 2% w/v propoxur 5% w/v sulphanilamide Negasunt, Bayer)	Topical dust onto feathers[38]	Most species/ectoparasites; useful for fly-blown wounds, contains carbamate propoxur
	20 mg/kg PO q14d × 3 treatments[38,432b,666]	Psitacines, raptors/trematodes, cestodes
Crotamiton (Eurax, Westwood-Squibb)	Topical to affected areas[38]	Most species/mites (i.e., *Knemidokoptes*); use in combination with ivermectin
Cypermethrin (5%) (Max Con, Y-Tex)	Spray or dip with 2% solution[38]	Pigeons, ostriches/lice, mites; treatment of premises infested with *Dermanyssus* spp.
Deltamethrin	50 mg/L topical spray[333]	Ostriches/lice; spray until runoff
Dichlorophene (Tapeworm tablets, Happy Jack)	100 mg PO q10d × 2 treatments, repeat in 10 days prn[402]	Pigeons/cestodes; administer after a 12-hr fast
Diclazuril (Protazil, Merck)	—	Benzene-acetonitrile anticoccidial; some *Eimeria* resistance in poultry documented recently;[4,640] rotation suggested for long-term prevention
	5 mg/L drinking water[194]	Passerines/*Toxoplasmosis*
	10 mg/kg PO q12h on days 0, 1, 2, 4, 6, 8, 10[194,502]	Passerines, including Hawaiian crows/*Toxoplasma*

TABLE 5-4 Antiparasitic Agents Used in Birds. (cont'd)

Agent	Dosage	Species/Comments
Dimetridazole (Emtryl 40% powder, MedPet)	—	Trichomonas, Giardia, Hexamita, Spironucleus, Histomonas; low therapeutic index; hepatotoxic to lories, some passerines (e.g., robins) and fledgling birds;[38] not recommended for finches; highly toxic to geese, ducks, and pigeons;[759] not available in many countries (United States, European Union) because of human health risks; Canada has banned use in food-producing animals;[548] do not give during breeding season
	50 mg/kg PO q24h × 10 days[534]	Falcons/Enterocytozoon bieneusi
	50 mg/kg PO or in drinking water q24h × 6 days[135]	Pigeons
	100 mg/L drinking water[201]	Canaries, finches
	200-400 mg/L drinking water × 5 days[194,333]	Psittacines/caution toxic if overdosed; do not use in finches and Pekin robins; use lower dose in lorikeets and mynahs[194]
	250 mg/L drinking water × 4-6 days[333]	Gouldian finches/Cochlostoma, Trichomonas
	265 mg/L drinking water[333]	Pigeons
	300 mg/L drinking water × 10 days[38]	Bustards/prevention of Trichomonas
	400 mg/L drinking water × 3 days[361]	Pigeons/PD; bioavailability reduced with feed
	666 mg/L drinking water × 7-12 days[38]	Pigeons/Trichomonas, Giardia, Hexamita
	900 mg/L drinking water × 5 days, followed by 700 mg/L × 10 days[38]	Bustards/treatment of choice for Trichomonas
	¼-½ tsp/gal drinking water × 3-5 days[320]	Pigeons/CNS symptoms if overdosed; because of variable water consumption, use lower dose in hot weather and higher dose in cool weather
	200-500 mg/kg feed[112]	Ostriches (≤3 mo of age)/Trichomonas
Doramectin (Dectomax, Zoetis)	1 mg/kg SC, IM,[38,432b] repeat in 2 wk[135]	Raptors, bustards/used to treat GI nematodes, lungworms, eyeworms, mites[38]
Doxycycline	20 mg/kg PO q12h × 10 days[295]	Humboldt penguins/Plasmodium
Febantel (Vercom, Bayer)	5 mg/kg PO[500]	Ostriches
	20 mg/kg PO[500]	Ostriches
	30 mg/kg PO once[34,194]	Pigeons/PD; ascarids; repeated doses required to eliminate Capillaria obsignata
	37.5 mg/kg PO once[38]	Pigeons

Continued

TABLE 5-4 Antiparasitic Agents Used in Birds. (cont'd)

Agent	Dosage	Species/Comments
Fenbendazole (Panacur, Merck)	—	Most species/anthelmintic effective against cestodes, nematodes, trematodes, *Giardia*, acanthocephalans; toxicity documented in pigeons and doves;[286,356,582,671] may be toxic for other species, including raptors,[685] vultures,[88,358] lories,[582] storks,[88,840] pelicans;[457] can cause feather abnormalities if administered during molting;[38] ineffective against finch ventricular worms;[38] can be toxic to bone marrow causing leukopenia[194]
	8-10 mg/kg q24h × 3-4 days[194]	Most species
	10-20 mg/kg PO q24h × 3 days[135]	Pigeons/nematodes
	10-50 mg/kg PO, repeat in 14 days[358,384]	Raptors/nematodes, trematodes
	15 mg/kg PO[149b,333]	Ostriches/"wire worms," nematodes, cestodes
	15 mg/kg PO q24h × 5 days[38]	Psittacines
	15 mg/kg PO × 5 days, then off 5 days × 4 treatment periods[510]	Umbrella cockatoos/proventricular Spiruroidea
	15 mg/kg PO q3wk[149b]	Ratite chicks/nematodes; administer at this frequency until 4 mo old, then at adult prophylaxis dosing intervals
	15-25 mg/kg PO × 4-5 days[740]	Tinamous
	15-45 mg/kg PO[333]	Ostriches
	20 mg/kg PO q24h × 10-14 days[149a]	Raptors/filarids
	20-25 mg/kg PO q24h × 5 days[149a,256,432b,650]	Raptors/*Capillaria*
	20-50 mg/kg PO q24h[38,333]	Psittacines, pigeons/ascarids in psittacines, treat once and repeat in 10 days; trematodes and microfilaria, treat for 3 days; *Capillaria*, treat for 5 days
	20-50 mg/kg PO q24h × 3 days, repeat in 2 wk[838]	Penguins[a]
	20-50 mg/kg PO q24h × 3 days, repeat in 21 days[358]	Raptors
	25 mg/kg PO, repeat in 14 days[144,749]	Most species, including owls/ascarids
	25 mg/kg PO q24h × 5 days,[135] repeat in 10-14 days[358]	Raptors/*Capillaria*, spirurids
	25 mg/kg PO q6wk[149b]	Ratites/cestode prophylaxis
	25-50 mg/kg PO once[194]	Most species
	30 mg/kg PO once[38]	Bustards
	30 mg/kg PO q24h × 5-8 days[16]	Falcons/eliminated *Serratospiculoides* fecal eggs and larvae

TABLE 5-4 Antiparasitic Agents Used in Birds. (cont'd)

Agent	Dosage	Species/Comments
Fenbendazole (Panacur, Merck) (cont'd)	33 mg/kg PO q24h × 3 days[148]	Psittacines, passerines, raptors/microfilaria, trematodes
	50 mg/kg PO q24h × 3-5 days[194,333,560,747]	Most species, including pigeons, Bali mynahs/nematodes, trematodes, *Giardia*
	50 mg/kg PO q24h × 5 days[482]	Cranes/*Capillaria*, gapeworms
	50 mg/kg PO q12h × 5 days[333]	Cockatoos/filarid adulticide treatment; use with ivermectin (0.2 mg/kg once)
	50 mg/kg q24h × 5 days[220]	Scops owls (fledglings)/treatment of *Gongylonema pulchrum* oral plaques
	50-100 mg/kg PO, repeat in 14 days[482]	Cranes/intestinal strongyles, ascarids
	100 mg/kg PO once, repeat in 10-14 days[432b]	Raptors/*Capillaria*, spirurids
	100 mg/kg PO q24h × 5 days[118]	Cranes/*Capillaria*
	50 mg/L drinking water × 5 days[333]	Finches
	125 mg/L drinking water × 5 days[333]	Most species/nematodes
Fipronil	—	Do not use spot-on preparation; use with caution in raptors, pigeons, passerines/ectoparasites; apply via pad to base of neck, tail base, and under each wing; avoid plumage during application; alcohol may create dry, brittle feathers; do not soak bird; do not exceed 7.5 mg/kg; in zebra finches[406] and wild[281] species; significant toxicity reported from mortality to sublethal effects such as cytotoxic effects,[189] impaired immune function,[464] and reduced growth and reproductive success,[407] often at concentrations well below those associated with mortality;[281,407] environmental contamination and secondary intoxication are of concern[281,405]
	3 mg/kg spray on skin once[194]	
	7.5 mg/kg; spray on skin once, repeat in 30 days prn[38,135,256,747]	
Flubendazole (Flutelmium 7.5%, Janssen-Cilag)	30-60 mg/kg feed × 7 days[333]	Tinamous; follow VFD guidelines
Hydroxychloroquine sulfate	—	Antimalarial
	830 mg/L drinking water × 6 wk[333]	Pigeons/*Plasmodium*
Hygromycin B (Hygromix 8, Elanco)	—	Aminoglycoside antibiotic used as anthelmintic feed additive; follow VFD guidelines

Continued

TABLE 5-4 Antiparasitic Agents Used in Birds. (cont'd)

Agent	Dosage	Species/Comments
Imidocarb dipropionate (Imizol, Merck)	—	Antiprotozoal effective against *Babesia*
	5-7 mg/kg IM once, repeat in 7 days[704,851]	Raptors/*Babesia*; some cases require a total of 3 treatments
Ipronidazole (Ipropran, Roche)	—	*Giardia, Trichomonas, Histomonas*; not available in the United States; 61 g/2.65 oz
	130 mg/L drinking water × 7 days[333]	Most species, including pigeons
	250 mg/L drinking water × 3-7 days[333]	Psittacines, pigeons
Ivermectin	—	All species/most nematodes, acanthocephalans, leeches, most ectoparasites (including *Knemidokoptes, Dermanyssus*); can dilute with water or saline for immediate use; dilute with propylene glycol for extended use; parenteral ivermectin may be toxic to finches and budgerigars;[333] brain inflammation detected as an adverse effect in king pigeons;[132] suspected toxicity reported in a nanday conure at 0.2 mg/kg[600]
	0.2 mg/kg PO, SC, IM once, can repeat in 10-14 days[38,135,320,375,482,571,747]	Most species, including psittacines, passerines, pigeons, raptors, guinea fowl, ratites, cranes/use in combination with fenbendazole at 50 mg/kg PO q12h × 5 days for microfilaria in cockatoos[333]
	0.2 mg/kg IM once[173,178]	Ostriches/only 60% effective against *Libyostrongylus dentatus* and *L. douglassii*
	0.2-0.4 mg/kg PO, SC, repeat 7-14 days[838]	Penguins
	0.2-1 mg/kg PO, SC, IM q14d × 2-3 treatments[432b]	Raptors
	0.2 mg/kg SC, topical on skin; can repeat 1-2 wk for 3-4 applications[135,171,205,738]	Canaries, finches/quill mites, *Knemidokoptes*; dilute to 0.02% solution with propylene glycol, can apply directly to lesions on cere, legs; also effective against the tracheal mite *Ptilonyssus morofskyi*[24]
	0.4 mg/kg SC once[333]	Raptors, passerines/*Capillaria* in towhees
	0.4 mg/kg IM q7d × 7 treatments[694]	Golden eagles/required additional treatment with selamectin to achieve eradication of a novel *Micknemidokoptes* spp. mite
	0.5-1 mg/kg PO, IM once[320]	Pigeons
	1 mg/kg SC, repeat in 7 days[700]	Falcons/*Serratospiculum*

TABLE 5-4 Antiparasitic Agents Used in Birds. (cont'd)

Agent	Dosage	Species/Comments
Ivermectin (cont'd)	2 mg/kg IM once[792]	Falcons/*Capillaria*; no adverse effects observed at this dose
	0.8-1 mg/L drinking water[201]	Canaries
	1 drop (0.05 mL) to skin q7d × 3 treatments[38]	Pigeons, passerines/*Knemidokoptes, Dermanyssus*
Levamisole (Tramisol, Schering-Plough)	—	Many species/nematodes; immunostimulant; low therapeutic index (toxic reactions, deaths reported); do not use in debilitated birds;[38] IM administration may cause severe toxicity; limb paralysis, vomiting, dyspnea reported in a parakeet; do not use in white-faced ibis or in lories; withhold food before treatment to prevent regurgitation[333]
	1.5 mg/kg split into 2 doses and administered topically in eyes[532]	Ostriches/PD; effective against *Philophthalmus gralli*
	2-5 mg/kg SC, IM, repeat in 10-14 days × 3 treatments[38]	Psittacines/immunostimulant
	7.5 mg/kg PO, SC[112]	Ostriches
	7.5 mg/kg IM once; can repeat in 7 days[38]	Pigeons
	10-20 mg/kg PO, SC q24h × 2 days[149a,358]	Raptors
	10-20 mg/kg SC once[38,333,432b]	Most species
	15-20 mg/bird PO once, repeat in 10 days[135]	Pigeons
	20 mg/kg PO once[38]	Psittacines, pigeons, raptors
	20-40 mg/kg IM once[194,432b]	Raptors
	20-50 mg/kg PO × 1-3 days[38]	Psittacines/low therapeutic index
	25 mg/kg PO once[482]	Crane chicks/*Capillaria*, intestinal strongyles, ascarids
	30 mg/kg PO q3wk[149b]	Ratite chicks/administer at this dosage until 4 mo of age, then reduce to adult prophylaxis interval thereafter
	30 mg/kg PO q10d[149b]	Ratites/cestodes, nematodes
	40 mg/kg PO once[38,432b,482]	Psittacines, pigeons, raptors, cranes/*Capillaria*, intestinal strongyles, ascarids
	100-200 mg/L drinking water × 3 days, repeat in 2 wk[135,194]	Psittacines, passerines, raptors
	264-396 mg/L drinking water × 1-3 days[333]	Most species, including pigeons
	300-400 mg/L drinking water for 24 hr, repeat in 7 days[38]	Pigeons/loft treatment for capillariasis, ascaridiasis
	375 mg/L drinking water as sole water source for 24 hr, repeat in 7 days[38]	Pigeons

Continued

TABLE 5-4 Antiparasitic Agents Used in Birds. (cont'd)

Agent	Dosage	Species/Comments
Mebendazole (Telmin Suspension, Telmintic Powder, Schering-Plough)	5-6 mg/kg PO q24h × 3-5 days, repeat in 21 days[333]	Pigeons
	5-7 mg/kg PO[806]	Ostriches
	10 mg/kg PO q12h × 5 days[333]	Canaries/avoid use during breeding season
	10-25 mg/kg q12h × 5 days[194]	Most species
	20 mg/kg PO q24h × 10-14 days[38,149a,432b]	Raptors/filarids
	25 mg/kg PO q12h × 5 days[159]	Psittacines, ramphastids (toucans)/nematodes; may not be effective for proventricular and ventricular parasites
	25 mg/kg PO q12h × 5 days, repeat q30d[358]	Raptors/intestinal nematodiasis
	50 mg/kg PO, repeat in 10-14 days[358]	Raptors/intestinal nematodiasis
	10-20 mg/L drinking water × 3-5 days[194,333]	Pigeons
Mefloquine HCl (Lariam, Hoffman-LaRoche)	—	Antimalarial; active against erythrocytic and tissue schizonts of some *Plasmodium*[659,793]
	30 mg/kg PO q12h × 1 day, then q24h × 1-2 days[385,432b,793,851]	Raptors
	30 mg/kg PO q12h × 1 day, then q24h × 2 days, then q7d[432b]	Raptors/long-term administration up to 6 mo reported
	30 mg/kg PO q7d[295]	Penguins/*Plasmodium* routine prevention during insect season
	50 mg/kg PO q24h[541]	Raptors/*Haemoproteus*; used in conjunction with chloroquine at doses up to 60 mg/kg
	50 mg/kg PO q24h × 7 days[135]	Raptors/*Plasmodium*
Melarsomine dihydrochloride (Immiticide, Merial)	—	Organic arsenical
	0.25 mg/kg IM q24h × 4 days[135]	Raptors/*Leucocytozoon*
Melarsomine dihydrochloride (M)/ivermectin (I)	(M) 0.25 mg/kg IM q24h × 2 days followed 10 days later with (I) 1 mg/kg IM[790]	Falcons/*Serratospiculum*; reduced clinical signs and eliminated shedding of embryonated eggs
Mepacrine HCl	—	Nonsteroidal antiinflammatory used as an antiprotozoal for *Giardia* in humans
	0.24 mg/kg PO q12h[194]	Canaries/*Plasmodium*
Metronidazole	—	Most species/antiprotozoal, including alimentary tract protozoa (especially flagellates such as *Giardia*, *Histomonas*, *Spironucleus*, *Trichomonas*); resistance identified in racing pigeons[682]
	10-20 mg/kg IM q12-24h × 2 days[333]	Pigeons, psittacines
	10-30 mg/kg PO, IM q12h × 10 days[38,808]	Psittacines

TABLE 5-4 Antiparasitic Agents Used in Birds. (cont'd)

Agent	Dosage	Species/Comments
Metronidazole (cont'd)	20-25 mg/kg PO q12h[806]	Ratites
	25 mg/kg PO q12h × 2-10 days[333]	Psittacine neonates
	25-50 mg/kg PO q12-24h × 5-10 days[333]	Companion birds/treatment, control, or prevention of *Giardia*, *Trichomonas*, and *Hexamita*
	25-50 mg/kg PO q12-24h[333]	Pigeons/use lower dose with twice daily dosing
	30 mg/kg PO via gavage once[228,747]	Passerines, including finches/*Cochlosoma*
	30 mg/kg PO q12h × 5-10 days[50]	Raptors, Gouldian finches, psittacines/*Trichomonas*
	30-50 mg/kg PO q24h × 3-5 days[654]	Raptors/*Trichomonas*
	40 mg/kg PO q24h[333]	Rheas
	40 mg/kg PO q24h × 7 days[333]	Budgerigars/*Trichomonas*
	40-50 mg/kg PO q24h × 5-7 days[135]	Pigeons
	50 mg/kg PO q12-24h[194]	Most species/*Trichomonas*, *Giardia*, *Cochlosoma*
	50 mg/kg PO q24h × 5-7 days[38,149a,256,358]	Raptors/*Trichomonas*, *Giardia*
	50 mg/kg PO q12h × 5 days[135,400]	Pigeons, passerines, raptors
	50-100 mg/kg PO q24h[432b]	Raptors
	100 mg/kg PO q24h × 3 days[702]	Falcons/*Trichomonas*
	100-150 mg PO total dose divided over 5 days[38]	Pigeons
	40 mg/L drinking water[228]	Finches/*Cochlosoma*
	40-80 mg/L drinking water × 3 days[194]	Most species/*Trichomonas*, *Giardia*, *Cochlosoma*
	100 mg/L drinking water[333]	Canaries
	200 mg/L drinking water × 7 days[135]	Passerines
	370 mg/L drinking water[333]	Passerines/protozoal sinusitis
	400 mg/L drinking water × 5-15 days[333]	Passerines/protozoal sinusitis
	1057 mg/L drinking water[333]	Pigeons
	1250 mg/L drinking water × 7-10 days[333]	Ratites
	100 mg/kg soft feed[333]	Canaries
Milbemycin oxime	2 mg/kg PO once[194]	Budgerigars, African finches, and European finches may be more sensitive
Monensin (Coban 45, Elanco)	—	Ionophore antibiotic anticoccidial feed additive
	94 mg/kg feed[121]	Cranes/coccidia (including disseminated visceral coccidiosis)
	99 mg/kg feed[122,482]	Sandhill cranes/prevented experimentally induced disseminated visceral coccidiosis

Continued

TABLE 5-4 Antiparasitic Agents Used in Birds. (cont'd)

Agent	Dosage	Species/Comments
Moxidectin (ProHeart, Zoetis)	—	Falcons/*Serratospiculum, Capillaria*, acanthocephalans, *Paraspiralatus sakeri*, and *Physaloptera alata*[38]
	0.2 mg/kg PO[135,700]	Raptors/nematodes
	0.2 mg/kg IM once[159]	Ramphastids (toucans)/repeat if necessary
	0.2 mg/kg IM once[178]	Ostriches/100% effective against *Libyostrongylus dentatus*, *L. douglassii*
	0.2-0.4 mg/kg PO, IM once[194]	
	0.5 mg/kg PO[38,432b]	Raptors
	0.5-1 mg/kg PO[135]	Raptors/*Capillaria*
	1 mg/bird topically once, or can repeat q10d × 2 treatments[333]	Budgerigars/*Knemidokoptes*; no adverse effects seen at this dose in this species
Niclosamide (Yomesan, Bayer)	—	Cestodes, trematodes; rarely used since praziquantel is more efficacious; may be toxic for geese and some Anseriformes; not available in the United States
	50-100 mg/kg PO, repeat in 10-14 days[194,333]	Ostriches
	100 mg/kg PO q6wk[149b]	Ostriches/cestode prophylaxis
	220 mg/kg PO, repeat in 10-14 days[333]	Most species
	250 mg/kg PO q14d prn[117]	Cranes
	500 mg/kg PO q7d × 4 wk[333]	Finches
Ormetoprim-sulfadimethoxine (Primor, Zoetis)	0.015% ormetoprim and 0.026% sulfadimethoxine in food × 3 wk[482]	Cranes/coccidiosis
Oxfendazole (Benzelmin, Syntex)	5 mg/kg PO once[333]	Ostriches/nematodes
	5 mg/kg PO q6wk[149b]	Ratites/cestode, nematode prophylaxis
	5 mg/kg PO q3wk[149b]	Ratite chicks/nematodes; administer at this frequency until 4 mo of age, then reduce to adult prophylactic dosing interval
	10-40 mg/kg PO once[194,494,768]	Most species, including finches/nematodes
	15-25 mg/kg PO once[159]	Ramphastids (toucans)/repeat in 15 days prn
	20 mg/kg PO once[340]	Raptors
Paromomycin	—	Highest efficacy of all drugs tested thus far against *Cryptosporidium*; oocyst output decreased by 67%-82% in chickens;[758] may result in secondary bacterial or mycotic infections; use with caution if ulcerative bowel lesions are suspected because renal toxicity may occur;[333] ineffective against *Histomonas*[357]

TABLE 5-4 Antiparasitic Agents Used in Birds. (cont'd)

Agent	Dosage	Species/Comments
Paromomycin (cont'd)	100 mg/kg PO q12h × 7 days[1,194,256]	Most species, including macaw chicks, falcons/mix a 250 mg capsule with 10 mL water to facilitate dosing; poorly absorbed
	1000 mg/kg soft food or hulled millet[333]	Gouldian finches/*Cryptosporidium*; may predispose to fungal infections
Permethrin	Dust plumage lightly[38]	Pigeons/lice, fleas
Permethrin, high-cis (Harker's Louse Powder, Harkers)	Topical application[38]	Raptors, psittacines/ectoparasites
Piperazine (Wazine, Fleming Laboratories)	—	Most species/ascarids, oxyurids; less efficacious than fenbendazole; seldom used in companion birds
	35 mg/kg PO q24h × 2 days[333]	Pigeons/ascarids
	50-100 mg/kg PO once[333,759]	Emus, ostriches
	100 mg/kg PO, repeat in 14 days[333,494]	Raptors
	100-250 mg/kg PO once[194]	Ascarids, resistance common
	250 mg/kg PO once[333]	Psittacines, pigeons
	79 mg/L drinking water × 2 days[333]	Pigeons/ascarids
	1000 mg/L drinking water × 3 days[333,494]	Raptors, pigeons
	1000-2000 mg/L drinking water × 1-2 days[135,333]	Game birds, pigeons
	3700 mg/L drinking water × 12 hr, repeat in 14-21 days[135]	Passerines
Piperonyl butoxide/pyrethrin (Ridmite Powder, Johnson)	Dust plumage, repeat in 10 days[38,194]	Psittacines
	Dust plumage, repeat in 21 days[38]	Raptors
Piperonyl butoxide/pyrethrin/methoprene (Avian Insect Liquidator, Vetafarm)	Apply to plumage, spray cages, aviaries, bird rooms, and surroundings[38]	Most species/fleas, lice, mosquitoes, moths, and some mites
Ponazuril (Marquis 5% paste; Bayer)	—	Triazine coccidiocidal drug; metabolite of toltrazuril
	20 mg/kg q24h × 7 days[825]	Falcons/respiratory *Cryptosporidium baileyi*
Praziquantel (Droncit, Bayer)	—	Most species/cestodes, trematodes; injectable form toxic in finches and associated with depression, death in some species[38,333]
	1 mg/kg PO[38]	Bustards/well tolerated
	5-10 mg/kg PO, repeat after 2-4 wk[38,149a,432b]	Psittacines, passerines, raptors
	5-10 mg/kg PO, SC q24h × 14 days[333,358]	Raptors/trematodes
	6 mg/kg PO, IM, repeat in 10-14 days[482]	Cranes/cestodes, trematodes
	7.5 mg/kg PO[525]	Ostriches

Continued

TABLE 5-4 Antiparasitic Agents Used in Birds. (cont'd)

Agent	Dosage	Species/Comments
Praziquantel (Droncit, Bayer) (cont'd)	7.5 mg/kg SC, IM repeat in 2-4 wk[135,148]	Most species, except finches
	9 mg/kg IM, repeat in 10 days[38,333]	Psittacines/cestodes
	10 mg/kg PO, SC, IM once; repeat in 7 days[256]	Raptors/cestodes, trematodes
	10 mg/kg SC, IM q24h × 3 days, then PO × 11 days[358,808]	Psittacines, raptors/trematodes
	10 mg/kg IM q24h × 3 days, then PO q24h × 11 days[282]	Toucans/trematodes
	10 mg/kg PO, SC, IM q24h × 14 days[159]	Toucans/trematodes; follow with 6 mg/kg PO q24h × 14 days[333]
	10-20 mg/kg PO, repeat in 10-14 days[38,135,194,321]	Most species
	15-20 mg/kg PO, SC, IM, repeat in 2 wk as necessary[838]	Penguins/user higher dose PO
	25 mg/kg PO, IM, repeat in 10-14 days[562,747]	Passerines, including Bali mynahs/cestodes
	30-50 mg/kg PO, SC, IM, repeat in 14 days[747,838]	Passerines, raptors/cestodes; use lower dose in passerines
	12 mg crushed and baked into 9″ × 9″ × 2″ cake[333]	Finches/withhold regular feed
Primaquine[a]	—	Pigeons, raptors, game birds, penguins[a]/hematozoa (i.e., *Plasmodium*, *Haemoproteus*, *Leucocytozoon*); use in conjunction with chloroquine; dosage based on amount of active base rather than total tablet weight
	0.3 mg/kg PO (at 24 hr following the initial chloroquine dose) q24h × 7 days[333]	Raptors/use with chloroquine (10 mg/kg at 0 hr, then 5 mg/kg at 6, 24, 48 hr)
	0.3 mg/kg PO q24h × 10 days[295,838]	Penguins[a]/*Plasmodium*; use with chloroquine (10 mg/kg at 0 hr, then 5 mg/kg at 6, 18, 24 hr)
	0.3-1 mg/kg PO q24h × 3-10 days[194]	Most species/*Atoxoplasma*, *Sarcocystis*; use with chloroquine
	0.75 mg/kg PO q3-7days[295]	African and Humboldt penguins[a]/during vector season, depending on institution
	0.75 mg/kg PO q24h × 5 days[791]	Falcons/*Haemoproteus tinnunculi*
	0.75-1 mg/kg PO once[750]	Raptors/*Plasmodium*; use with chloroquine (25 mg/kg at 0 hr, then 15 mg/kg at 12, 24, and 48 hr); palliative therapy
	1 mg/kg PO on day 2, then q24h × 3 days[106]	Magellanic penguins[a]/*Plasmodium*, use with chloroquine (10 mg/kg at 0, 6, 12, 18, 24 hr on day 1, then 5 mg/kg q24h × 3 days)

TABLE 5-4 Antiparasitic Agents Used in Birds. (cont'd)

Agent	Dosage	Species/Comments
Primaquine[a] (cont'd)	1 mg/kg PO q7d[655]	Most species/use with chloroquine (10 mg/kg q7d) as a preventive regimen for birds recovering from *Plasmodium* infection
	1 mg/kg PO q24h × 2 days, repeat q7d × 3-5 treatments to prevent relapse[655]	Raptors/*Plasmodium*; use with chloroquine (20 mg/kg IV initially, followed by 10 mg/kg PO at 6, 18, 24 hr)
	1 mg/kg at 0, 24 hr then q24h × 10-14 days[295,851]	African penguins,[a] raptors/upon diagnosis of *Plasmodium*, administer with mefloquine 30 mg/kg PO at 0, 12, 24, 48 hr
	1 mg/kg PO q24h × 45 days[845]	Psittacines (keas)/*Sarcocystis*; use in combination with amprolium, enrofloxacin, and pyrimethamine
	1.25 mg/kg PO q24h × 10-14 days[598]	Medium sized (3-5 kg) penguins[a]/upon diagnosis with *Plasmodium* with chloroquine 10 mg/kg PO q24h × 10-14 days; then 5 mg/kg PO q12h × 3 days; some institutions stop here, others continue primaquine and chloroquine 5 mg/kg PO q24h
	1.25 mg/kg PO q24h (March until October, Northern hemisphere)[295,838]	African and Humboldt penguins[a]/prophylactic therapy against *Plasmodium*
	3.75 mg/kg PO q3-7days (March until October; Northern hemisphere)[295]	African and Humboldt penguins[a]/prophylactic therapy against *Plasmodium*
	4 mg PO q48h[838]	Medium sized (3-5 kg) penguins[a]/during vector season (or year round, depending on location of institution) in capsule with sulfadiazine 125 mg and folic acid 0.4 mg
Pyrantel pamoate	—	Intestinal nematodes; poorly absorbed, so increased safety margin[194]
	4.5 mg/kg PO, repeat in 10-14 days[38,482,856]	Cranes, psittacines, including cockatoo chicks[856]
	5-7 mg/kg PO[806]	Ostriches
	7 mg/kg PO, repeat in 14 days[144]	Most species
	7-20 mg/kg PO, repeat in 14 days[358]	Raptors
	7-25 mg/kg PO once[194]	Nematodes
	20 mg/kg PO once[38,149a,432b]	Raptors
	20-25 mg/kg PO[321]	Pigeons
	70 mg/kg PO once[159]	Ramphastids (toucans)/repeat if necessary
	148 mg/L drinking water[333]	Psittacines, pigeons/medication floats

Continued

TABLE 5-4 Antiparasitic Agents Used in Birds. (cont'd)

Agent	Dosage	Species/Comments
Pyrethrins (0.15%) (Adams, Pfizer)	Dust plumage lightly to moderately prn[194,333,482]	Most species, including psittacines, pigeons/ectoparasites
Pyrimethamine	—	Toxoplasma, Atoxoplasma, Sarcocystis; may be effective for Leucocytozoon; supplement with folic or folinic acid
	0.25-0.5 mg/kg PO q12h[432b]	Raptors
	0.25-0.5 mg/kg PO q12h × 30 days[38,149a]	Raptors/Sarcocystis, Toxoplasma
	0.5 mg/kg PO q12h × 14-28 days[135,194]	Most species/use for 28 days for Leucocytozoon in raptors
	0.5 mg/kg PO q12h × 45 days[845]	Psittacines (keas)/Sarcocystis; use in combination with amprolium and primaquine
	0.5-1 mg/kg PO q12h × 2-4 days, then 0.25 mg/kg PO q12h × 30 days[333]	Companion birds/Sarcocystis; use in combination with trimethoprim-sulfa 5 mg/kg IM q12h or 30-100 mg/kg PO q12h × 7 days
	0.5-1 mg/kg PO q12h × 30 days[580]	Eclectus, Amazon parrots/use with trimethoprim-sulfadiazine (30 mg/kg)
	100 mg/kg feed[333]	Most species
Quinacrine HCl[a] (Atabrine, Sanofi)	—	Most species/Atoxoplasma, Plasmodium; chloroquine and primaquine are preferred; overdosage may cause hepatoxicity
	5-10 mg/kg PO, IM q24h[432b]	Raptors/Plasmodium
	5-10 mg/kg PO q24h × 7-10 days[38,194,382]	Most species/use higher doses for Lankesterella, Plasmodium
	7.5 mg/kg PO q24h × 10 days[38,333]	Most species/Atoxoplasma
	26-79 mg/L drinking water × 10-21 days[38,321]	Pigeons
Rafoxanide (Flukex, Univet; Ranide, MSD)	10 mg/kg PO[194]	Raptors/trematodes, cestodes; not available in the United States
Resorantel (Terenol-S, Intervet)	130 mg/kg PO[149b,333]	Ostriches/highly effective against H. struthionis when administered with or without fenbendazole
Ronidazole (Ronivet-S, Vetafarm)	—	Antiprotozoal used against trichomoniasis; toxicity documented with overdose in drinking water in society finches[861]
	2.5 mg/kg PO × 6 days[321]	Pigeons
	6-10 mg/kg PO q24h × 6-10 days[333]	Most species
	10-20 mg/kg PO q24h × 7 days[135]	Pigeons
	12.5 mg/kg PO q24h × 6 days[38]	Pigeons
	50-400 mg/L drinking water × 5 days[135]	Passerines
	60 mg/L drinking water[228]	Finches/Cochlosoma

TABLE 5-4 Antiparasitic Agents Used in Birds. (cont'd)

Agent	Dosage	Species/Comments
Ronidazole (Ronivet-S, Vetafarm) (cont'd)	100-200 mg/L drinking water × 7 days[333]	Cockatiels, pigeons/higher dosage required for resistant strains in pigeons
	100-600 mg/L drinking water × 3-5 days[321]	Pigeons
	400 mg/L drinking water × 5-7 days (Bailey, 2016)[201]	Canaries, pigeons/flock treatment; *Trichomonas*; preventive dose[38]
	600 mg/L drinking water × 5-7 days[38]	Pigeons/*Trichomonas*; flock treatment
	1000 mg/L drinking water q24h[135]	Pigeons/equivalent to 12.5 mg/kg/day
	400 mg/kg soft feed[201]	Canaries
Selamectin (Revolution, Zoetis)	—	No adverse effects, including neurologic signs, were seen in healthy zebra finches with doses up to 92 mg/kg[84]
	23 mg/kg topically, repeat in 3-4 wk[83]	Budgerigars/*Knemidokoptes* improvement in 13/14 birds at 4 wk, with no neurologic signs identified but monitor for weight loss
	23 mg/kg topically q7d × 4 treatments[694]	Golden eagle/treatment for *Micnemidocoptes* spp.; no evidence of toxicity at this dosage
Sulfachlorpyrazine (ESB3, Novartis)	—	Coccidiostat; affects the intestinal stages of *Atoxoplasma*;[201] not available in the United States, but can be obtained through the Bali mynah Species Survival Plan[562]
	1 g of 30% powder/L drinking water × 5 days, off 3 days, on 5 days, then repeat cycle × 4 treatments; administer treatment 3× annually[562]	Bali mynahs/*Atoxoplasma*; significantly reduced or totally cleared oocyst shedding for extended time; it is uncertain if the drug is safe to use when parents are feeding chicks; supplement with vitamin B_6
Sulfachlorpyridazine (Vetisulid, Boehringer-Ingelheim)	—	Coccidiostat; used as replacement for sulfachlorpyrazine in the United States; contraindicated with dehydration, liver disease, renal disease;[194] treatment >2 wk may require folic acid supplementation[194]
	100-400 mg/L drinking water × 3-5 days/wk; repeat[194]	Passerines/repeat after 5 days to allow for prepatent period of coccidia
	150-300 mg/L drinking water;[201] 5 days/wk × 2-3 wk[171]	Passerines, including canaries/may need to treat for months for systemic coccidiosis
	300 mg/L drinking water × 5 days, off 3 days, on 5 days, then repeat cycle × 4 treatments; administer treatment 3× annually[562,747]	Passerines, including Bali mynahs/ *Atoxoplasma*

Continued

TABLE 5-4 Antiparasitic Agents Used in Birds. (cont'd)

Agent	Dosage	Species/Comments
Sulfachlorpyridazine (Vetisulid, Boehringer-Ingelheim) (cont'd)	300 mg/L drinking water × 7-10 days[321]	Pigeons
	300-1000 mg/L drinking water × 3 days, off 2 days, then repeat course[135]	Pigeons
	400 mg/L drinking water × 30 days[333]	Cockatiels, budgerigars/mixture is stable for up to 5 days if refrigerated; change daily; mix well
	400-500 mg/L drinking water × 5 days, off 2 days, on 5 days[333]	Most species
Sulfadimethoxine (12.5%)	20 mg/kg PO q12h[333]	Most species/treatment and prophylaxis of coccidian; contraindicated with dehydration, liver disease, renal disease;[194] treatment >2 wk may require folic acid supplementation[194]
	20-50 mg/kg PO q12h × 3-5 days/wk; repeat treatment[194]	Passerines/repeat after 5 days to allow for prepatent period of coccidia[194]
	25 mg/kg PO q12h × 5 days[321]	Most species
	25-50 mg/kg PO q24h × 3 days[333]	Raptors
	25-50 mg/kg PO q24h × 3 days, off 2 days, then q24h × 3 days[358]	Raptors
	25-55 mg/kg PO q24h × 3-7 days[652]	Raptors/*Eimeria, Sarcocystis*
	50 mg/kg PO once, then 25 mg/kg PO q24h × 7-10 days[358]	Raptors
	50 mg/kg PO q24h × 5 days, off 3 days, on 5 days[808]	Psittacines
	50 mg/kg PO q24h × 14 days[482]	Cranes/coccidiosis
	250 mg/kg IM q24h × 3 days, off 2 days, on 3 days[105]	Pigeons/PK, PD; close to toxic level
	250-500 mg/L drinking water × 5-7 days/week; repeat treatment[194]	Passerines/repeat after 5 days to allow for coccidial prepatent period[194]
	330-400 mg/L drinking water × 1 day then 200 mg/L × 4 days[321]	Pigeons/supplement with vitamin B for 5 days
Sulfadimidine sodium (33.3%)	—	Contraindicated with dehydration, liver disease, renal disease;[194] treatment >2 wk may require folic acid supplementation[194]
	40-50 mg/kg PO q24h × 7 days or 3 days on, 2 days off[135]	Pigeons
	50-150 mg/kg PO, IM q12h × 3-5 days/wk; repeat treatment[194]	Passerines/repeat after 5 days to allow for coccidial prepatent period[194]
	50-150 mg/kg PO, IM q24h × 5-7 days[333]	Raptors/coccidia; lack of efficacy reported in merlins[333]
	3300-6600 mg/L drinking water × 5 days[194]	Passerines/repeat after 5 days to allow for coccidial prepatent period[194]
	3330-6660 mg/L drinking water × 3-5 days on, 2 days off repeated twice[38]	Pigeons/coccidia; may be effective against *Toxoplasma*

TABLE 5-4 Antiparasitic Agents Used in Birds. (cont'd)

Agent	Dosage	Species/Comments
Sulfamethazine (Sulmet, Boehringer-Ingelheim)	—	See sulfonamides; coccidiostat; contraindicated with dehydration, liver disease, renal disease;[194] treatment >2 wk may require folic acid supplementation[194]
	50-65 mg/pigeon PO × 3 days, off 2-3 days, repeat × 2-3 days[426]	Pigeons
	50-65 mg/pigeon PO × 5 days[321,426]	Pigeons/supplement vitamin B for 5 days[321]
	75 mg/kg PO q24h × 3 days, off 2 days, on 3 days[333]	Parakeets
	75-185 mg/kg PO q24h × 3 days[194]	Passerines/repeat after 5 days to allow for prepatent period[194]
	125 mg/L drinking water × 3 days, off 2 days, on 3 days[333]	Most species
	400 mg/L drinking water once, then 200-270 mg/L × 4 days[321]	Pigeons
Sulfaquinoxaline (Sulquin 6-50, Zoetis)	—	Sulfonamide used for prevention and treatment of coccidiosis; contraindicated with dehydration, liver disease, renal disease;[194] treatment >2 wk may require folic acid supplementation[194]
	100 mg/kg PO q24h × 3 days, off 2 days, on 3 days[194,333]	Lories, pigeons, passerines
	250 mg/L drinking water × 5-7 days[194]	Passerines/repeat after 5 days to allow for prepatent period of coccidia
	500 mg/L (1.8 mL/L) drinking water × 6 days, off 2 days, on 6 days[686]	Pigeons
Sulfonamides	—	Competitvely inhibit para-aminobenzoic acid, required by schizonts for folic acid synthesis;[426] contraindicated with dehydration, liver disease, or bone marrow suppression; gastrointestinal upset, regurgitation are common, especially in macaws; use for longer than 2 wk may require vitamin B (folic acid) supplementation
Tetracycline (T)/ furaltadone (F)	400 mg (T) + 400 mg (F)/L drinking water for 7 days	Pigeons/indicated for trichomoniasis, hexamitiasis; avoid in adults feeding young less than 10 days of age
Thiabendazole	—	Most species/nematodes (especially *Syngamus trachea*), acanthocephalans; generally less efficacious than fenbendazole; may be toxic to cranes and ratites[38]
	40-100 mg/kg PO q24h × 7 days[38,194,333]	Most species

Continued

TABLE 5-4 Antiparasitic Agents Used in Birds. (cont'd)

Agent	Dosage	Species/Comments
Thiabendazole (cont'd)	50 mg/kg PO, repeat in 14 days[333]	Ostriches
	100 mg/kg PO once, repeat in 10-14 days[38,333,482]	Raptors, cranes/intestinal strongyles, ascarids
	100 mg/kg PO q24h × 7-10 days[333]	Most species/gapeworms, ascarids
	100-200 mg/kg PO q12h × 10 days[149a]	Raptors/nematodes; may interfere with egg laying
	100-500 mg/kg PO once[38,194,333]	Most species
	250-500 mg/kg PO, repeat in 10-14 days[38,808]	Most species, including psittacines/ascarids
	425 mg/kg feed × 14 days[120]	Cranes
Toltrazuril (Baycox, Bayer)	—	Coccidiocidal;[426] efficacious for refractory coccidiosis; has been successful in reducing mortality from *Atoxoplasma* in canaries and other passerines and may affect systemic stages of the disease;[562] not very effective against *Atoxoplasma* when given in water; bitter taste, mixing with soft drink (i.e., cola) increases palatability;[38] 2.5% solution is very alkaline and should not be gavaged directly into the crop[426]
	7 mg/kg PO q24h × 2-3 days[350,384]	Budgerigars, raptors
	7-15 mg/kg q24h × 3 days[194]	Passerines/*Atoxoplasmosis*
	10 mg/kg PO q24h × 2 days[652]	Raptors/preferred treatment for *Caryospora*
	10 mg/kg PO q48h × 3 treatments[38]	Raptors/treatment of choice for coccidiosis in falcons
	12.5 mg/kg PO q24h × 14 days[562,747]	Passerines including Bali mynahs/*Atoxoplasma*; dosage is based on a limited number of clinical cases
	12.5 mg/kg PO q24h × 2 days, off 5 days, repeat prn[368]	Blue-crowned laughing thrush/PD; reduced clinical signs and all intestinal stages of *Isospora* spp. within 7 days, white blood cell effects within 3 mo
	12.5 mg/kg PO q24h × 2 days in hand-feeding, then 45 mg/L drinking water × 2 days, repeat prn[509]	Cirl buntings/PD; reduced intestinal stages of *Isospora* spp., 72/75 affected birds released
	15-25 mg/kg PO q24h × 2 days[38,432b]	Raptors
	15-25 mg/kg PO q48h × 3 treatments[432b]	Raptors
	20-35 mg/kg PO once[194,827a]	Pigeons/higher dose prevents shedding up to 4 wk; lower dose is minimum dose required to suppress oocyst shedding

TABLE 5-4 Antiparasitic Agents Used in Birds. (cont'd)

Agent	Dosage	Species/Comments
Toltrazuril (Baycox, Bayer) (cont'd)	25 mg/kg q24h × 2 days[486]	Pigeons/PD; not effective against *S. chalchasi* when administered on day 0, 10, or 40 postinoculation
	25 mg/kg PO q7d × 3 treatments[135,256]	Raptors/*Caryospora*, coccidiosis
	2 mg/L drinking water × 2 consecutive days/wk[148]	Psittacines
	5 mg/L drinking water × 2 days, repeat in 14-21 days[463]	Lories/10 mg/L administered during second course of treatment
	20 mg/kg in drinking water × 2 days[426]	Pigeons
	25 mg/L drinking water × 2 days, repeat in 14-21 days[463]	Cockatiels, passerines, including goldfinches, manikins, siskins/coccidia
	25-75 mg/L drinking water × 5 days[194]	Canaries/*Atoxoplasma* spp.
	75 mg/L drinking water × 2 days/wk × 4 wk[171]	Passerines
	75 mg/L drinking water × 5 days[323]	Pigeons
	125 mg/L drinking water × 5 days[38]	Pigeons
Trimethoprim/sulfadiazine	—	See sulfonamides
	5 mg/kg IM q12h[333]	Companion birds/*Sarcocystis*; use in conjunction with pyrimethamine (0.5-1 mg/kg PO q12h × 2 days, then 0.25 mg/kg PO q12h × 30 days)
	30 mg/kg PO q8-12h[78,358]	Most species, including psittacines, raptors/*Sarcocystis* (treat for at least 6 wk); coccidia
	30-100 mg/kg PO q12h × 7 days[333]	Companion birds/*Sarcocystis*; use in conjunction with pyrimethamine (0.5-1 mg/kg PO q12h × 2 days, then 0.25 mg/kg PO q12h × 30 days)
	60 mg/kg PO, SC q12h × 3 days, off 2 days, on 3 days[38]	Raptors/coccidia
	80 mg (trimethoprim) + 40 mg (sulfadiazine)/mL drinking water[854]	Canaries/*Toxoplasma gondii*
Trimethoprim/sulfamethoxazole	10-50 mg/kg q24h[747]	Passerines
	16-24 mg/kg (based on trimethoprim) PO q12-24h[482]	Cranes/coccidiosis
	25 mg/kg PO q24h[333]	Toucans, mynahs/coccidia
	30 mg/kg PO q12-24h[135]	Passerines/antiprotozoal
	480 mg/L drinking water q24h[135]	Pigeons/antiprotozoal

[a]Because adult penguins regurgitate food to chicks, usage of these regimens must be considered carefully during chick rearing.

TABLE 5-5 Chemical Restraint/Anesthetic/Analgesic Agents Used in Birds.[a,b]

Agent	Dosage	Species/Comments
Acepromazine	—	Phenothiazine tranquilizer; see etorphine and ketamine for combinations
	0.1-0.2 mg/kg IV[333]	Ratites/most commonly used in combination with other anesthetics; rarely used in other bird species
	0.25-0.5 mg/kg IM[333]	
Alfaxalone (Alfaxan, Jurox)	—	Not to be confused with dosing information for alfaxalone/alfadalone (Saffan, Schering-Plough); this is a completely new formulation, so doses cannot be extrapolated from older literature using alfaxalone/alfadalone; see dexmedetomidine for combination
	2 mg/kg IV[831]	Flamingos/induction; induction significantly shorter and quality smoother than with isoflurane alone; decreased isoflurane maintenance requirements but produced moderate cardiorespiratory effects not seen in isoflurane-only group; recovery times similar with both groups, without significant differences in quality or length
	10 mg/kg IM[847]	Quaker parrots/lower dose significantly longer induction time (13.5 ± 4.5 min) compared to higher dose (6.0 ± 1.3 min), while recovery time significantly longer in the high-dose group (86.2 ± 13.4 min) than the low-dose group (44.4 ±10.8 min); muscle tremors and hyperexcitation evident in both groups
	25 mg/kg IM[847]	
	20 mg/kg IM[579]	Yellow legged gulls/loss of righting reflex only achieved in 1/6 birds after 20 min; could not intubate; some birds manifested adverse effects like muscle twitches, wing and tail flapping, and opisthotonus
Alfaxalone (A)/fentanyl (F)	(A) 20 mg/kg + (F) 20 μg/kg IM[579]	Yellow legged gulls/loss of righting reflex only achieved in 2/6 birds after 12.5 min; could not intubate; significant reduction in respiratory rate; some birds manifested adverse effects like muscle twitches, wing and tail flapping, and opisthotonus
Alfaxalone (A)/fentanyl (F)/ midazolam (Mi)	(A) 20 mg/kg + (F) 20 μg/kg + (Mi) 1 mg/kg IM[579]	Yellow legged gulls/loss of righting reflex achieved in 6/6 birds after 20 min; could not intubate; significant heart rate and respiratory rate reduction; a number of birds manifested adverse effects like muscle twitches, wings and tail flapping, and opisthotonus

TABLE 5-5 Chemical Restraint/Anesthetic/Analgesic Agents Used in Birds. (cont'd)

Agent	Dosage	Species/Comments
Alfaxalone (A)/ midazolam (Mi)	(A) 10 mg/kg + (Mi) 1 mg/kg IM[847]	Quaker parrots/lower induction time than same dose (A) alone (6.5 ± 2.9 min) but significantly longer recovery time (103.5 ± 15.1 min); reduced muscle tremors and hyperexcitability
	(A) 20 mg/kg + (Mi) 1 mg/kg IM[579]	Yellow legged gulls/loss of righting reflex in 5/6 birds after 8 min; a number of birds manifested adverse effects like muscle twitches, wings and tail flapping, and opisthotonus
Alphachloralose (Fisher Scientific)	—	Chloral derivative of glucose which depresses cortical centers of the brain; induces hypothermia; low therapeutic index in chickens suggests only marginally safe in domestic species or for field applications where dosage difficult to control[333]
	250-430 mg/cup of bait[333]	Cranes, American crows/immobilization; 160-210 mg/4.5 kg sandhill crane; cranes could generally be approached within 1-2 hr of feeding and releasable 8-22 hr later
Atipamezole (Antisedan, Zoetis)	—	α_2-adrenergic antagonist; 1:1 volume reversal of dexmedetomidine is general rule; although the same effect is expected as with medetomidine (no longer available)[799]
	2.5-5 × medetomidine dose IM, IV[711,713]	Psittacines, pigeons, raptors/righting reflex regained 2-10 min after administration
	0.25-0.5 mg/kg IM[333,355,618,711,713]	Most species, including psittacines, pigeons
	0.4 mg/kg ½ IV, ½ SC[435]	Ostriches
	6 mg/kg intranasally[829]	Ring-necked parakeets/dose divided evenly between nares and given slowly; significantly reduced recumbency time after detomidine administration
Atropine sulfate	—	Anticholinergic agent
	0.01-0.02 mg/kg SC, IM, IV[333]	Most species/preanesthetic
	0.04-0.1 mg/kg SC, IM, IV, IO, intratracheal[333]	Most species/bradycardia; higher doses with CPR
Azaperone (Stresnil, Elanco)	—	Butyrophenone neuroleptic agent; see metomidate for combination; not available in the United States
	0.73 mg/kg IM[806]	Ratites/sedation
	1-4 mg/kg IM, IV[333]	Ostriches/premedication, sedation
Benzocaine	Topical anesthesia[333]	Small birds/minor wound repair

Continued

TABLE 5-5 Chemical Restraint/Anesthetic/Analgesic Agents Used in Birds. (cont'd)

Agent	Dosage	Species/Comments
Bupivacaine HCl	—	Local anesthetic agent; 4-6 hr duration of action in mammals; may be shorter acting in some birds; recommend minimizing dose to limit potential toxic effects; see bupivacaine combination[333]
	2 mg/kg infused SC[333]	
Buprenorphine HCl	—	Partial μ-opioid agonist[c]
	0.1 mg/kg IM[588]	African grey parrots/PD; ineffective for analgesia
	0.1-0.6 mg/kg IM[128,300]	American kestrels/PK, PD; resulted in thermal antinociception for ≥6 hr
	0.25 mg/kg IM q7h[589]	African grey parrots/PD; dose required to reach human analgesic plasma concentrations; analgesic effect not evaluated at this dose
	0.25 mg/kg IM[505]	Red-tailed hawks/PD; did not change any scored pain behaviors
	0.25-0.5 mg/kg IM[270]	Pigeons/PD; dose-dependent increased withdrawal time from noxious stimulus for 2-5 hr
Buprenorphine (Simbadol, Zoetis)		Concentrated formulation; not to be confused with compounded sustained-release product, as dosing may differ
	0.3 mg/kg SC q24h[332b]	Red-tailed hawks/PK; plasma concentrations of >1 ng/mL were maintained for these time periods
	1.8 mg/kg SC q48h[332b]	
Buprenorphine sustained release (Bup-SR, ZooPharm)		Compounded sustained-release product; not to be confused with concentrated formulation, as dosing may differ
	1.8 mg/kg SC, IM q24h[709]	American kestrels/PK, PD; thermal anti-nociceptive response for 12-24 hr
Butorphanol tartrate	—	Opioid agonist-antagonist;[c] PO bioavailability <10% in Hispaniolan Amazon parrots; PO route not recommended;[707] butorphanol combination follows; see dexmedetomidine, ketamine, and xylazine for combinations
	0.05-0.25 mg/kg IV[806]	Ratites
	0.5 mg/kg IM, IV q1-4h[663]	Raptors/PK: $t_{1/2}$ IM, IV very short (approx. 1-2 hr); more rapid clearance and shorter $t_{1/2}$ when given IV medial metatarsal vein than IV median ulnar vein
	0.5-4 mg/kg IM, IV q1-4h[162,270,410,588,663,707,746]	Most species, including psittacines/no isoflurane-sparing effects detected in harlequin ducks when administered IM 15 min prior to induction[533]

TABLE 5-5 Chemical Restraint/Anesthetic/Analgesic Agents Used in Birds. (cont'd)

Agent	Dosage	Species/Comments
Butorphanol tartrate (cont'd)	1-2 mg/kg IM[161,162]	African grey parrots, cockatoos, blue-fronted Amazon parrots/PD; significantly reduced ED_{50} of isoflurane for African greys and cockatoos but not for Amazon parrots; African grey parrots had more significant reduction of withdrawal response to electrical stimulus at 2 mg/kg
	1-6 mg/kg IM[303a]	American kestrels/PD; did not cause thermal antinociception suggestive of analgesia; sex-dependent responses were identified
	2-5 mg/kg IM, IV q2-3h[410,707,746]	Hispaniolan Amazon parrots/PK; low mean plasma concentrations at 2 hr postinjection; PD: withdrawal from electrical stimuli reduced after 2 mg/kg IM; effective pre-emptive analgesia with sevoflurane anesthesia for endoscopy[410]
	3 mg/kg (premedication) + 75 µg/kg/min IV CRI (maintenance)[453]	Psittacines/PD; significantly reduced isoflurane MAC
	3-6 mg/kg IM[588]	Hispaniolan Amazon parrots/PD; electrical stimuli to assess withdrawal thresholds
Butorphanol (B)/ midazolam (Mi)	(B) 1 mg/kg IM + (Mi) 0.5 mg/kg IM[429]	Psittacines/induction time and isoflurane concentration were reduced in the B + Mi group; induction quality scores were improved in the B + Mi group and no adverse effects on anesthesia and cardiovascular stability were observed
Carfentanil (Wildnil, Wildlife Pharmaceuticals)	—	Super-potent opioid agonist;[c] carfentanil combination follows; not generally recommended for use in birds; no longer commercially available in the United States
	0.024 mg/kg IM[333]	Ostriches (free-ranging)/darted from helicopter
	0.03 mg/kg IM[333]	Ratites
Carfentanil (C)/xylazine (X)	(C) 3 mg + (X) 150 mg IM per ostrich[630]	Ostriches (free-ranging)/darted from helicopter
Desflurane (Suprane, Baxter)	—	Fluorine halogenated ether; fast induction, rapid recovery;[337] currently no studies evaluating its use in any avian species
Detomidine (Dormosedan, Zoetis)	—	α_2-adrenergic agonist
	12 mg/kg intranasally[829]	Ring-necked parakeets/dose divided into each nare and given slowly; sedation <3 min but did not allow dorsal recumbency or manipulation; reversal with atipamezole significantly reduced time to recovery

Continued

TABLE 5-5 Chemical Restraint/Anesthetic/Analgesic Agents Used in Birds. (cont'd)

Agent	Dosage	Species/Comments
Detomidine (Dormosedan, Zoetis) (cont'd)	12-15 mg intranasally[830]	Canaries/dose divided into each nare and given slowly; higher dose prolonged sedation but could not place in dorsal recumbency; prolonged duration of effect (257.5 ± 1.5 min); completely reversed with yohimbine intranasally
Dexmedetomidine HCl (Dexdomitor, Zoetis)	—	α_2 agonist; active optical enantiomer of racemic compound medetomidine; ½ the dose of medetomidine but same volume due to concentration has been used as a general guideline;[d] although the same effects would be expected as with medetomidine (not commercially available, but can be compounded); limited data on the efficacy and safety of dexmedetomidine in birds to date; dexmedetomidine combinations follow
	25 μg/kg IM[713]	Common buzzards/adequate restraint to prevent reaction to handling but did not allow for intubation; loss of righting reflex = 3.5 ± 1 min; no arrhythmias, excitement, or major adverse effects noted; complete reversal with atipamezole
	75 μg/kg IM[713]	Common kestrels/adequate restraint to prevent reaction to handling but did not allow for intubation; loss of righting reflex = 7 ± 1.2 min; no arrhythmias, excitement, or major adverse effects noted; complete reversal with atipamezole
Dexmedetomidine (D)/ alfaxalone (A)	(D) 0.4 mg/kg + (A) 20 mg/kg IM[872]	Domestic doves/time to loss of consciousness = 102 ± 48 sec, loss of righting reflex = 240 ± 135 sec; 2 birds could not undergo endoscopic procedure; 1 bird died due to prolonged recovery; significant variability in heart rate and respiratory rate; not recommended at these doses for minimally invasive procedures
Dexmedetomidine (D)/ midazolam (Mi)	(D) 80 μg/kg + (Mi) 5 mg/kg intranasally[355]	Pigeons/PD; effective immobilization 20 to 30 min after intranasal administration; birds tolerated postural changes without resistance; significant decreases in heart rate and respiratory rate that persisted until the end of sedation; atipamezole antagonized sedation and cardiorespiratory side effects within 10 min
Dexmedetomidine (D)/ ketamine (K)/ butorphanol (B)	(D) 0.4 mg/kg + (K) 40 mg/kg + (B) 1 mg/kg IM[872]	Domestic doves/mean time to loss of consciousness and loss of righting reflex was 79.6 ± 44.4 sec and 162.6 ± 102.3 sec, respectively; all birds experienced a prolonged recovery period (>1 hr); significant variability in heart rate and respiratory rate; not recommended at these doses for minimally invasive procedures

TABLE 5-5	Chemical Restraint/Anesthetic/Analgesic Agents Used in Birds. (cont'd)	
Agent	Dosage	Species/Comments
Dexmedetomidine (D)/ thiafentanil oxalate (Th)/ tiletamine-zolazepam (Tz)	—	Ultra-short-acting opioid agonist (Th) not currently available in the United States; α_2 agonist (D); dissociative anesthetic (Tz)
	(D) 0.2 mg +(Th) 7 mg +(Tz) 100 mg IM per bird[798]	Greater rheas/anesthesia administered via remote injection; smooth induction/ recovery; respiratory depression in 1/8 birds but recovered with reversal
Diazepam	—	Benzodiazepine; used alone for sedation, seizure control, tranquilization, and/or appetite stimulation; IM administration may cause severe muscle irritation and absorption may be delayed; reversal with flumazenil; see ketamine for combinations
	0.05-0.5 mg/kg IV[333]	Most species
	0.1-0.3 mg/kg IV[333,375]	Ratites/tranquilization; smooth anesthetic recovery
	0.2-0.5 mg/kg IM[195]	Most species/premedication; onset in 15-20 min
	0.25-0.5 mg/kg IM, IV q24h × 2-3 days[779]	Raptors/appetite stimulant
	0.5 mg/kg PO[333]	Passerines/calms fractious species while improving acceptance to a novel captive diet; oral solution (1 mg/mL, Roxane Laboratories) works best
	0.5-1 mg/kg IM, IV q8-12h[38]	Raptors/sedation; anticonvulsant
	0.8 mg/kg intranasally[25]	Ostriches (juvenile)/slower onset (4.3 ± 0.4 min) than midazolam (2.9 ± 1.2 min); moderate sedation was achieved for standing chemical restraint, with the maximum duration effect of 9.2 ± 2.5 min
	1-2 mg/kg IV[333]	Ostriches/administer just prior to recovery from teletamine/zolazepam to counter its undesirable effects
	2.5-4 mg/kg PO[333]	Most species/sedation
	5 mg/kg PO[333]	Ostriches/standing sedation
	5 mg/kg IV[262,333]	Emus, rheas/sedation
	6 mg/kg IM[812]	Rock partridges/decrease in cloacal temperature; prolonged recoveries (149 ± 8.3 min)
	10 mg/kg IM[623]	Zebra finches/deep sedation, dorsal recumbency achieved in minutes and lasted for several hours; reversed completely with flumazenil

Continued

TABLE 5-5 Chemical Restraint/Anesthetic/Analgesic Agents Used in Birds. (cont'd)

Agent	Dosage	Species/Comments
Diazepam (cont'd)	12 mg/kg intranasally[829]	Ring-necked parakeets/dose divided into each nare and given slowly; time to onset 3.5 ± 1.2 min, dorsal recumbency 11.0 ± 6.4 min; not sedate enough for any manipulation; flumazenil intranasally significantly reduced recumbency time
	12.5-15.6 mg/kg intranasally[830]	Canaries/dose divided into each nare and given slowly; dorsal recumbency for approx. 35 min; flumazenil intranasally significantly reduced recumbency time
	13 ± 1 mg/kg intranasally[80]	Finches/onset of sedation significantly slower (1.8 ± 0.2 min) compared with midazolam (1.0 ± 0.3 min); longer duration of dorsal recumbency observed after diazepam (68 ± 12.7 min) than with midazolam (32.0 ± 8.1 min); diazepam produced significantly longer duration of sedation (182.0 ± 18.4) than midazolam (74.2 ± 8.7)
	13.6 ± 1.1 mg/kg intranasally[695]	Budgerigars/onset of sedation significantly longer after diazepam (2.8 ± 0.88 min) than midazolam (1.3 ± 0.44 min); diazepam produced significantly longer duration of sedation (165.4 ± 19.2 min) than midazolam (71.6 ± 8.9 min); adequate sedation for diagnostic, minor therapeutic procedures
Diprenorphine	0.04-0.06 mg/kg IV[703]	Ostriches/opioid antagonist
Dobutamine	—	β_1-adrenergic agonist, with weak β_2 activity, and selective α_1 activity; used to treat anesthetic-induced hypotension
	15 µg/kg/min IV[718]	Hispaniolan Amazon parrots/PD; significant increase in direct arterial pressure within 4-7 min
Dopamine HCl	—	Catecholamine neurotransmitter activating dopamine receptors; inotropic vasopressor used to treat anesthetic-induced hypotension
	7-10 µg/kg/min IV[718]	Hispaniolan Amazon parrots/PD; significant increase in direct arterial pressure within 4-7 min; greater effects on direct arterial pressures than dobutamine
Etorphine HCl (M-99, Wildlife Pharmaceuticals)	—	Super-potent opioid agonist;[c] may be inadequate when used as sole agent;[375] see etorphine combinations
	0.025 mg/kg IM[333]	Ostriches
Etorphine (E)/ acepromazine (A)	(E) 0.04-0.07 mg/kg + (A) 0.19 mg/kg IM[703]	Ostriches (10-12 mo of age)
	(E) 3.6 mg/bird + (A) 15 mg/bird IM[703]	Ostriches

TABLE 5-5 Chemical Restraint/Anesthetic/Analgesic Agents Used in Birds. (cont'd)

Agent	Dosage	Species/Comments
Etorphine (E)/ acepromazine (A)/ xylazine (X)	(E) 0.04 mg/kg + (A) 0.16 mg/kg + (X) 0.66 mg/kg IM[703]	Ostriches/sedation for simple procedures lasting 10-20 min
Etorphine (E)/ketamine (K)	(E) 6-12 mg/bird IM + (K) 200-300 mg/bird IM[333]	Ostriches (adults)
Fentanyl citrate	—	Short-acting μ-opioid agonist[c]
	20 μg bolus + 0.2-0.5 μg/kg/min IV CRI[332b,593]	Red-tailed hawks/PD; reduced isoflurane MAC 31%-55% in a dose-related manner, without significant effects on heart rate, blood pressure, $paCO_2$, or paO_2
	20 μg bolus + 1.5-6 μg/kg/min IV CRI[332b]	Hispaniolan Amazon parrots/PK; PD; reduced isoflurane in a dose-related manner similar to red-tailed hawks but with much higher dosages; significant decreases in heart rate, indirect blood pressure; monitor closely
	0.02 mg/kg IM[351]	Cockatoos/PK; PD; rapid absorption, elimination; no effect withdrawal to thermal, electrical stimulus
	0.2 mg/kg SC[351]	Cockatoos/PK; PD; some analgesia; large dose and volume; hyperactivity first 15-30 min in some birds
Fentanyl (F)/midazolam (M)	(F) 30 μg bolus + (M) 1-2 mg/kg IM then (F) 30 μg/kg/h IV CRI + (M) 1 mg/kg/h IV CRI[578]	Wild birds/partial IV anesthesia (PIVA) with isoflurane anesthesia for orthopedic surgery; recovery = 63.2 ± 24.0 min with excellent quality; no significant change in HR detected
Flumazenil	—	Benzodiazepene antagonist
	0.02-0.1 mg/kg IM, IV[6,333]	Most species
	0.05 mg/kg intranasally[490]	Hispaniolan Amazon parrots
	0.13 mg/kg intranasally[829]	Ring-necked parakeets/dose divided evenly between nares and given slowly; significantly reduced recumbency time
	0.25-0.31 mg/kg intranasally[830]	Canaries/dose divided evenly between nares and given slowly; significantly reduced recumbency time
	0.3 mg/kg IM[623]	Zebra finches/smooth, complete recovery after deep sedation with diazepam
Gabapentin	—	GABA analogue; used to treat human neuropathic pain
	3 mg/kg PO q24h[745]	Senegal parrots/analgesia; used with fluoxetine so difficult to determine sole efficacy; bird appeared sedated 3 days after initiation of administration
	10 mg/kg PO q12h[193,194]	Little corella/long-term (>90 days) analgesia; sole analgesic for self-mutilation; no adverse effects noted

Continued

TABLE 5-5 Chemical Restraint/Anesthetic/Analgesic Agents Used in Birds. (cont'd)

Agent	Dosage	Species/Comments
Gabapentin (cont'd)	11 mg/kg PO q12h[734]	Prairie falcons/long-term (>90 days) analgesia; adjunct to multimodal therapy for self-mutilation; bird exhibited neurologic signs, diarrhea when dosed at 110 mg/kg, but no adverse effects at 82 mg/kg
	11 mg/kg PO q8h[864]	Great horned owls/PK; maintained plasma concentrations >2 µg/mL approx. 8 hr
	15 mg/kg PO q8h[43]	Hispaniolan Amazon parrots/PK; maintained plasma concentrations ≥ human analgesic concentration approx. 8 hr
Glycopyrrolate	—	Anticholinergic agent; slower onset than atropine
	0.01-0.02 mg/kg IM, IV[333]	Most species/preanesthetic; rarely indicated
	0.04 mg/kg IV[806]	Ratites
Hydromorphone	0.1-0.6 mg/kg IM q3-6h[303b,304]	American kestrels/PK; PD: doses of 0.1, 0.3, and 0.6 mg/kg IM significantly increased thermal foot withdrawal responses; appreciable sedation with 0.6 mg/kg
	0.1, 0.3, and 0.6 mg/kg IM[708]	Cockatiels/PD; doses did not significantly increase thermal foot withdrawal responses; 0.3 and 0.6 mg/kg produced mild sedation[708]
Isoflurane	—	Inhalant anesthetic agent of choice in birds; dose-dependent hypotension with all inhalants; raptors, macaws may be more likely to exhibit isoflurane-induced arrhythmias;[333] no significant differences in ventilation or O_2 transport between dorsal and lateral recumbency in red-tailed hawks[334]
	0.5%-4% (usually 1.5%-2%)[333]	Ostriches/use following preanesthetic medication
	1%-3%[732]	Cinereous vultures/dose-dependent increases in heart rate and $ETCO_2$ and decreases in direct blood pressure and respiratory acidosis during spontaneous ventilation
	1.115%[748]	Emus/PD; minimum anesthetic concentration
	1.3%[470,471]	Cranes, ducks/minimum anesthetic concentration
	1.46 ± 0.30%[130]	Crested serpent eagles/minimum anesthetic concentration; time-related increase in $ETCO_2$ and decreases in body temperature and respiratory rates

TABLE 5-5 Chemical Restraint/Anesthetic/Analgesic Agents Used in Birds. (cont'd)

Agent	Dosage	Species/Comments
Isoflurane (cont'd)	$1.44 \pm 0.07\%$[162]	Cockatoos/PD; ED_{50}
	$1.8 \pm 0.4\%$[93]	Pigeons/PD; minimum anesthetic concentration; dose-dependent hypercapnia, hypotension, mild hypothermia and 2nd- and 3rd-degree atrioventricular blocks
	$2.05 \pm 0.45\%$[593]	Red-tailed hawks/PD; minimum anesthetic concentration
	3%-5%[333]	Ostriches/when used without preanesthetic medication
	3%-5% induction, 1.5%-2.5% maintenance[333]	Most species
Ketamine HCl	—	Dissociative anesthetic; seldom used as sole agent because of poor muscle relaxation and prolonged (up to 3 hr), violent recovery; may produce excitation or convulsions in pigeons, gallinules, water rails, golden pheasants, Hartlaub's turacoes, ratites, and vultures;[375,705] may fail to produce general anesthesia in some species including great horned owls, snowy owls, Cooper's hawks, sharp-shinned hawks; See dexmedetomidine and etorphine for combinations; ketamine combinations follow
	5 mg/kg IV q10min prn[375]	Ratites/maintenance
	5-30 mg/kg IM, IV[38,333]	Raptors/sedation
	10-50 mg/kg SC, IM, IV[195,333]	Psittacines, pigeons, ratites, waterfowl/restraint 30-60 min; smaller species require a higher dose; large birds tend to recover more slowly
	25 mg/kg IM[333]	Emus/may need to supplement 5-9 mg/kg IV q10min
	50 mg/kg IO[393]	Pigeons/provided effective anesthesia
	50-100 mg/kg PO in bait[33,76,149a]	Raptors/sedation to catch an escaped bird; place in a 30 g piece of meat
Ketamine (K)/ acepromazine (A)	(K) 10-25 mg/kg + (A) 0.5-1 mg/kg IM[846]	Most species/high dose for birds <250 g
Ketamine (K)/diazepam (D)	(K) 2-5 mg/kg IV + (D) 0.25 mg/kg IV[333]	Ostriches/ketamine may be given 15-30 min after diazepam
	(K) 3-8 mg/kg + (D) 0.5-1 mg/kg IM[340]	Eagles, vultures
	(K) 5-30 mg/kg + (D) 0.5-2 mg/kg IV[333]	Most species/psittacines and pigeons lower end of range is preferred
	(K) 8-15 mg/kg + (D) 0.5-1 mg/kg IM[340]	Falcons

Continued

TABLE 5-5 Chemical Restraint/Anesthetic/Analgesic Agents Used in Birds. (cont'd)

Agent	Dosage	Species/Comments
Ketamine (K)/diazepam (D) (cont'd)	(K) 10 mg/kg + (D) 0.2 mg/kg IM[31]	Pigeons/rapid induction with an increase in anesthesia duration; good muscle relaxation and a smooth, slow recovery
	(K) 10 mg/kg + (D) 0.5 mg/kg IM[586]	Amazon parrots/PD; significantly reduced sevoflurane MAC
	(K) 10-40 mg/kg IV + (D) 1-1.5 mg/kg IM, IV[653]	Raptors, waterfowl/induction or surgical anesthesia (rapid bolus may produce apnea, arrhythmia, and increased risk of death)
	(K) 20-40 mg/kg IM + (D) 1-1.5 mg/kg IM[531]	Birds >250 g
	(K) 20 mg/kg + (D) 1 mg/kg IV[159]	Toucans/short procedures (15-20 min)
Ketamine (K)/butorphanol (B)/medetomidine (Me)	—	Medetomidine no longer available, but can be compounded; see dexmedetomidine
	(K) 3 mg/kg + (B) 1 mg/kg + (Me) 40 μg/kg IM[865]	Psittacines/premedication or supplement to isoflurane; reduces isoflurane requirement and improves ventilation
	(K) 50 mg + (B) 50 μg + (Me) 50 μg IM per pigeon[29]	Pigeons/PD; satisfactory anesthesia in 7/8 pigeons; heart rate, respiratory rate decreased within 10 min following Me + B injection; arrhythmias in 3/8 pigeons; cloacal temperature decreased gradually during anesthesia
Ketamine (K)/medetomidine (Me)	—	Unreliable level of sedation in pigeons at (K) 5 mg/kg + (Me) 80 μg/kg IM;[618] medetomidine not currently available, but can be compounded
	(K) 1.5-2 mg/kg + (Me) 60-85 μg/kg IM, IV[333]	Pigeons/sedation
	(K) 2 mg/kg + (Me) 80 μg/kg IM[435]	Ostriches/sedation
	(K) 2-4 mg/kg + (Me) 25-75 μg/kg IV[366]	Raptors
	(K) 2.5-7 mg/kg + (Me) 50-100 μg/kg IV[367]	Large psittacines
	(K) 3-5 mg/kg + (Me) 50-100 μg/kg IM[366]	Raptors
	(K) 3-7 mg/kg + (Me) 75-150 μg/kg IM[367]	Large psittacines
	(K) 25 mg/kg + (Me) 100 μg/kg IM[658]	Psittacines/anesthesia
Ketamine (K)/midazolam (Mi)	(K) 10-40 mg/kg + (Mi) 0.2-4 mg/kg SC, IM[194,333,531]	Most species, including psittacines
	(K) 40-50 mg/kg + (Mi) 3.65 mg/kg intranasally[829]	Ring-necked parakeets/dose divided into each nare and given slowly; onset of action <3 min, dorsal recumbency for 70.7 ± 46.7 min recovery times reduced with flumazenil intranasally

TABLE 5-5 Chemical Restraint/Anesthetic/Analgesic Agents Used in Birds. (cont'd)

Agent	Dosage	Species/Comments
Ketamine (K)/midazolam (Mi)/butorphanol (B)	(Mi) 0.2 mg/kg + (B) 0.4 mg/kg IM followed by (K) 8.7 ± 0.5 mg/kg IV[36]	Ostriches/PD; anesthesia; followed by intubation and isoflurane anesthesia
Ketamine (K)/tiletamine/zolazepam (Tz)	(K) 15 mg/kg + (Tz) 10 mg/kg IM[427]	Raptors/anesthesia
Ketamine (K)/xylazine (X)	—	Often associated with cardiac depressive effects and rough recoveries
	(K) 0.45 mg/kg + (X) 25 mg/kg IM[500]	Ostriches
	(K) 2-3 mg/kg IV + (X) 5-10 mg/kg IM[112]	Ostriches
	(K) 2-5 mg/kg IV + (X) 0.25 mg/kg IV[112]	Ostriches
	(K) 2.2-3.3 mg/kg + (X) 2.2 mg/kg IM[375]	Ratites/administer xylazine 10-15 min before ketamine
	(K) 4.4 mg/kg + (X) 2.2 mg/kg IV[358,440]	Psittacines, raptors
	(K) 5 mg/kg + (X) 1 mg/kg IM[85]	Ostriches
	(K) 8 mg/kg IV + (X) 4 mg/kg IM[15]	Ostriches/ketamine administered 20 min after xylazine; as an adjunct to isoflurane anesthesia produced sufficient surgical plane of anesthesia
	(K) 10 mg/kg + (X) 0.5-1 mg/kg IM[14,503]	Ratites, turkey vultures
	(K) 10-15 mg/kg + (X) 2 mg/kg IM[531]	Owls
	(K) 10-30 mg/kg + (X) 2-6 mg/kg IM[531]	Psittacines/birds <250 g require dose at higher end of range
	(K) 20 mg/kg + (X) 1-2 mg/kg IV slow bolus[159]	Toucans
	(K) 25 mg/kg + (X) 2.5 mg/kg IM[531]	Cockatiels
	(K) 25-30 mg/kg + (X) 2 mg/kg IM[531]	Falcons, hawks
	(K) 30 mg/kg + (X) 6.5 mg/kg IM[531]	Budgerigars
	(K) 40-50 mg/kg + (X) 10 mg/kg intranasally[829]	Ring-necked parakeets/dose divided evenly between nares and given slowly; time to sedation, 7.7 ± 1.4 min; dorsal recumbency, 12.2 ± 14.1 min; yohimbine IM shortened recovery
Ketamine (K)/xylazine (X)/acepromazine (A)	(K) 34 mg/kg + (X) 0.2 mg/kg + (A) 0.1 mg/kg IM[375]	Ostriches
Lidocaine	—	Local anesthetic agent with a duration of action in mammals of 90-200 min;[152] previous reports state that the dose of lidocaine used in birds should be ≤3.3 mg kg;[333] a recent study in chickens showed 6 mg/kg IV was not associated with adverse cardiovascular effects[100]

Continued

TABLE 5-5 Chemical Restraint/Anesthetic/Analgesic Agents Used in Birds. (cont'd)

Agent	Dosage	Species/Comments
Lidocaine (cont'd)	1-3 mg/kg[333]	Most species
	1 mg/kg perineurally each nerve[208]	Raptors/sciatic-femoral nerve block under inhalant anesthesia
	2 mg/kg perineurally[167]	Hispaniolan Amazon parrots/brachial plexus block via palpation or ultrasound-guided; onset of block tended to be faster when ultrasonography was used but neither technique produced an effective block
Medetomidine[d] (Domitor, Pfizer)	—	No longer commercially available; can be compounded; dosages listed here as a general guide for possible dexmedetomidine dosing; α_2-adrenergic agonist; 80-2000 μg/kg IM was associated with inadequate sedation in the pigeon;[618,711] 100 μg/kg IM did not immobilize ostrich chicks;[824] see ketamine and thiafentanil for combinations; see dexmedetomidine for more details
	60-85 μg/kg IM[4]	Psittacines
	150-350 μg/kg IM[39]	Raptors
Meperidine HCl	—	Short-acting opioid agonist[c]
	1-4 mg/kg IM[667,806]	Most species, including ratites (at 1 mg/kg)/sedation; analgesia
Midazolam HCl	—	Benzodiazepine; shorter acting than diazepam, water soluble; see butorphanol, dexmedetomidine, and ketamine for combinations
	0.1-2 mg/kg IM, IV[6]	Most species/premedication at lower doses, onset approx. 15 min when administered IM
	0.15 mg/kg IV[375]	Ostriches/rapid sternal recumbency in adults
	0.2 mg/kg SC, IM[38]	Psittacines/for use in combination with ketamine
	0.3-0.4 mg/kg IM[375,503]	Ostriches, emus/premedication; sedation of adult emus
	0.4 mg/kg intranasally[25]	Ostrich (juvenile)/significantly shorter onset time (2.9 ± 1.2 min) compared with diazepam (4.3 ± 0.4 min) with longer duration of sedation; moderate sedation for standing chemical restraint, with maximum duration effects of 7.0 ± 1.4 min; deep sedation achieved with 0.8 mg/kg intranasally with sternal recumbency for 21.7 ± 4.9 min
	0.4 mg/kg IV[375]	Emus

TABLE 5-5 Chemical Restraint/Anesthetic/Analgesic Agents Used in Birds. (cont'd)

Agent	Dosage	Species/Comments
Midazolam HCl (cont'd)	0.5-1 mg/kg IM, IV q8h[38]	Raptors/anticonvulsant
	2 mg/kg intranasally[491]	Hispaniolan Amazon parrots/mild to moderate sedation in 3 min; reduced vocalizations, struggling and defensive behaviors for 15 min; reversed with flumazenil intranasally
	2 mg/kg IM[814]	Canada geese/sedation for 15-20 min
	5 mg/kg intranasally[355]	Pigeons/PD; minimal side effects on vital functions but caused inadequate immobilization of pigeons for restraint in dorsal recumbency
	2 mg/kg intranasally[714b]	Wild macaws/PD; provided approximately 20 min of sedation in 80% of macaws
	7.3-8.8 mg/kg intranasally[829,830]	Ring-necked parakeets/dose divided into each nare and given slowly; time to onset, 3 min; dorsal recumbency, 57.7 ± 24.4 min; flumazenil intranasally significantly reduced recovery time
	12.5-15.6 mg/kg intranasally[830]	Canaries/dose divided into each nare and given slowly; time to onset, <3 min; dorsal recumbency, 17.1 ± 5 min; flumazenil intranasally significantly reduced recovery time
	13 ± 1 mg/kg intranasally[80]	Finches/time to onset of sedation significantly faster (1.0 ± 0.3 min) than xylazine or diazepam; shorter duration of dorsal recumbency observed (32.00 ± 8.09 min) compared with diazepam (68.2 ± 12.7 min); significantly shorter duration of sedation (74.2 ± 8.7 min) than diazepam (182.00 ± 18.37 min) and xylazine (360.2 ± 41.31 min); no complications noted
	13.2 ± 1.3 mg/kg intranasally[695]	Budgerigars/time to onset of sedation significantly shorter (1.3 ± 0.44 min) than xylazine (2.6 ± 0.89 min) and diazepam (2.8 ± 0.88 min); sedation significantly shorter (71.60 ± 8.9 min) than with xylazine and diazepam; adequate sedation for diagnostic and minor therapeutic procedures
Morphine sulfate	—	Opioid agonist;[c] early work in chickens demonstrated confusing clinical dosage results
Nalbuphine HCl	—	Opioid partial κ-agonist and partial μ-antagonist;[c] due to its low abuse potential, this opioid is currently not a DEA scheduled substance at the time of writing

Continued

TABLE 5-5 Chemical Restraint/Anesthetic/Analgesic Agents Used in Birds. (cont'd)

Agent	Dosage	Species/Comments
Nalbuphine HCl (cont'd)	12.5 mg/kg IM q2-3h[397,710a]	Hispaniolan Amazon parrots/PK; PD; excellent IM bioavailability; little sedation and no adverse effects; rapidly cleared after IM and IV dosing; thermal foot withdrawal threshold values increased ≥3 hr; higher dosages (25, 50 mg/kg IM) did not significantly increase withdrawal values
Naloxone HCl	—	Opioid antagonist; shorter acting than naltrexone
	0.01 mg/kg IV[36]	Ostriches
	2 mg IV q14-21h[333]	Most species, including psittacines
Naltrexone HCl	—	Opioid antagonist; longer acting than naloxone
	300-330 mg IM, IV[396,500,630]	Ostriches/opioid antagonist
Nitrous oxide	—	Sufficient oxygen must be provided to avoid hypoxic mixtures; may cause some cardiovascular depression;[337] do not use in birds with normal subcutaneous air pockets (e.g., pelicans, hornbills) or in birds with marginal respiratory reserves[6,337]
Nitrous oxide (N)/ isoflurane (I)/ vecuronium (V)	(N) 0.3 L/kg/min of oxygen and (1:1, min 33% O_2) + (I) 1-2.4% + (V) 0.2 mg/kg IV[416,418a]	Most species/mydriasis and anesthesia; gases are administered via air sac cannulation; vecuronium effective up to 256 min in pigeons
Pentobarbital sodium	—	Short-acting barbiturate; see Table 5-17 for other indications
	13.3 mg/kg IV[500]	Emus/premedicate with diazepam
Propofol	—	IV sedative-hypnotic agent; intubation, ventilation, and supplemental oxygen is strongly recommended[479,723]
	1-5 mg/kg IV[195]	Many species/give slowly for induction to minimize apnea; intubation and IPPV required
	1.33 mg/kg IV[38,358]	Psittacines, raptors
	2.9-4.7 mg/kg IV (induction); 0.4-0.55 mg/kg/min IV (maintenance)[335]	Red-tailed hawks, great horned owls/PK; PD; minimal blood pressure effects, but ventilation significantly reduced; prolonged recoveries with moderate-to-severe excitatory CNS signs may occur in these species at these doses
	3 mg/kg IV (induction); 0.2 mg/kg/min IV (maintenance)[435]	Ostriches/PD; anesthesia
	3.7 mg/kg IV (induction); 0.3 mg/kg/min IV (maintenance)[79]	King penguins/rapid and smooth induction and calm recovery

TABLE 5-5 Chemical Restraint/Anesthetic/Analgesic Agents Used in Birds. (cont'd)

Agent	Dosage	Species/Comments
Propofol (cont'd)	4 mg/kg IV (induction); 0.5 mg/kg/min IV (maintenance)[488]	Barn owls/anesthesia
	5 mg/kg IV (induction); 0.5 mg/kg/min IV (maintenance)[723]	Wild turkeys/PD; anesthesia
	5 mg/kg IV (induction); 1 mg/kg/min IV (maintenance)[437]	Hispaniolan Amazon parrots/PD; recovery times (15.4 ± 15.2 min) were prolonged when compared with isoflurane; 6/10 birds had agitated recoveries; light anesthetic plane in 8/10 birds
	14 mg/kg IV[235,358]	Pigeons, raptors/anesthesia; 2-7 min duration; severe respiratory depression and apnea documented in pigeons
Sevoflurane	2.35%[605]	Thick-billed parrots/PD; minimum anesthetic concentration when using mechanical stimulation; minimum anesthetic concentration was much higher (4.24%) when using electrical stimulus
	3 ± 0.6%[94]	Pigeons/PD; minimum anesthetic concentration; SAP decreased significantly, $PECO_2$ increased significantly despite an increase in respiratory rate; sinus arrhythmias were detected in 2 birds; time to tracheal intubation and recovery were 2.5 ± 0.7 and 6.4 ± 1.7 min, respectively; recovery was rapid and uneventful in all birds
	6% induction; 3.5% maintenance[219]	Crested caracara/PD; smooth induction/recovery; reduced respiratory rate and arterial blood pressures
	Incremental increases up to 7% prn (induction)[410,627]	Psittacines/anesthesia; similar to isoflurane; provides more rapid recovery; less incidence of ataxia during recovery[337,416,627]
Thiafentanil oxalate (T)/medetomidine (Me)	—	Ultra-short-acting opioid agonist[c] (T); α_2 agonist (Me); neither drug currently available in the United States
	(T) 0.175 mg/kg + (Me) 0.092 mg/kg IM[163]	Emus (adults)/anesthesia via remote injection; rapid induction (6.8 min) and recovery (3.2 min)
Tiletamine/zolaze-pam (Telazol, Zoetis)	—	Dissociative anesthetic associated with prolonged, rough recoveries; see dexmedetomidine and ketamine for combinations; tiletamine/zolazepam combinations follow

Continued

TABLE 5-5 Chemical Restraint/Anesthetic/Analgesic Agents Used in Birds. (cont'd)

Agent	Dosage	Species/Comments
Tiletamine/zolaze-pam (Telazol, Zoetis) (cont'd)	1-8 mg/kg IV[375,531]	Ratites (adults)/induction and/or short procedures
	2-12 mg/kg IM[455,770]	Ratites (adults)/induction and/or short procedures;[263] recommend 3-5 mg/kg IM for captive birds and 5 mg/kg IM for free-ranging birds
	4-25 mg/kg IM[149a,719,824]	Most species, including psittacines, raptors, ostriches, flamingos/sedation
	5-10 mg/kg IM[38,76,358,396,427,440,441]	Ostrich (chicks), raptors, psittacines/good immobilization
	9-30 mg/kg IM[719]	Owls, wood partridges/restraint
	10 mg/kg IM[427,719]	Raptors
	15-22 mg/kg IM[531,719]	Budgerigars, emus
	40-80 mg/kg PO[149a]	Raptors
	80 mg/kg in feed[370,870]	Eurasian buzzards/sufficient in most birds to allow safe handling after 30-60 min; birds receiving drug in powder form reached a deeper plane of anesthesia more quickly
Tiletamine-zolazepam (Tz) thiafentanil oxalate (Th)/ dexmedetomidine (D	—	Ultra-short-acting opioid agonist[c] (Th) not currently available in the United States; α_2 agonist (D); dissociative anesthetic (Tz)
	(Th) 7 mg + (D) 0.2 mg + (Tz) 100 mg IM per bird[799]	Greater rheas/anesthesia administered via remote injection, smooth induction/recovery; respiratory depression in 1/8 birds but recovered when reversed
Tolazoline HCl (Tolazine, Akorn)	—	α_2-adrenergic antagonist
	1 mg/kg IV[396]	Ostriches
	15 mg/kg IV[14]	Turkey vultures
Tramadol HCl	—	Synthetic analog of codeine with opioid, α-adrenergic, and serotonergic receptor activity; O-desmethyltramadol (M1) metabolite is more potent μ-opiate agonist in mammals
	5 mg/kg PO, IV q12h[755a,756]	Bald eagles/PK; similar plasma concentrations to humans for analgesia but analgesia not evaluated; PO bioavailability in bald eagles higher than in humans, dogs;[756] sedation evident after multiple dosing; monitor for sedation and reduce dose and/or frequency prn
	5 mg/kg PO q2-9h[303c]	American kestrels/PD

TABLE 5-5 Chemical Restraint/Anesthetic/Analgesic Agents Used in Birds. (cont'd)

Agent	Dosage	Species/Comments
Tramadol HCl (cont'd)	8-11 mg/kg PO q12h[755a,757]	Red-tailed hawks/PK; only 3 birds; 15 mg/kg PO q12h data model suggested more frequent dosing to achieve human analgesic plasma tramadol concentrations; analgesia not evaluated;[755a] birds sedated after multiple dosing; monitor for sedation and reduce dose and/or frequency prn[755a]
	10 mg/kg PO q24h[403b]	African penguins/PK: maintained plasma concentrations for 24 hr
	30 mg/kg PO q6h[710b,755b]	Hispaniolan Amazon parrots/PK; PD; similar plasma concentrations to humans for analgesia; effectively reduced thermal withdrawal response for 6 hr
Xylazine	—	α_2-adrenergic agonist; not recommended by itself for tranquilization and seldom used in pet birds due to adverse effects—excitement, convulsions, bradycardia, arrhythmias, bradypnea, hypoxemia, hypercarbia, and death when used alone; reversible with yohimbine, atipamezole; most useful in ratites;[705] see carfentanil, etorphine, and ketamine for combinations
	0.2-1 mg/kg IM[375,630]	Ratites/calming sedation
	1-2.2 mg/kg IM, IV[38]	Raptors, psittacines/in combination with ketamine (1:3 or 1:5); still widely used in raptors in some countries
	1-20 mg/kg IM, IV[358]	Raptors/sedation
	20 mg intranasally[829]	Ring-necked parakeets/time to onset, 7.9 ± 2.8 min but sedation not adequate for manipulation; reversed with yohimbine intranasally
	24-30 mg intranasally[830]	Canaries/heavy sedation; prolonged sedation but could not place in dorsal recumbency at either dose; reversed with yohimbine intranasally
	25.6 ± 2.2 mg/kg intranasally[695]	Budgerigars/time to onset 2.6 ± 0.9 min; significantly longer sedation that midazolam or diazepam; quality of sedation insufficient to perform clinical procedures
Xylazine (X)/butorphanol (B)	(X) 1.06-2.75 mg/kg + (B) 0.1-0.55 mg/kg IM[455]	Ratites, including rheas/sedation, premedication; higher doses were needed in rheas
Yohimbine HCl (Yobine, Akorn)	—	α_2-adrenergic antagonist; excitement and mortality observed at doses >1 mg/kg[337]

Continued

TABLE 5-5 Chemical Restraint/Anesthetic/Analgesic Agents Used in Birds. (cont'd)

Agent	Dosage	Species/Comments
Yohimbine HCl (Yobine, Akorn) (cont'd)	0.1-0.2 mg/kg IV[38]	Psittacines, raptors
	0.1-0.2 mg/kg IM, IV[358]	Raptors
	0.1-1 mg/kg[333]	Most species
	0.11-0.275 mg/kg IM, IV once[339]	Budgerigars
	0.125 mg/kg IV[375,396,630]	Ratites
	12 mg/kg intranasally[829]	Ring-necked parakeets/dose divided evenly between nares and administered slowly; successful reversal of xylazine intranasally
	12-15 mg/kg intranasally[830]	Canaries/dose divided evenly between nares and administered slowly; successful reversal of xylazine and detomidine

[a]For other analgesic recommendations, refer to Table 5-6 (nonsteroidal antiinflammatory agents).
[b]The anesthetic agents of choice in most avian species are the inhalant agents, isoflurane and sevoflurane.
[c]All opioid agonists and agonist-antagonists may cause respiratory depression; profound bradypnea may occur with potent opioid agonists.
[d]The effects of the volume:volume use of the dexmedetomidine and medetomidine may not be equivalent, so the dose of dexmedetomidine may need to be adjusted based on clinical response.

TABLE 5-6 Nonsteroidal Antiinflammatory Agents Used in Birds.[a-c]

Agent	Dosage	Species/Comments
Acetaminophen	5 mg/L drinking water[333]	Most species/antipyretic, analgesic; overdosage may be associated with hepatotoxicity
Aspirin (acetylsalicylic acid)	—	Contraindicated with tetracycline, insulin, or allopurinol therapy[5]
	5 mg/kg PO q8h[333]	Most species
	25 mg/kg IV[32,33]	Ostriches, pigeons/PK; rapid clearance except longer $t_{1/2}$ in pigeon
	50 mg/kg PO q8h[212]	Psittacines
	150 mg/kg PO[333]	Psittacines
	325 mg/250 mL drinking water[333]	Most species/make fresh q8-12h; alters taste of water (may not be well accepted)
Carprofen	—	Caution should be used when administering to *Gyps* vultures[165,261] and pigeons[874]
	1-2 mg/kg PO, IM, IV q12-24h[149a,358]	Most species, including raptors

TABLE 5-6 Nonsteroidal Antiinflammatory Agents Used in Birds. (cont'd)

Agent	Dosage	Species/Comments
Carprofen (cont'd)	2-10 mg/kg IM q24h up to 7 days[874]	Pigeons/PD; 2, 5, and 10 mg/kg associated with increases in plasma AST, ALT, mottled yellow livers, pale muscle injection sites, and histologic changes in the kidney, liver (lipidosis, necrosis, portal hepatitis), and muscle injection sites
	2-10 mg/kg SC, IM[38,212,333]	Psittacines, passerines, raptors
	3 mg/kg IM q12h[592]	Hispaniolan Amazon parrots/PD; markedly reduced arthritis pain 2 hr postadministration, but short-term effect thus more frequent dosing recommended
	5-10 mg/kg PO, IM[333]	Raptors/postoperative analgesia
Celecoxib (Celebrex, Pfizer)	10-20 mg/kg PO q24h × 6-24 wk[140,168]	Psittacines/clinical proventricular dilatation disease; clinical improvement may be seen within 7-14 days; compounded formulation of 10 mg/mL stable for approximately 90 days at room temperature[196]
Diclofenac	—	Recent massive mortalities in three vulture species lead to banning of diclofenac in India, Pakistan, and Nepal; severe renal lesions suggested toxicity of the kidneys or the renal supportive vascular system;[165,514,543,564,786] diclofenac toxicity has also been reported in Steppe eagles in India[733] and is suspected in other species; aceclofenac is rapidly metabolized to diclofenac in cattle, thus should also be avoided for its potential toxicity[272]
	12.5 mg PO once[38]	Pigeons/arthritis
Dimethylsulfoxide (DMSO) (90%) (Domoso, Zoetis)	1 mL/kg topical to affected area q4-7d[333]	Most species/antiinflammatory, analgesic; systemic absorption; use gloves during application
Dipyrone	20-25 mg/kg SC, IM, IV q8-12h[806]	Ratites/analgesic for intestinal disorders; antipyretic
Flunixin meglumine	—	Potential nephrotoxicity; hydration is essential; use only for short duration (<5 days);[149b] 5 mg/kg led to renal ischemia and necrosis in Siberian cranes;[587] histologic lesions occurred in budgerigars administered 5.5 mg/kg and severity increased with duration of therapy;[599] histologic glomerular changes were demonstrated in bobwhite quail given doses as low as 0.1 mg/kg (severity of lesions was directly correlated to dose);[411] avoid in *Gyps* vultures;[165,261] IM administration caused muscle necrosis in ducks;[481] regurgitation may occur after administration[385]
	0.2 mg/kg IM[806]	Ratites
	0.5 mg/kg IM[337]	Most species, including psittacines
	1-10 mg/kg IM, IV q24h[331,358,371,649]	Most species, including raptors, psittacines
	1.1 mg/kg IV[32,33]	Ostriches, pigeons/PK; ostrich $t_{1/2} = 10$ min
	1.1 mg/kg IM q12h[1,3]	Ostriches/myositis[3]

Continued

TABLE 5-6   Nonsteroidal Antiinflammatory Agents Used in Birds. (cont'd)

Agent	Dosage	Species/Comments
Flunixin meglumine (cont'd)	1.5 mg/kg IM q24h × 3 days[112]	Ostriches
	5 mg/kg IV[540]	Budgerigars, Patagonian conures/PK: elimination half-life and mean residence time rapid and similar in both spp.
	5.5 mg/kg IM q24h × 3 or 7 days[599]	Budgerigars/some renal changes at 3 days; 6/8 birds had tubular necrosis at 7 days
Ibuprofen	—	Avoid in *Gyps* vultures[165]
	5-10 mg/kg PO q8-12h[212]	Psittacines/use pediatric suspension for small birds
Ketoprofen	—	Avoid in *Gyps* vultures, mortalities reported at clinical doses;[261,544] 7/11 Cape Griffon vultures administered 5 mg/kg PO died within 48 hr[546]
	1 mg/kg IM q24h × 1-10 days[38,76]	Raptors
	1-5 mg/kg IM q12h[648]	Raptors
	2.5 mg/kg IM q24h × 3 or 7 days[599]	Budgerigars/low frequency of glomerular congestion, degeneration/dilation of tubules occurred at 3-7 day treatment
Meloxicam	—	No reported mortalities in over 700 cases of 60 species of birds, including *Gyps* vultures,[165,786,787] but few studies to date evaluating renal effects of higher doses;[190,524b,744] the combination of avian bornavirus challenge and meloxicam treatment resulted in severe disease and death in cockatiels, whereas challenge alone or meloxicam treatment alone were not lethal within the duration of this study[352,353]
	0.1 mg/kg IM q24h × 3 or 7 days[599]	Budgerigars/mild glomerular congestion and tubular degeneration at 3 and 7 days
	0.5 mg/kg PO q12h × 14 days[524b]	African grey parrots/PD; mild to no hematological or biochemical changes, and no histologic lesions in 9 of 10 birds after 14 days of treatment
	0.5 mg/kg IV[32]	Ostriches, pigeons/PK; variable distribution, ostrich had more rapid $t_{1/2}$ (0.5 hr) than other species studied
	0.5 mg/kg PO, IV[433]	Red-tailed hawks, great horned owls/PK; significant differences in pharmacokinetics between species strongly discourages extrapolation between species; hawks had shortest half-life (0.49 hr) of any species recorded to date; once daily dosing not applicable at this dose in these species
	0.5 mg/kg PO, IM q8-12h[875]	Lesser flamingos/PK; PO had higher bioavailability and longer elimination half-life than IM, but the plasma concentrations may be insufficient to provide analgesia; IM administration achieved the desired plasma concentration but would require more frequent administration

TABLE 5-6 Nonsteroidal Antiinflammatory Agents Used in Birds. (cont'd)

Agent	Dosage	Species/Comments
Meloxicam (cont'd)	0.5-1 mg/kg PO q12h[857]	Ring-necked parakeets/PK; no analgesic evaluation
	0.5 mg/kg IM q6-8h[89] – 1.5 mg/kg SC q8-12h[456]	Caribbean (American) flamingos/PK
	0.5-2 mg/kg PO, IM q12h × 9 days[188]	Pigeons/PD; 0.5 mg/kg dose ineffective in minimizing postoperative orthopedic pain; 2 mg/kg provided quantifiable analgesia that appeared safe under experimental conditions
	0.5-3 mg/kg PO q8-12h[89,456]	Caribbean (American) flamingos/PK; oral bioavailability only 45% when compared with SC administration; fasting status may change absorption;[456] results in these two studies differ significantly (possibly associated with fasting vs. nonfasting or other differences in the population); higher dose than 0.5 mg/kg may be required for PO administration;[89] selecting a dose midway between the two extremes may be the most reasonable
	1 mg/kg PO, IM, IV[524a]	African grey parrots/PK; slower absorption and lower bioavailability than IM (40%)
	1 mg/kg PO, IM, IV q12h[146,521]	Hispaniolan Amazon parrots/PD; improved weight-bearing on arthritic limb compared with lower doses; PO lower bioavailability than parenteral; PO did not attain plasma concentrations similar to humans for analgesia; concentrations similar to humans for analgesia for IM, IV for 6 hr
	1.6 mg/kg PO q12h × 15 days[190]	Hispaniolan Amazon parrots/PD; no apparent negative changes in several renal, gastrointestinal, or hemostatic variables in healthy birds
	2 mg/kg PO, IM[545]	Cape Griffon vultures/PD; rapid metabolism and short elimination $t_{1/2}$ (<45 min) suggests low potential for drug accumulation
	2, 10, 20 mg/kg PO q12h × 7 days[785]	American kestrels; histologic evaluation showed a significant correlation between hepatic lipidosis and meloxicam dose; 2/9 birds developed gastric ulcers at highest dose
Phenylbutazone	—	Caution with use in *Gyps* vultures; mortalities associated with use[165,261]
	3.5-7 mg/kg PO q8-12h[212]	Psittacines
	10-14 mg/kg PO q12h[806]	Ratites
	20 mg/kg PO q8h[333]	Raptors
Piroxicam	—	Indicated for chronic osteoarthritis; has been used to treat pain associated with chronic degenerative joint disease in cranes and other species
	0.5 mg/kg PO q12h[333]	Psittacines
	0.5-0.8 mg/kg PO q12h[333]	Whooping cranes/acute myopathy, chronic degenerative joint disease

[a]Unless otherwise noted, drugs provide analgesic, antipyretic, and antiinflammatory effects.
[b]Nonsteroidal antiinflammatory agents may potentially cause gastrointestinal upset and hemorrhage, as well as adverse renal effects ranging from fluid retention to renal failure.
[c]For other analgesic recommendations, refer to Table 5-5.

TABLE 5-7 Hormones and Steroids Used in Birds.

Agent	Dosage	Species/Comments
Adrenocorticotropic hormone (ACTH)	1-2 U/kg IM[333]	Psittacines/ACTH stimulation test
	16-26 U/bird IM[466,871]	Psittacines/obtain baseline sample, administer ACTH, then sample in 1-2 hr; stress of handling and venipuncture may invalidate results
	50-125 µg/bird IM[333]	Pigeons
Boldenone undecylenate (Equipoise, Zoetis)	1.1 mg/kg IM q21d[806]	Ratites/anabolic steroid
Buserelin (Receptal, Intervet India)	0.5-1 µg/kg q48h up to 3 treatments[38]	Psittacines/used to suppress chronic egg-laying
	8 µg/kg IM[467]	Cockatiels, sulfur-crested cockatoos/increased circulating testosterone after single injection
Buserelin acetate depot (Suprefact, Sanofi Aventis Canada)	10 µg/kg SC implant[153]	Budgerigars/when administered in inguinal region increased reproductive activity and egg laying
Cabergoline	10-50 µg/kg q12-24h[38]	Psittacines/egg laying
Calcitonin	4 U/kg IM q12h × 14 days[333]	Most species/reduce hypercalcemia (caused by cholecalciferol rodenticide toxicity)
	10 µg/kg IM[863]	Pigeons/significant reduction in plasma calcium over 5 days
Chorionic gonadotropin (hCG)	500-1000 U/kg IM on day 1, 3, 7 q3-6wk prn[333]	Most species/inhibits egg laying; administer on days 3 and 7 if hen lays after day 1
Delmadinone	1 mg/kg[38]	Antiandrogen sometimes effective for neurotic regurgitation in budgerigars
Deslorelin (Suprelorin, Virbac)	—	GnRH agonist available as 4.7 mg and 9.4 mg long-term implants; also used for long-term management of ovarian neoplasia in cockatiels[399,551] and Sertoli cell tumors in budgerigars;[774] anecdotal evidence of decreased efficacy over time with repeated administration;[27] to date, only approved for use in adrenocortical disease in ferrets in the United States
	4.7 mg implant placed SC intrascapularly[784]	Cockatiels/suppressed egg laying for ≥180 days; 5/13 implanted birds laid first egg between 192 and 230 days following implant placement; no difference in egg shape, color, shell quality or number of eggs per clutch was observed between treated and control groups

TABLE 5-7　Hormones and Steroids Used in Birds. (cont'd)

Agent	Dosage	Species/Comments
Deslorelin (Suprelorin, Virbac) (cont'd)	4.7 mg implant placed IM[154]	Domestic pigeons/effectively controlled egg laying for at least 49 days; significantly reduced serum LH concentrations in males and females compared to pretreatment levels for 56 and 84 days, respectively
	5 mg/kg implant SC[537]	Male zebra finches/transiently suppressed testosterone concentrations, reversible when implant removed
Desmopressin	4.6 µg/kg IM q12h[766]	African grey parrots/long-term treatment of central diabetes insipidus; dosage adjusted as needed up to 24 µg/kg 16 mo after initial diagnosis
Dexamethasone[a]	0.2-1 mg/kg IM, IV once or q12-24h × 2-7 days, then q48h × 5 days[38,333]	Most species
	2-4 mg/kg IM, IV q12-24h[38,333]	Most species, including ratites/shock, trauma
	2-8 mg/kg SC, IM, IV q12-24h[566]	Cranes/reduce doses for long-term therapy
Dexamethasone sodium phosphate[a]	2-4 mg/kg SC, IM, IV q6-24h[38,333]	Most species, including raptors/head trauma, shock, hyperthermia; higher dose for shock, head trauma, and endotoxemia
Diethylstilbestrol diphosphate (Stilphostrol, Bayer)	0.025-0.075 mg/kg IM[333]	Most species/narrow therapeutic index
	0.4 mg/L drinking water[333]	Most species
Dinoprost tromethamine	—	See prostaglandin $F_{2\alpha}$
Dinoprostone	—	See prostaglandin E_2
Estradiol benzoate	—	Estrogens have been associated with severe adverse reactions in mammals;[615] anemia, hypercholesterolemia, and hyperlipidemia were observed in penguins[345]
	0.3-0.5 mg/kg PO q24h × 1 mo[345]	Penguins/induces molt
	10-15 mg/kg IM q7d × 4 treatments[345]	Penguins/induces molt
Flumethasone (Flucort, Glenmark)[a]	1-1.5 mg/kg PO, SC, IM, IV[806]	Ratites/glucocorticoid; antiinflammatory
Glipizide	1 mg/kg PO q12h[359a]	Most species
Hydrocortisone[a]	3-4.5 mg/kg PO q12h[806]	Ratites
	10 mg/kg IM, IV[333]	Psittacines, passerines, raptors
	40-50 mg/kg IV q24h[806]	Ratites

Continued

TABLE 5-7 Hormones and Steroids Used in Birds. (cont'd)

Agent	Dosage	Species/Comments
Insulin	0.002 U/bird IM q12-48h[333]	Budgerigars/NPH insulin
	0.01-0.1 U/bird IM q12-48h[333]	Amazon parrots/NPH insulin
	0.1-0.5 U/bird IM q24h or prn[333]	Toco toucans
	0.2-10.7 U/kg SC, IM q12h[48]	Bali mynah/PZI insulin: commercial and compounded products used with differing results, so increase/change dose/product with caution
	0.5-3 U/kg IM[333]	Psittacines/NPH insulin
	1.4 U/kg IM q12-24h[333,377]	Cockatiels, toco toucans/NPH insulin
	2 U/bird IM[333]	Toco toucans/ultralente or PZI insulin; adjust dose or frequency based on glucose curves
Lecirelin (Dalmarelin; Selecta, Germany; Vetcare, Finland; Fatro, Ireland, Israel, Italy, Netherlands; Ufamed, Switzerland; Reprorelin: Vetoquinol, France)	5-21 µg/kg transcutaneous (combined with cream vehicle) administered skin over right jugular[672]	Canaries/time from start of treatment to onset of egg laying was significantly shorter for treated birds than controls, irrespective of photoperiod given
Leuprolide acetate (Lupron Depot, TAP Pharmaceuticals; Lupron Kit, Florida Infusion Pharmacy [single-dose leuprolide acetate available from Professional ArtsPharmacy, Baltimore, MD])	—	Synthetic GnRH agonist depot drug; prevents ovulation; may be indicated in some cases of sexually related feather picking or mutilation;[285] variable results obtained; in treating reproductive diseases, administration before onset of egg laying may be more successful than treatment during breeding; single report of anaphylaxis following chronic administration in 2 elf owls;[777] rarely seen in humans unless impurities in formulation
	(No. of days for desired effect) × (52 or 156 µg/kg) = dosage IM[517]	Cockatiels/PD
	100 µg/kg q14d × 3 treatments[333,372]	Most species/feather-damaging behavior
	200-800 µg/kg IM q2-6wk[333,378]	Most species
	375 µg/bird IM[39,518]	Cockatiels/inhibits ovulation
	400-1000 µg/kg IM q2-3 wk[489]	Psittacines
	500 µg/kg IM q14d[867]	Psittacines (>300 g)/for most problems, begin with 3 treatments
	750 µg/kg IM q14d[867]	Psittacines (≤300 g)/for most problems, begin with 3 treatments

TABLE 5-7 Hormones and Steroids Used in Birds. (cont'd)

Agent	Dosage	Species/Comments
Leuprolide acetate (cont'd)	800 µg/kg IM[409]	Hispaniolan Amazon parrots/hormonal effects may taper off between 7 and 21 days after administration
	1250 µg/kg IM once[345]	Penguins/induced molt in 1 of 2 birds dosed
Levothyroxine (l-thyroxine)	—	May induce molt; monitor blood levels and body weight
	5-200 µg/kg PO q12h[678]	Amazon parrots
	20 µg/kg PO q12-24h[38,135,333]	Most species, including psittacines, pigeons, and raptors
	25 µg q24h × 7 days, then 50 µg q24h × 7 days, then 75 µg q24h × 7 days, then 50 µg q24h × 7 days, then 25 µg q24h × 7 days[358]	Raptors (750-1000 g)/induces molt; scale dose up or down by up to 50% for larger or smaller birds
Medroxyprogesterone acetate	—	This agent is not recommended; previously used for sexually related feather picking or chronic egg laying; high incidence of adverse effects, including lethargy, polydipsia, polyphagia, polyuria, immunosuppression, weight gain, liver disease, thromboembolism, diabetes mellitus, salpingitis, sudden death[285]
	5-25 mg/kg SC, IM, repeat q4-6wk prn[316,333]	Psittacines/suppresses ovulation; antipruritic (feather picking in male parrots)
	5-50 mg/kg SC, IM q4-6wk[38]	Psittacines/higher dosages recommended for smaller birds (e.g., 50 mg/kg for 150 g bird)[500]
	15-30 mg/kg IM q7d × 4-5 treatments[656]	Penguins/induces molt 60-90 days postinjection
	30 mg/kg SC, repeat in 90 days prn[333]	Most species
	1000 mg/kg feed[333]	Pigeons/inhibits ovulation
Megestrol acetate	—	Progestin; adverse effects can be severe (diabetic-like); not generally recommended, so dosages are not provided
Methylprednisolone acetate[a]	0.5-1 mg/kg PO, IM[333]	Most species/allergies (Amazon foot necrosis);[666] use orally once weekly, then taper to once monthly, then stop
	200 mg/bird IM, repeat prn[806]	Ratites (adults)

Continued

TABLE 5-7 Hormones and Steroids Used in Birds. (cont'd)

Agent	Dosage	Species/Comments
Nandrolene laurate (Laurabolin, Intervet)	—	Testosterone derivative; used in the treatment of chronic, debilitating disease; may be hepatotoxic
	0.2-2 mg/kg IM once[333]	Most species
	0.4 mg/kg SC, IM q21d[38]	Psittcines, raptors, bustards
Oxytocin	—	Use of oxytocin should be preceeded by calcium administration for egg binding; contraindicated unless uterovaginal sphincter is well dilated and uterus is free of adhesions; used alone to stop uterine bleeding[333]
	0.5-5 U/kg, may repeat q30min[333]	Most species, including raptors
	5-10 U/kg IM once[333]	Psittacines/in some cases, multiple injections are recommended
	20-30 U/bird IM q24h × 2 treatments[806]	Ratites (adults)/egg binding
Prednisolone (prednisone)[a]	0.5-1 mg/kg IM, IV[333]	Most species
	1-1.25 mg/kg PO q48h[806]	Ratites
	2 mg/kg IM, IV q12-24h[566]	Cranes/shock, trauma, chronic lameness
	2-4 mg/kg IM, IV[358]	Raptors/shock
Prednisolone sodium succinate (Solu-Delta-Cortef, Zoetis)[a]	0.5-1 mg/kg IM, IV[333]	Psittacines/antiinflammatory
	1.5-2 mg/kg IM q12h[806]	Ratites/immunosuppression (see prednisolone for prolonged therapy)
	2-4 mg/kg IM, IV once[333]	Psittacines/shock; trauma; endotoxemia; immunosuppression
	5-8.5 mg/kg IV q1h[806]	Ratites/shock
	10-20 mg/kg IM, IV q15min prn[333]	Most species/head trauma; cardiopulmonary resuscitation
Prednisone	—	See prednisolone
Prostaglandin E_2 (dinoprostone) (Prepidil Gel, Pfizer)	0.02-0.1 mg/kg applied topically to uterovaginal sphincter[333]	Most species, including psittacines, raptors/dystocia; relaxes uterovaginal sphincter; lower dosage may be effective; freeze into aliquots
Prostaglandin $F_{2\alpha}$ (Dinoprost tromethamine) (Lutalyse, Zoetis)	0.02-0.1 mg/kg IM, intracloacal once[697]	Most species, including psittacines, raptors, and waterfowl/dystocia; may be helpful when the egg is located distally and the uterovaginal sphincter is dilated; can result in uterine rupture, bronchoconstriction, hypertension, death

TABLE 5-7 Hormones and Steroids Used in Birds. (cont'd)

Agent	Dosage	Species/Comments
Somatostatin	0.003 mg/kg SC q12h[391]	Toucans (sulfur-breasted)/diabetes mellitus; some clinical improvement observed, hyperglycemia and elevated glucagon levels persisted
Tamoxifen citrate	—	Nonsteroidal antiestrogen
	2 mg/kg PO q24h given on 2 consecutive days per wk for 38-46 wk[478]	Budgerigars/effects suggested by change in cere color from white/brown to blue; leukopenia was the most significant adverse effect
	40 mg/kg IM[345]	Penguins/induces molt
Testosterone	—	Anabolic steroid; may adversely affect spermatogenesis; contraindicated with hepatic or renal disease[138]
	2-8 mg/kg SC, IM once[38]	Most species/stimulates sexual behavior in the male; baldness in canaries
	8-8.5 mg/kg IM q7d prn[13]	Most species, including psittacines/anemia due to debilitation; increases libido; use with caution
	10-15 mL stock solution/L drinking water × 5 days-2 mo[333]	Canaries/finish molt or regain singing; stock solution: 100 mg parenteral suspension/30 mL drinking water (3333 mg/L); mix fresh daily
Thyroid releasing hormone	15 μg/kg IM once[333]	Most species
Thyroid stimulating hormone (thyrotropin; TSH)	0.1 U/bird IM (Bovine)[322]	Cockatiels/3-24-fold higher T_4 6 hr after receiving TSH
	0.2 U/kg IM (Human)[291]	Macaws/PD; T_4 doubled in 6/11 birds 4 hr after receiving TSH
	1 U/kg IM (Human)[290,291,871]	Hispaniolan parrots, blue-fronted Amazon parrots, African grey parrots, pigeons/PD; T_4 doubled in Hispaniolan and blue-fronted parrots 6 hr after receiving TSH
	1-2 U/kg IM (Human)[465]	Psittacines/obtain blood at 0 hr, then 4-6 hr after TSH stimulation

[a]Steroid administration may predispose birds to aspergillosis and other mycoses.[358] Administration may also be associated with the development of polyuria/polydipsia/polyphagia, increased protein catabolism, glucosuria, and diabetes mellitus. Toxic levels may be attained even with topical application.[344] Administration should ideally not exceed 5 days. Rapid onset, shorter-acting drugs are generally less likely to cause serious adverse effects.

TABLE 5-8 Nebulization Agents Used in Birds.[a]

Agent	Dosage	Species/Comments
N-acetyl-L-cysteine 10%-20% (Mucomyst, Bristol)	—	See other antimicrobials and drugs for combinations
	22 mg/mL sterile water until dissipated[333]	Most species/mucolytic agent; tracheal irritation and reflex bronchoconstriction reported in mammals; use is preceded by bronchodilators in mammals[662]
Amikacin	5-6 mg/mL sterile water or saline × 15 min q8-12h[333]	Most species/discontinue if polyuria develops
Aminophylline	3 mg/mL sterile water or saline × 15 min[333]	Most species/bronchial and pulmonary vasculature smooth muscle relaxation; incompatible with amikacin, cephalothin, clindamycin, erythromycin, oxytetracycline, methylprednisone, penicillin G, tetracycline; consult with specialized references for more information[615]
Amphotericin B (Fungizone, Squibb)	—	May lead to hypokalemia; corticosteroids may exacerbate this effect;[615] minor systemic absorption with aerosol administration; can be nebulized long-term;[615] mix with sterile water, may precipitate with saline and other electrolytic solutions
	0.1-1 mg/mL sterile water × 15-60 min q12-24h[37,53,333,838]	Most species including birds of prey, penguins, and parrots (0.5-1 mg/mL q30-40 min is usually used)
	0.25 mg/mL saline × 15 min q12h[329]	Hummingbirds/low efficacy; may cause weight loss
Amphotericin B liposome (AmBisome, Astellas Pharma)	1-4 mg/mL sterile water × 15-60 min[55]	Most species; do not mix with saline or other drugs
Carbenicillin (Geocillin, Roerig)	20 mg/mL saline × 15 min q12h[333]	Psittacines
Cefotaxime	10 mg/mL saline × 10-30 min q6-12h[53]	Most species
Chloramphenicol	13 mg/mL saline[333]	Most species/human health concerns; the development of aplastic anemia reported in humans; prohibited by the FDA for use in food animals
Clotrimazole (1%) (Lotrimin, Schering)	10 mg/mL propylene glycol or polyethylene glycol × 30-45 min q24h × 3 days, off 2 days, repeat prn for up to 4 mo[53,333]	Most species/treatment of aspergillosis; can be toxic to psittacines at this dose
	10 mg/mL polyethylene glycol × 30-60 min[333]	Raptors, psittacines/used in combination with systemic antifungals
	5%-10% clotrimazole in propylene glycol with 5% DMSO × 1 hr[645]	Raptors
Dexamethasone sodium phosphate	0.16 mg/mL in saline[511]	Eclectus parrot/tracheal stent placement

TABLE 5-8 Nebulization Agents Used in Birds. (cont'd)

Agent	Dosage	Species/Comments
Doxycycline hyclate (Vibramycin, Zoetis)	13 mg/mL saline[53,333]	Psittacines
Enilconazole (Imaverol, Janssen; Clinafarm, Schering)	0.2 mg/5 mL saline q12h × 21 day[333]	Most species, including raptors, psittacines
	10 mg/mL sterile water[53,333]	Most species/antifungal
	50 mg in 25 mL saline × 30-45 min q12h[37]	Raptors
Enrofloxacin	10 mg/mL saline[37,53,333]	Most species
Erythromycin	5-20 mg/mL saline × 15 min q8h[333]	Most species
F10	1:250 dilution[37]	Raptors/prevention and treatment of aspergillosis
	0.2% superconcentrate[828]	Falcons/using a fogging system, prevention and treatment of aspergillosis
Gentamicin	3-6 mg/mL saline or sterile water and 1-2 mL acetylcysteine (20%) × 20 min q8h[37,53,333]	Most species, including cranes and raptors
Itraconazole	1%-10% nanoparticulate suspension × 30 min[683]	Japanese quail/PD; reached high lung levels
	4% nanoparticulate suspension × 30 min q24h[860]	Japanese quail/PD; less effective than 10% in experimental aspergillosis
	10% nanoparticulate suspension × 30 min q24h[860]	Japanese quail/PD; experimental aspergillosis, blocked lethality in low spore load group and delayed disease progression in high spore load group
Lincomycin	250 mg/mL water[333]	Most species
	250 mg aerosolized drug/m³ chamber × 15-30 min[129]	Chickens/PD; antibiotic; therapeutic concentrations in blood, lungs, and trachea for up to 24 hr
Miconazole (Daktarin, Janssen)	Nebulize 15 min q8h × 10 days[333]	Raptors/aspergillosis
Oxytetracycline	2 mg/mL × 60 min q4-6h[333]	Parakeets/PD; therapeutic concentrations in lungs and trachea, low plasma concentrations
Piperacillin	10 mg/mL saline × 10-30 min q6-12h[37,53,333]	Most species
Polymyxin B sulfate	66,000 U/mL saline[333]	Psittacines/poorly absorbed from respiratory epithelium
Praziquantel	56.8-85.2 mg in 100% oxygen × 5-15 min q24h[185]	Blue-crowned motmots, fairy bluebirds/treatment of air sac flukes, decreased parasite burden
Sodium chloride	0.9% or 3% (hypertonic)	Viscosity of respiratory secretions may be decreased by hydration, mucolytic properties[333]
Spectinomycin (Spectam, Ceva)	13 mg/mL saline[333]	Most species
Sterile water	—	Viscosity of respiratory secretions may be decreased by hydration[333]

Continued

TABLE 5-8 Nebulization Agents Used in Birds. (cont'd)

Agent	Dosage	Species/Comments
Sulfadimethoxine	13 mg/mL saline[333]	Most species
Terbinafine	1 mg/mL crushed pills in sterile water × 15 min[216]	Hispaniolan Amazon parrots/PD; plasma levels above MIC for 1 hr; solution concentration was lower than expected at 0.9 mg/mL
	1 mg/mL raw powder in sterile water × 15 min[216]	Hispaniolan Amazon parrots/PD; plasma levels above MIC for 4 hr
Terbutaline	0.01 mg/kg with 9 mL saline[53,333]	Psittacines/bronchodilation
Tylosin	10 mg/mL saline × 10-60 min q12h[333]	Most species
	20 mg/mL DMSO or distilled water × 1 hr[460,461]	Most species, pigeons, quail/PD
	20 mg/mL DMSO and 0.5 mL saline[333]	Psittacines
Voriconazole	10 mg/mL of saline 0.9% × 15 min[71]	Pigeons/PD; low plasma concentrations; no measurable drug in the lungs 1 hr after nebulization; plasma and lung levels below MIC for *Aspergillus*
	10 mg/mL saline × 15-30 min q8-12h[53]	Most species

aNebulization is an adjunctive therapy indicated for rhinitis, sinusitis, tracheitis, pneumonia, airsacculitis, and syringeal aspergilloma, where there is air movement occurring in the patient's disease state; optimal particle size for deposition in the trachea is 2-10 µm; optimal particle size for peripheral airways and air sacs is 0.5-5 µm; treatments of 30-45 min repeated q4-12h are recommended (longer nebulization periods of 1 to several hours may be required[720,796]); caution: do not overhydrate airways.[333] Saline or propylene glycol can be used as a carrier.[720] A variety of nebulizers exist, including air jet nebulizer (most commonly used) and ultrasonic nebulizers. Air jet nebulizers are better to nebulize viscous liquid.[53] Pressurized metered-dose inhalers are air jet nebulizers and should be used with a holding chamber (e.g., Aerokat®).[53]

TABLE 5-9 Agents Used in the Treatment of Toxicologic Conditions of Birds.

Agent	Dosage	Species/Comments
Atropine sulfate	—	Antidote for muscarinic effects of organophosphate/carbamate (acetylcholinesterase inhibitors) toxicosis; does not treat nicotinic effects
	0.01-0.02 mg/kg SC, IM[333]	Most species/facilitates bronchodilation in acutely dyspneic animals; treatment of choice for anticholinesterase-induced respiratory distress
	0.03-0.05 mg/kg SC, IM, IV q8h[806]	Ratites
	0.04-0.1 mg/kg IM[333]	Psittacines/bronchodilation in acutely dyspneic animals; treatment of choice for anticholinesterase-induced respiratory distress
	0.1 mg/kg IM, IV q3-4h[333]	Raptors, waterfowl

TABLE 5-9 Agents Used in the Treatment of Toxicologic Conditions of Birds. (cont'd)

Agent	Dosage	Species/Comments
Atropine sulfate (cont'd)	0.2-0.5 mg/kg IM, IV q3-4h[333]	Most species, including pigeons, raptors/cholinesterase inhibitors toxicosis
	0.5 mg/kg IM, IV q6-8h[651]	Raptors/cholinesterase inhibitors toxicosis
Bismuth sulfate (Bismusal, Bimeda)	1-2 mL/kg PO[333]	Most species/weak adsorbent, demulcent; may be useful for toxin removal
Botulinum type C antitoxin (100 U/mL) (National Wildlife Health Center)	1 mL IP[498] once	Waterfowl/not commercially available; produced for experimental use in migratory birds
Botulinum antitoxin	0.05-1 mL/day[699]	Most species
Calcium EDTA (edetate calcium disodium)	—	Preferred initial chelator for lead and zinc toxicosis; may cause renal tubular necrosis in mammals; maintain hydration and monitor patient for PU/PD; SC, IM absorbed well;[615] poorly effective at removing lead in soft tissues; combine with DMSA in severe cases[651]
	10-40 mg/kg IM q12h × 5-10 days[699]	Raptors, most species
	20-70 mg/kg IV[174]	Most species/empirical diagnosis; signs should resolve for up to 48 hr; diluted 1:4 in saline
	30 mg/kg SC q24h × 5 days[613]	Vultures
	30-35 mg/kg IM q12h × 3-5 days, off 3-4 days, repeat prn[333]	Most species
	35-50 mg/kg SC diluted with saline[651]	Raptors
	40 mg/kg IM q12h[187]	Cockatiels/PD; reduces lead levels when used alone or with DMSA
	50 mg/kg IM q12h × up to 23 days[701]	Raptors/no deleterious effects observed
	100 mg/kg IM q12h × 5-25 days[699]	Falcons/no observed deleterious effects
Charcoal, activated	—	Adsorbs toxins from the intestinal tract; may be mixed with hemicellulose to act as a bulk laxative to aid in the passage of ingested toxins; administration prior to cathartic use may help bind small particles of heavy metal;[613] see magnesium hydroxide for combination

Continued

TABLE 5-9 Agents Used in the Treatment of Toxicologic Conditions of Birds. (cont'd)

Agent	Dosage	Species/Comments
Charcoal, activated (cont'd)	52 mg/kg PO once[519]	A component of oiled bird treatment; alternatively, may use bismuth
	1-3 g/kg[859]	Most species
	2-8 g/kg PO[333]	Most species
Deferiprone (Ferriprox, Apotex)	50 mg/kg PO q12h × 30 days[333,849]	Toucans, pigeons/iron chelation; may produce rust-colored urates
	50 mg/kg PO q12h[848]	Pigeons/PK
	75 mg/kg PO q24h × 90 days[712]	Hornbills/PD; $n = 3$
Deferoxamine mesylate	—	Iron chelator for hemochromatosis; may take 3 mo to see response; may cause reddish discoloration of urine; avoid in birds with renal disease; combine with a low-iron diet;[333,438] poorly absorbed from the gastrointestinal tract[615]
	20 mg/kg PO, IM q4h until recovery[333]	Most species
	40 mg/kg IM q24h × 7 days[559]	Bali mynahs
	50 mg/kg IM q12h × 14 days[274]	Macaws
	100 mg/kg SC, IM q24h up to 3.5 mo[151,438,789]	Most species, including toucans
	100 mg/kg SC q24h × 16 wk[569]	European starlings/PD
Dimercaprol (BAL in Oil, Becton Dickinson)	2.5-5 mg/kg IM q4h × 2 days, then q12h × 10 days or until recovery[333]	Most species/heavy metal toxicosis; arsenical compound toxicosis; occasionally used for lead, mercury, and gold intoxication (if ingestion <2 hr);[333,615] crosses blood-brain barrier, nephrotoxic, and painful upon injection[651,859]
	25-35 mg/kg PO q12h × 3-5 wk[333]	Most species/give 5 days/wk
Dimercaptosuccinic acid (DMSA or succimer) (DMSA, Aldrich; Chemet, Bock Pharmacal)	—	Oral chelator for lead or zinc; may be effective for mercury toxicity; does not chelate lead from bones; combine with Ca-EDTA in severe cases[333,859]
	25-35 mg/kg PO q12h × 5 day/wk × 3-5 wk[333]	Most species, including raptors/lead toxicosis
	25-35 mg/kg PO q24h × 10 days[333]	Psittacines, raptors/lead and zinc toxicosis
	30 mg/kg PO q12h × ≥7 days[349]	Most species/lead toxicosis

TABLE 5-9 Agents Used in the Treatment of Toxicologic Conditions of Birds. (cont'd)

Agent	Dosage	Species/Comments
Dimercaptosuccinic acid (DMSA or succimer) (DMSA, Aldrich; Chemet, Bock Pharmacal) (cont'd)	35 mg/kg PO q12h × 34 weeks[477]	Budgerigars/PD; prevented experimental lead toxicosis
	40 mg/kg PO q12h × 21 days[187]	Cockatiels/PD; lead toxicosis; reduces lead levels when used alone or in combination with CaEDTA; 80 mg/kg resulted in death in >60% of cockatiels
Diphenhydramine	2 mg/kg PO, IM q12h[765]	Macaws/used to treat extrapyramidal effects of clomipramine/haloperidol
Grit	3-5 pieces[210]	Most species/reduce size of metal particles
	80 particles of fine grit (silica 0.2 mm) or 20 particles of coarse grit (silica, 1-2 mm)[477]	Budgerigars/PD; experimental lead particle administration, faster elimination time than controls but not statistically significant
Magnesium hydroxide (M)/ activated charcoal (C)	(M) 10-12 mL + (C) 1 tsp powder[333]	Most species/cathartic;[a] adsorbent
Magnesium sulfate (Epsom salts)	500-1000 mg/kg PO q12-24h × 1-3 days[333]	Raptors, waterfowl/cathartic used in lead toxicosis to reduce lead absorption;[a] give 30 min after activated charcoal treatment or can cause lethargy[333]
Peanut butter	1 mL combined with mineral oil (2:1)[477]	Budgerigars/PD; cathartic;[a] experimental lead particle administration, faster elimination time than controls but not statistically significant
Penicillamine (Cuprimine, Merck)	—	Preferred chelator for copper toxicosis; may be used for lead, zinc, and mercury toxicosis;[333] significant gastrointestinal side effects (emesis)[615]
	30 mg/kg PO q12h × ≥7 days[349]	Most species/initially supplemented with CaEDTA once in severe neurologic disease
	30-55 mg/kg PO q12h × 7-14 days[333]	Most species, including raptors, waterfowl
	50-55 mg/kg PO q24h × 1-6 wk[333]	Most species, including psittacines, raptors/use in combination with CaEDTA for several days followed by penicillamine × 3-6 wk[713]
	55 mg/kg PO q12h × 10 days[699]	Most species
Phytonadione	—	See vitamin K

Continued

TABLE 5-9 Agents Used in the Treatment of Toxicologic Conditions of Birds. (cont'd)

Agent	Dosage	Species/Comments
Pralidoxime (2-PAM) (Protopam, Wyeth-Ayerst)	—	Administer within 24-36 hr of organophosphate intoxication; use lower dose in combination with atropine;[333] contraindicated for some carbamate poisoning[651]
	10-100 mg/kg IM q24-48h or repeat once q6h[333]	Psittacines, raptors, waterfowl
	100 mg/kg IM once[735]	Raptors/monocrotophos toxicosis
	100 mg/kg IM once[736]	Goslings/PD; experimental diazinon toxicosis; lower dosages (25-50 mg/kg) were less effective
Psyllium (Metamucil)	1 mL of a solution made of ½ tsp diluted in 60 mL of water[477]	Budgerigars/PD; cathartic;[a] experimental lead particle administration, similar elimination time than controls
Sodium sulfate (Glauber's salt) (GoLytely, Braintree; Anydrous sodium sulfate, ACS Grade, Fisher Scientific)	—	Cathartic;[a] contraindicated with impaired gastrointestinal function; maintain hydration[333]
	500 mg/kg PO q48h[187]	Cockatiels/PD; did not result in further decrease in lead concentrations when given to birds receiving CaEDTA alone or in combination with DMSA
	500-2000 mg/kg PO[333]	Most species
	2000 mg/kg PO q24h × 2 days[333]	Most species
Succimer (Chemet, Bock Pharmacal)	—	See dimercaptosuccinic acid (DMSA)
Tea (black tea leaves) (Ceylon CO_2-decaffeinated tea leaves, Frontier Natural)	8 g/kg diet[727]	Starlings/hepatic iron concentrations did not increase significantly in starlings on an iron-enriched diet when supplemented with tea leaves; tea containing approximately 20% (by weight) condensed tannins were blended directly into the food mixture (8 g/kg diet)
Tetanus antitoxin (equine)	50 U IV over 15 min[61]	Falcons/tetanus
Vitamin K_1	0.2-2.2 mg/kg IM q4-8h until stable, then q24h PO, IM × 14-28 days[333,651]	Most species, including raptors/rodenticide anticoagulant toxicosis
	2.5 mg/kg SC q12h[538]	Red-tailed hawks/secondary brodifacoum toxicosis

[a]Cathartics increase gastrointestinal motility and are used to evacuate the gut and prevent absorption of toxins.

TABLE 5-10 Psychotropic and Antiepileptic Agents Used in Birds.[a]

Agent	Dosage	Species/Comments
Amitriptyline	—	Tricyclic antidepressant; inhibits serotonin and norepinephrine reuptake; strong antihistamine effect[497,818]
	1-5 mg/kg PO q12-24h[333]	Most species/feather-damaging behavior, anxiety, phobia;[497] severe extrapyramidal side effects encountered in a blue and gold macaw at 5 mg/kg PO[55]
	1.5-4.5 mg/kg[835]	African grey parrots, cockatoos/PK; erratic plasma concentrations generally below therapeutic levels
	2 mg/kg PO q24h[223]	Psittacines/minimum of 30 days
	9 mg/kg[835]	African grey parrots, cockatoos/PK; good levels but unpredictable half-life, toxicity in 1/3 African grey parrots
Buspirone HCl	0.5 mg/kg PO q12h[389]	Anxiolytic; used to control behavior interpreted as paradoxical anxiety caused by clomipramine
Carbamazepine	3-10 mg/kg PO q24h[333]	Most species/anticonvulsant, analgesic; may cause bone marrow suppression (including aplastic anemia and agranulocytosis) and hepatotoxicity; combination with chlorpromazine or haloperidol recommended for initial treatment during the first 2 wk[333]
	166 mg/L drinking water[333]	
Chlorpromazine	—	Phenothiazine; dopamine antagonist[333] used in some cases of feather picking; correct underlying problems and discontinue within 30 days; efficacy diminishes in 14-30 days when given PO; may cause ataxia, regurgitation, drowsiness[333]
	0.1-0.2 mg/kg IM once[333]	Cockatoos, ringneck parakeets/use with carbamazepine following removal of Elizabethan collar; mild sedation and decreases obsessive behaviors
	Mix 1 mL stock solution/120 mL drinking water or 0.2-1 mL/kg stock PO q12-24h prn[333]	Most species/stock solution: crush five 25 mg tablets and mix with 31 mL simple syrup; start at low dose initially; mild sedation
Clomipramine	—	Most selective for serotonin reuptake inhibition among tricyclic antidepressants; antihistamine; may cause regurgitation, drowsiness; adverse effects in mammals include cardiac conduction abnormalities, tachyarrhythmias, postural hypotension, dry mucous membranes, urinary retention, constipation, and lowering of the seizure threshold;[389] anecdotal reports of death in birds possibly associated with preexisting arrhythmias;[333] wait 2-3 wk before adjusting dose;[333] reports of illness, extrapyramidal signs, and death reported in macaws;[765] indicated for compulsive disorders, feather-damaging behavior, and anxiety;[497,818] contraindicated for aggressive behaviors[497]

Continued

TABLE 5-10 Psychotropic and Antiepileptic Agents Used in Birds. (cont'd)

Agent	Dosage	Species/Comments
Clomipramine (cont'd)	0.5-1 mg/kg PO q12-24h[333]	Psittacines/feather-damaging behavior; self-mutilation; start with low dose and gradually increase over 4-5 days
	1 mg/kg PO q24h or divided q12h × 6 wk[636]	Psittacines/feather-damaging behavior; occasional regurgitation and drowsiness observed; 2/11 birds decreased feather picking[636]
	1-2 mg/kg PO q24h[333]	Psittacines/begin with 1 mg/kg and increase if needed
	3 mg/kg PO q12h[730]	Cockatoos/PD; placebo-controlled clinical trial; no appreciable deleterious side effects; no significant differences between baseline and post-treatment bloodwork or body weight; significant decrease in feather-damaging behavior at 3 and 6 wk
	4-8 mg/kg PO q12h[389]	African grey parrots/behavior interpreted as paradoxical anxiety; combine with anxiolytic therapy (buspirone)
Clonazepam	0.5 mg/kg PO q12h[62]	African grey parrot/antiepileptic; developed tolerance after 7 mo
Delmadinone (Tardak, Pfizer)	1 mg/kg IM once[333]	Psittacines/sexual behavior problems; not available in the United States
Deslorelin (Suprelorin, Virbac)	4.7 mg implant[254]	Parrots, birds of prey/decrease reproduction-related behavior
Diazepam	—	Benzodiazepine sedative; anxiolytic/stress-associated feather picking; useful as sole agent or in combination with phenobarbital for seizure control
	0.25-0.5 mg/kg IM, IV q24h × 2-3 days[779]	Raptors/appetite stimulant
	0.5 mg/kg PO[280]	'Amakihi/calm fractious species while improving acceptance to a novel captive diet; oral solution (1 mg/mL; Roxane Laboratories) worked best
	0.5-0.6 mg/kg IM[333]	Most species/facilitates acceptance of Elizabethan collar, especially in lovebirds
	0.5-1.5 mg/kg IM, IV q8-12h[333]	Most species/control of seizures
	2.5-4 mg/kg PO q6-8h[333]	Psittacines/sedation
	10-20 mg/L drinking water[333]	Most species
	1 mg/kg/h IV, CRI, decrease after 12-24 hr without seizures[186]	Most species
Diphenhydramine	—	Antihistamine; mild hypnotic effects; suspected allergic feather picking
	2 mg/kg PO, IM q12h[765]	Blue and gold macaw/treatment of extrapyramidal side effects of a haloperidol/clomipramine combination
	2-4 mg/kg PO q12h[333,497]	Most species
	2 mg/L drinking water[333,497]	Most species

TABLE 5-10 Psychotropic and Antiepileptic Agents Used in Birds. (cont'd)

Agent	Dosage	Species/Comments
Doxepin	—	Tricyclic antidepressant; antihistamine; dose may be increased at 14-day intervals;[333] may cause sedation[333]
	0.5-1 mg/kg PO q12h[333]	Most species/feather picking
	1-2 mg/kg PO q12h[333]	Psittacines/anxiety; pruritus
Fluoxetine	—	Selective serotonin reuptake inhibitor; antidepressant; adjunctive treatment for depression-induced feather picking, compulsive disorders, phobia, aggression[497]
	0.4-4 mg/kg PO q24h[333]	Psittacines/compulsive feather picking
	1 mg/kg PO q24h[333,728]	Psittacines
	1-4 mg/kg q24h, up to 20 mg/kg[497]	Parrots
	2-3 mg/kg PO q12-24h[333]	Most species, including psittacines
Gabapentin	11 mg/kg PO q8h[864]	Great horned owl/PK
	15 mg/kg PO q8h[43]	Hispaniolan Amazon parrots/PK
	20 mg/kg PO q12h[62]	African grey parrot/seizures
Haloperidol (Haldol, McNeil)	—	Butyrophenone dopamine antagonist tranquilizer; may work best with self-mutilators;[818] may cause anorexia, depression, hypotension, bradycardia, ataxia, sedation;[818] extrapyramidal signs and/or death reported in various species of macaw;[447,765] Quaker parrots and cockatoos may be more sensitive to side effects[818]
	0.1-0.2 mg/kg PO q12-24h[333]	Birds weighing >1 kg
	0.1-0.4 mg/kg PO q12-24h[333]	Psittacines/dose may be increased in increments of 0.1 mg/kg if no response is seen in 5-7 days and no adverse effects are observed
	0.2-0.9 mg/kg PO q24h[333,497]	Most species/stereotypic preening behavior
	1-2 mg/kg IM q14-21d[333]	Most species, including psittacines
	6.4 mg/L drinking water × 7 mo[360]	African grey parrots/feather picking
Hydroxyzine	—	Antihistamine with mild sedative effects
	2 mg/kg PO q12h[333]	Most species/pruritus
	2-2.2 mg/kg PO q8h[333,428,497]	Most species/feather picking
	30-40 mg/L drinking water[333]	Most species
Leuprolide acetate	100-1000 μg/kg q2wk for 3 treatments[497]	Parrots/hormonal feather-damaging behavior
	500 μg/kg; BW >300 g[497]	Parrots/sexual behaviors
	750 μg/kg; BW ≤300 g[497]	Parrots/sexual behaviors
Levetiracetam	5.4-190 mg/kg PO q8-12h[834]	African grey parrots/PK; population PK; short half-life (2.3 hr); no dose recommendation, but q8h recommended
	50 mg/kg PO q8h[717] or 100 mg/kg PO q12h[717]	Hispaniolan Amazon parrots/PK
	50-100 mg/kg PO q8h[62]	African grey parrot/seizures; therapeutic drug monitoring was performed

Continued

TABLE 5-10 Psychotropic and Antiepileptic Agents Used in Birds. (cont'd)

Agent	Dosage	Species/Comments
Lorazepam	—	Benzodiazepine with anxiolytic and sedative effects
	0.1 mg/kg PO q12h[333]	Macaws/aggression; feather picking; use alone or with haloperidol
Megestrol acetate (Ovaban, Schering)	—	Progestin providing nonspecific calming effects; side effects can be severe (diabetic-like); seldom used[333]
	2.5 mg/kg PO q24h × 7 days then 1-2 ×/wk[333]	Psittacines/feather picking; reproductively associated behavior problems
Naloxone HCl	2 mg/kg IV[333]	Psittacines/opioid antagonist; may be used to determine the response of stereotypic behavior to antagonist therapy; reduction of the behavior should be observed within 20 min
Naltrexone HCl	1.5 mg/kg PO q8-12h × 1-18 mo[333]	Most species/opioid antagonist; feather-damaging behavior; self-mutilation; contraindicated in patients with liver disease; may need to increase dosage 2-6 × to be effective; dissolve tablet in 10 mL sterile water; preservative does not go into solution
Nortriptyline (Pamelor, Sandoz)	16 mg/L drinking water (2 mg/120 mL)[333,497]	Most species/tricyclic antidepressant; feather-damaging behavior; seldom used; decrease dose or discontinue if hyperactivity develops; taper dose to discontinue
Paroxetine	1-2 mg/kg PO q24h[333,497]	Macaws, ibis/selective serotonin reuptake inhibitor (SSRI); feather-damaging behavior; self-mutilation; generally requires long-term therapy; fewer side effects than tricyclic antidepressants and other SSRIs[818]
	3 mg/kg PO q24h[395]	Waldrapp ibis
	4 mg/kg PO q12h, bulk chemical compounded in water[820]	African grey parrots/PK; slow absorption and low oral bioavailability; bioavailability increased with repeated dosing; commercial oral suspension (Seroxat) resulted in nondetectable plasma levels; large individual differences
Phenobarbital sodium	—	Barbiturate anticonvulsant; mild sedative effect; long-term seizure management; adjust dosage based on blood levels; may cause deep sedation and inability to perch; hepatotoxic; oral formulations may not reach therapeutic plasma levels in parrots[62,620]
	1-5 mg/kg IV bolus[333]	Most species/status epilepticus; begin at low end of dosage range and increase for refractory seizures

TABLE 5-10 Psychotropic and Antiepileptic Agents Used in Birds. (cont'd)

Agent	Dosage	Species/Comments
Phenobarbital sodium (cont'd)	1-7 mg/kg PO q8-12h[333]	Most species/feather picking; mild sedative effect
	2 mg/kg PO q12h[62]	African grey parrot/antiseizure, therapeutic drug monitoring did not show detectable plasma level
	2-7 mg/kg PO q12h[333]	Most species, including Amazon parrots/seizures; self-mutilation
	17 mg/kg PO[620]	African grey parrots/PD; used diluted commercial intravenous solution and compounded suspension, plasma levels below therapeutic levels
	50-80 mg/L drinking water[333]	Most species, including Amazon parrots/idiopathic epilepsy
Potassium bromide	—	Long-term seizure management; use as sole agent or in conjunction with phenobarbital; monitor blood levels which may take up to several weeks to establish steady state; not available in approved dosage forms in North America; may be obtained from chemical companies or compounding pharmacies; for a concentration of 250 mg/mL, add distilled water as needed to 25 g of potassium bromide for a final volume of 100 mL
	25 mg/kg PO q24h[333]	Most species
	50-80 mg/kg PO q24h[333]	Pigeons
	75 mg/kg PO[333]	Psittacines
	80 mg/kg PO q24h[95]	Umbrella cockatoo/serum drug levels ranged from 1.7-2.2 mg/mL
	80 mg/kg PO q12h × 3 days, then 20-200 mg/kg PO q12h[62]	African grey parrot/antiseizure; therapeutic drug monitoring showed plasma level below therapeutic levels (<0.7 mg/mL)
Zonisamide	20 mg/kg PO q8h[62]	African grey parrot/antiseizure; therapeutic drug monitoring performed
	20 mg/kg PO q12h[706]	Hispaniolan Amazon parrots, chickens/PD; 2/8 chickens of multiple escalating dose study developed immune-mediated anemia
	19.8-80 mg/kg PO q8-12h[834]	African grey parrots/PK; population PK; half-life was highly variable (10.9 ± 18 hr), no dose recommendation but q8-12h recommended

[a]The use of psychotropic agents in birds is controversial because safety, efficacy, and pharmacologic effects are poorly documented;[818] anxiolytics or tricyclic antidepressants may be useful for stereotypic behaviors or mutilation; selective serotonin reuptake inhibitors may prove helpful for compulsive behaviors; consider metabolic scaling when calculating dosages; these treatments should be used as components of a structured behavior-change strategy.

TABLE 5-11 Nutritional/Mineral Support and Supplementation Used in Birds.

Agent	Dosage	Species/Comments
Biotin	0.05 mg/kg PO q24h × 30-60 days[333]	Raptors/beak and nail regrowth
Brewer's yeast	30 mg/bird in feed[333]	Pigeons/brittle plumage; use daily during molt
Calcium	—	Recommended dietary levels;[a] higher dietary levels than in commercial food were found in wild macaw chicks (1.4%)[103]
	3-7 mg/kg feed (0.3%-0.7%)[177]	Maintenance diet for most birds
	3-10 mg/kg feed (0.3%-1%)[333]	Laying parrots
	3.5 mg/kg feed (0.35%)[422]	Egg-laying cockatiels
	8.5 mg/kg feed (0.85%)[422]	Egg-laying budgerigars
Calcium borogluconate (10%)	10 mg/kg PO q24h[764]	African grey parrots/hypocalcemia; in addition to UV_b supplementation and diet correction
	50-100 mg/kg IM, IV[333]	Psittacines/20% solution
	100-500 mg/kg SC, IV (slow) once[333]	Raptors/hypocalcemia
	300 mg/kg IV[333]	Goshawks
Calcium chloride	150-200 mg/kg IM, IV (slow) q8h[333]	Hypocalcemia; seldom used
Calcium glubionate	—	Most species/hypocalcemia, calcium supplementation
	23 mg/kg PO q24h[333]	Psittacines (neonates)
	25 mg/kg PO[333]	Most species, including raptors
	150 mg/kg PO q12h[333]	Most species
	750 mg/L drinking water[333]	Most species
Calcium gluconate (10%)	—	Hypocalcemia; dilute 1:1 with saline or sterile water for IM or IV injections
	5-10 mg/kg IV slowly to effect[333]	Psittacines/hypocalcemic tetany
	5-10 mg/kg SC, IM q12h prn[333]	Psittacines
	10-100 mg/kg IM[333]	Psittacines/acute presentation of hypocalcemia
	25-50 mg/kg SC, IV (slow)[333]	Pigeons
	50-100 mg/kg IM (diluted), IV (slow)[333]	Most species, including psittacines, pigeons, raptors
	50-150 mg/kg IV over 15-20 minutes[54]	Ionized hypocalcemia, hyperkalemia
	100-300 mg/kg SC diluted 1:1-2 with fluids[55]	Most species
	100-500 mg/kg SC, IV (slow) once[333]	Raptors/hypocalcemia
	1 mL/30 mL (3300 mg/L) drinking water[333]	Psittacines/calcium supplementation
Calcium lactate/calcium glycerophosphate (Calphosan, Glenwood)	5-10 mg/kg IM q7d prn[333]	Most species, including raptors/hypocalcemia
	50-100 mg/kg IV (slow bolus) once[333]	African grey parrots

TABLE 5-11 Nutritional/Mineral Support and Supplementation Used in Birds. (cont'd)

Agent	Dosage	Species/Comments
Calcium levulinate	75-100 mg/kg IM, IV[333]	Most species/hypocalcemia
L-carnitine	1000 mg/kg feed[179]	Budgerigars/PD; lipomas; average lipoma size decreased significantly
Dextrose (50%)	50-100 mg/kg IV (slow bolus) to effect[333]	Psittacines/hypoglycemia; can dilute with fluids
	500-1000 mg/kg IV (slow bolus)[333]	Hypoglycemia; can dilute with fluids
Diatrizoate meglumine sodium (37% iodine) (Renografin-76, Solvay)	—	Parenteral treatment of goiter is generally reserved for emergency situations
	122 mg/kg IM[333]	Budgerigars/thyroid hyperplasia
Essential fatty acids	0.5 mL/kg PO q24h × 50 days or indefinitely[333]	Raptors/pruritic dermatitis (atopy)
Fatty acids (omega-3, omega-6)	0.1-0.2 mL/kg of flaxseed oil to corn oil mixed at a ratio of 1:4 PO or added to food; ratio of omega-6:omega-3 is 4-5:1[333]	Psittacines, pigeons/glomerular disease; used to reduce thromboxane A_2 synthesis in platelets and glomerular cells; adjunct therapy for arthritis, feather picking, mutilators, and neoplasia; 2-4 wk of therapy are required to recognize effects; may increase dietary vitamin E requirements; consider supplementation with chronic use
	0.11 mL/kg q24h in a 5:1 ratio of omega-6:omega-3[333]	Psittacines/glomerulonephritis, pancreatitis
	10% flaxseeds[604]	Quaker parrots/PD; shift in HDL subgroups, higher plasma phospholipid omega-3 fatty acids
	α-linolenic acid, 0.2%-4% of daily energy[603]	Quaker parrots/PD; no change in blood cholesterol compared to control group, changes in polyunsaturated fatty acid blood profile
Hemicellulose (Metamucil, Searle)	—	For bulk in diet; facilitates defecation in bowel deficit disorders and other conditions
	0.5 tsp/60 mL hand-feeding formula or baby food gruel[333]	Psittacines/bulk diet to delay absorption of an ingested toxin
	1 Tbs/60 mL water q24h[806]	Ostrich chicks/impaction
	1 mL of solution of ½ tsp diluted in 60 mL of water[477]	Budgerigars/no difference from controls in elimination rate of ventricular lead particles
Inositol	20 g/kg of food[569,570]	Starlings/PD; not effective to decrease liver stored iron but prevented an increase in stored iron concentration

Continued

TABLE 5-11 Nutritional/Mineral Support and Supplementation Used in Birds. (cont'd)

Agent	Dosage	Species/Comments
Iodine (Lugol's iodine)	0.2 mL/L drinking water daily[333]	Most species/thyroid hyperplasia
	2 parts iodine + 28 parts water; 3 drops into 100 mL drinking water[333]	Budgerigars/thyroid hyperplasia
Iodine (sodium iodide 20%)	—	Parenteral treatment of goiter is generally reserved for emergency situations or initial treatment of severe thyroid dysplasia; continue with oral therapy when improvement is noted
	2 mg (0.01 mL)/bird IM prn[333]	Budgerigars
	60 mg (0.3 mL)/kg IM[333]	Most species/thyroid hyperplasia
Iron	20-60 mg/kg feed[333,438,468,569]	Species susceptible to iron storage disease/levels recommended for a low-iron diet
Iron dextran	10 mg/kg IM, repeat in 7-10 days prn[333]	Most species, including raptors, waterfowl/iron deficiency anemia; use cautiously in species in which iron storage disease is common (e.g., toucans, mynahs, starlings, birds of paradise, other passerines)
Lactobacillus (Bene-Bac, Pet-Ag)	1 pinch/day/bird[333]	Psittacines/stimulation of normal gastrointestinal flora regrowth
Lactobacillus acidophilus	0.25 g/dose mixed with diet, $2.5\text{-}6 \times 10^6$ CFU/dose[805]	Neonatal cockatiels/PD; increased growth rate in birds receiving the gel form, no effect in birds receiving the powder form; no overall benefit noted
	1 tsp/L hand-feeding formula[333]	Most species
Magnesium sulfate	20 mg/kg IM[404]	African grey parrot/dietary hypomagnesemia and seizures
Niacin (nicotinic acid)	50 mg/kg PO q8h[333]	Psittacines/yolk emboli; give with gemfibrozil (30 mg/kg PO)
Pancreatic enzyme powder (Viokase-V Powder, Fort Dodge)	—	Most species/exocrine pancreatic insufficiency; maldigestion; mix with food and let stand 30 min[333]
	2-5 g/kg[333]	Most species
	⅛ tsp/kg feed[333]	Most species
	⅛ tsp/60-120 g lightly oil-coated seed[333]	Most species
	⅛ tsp/30-120 mL hand-feeding formula prn[333]	Psittacine neonates
Phytonadione	—	See vitamin K_1
Potassium chloride (KCl)	0.5 mEq/kg PO q12h[55]	Most species/hypokalemia
Selenium (Seletoc, Schering)	0.05-0.1 mg Se/kg IM q14d[333]	Most species/neuromuscular diseases (capture myopathy, white muscle disease, some cardiomyopathies); may be useful in some cockatiels with jaw, eyelid, and tongue paralysis
	0.06 mg Se/kg IM q3-14d[333]	

TABLE 5-11 Nutritional/Mineral Support and Supplementation Used in Birds. (cont'd)

Agent	Dosage	Species/Comments
Sodium chloride (buffered salt tablet)	450 mg PO daily[333]	Penguins/prevents atrophy of salt gland; may not be needed[838]
Tannic acid	20 g/kg feed[569,570]	Starlings/PD; not effective to decrease liver-stored iron but prevented an increase in stored iron concentration
Tea (black Ceylon decaffeinated)	8 g/kg feed[727]	Starlings/PD; effectively limited iron absorption
Vitamin A (Aquasol A Parenteral, Astra)	—	1 µg = 14 U; 1 µg retinol = 3.3 U; 1 µg beta-carotene = 1.7 U; 3000 µg/kg dietary vitamin A after 269 days induced increased plasma retinol, splenic hemosiderosis and altered vocalization patterns in cockatiels;[423] toxicosis may follow oversupplementation[423,583]
	200 U/kg IM[333]	Raptor juveniles/supplemental therapy for pox infection
	2000 U/kg PO, IM[333]	Psittacines/adjunctive therapy for pox infection
	5000 U/kg IM q24h × 14 days, then 250-1000 U/kg q24h PO[333]	Psittacines/adjunctive therapy for respiratory or epithelial disease
	20,000 U/kg IM[333]	Most species/hypovitaminosis A; maximum dose; improves skin healing
	33,000 U/kg (10,000 U/300 g) IM q7d[333]	Most species/hypovitaminosis A
	50,000 U/kg IM q7d[333]	Psittacine neonates
	1 mL/135 kg IM[333]	Ostriches/hypovitaminosis A
Vitamin B1 (thiamine)	—	Thiamine deficiency; requirements may be higher if thiaminase is present in diet[b]
	1-2 mg/kg PO q24h[333]	Raptors, penguins, cranes/daily supplement
	1-2 mg/kg IM q24h[333]	Vultures, raptors, cranes, penguins/CNS signs
	1-3 mg/kg IM q7d[333]	Most species, including raptors
	1-50 mg/kg PO q24h × 7 days or indefinitely[333]	Raptors
	2 mg/kg IM[806]	Ratites/curly toe paralysis
	3-30 mg/kg IM q7d[333]	Raptors/stimulates appetite, hematopoiesis; neuromuscular disease; liver disease; supportive therapy; adjunct to sulfa therapy
	4 mg/kg IM once, then 2 mg/kg PO q12h × 5 days[116]	Juvenile goshawks/thiamine deficiency with neurologic signs

Continued

TABLE 5-11 Nutritional/Mineral Support and Supplementation Used in Birds. (cont'd)

Agent	Dosage	Species/Comments
Vitamin B1 (thiamine) (cont'd)	1-2 mg/kg feed[333]	Vultures
	25-30 mg/kg fish (wet basis)[74]	Piscivorous species/recommended level of supplementation
	2850 mg/L drinking water q7d[333]	Pigeons
Vitamin B_{12} (cyanocobalamin)	0.25-0.5 mg/kg IM q7d[333]	Most species, including psittacines, raptors/anemia
	2-5 mg/bird SC	Pigeons/vitamin B_{12} deficiency
Vitamin B complex	—	Usually dosed based on thiamine (see vitamin B_1); death has been reported in falcons following injections, which was attributed to an overdose of vitamin B_6 (pyridoxine);[699] has been used to treat folate and cobalamin dietary deficiency in a hyacinth macaw[299]
Vitamin C (ascorbic acid)	20-50 mg/kg IM q1-7d[333]	Most species, including raptors/nutritional support; supplemental therapy for pox infection
	150 mg/kg PO q24h[313]	Willow ptarmigan chicks/PD; supplemental daily requirements over 265 mg/kg diet
Vitamin D_3 (Vital E-A + D, Schering)		1 µg = 40 U; macaws are more susceptible to toxic side effects; vitamin D_2 is poorly effective in birds[177]
	3300 U/kg (1000 U/300 g) IM q7d prn[333]	Most species/hypovitaminosis D_3; hypervitaminosis D may occur with excessive use
	5000 U IM once, then 200 U PO q24h × 88d[424]	Red-legged seriema chicks/hypovitaminosis D, in combination with UV_b supplementation
	6600 U/kg IM once[333]	Most species
Vitamin E (Vitamin E20, Horse Health Products; Bo-SE, Schering Plough)	—	1 mg d α-tocopherol acetate = 1.5 U; 1 mg dL α-tocopherol acetate = 1.1 U; injectable vitamin E may have lower efficacy than oral[487]
	0.06 mg/kg IM q7d[333]	Psittacines/hypovitaminosis E
	0.06 mg/kg IM[2806]	Ratites/prevention or treatment of capture myopathy
	15 mg/kg PO once[487]	Swainson's hawks/PK; administer without food
	70 mg/kg IM q24h for up to 5 days[873]	Pelicans/hypovitaminosis E; steatitis
	200-300 mg/kg IM[333]	Ostrich chicks
	200-400 mg/bird PO q24h[333]	Great blue herons

TABLE 5-11 Nutritional/Mineral Support and Supplementation Used in Birds. (cont'd)

Agent	Dosage	Species/Comments
Vitamin E (Vitamin E20, Horse Health Products; Bo-SE, Schering Plough) (cont'd)	73.5 mg/kg fish (wet basis)[873]	Pelicans/supplementation; excessive supplementation (550-10,560 U/kg) has been associated with coagulopathy in pink-backed pelicans[557]
	100 mg/kg fish (wet basis)[74,873]	Piscivorous species/recommended level of supplementation
	4400-8800 mg/kg feed[333]	Ostrich chicks/hypovitaminosis E
Vitamin E/γ-linolenic acid (2%), linoleic acid (71%) (Derm Caps, DVM Pharmaceuticals)	0.1 mL/kg PO q24h[333]	Most species/feather picking; use liquid from gel caps
Vitamin K1 (phytonadione)	0.025-2.5 mg/kg IM q12h[333]	Most species
	0.2-2.2 mg/kg IM q4-8h until stable, then q24h × 14 days[333]	Most species, including raptors/rodenticide toxicity
	2.5 mg/kg SC q12h[538]	Red-tailed hawk/treatment of brodifacoum toxicosis
	2.5 mg/kg IM q24h until hemostasis, then q7d prn[333]	Psittacines/vitamin K responsive disorders; hematochezia; coagulopathy
	5 mg/kg IM q24h for several days[806]	Ratites/coagulopathy
	10-12.5 mg/kg SC q12h × 4 days[873]	Pelicans/coagulopathy
	10-20 mg/kg IM q12-24h[333]	Psittacines
	0.1 mg/kg feed[333]	Turkeys/PD; as effective as 1-2 mg/kg in reducing plasma prothrombin time
	5 mg/kg feed[333]	Budgerigars/vitamin K responsive bleeding disorders; mix contents of gel cap into small grain seed mix and coat seed lightly

[a]Grains and seeds commonly fed to parrots contain calcium levels of approximately 0.02%-0.1% DM.
[b]Food items known to contain appreciable amounts of thiaminase include clams, herring, smelt, and mackerel.[74]

TABLE 5-12 Ophthalmologic Agents Used in Birds.[a]

Agent	Dosage	Species/Comments
Amphotericin B	125 μg/5 mL sterile water subconjunctival[156]	Ducks (ornamental)/candidiasis of third eyelid
Amphotericin B ointment (4%) (formulated)	Topical q24h[156]	Ducks (ornamental)/candidiasis of third eyelid; administered in conjunction with systemic antifungal therapy
Atracurium	0.05 μL intracameral[127]	Great horned owls/mydriasis for cataract surgery
	0.01 mg intracameral[55]	Parrots/mydriasis for cataract surgery

Continued

TABLE 5-12 Ophthalmologic Agents Used in Birds. (cont'd)

Agent	Dosage	Species/Comments
Atropine (0.4%-0.5%)	0.6 mg/bird topical[633]	Cockatoos/PD; partial mydriasis; some birds have iridal smooth muscle; may cause ocular irritation, weakness, shallow breathing; dilute with 0.9% saline[a]
	Topical[333]	Ratites/partial mydriasis; use in combination with curariform drugs; some ratites have iridal smooth muscle[a]
Atropine (1%)	1 drop topical[462]	Double-crested cormorants/PD; no mydriasis when used alone
Bacitracin/neomycin/ polymyxin B sulfate	Small bead topical[333]	Most species/antibiotic; corneal ulcers, conjunctivitis; excessive amounts will cause eye wiping and soiled plumage
Chloramphenicol ophthalmic drops	1 drop topical q6-8h[333]	Pigeons/antibiotic
Ciprofloxacin HCl (0.3%) (Ciloxan, Alcon)	1 drop topical q4-8h[333]	Most species/antibiotic; corneal ulcers, conjunctivitis (e.g., *Chlamydia*, *Mycoplasma*)
	1 drop topical q12h; use in conjunction with tylosin 1 mg/mL drinking water × 21-77 days[501]	House finches/PD; *Mycoplasma gallisepticum* conjunctivitis
Demecarium bromide (0.125%)	1 drop topical[333]	Most species/topical anesthetic; allows removal of *Thelazia*
Dexamethasone (0.1%) ophthalmic drops	—	Pigeons/PD; ophthalmic administration results in significant adrenocortical suppression for 24 hours at 4 μg/drop[844]
	1 drop topical q4-8h[333]	Raptors/traumatic anterior uveitis without corneal ulceration
Diclofenac	1 drop topical q12h[55]	Most species/caution in species susceptible to toxicosis (*Gyps* vultures, pigeons)[563]
Edetate disodium ophthalmic drops	1 drop several times daily[333]	Most species/used to treat calcific keratopathy
Fumagillin (Fumidil B; Mid-Continent Agrimarketing)	1 drop topical q2h[115]	Amazon parrots/fungal and microsporidial keratoconjunctivitis in combination with oral albendazole
	0.114 mg/mL drops q2-3h until 1 wk postclinical signs[751]	Lovebirds/*Encephalitozoon hellem* conjunctivitis; use in combination with albendazole
	60 mg in sterile water topical[751]	Most species/filter solution to remove bacteria before applying
Gentamicin sulfate	1 drop topical q4-8h[333]	Most species/antibiotic; corneal ulcers; causes irritation
	1 drop topical q12h × 21 days[842]	House finches/PD; mycoplasmosis treatment, in combination with oral enrofloxacin, was not effective
Isoflurane	1%-2% maintenance[333]	Most species/mydriasis[a]
	1%-2.4% maintenance by air sac perfusion[120,418b]	Most species/mydriasis,[a] ocular surgery

TABLE 5-12 Ophthalmologic Agents Used in Birds. (cont'd)

Agent	Dosage	Species/Comments
Miconazole (Monistat IV, Janssen)	1 drop topical q2h[115]	Amazon parrots/fungal keratitis
Miconazole vaginal cream (2%) (Monistat, Ortho-McNeal)	Topical[7] Topical q24h × 7d[401]	Most species/antifungal Ring-billed gulls/third eyelid candidiasis
Natamycin (Natacyn, Alcon)	1 drop topical q6h[333]	Most species/antifungal; gradually taper off
Neomycin/polymixin B/dexamethasone (0.1%)	1 drop topical q8-24h[127]	Great horned owl/post cataract surgery
Neomycin/polymyxin B/gramicidin	1 drop topical q2-8h[333]	Most species/antibiotic; corneal ulcers; conjunctivitis
Oxybuprocaine (0.45%)	Topical[421]	Pigeons, buzzards/topical anesthetic of choice due to reliable effect with minimal side effects
Oxytetracycline/polymyxin B (Terramycin, Zoetis)	Small bead topical[333]	Most species/antibiotic; conjunctivitis; excessive amounts will cause eye-wiping and soiled plumage
Phenylephrine (2.5%)	Topical[333]	Ratites/partial mydriasis; use in combination with curariform drugs; some ratites have iridal smooth muscle[a]
Phenylephrine (4%-5%)	— 6 mg/bird topical[633] Topical[462]	4%-5% ophthalmic solution is not available in the United States Cockatoos/PD; partial mydriasis;[a] some birds have iridal smooth muscle; may cause ocular irritation, weakness, shallow breathing; dilute with 0.9% saline Cormorants/PD; mydriasis; use in combination with vecuronium bromide and atropine
Phenylephrine (10%)	2 drops topical, diluted to 1%[275,276,852]	Various species/diagnosis of Horner's syndrome
Pimaricin (Natacyn, Alcon)	1 drop topical q6h, taper after 14-21 days[333]	Most species/polyene antifungal
Prednisolone acetate	—	Pigeons/PD; ophthalmic administration results in significant adrenocortical suppression for 4 hr at 35 μg/drop[844]
Prednisolone acetate (1%)	1 drop topical q4-8h[333]	Raptors/traumatic anterior uveitis without corneal ulceration
Prednisolone acetate (0.12%)	1 drop topical q4h[330]	Macaw/treatment of uveitis and hyphema secondary to lymphoma
Proxymetacaine (proparacaine) (0.5%)	Topical[421] 1 drop/eye topical[773]	Topical anesthetic Hispaniolan Amazon parrots/PD; at 10 minutes: no difference in phenol red thread test values, lower Schirmer tear test values

Continued

TABLE 5-12 Ophthalmologic Agents Used in Birds. (cont'd)

Agent	Dosage	Species/Comments
Rocuronium bromide (1%)	20 μL/eye[602]	Hispaniolan Amazon parrots/PD; mydriasis from 20 to 360 min; some birds had transient palpebral paresis
	0.12 mg/eye[47]	European kestrels/PD; maximal mydriasis at 90 min, onset of action 20 min, duration of action 250 min
	0.15 mg/eye[41]	Hispaniolan Amazon parrots/PD; mydriasis starting at 5-10 min and lasting 360 min
	0.2 mg/eye[45]	Little owls/PD; maximal mydriasis at 40 min, onset of action 20 min, duration of action 290 min
	0.35-0.7 mg/eye[46]	Tawny owls/PD; maximal mydriasis at 60-80 min (depending on dose), onset of action 20 min, duration of action 240 min
	0.4 mg/eye[45]	Common buzzards/PD; maximal mydriasis at 90 min, onset of action 20 min, duration of action 240 min
Tetracaine (6%)	Topical[421]	Topical anesthetic
Tissue plasminogen activator (rTPA) (activase)	400 μL via injection[22] 25 μg intracameral[55]	Great horned owls/hyphema Prevention of hyphema post-cataract surgery
Tissue plasminogen activator (rTPA) (TNKase Tenecteplase, Genetech)	50 μg via injection[419]	Raptors/hyphema (use paracentesis into the anterior eye chamber); intraocular hemorrhage (use intravitreous injection)
Tobramycin	1 drop topical q6-12h[55]	Most species
Triamcinolone (Vetalog, Fort Dodge)	0.075 mg/kg subconjunctival[127] 0.1-0.25 mL subconjunctival[333]	Great horned owls/cataract surgery Raptors/traumatic anterior uveitis without corneal ulceration in patients where restraint is a concern
d-Tubocurarine (Curarin-Asta, Asta-Werke)	—	Mydriatic agent;[a] recommended for therapeutic use only; administer into anterior chamber; high risk of intraocular injury; topical application has no effect[418a]
	0.01-0.03 mL of 0.3% solution, intracameral[120,418b,536]	Most species, including pigeons, raptors/dilation within 15 min, duration 4-12 hr
Tylosin	Topical (mix powder 1:10 with sterile water)[7]	Cockatiels/conjunctivitis; use in conjunction with systemic treatment
Vecuronium bromide	—	Mydriatic agent; may cause respiratory paralysis or shallow breathing, ataxia, death (especially when applied bilaterally);[516] neostigmine may counteract systemic effects[a]
	0.096 mg/bird of 0.08% solution topical[633]	Cockatoos, blue-fronted Amazon parrots, African grey parrots/PD

TABLE 5-12 Ophthalmologic Agents Used in Birds. (cont'd)

Agent	Dosage	Species/Comments
Vecuronium bromide (cont'd)	0.16 mg/eye (0.4% solution)[462]	Doubled crested cormorants/PD; mydriasis; combination with atropine and phenylephrine provided more consistent and longer mydriasis
	0.18-0.22 mg/kg topical[633]	African grey parrots/PD
	0.18-0.29 mg/kg topical[633]	Cockatoos/PD
	0.24-0.28 mg/kg topical[633]	Blue-fronted Amazon parrots/PD
	0.96 mg/bird topical[633]	Cockatoos/use caution with bilateral application
	1 drop of 0.4% solution topical[853]	Cormorants, loons/dilation at 30-45 min; duration >2 hr
	2 drops of 0.4% solution topical q15min × 3 treatments[516]	Kestrels/PD; maximal effect in 65 ± 12 min
	0.5% solution topical[333,516]	Raptors/duration 1 hr
Vecuronium (V)/nitrous oxide (N)/isoflurane (I)	(V) 0.2 mg/kg IV + 1:1 ratio of oxygen to 33% (N) at 0.3 L/kg/min + (I) 1%-2.4%[333]	Most species/mydriasis and anesthesia; gases are administered via air sac cannulation; vecuronium effective up to 256 min in pigeons[a]

[a]Variable amounts of skeletal muscle are present in the avian iris, giving birds voluntary control over pupil dilation. In many avian patients, the pupils are best dilated by restraining the animal in a dark room. Consensual pupillary light reflex is generally absent in birds.

TABLE 5-13 Oncologic Agents and Radiation Therapy Used in Birds.

Agent	Dosage	Species/Comments
Acemannan	2 mg/kg intralesional q7d × 4 treatments[333]	Cockatoos/use prior to surgical debulking in fibrosarcoma
Asparaginase (Elspar, Merck)	400 U/kg IM q7d[333]	Cockatoos/lymphosarcoma; premedicate with diphenhydramine
	1650 U/kg SC once[692]	Great horned owl/sarcoma; associated with severe bone marrow suppression
Carboplatin	5 mg/kg IV, IO over 3 min[233,484]	Sulphur-crested cockatoos (PD), budgerigars/mix with 5% dextrose to 400 mg/L; renal adenocarcinoma (leg paresis showed improvement over 2 mo; mass continued to grow); mix with saline
	5 mg/kg intralesional[333]	Amazon parrots/squamous cell carcinoma; mix with sesame oil or plasma at a concentration of 10 mg/mL
	5 mg/kg IO q4wk × 3 doses[868]	Green-winged macaw/pancreatic adenocarcinoma
	15 mg/kg IV q5wk × 4 doses[133]	Mallard duck/sertoli cell tumor, survival of 13 months
	17.2 mg/kg q3-10wk × 4 doses[868]	Amazon parrot/choanal squamous cell carcinoma, survival of 9 months

Continued

TABLE 5-13 Oncologic Agents and Radiation Therapy Used in Birds. (cont'd)

Agent	Dosage	Species/Comments
Carboplatin (cont'd)	24 mg/kg q4wk × 4 doses[868]	Amazon parrot/cutaneous squamous cell carcinoma, survival of 1 year
	27 mg/kg q4wk × 4 doses[868]	Cockatiel/cutaneous squamous cell carcinoma, survival of 3 mo
	125 mg/m² IV (slow bolus) q14-21d[866]	Amazon parrot/bile duct carcinoma; dilute with 5% dextrose[a]
Chlorambucil (Leukeran, GlaxoSmithKline)	1 mg/bird PO 2×/wk[555]	Pekin duck/lymphocytic leukemia or lymphosarcoma; responded to treatment initially, but was euthanatized 1 mo after presentation because of respiratory distress and hemorrhages
	1 mg/kg PO 2×/wk[310]	Green-winged macaw/chronic lymphocytic leukemia, in combination with chlorambucil, died after 29 weeks
	1.5 mg/kg PO q72h[271]	Starling/chronic lymphocytic leukemia; follow up of 6 mo
	2 mg/kg PO 2×/wk[673]	Umbrella cockatoo/cutaneous lymphosarcoma
Cisplatin	0.2 mg/kg intralesional[227]	Black-footed penguin/choanal squamous cell carcinoma; remission for 13 mo
	Intralesional (undisclosed dose)[635]	Blue and gold macaw/facial fibrosarcoma; in combination with radiation therapy; remission for 29 mo
	1 mg/kg IV over 1 hr[231,232]	Cockatoos/PK; may cause nephrotoxicity; administer IV fluids 1 hr before and 2 hr after infusion
	17.5 mg/m² intralesional q7d × 4 treatments[408]	African grey parrot/multiple integumentary squamous cell carcinomas, did not seem effective
Cyclophosphamide	200 mg/m² IO q7d[333]	Cockatoo/lymphosarcoma[a]
	300 mg/m² PO once[692]	Great horned owl/sarcoma;[a] dose associated with severe bone marrow suppression
Deslorelin implant	4.6 mg SC q4-6mo[399]	Cockatiels/ovarian adenocarcinoma
Diphenhydramine	2 mg/kg IO once[333]	Cockatoo/before chemotherapy
Doxorubicin	2 mg/kg IV[283,284]	Cockatoos/PD; may produce mild transient inappetence; frequency was not determined; PK of metabolite doxorubicinol showed no toxicity[284]
	30 mg/m² IO q2d[333]	Cockatoo/lymphosarcoma;[a] premedicate with diphenhydramine
	60 mg/m² IV q30d[197]	Blue-fronted Amazon parrot/osteosarcoma;[a] premedicate with diphenhydramine 30 min before; dilute with saline and give over 30 min (anesthesia recommended); remission for 20 mo

TABLE 5-13 Oncologic Agents and Radiation Therapy Used in Birds. (cont'd)

Agent	Dosage	Species/Comments
Hexyl ether pyropheophorbide-a (Photochlor, Roswell Park Cancer Institute)	0.3 mg/kg IV[780,783]	African rose-ringed parakeet, hornbill/photosensitizing agent; use 24 hr prior to photodynamic therapy
L-carnitine	1000 mg/kg of food[179]	Budgerigars/PD; lipoma size decrease
Leuprolide acetate	1500-3000 µg/kg IM q2-3wk[399]	Cockatiels/ovarian adenocarcinoma
Methylprednisolone	2 mg IM once[21]	African grey parrot/bronchial carcinoma
Porfimer sodium (Photofrin, QLT PhotoTherapeutics)	3 mg/kg IV[680]	Cockatiel/photodynamic therapy
Prednisone	1 mg/kg PO q24h[310]	Green-winged macaw/chronic lymphocytic leukemia; in combination with prednisone; drug was discontinued after 6 wk because of thrombocytopenia
	1.6 mg/kg PO q24h[692]	Great horned owl/sarcoma
Radiation therapy	1 Gy at 2.5 Gy/min × 3-4 doses[166]	Military macaws/PD; radiation of normal choana; delivered dose was slightly lower (0.94-0.97 Gy) than calculated
	2.5 Gy fractions, total dose of 50 Gy[301]	Thick-billed parrot/beak melanoma; 2.5 mo survival
	4 Gy fractions, total doses of 48, 60, or 72 Gy[44]	Ring necked parakeets/PD; radiation of normal skin and crop; no adverse radiation effects detected
	4 Gy fractions q48h over 22 days, total dose of 40 Gy[434]	Blue and gold macaw/wing fibrosarcoma; in combination with cisplatin chemotherapy; remission observed over 2 mo until 15 mo
	4 Gy fractions 3d/wk × 4 wk, total dose of 48 Gy; then booster dose of 8 Gy 5 wk later[492]	Buffon's macaw/squamous cell carcinoma of the beak; no evidence of tissue or tumor damage
	4 Gy fractions 4d/wk, total dose of 40 Gy[266]	Budgerigar/metacarpal hemangiosarcoma; complete tumor regression observed; death 8 wk later from metastasis
	4 Gy fractions 3d/wk, total dose of 44 Gy[635]	Blue and gold macaw/facial fibrosarcoma; in combination with intralesional cisplatin; erythema over the tumor site; 29 mo remission
	4 Gy fractions 3d/wk, total dose of 40 Gy[590]	African grey parrot/periocular lymphoma; 2 mo survival
	4 Gy fractions 3d/wk × 6 wk, total dose of 68 Gy[259]	Umbrella cockatoo/intraocular osteosarcoma; 2 mo survival time
	5 Gy fractions q3-4d over 3 wk, total dose of 30 Gy[12b]	Blue and gold macaw/periorbital lymphoma; mass regression; 3 mo survival time
	8 Gy fraction q7d × 4 treatments, total dose of 32 Gy[788b]	African grey parrot/beak squamous cell carcinoma; 4 mo survival time
	10 Gy fractions at 0, 7, and 21 days, 2 additional doses 1 mo later, total dose of 50 Gy[8]	American flamingo/cutaneous squamous cell carcinoma; no tumor reduction

Continued

TABLE 5-13 Oncologic Agents and Radiation Therapy Used in Birds. (cont'd)

Agent	Dosage	Species/Comments
Silymarin (milk thistle)	100-150 mg/kg PO divided q8-12h[333]	Hepatic antioxidant/protectant; use in patients with liver disease and as ancillary to chemotherapy; use a low-alcohol or alcohol-free liquid formulation
Strontium (Sr-90 ophthalmic applicator)	100 Gy/area × 1-3 areas[552]	Budgerigars, cockatiels/uropygial squamous cell carcinoma; good response at 2-9 mo follow up
	100 Gy/area × 4 areas, repeated 1 wk later[612]	African grey parrots/uropygial squamous cell carcinoma; good response at 6 mo
Vincristine sulfate	0.1 mg/kg IV q7-14d[673]	Cockatoo/monitor CBC weekly; complete remission
	0.5 mg/m² IV, then 0.75 mg/m² q7d × 3 treatments[555]	Pekin duck/lymphoma; lymphocytic leukemia[a]
	0.75 mg/m² IO q7d × 3 treatments[333]	Cockatoo/lymphosarcoma[a]

[a]Body weight (kg) = surface area (m²); 0.5 kg = 0.06 m²; 1 kg = 0.1 m²; 2 kg = 0.15 m²; 3 kg = 0.2 m²; 4 kg = 0.25 m²; 5 kg = 0.29 m².

TABLE 5-14 Antimicrobial-Impregnated Polymethylmethacrylate (PMMA) Agents Used in Birds.[a,333,484]

Agent	Dosage	Species/Comments
Amikacin	1.25-2.5 g/20 g polymer powder[222]	PD/elution of amikacin from PMMA beads was greater when the powdered form was used compared with liquid amikacin
Bone cement (Surgical Simplex P Radiopaque Bone Cement, Howmedica)	—	Polymer powder and liquid monomer for use in making antibiotic impregnated beads
Cefazolin	1-2 g/20 g polymer powder[333]	
Cefotaxime	2 g/20 g polymer powder[333]	
Ceftazidime	2 g/20 g polymer powder[333]	
Ceftiofur (Naxcel, Pfizer)	2 g/20 g polymer powder[222]	Studies show elution for approximately 7 days only[145]
Ciprofloxacin	—	Release for 360 days[803]
Clindamycin	—	PMMA beads with clindamycin had adequate drug levels for more than 90 days[485,660]
Enrofloxacin	—	Raptors/pododermatitis[660]
Gentamicin	1 g powder or solution/20 g polymer powder[222]	PD/elution concentration remained greater than MIC for common pathogens for 30 days; powder and liquid forms of gentamicin had similar elution rates from PMMA

TABLE 5-14	Antimicrobial-Impregnated Polymethylmethacrylate (PMMA) Agents Used in Birds. (cont'd)	
Agent	Dosage	Species/Comments
Gentamicin (cont'd)	1 mL of 50 mg/mL solution/20 g polymer powder[660]	Raptors/pododermatitis
	Ratio PMMA:gentamicin of 20[634]	Good elution for at least 21 days
Gentamicin (Septopal, Merck)	Premade beads[333]	Commercially available in Europe; not available in the United States
Hydroxyapatite cement (BoneSource, Osteogenics)	—	Polymer powder used as an alternative to bone cement; absorbs into muscle and tissue; osteoconductive in bone; fabricates with water which aids in formulation with liquid antibiotics[222]
Itraconazole	16% intraconazole-impregnated PMMA fed as grit stones[769]	Indian peafowl/PD; antifungal agent; when used as grit, therapeutic levels achieved in 2 days and decreased over 7 days; beads from capsules mix into PMMA uniformly before hardening; PMMA cut into 1-g size pieces (grit stone size) after hardening
Meropenem	Ratio PMMA:meropenem of 5:1[35]	Elution for 15 days
Metronidazole	Ratio PMMA:metronidazole of 20-40:1[634]	Good elution for at least 21 days
Oxytetracycline	4.5 mL of 200 mg/mL solution/20 g polymer powder[660]	Raptors/pododermatitis
(R) Rifampin/(P) pefloxacin (Pelwin, 5% soluble powder, Wockhardt)	1 part (R) + 1 part (P) is finely ground in equal volumes in a mortar and pestle; thoroughly mix with 5 parts PMMA powder[660]	Rifampin powder taken from oral capsules; pefloxacin powder obtained from the preparation intended for oral use in poultry
(R) Rifampin/(P) piperacillin	1 part (R) + 1 part (P) is combined and finely ground in a mortar and pestle; thoroughly mix with 5 parts PMMA powder[660]	Rifampin powder taken from oral capsules; piperacillin powder taken from parenteral preparation prior to reconstitution
Tobramycin	—	Release for 220 days[485]

[a]Antimicrobial-impregnated polymethylmethacrylate (PMMA) is used to elute antimicrobial agents for long-term treatment of infected lesions. Following are guidelines for its use and preparation:
- Choose antibiotic based on culture and sensitivity.
- Mix 1-2 g of sterile antibiotic powder with 40-60 g of PMMA powder. Add approximately 2 Tbs to antibiotic at a time. The use of liquid antibiotic reduces the mechanical strength of the bead.
- Shake mixture well (for at least 2 min) to make it homogeneous.
- Add liquid monomer as usual.
- The dough is placed in a catheter tip syringe and extruded, rolled into beads, and placed onto steel surgical wire. Dough may also be injected into a red rubber catheter that may be cut into variable sizes. The smaller the bead, the greater the elution of antibiotic.
- Gas sterilization or UV radiation is recommended; beads are aerated for at least 24 hr at room temperature.
- The wound is aggressively debrided and beads are placed within it; the wound is then closed and the beads are left within the site until the wound is no longer infected.[333]
- In human medicine, beads are removed after 2-6 wk. Despite their antibiotic release, beads act as a surface to which bacteria preferentially adhere, grow, and potentially develop antibiotic resistance.[156] Beads are difficult to remove if left in place for more than 14 days.[581]

TABLE 5-15 Agents Used in the Treatment of Oiled Birds.

Agent	Dosage	Species/Comments
Bismuth subsalicylate	2-5 mg/kg PO once[519]	Adsorbent; gavage; alternatively, can use activated charcoal
Charcoal, activated (Toxiban, Vet-A-Mix)	52 mg/kg PO once[519]	Adsorbent; gavage; alternatively, can use bismuth subsalicylate
Charcoal, activated/electrolyte slurry (Toxiban, Vet-A-Mix)	50 mL/kg by gavage[802]	3 bottles of charcoal slurry (3.75 g/kg) added to 250 mL of electrolyte solution
Detergent (Dawn, Procter & Gamblc)	1%-5% bath[519]	Submerse bird up to mid-neck region; rinse with water; use water at 103-105°F (39-41°C) and 40-60 psi (pounds per square inch); water should be soft(ened);[519,527] sea water may also be used[506]
Fluid therapy	—	See Table 5-36 for guidelines
Iron dextran	10 mg/kg IM q5-7d[519]	If PCV <25%
Lactulose	0.3 mL/kg PO q12h[504]	Prophylactic laxative
Oral electrolyte solutions (Pedialyte; Ross Labs)	30 mL/kg by gavage[802]	Most species/at field stabilization site
Papaya enzyme	1 tablet PO q12h[504]	Prophylactic laxative
Thiamine (vitamin B_1)	25-30 mg/kg fish[519]	Piscivorous species

TABLE 5-16 Agents Used in Bird Emergencies.[a]

Agent	Dosage	Species/Comments
Aminophylline	4 mg/kg PO q6-12h[333]	Can give orally after initial response
	4 mg/kg IM q12h[742]	Pionus parrots/smoke inhalation injury
	10 mg/kg IV q3h[333]	Use for pulmonary edema
Atropine sulfate	0.02 mg/kg IM, IV, IO[452]	CPR, bradycardia
	0.2 mg/kg IM, IV, IO[333]	Bradycardia
	0.5 mg/kg IM, IV, IO, intratracheal[333]	CPR
Blood homologous transfusion	—	Administer over 1-4 hr; use filter;[109] half-life of 8-10 days; heterologous blood transfusion may not be effective[181,184]
Calcium gluconate	1-5 mg elemental calcium/kg/h[54]	CRI for ionized hypocalcemia
	50-150 mg/kg IM, IV (slow bolus)[54,333,452]	Hypocalcemia; dilute 50 mg/mL; hyperkalemia; facilitates potassium movement across cell membranes
Dexamethasone Na phosphate	2-6 mg/kg IM, IV q12-24h[333]	Head trauma (until signs abate); shock (one dose); hyperthermia (until stable)

TABLE 5-16 Agents Used in Bird Emergencies. (cont'd)

Agent	Dosage	Species/Comments
Dextrose (50%)	50-100 mg/kg IV (slow bolus to effect)[333]	Hypoglycemia; can dilute with fluids
	500-1000 mg/kg IV (slow bolus)[333,628]	Hypoglycemia; can dilute with fluids
	0.25 mL/kg after 1:1 dilution with saline[452]	Hypoglycemia
	0.5 mL/kg over 15 min[54]	Hypoglycemia
Dextran 70	10-20 mL/kg IV[333]	Most species/colloid for the adjunctive treatment of hypovolemic shock
Dobutamine	5-15 µg/kg/min[718]	Hispaniolan Amazon parrots/PD; less effective than dopamine
Dopamine	5-10 µg/kg/min[718]	Hispaniolan Amazon parrots/PD; more effective than dobutamine
Doxapram	2 mg/kg IV, IO[452]	CPR, respiratory arrest
	5-10 mg/kg IM, IV once[333]	Raptors/respiratory depression or arrest
	20 mg/kg IM, IV, IO[333]	CPR; respiratory depression
Epinephrine (1:1000)	0.01 mg/kg[452]	CPR
	0.5-1 mL/kg IM, IV, IO, intratracheal[333]	CPR; bradycardia
Fluids	10-25 mL/kg IV, IO[333]	Bolus over 5-7 min, see Table 5-37 (fluid therapy)
Hemoglobin glutamer-200 (Oxyglobin, OPK Biotech)	—	Hemoglobin polymer; hemoglobin replacement product; anemia treatment; currently unavailable, but under FDA testing by new manufacturer (Dechra)
	3-10 mL/kg IV (slow)[333]	Most species
	5 mL/kg IV[454]	Mallard ducks/PD; no difference in mortality rate from crystalloid fluids in a hemorrhagic shock model (but a trend of decreased mortality)
	10 mL/kg IV[333]	Raptors
Hetastarch	5 mL/kg IV[454]	Mallard ducks/PD; no difference in mortality rate from crystalloid fluids in a hemorrhagic shock model
	10-15 mL/kg IV (slow) q8h[333] × 1-4 treatments	Most species, including raptors/hypoproteinemia; hypovolemia
	20 mL/kg/day; 5 mL/kg bolus may be repeated twice[54]	Hypovolemia; half-life: 25 hr
Insulin/dextrose 50%	0.5 U/kg + 2 g dextrose/insulin unit[54]	Hyperkalemia
Mannitol	0.25-2 g/kg IV (slow bolus) q24h[333]	Raptors/cerebral edema; anuric renal failure
Oxyglobin	—	See Hemoglobin glutamer-200
Pentastarch	20 mL/kg/day; 5 mL/kg IV bolus[54]	Hypovolemia, half-life: 2.5 hr

Continued

TABLE 5-16 Agents Used in Bird Emergencies. (cont'd)

Agent	Dosage	Species/Comments
Potassium chloride (KCl)	Maintenance: 15-20 mEq/L Moderate hypoK: 40 mEq/L Severe hypoK: 60 mEq/L[54]	Supplement IV/IO fluids; hypokalemia; do not exceed 0.5 mEq/kg/h
Prednisolone Na succinate (Solu-Delta-Cortef, Upjohn)	10-20 mg/kg IM, IV q15min prn[333] 15-30 mg/kg IV[333]	Head trauma; CPR Raptors
Sodium bicarbonate	1 mEq/kg IV q15-30min to maximum of 4 mEq/kg total dose[333]	Metabolic acidosis
	5 mEq/kg IV, IO once[333]	CPR
	0.3 × BW(kg) × Base excess, IV bolus[54]	Most species/metabolic acidosis; give over 30-60 min
Terbutaline	0.01 mg/kg PO, IM q6h[333]	Psittacines/α_2-selective smooth muscle bronchodilator
	0.1 mg/kg PO q12-24h[333]	Macaws, Amazon parrots/bronchodilator; obstructive pulmonary disease, pneumonitis
Vasopressin	0.8 U/kg[452]	CPR

[a]Because of the presence of peripheral vasoconstriction, subcutaneous administration is not adequate for patients in shock.

TABLE 5-17 Euthanasia Agents Used in Birds.[a]

Agent	Dosage	Species/Comments
Carbon dioxide (CO_2)	70%[333]	Most species/danger to person administering gas; compressed gas is the only recommended source[442]
Carbon monoxide (CO)	Minimum 6% concentration in a closed container[333]	Most species/unconsciousness occurs rapidly; inexpensive;[333] danger to person administering gas; compressed gas recommended
Isoflurane	Saturated cotton ball in closed container or face mask[333]	Most species/very rapid induction; wing flapping and vocalizing may occur
Methoxyflurane	Saturated cotton ball in closed container or face mask[333]	Most species/induction may be slower than with isoflurane
Pentobarbital sodium	0.2-1 mL/kg IV, ICe[333]	Most species/birds may react unpredictably with IV administration; ICe administration is smooth, quiet; proper carcass disposal is advised as secondary poisoning of wild scavenging birds may occur;[336,690,832] induces significant histopathologic changes that may impair interpretation (especially for lungs)[294,632]
Potassium chloride	1-2 mEq/kg IV[442]	Most species/must be provided in conjunction with prior general anesthesia
	3-10 mEq/kg[632]	Parrots/PD; no histologic artifacts; death in 0.5-1.1 min; performed under isoflurane anesthesia

[a]The American Veterinary Medical Association accepts inhalant anesthetic overdose, carbon monoxide, carbon dioxide, KCl (after anesthesia), and barbiturate overdose as humane euthanasia methods.[442] Cervical dislocation and decapitation are conditionally acceptable for research and poultry. Thoracic compression is commonly used for wild passerine birds.[591]

TABLE 5-18 Miscellaneous Agents Used in Birds.

Agent	Dosage	Species/Comments
2-deoxy-2-fluoro-d-glucose (fluodeooxyglucose F18 injection, Siemens)	128.5 ± 20.2 MBq (3.5 ± 0.5 mCi)[380]	Bald eagles/PD; PET scan
	37 MBq (1 mCi)[754]	Amazon parrots/PD; PET scan
Acetic acid (apple cider vinegar)	15 mL/qt drinking water	Most species/intestinal dysbiosis
Acetylsalicylic acid (aspirin)	5 mg/kg PO q48h[62]	Most species, African grey parrots/anti-thrombotic agent
Allopurinol	—	Xanthine oxidase inhibitor/use in treatment of gout is controversial: 50 mg/kg given to red-tailed hawks was toxic leading to marked elevations in plasma oxypurinol, xanthine, and hypoxanthine with secondary renal dysfunction[476]
	10-30 mg/kg PO q12-24h[333]	Most species/gout
	25 mg/kg PO q24h[476,617]	Red-tailed hawks/PD; no significant effect on plasma uric acid levels
	830 mg/L drinking water[333]	Most species
	1 mL stock solution/30 mL drinking water mixed fresh several times daily (300 mg/L)[333]	Budgerigars/decrease initial dose to 25% recommended dose in severe cases and gradually increase over several days; use with colchicine in severe cases; stock solution: 100 mg tablet/10 mL sterile water
Aloe vera	Topical[333]	Most species/antiinflammatory; antithromboxane activity; beneficial in treating burns, electrical injury, or dying skin flaps;[a] see heparin for combination
Aluminum hydroxide	30-90 mg/kg PO q12h[333]	Most species/antacid; phosphate binder
Aminoloid (Aminoloid, Schering)	0.25-0.75 mg/kg IM, repeat in 10-14 days[333]	Raptors/induction of molt
Aminopentamide hydrogen sulfate (Centrine, Fort Dodge)	0.05 mg/kg SC, IM q12h up to 5 doses[333]	Most species/regurgitation
	0.11 mg/kg SC, IM q8-12h × 1 day, then q12h × 1 day, then q24h × 1 day[333]	Most species/regurgitation
Aminophylline	4 mg/kg PO, IM q6-12h[333]	Most species/bronchodilator; need to prepare as a suspension daily
	5 mg/kg PO, IV q12h[450]	Psittacines
	8-10 mg/kg PO, IM, IV q6-8h[333,806]	Most species, including ratites/may be diluted prior to injection; initial doses may be given IV; subsequent doses given PO once response is observed
Ammonium solution	Topical prn[333]	Most species/analgesic; antipruritic; antiinflammatory; can use on fresh wounds; avoid overuse[a]

Continued

TABLE 5-18   Miscellaneous Agents Used in Birds. (cont'd)

Agent	Dosage	Species/Comments
Arginine vasopressin	24 µg/kg IM q12h[766]	African grey parrots/central diabetes insipidus; oral administration was not effective
Arginine vasotocin	0.5-4 µg/kg intranasal q12h[439]	African grey parrots/central diabetes insipidus
Armor All Protectant (Armor All Protectant Corp)	Topical to affected plumage[333]	Most species/soften sticky-trap glue covered plumage; use detergent (Dawn) to remove Armor All
Atenolol	5-10 mg/kg PO q12-24h[58]	Most species
Atorvastatin (Lipitor, Pfizer)	10-20 mg/kg PO q12h[55]	Parrots/hypercholesterolemia; needs to be compounded from tablets
Barium sulfate	—	Dilute 72% suspension 1:1 with water; dilute 92% suspension 1:2 with water; 60% suspension effective in Amazon parrots;[63,218] more dilute concentrations (20%-25%) can also be used;[833] administer ½ volume diluted barium and ½ volume air for double contrast study of crop[333]
	15 mL/kg PO of 1:1 barium 60% and hand feeding formula[63]	Amazon parrots/PD; contrast fluoroscopy
	20 mL/kg PO of barium 25%[833]	Amazon parrots/PD; contrast fluoroscopy, radiography
	20-25 mL/kg PO via gavage[333]	Most species
	25-50 mL/kg PO[333]	Most species/smaller species require relatively more contrast media; African grey parrots, 25 mL/kg; Quaker parakeets and budgerigars, 50 mL/kg
		Amazon parrots/PD; contrast fluoroscopy, radiography
Benazepril	0.5 mg/kg PO q24h[18b,206]	Parrots
Bismuth subsalicylate	1-2 mL/kg PO q12h[333]	Most species/weak adsorbent, demulcent
Bromhexine HCl	1.5 mg/kg IM q12-24h[333]	Most species/expectorant
	3-6 mg/kg IM[333]	Most species, including psittacines, passerines, raptors
	6.5 mg/L drinking water[333]	Psittacines
	1200 mg/L drinking water[333]	Most species
Cimetidine	—	Prototype histamine-2 blocker used to reduce gastrointestinal acid production
	3-5 mg/kg PO, IV q8h[806]	Ratites
	5 mg/kg PO, IM q8-12h[333]	Psittacines/proventriculitis; gastric ulceration
	5-10 mg/kg IM q12h[806]	Ratites

TABLE 5-18 Miscellaneous Agents Used in Birds. (cont'd)

Agent	Dosage	Species/Comments
Cisapride	—	Gastrointestinal prokinetic agent, stimulates motility in mammals;[615] not commercially available in the United States; can be compounded
	0.5-1.5 mg/kg PO q8-12h[333]	Most species
Citrate phosphate dextrose adenine solution (CPDA)	1 part CPDA:5-6 parts whole blood[288,333,530]	Most species/anticoagulant for blood collection for transfusion; not for extended storage of whole blood;[530] a cryopreservation study has also been published[288]
Citric acid	5000 mg/L drinking water[333]	Most species/reduces the effect of calcium and magnesium on the absorption of tetracyclines
Colchicine	—	Unique antiinflammatory used in the treatment of gout or hepatic fibrosis/cirrhosis;[615] may potentiate gout formation in some cases[333]
	0.01 mg/kg PO q12h[333]	Juvenile macaws/gout
	0.04 mg/kg PO q12-24h[347]	Most species/gradually increase to q12h
	0.2 mg/kg PO q12h[333]	Psittacines
Copper sulfate (Cu-7, Searle)	Topical[333]	Most species/ulcerative dermatitis[a]
Cyclosporine	10 mg/kg PO q12h[353]	Cockatiels/PD; ineffective at preventing avian bornaviral lesions
	10 mg/kg IV[813]	Pekin ducks/PK; low plasma levels and high clearance
	10-20 mg/kg PO q24h[55]	Most species/no detectable plasma level in a single African grey parrot case
Digoxin	—	Toxic reactions include depression, ataxia, vomiting, diarrhea; contraindicated with renal or liver disease; monitoring of serum digoxin, potassium, magnesium, calcium, and ECG is recommended; induced arrythmias in pigeons at 0.2 mg/kg/day[333]
	0.01-0.02 mg/kg PO q12h[333]	Psittacines, passerines, raptors/congestive heart disease
	0.02 mg/kg PO q24h × 5 days[309]	Budgerigars, sparrows (PD)/produces a plasma concentration of 1.6 μg/mL (within mammalian therapeutic range); this dose led to signs of toxicity in a mynah[679]
	0.05 mg/kg PO q24h[858]	Quaker parakeets/PK; congestive heart failure; cardiomyopathy
	0.066 mg/kg IV q12h[594]	Pekin ducks/PK; short half-life
	0.13 mg/L drinking water[333]	Psittacines, passerines, raptors/congestive heart disease

Continued

TABLE 5-18 Miscellaneous Agents Used in Birds. (cont'd)

Agent	Dosage	Species/Comments
Dimethylsulfoxide (90%)	1 mL/kg topical to affected area q4-7d[333]	Most species/antiinflammatory, analgesic; systemic absorption; use gloves during application[a]
Dioctyl sodium sulfosuccinate	33 mL/L drinking water[333]	Psittacine chicks/constipation; use only if chick is drinking
Diphenhydramine	1-4 mg/kg PO q8-12h[333]	Most species/hypersensitivity; pruritus; anxiety; may cause hypotension
	2 mg/kg IV, IO once[333]	Cockatoos/use prior to chemotherapy
	20-40 mg/L drinking water[333]	Most species
Diphenoxylate with atropine (Lomotil, Searle)	2-2.5 mg/kg PO q8h[806]	Ratites/opiate; gastrointestinal motility modifier
EDTA-tromethamine or EDTA-Tris	IT, intranasal, or wound lavage[333]	Most species/potentiates the effect of antibiotics on resistant bacteria;[225] 1.2 g EDTA + 6.05 g Tris added to 1 L sterile water, pH adjusted to 8 with a dilute solution of sodium hydroxide, autoclaved × 15 min; Tris-EDTA may also be added to chlorhexidine solution[28]
Enalapril	0.2-0.5 mg/kg q24h[333]	Most species
	1.25 mg/kg PO q8-12h[596]	Pigeons, Amazon parrots/PD
	2.5-5 mg/kg PO q12h[597]	Amazon parrot/right-sided heart failure; long-term therapy
	5 mg/kg PO q24h[333]	Lovebirds
Ferric subsulfate	Topical[333]	Most species/hemostasis of bleeding nail or beak tip; will cause necrosis if used on open skin lesions
Furosemide	—	Diuretic; overdose can cause dehydration and electrolyte abnormalities
	0.1-2 mg/kg PO, SC, IM, IV q6-24h[58,333,595,806]	Most species, including psittacines, raptors, pigeons, mynahs, ratites; lories are extremely sensitive[333]
	0.15 mg/kg IM[333]	Psittacine neonates/pulmonary congestion
	1-5 mg/kg IM q2-12h[234]	Parrots/acute treatment of congestive heart failure
	1-10 mg/kg PO q8-12h[234]	Parrots/maintenance treatment of congestive heart failure
	2-6 mg/kg PO, IM[333]	Raptors
	40 mg/L drinking water[333]	Most species/congestive heart failure; can be used with digoxin and ACE inhibitors
Gadopentate dimeglumine (Magnevist, Berlex)	0.25 mmol/kg IV[677]	Pigeons/PD; contrast agent for magnetic resonance imaging
Gallium-67 citrate (Ga-67)	0.5 mCi (microcuries)/bird IV[392]	Green-winged macaws/radiopharmaceutical used for detection of infection and inflammatory lesions; requires a gamma camera for imaging

TABLE 5-18 Miscellaneous Agents Used in Birds. (cont'd)

Agent	Dosage	Species/Comments
Gemfibrozil	30 mg/kg PO q8h[333]	Psittacines/lipid regulating agent; yolk emboli; sometimes effective in controlling signs; gradual improvement may be seen over weeks to months; give with niacin
Gentian violet (crystal violet)	Topical[333]	Raptors/wound management[a]
Glipizide	—	Sulfonylurea antidiabetic; contraindicated in ketotic patients; patients should be maintained at trace glucosuria to prevent hypoglycemia[333]
	0.5 mg/kg PO q12h[333]	Cockatiels/diabetes mellitus; did not reduce blood glucose in a Bali mynah[48]
	1.25 mg/kg PO q24h[333]	Most species/diabetes mellitus; did not reduce blood glucose in a macaw[274]
	2 mg/kg PO q8-12h[55]	Cockatiels/diabetes mellitus; reduced blood glucose and fructosamine in one case
Glycosaminoglycan	—	See polysulfated glycosaminoglycan
Guaifenesin	0.8 mg/kg PO q12h[611]	Severe macaws/expectorant, bronchodilation
Heparin	2 U/mL whole blood[181]	Cockatiels, conures/anticoagulant for blood transfusions
Heparin/aloe vera	Topical to affected area[333]	Most species/antiinflammatory; dilute 1000 U heparin/150 mg aloe vera[a]
Hyaluronidase	5 U/kg IV q12h × 1-3 days then 2 ×/wk prn[333]	Psittacines/egg-yolk related disease; egg yolk visually apparent in blood or serum; dilute with an equal or greater quantity of isotonic NaCl
	75-150 U/L fluids[333]	Most species/increases absorption rate of fluids
	Few drops to the lumen of feather shaft at the base[340]	Raptors/flight feather pulling
Hydroxyzine	2-2.2 mg/kg PO q8h[333]	Amazon parrots/allergic pruritus; feather picking; self-mutilation
	34-40 mg/L drinking water[333]	Most species/respiratory allergy; feather picking
Iohexol (Omnipaque, Sanofi Winthrop)	2-3 mL/kg IV over 3-5 sec[66,67]	Most parrots/PD; angiography; CT contrast; distribution of contrast is extremely fast in vascular system
	25-30 mL/kg PO[218]	Cockatoos, Amazon parrots/gavage; radiographic gastrointestinal iodinated contrast media; 1:1 dilution with water can also be used
	50 mL/kg PO[333]	Quaker parakeets, budgerigars
Isoxsuprine	5-10 mg/kg PO q24h × 20-40 days[333]	Raptors/peripheral vasodilator; wingtip edema
	10 mg/kg PO q24h[741]	Amazon parrots/atherosclerosis

Continued

TABLE 5-18 Miscellaneous Agents Used in Birds. (cont'd)

Agent	Dosage	Species/Comments
Kaolin/pectin	2 mL/kg PO q6-12h[333]	Psittacine neonates/intestinal protectant, antidiarrheal
	≤15 mL/kg PO, repeat prn[333]	Raptors
Lactulose	—	Does not treat liver disease; reduces blood ammonia levels; exerts osmotic effect in birds with caeca through fermentation to acetic and lactic acid[615]
	150-650 mg/kg (0.2-1 mL/kg) PO q8-12h[333]	Most species, including psittacines/hepatic encephalopathy
	200 mg/kg (0.3 mL/kg) PO q8-12h[333]	Psittacine neonates
Magnesium hydroxide (M)/ activated charcoal (C)	(M) 10-12 mL + (C) 1 tsp powder PO[333]	Most species/cathartic; adsorbent
Magnesium sulfate (Epsom salts)	—	Purgative, cathartic; may cause lethargy;[333] see peanut butter for combination
	0.25-1 g/kg PO q24h × 1-2 days[333]	Most species, including raptors
	¼ tsp/bird PO[806]	Ratite juveniles/obstipation
	2 Tbs/bird PO[806]	Ratite adults/obstipation
Mannitol	—	Osmotic diuretic used to treat cerebral edema, especially after head trauma; may be used with furosemide; also used to treat glaucoma
	0.25-2 g/kg q24h IV (slow bolus)[333]	Most species, including raptors
	1500 mg/kg IV q6h[806]	Ratites
Maropitant	1 mg/kg SC, IM[55]	Parrots
Methocarbamol	32.5 mg/kg PO q12h[333]	Cranes (desmoiselle), swans/capture myopathy
	50 mg/kg IV (slow bolus)[333]	Most species, including demoiselle cranes, swans/muscle relaxation; capture myopathy; may be given q12h for muscle relaxation
Metoclopramide	—	Gastrointestinal motility disorders; regurgitation; slow crop motility; extrapyramidal signs may be seen as an adverse effect[55]
	0.1 mg/kg IV[806]	Ostriches
	0.5-1 mg/kg PO, IM, IV q8-12h[333]	Most species, including psittacines/gastrointestinal ileus; regurgitation
	1 mg/kg IM[97]	Amazon parrots/PD; no alterations in motility observed
	2 mg/kg IM, IV q8-12h[333]	Raptors, waterfowl/crop stasis; ileus
	12.5 mg/kg PO[806]	Ratites/gastrointestinal disorders
Mexiletine	4-8 mg/kg PO q12-24h[55]	Parrots

TABLE 5-18 Miscellaneous Agents Used in Birds. (cont'd)

Agent	Dosage	Species/Comments
Mineral oil	—	Cathartic; used to aid passage of grit and other foreign bodies; administer directly into the crop because oral administration may result in aspiration pneumonia; see peanut butter for combination
	≤5 mL/kg via gavage or per cloaca[333]	Most species, including psittacines, raptors
	5-10 mL/kg PO via gavage[333]	Most species, including psittacines/cathartic
	15 mL/kg PO via gavage[806]	Ratite adults/impaction
Nicarbazin (Ovocontrol, Innolytics)	—	Inhibits sperm receptor sites on the vitelline membrane to prevent fertilization of eggs; check federal and state permit requirements prior to use
	Formulated pellets provided at baiting stations[333]	Pigeons, waterfowl/egg hatch control
Peanut butter	Peanut butter and mineral oil (2:1)[333]	Most species/add to diet; cathartic
	Dilute peanut butter and magnesium sulfate[333]	Most species/add to diet; cathartic; dilute with water
	1 mL combined with mineral oil (2:1)[477]	Budgerigars/PD; cathartic;[a] experimental lead particles administration; faster elimination time than controls but not statistically significant
Pentoxifylline	15-25 mg/kg PO q8-12h[495,841]	Most species/frostbite
	30 mg/kg PO q12h × 5 days[55,60]	Most species/improve peripheral perfusion; peripheral arterial disease; raptor wingtip edema
Perflutren lipid microspheres (Definity, Lantheus Medical)	0.1 mL/bird IV[67]	Most birds/ultrasound contrast agent; necessitates a mechanical activating device
	0.1 mL/bird IV diluted with 0.9 mL NaCl[65]	Red-tailed hawks/PD; lasted several min in cardiac chambers
Pimobendan	0.25 mg/kg PO q12h[101]	Harris hawks/congestive heart failure; therapeutic drug monitoring performed
	0.25 mg/kg PO q12h[57,726,819]	Parrots
	6-10 mg/kg PO q12h[234]	Parrots
	10 mg/kg PO q12h[302]	Hispaniolan Amazon parrots/PK
Policosanol	0.3-2 mg PO q25h[253]	Psittacines/hyperlipidemia; use was reported in 2 birds
Polysulfated glycosaminoglycan (PSGAG) (Adequan, Luitpold)	—	Used for osteoarthritis in a variety of birds; coagulopathies including 3 deaths reported in 4 birds following IM injection[4]
	5 mg/kg IM q7d[333]	Pekin ducks/degenerative joint disease

Continued

TABLE 5-18 Miscellaneous Agents Used in Birds. (cont'd)

Agent	Dosage	Species/Comments
Polysulfated glycosaminoglycan (PSGAG) (Adequan, Luitpold) (cont'd)	10 mg/kg IM, intrarticular q7d × 3 mo[333,781]	Most species, including pheasants, vultures, cranes/noninfectious or traumatic joint dysfunction; 250 mg/mL for intraarticular use; 500 mg/mL for IM use
	500 mg/bird IM q4d × 7 treatments[806]	Ratites
Povidone-iodine	Topical, wash off within 5 min[333]	Raptors/wound cleansing
Probenecid	—	Not currently recommended for the treatment of gout; may exacerbate the condition[333]
	125 mg/kg PO q6h[333]	Macaw chicks/antigout
Probucol (Lorelco, Marion Merrell Dow)	1 drop stock/300 g PO q12h × 2-4 mo[333]	Most species/low density lipoprotein-cholesterolemia; contains iron: use cautiously in species susceptible to hemochromatosis; may increase bile acids; use with low-fat diet; prepare stock: crush 250-mg tablet/7.5 mL lactulose
Propentofylline (Vivitonin, Hoechst)	5 mgP/kg PO q12h × 20-40 days[333]	Raptors/wingtip edema; dry gangrene syndrome
Propranolol	0.04 mg/kg IV (slow)[333] 0.2 mg/kg IM[333]	Most species/supraventricular arrhythmia, atrial flutter, fibrillation
Psyllium (Metamucil, Procter & Gamble)	0.5 tsp/60 mL hand feeding formula[333]	Most species/bulk diet; can use mineral oil as alternative or in addition to psyllium
	1 mL of a solution made of ½ tsp diluted in 60 mL of water[477]	Budgerigars/PD; cathartic;[a] experimental lead particles administration, similar elimination time than controls
	1 Tbs/60 mL water/bird PO, up to 120 mL/day[806]	Ratite chicks/impaction
Rosuvastatin	10-25 mg/kg PO[64]	Hispaniolan Amazon parrots/PD; low plasma levels
Sodium benzoate	1 tsp/L (5 mL/L)[354]	Budgerigars/treatment of macrorhabdosis; may be toxic to chicks and breeding birds due to increase water consumption
Sildenafil	2.5 mg/kg PO q8h[99]	Amazon parrots/pulmonary hypertension treatment
Silymarin (milk thistle)	10-100 mg/kg PO q24h × 21 days[297]	Pigeons/PD; no demonstrable hepatoprotective effect in experimental hepatitis
	50-75 mg/kg PO q12h[333]	Most species
	100-150 mg/kg PO divided q8-12h[333]	Most species/hepatic antioxidant; use in patients with liver disease and as ancillary to chemotherapy; use a low-alcohol or alcohol-free liquid formulation

TABLE 5-18 Miscellaneous Agents Used in Birds. (cont'd)

Agent	Dosage	Species/Comments
Skin-So-Soft (Avon)	Topical to affected plumage[333]	Most species/softens and removes sticky-trap glue from plumage; use Dawn dish detergent to remove Skin-So-Soft product[a]
Sodium tetradecyl sulfate	2 mg/kg diluted at 5% topical[59]	Most species/fibrotic agent; topical administration in cervicocephalic diverticulum in case of hyperinflation
Spironolactone	1 mg/kg PO q12h[58,726]	Parrots/diuretic
Sucralfate	25 mg/kg PO q8h[333]	Most species, including raptors/oral, esophageal, gastric, duodenal ulcers; give 1 hr before food or other drugs[333]
^{99m}Technetium-disofenin	1 mCi (microcuries)[183] in a commercial liquid or solid diet PO	African grey parrots/radionucleotide used for gastrointestinal scintigraphy
^{99m}Technetium-mebrofenin	1.5-2 mCi[297,307]	Pigeons/PD; liver scintigraphy
^{99m}Technetium-diethylene-triaminepenta-acetic acid (DTPA)	42 ± 0.16 MBq (1.158 $\pm$ 0.164 mCi [microcuries])/bird IV[493]	Pigeons/PD; radiopharmaceutical agent of choice for the assessment of renal function
Terbutaline	0.01 mg/kg PO, IM q6h[450]	Psittacines/α_2-selective smooth muscle bronchodilator
	0.1 mg/kg PO q12-24h[333]	Macaws, Amazon parrots/bronchodilator; obstructive pulmonary disease; pneumonitis
Theophylline	2 mg/kg PO q12h[611]	Severe macaws/bronchodilation
	5-10 mg/kg PO q12h[55]	Blue and gold macaws/chronic obstructive pulmonary disease
	10 mg/kg PO q12h[55]	Amazon parrots/syringeal masses
Tincture of iodine	Topical[333]	Raptors/wounds; inexpensive; readily available in developing countries[a]
Trilostane	1 mg/kg PO q24h[817]	Senegal parrots/Cushing's disease
Trypsin-balsam of Peru-castor oil (Granulex, Pfizer)	Topical[333]	Most species/digests necrotic tissue (may have debriding action); may have analgesic effects; may cause local inflammation and pyogenic reaction; do not use for long-term management[a]
Tyrode's solution	Offer in place of drinking water[333]	Cockatiels/restores renal-medullary gradient; add 8 g NaCl, 0.13 g $CaCl_2$, 0.2 g KCl, 0.1 g $MgCl_2$, 0.05 g Na_2HPO_4, 1 g $NaHCO_3$, 1 g glucose to 1 L water
Urate oxidase (Uricozyme, Sanofi Winthrop)	100-200 U/kg IM q24h[616,617]	Red-tailed hawks, pigeons/PD; significantly lowered plasma uric acid, including postprandial plasma uric acid
Ursodeoxycholic acid	15 mg/kg PO q24h[55]	Most species
Vegetable oil	15 mL/kg PO[806]	Ratites/impaction
Yeast cell derivatives (Preparation H, WhiteHall)	Topical q24h[333]	Most species/pododermatitis; stimulation of epithelialization; one of the four commercial products contains 1% hydrocortisone[a]

[a]Many topical agents contain oils that adhere to plumage. These agents should be used sparingly and generally in nonfeathered regions to prevent losing the insulative properties of the plumage.

TABLE 5-19 Hematologic and Biochemical Values of Selected Psittaciformes.

Measurement	African Grey Parrot (*Psittacus* spp.)[155,269]	Amazon Parrots (*Amazona* spp.)[155,269]	Orange-winged Amazon Parrot (*Amazona amazonica*)[827b]
Hematology			
PCV (%)	45-53	41-53	51 (42-60)
RBC ($10^6/\mu L$)	2.84-3.62	2.45-3.18	2.47 (2.40-3.67)
Hgb (g/dL)	12.7-15.9	12.2-15.9	—
MCV (fL)	144-155	160-175	166 (138-193)
MCH (pg)	36.4-43.9	47.2-56.8	—
MCHC (g/dL)	25.4-28.1	29.1-31.9	—
WBC ($10^3/\mu L$)	6-13	6-17	8 (0.7-16)
Heterophils $10^3/\mu L$ (%)	4.64-7.52	3.81-8.73	3.07 (0.71-7.24)
	45-73	31-71	—
Lymphocytes $10^3/\mu L$ (%)	1.96-5.15	2.40-6.48	4.55 (0-10.8)
	19-50	20-54	—
Monocytes $10^3/\mu L$ (%)	0-0.21	0.12-0.36	0.38 (0.09-0.86)
	0-2	1-3	—
Eosinophils $10^3/\mu L$ (%)	0-0.10	0.12-0.24	0.05
	0-1	1-2	—
Basophils $10^3/\mu L$ (%)	0-0.1	0-0.12	—
	0-1	0-1	—
H:L ratio	—	—	—
Chemistries			
ALP (U/L)	20-160	15-150	46 (18-120)
ALT (U/L)	5-12	5-11	—
Amylase (U/L)	210-530	205-510	—
AST (U/L)	109-305	141-437	168 (125-375)
Bile acid ($\mu mol/L$)			
RIA	13.7-73.6	10.3-79.3	—
Colorimetric	12-96	33-154	20 (8-88)
BUN (mg/dL)	3-5.4	—	1 (0-2)
Calcium (mg/dL)	7.7-11.3	8.2-10.9	9.1 (7.7-10.4)
Chloride (mEq/L)	—	—	110 (105-114)
Cholesterol (mg/dL)	160-425	180-305	237 (110-363)
CK (U/L)	228-322	125-345	341 (182-1459)
Creatinine (mg/dL)	0.1-0.4	0.1-0.4	—
GGT (U/L)	1-10	—	—
Glucose (mg/dL)	206-275	221-302	266 (213-371)
LDH (U/L)	145-465	155-425	—

TABLE 5-19 Hematologic and Biochemical Values of Selected Psittaciformes. (cont'd)

Measurement	African Grey Parrot (*Psittacus* spp.)	Amazon Parrots (*Amazona* spp.)	Orange-winged Amazon Parrot (*Amazona amazonica*)
Lipase (U/L)	35-350	35-225	—
Phosphorus (mg/dL)	3.2-5.4	3.1-5.5	3.1 (1.2-5.0)
Potassium (mEq/L)	2.9-4.6	3-4.5	3.2 (1.3-5.0)
Protein, total (g/dL)	3.2-5.2	3-5.2	4.2 (3.4-4.9)
Albumin (g/dL)	1.22-2.52	1.79-2.81	—
Globulin (g/dL)	—	—	—
A:G ratio	1.02-2.59	1.21-2.29	—
Prealbumin (g/dL)	0.30-0.92	0.6-1.23	—
α-globulin (g/dL)	0.06-0.20 (α_1)	0.09-0.23 (α_1)	—
	0.10-0.28 (α_2)	0.20-0.42 (α_2)	—
β-globulin (g/dL)	0.49-0.88	0.33-0.89	—
γ-globulin (g/dL)	0.21-0.81	0.21-0.72	—
Sodium (mEq/L)	157-165	125-155	150 (146-154)
Triglycerides (mg/dL)	45-145	49-190	14 (69-234)
Uric acid (mg/dL)	2.7-8.8	2.1-8.7	1.6 (1.9-12.7)

Measurement	Budgerigar Parakeet (*Melopsittacus undulatus*)[155,269,346]	Caique (*Pionites* spp.)[155,269]	Cockatiel (*Nymphicus hollandicus*)[155,269]
Hematology			
PCV (%)	44-58	47-55	43-57
RBC (10^6/μL)	3.77-4.6	—	3.1-4.4
Hgb (g/dL)	12.4-16.9	—	10.2-14.7
MCV (fL)	116-127	—	126-142
MCH (pg)	23.1-30.9	—	26.4-35.8
MCHC (g/dL)	19.8-23.9	—	20.4-25.2
WBC (10^3/μL)	3-10	8-15	5-11
Heterophils 10^3/μL (%)	2.68-4.55	4.68-8.64	3.68-5.76
	40-75	39-72	46-72
Lymphocytes 10^3/μL (%)	1.47-4.02	2.4-7.32	2.08-4.8
	20-45	20-61	26-60
Monocytes 10^3/μL (%)	0-0.13	0-0.24	0-0.08
	0-2	0-2	0-1
Eosinophils 10^3/μL (%)	0	0-0.12	0-0.16
	0	0-1	0-2
Basophils 10^3/μL (%)	0-0.13	0-0.12	0-0.08
	0-1	0-1	0-1
H:L ratio	—	—	—

Continued

TABLE 5-19   Hematologic and Biochemical Values of Selected Psittaciformes. (cont'd)

Measurement	Budgerigar Parakeet (Melopsittacus undulatus)	Caique (Pionites spp.)	Cockatiel (Nymphicus hollandicus)
Chemistries			
ALP (U/L)	10-80	—	20-250
ALT (U/L)	—	—	5-11
Amylase (U/L)	302-560	244-290	205-490
AST (U/L)	55-154	193-399	160-383
Bile acid (μmol/L)			
RIA	20-65	11.8-56.7	11.7-80.7
Colorimetric	32-117	12-112	44-108
BUN (mg/dL)	3-5.2	—	2.9-5
Calcium (mg/dL)	6.4-11.2	7.1-11.5	7.3-10.7
Chloride (mEq/L)	—	—	—
Cholesterol (mg/dL)	145-275	—	140-360
CK (U/L)	54-252	134-427	58-245
Creatinine (mg/dL)	0.1-0.4	—	0.1-0.4
GGT (U/L)	1-10	—	1-30
Glucose (mg/dL)	254-399	167-366	249-363
LDH (U/L)	154-271	—	120-455
Lipase (U/L)	—	—	30-280
Phosphorus (mg/dL)	3-5.2	—	3.2-4.8
Potassium (mEq/L)	2.2-3.7	—	2.4-4.6
Protein, total (g/dL)	2-3	2.4-4.6	2.4-4.8
Albumin (g/dL)	—	0.96-2.04	0.78-1.75
Globulin (g/dL)	—	—	—
A:G ratio	—	1.09-2.76	1.01-2.19
Prealbumin (g/dL)	—	0.33-0.89	0.59-1.24
α-globulin (g/dL)	—	0.05-0.17 (α_1)	0.05-0.32 (α_1)
	—	0.13-0.38 (α_2)	0.07-0.39 (α_2)
β-globulin (g/dL)	—	0.34-0.99	0.34-0.81
γ-globulin (g/dL)	—	0.13-0.50	0.15-0.60
Sodium (mEq/L)	139-159	—	130-153
Triglycerides (mg/dL)	—	—	45-200
Uric acid (mg/dL)	3-8.6	3.4-12.2	3.5-11

TABLE 5-19 Hematologic and Biochemical Values of Selected Psittaciformes. (cont'd)

Measurement	Cockatoos (Cacatuidae)[269,365]	Conures (*Aratinga* and *Pyrrhura* spp.)[155,269]	Eclectus Parrot (*Eclectus roratus*)[155,269]
Hematology			
PCV (%)	40-54	42-54	45-55
RBC ($10^6/\mu L$)	2.44-3.34	2.9-4.5	2.5-3.7
Hgb (g/dL)	11.1-16.0	12-16	11.1-13.9
MCV (fL)	158-175	90-190	157-170
MCH (pg)	40.4-53.7	28-55	37.5-44.6
MCHC (g/dL)	25.8-31.5	—	22.69-27.53
WBC ($10^3/\mu L$)	5-13	5-13	9-15
Heterophils $10^3/\mu L$ (%)	4.68-7.49	4.22-6.91	5.75-8.75
	45-72	44-72	46-70
Lymphocytes $10^3/\mu L$ (%)	2.08-5.20	2.11-4.89	2.87-7.12
	20-50	22-51	23-57
Monocytes $10^3/\mu L$ (%)	0-0.2	0-0.09	0-0.12
	0-2	0-1	0-1
Eosinophils $10^3/\mu L$ (%)	0-0.2	0-0.09	0-0.12
	0-2	0-1	0-1
Basophils $10^3/\mu L$ (%)	0-0.1	0-0.09	0-0.12
	0-1	0-1	0-1
H:L ratio	—	—	1-2
Chemistries			
ALP (U/L)	15-255	80-250	—
ALT (U/L)	6-12	5-13	5-11
Amylase (U/L)	200-510	100-450	200-645
AST (U/L)	117-314	178-307	148-378
Bile acid ($\mu mol/L$)			
RIA	10.3-79.1	8.3-85.2	9.7-87.5
Colorimetric	34-112	32-105	30-110
BUN (mg/dL)	3-5.1	2.5-5.4	3.5-5
Calcium (mg/dL)	8.3-10.8	7.9-10.8	7.9-11.4
Chloride (mEq/L)	—	—	—
Cholesterol (mg/dL)	135-355	120-400	130-350
CK (U/L)	106-305	154-355	118-345
Creatinine (mg/dL)	0.1-0.4	0.1-0.4	0.1-0.4
GGT (U/L)	1-45	1-15	1-20
Glucose (mg/dL)	214-302	217-323	220-294
LDH (U/L)	220-550	120-390	200-425
Phosphorus (mg/dL)	2.5-5.5	2-10	2.9-6.5
Potassium (mEq/L)	2.5-4.5	3.4-5	3.5-4.3

Continued

TABLE 5-19 Hematologic and Biochemical Values of Selected Psittaciformes. (cont'd)

Measurement	Cockatoos (Cacatuidae)	Conures (Aratinga and Pyrrhura spp.)	Eclectus Parrot (Eclectus roratus)
Protein, total (g/dL)	3-5	2.8-4.6	3-5
Albumin (g/dL)	1.11-2.28	1.01-1.94	1.23-2.26
Globulin (g/dL)	—	—	—
A:G ratio	1.06-2.54	1.08-2.73	1.09-2.50
Prealbumin (g/dL)	0.29-0.83	0.39-1.12	0.31-1.18
α-globulin (g/dL)	0.07-0.16 (α_1)	0.07-0.17 (α_1)	0.08-0.19 (α_1)
	0.09-0.26 (α_2)	0.18-0.43 (α_2)	0.10-0.30 (α_2)
β-globulin (g/dL)	0.39-0.89	0.30-0.81	0.46-0.89
γ-globulin (g/dL)	0.18-0.61	0.12-0.55	0.17-0.63
Sodium (mEq/L)	130-155	135-149	130-145
Triglycerides (mg/dL)	45-200	50-300	—
Uric acid (mg/dL)	2.9-11.0	3.0-11.4	2.5-8.7

Measurement	Grey-Cheeked Parakeet (Brotogeris pyrrhoptera)[269]	Jardine's Parrot (Poicephalus gulielmi)[155]	Lories and Lorikeets[155,269]
Hematology			
PCV (%)	45-56	41-53	47-55
RBC (10^6/μL)	—	3.03-4.47	3.3-4
Hgb (g/dL)	—	—	10.8-14.8
MCV (fL)	—	—	128-140
MCH (pg)	—	—	27.5-31.4
MCHC (g/dL)	—	—	20.3-23.1
WBC (10^3/μL)	4-12	4.1-12.6	8-13
Heterophils 10^3/μL (%)	3.74-5.64	—	4.21-6.48
	45-68	55-75	39-60
Lymphocytes 10^3/μL (%)	1.83-3.98	—	2.38-7.45
	22-48	25-45	22-69
Monocytes 10^3/μL (%)	0-0.08	—	0-0.22
	0-1	0-2	0-2
Eosinophils 10^3/μL (%)	0-0.08	—	0-0.11
	0-1	0-1	0-1
Basophils 10^3/μL (%)	0-0.08	—	—
	0-1	0-1	0-1
H:L ratio	—	—	—
Chemistries			
ALP (U/L)	—	80-156	—
ALT (U/L)	—	5-12	—
Amylase (U/L)	—	100-425	20-65
AST (U/L)	189-388	150-278	141-369

TABLE 5-19 Hematologic and Biochemical Values of Selected Psittaciformes. (cont'd)

Measurement	Grey-Cheeked Parakeet (*Brotogeris pyrrhoptera*)	Jardine's Parrot (*Poicephalus gulielmi*)	Lories and Lorikeets
Bile acid (μmol/L)			
RIA	—	10.2-61.7	20-65
Colorimetric	15-81	—	20-97
BUN (mg/dL)	—	2.8-5.6	—
Calcium (mg/dL)	8.0-11.6	7.0-12.8	8-12
Chloride (mEq/L)	—	—	—
Cholesterol (mg/dL)	96-249	100-300	100-257
CK (U/L)	164-378	110-310	178-396
Creatinine (mg/dL)	—	—	—
GGT (U/L)	—	1-15	—
Glucose (mg/dL)	210-385	199-348	200-400
LDH (U/L)	154-356	119-335	124-302
Phosphorus (mg/dL)	—	2-6.8	—
Potassium (mEq/L)	—	3-4.5	—
Protein, total (g/dL)	2.5-4.5	2.8-4	1.9-4.1
Albumin (g/dL)	—	1.17-1.92	1.3-2.1
Globulin (g/dL)	—	—	0.9-2.4
A:G ratio	—	1.32-2.56	1-2.3
Prealbumin (g/dL)	—	0.12-0.42	—
α-globulin (g/dL)	—	0.07-0.16 (α_1)	—
	—	0.08-0.22 (α_2)	—
β-globulin (g/dL)	—	0.38-0.84	—
γ-globulin (g/dL)	—	0.12-0.47	—
Sodium (mEq/L)	—	133-153	—
Tryglycerides (mg/dL)	—	60-130	—
Uric acid (mg/dL)	0.3-12	2.5-12	2-11.9

Measurement	Lovebirds (*Agapornis* spp.)[155,269]	Macaws (*Ara* and *Anodorhynchus* spp.)[155,269]	Parrotlets (*Forpus* spp.)[269]
Hematology			
PCV (%)	44-55	42-56	48-55
RBC (10^6/μL)	3.25-3.95	2.7-4.5	—
Hgb (g/dL)	10.8-14.8	15-17	—
MCV (fL)	128-140	125-170	—
MCH (pg)	27.5-31.4	36-55	—
MCHC (g/dL)	20.3-23.1	29-35	—

Continued

TABLE 5-19 Hematologic and Biochemical Values of Selected Psittaciformes. (cont'd)

Measurement	Lovebirds (*Agapornis* spp.)	Macaws (*Ara* and *Anodorhynchus* spp.)	Parrotlets (*Forpus* spp.)
WBC ($10^3/\mu L$)	7-16	10-20	5-13
Heterophils $10^3/\mu L$ (%)	3.33-9.21	7.6-11.4	4.84-6.51
	40-75	50-75	55-74
Lymphocytes $10^3/\mu L$ (%)	3.34-6.20	3.50-8.06	2.11-4.4
	20-53	23-53	19-70
Monocytes $10^3/\mu L$ (%)	0-0.12	0-0.15	0-0.09
	0-1	0-1	0-1
Eosinophils $10^3/\mu L$ (%)	0-0.23	0	0-0.09
	0-2	0	0-1
Basophils $10^3/\mu L$ (%)	0-0.23	0-0.15	0-0.09
	0-6	0-1	0-1
H:L ratio	—	—	—
Chemistries			
ALP (U/L)	10-90	20-230	—
ALT (U/L)	5-13	5-12	—
Amylase (U/L)	90-400	150-550	—
AST (U/L)	125-377	105-324	110-224
Bile acid ($\mu mol/L$)			
RIA	8.5-77.1	7.6-60	—
Colorimetric	12-90	7-100	—
BUN (mg/dL)	2.8-5.5	3-5.6	—
Calcium (mg/dL)	7.2-10.6	8.2-10.9	—
Chloride (mEq/L)	—	—	—
Cholesterol (mg/dL)	95-335	100-390	—
CK (U/L)	58-337	101-300	—
Creatinine (mg/dL)	0.1-0.4	0.5-0.6	—
GGT (U/L)	2.5-18	1-30	—
Glucose (mg/dL)	246-381	228-325	252-384
LDH (U/L)	105-355	70-350	—
Lipase (U/L)	30-320	30-250	—
Phosphorus (mg/dL)	2.8-4.9	—	—
Potassium (mEq/L)	2.1-4.8	2-5	—
Protein, total (g/dL)	2.4-3.6	2.6-5.0	—
Albumin (g/dL)	0.98-1.68	1.12-2.43	—
Globulin (g/dL)	—	—	—
A:G ratio	1.06-2.09	1.08-2.55	—
Prealbumin (g/dL)	0.37-0.68	0.24-0.80	—
α-globulin (g/dL)	0.08-0.17 (α_1)	0.07-0.18 (α_1)	—
	0.12-0.37 (α_2)	0.15-0.45 (α_2)	—
β-globulin (g/dL)	0.33-0.78	0.34-0.85	—
γ-globulin (g/dL)	0.12-0.38	0.15-0.58	—

TABLE 5-19 Hematologic and Biochemical Values of Selected Psittaciformes. (cont'd)

Measurement	Lovebirds (*Agapornis* spp.)	Macaws (*Ara* and *Anodorhynchus* spp.)	Parrotlets (*Forpus* spp.)
Sodium (mEq/L)	125-155	140-165	—
Triglycerides (g/L)	45-200	—	—
Uric acid (mg/dL)	2.5-12	2.9-10.6	4.1-12

Measurement	Pionus Parrots (*Pionus* spp.)[155,269]	Quaker Parakeet (*Myopsitta monachus*)[155,269]	Senegal Parrot (*Poicephalus senegalus*)[155,269]
Hematology			
PCV (%)	44-54	30-58	45-60
RBC (10^6/μL)	2.4-4	—	2.4-4
Hgb (g/dL)	11-16	—	12.3-14.0
MCV (fL)	85-210	—	139-151
MCH (pg)	26-54	—	33.1-39.4
MCHC (g/dL)	24-31	—	23.4-27.4
WBC (10^3/μL)	5-13	8-17	6-14
Heterophils 10^3/μL (%)	0.48-7.10	—	4.70-7.81
	55-74	0-24	44-73
Lymphocytes 10^3/μL (%)	1.82-6.72	—	2.35-7.49
	19-70	74-90	22-70
Monocytes 10^3/μL (%)	0-0.10	—	0-0.11
	0-1	1-4	0-1
Eosinophils 10^3/μL (%)	0-0.10	—	0-0.21
	0-1	0-2	0-2
Basophils 10^3/μL (%)	0-0.10	—	0-0.11
	0-1	0-6	0-1
H:L ratio	—	—	—
Chemistries			
ALP (U/L)	80-290	70-300	70-300
ALT (U/L)	5-12	5-11	5-11
Amylase (U/L)	200-500	100-400	190-550
AST (U/L)	140-359	225-375	183-352
Bile acid (μmol/L)			
RIA	6.1-62.7	9.6-83.2	13.8-87.4
Colorimetric	15-92	21-90	20-94
BUN (mg/dL)	3-5.4	2.9-5.4	2.9-5.4
Calcium (mg/dL)	7.8-10.8	7-10.0	7.6-10.7
Chloride (mEq/L)	—	—	—
Cholesterol (mg/dL)	130-295	110-295	130-340
CK (U/L)	169-354	110-311	100-330
Creatinine (mg/dL)	0.1-0.4	0.1-0.4	0.1-0.4

Continued

TABLE 5-19 Hematologic and Biochemical Values of Selected Psittaciformes. (cont'd)

Measurement	Pionus Parrots (*Pionus* spp.)	Quaker Parakeet (*Myopsitta monachus*)	Senegal Parrot (*Poicephalus senegalus*)
GGT (U/L)	1-18	1-15	1-15
Glucose (mg/dL)	228-312	229-318	220-284
LDH (U/L)	125-380	120-300	150-350
Lipase (U/L)	30-250	25-225	32-250
Phosphorus (mg/dL)	2.9-6.6	2.9-6.5	—
Potassium (mEq/L)	3.5-4.6	2.8-4.6	3-5
Protein, total (g/dL)	3.6-5.2	3.0-4.8	2.8-4.2
Albumin (g/dL)	—	0.92-2.48	1.19-1.81
Globulin (g/dL)	—	—	—
A:G ratio	0.6-1.9	1.07-2.38	1.41-2.66
Prealbumin (g/dL)	1.52-2.37	0.91-2.46	0.55-0.99
α-globulin (g/dL)	0.08-0.23 (α_1)	0.08-0.21 (α_1)	0.08-0.15 (α_1)
	0.11-0.36 (α_2)	0.22-0.45 (α_2)	0.11-0.25 (α_2)
β-globulin (g/dL)	0.40-0.95	0.37-0.79	0.32-0.87
γ-globulin (g/dL)	0.23-0.69	0.19-0.77	0.15-0.45
Sodium (mEq/L)	145-155	140-155	130-155
Triglycerides (mg/dL)	60-225	50-200	45-145
Uric acid (mg/dL)	2.0-7.9	3.5-11.5	2.5-7.8

TABLE 5-20 Hematologic and Biochemical Values for Juveniles of Selected Psittaciformes.

Measurement	Cockatoos (*Cacatua* spp.)[142] (9 species) ($n = 152$)[a]	Umbrella Cockatoo (*Cacatua alba*)[142] ($n = 111$)[a]	Macaws (*Ara* spp.)[143] (7 species) ($n = 113$)[a]	Blue and Gold Macaw (*Ara ararauna*)[143] ($n = 43$)[a]	Eclectus Parrot (*Eclectus roratus*)[141] ($n = 111$)[a]
Hematology					
PCV (%)	39.7 ± 9 (25-59)	39.3	41.7 ± 8.4 (25-55)	40 ± 7.7	43.8 ± 8.4 (26-58)
RBC (10^6/μL)	2.53 ± 0.63 (1.5-4)	2.54	2.9 ± 0.8 (1.5-4.5)	2.7 ± 0.7	2.69 ± 0.67 (1.5-4)
Hgb (g/dL)	11.4 ± 2.9 (6.5-17)	11.6	12.3 ± 3.3 (7-17)	11 ± 2.9	12.5 ± 3 (6.5-18)
WBC (10^3/μL)	12.9 ± 6.3 (5.5-25)	16.6	19.2 ± 6.9 (7-30)	18.9 ± 5.6	13.7 ± 6.3 (5.5-25)
Heterophils (%)	50.8 ± 11.7 (27-74)	54.1	55.3 ± 10 (37-75)	52 ± 10	53.9 ± 11.4 (35-75)
Bands (%)	1.3 ± 2.3 (0-7)	1.31	0.6 ± 1.7 (0-5)	0.1 ± 0.7	0.5 ± 1.5 (0-5)
Lymphocytes (%)	41.2 ± 11.9 (17-65)	38.1	39 ± 10 (20-60)	42 ± 10	39.5 ± 11.5 (20-65)
Monocytes (%)	5.8 ± 3.4 (0-12)	5.35	4.4 ± 2.9 (1-10)	4.3 ± 2.7	5 ± 2.7 (1-11)
Eosinophils (%)	0	0.02	0 ± 0.2 (0-1)	0	0.1 ± 0.3 (0-1)
Basophils (%)	0.9 ± 1.1 (0-4)	1.03	0.5 ± 1 (0-3)	0.9 ± 1.3	1.1 ± 1 (0-3)

Continued

TABLE 5-20 Hematologic and Biochemical Values for Juveniles of Selected Psittaciformes. (cont'd)

Measurement	Cockatoos (Cacatua spp.) (9 species) (n = 152)	Umbrella Cockatoo (Cacatua alba) (n = 111)	Macaws (Ara spp.) (7 species) (n = 113)	Blue and Gold Macaw (Ara ararauna) (n = 43)	Eclectus Parrot (Eclectus roratus) (n = 111)
Chemistries					
ALP (U/L)	579 ± 239 (200-1000)	440	970 ± 397 (290-1600)	1200 ± 390	489 ± 159 (200-900)
ALT (U/L)	2 ± 3 (0-13)	2.1	3 ± 2 (0-9)	4 ± 3	4 ± 3 (0-10)
AST (U/L)	143 ± 79 (50-400)	136	104 ± 31 (60-180)	101 ± 24	140 ± 58 (65-260)
BUN (mg/dL)	2 ± 2 (0-6)	1.6	2.4 ± 2.3 (0-6)	1.9 ± 2.2	1.7 ± 2.4 (0-6)
Calcium (mg/dL)	9.6 ± 0.7 (8-11)	9.8	9.9 ± 0.5 (8.5-10.8)	10 ± 0.5	9.3 ± 0.4 (8.5-10.2)
Chloride (mEq/L)	110 ± 6 (97-120)	111	106 ± 6 (96-118)	104 ± 5	111 ± 5 (100-120)
Cholesterol (mg/dL)	251 ± 105 (100-500)	291	165 ± 62 (75-300)	164 ± 67	268 ± 80 (125-450)
CK (U/L)	510 ± 235 (140-1000)	517	550 ± 312 (180-1100)	540 ± 267	616 ± 472 (200-1600)
Creatinine (mg/dL)	0.4 ± 0.1 (0.2-0.7)	0.4	0.4 ± 0.1 (0.3-0.6)	0.4 ± 0.1	0.4 ± 0.1 (0.2-0.5)
GGT (U/L)	2.6 ± 1.7 (0-6)	2.7	1.8 ± 1.2 (0-4)	1.7 ± 1.2	4 ± 2 (0-7)
Glucose (mg/dL)	253 ± 24 (200-300)	244	281 ± 30 (225-330)	288 ± 31	258 ± 18 (220-300)
LDH (U/L)	371 ± 285 (150-1000)	325	138 ± 84 (35-275)	144 ± 98	228 ± 101 (100-400)
Phosphorus (mg/dL)	6.1 ± 1.1 (3.5-8)	5.6	6.5 ± 1 (4.6-6.9)	6.6 ± 0.9	6.8 ± 1.2 (4.5-9)
Potassium (mEq/L)	3.6 ± 0.7 (2.5-5.5)	3.5	2.9 ± 0.8 (2-4.2)	2.7 ± 0.6	2.8 ± 0.7 (2-4.6)
Protein, total (g/dL)	2.8 ± 0.7 (1.5-4)	3	2.6 ± 0.6 (1.5-3.5)	2.5 ± 0.7	2.9 ± 0.5 (1.8-3.8)
Albumin (g/dL)	1.1 ± 0.3 (0.3-1.6)	1.7	1.2 ± 0.3 (0.6-1.7)	1.2 ± 0.3	1.3 ± 0.3 (0.8-1.8)
Globulin (g/dL)	1.7 ± 0.5 (0.8-2.5)	0.9	1.3 ± 0.6 (0.8-1.9)	1.3 ± 0.6	1.5 ± 0.3 (0.8-2.2)
A:G ratio	0.6 ± 0.2 (0.4-1)	0.6	0.8 ± 0.3 (0.5-1)	0.8 ± 0.2	0.9 ± 0.2 (0.6-1.1)
Sodium (mEq/L)	145 ± 6 (135-155)	145	145 ± 6 (135-156)	142 ± 6	148 ± 6 (138-158)
Uric acid (mg/dL)	2.9 ± 2.3 (0.2-8.5)	2.7	2.3 ± 2.1 (0.2-6)	1.9 ± 2.5	2 ± 1.6 (0.2-6.5)

CHAPTER 5 Birds

TABLE 5-21 Hematologic and Biochemical Values of Selected Passeriformes.

Measurement	Canary (*Serinus canaria*)[267]	Mynah[a] (*Gracula religiosa*)[26]
PCV (%)	45-56	47.6 ± 4.9
RBC (10^6/μL)	2.5-3.8	3.8 ± 0.4
Hgb (g/dL)	12-16	14.3 ± 1.2
MCV (fL)	90-210	126 ± 11.7
MCH (pg)	26-55	38.4 ± 3.6
MCHC (g/dL)	22-32	30.1 ± 1.5
WBC (10^3/μL)	3-10	20.8 ± 5.8
Heterophils 10^3/μL	—	—
(%)	50-80	43.8 ± 8
Lymphocytes 10^3/μL	—	—
(%)	20-45	48.7 ± 7.5
Monocytes 10^3/μL	—	4.6 ± 4.1
(%)	0-1	—
Eosinophils 10^3/μL	—	4.1 ± 2.5
(%)	0-2	—
Basophils 10^3/μL	—	0.8 ± 0.7
(%)	0-1	—
H:L ratio	—	—
ALP (U/L)	20-135	—
ALT (U/L)	—	—
AST (U/L)	14-345	130-350
Bile acid (μmol/L)		
RIA	23-90	—
Colorimetric	—	—
Calcium (mg/dL)	5.5-13.5	9-13
Chloride (mEq/L)	—	—
Cholesterol (mg/dL)	150-400	—
CK (U/L)	55-350	—
Creatinine (mg/dL)	0.1-0.4	0.1-0.6
GGT (U/L)	1-14	—
Glucose (mg/dL)	205-435	190-350
LDH (U/L)	120-450	600-1000
Phosphorus (mg/dL)	2.9-4.9	—
Potassium (mEq/L)	2.2-4.5	0.3-5.1
Protein, total (g/dL)	2.8-4.5	2.3-4.5
Albumin (g/dL)	—	—
Globulin (g/dL)	—	—
A:G ratio	—	—
Sodium (mEq/L)	135-165	136-152
Uric acid (mg/dL)	4-12	4-10

[a]Values reported in captive adult males.

TABLE 5-22 Hematologic and Biochemical Values of Selected Ratites.

Measurement	Emu (Dromaius novaehollandiae)[375,668]	Ostrich (Struthio camelus)[448,449]	Rhea (Rhea spp.)[a,192]
Hematology			
PCV (%)	40-60	32 ± 3	29-59
RBC (10⁶/μL)	2.5-4.5	1.7 ± 0.4	—
Hgb (g/dL)	—	12.2 ± 2.0	64-170 (126)
MCV (fL)	—	174 ± 42	—
MCH (pg)	—	—	—
MCHC (g/dL)	—	33 ± 5	44.4-45.7 (45.1)
WBC (10³/μL)	8-25	5.5 ± 1.9	4.1-25.7 (11.8)
Heterophils 10³/μL (%)	—	—	—
	45-75	63 ± 8	—
Lymphocytes 10³/μL (%)	—	—	—
	20-40	34 ± 7	—
Monocytes 10³/μL (%)	—	—	—
	0-2	3 ± 1	—
Eosinophils 10³/μL (%)	—	—	—
	0-1	0.3 ± 0.5	—
Basophils 10³/μL (%)	—	—	—
	0-1	0.2 ± 0.5	—
H:L ratio	—	—	—
Chemistries			
ALP (U/L)	—	575 ± 248	—
AST (U/L)	80-380	131 ± 31	20-192
Bile acid (μmol/L)			
RIA	6-45	—	—
Colorimetric	—	—	—
Calcium (mg/dL)	8.8-12.5	9.2	2.6-8.2
Chloride (mEq/L)	—	100 ± 16	—
Cholesterol (mg/dL)	68-170	108	—
CK (U/L)	100-750	688 ± 208	0-2640
Creatinine (mg/dL)	0.22	0.32	—
GGT (U/L)	—	1.5 ± 2.9	—
Glucose (mg/dL)	100-290	250	37.8-158.6
LDH (U/L)	310-1200	1565 ± 660	269-1640
Phosphorus (mg/dL)	3.8-7.2	3.7	—
Potassium (mEq/L)	3.5-6.5	3 ± 0.8	—
Protein, total (g/dL)	3.4-5.6	3.7 ± 0.7	3.4-6.2
Albumin (g/dL)	1-2.5	—	—
Sodium (mEq/L)	—	147 ± 34	—
Uric acid (mg/dL)	4.5-14	8.2	—

[a]Numbers in parentheses represent the mean.

TABLE 5-23 Hematologic and Biochemical Values of Selected Piciformes and Columbiformes.

Measurement	Toco Toucan (*Ramphastos toco*)[a,160,269]	Pigeon (*Columba livia*)[474,724]
Hematology		
PCV (%)	45-60 (46)	49 ± 3.8
RBC (10^6/μL)	2.5-4.5 (2.5)	—
Hgb (g/dL)	14.6-18.2 (16.4)	—
MCV (fL)	176-214 (196)	—
MCH (pg)	53-76 (65)	—
MCHC (g/dL)	31-39 (35)	—
WBC (10^3/μL)	4-10 (5.5)	8348 ± 4813
Heterophils 10^3/μL (%)	—	1369 ± 1031
	35-65	—
Lymphocytes 10^3/μL (%)	—	5877 ± 4099
	25-50	—
Monocytes 10^3/μL (%)	—	225 ± 232
	—	—
Eosinophils 10^3/μL (%)	—	9 ± 25
	0-4	—
Basophils 10^3/μL (%)	—	120 ± 130
	0-5	—
H:L ratio	—	—
	—	—
Chemistries		
ALP (U/L)	—	160-780
ALT (U/L)	—	19-48
AST (U/L)	130-330	45-123
Bile acid (μmol/L)		
RIA	—	—
Colorimetric	20-40	22-60
BUN (mg/dL)	—	2.4-4.2
Calcium (mg/dL)	10-15	7.6-10.4
Chloride (mEq/L)	—	101-113
Cholesterol (mg/dL)	—	—
CK (U/L)	—	110-480
Creatinine (mg/dL)	0.1-0.4	0.3-0.4
GGT (U/L)	—	0-2.9
Glucose (mg/dL)	220-350	232-369
LDH (U/L)	200-400	30-205
Phosphorus (mg/dL)	—	1.8-4.1
Potassium (mEq/L)	—	3.9-4.7

Continued

TABLE 5-23 Hematologic and Biochemical Values of Selected Piciformes and Columbiformes. (cont'd)

Measurement	Toco Toucan (*Ramphastos toco*)	Pigeon (*Columba livia*)
Protein, total (g/dL)	3-5	2.1-3.3
Albumin (g/dL)	—	1.3-2.2
Globulin (g/dL)	—	0.6-1.2
A:G ratio	—	1.5-3.6
Sodium (mEq/L)	—	141-149
Uric acid (mg/dL)	4-14	2.5-12.9

[a]Numbers in parentheses represent the mean.

TABLE 5-24 Hematologic and Biochemical Values of Selected Raptors.

Measurement	Bald Eagle (*Haliaeetus leucocephalus*)[379]	Golden Eagle (*Aquila chrysaetos*)[a,332a,550]
Hematology		
PCV (%)	35-57	35-47 (41)
RBC ($10^6/\mu L$)	2.60-4.05	1.9-2.7 (2.4)
Hgb (g/dL)	—	12.1-15.2 (13.8)
MCV (fL)	—	160-184 (174)
MCH (pg)	—	56.3-62.7 (58.9)
MCHC (g/dL)	—	32.3-35.9 (34)
WBC ($10^3/\mu L$)	4.1-27.3	5.9-24 (12.3)
Heterophils $10^3/\mu L$ (%)	50-93	—
	—	49-86
Lymphocytes $10^3/\mu L$ (%)	4-38	—
	—	14-38
Monocytes $10^3/\mu L$ (%)	0-4	—
	—	0-9
Eosinophils $10^3/\mu L$ (%)	—	—
	0-9	1-5
Basophils $10^3/\mu L$ (%)	—	—
	0-1	0-1
H:L ratio	—	—
Fibrinogen (g/L)	—	2-4.1 (2.9)
Chemistries		
ALP (U/L)	—	15-36
ALT (U/L)	—	—
AST (U/L)	131-956	95-210

TABLE 5-24 Hematologic and Biochemical Values of Selected Raptors. (cont'd)

Measurement	Bald Eagle (*Haliaeetus leucocephalus*)	Golden Eagle (*Aquila chrysaetos*)
Bile acid (μmol/L)		
RIA	—	—
Calcium (mg/dL)	8.2-10.4	7.4-9.5
Chloride (mEq/L)	—	—
Cholesterol (mg/dL)	—	—
CK (U/L)	190-1797	—
GGT (U/L)	—	—
Glucose (mg/dL)	246-431	250-408
LDH (U/L)	—	320-690
Phosphorus (mg/dL)	—	1.9-3.6
Potassium (mEq/L)	—	—
Protein, total (g/dL)	2.2-4.6	2.5-3.9
Albumin (g/dL)	1.09-2.05	1-1.4
Globulin (g/dL)	0.19-0.59	—
A:G ratio	0.57-1.59	—
Sodium (mEq/L)	—	—
Uric acid (mg/dL)	1.8-15.3	4.4-12

[a]Numbers in parentheses represent the mean.

Measurement	Red-tailed Hawk (*Buteo jamaicensis*)[698]	Harris Hawk (*Parabuteo unicinctus*)[b,114,373,698]
PCV (%)	31-43	32-44
RBC ($10^6/\mu L$)	2.4-3.6	2.13-2.76
Hgb (g/dL)	10.7-16.6	10.1-16.7
MCV (fL)	150-178	147-163
MCH (pg)	46-57.4	45.4-51.1
MCHC (g/dL)	297-345	30.1-33.0
WBC ($10^3/\mu L$)	19.1-33.4	4.8-10
Heterophils $10^3/\mu L$ (%)	—	—
	35 ± 11	2.3-6.7
Lymphocytes $10^3/\mu L$ (%)	—	—
	44 ± 9	0.6-2.4
Monocytes $10^3/\mu L$ (%)	—	—
	6 ± 3	0.2-1.5
Eosinophils $10^3/\mu L$ (%)	—	—
	13 ± 4	0-0.8
Basophils $10^3/\mu L$ (%)	—	—
	Rare	0-1.6
H:L ratio	—	—
Fibrinogen (g/L)	—	—

Continued

TABLE 5-24 Hematologic and Biochemical Values of Selected Raptors. (cont'd)

Measurement	Red-tailed Hawk (*Buteo jamaicensis*)	Harris Hawk (*Parabuteo unicinctus*)
Chemistries		
ALP (U/L)	22-138	15-36
ALT (U/L)	3-50	—
AST (U/L)	76-492	95-210
Bile acid (µmol/L)		
RIA	8.4-10.2	—
Calcium (mg/dL)	10-12.8	8.4-10.6
Chloride (mEq/L)	118-129	113-119
Cholesterol (mg/dL)	—	—
CK (U/L)	—	224-650
GGT (U/L)	0-20	2-6.9
Glucose (mg/dL)	292-390	220-283
LDH (U/L)	0-2640	160-563
Phosphorus (mg/dL)	1.9-4	3-4.4
Potassium (mEq/L)	2.6-4.3	0.8-2.3
Protein, total (g/dL)	3.9-6.7	3.1-4.6
Albumin (g/dL)	—	1.4-1.7
Globulin (g/dL)	—	2.1-2.9
A:G ratio	—	0.45-0.55
Sodium (mEq/L)	143-162	155-171
Uric acid (mg/dL)	8.1-16.8	9-13.2

Measurement	Sharp-shinned Hawk (*Accipiter striatus*)[322]	Turkey Vulture (*Cathartes aura*)[a,698]
Hematology		
PCV (%)	44-52	51-58 (54)
RBC (10^6/µL)	—	2.4-2.9 (2.7)
Hgb (g/dL)	—	15.7-17.3 (16.3)
MCV (fL)	—	194-224 (204)
MCH (pg)	—	58.6-65 (61.7)
MCHC (g/dL)	—	28.6-32 (30.2)
WBC (10^3/µL)	7.7-16.8	10.5-31.9 (20.1)
Heterophils 10^3/µL (%)	—	—
	16-24	59-64
Lymphocytes 10^3/µL (%)	—	—
	54-75	8-18
Monocytes 10^3/µL (%)	—	—
	0-3	0-1
Eosinophils 10^3/µL (%)	—	—
	5-11	3-4
Basophils 10^3/µL (%)	—	—
	0-1	0
H:L ratio	—	—

TABLE 5-24 Hematologic and Biochemical Values of Selected Raptors. (cont'd)

Measurement	Sharp-shinned Hawk (*Accipiter striatus*)	Turkey Vulture (*Cathartes aura*)
Chemistries		
ALP (U/L)	—	—
ALT (U/L)	—	—
AST (U/L)	—	—
Bile acid (μmol/L)		
RIA	—	—
Calcium (mg/dL)	—	—
Chloride (mEq/L)	—	—
Cholesterol (mg/dL)	—	—
CK (U/L)	—	—
GGT (U/L)	—	—
Glucose (mg/dL)	—	—
LDH (U/L)	—	—
Phosphorus (mg/dL)	—	—
Potassium (mEq/L)	—	—
Protein, total (g/dL)	2.4-3.2	—
Albumin (g/dL)	—	—
Globulin (g/dL)	—	—
A:G ratio	—	—
Sodium (mEq/L)	—	—
Uric acid (mg/dL)	—	—

Measurement	American Kestrel (*Falco sparverius*)[209]	Gyrfalcon (*Falco rusticolus*)[698]	Peregrine Falcon (*Falco peregrinus*)[373,629,698]
Hematology			
PCV (%)	43 ± 3.2	49 ± 2	37-53
RBC (10^6/μL)	—	—	3-4
Hgb (g/dL)	—	—	118-188
MCV (fL)	14.5-57	—	118-176
MCH (pg)	11-33	—	40-48.4
MCHC (g/dL)	24-58	—	319-352
WBC (10^3/μL)	9.8 ± 4.9	4.6 ± 1.7	3.3-21 (13 ± 3)
Heterophils 10^3/μL	—	—	—
Heterophils (%)	47 ± 3	51 ± 5	65 ± 12
Lymphocytes 10^3/μL	—	—	—
Lymphocytes (%)	46 ± 3	45 ± 5	35 ± 13
Monocytes 10^3/μL	—	—	—
Monocytes (%)	2 ± 0.2	1 ± 1	0
Eosinophils 10^3/μL	—	—	—
Eosinophils (%)	1 ± 0.2	1 ± 1	0
Basophils 10^3/μL	—	—	—
Basophils (%)	2 ± 0.2	Rare	0

Continued

TABLE 5-24 Hematologic and Biochemical Values of Selected Raptors. (cont'd)

Measurement	American Kestrel (Falco sparverius)	Gyrfalcon (Falco rusticolus)	Peregrine Falcon (Falco peregrinus)
Chemistries			
ALP (U/L)	232 ± 72	257	97-350
ALT (U/L)	41 ± 33	—	19-54
AST (U/L)	77 ± 29	97	20-52
Bile acid (μmol/L)			
RIA	—	—	20-118
Calcium (mg/dL)	7.1 ± 0.8	9.6	8.4-10.2
Chloride (mEq/L)	108 ± 33	125	121-134
Cholesterol (mg/dL)	—	—	175-401
CK (U/L)	1739 ± 734	402	357-850
GGT (U/L)	—	—	0-7
Glucose (mg/dL)	305 ± 40	318	11-16
LDH (U/L)	—	—	625-1210
Phosphorus (mg/dL)	3 ± 0.9	—	3.4
Potassium (mEq/L)	2.2 ± 0.7	—	1.6-3.2
Protein, total (g/dL)	3.2 ± 0.5	2.89	2.5-4
Albumin (g/dL)	1 ± 0.2	—	0.8-1.3
Globulin (g/dL)	1.2 ± 0.4	—	1.6-2.8
A:G ratio	0.9 ± 0.4	—	0.4-0.6
Sodium (mEq/L)	158 ± 3	160	152-168
Uric acid (mg/dL)	9 ± 6	13.9	4.4-22

Measurement	Barn Owl (Tyto alba)[c,17,18a]	Barred Owl (Strix varia)[c,17,18a]	Great-horned Owl (Bubo virginianus)[c,17,18a]
Hematology			
PCV (%)	48 ± 4 (41-57)	44 ± 4 (38-52)	43 ± 4
RBC (10^6/μL)	2.4 ± 0.4 (1.6-3.3)	3.0 ± 0.9 (1.0-4.7)	2.6 ± 0.5
Hgb (g/dL)	—	—	—
MCV (fL)	202 ± 29 (135-270)	156 ± 38 (77-236)	164 ± 28
MCH (pg)	—	—	—
MCHC (g/dL)	—	—	—
WBC (10^3/μL) PBT	13.1 ± 5.9 (5.0-28.8)	18.9 ± 7.4 (2.6-33.7)	18.3 ± 9.2 (4.2-42.4)
NHT	8.3 ± 5.0 (2.5-22.1)	6.6 ± 2.9 (2.3-13.9)	17.1 ± 9.6 (4.8-42.6)
EST	12.4 ± 6.1 (3.8-28.6)	16.5 ± 3.6 (8.8-23.0)	20.0 ± 6.2 (7.2-33.0)
Heterophils 10^3/μL (%)	6.9 ± 2.8 (3.2-15.0)	4.7 ± 1.8 (0.5-8.6)	9.9 ± 5.8 (2.0-25.5)
	56 ± 15 (26-85)	28 ± 12.5 (10-52)	54 ± 12 (28-79)
Lymphocytes 10^3/μL (%)	3.1 ± 2.1 (0.3-8.6)	9.6 ± 5.5 (0.9-22.7)	3.4 ± 2.3 (0.4-9.7)
	23 ± 10 (2-41)	48 ± 15 (18-80)	18 ± 8 (4-37)

TABLE 5-24 Hematologic and Biochemical Values of Selected Raptors. (cont'd)

Measurement	Barn Owl (*Tyto alba*)	Barred Owl (*Strix varia*)	Great-horned Owl (*Bubo virginianus*)
Monocytes $10^3/\mu L$ (%)	1.0 (0.1-1.3)	2.5 ± 1.8 (0.2-7.6)	2.1 ± 1.4 (0.2-6.7)
	7 ± 5 (0-17)	12 ± 6 (3-29)	11 ± 4 (2-20)
Eosinophils $10^3/\mu L$ (%)	1.6 ± 1.5 (0.2-7.4)	2.1 ± 2.2 (0.4-4.3)	2.6 ± 2.4 (0.4-8.2)
	12 ± 7 (2-34)	11 ± 4 (1-20)	15 ± 8 (2-33)
Basophils $10^3/\mu L$ (%)	0.3 ± 0.3 (0.0-1.1)	0.2 ± 0.2 (0.0-4.4)	0.3 ± 0.4 (0.2-2.9)
	2 ± 2 (2-34)	1 ± 1 (1-3)	2 ± 2 (2-33)
H:L ratio	38 ± 4.5 (0.8-22.2)	0.7 ± 0.7 (0.1-2.7)	4.2 ± 4.2 (1.0-19.8)
Fibrinogen (g/L)	—	—	—
Chemistries			
ALP (U/L)	—	—	—
ALT (U/L)	—	—	—
AST (U/L)	151 (93-263)*	88-358†	55-277†
Bile acid (μmol/L)			
Colorometric	17.0 (1.0-55.0)*	6.4-54‡	4.2-48.9‡
Calcium (mg/dL)	9.16 (4.80-18.8)*	7.44-12.24†	6.4-12‡
Chloride (mEq/L)	115 (112-120)*	108-122‡	111-127†
Cholesterol (mg/dL)	262 (190-352)*	159-267†	117-281†
CK (U/L)	1243 (158-3415)*	22-3657‡	27-1544‡
GGT (U/L)	0 (0-388)*	0-2‡	0-6‡
Glucose (mg/dL)	245 (187-425)*	283-405†	292-448†
LDH (U/L)	173 (76-640)*	63-2103‡	106-747‡
Phosphorus (mg/dL)	3.12 (1.85-4.39)*	2.78-8.02‡	1.76-8.23‡
Potassium (mEq/L)	4.1 (2.2-6.7)*	1.7-4.9†	2.3-5.7†
Protein, total (g/dL)	3.4 (2.4-4.6)*	2.9-5.0‡	3.0-5.1‡
Albumin (g/dL)	1.9 (1.3-2.3)*	1.2-1.8‡	1.2-1.8‡
Globulin (g/dL)	1.5 (1.0-2.4)*	1.7-3.4‡	1.5-3.3‡
A:G ratio	1.4 (0.7-1.6)*	0.5-0.8‡	0.4-1.0‡
Sodium (mEq/L)	158 (153-166)*	154-169†	151-172†
Uric acid (mg/dL)	11.74 (5.49-18.06)*	1.29-18.05†	3.09-17.80‡

Measurement	Eastern Screech Owl (*Megascops asio*)[c,17,18a]	Eurasian Eagle Owl (*Bubo bubo*)[c,17,18a]	Northern Saw-whet Owl (*Aegolius acadicus*)[c,17,18a]
Hematology			
PCV (%)	47 ± 3 (40-54)	50 ± 9 (NA)	48 ± 5 (NA)
RBC ($10^6/\mu L$)	3.4 ± 7 (1.7-4.8)	2.0 ± 0.3 (NA)	2.8 ± 0.5 (NA)
Hgb (g/dL)	—	—	—
MCV (fL)	145 ± 26 (89-200)	—	176 ± 29 (NA)

Continued

TABLE 5-24 Hematologic and Biochemical Values of Selected Raptors. (cont'd)

Measurement	Eastern Screech Owl (*Megascops asio*)	Eurasian Eagle Owl (*Bubo bubo*)	Northern Saw-whet Owl (*Aegolius acadicus*)
MCH (pg)	—	—	—
MCHC (g/dL)	—	—	—
WBC ($10^3/\mu L$) PBT	15.4 ± 6.3 (1.2-28.1)	20.9 ± 14.4 (6.6-64.7)	6.3 ± 3.1 (NA)
NHT	8.4 ± 3.9 (3.1-19.8)	17.2 ± 11.6 (3.0-56.6)	5.7 ± 2.5 (NA)
EST	15.2 ± 6.3 (1.8-28.5)	20.4 ± 12.6 (6.2-65.8)	11.6 ± 3.6 (NA)
Heterophils $10^3/\mu L$ (%)	4.0 ± 1.6 (0.4-7.3)	10.9 ± 8.3 (2.3-48.9)	1.8 ± 0.8 (NA)
	27 ± 10 (6-47)	51 ± 12 (24-76)	29 ± 10 (NA)
Lymphocytes $10^3/\mu L$ (%)	6.0 ± 3.6 (0.9-15.9)	4.0 ± 2.1 (1.5-12.0)	2.4 ± 1.9 (NA)
	38 ± 13 (12-65)	23 ± 11 (5-50)	35 ± 15 (NA)
Monocytes $10^3/\mu L$ (%)	2.3 ± 1.1 (0.5-5.0)	1.7 ± 1.3 (0.3-5.6)	0.8 ± 0.4 (NA)
	15 ± 6 (3-27)	9 ± 4 (0-17)	13 ± 3 (NA)
Eosinophils $10^3/\mu L$ (%)	2.8 ± 1.8 (0.4-7.9)	4.0 ± 5.9 (NA)	±0.7 (NA)
	18 ± 8 (5-39)	16 ± 10 (4-46)	22 ± 10 (NA)
Basophils $10^3/\mu L$ (%)	0.3 ± 0.4 (0.0-1.3)	0.2 ± 0.3 (0.0-0.9)	±0.1
	2 ± 2 (0-6)	1 ± 1 (NA)	1 ± 2
H:L ratio	0.9 ± 0.8 (0.8-15.8)	2.9 ± 1.9 (0.6-9.9)	1.2 ± 1.2
Fibrinogen (g/L)	—	—	—

Chemistries

Measurement	Eastern Screech Owl (*Megascops asio*)	Eurasian Eagle Owl (*Bubo bubo*)	Northern Saw-whet Owl (*Aegolius acadicus*)
ALP (U/L)	—	—	—
ALT (U/L)	—	—	—
AST (U/L)	108-647‡	—	248 (127-411)*
Bile acid (μmol/L)			
Colorometric	4-59‡	—	50 (21-61)*
Calcium (mg/dL)	4.9-12.4†	—	9.4 (5.6-10.4)*
Chloride (mEq/L)	106-119†	—	113 (92-114)*
Cholesterol (mg/dL)	168-336.3†	—	307.67 (193.5-491.5)*
CK (U/L)	5-1174‡	—	377 (19-4299) *
GGT (U/L)	0-10‡	—	0 (0-4)*
Glucose (mg/dL)	282.6-455.4†	—	318.6 (271.8-347.4)*
LDH (U/L)	62-2984‡	—	140 (6-308)*
Phosphorus (mg/dL)	1.2-8.5‡	—	3.96 (2.79-5.26)*
Potassium (mEq/L)	1.2-6.2†	—	3.0 (2.6-3.6)*
Protein, total (g/dL)	2.5-4.3‡	—	3.0 (2.7-3.7)*
Albumin (g/dL)	1.3-2.6†	—	2.1 (1.9-2.7)*
Globulin (g/dL)	0.9-2.2†	—	0.9 (0.4-1.5)*
A:G ratio	0.6-1.9†	—	2.3 (1.3-6.5)*
Sodium (mEq/L)	152-165†	—	153 (129-155)*
Uric acid (mg/dL)	2.84-26.30‡	—	9 (2.63-12.6)*

TABLE 5-24 Hematologic and Biochemical Values of Selected Raptors. (cont'd)

Measurement	Great Gray Owl (*Strix nebulosa*)[c,17,18a]	Short-eared Owl (*Asio flammeus*)[c,17,18a]	Snowy Owl (*Bubo scandiaca*)[c,17,18a]
Hematology			
PCV (%)	50 ± 5 (39-61)	48 ± 6 (NA)	49 ± 6 (NA)
RBC (10^6/μL)	2.8 ± 0.3 (2.1-3.4)	2.6 ± 0.6 (NA)	3.3 ± 0.7 (NA)
Hgb (g/dL)	—	—	—
MCV (fL)	181 ± 26 (127-236)	181 ± 29 (NA)	142 ± 23 (NA)
MCH (pg)	—	—	—
MCHC (g/dL)	—	—	—
WBC (10^3/μL) PBT	11.1 ± 6.0 (1.8-26)	11.0 ± 7.3 (NA)	9.6 ± 5.4 (NA)
NHT	4.8 ± 2.5 (1.7-11.4)	6.0 ± 3.6 (NA)	6.7 ± 6.5 (NA)
EST	13.0 ± 4.6 (2.7-21.7)	12.4 ± 5.5 (NA)	10.2 ± 5.7 (NA)
Heterophils 10^3/μL (%)	3.6 ± 2.6 (1.0-12.2)	3.5 ± 2.9 (NA)	4.5 ± 3.4 (NA)
	34 ± 12 (9-58)	30 ± 14 (NA)	46 ± 19 (NA)
Lymphocytes 10^3/μL (%)	4.3 ± 3.0 (0.4-12.3)	5.0 ± 3.4 (NA)	3.3 ± 2.8 (NA)
	37 ± 15 (5-69)	47 ± 15 (NA)	34 ± 17 (NA)
Monocytes 10^3/μL (%)	1.6 ± 1.0 (0.2-4.7)	1.1 ± 1.1 (NA)	0.9 ± 0.4 (NA)
	14 ± 4 (5-23)	9 ± 5 (NA)	11 ± 5 (NA)
Eosinophils 10^3/μL (%)	1.4 ± 1.6 (0.7-11.9)	1.2 ± 0.8 (NA)	0.8 ± 1.0 (NA)
	12 ± 8 (0-42)	13 ± 8 (NA)	8 ± 5 (NA)
Basophils 10^3/μL (%)	0.2 ± 0.2 (0.0-0.9)	0.2 ± 0.3 (NA)	0.0 ± 0.1 (NA)
	2 ± 2 (0-7)	2 ± 2 (NA)	1 ± 2 (NA)
H:L ratio	1.3 ± 1.1 (0.2-5.8)	0.9 ± 1.0 (NA)	2.6 ± 3.6 (NA)
Fibrinogen (g/L)	—	—	—
Chemistries			
ALP (U/L)	—	—	—
ALT (U/L)	—	—	—
AST (U/L)	125-467[‡]	213 (121-431)*	215 (171-301)*
Bile acid (μmol/L)			
Colorometric	6-81[‡]	19 (4-94)*	27 (8-78)*
Calcium (mg/dL)	2.88-11.88[†]	6.72 (3.6-9.6)*	8.84 (7.32-11.12)*
Chloride (mEq/L)	107-121[†]	114 (104-122)*	113 (109-121)*
Cholesterol (mg/dL)	139.32-284.06[†]	206.3 (174.2-278.6)*	261.6 (152.48-839.8)*
CK (U/L)	1-574[‡]	29 (0-265)*	203 (20-3338)*
GGT (U/L)	0-10[‡]	0 (0-3)*	0 (0-5)*
Glucose (mg/dL)	245-378[†]	319 (261-360)*	338 (218-468)*
LDH (U/L)	65-353[‡]	180 (92-530)*	209 (132-861)*

Continued

TABLE 5-24 Hematologic and Biochemical Values of Selected Raptors. (cont'd)

Measurement	Great Gray Owl (*Strix nebulosa*)	Short-eared Owl (*Asio flammeus*)	Snowy Owl (*Bubo scandiaca*)
Phosphorus (mg/dL)	0.50-8.18[†]	2.60 (0.93-7.12)*	5.51 (1.64-7.77)*
Potassium (mEq/L)	2.1-4.8[†]	3.7 (2.9-5.3)*	3.8 (1.5-5.5)*
Protein, total (g/dL)	2.7-4.1[‡]	2.7 (2.1-3.3)*	3.6 (2.6-4.7)*
Albumin (g/dL)	1.5-2.4[†]	1.4 (1.0-1.7)*	1.4 (0.8-1.9)*
Globulin (g/dL)	1.0-2.6[‡]	1.3 (1.0-1.6)*	1.8 (1.3-3.4)*
A:G ratio	0.6-1.9[‡]	1.1 (0.8-1.4)*	0.8 (0.4-1.3)*
Sodium (mEq/L)	152-168[‡]	157 (151-161)*	158 (156-170)*
Uric acid (mg/dL)	3.33-21.37[‡]	7.09 (2.56-25.28)*	11.42 (5.51-22.33)*

[a]Numbers in parentheses represent the mean.
[b]WBC count and differentials for Harris hawk are absolute values.
[c]Hematology: Mean and SD (reference interval); *PBT*, phloxine B technique; *NHT*, Natt and Herrick technique; *EST*, estimation from the smear technique. Differential counts were computed from the phloxine B technique. Reference intervals were calculated by the robust method or robust method after Box–Cox transformation; *NA*, insufficient sample size for reference interval calculation ($n < 20$). Biochemistry:
*Median (range) ($10 < n < 20$). Reference intervals were not reported when $n < 10$.
[†]Robust technique ($n > 20$, Gaussian distribution). [‡]Robust technique with Box–Cox transformation ($n > 20$, non-Gaussian distribution).

CHAPTER 5 Birds   307

TABLE 5-25 Biologic and Physiologic Values of Selected Avian Species.[a,12a,30,142,143,191,192,214,260,327,328,377,414,542,675,737,778,836]

Species	Incubation Period (days)[b]	Fledgling Age (days)	Weaning Age (days) Parent-raised	Weaning Age (days) Hand-reared	Sexual Maturity	Lifespan in Captivity (Maximum) (years)	Body Weight (g)[c]
Psittaciformes							
African grey parrot	26-28[d]	50-65	100-120	75-90	4-6 yr	50-60	454 (370-534)
Amazon parrot	24-29[e]	45-60	90-120	75-90	4-6 yr	>50 (80)	[f]
Australian parakeet	18-19	30-45	50-65	—	1-3 yr	10-12	30-110
Budgerigar parakeet	16-18	22-26	30-40	30	6-9 mo	5-10 (18)	30
Cockatiel	18-20	32-38	47-52	42-49	6-12 mo	10-12 (30)	80-90
Cockatoo, galah	22-24	45-55	90-120	80-90	1 yr	40-60	[g]
Cockatoo, large	[h]	60-80	120-150	95-120	5-6 yr	50-60	[g]
Cockatoo, medium	[h]	45-60	90-120	75-100	3-4 yr	40-60	[g]
Conure	[i]	35-40	45-70	60	2-3 yr	25-40	80-100[j]
Eclectus parrot	26-28	72-80	120-150	100-110	4 yr	20-40 (80)	432 (347-512)
Lory/lorikeet	21-27	42-50	62-70	50-60	2 yr	20-30	—
Lovebirds	18-24	30-35	45-55	40-45	6-12 mo	15-30	42-48
Macaw, large	26-28	70-80	120-150	95-120	5-7 yr	75-100	[k]
Macaw, small	23-26	45-60	90-120	75-90	4-6 yr	50-80	[k]
Ring-neck parakeet, Indian	22-23	40-45	55-65	—	3 yr	18-25	115

Continued

TABLE 5-25 Biologic and Physiologic Values of Selected Avian Species. (cont'd)

Species	Incubation Period (days)	Fledgling Age (days)	Weaning Age (days) Parent-raised	Weaning Age (days) Hand-reared	Sexual Maturity	Lifespan in Captivity (Maximum) (years)	Body Weight (g)
Passeriformes							
Canary	12-14	14	21	—	<1 yr	6-12	12-30
Mynah	14-15	30	60	—	2-3 yr	12	180-260
Zebra or society finch	12-16	18-20	25-28	—	9-10 mo	4-7	10-16
Columbiformes							
Dove, common ground	12->14	18	—	—	1 yr	4-8	30
Dove, mourning	13-14	12-14	—	—	—	—	120
Pigeon (rock dove)	16-19	28-35	35	—	1 yr	4-8 (>20)	240-300
Ratites							
Emu	50-57	—	Precocial	—	3-5 yr	30	40-45 kg
Ostrich	41-43	—	Precocial	—	4 yr	80	120-160 kg
Rhea	36-41	—	Precocial	—	1.5-2 yr	—	25 kg

aGuidelines only; data vary between references. For raptors, see Table 5-26.
bBrotogeris parakeets, 22; Pionus parrot, 25-26; Psittacula parakeets, 23-26; Quaker parakeet, 23; Senegal parrot, 24-25.
cBourke's parakeet, 40 (35-50); kakariki parakeet, 95-100; Princess of Wales parakeet, 108 (100-129); red-rumped parakeet, 65 (60-69).
dCongo, 28; Timneh, 26.
eGreen-cheeked, blue-fronted, 26; spectacled (white-fronted), 24; yellow-naped, yellow-fronted, yellow-crowned, double yellow-headed, 28-29.
fBlue-crowned, 740 (618-998); blue-fronted, 432 (361-485); double yellow-headed, 568 (463-694); Mexican red-headed, 360 (343-377); yellow-naped, 596 (476-795).
gBare-eyed, 331; greater sulphur-crested, 806; Leadbeater's (Major Mitchell's), 423 (381-474); lesser sulphur-crested, 303; Moluccan, 808; rose-breasted, 299; tri-ton, 559; umbrella, 552.
hBare-eyed, 23-24; citron-crested, 25-26; greater sulphur-crested, 27-28; Leadbeater's (Major Mitchell's), 26; lesser sulphur-crested, 24-25; Moluccan, 28-29; palm, 28-30; triton, 27-28; umbrella, 28.
iBlue-crowned, 23-24; orange-fronted, 30; Nanday, 21-23; Patagonian, 24-25; sun, 27-28.
jQueen of Bavaria, 262 (252-276).

TABLE 5-26 Biologic and Physiologic Values of Selected Raptors.[75,134,214,257,317,698,737]

Species	Clutch Size	Incubation Period (days)	Interval Between Eggs (days)	Start of Incubation	Fledging (days)	Sexual Maturity (yr)	Longevity (yr)	Body Weight Male	Body Weight Female
American kestrel	3-7	29-31	—	—	30-31	—	2-7	103-120 g	126-166 g
Bald eagle	1-3	34-36	—	—	70-98	—	—	4.1 kg	5.8 kg
Barn owl	2-9	30-31	2-3	First egg	70-75	7	—	441-470 g	490-570 g
Barred owl	2-4	28-33	—	—	6	—	—	630 g	800 g
Black vulture	1-3	37-48	—	—	80-94	—	—	a	a
Common kestrel	3-6	27-29	1-2	Second to third egg	—	7	—	136-252 g	154-314 g
Cooper's hawk	3-6	32-36	—	—	27-34	—	—	220-410 g	330-680 g
Eurasian buzzard	2-4	36-38	4	First to second egg	—	2-3	—	0.55-0.85 kg	0.7-1.2 kg
Eurasian eagle owl	2-4	34-36	2-3	First to second egg	6	2-3	50-60	1.5-2.8 kg	1.8-4.2 kg
Golden eagle	1-3	43-45	—	—	6	>5	50-60	2.5-4 kg	3.25-6.35 kg
Gyrfalcon	3-5	34-36	—	—	49-56	—	—	0.96-1.3 kg	1.3-2.1 kg
Harris hawk	2-5	3	2-3	Penultimate or last egg	43-49	>3	20-30	0.7 kg	1 kg
Merlin	2-7	28-32	—	—	30-35	7	10-14	150-210 g	189-255 g
Northern goshawk	3-5	35-38	2-3	First to second egg	35-42	>3	15-20	0.5-1.2 kg	0.8-1.5 kg
Northern sparrow hawk	4-6	3	2-3	Third to fourth egg	—	1-2	—	—	—

Continued

TABLE 5-26 Biologic and Physiologic Values of Selected Raptors. (cont'd)

Species	Clutch Size	Incubation Period (days)	Interval Between Eggs (days)	Start of Incubation	Fledging (days)	Sexual Maturity (yr)	Longevity (yr)	Body Weight Male	Body Weight Female
Osprey	2-4	32-43	—	—	48-59	—	—	[b]	[b]
Peregrine falcon	3-4	29-32	2-3	Penultimate or last egg	35-42	>3	15-20	440-750 g	910-1500 g
Prairie falcon	2-7	29-33	—	—	35-42	—	—	500-650 g	700-975 g
Screech owl, eastern	3-4	—	—	—	—	—	—	158-184 g	180-220 g
Screech owl, western	2-6	21-30	—	—	6	—	—	131-210 g	157-250 g
Sharp-shinned hawk	3-8	32-35	—	—	24-27	—	—	82-125 g	144-208 g
Snowy owl	3-9	30-33	2-3	First egg	6	7	—	1.6 kg	1.1-2 kg
Turkey vulture	1-3	38-41	—	—	66-88	—	—	[c]	[c]

[a]1.7-2.3 kg; weights of males and females were not listed separately.
[b]1-2.1 kg; weights of males and females were not listed separately, but females are generally 25% heavier than males.
[c]0.8-2.3 kg; weights of males and females were not listed separately, but females are slightly heavier than males.

TABLE 5-27 Quick Reference to Abnormalities of the Standard Avian Hematology Profile.[268]

Parameter	Increases	Decreases
PCV/RBC	Dehydration • Increased total protein Erythrocytosis (polycythemia) • Normal or low total protein • Primary rare • Secondary to respiratory or cardiovascular disease	Regenerative anemia • Polychromasia (10%), reticulocytes, immature RBC • Hemorrhagic: Trauma, parasites, coagulopathies, ulcerated neoplasms, gastrointestinal ulcers • Hemolytic: Septicemia, hemoparasites, toxicities, immune-mediated • Presence of Heinz bodies, agglutination of RBC Nonregenerative anemia • Hypoplastic: Inflammatory infectious, myelosuppresive drugs, iron deficiency, food restriction, folic acid deficiency

Heterophils	Inflammatory processes
	• Bacterial (including Mycobacterium) and fungal infections
	• Excess corticosteroids
	  ○ Endogenous production
	  ○ Exogenous administration
	Birds with a high heterophil: lymphocyte ratio may mount a greater leukocytic response
		Infection
		• Bacterial and viral (i.e., PBFD)
		Poor sample preparation, collection, and storage

Lymphocytes	Chronic antigenic stimulation Neoplasia: lymphocytic leukemia Stress response (acute)	Stress response (chronic) Immunosuppresive drugs Viral infection Endotoxemia/septicemia
Monocytes	Granulomatous and/or chronic inflammation (e.g., bacterial, fungal, parasitic) Neoplasia	—
Eosinophils	Gastrointestinal parasitism Type IV hypersensitivity reactions	Corticosteroids Stress response (chronic)
Basophils	Early inflammatory responses Type I hypersensitivity reaction Anaphylactic reaction Induced molting	—
Thrombocytes	—	Vitamin K deficiency Rodenticide toxicity Aflatoxicosis Septicemia-associated DIC (as with polyomavirus and reovirus) Hepatic disease or failure

TABLE 5-28 Quick Reference to Abnormalities of the Standard Avian Biochemical Profile.[a,269]

Parameter	Increases Nonmedical	Increases Medical	Decreases Nonmedical	Decreases Medical
ALP (U/L)	Juveniles have higher levels	Hyperparathyroidism induced osteoclastic activity (fractures); egg laying; hepatic disease; enteritis; aflatoxicosis	—	Dietary zinc deficiency
ALT (U/L)	Seasonal variation in raptors; sample hemolysis	—	Seasonal variation in raptors	—
Amylase (U/L)	—	Pancreatitis; gastrointestinal disease; zinc toxicity	—	—
AST (U/L)	Rare; severe lipemia; 300-1000	Liver, muscle, or heart damage; vitamin E/selenium, methionine deficiency; 300-15,000	—	<50; end-stage liver disease
Bile acids (µmol/L)	Lipemia; sample hemolysis, such samples should not be analyzed	Loss of liver function, even with normal enzymes	Lipemic samples that are chemically treated	Response to therapy; liver cirrhosis; microhepatica
Calcium (mg/dL)	Lipemia (or cloudy from other causes); protein elevations; bacterial contamination	Hormonal disorders; egg production; metabolic disease; excess dietary vitamin D; dehydration; osteolytic neoplasia	EDTA; bacterial contamination; young birds have lower levels	<8; metabolic and nutritional disorders; lead poisoning; glucocorticoid administration; low albumin; African grey parrot hypocalcemia
Cholesterol (mg/dL)	Postprandial;[530] high fat diet; carnivorous diet	Metabolic disease; hepatic lipidosis; bile duct obstruction; hypothyroidism; starvation	—	Liver, metabolic disease
CK (U/L)	>300; healthy birds up to 1000	600-25,000; muscle or heart damage; CNS disease (seizures); vitamin E/selenium deficiency; chlamydiosis; lead toxicity; IM injections	<10; bacterial contamination	Rare
Creatinine (mg/dL)	—	Not useful in birds	—	Not useful in birds
Glucose (mg/dL)	Improper dilution; postprandial; posthandling	Stress, 400-600; diabetes, 800-1500; corticosteroids	<100; unseparated blood; bacterial contamination	<100; hepatic dysfunction; septicemia; neoplasia; aspergillosis
LDH (U/L)	Sample hemolysis	300-15,000; liver, heart, or muscle damage; hepatitis; muscle damage	<50	End-stage liver disease

Analyte		Increased		Decreased
Lipase (U/L)	—	Acute pancreatitis		
Phosphorus (mg/dL)	Postprandial; sample hemolysis	Severe renal disease; nutritional secondary hyperparathyroidism; hypoparathyroidism	EDTA	Hypovitaminosis D; malabsorption; chronic glucocorticoid therapy
Potassium (mEq/L)	Hemolysis; dietary supplementation	Adrenal disease; metabolic disease; severe tissue damage; renal disease; acidosis; dehydration; hemolytic anemia	—	Adrenal disease; metabolic disease; diuretic therapy; alkalosis; overhydration; dietary deficiency
Protein, total (g/dL)	Lipemia; non–temperature compensated refractometer	Inflammation; dehydration; chronic infection; gamma globulinopathy; lympho-proliferative disease; myelosis	Non–temperature compensated refractometer	Chronic hepatopathy; malabsorption; renal disease; blood loss; neoplasia; starvation/malnutrition
Sodium (mEq/L)	Dietary supplementation	Dehydration; salt poisoning	—	Renal disease; overhydration
Sorbitol dehydrogenase (U/L)	—	Hepatitis	—	—
Uric acid (mg/dL)	5-15; severe lipemia; dirty nail clip; carnivorous birds have higher levels	Renal disease; gout; dehydration; postprandial; ovulation; tissue damage; starvation; hypervitaminosis D	Overhydration of patient; juvenile levels are lower	End-stage liver disease

aThe ranges given are not absolute and are to be used as a guide for interpretation of a wide range of avian species.

TABLE 5-29 Blood Gases of Selected Avian Species.[a]

Parameter	Amazona aestiva[b] (n = 35)[585]	Falco rusticolus[c] (n = 30)[631]	Psittacus spp.[d] (n = 46)[523]
$pH_{37°C}$	7.45 ± 0.05	7.49 ± 0.08	7.32 ± 0.08
PCO_2 (mmHg)	22.1 ± 4	35.5 ± 6.1	29.3 ± 6.1
PO_2 (mmHg)	98.1 ± 7.6	111.8 ± 20.5	37.9 ± 3.8
HCO_3 (mmol/L)	14.8 ± 2.8	22.5 ± 4.0	15 ± 2.4
TCO_2 (mmol/L)	—	23.3 ± 4.0	16.0 ± 2.7
BEecf (mmol/L)	7.9 ± 3.1	0.9 ± 4.9	17 0
Na (mmol/L)	147.4 ± 2.2	148 ± 1.8	141-159
K (mmol/L)	3.5 ± 0.5	3.3 ± 0.3	3.6 ± 0.5
iCa (mmol/L)	0.8 ± 0.3	1.0 ± 0.1	1.1 ± 0.1
SO_2 (%)	96.2 ± 1.1	98.6 ± 1.0	68.4 ± 10.1
Hct (%)	38.7 ± 6.2	42.1 ± 4.0	—
Hgb (g/dL)	13.2 ± 2.1	14.3 ± 1.4	—
Glu (mg/dL)	—	317 ± 17	247 ± 25
Temperature (°C)	41.8 ± 0.6	41.2 ± 0.5	41.6 ± 0.4
$pH_{Temp°C}$	—	7.4 ± 0.1	7.3 ± 0.1
PCO_2 (mmHg) $_{Temp°C}$	—	35.5 ± 6.1	35.7 ± 7.5
PO_2 (mmHg) $_{Temp°C}$	—	140.3 ± 21.1	52.5 ± 5.6

[a]PCO_2, partial pressure carbon dioxide; PO_2, partial pressure of oxygen; HCO_3, bicarbonate concentration; TCO_2, total carbon dioxide concentration; SO_2, hemoglobin saturated with oxygen.
[b]i-STAT EC7+ cartridges. Mean and SD. Arterial sample under manual restraint.
[c]i-STAT CG8+ cartridges. Mean and SD. Venous sample under isoflurane anesthesia with O_2.
[d]i-STAT EC8+ and CG8+ cartridges. Mean and SD, or range. Venous sample under manual restraint.

TABLE 5-30 Lipoprotein Panel of Selected Avian Species.

Parameter[a]	Amazona spp.[b] (n = 29)[642]	African grey parrot (n = 20)[763]	Pionus parrot (n = 29)[763]
Cholesterol (mg/dL)	238 (87-364)	222-297	100-116
Triglycerides (mg/dL)	156 (10-300)	104-190	270-301
HDL (mg/dL)	109 (75-148)	161-176	172-177
LDL (mg/dL)	92 (2-182)	24-100	75-103
VLDL (mg/dL)	31 (2-60)	—	—
LDL:HDL (mg/dL)	0.75 (0.18-1.28)	—	—
Non-HDL-LDL (mg/dL)	1.08 (0.24-1.82)	—	—

[a]HDL, high-density lipoprotein; LDL, low-density lipoprotein; VLDL, very low-density lipoprotein.
[b]Mean and 90% confidence intervals.

TABLE 5-31 T_4 Values of Selected Avian Species.[a,155,465,472,871]

Species	Baseline T_4 (nmol/L)[b]	Post-TSH (nmol/L)[c,d]
African grey parrot	3.83-27.03[155,377]	—
	1.83 ± 0.57[465]	11.97 ± 3.73[465]
	≤1.93[871]	23.04 ± 13.26[871]
Amazon parrot	1.29-14.16[155]	—
	10.54 ± 8.88[465]	35.26 ± 20.5[465]
	5.53 ± 0.36 (red-lored)[871]	78.64 ± 44.79[871]
	≤1.93 (blue-fronted)[871]	98.33 ± 26.38[871]
Budgerigar	6.44-27.03[155]	—
Canary	9.01-41.18[155]	—
Cockatiel	9.01-30.89[155]	—
	15.24 ± 8.7[465]	50.19 ± 7.28[465]
Cockatoo	17.54 ± 8.4[465]	45.17 ± 16.94[465]
Conure	6.44-25.74[155]	—
	2.27 ± 0.99[465]	17.37 ± 9.92[465]
Eclectus parrot	3.86-25.74[155]	—
Jardine's parrot	2.57-19.31[155]	—
Lory	3.86-15.44[155]	—
Lovebird	2.57-55.34[155,377]	—
Macaw, blue and gold	4.39 ± 2.29[465]	15.91 ± 8.16[465]
Macaw, scarlet	1.72 ± 0.66[465]	8.31 ± 3.99[465]
Pigeon	6.05-35.01[155,377,472]	—
Pionus parrot	6.44-24.45[155]	—
Quaker parrot	5.15-27.03[155]	—
Senegal parrot	6.44-29.6[155]	—

[a]0.5 μg/dL = 6.5 nmol/L = 5 ng/mL.[291] To convert thyroxine from μg/dL to nmol/L, multiply by 12.87.[472]
[b]T_4 levels will vary with the time of day and year, with higher levels measured in the winter. Physiologic states such as molting or reproductive activity may also alter the ratio of T_4 to T_3 released. The half-life of thyroid hormones is much shorter in birds than in mammals; therefore it is difficult to accurately measure single hormone levels.[513]
[c]The canine radioimmunoassay (RIA) kit does not accurately measure total T_4 below 6.5 nmol/L.[291] Results of high-sensitivity total T_4 testing in parrots ranged from 2 to 6 nmol/L. This high sensitivity test is available through the University of Tennessee Clinical Endocrinology Laboratory (865-974-5638).[292]
[d]Low-dose TSH (0.2 U/kg).

TABLE 5-32 Approximate Resting Respiratory Rates of Selected Avian Species and by Weight.[149a,257,688]

Species	Respiratory Rate (breaths/min)[a]
Amazon parrot	15-45
Budgerigar	60-75
Canary	60-80
Cockatiel	40-50
Cockatoo	15-40
Conure, large	30-45
Conure, small	40-50
Finch	90-110
Lovebird	50-60
Macaw	20-25
Raptor	10-20
Toucan	15-45

Weight (g)	Respiratory Rate (breaths/min)[a]
100	40-52
200	35-50
300	30-45
400	25-30
500	20-30
1000	15-20

[a]Restraint can increase respiratory rate 1.5-2 × the resting rate.

TABLE 5-33 Urinalysis Values Reported in Birds.[102,606]

Parameter	Reference Range	Pigeon[a,308]	Falcon[801]	Ostrich[539]
Specific gravity (g/mL)	1.005-1.020	—	—	—
pH	6.4-8	5.5-6.9	5-7	7.6 ± 1.5
	Laying hens and carnivorous birds may have more acidic urine; cloacal contents may alter urine pH			
Protein (g/dL)	Negative to trace	0.11-1.99	0.3 ± 0.2	2.6 ± 1.5
Glucose (mg/dL)	Negative to trace	—	24.3 ± 39.6	Negative
Ketones	Negative; ketonuria is sometimes present in migratory birds	—	Negative	Negative
Bilirubin	Negative	—	—	Negative
Urobilinogen	Negative	—	—	Negative

[a]95% confident interval.

TABLE 5-34 Values Reported for Selected Ophthalmic Diagnostic Tests in Avian Species.[a,b,70,376,430,432a,522,661,771,773,855]

Species	Tear Production		Intraocular Pressure (mmHg)	
	Phenol Red Thread Test (mm/15 sec)	Schirmer Tear Test (mm/min)	Applanation Tonometry	Rebound Tonometry
Psittacine birds				
Amazon parrots, blue-fronted	21.9 ± 2.3[c]	—	8.3 ± 1.1[c]	—
Amazon parrots, Hispaniolan	12.5 ± 5.0	7.9 ± 2.6	—	—
Amazon parrots, orange-winged	12.6 ± 2.6[c]	—	9.7 ± 1.7[c]	—
Raptors				
Bald eagle	—	14 ± 2	21.5 ± 1.7	—
Barn owl	19.5 ± 7.2	3.6 ± 2.2	18.0 ± 6.6	11.5 ± 4.7
Common buzzard	16.0 ± 7.7	13.7 ± 4.4	19.4 ± 3.9	29.9 ± 6.1
Cooper's hawk	—	—	16.0 ± 1.8	10.7 ± 1.4
Eastern screech owl	—	—	9.3 ± 2.6	6.3 ± 1.3
Eurasian eagle owl	—	—	9.3 ± 1.8	10.5 ± 1.6
Eurasian scops owl	11.8 ± 5	1.0 ± 0.5	14.5 ± 3.9	—
Golden eagle	—	—	21.5 ± 3	—
Great horned owl	—	—	9.9 ± 2.4	9.9 ± 2.4
Kestrel, American	—	—	8.5 ± 4.4	6.8 ± 1.7
Kestrel, common	29.6 ± 4.7	5.8 ± 4	11.9 ± 3.3	11.6 ± 2.7
Northern goshawk	—	—	—	21.2 ± 2.4
Peregrine falcon	—	—	—	15.3 ± 6.1
Red-tailed hawk	—	—	20.3 ± 2.8	19.8 ± 4.9
Snowy owl	—	9.8 ± 2.4	—	9.1 ± 1.9
Swainson's hawk	—	—	20.8 ± 2.3	—
Tawny owl	—	4.3	9.4 ± 1.8	11.1 ± 3.1
Turkey vulture	—	—	15.0 ± 2.1	11.7 ± 1.0

[a]Mean ± SD values reported.
[b]For ultrasonographic ocular measurements, see references.
[c]Median ± S-IQR.

TABLE 5-35 Checklist of Supportive Care Procedures Used in Companion Bird Medicine.[96]

Supportive care is an essential component of companion bird medicine.
1. **Minimize handling and other stressors**
2. House the bird in a **warm, quiet,** well-ventilated environment
   - Ensure minimal to no disturbance
   - Debilitated birds are often fluffed and ruffled and require supplemental heat 86°F (30°C)
3. **Fluid therapy** (see Table 5-36 and Table 5-37)
4. Provide analgesia when indicated (see Table 5-5 and Table 5-6)
5. Supplement vitamins as needed
   - Vitamin A, vitamin E/selenium
   - Vitamin B complex in selected cases of injury, anorexia, cachexia, CNS disorders, or blood loss
6. Antibiotics (see Table 5-1)
   - To control primary infections and for injured or debilitated birds where secondary infections may result
7. Iron dextran
   - Iron deficiency or following hemorrhage
8. Normal photoperiod (or subdued lighting, if needed)
9. Oxygen
   - Dyspnea, hypoxia, or severe pneumonia and air sacculitis
10. Maintain body weight
    - Weigh once or twice daily if possible
    - Offer favorite foods and avoid changing diet while ill
11. Gavage or tube feeding[a]
    - Malnourishment, anorexia, cachexia, and dehydration
    - High carbohydrate formula is initially recommended
    - High-protein/high-calorie formulas may be used to increase body weight during recovery

[a]Crop volume may be estimated as 5% BW or 50 mL/kg.

TABLE 5-36 Fluid Therapy Recommendations for Birds.

When evaluating a patient for fluid therapy, the following factors should ideally be considered: hydration status, electrolyte balance, acid-base status, hematologic and biochemical values, and caloric balance.
- Warm fluids to 100-102°F (38-39°C) to help prevent or correct hypothermia
- Use caution when giving dextrose parenterally; 5% dextrose is a good choice for simple dehydration; however, it can exacerbate problems significantly if used concurrent with significant electrolyte loss[496,767]
- When given orally, dextrose is rapidly absorbed from the intestinal tract without creating an influx of fluid into the intestinal lumen and secondary dehydration[496,767]
- Potassium chloride can be diluted in fluids to correct for potassium depletion based on electrolyte analysis (0.1-0.3 mEq/kg)[808]
- Hetastarch at 10-15 mL/kg IV q8h for up to four treatments or dextrans may be effective for hypoproteinemia; synthetic colloids should be used with caution in patients suffering from congestive heart failure or renal failure[529,772]

Total parenteral nutrition may also be considered.[180,182]

Maintenance and Deficit Replacement[289,358,529,628]

- Determine fluid deficit:
  Fluid deficit (mL) = body weight (g) × % dehydration
- Determine daily maintenance:
  Daily maintenance is estimated at 50 mL (range: 40-60 mL/kg/day in many avian species); the smallest passerines drink 250-300 mL/kg daily[483]
- If possible, replace 50% of the deficit in the first 12-24 hr, and the remainder over the next 24-48 hr; some clinicians recommend replacing 20%-25% of the deficit in the first 4-6 hr, and the remaining volume during the next 24-72 hr

TABLE 5-37 Routes of Administration and Maximum Suggested Volumes of Fluids Which Can Be Administered to Psittacines.[326,646,767]

Route	Maximum Suggested Volume of Fluid[a]
Gavage	• Administer up to 5 mL/100 g bird[b] • Initial volume should be much less in critically ill and anorectic patients (begin with ½ - ⅓ of estimated crop volume) • Crop volume may be up to 10% BW in neonatal birds
Subcutaneous	50 mL/kg[c,d]
Intravenous or intraosseous bolus	Administer up to 10 mL/kg (ideally over a 5-10 min period); in emergencies, could go as high as 25 mL/kg (see Table 5-16)

[a]Combinations of routes (PO, SC, and IV/IO) are recommended if large fluid volumes are administered.
[b]Crop volume may be estimated at 5% of body weight (BW).
[c]Volumes of 10-15 mL/kg may be comfortably given per subcutaneous injection site, although up to 25 mL/kg per site may be given. Overdistension of the area may compromise blood supply to the area and reduce absorption.[767]
[d]Hyaluronidase (Wydase, Wyeth-Ayerst) (1 mL [150 U]/L fluids) may be used in most species to increase the absorption rate of fluids.[385]

TABLE 5-38 Suggested Volumes and Frequency of Gavage Feeding in Anorectic Birds.[628,689]

Species	Volume (mL)[a,b]	Frequency[a]
Finch	0.1-0.5	q4h
Budgerigar	0.5-3	q6h
Lovebird	1-3	q6h
Cockatiel	1-8	q6h
Conure, small	3-12	q6h
Conure, large	7-24	q6-8h
Amazon parrot	5-35	q8h
Cockatoo	10-40	q8-12h
Macaw	20-60	q8-12h

[a]Adjust volume and frequency as crop accommodates larger volumes.
[b]Generally 3%-5% of body weight.[325]

TABLE 5-39 Calculation of Enteral Feeding Requirements for Birds.[624]

When dealing with a debilitated patient that must be tube fed more than once or twice, it is always prudent to make sure you are meeting its caloric requirements.
Basal metabolic rate (BMR) (kcal/day) = $kW^{0.75}$
Maintenance energy requirements (MER) (kcal/day) = $(1.5 \times BMR)$
k = kcal/kg/day constant (nonpasserines = 78, passerines = 129)
- Calculate MER
- Adjust the MER value for debilitated patients, taking their specific clinical condition into account. For instance, an adjustment for sepsis is made by multiplying by 1.5.

Most manufacturers of critical care diets provide information on caloric content (see below); if they do not, call them and ask (see Table 5-41).

Product (Manufacturer)	Protein (%) Label Claim (min)	Protein (%) Dry Matter Basis	Fat (%) Label Claim (min)	Fat (%) Dry Matter Basis	Fiber (%) Label Claim (max)	Fiber (%) Dry Matter Basis	CHO (NFE)[a] (%) Dry Matter Basis	Caloric Content (kcal)
a/d Canine/Feline Critical Care (Hill's)	8.5	44.2	6.6	30.4	0.5	1.3	15.4	1.3/mL
Carnivore Care (Oxbow)	45	—	32	—	3	—	—	0.8/mL[b]
CliniCare Canine/Feline Liquid Diet (Abbott)	8.2	35.1	5.1	22.2	0.1	0.4	29.5	1/mL
Emeraid Carnivore (Lafeber)	37.8	—	34	—	4.5	—	—	5.14 kcal/g dry weight; 1.67 kcal/mL when prepared as directed
Emeraid Herbivore (Lafeber)[c]	19	—	9.5	—	32	—	—	3.04 kcal/g dry weight; 1 kcal/mL when prepared as directed
Emeraid Omnivore (Lafeber)	20	—	9.5	—	0.5	—	—	4.06 kcal/g dry weight; 2.39 kcal/mL when prepared as directed
Emeraid Nutri-Support (Lafeber)	18.5	—	5	—	1	—	—	2.5
Exact Baby Bird Hand Feeding Formula (Kaytee)	22	—	9	—	5	—	—	3.9/g
Exact Macaw Hand Feeding Formula (Kaytee)	19	—	13	—	5	—	—	4.1/g
Formula AA Acute Care (Roudybush)	20	—	10	—	5	—	—	3.5/g DW
Maximum-Calorie Veterinary Formula (Iams)	14	—	12	—	1	—	—	2.1/mL
Recovery Formula (Harrison's)	35	—	19	—	1	—	—	3.9/g

[a]Carbohydrate nitrogen-free extract.
[b]24 kcal/Tbs of powder.
[c]Fed in combination with Emeraid Omnivore to geese and swans.

TABLE 5-40 Doxycycline Recipes Used in Psittacines.[241,621]

Medicated water for cockatiels:
1. Mix doxycycline with tap water to a final concentration of 280 mg/L (0.28 mg/mL) using a magnetic stir bar and plate
2. Prepare daily for 45 days
3. No calcium supplementation should be provided

Medicated seed for cockatiels:
1. Combine 60% hulled millet and 40% hulled sunflower seed with 6.25 mL sunflower oil/kg seed; mix well
2. Mix doxycycline with seeds at 500 mg/kg wet weight using an electric mixer
3. Prepare daily for 45 days
4. No calcium supplementation should be provided

Medicated seed for budgerigars:
1. Create a 1:4 mixture of hulled oat groat and hulled millet
2. Mix well
3. Add approximately 6 mL sunflower oil/kg seed (enough to coat seeds, but not dripping)
4. Mix well
5. Add the contents of doxycycline hyclate capsules aseptically (300 mg drug/kg seed)
6. Prepare daily for 45 days
7. No calcium supplementation should be provided

TABLE 5-41 Selected Sources of Formulated and Medicated Diets for Companion and Aviary Birds

Avi-Sci, Inc[a] 4477 South Williams Road St. Johns, MI 48879, USA www.avi-sci.com	Pretty Bird International, Inc[a] 31008 Fox Hill Ave Stacy, MN 55079, USA www.prettybird.com/
Harrison's Bird Foods 7108 Crossroads Blvd, Suite 325 Brentwood, TN 37027, USA www.harrisonsbirdfoods.com/	Rolf C. Hagen, Inc[a] 50 Hampden Rd Mansfield, MA 02048, USA www.hagen.com/usa/index
Kaytee Products, Inc 521 Clay St, PO Box 230 Chilton, WI 53014, USA www.kaytee.com/	Roudybush Foods[a] 340 Hanson Way Woodland, CA 95776, USA www.roudybush.com/
Lafeber Co 24981 N 1400 East Rd Cornell, IL 61319, USA www.lafebervet.com/	Scenic Bird Food Marion Zoological 2003 E. Center Circle Plymouth, MN 55441, USA www.marionzoological.com/bird/
L'Avian Plus D & D Commodities Ltd. PO Box 359 Stephen, MN 56757, USA www.lavianplus.com	Zeigler Bros, Inc[a] PO Box 95 Gardners, PA 17324, USA www.zeiglerfeed.com
Mazuri Diets PMI Nutrition International LLC PO Box 66812 St. Louis, MO 63166-6812, USA www.mazuri.com/	ZuPreem Diets Premium Nutritional Products, Inc PO Box 2094 Mission, KS 66201, USA www.zupreem.com/

[a]Source of medicated feeds.

TABLE 5-42 Selected Nutritional Recommendations for Wild Bird Rehabilitation.[104,214,215,258,737,a]

Aquatic Birds, Including Wading Birds and Seabirds

- Live-prey eating birds like pelicans and herons may not recognize familiar food in an unfamiliar presentation; offer live fish in large tubs, such as a small child's pool, but be prepared to force-feed as needed

Hummingbirds

- It is extremely challenging to meet the nutritional needs of hummingbirds; hummingbirds must constantly replenish energy sources to survive; nectar from plants as well as protein from insects (an estimated 100 mg) are both critical daily dietary requirements
- Nektar-Plus (Nekton) will provide adequate nutritional support, including protein
- Insects, such as *Drosophila* fruit flies, may be released into the enclosure[576]

Raptors

- Rehydrate first (see Table 5-36 and Table 5-37); this is particularly important in birds of prey because the raptor's digestive process requires copious secretions
- For debilitated birds, tube feed a diet rich in protein and fat; offer an enteral tube feeding product (see Table 5-39), ground whole prey (less feet, fur or feathers, gastrointestinal tract), or small amounts of quail breast meat soaked in oral electrolytes
- Feed whole prey after establishing normal gastrointestinal time; offer food the bird will recognize as prey such as eviscerated fish, rats, mice, and/or quail; to increase the chances of self-feeding, offer a variety of foods
- Feed juvenile raptors a whole animal diet of mice or rats supplemented with vitamins; for young nestlings, remove the fur, toenails, and the gastrointestinal tract, then dice the remainder of the body to create a fine "mush"

Songbirds

- Determine if the bird is an omnivore, herbivore, nectarivore, or insectivore and offer a variety of foods; use a good identification book like *The Sibley Guide to Birds*[737] paired with a resource like *The Birder's Handbook*[214] to determine preferred foods
- Offer a variety of foods, such as high-quality birdseed, mealworms, and tiny pieces of fresh fruit and vegetables, in a shallow container or lid
- Presentation of food promotes self-feeding; place earthworms in a pan of soil for thrushes, offer berries still attached to a branch to a mockingbird
- Swifts and swallows may take a live insect on a forcep
- Woodpeckers may eat mealworms trapped in peanut butter spread on bark

[a]See Tables 14-1 for more details.

TABLE 5-43 Management of Dystocia or Egg Binding in Birds.

Definition
- Dystocia or egg binding—obstructive or nonobstructive abnormal oviposition

Etiology—Often Multifactorial
- Environmental stressors
- Nutritional: dehydration, hypocalcemia, low-protein diet, and/or general malnutrition
- Egg-related: abnormal egg size and shape or position
- Hen-related: systemic disease, salpingitis, oviduct perforation, torsion or scarring, and/or neoplasia

Diagnosis
- History/clinical signs/physical findings: nonspecific signs of illness, respiratory distress, persistent tail bobbing, ± blood from vent or in droppings, coelomic distension ± palpable egg
- Complete blood/chemistry panel
- Radiography/ultrasonography

Treatment
- Stabilize the patient
    - Warm, dark, humidified environment
    - Administer warmed fluids, SC, IV, or IO if dehydrated
    - Dextrose: 50% bolus IV or IO; 2.5% in fluids SC if hypoglycemic
    - Calcium gluconate: 50-100 mg/kg IM or SC if hypocalcemic
    - Nutritional support required in most cases
- Medical management
    - Oxytocin: 5 U/kg IM, may repeat q30min
    - Prostaglandin E_2: 0.1 mL/100 g (1 mL/kg) intracloacal on uterovaginal sphincter
- Surgical management
    - Attempt after 12-24 hr unless patient is obstructed and requires faster intervention
    - Sedation with oxygen supplementation or general anesthesia must be used
    - Use caution when manipulating egg; do not press cranially when stabilizing the egg, as this will compromise respiration; instead, gentle laterolateral digital pressure to direct egg caudally
    - Cloacal ovocentesis
        - 18g-20g needle regardless of patient size
        - Visualize egg/oviductal opening using lubricated speculum or cotton applicators and focal light source
        - Insert needle into egg and aspirate contents while stabilizing egg
        - Gently implode egg with laterolateral digital pressure
        - Extract fragments with curved hemostats
    - Percutaneous ovocentesis
        - 18g-20g needle
        - Stabilize egg against left side of body, then aseptically prepare area
        - Insert needle and aspirate contents
        - Gently implode egg with laterolateral digital pressure if it does not collapse
        - Salpingotomy or salpingohysterectomy

TABLE 5-44 Protocols Used in Treating Mycobacteriosis in Birds.[a,b]

Agent	1[c,821]	2[51]	3[821]	4[821]	5[821]	6[d,76]	7[444]	8[202]	9[822]	10[688]
Azithromycin	—	—	—	—	—	—	—	45 mg/kg PO q24h	—	43 mg/kg PO q24h
Ciprofloxacin	—	10 mg/kg PO q12h	—	—	80 mg/kg PO q24h	—	—	—	—	15 mg/kg PO q12h[e]
Clarithromycin	—	—	—	—	—	—	55 mg/kg PO q24h	85 mg/kg PO q24h	—	—
Clofazimine	—	—	—	—	—	1.5 mg/kg PO q24h	—	—	6 mg/kg PO q24h	—
Cycloserine	—	—	—	—	—	5 mg/kg PO q12h	—	—	—	—
Enrofloxacin	—	—	30 mg/kg PO q24h	30 mg/kg PO q24h	—	10-15 mg/kg PO, IM q12h	6 mg/kg PO q24h	—	—	—
Ethambutol	30 mg/kg PO q24h	—	30 mg/kg PO q24h	30 mg/kg PO q24h	30 mg/kg PO q24h	20 mg/kg PO q24h	30 mg/kg PO q24h	15-30 mg/kg PO q12-24h	30 mg/kg PO q24h	30 mg/kg PO q24h
Isoniazid	30 mg/kg PO q24h	—	15 mg/kg PO q24h	—	—	—	—	—	—	—
Rifabutin	—	—	—	—	—	—	45 mg/kg PO q24h	15-45 mg/kg PO q24h	—	—
Rifampin	45 mg/kg PO q24h	15 mg/kg PO q12h	—	45 mg/kg PO q24h	45 mg/kg PO q24h	—	—	—	45 mg/kg PO q24h	15 mg/kg PO q24h
Streptomycin	—	30 mg/kg IM q12h	—	—	—	—	—	—	—	—

[a]Because of its zoonotic potential, controversy exists concerning whether to treat pet and aviary birds for *Mycobacterium avium*. Because *M. avium* isolates from birds differ from human isolates in antibiotic susceptibility, serovars, and genetic sequencing, pet birds are an unlikely source of *M. avium* in people (except immunosuppressed individuals). Nevertheless, veterinarians who treat birds with this disease do so at their own risk. The veterinarian should be aware that treatment is often lifelong for the bird and that treatment does not necessarily prevent shedding.[51,76,202,444,688,821]

[b]Empirical evaluation of multidrug therapy found that azithromycin (43 mg/kg), rifampin (45 mg/kg), and ethambutol (30 mg/kg) were ineffective in ring-necked doves (*Streptopelia risoria*) naturally infected with avian mycobacteriosis. Culture and sensitivity results indicated resistance to all drugs except for azithromycin.[696]

[c]Mix into dextrose powder, administered with a small amount of food.[821]

[d]Recommended for use in raptors.[76]

TABLE 5-45 Suggested Chemotherapeutic Protocols Used in Birds.

C.O.P. PROTOCOL FOR LYMPHOSARCOMA[264]
- Prednisone 25 mg/m^2 PO q24h
- Cyclophosphamide 200 mg/m^2 IO q7d
- Vincristine 0.75 mg/m^2 IO q7d × 3 treatments
- Doxorubicin 30 mg/m^2 IO q21d
- L-asparaginase 400 U/kg IM q7d
- Interferon α 15,000 U/m^2 SC q2d × 3 treatments
- Diphenhydramine 2 mg/kg IO before doxorubicin and L-asparaginase treatments
- Dexamethasone 1 mg/kg IM before doxorubicin and L-asparaginase treatments

PROTOCOL FOR LYMPHOCYTIC LEUKEMIA OR LYMPHOSARCOMA[a,555]
- Vincristine sulfate 0.5 mg/m^2 IV initial dose, then 0.75 mg/m^2 q7d × 3 treatments
- Prednisone 1 mg/454 g PO q12h
- Chlorambucil 1 mg/bird PO 2 ×/wk

PROTOCOL FOR CUTANEOUS LYMPHOSARCOMA[b,673]
- Vincristine 0.1 mg/kg IV q7-14d
- Chlorambucil 2 mg/kg PO 2 ×/wk

PROTOCOL FOR OSTEOSARCOMA[c,197]
- Diphenhydramine 30 min before doxorubicin treatment (route and dose not given)
- Doxorubicin 60 mg/m^2 is diluted into 6 mL sterile saline and administered IV over 30 min in an anesthetized patient via an angiocatheter in the jugular vein q30d
- Do not extravasate doxorubicin; doxorubicin may cause myelosuppression and cardiac toxicity; monitor the CBC
- Electrocardiography during treatment is recommended

[a]Dosages are for a Pekin duck (*Anas platyrhynchos domesticus*).
[b]Dosages are for an umbrella cockatoo (*Cacatua alba*).
[c]Dosages are for a blue-fronted Amazon parrot (*Amazona aestiva*).

TABLE 5-46 Drug Dosages and Volumes Suggested for Cardiopulmonary Resuscitation (CPR) and in Critical Birds.[a]

Emergency Drug	Dose	15 g (Canary; Finch)	30 g (Budgerigar)	40-50 g (Lovebird)	100 g (Conure; Cockatiel)	200 g (Mynah)	300 g (Pigeon; Sulphur-crested Cockatoo)	400 g (African Grey Parrot; Eclectus Parrot)	500 g (Umbrella Cockatoo)	750 g (Greater Sulphur-crested Cockatoo)	1 kg (Blue and Gold Macaw)
Atropine (0.2-0.5 mg/mL)	0.5 mg/kg	0.006-0.015 mL	0.012-0.03 mL	0.015-0.05 mL	0.04-0.1 mL	0.08-0.2 mL	0.12-0.3 mL	0.16-0.4 mL	0.2-0.5 mL	0.3-0.75 mL	0.4-1 mL
Calcium gluconate (10%) (100 mg/mL)	50-100 mg/kg	0.007-0.015 mL	0.015-0.03 mL	0.02-0.05 mL	0.05-0.1 mL	0.1-0.2 mL	0.15-0.3 mL	0.2-0.4 mL	0.25-0.5 mL	0.375-0.75 mL	0.5-1 mL
Dexamethasone sodium phosphate (4 mg/mL)	2-4 mg/kg	0.007-0.015 mL	0.015-0.03 mL	0.02-0.05 mL	0.05-0.1 mL	0.1-0.2 mL	0.15-0.3 mL	0.2-0.4 mL	0.25-0.5 mL	0.375-0.75 mL	0.5-1 mL
Dextrose (50%) (diluted with saline)	0.25 mL/kg (slow)	0.004 mL	0.008 mL	0.01-0.125 mL	0.025 mL	0.05 mL	0.075 mL	0.1 mL	0.12 mL	0.18 mL	0.25 mL
Epinephrine (1:1000; 1 mg/mL)	0.1 mg/kg	0.001 mL	0.003 mL	0.005 mL	0.01 mL	0.02 mL	0.03 mL	0.04 mL	0.05 mL	0.075 mL	0.1 mL
Isotonic crystalloid fluids (bolus)	10 mL/kg	0.15 mL	0.3 mL	0.4-0.5 mL	1 mL	2 mL	3 mL	4 mL	5 mL	7.5 mL	10 mL
7.5% NaCl	3 mL/kg	0.04 mL	0.09 mL	0.12-0.15 mL	0.3 mL	0.6 mL	0.9 mL	1.2 mL	1.5 mL	2.1 mL	3 mL
6% Hetastarch	5 mL/kg bolus (20 mL/kg/day)	0.07 mL	0.15 mL	0.2-0.25 mL	0.5 mL	1 mL	1.5 mL	2 mL	2.5 mL	3.75 mL	5 mL

Mannitol (20%) (200 mg/mL)	0.5-2 mL/kg	0.0075-0.03 mL	0.015-0.06 mL	0.02-0.1 mL	0.05-0.2 mL	0.1-0.4 mL	0.15-0.6 mL	0.2-0.8 mL	0.25-1 mL	0.375-1.5 mL	0.5-2 mL
Prednisolone sodium succinate (10 mg/mL)	10-20 mg/kg	0.015-0.03 mL	0.03-0.06 mL	0.04-0.1 mL	0.1-0.2 mL	0.2-0.4 mL	0.3-0.6 mL	0.4-0.8 mL	0.5-1 mL	0.75-1.5 mL	1-2 mL
Sodium bicarbonate (1 mEq/mL)	5 mEq/kg	0.075 mL	0.15 mL	0.2-0.25 mL	0.5 mL	1 mL	1.5 mL	2 mL	2.5 mL	3.75 mL	5 mL
Vasopressin (20 U/mL)	0.8 U/kg IV, IO	—	—	—	0.004 mL	0.008 mL	0.012 mL	0.016 mL	0.02 mL	0.03 mL	0.04 mL

[a]Dose in mL/kg body weight, IV, IO, or IM. If weight is not available, base CPR on approximate weight of species closest in size.

TABLE 5-47 Vaccines Used in Birds (Non-Poultry).[113,126,320,381,396,478,498,528,567,608,664,670,676,808,862]

Species	Agent	Dosage	Initial	Booster	Comments
See comments	West Nile virus (West Nile-Innovator, Zoetis; Equine killed vaccine; (Recombitek-equine rWNV vaccine, Merial; equine recombinant DNA vaccine)	0.5-1 mL IM	Repeat q3-4wk for 2-3 treatments	3 wk	Environmental control is generally considered most important; however, West Nile virus vaccine has been administered to many types of birds, including Ciconiiformes, Columbiformes, Coraciiformes, Passeriformes, Phoenicopteriformes, Psittaciformes, and raptors (including falcons); an antibody response has been documented inconsistently (flamingos, penguins);[131,172,565,568,739] hemolytic anemia reported in lories immunized a year after first set of immunizations[609]
Raptors	Paramyxovirus-1 (V.P. Vaccin Nobilis Lasota, Intervet)	Intranasally or added to drinking water	—	Booster in 3-4 wk; protects approximately 6 mo	Hitchner B1 and Lasota strain poultry vaccines in drinking water appear to be effective; may see mild palpebral swelling for a few days[381]
Pigeons, racing	Paramyxovirus-1 (V.P. Vaccin Nobilis Lasota, Intervet)	Apply 1-2 drops in nostrils or eyes	2-4 wk before shows/races	6-8 wk	MLV; poor immune response
	—	Add to drinking water	—	8 wk	1 bottle is administered to entire flock (>100 birds), divided evenly in drinking water for 24 hr; poor immune response
	Paramyxovirus-1/Pox, pigeon (Columbovac, Solvay Duphar)	0.2 mL SC[a,76]	4 wk of age	—	Killed vaccine; poor immunologic response to pox

Psittacines	Polyomavirus (Psittimune APV, Creative Science)	0.25 mL/bird (that will weigh <200 g at maturity) SC[624] 0.5 mL/bird (that will weigh >200 g at maturity) SC[624]	35-50 days of age; chicks may be safely vaccinated as young as 10-20 days of age, degree of protection uncertain[670]	2-3 wk, then annually	May cause discoloration, thickening, or granuloma of skin at vaccination site
	—	—	—	Last booster should be given at least 2 wk before leaving aviary[669]	May be indicated in the face of an outbreak;[b,670] registered with the United States Department of Agriculture[676]
Emus[797]	Eastern and western equine encephalitis and tetanus (Equiloid, Fort Dodge)	Same dosage as recommended for the target species (horses) IM	6 wk to 3 mo of age	Repeat 3-4 wk later, then booster annually or biannually before and after breeding season (March/Sept)[797]	—

[a]Vaccinating birds during an outbreak may allow humans to theoretically serve as mechanical vectors.[664]
[b]Choose subcutaneous injection site carefully in pigeons to avoid bleeding; cranial to thigh or lower ⅓ of neck on dorsal midline.

TABLE 5-48 Blood Pressure Values Reported in Birds.

Species	Direct or Indirect	Mean Arterial Pressure (mmHg)	Systolic Arterial Pressure (mmHg)	Diastolic Arterial Pressure (mmHg)
Psittacines	Indirect in conscious birds[451]	—	120-180	—
	Indirect in birds under isoflurane anesthesia[451]	—	90-180	—
Hispaniolan Amazon parrots[a] (n = 16)	Direct in birds under isoflurane anesthesia using the wing[9]	155 ± 18 (112-185)	163 ± 18 (119-200)	148 ± 18 (106-171)
	Direct in birds under isoflurane anesthesia using the leg[9]	152 ± 28 (97-190)	159 ± 28 (113-206)	144 ± 30 (83-181)
	Indirect in birds under isoflurane anesthesia using the wing[9]	140 ± 25 (104-197)	—	—
	Indirect in birds under isoflurane anesthesia using the leg[9]	145 ± 28 (96-196)	—	—
Falcons (n = 45)	Indirect in birds under isoflurane anesthesia[459]	202 ± 27.57	—	—
Red-tailed hawks (n = 6)	Indirect in birds under sevoflurane anesthesia[b,869]	155 ± 27	181 ± 25	—
	Indirect in conscious birds[869]	190 ± 38	236 ± 42	—
	Direct in birds under sevoflurane anesthesia[869]	159 ± 25 (102-216)	178 ± 27 (124-251)	143 ± 24 (78-198)
	Direct in conscious birds[869]	201 ± 29 (154-262)	238 ± 39 (161-301)	180 ± 31 (142-254)
Bald eagles (n = 17)	Direct in spontaneously breathing birds under general anesthesia[388]	MAP was significantly elevated with isoflurane when compared to sevoflurane	176 ± 14.4-209.3 ± 14.4 on isoflurane over 40 min	139.2 ± 14.5-171.6 ± 14.4 on isoflurane over 40 min
			128.8 ± 15-163 ± 13.5 on sevoflurane over 40 min	129.2 ± 15.2-147.1 ± 13.8 on sevoflurane over 40 min
	Indirect in conscious birds[11]	123.5 ± 61.9	—	—
Pigeons (n = 7)	Indirect in conscious birds[93]	—	155 ± 21	—
	Indirect under isoflurane anesthesia	—	87 ± 11	—
Chicken (n = 40)	Direct in birds under general anesthesia[413]	136 (114-158)	141 (118-163)	131 (109-153)
Pekin ducks (n = 72)	Direct in birds under general anesthesia[436]	143 (111–174)	165 (138–192)	121 (85–157)

[a]There was substantial disagreement between direct systolic arterial blood pressure and indirect blood pressure measurements obtained with the Doppler probe from the wing and from the leg of the Hispaniolan parrot (*Amazona ventralis*); attempts to obtain indirect blood pressure measurements with an oscillometric unit were unsuccessful.[9]

[b]Indirect blood pressure measured using an oscillometric unit was unreliable; indirect blood pressure measurements using a Doppler probe and cuff 3 were closer to direct mean arterial pressure measured from the superficial ulnar artery.

TABLE 5-49 Selected Arrhythmias and Some Documented Causes in Birds.[56]

Arrhythmias	ECG Changes	Causes
Excitability Disturbances		
Respiratory sinus arrhythmia	Slowing of HR during expiration	Physiologic
Sinus bradycardia	Low HR, normal sinus rhythm	Vagal stimulation, atropine, anesthesia, hypokalemia, hyperkalemia, vitamin E deficiency, vitamin B_1 deficiency, acetylcholinesterase inhibitors
Sinus tachycardia	High HR, normal sinus rhythm	Sympathetic, catecholamine stimulation
Atrial tachycardia	Series of fast atrial extrasystoles	Atrial distension, ectopic foci
Atrial fibrillation	No normal P waves, irregular SS intervals	Atrial enlargements, cardiac disease
Ventricular premature contraction (VPC)	Wide, bizarre QRS unrelated to P	Ectopic foci, hypokalemia, vitamin B_1 deficiency, vitamin E deficiency, PMV-1, AI, myocardial infarction
Ventricular tachycardia	Series of VPC	Similar causes as for VPCs
Ventricular fibrillation	Chaotic ventricular depolarization	Myocardial hypoxia, shock, severe disorders
Conduction Disturbances		
1st-degree AV block	Long PR intervals	Anesthetics, increased vagal tone
2nd-degree AV block	Long PR intervals, some P without QRS	Anesthetics, increased vagal tone, occasionally normal in pigeons, parrots, raptors
3rd-degree AV block	Escape ventricular rhythm (slow and bizarre QRS), no consistent PR	Severe cardiomegaly
Bundle branch block	Short PR, bizarre and widened QRS	Lead, myopathy, myocarditis, uncommon in birds

TABLE 5-50 ECG Measurements Reference Values on Lead II in Selected Avian Species (Amplitude in mV, Interval/Duration in Sec).[a,58]

Species	African Grey parrot	Amazon Parrot	Bald Eagle	Chicken	Cockatoo	Macaw	Pekin Duck	Racing Pigeon	Red-tailed Hawk
n	45	37	20	72	31	41	50	60	11
Heart rate	340-600	340-600	50-160	180-340	259-575	255-555	200-360	160-300	80-220
P amplitude	0.25-0.55	0.25-0.60	0.050-0.325	—	0.13-0.53	0.03-0.47	—	0.4-0.6	-0.1-0.175
P duration	0.012-0.018	0.008-0.017	0.030-0.060	0.035-0.043	0.009-0.025	0.009-0.021	0.015-0.035	0.015-0.020	0.020-0.035
PR interval	0.040-0.055	0.042-0.055	0.070-0.110	0.073-0.089	0.039-0.071	0.040-0.068	0.04-0.08	0.045-0.070	0.050-0.090
S amplitude	0.9-2.2	0.7-2.3	0.150-1.450	0.10-1.0	0.27-1.59	0.27-1.43	0.35-1.03	1.5-2.8	0.300-0.900
QRS duration	0.010-0.016	0.010-0.015	0.020-0.040	0.02-0.028	0.014-0.026	0.002-0.030	0.028-0.044	0.013-0.016	0.020-0.030
T amplitude	0.18-0.6	0.3-0.8	0.050-0.200	0.03-0.28	0.17-0.97	0.12-0.80	0.04-0.40	0.3-0.8	0.000-0.300
QT interval	0.048-0.080	0.050-0.095	0.110-0.165	—	0.065-0.125	0.053-0.109	0.08-0.12	0.060-0.075	0.080-0.165
MEA	−79 to −103	−90 to −107	−30 to −150	−91 to −120	−73 to −89	−76 to −87	−160 to 95	−83 to −99	−50 to −110

[a]To obtain a 95% reference interval, all published results in the form of mean ± SD were reported as mean ± 2SD and in the form of mean ± sem were reported as mean ±2 sem √n, when only the range or a 95% reference interval was published, it was reported as is.

TABLE 5-51 Echocardiographic Reference Intervals (mm) in Selected Avian Species Obtained in the Horizontal Four-Chamber View.[a,58]

Parameter	African Grey Parrots	Amazon Parrots	Cockatoos	Diurnal Raptors[b]	Pigeons (Parasternal)
n	60	10	10	100	50
Left ventricle					
Systole length	18.4-26	16.5-25.7	16.4-21.6	9.1-20.3	15.9-19.9
Systole width	4.8-8.8	4.3-9.1	3.0-9.8	4.1-8.5	4.4-6.0
Diastole length	20.2-27.8	17.7-26.5	16.7-23.1	11.0-21.8	17.3-22.9
Diastole width	6.6-10.6	6.4-10.4	5.3-11.3	5.3-10.1	6.2-8.6
FS (%)	13.8-31.4	14.4-31.2	11.6-39.6	—	—
Right ventricle					
Systole length	6.4-12.0	5.8-13.0	7.9-12.7	7.3-18.1	—
Systole width	1.0-4.6	1.7-4.5	7.9-12.7	0.9-3.3	—
Diastole length	7.7-15.3	7.7-12.9	6.7-15.9	8.9-18.9	8.3-11.5
Diastole width	2.6-7.0	2.6-7.8	2.5-4.5	0.9-4.1	3.0-5.0
FS (%)	17.0-64.6	26.7-41.5	12.7-53.9	—	—
Aorta					
Systole diameter	2.8-4.4	2.0-4.0	—	—	—
Diastole diameter	2.8-5.2	2.2-4.6	—	2-3.6	2.8-3.2

[a]To obtain a 95% reference interval, all published results in the form of mean ± SD were reported as mean ± 2SD and in the form of mean ± sem were reported as mean ± 2sem$\sqrt{n}$, when only the range or a 95% reference interval was published, it was reported as is. FS, fractional shortening. Echocardiographic measurements may not be reliable and clinically useful.
[b]European diurnal raptors included common buzzard, European sparrowhawk, northern goshawk, and black kite.

TABLE 5-52 Spectral Doppler Echocardiographic Reference Intervals (m/s) in Selected Avian Species Obtained in the Horizontal Four-Chamber View.[a,28,595,775,776]

Species	n	Left Diastolic Inflow	Right Diastolic Inflow	Aortic Systolic Outflow
African grey parrots	—	0.27-0.51	—	0.63-1.15
Amazon parrots	—	0.12-.24	0.12-0.32	0.67-0.99
Barn owls	10	0.14-0.26	0.10-0.34	0.84-1.32
Cockatoos	—	0.02-0.62	—	0.40-1.16
Common buzzard	10	0.16-0.28	0.13-0.25	1.04-1.68
Falcons	15	0.18-0.38	0.17-0.37	1.07-1.43
Harris' hawks	10	0.13-0.25	0.15-0.27	0.75-1.43
Macaws	—	0.40-0.68	—	0.55-1.07

[a]To obtain a 95% reference interval, all published results in the form of mean ± SD were reported as mean ± 2SD and in the form of mean ± sem were reported as mean ± 2sem$\sqrt{n}$, when only the range or a 95% reference interval was published, it was reported as is. Parrots were anesthetized; raptors were awake.

TABLE 5-53 Guidelines for Selection of Psychotherapeutic Agents for Birds.[92,497,729,743]

1. Perform a complete medical and behavioral workup:
   - Obtain a detailed medical and behavioral history.
   - Perform careful physical examination, looking for evidence of feather dysplasia or skin abnormalities.
   - Collect a minimum database that includes complete blood count, plasma biochemistry panel, radiographs, psittacine beak and feather disease testing, as well as paired (affected/nonaffected) skin/feather follicle biopsy when indicated.
2. Once a medical problem has been ruled out or treated, assuming the problem does not abate, form a **behavioral diagnosis:**
   - It is not enough to determine the bird is feather picking; identify "why" the bird is feather picking; use of "antecedent, behavior, and consequence" data can be particularly helpful.
   - Many behavioral problems are multifactorial in origin.
3. Formulate a treatment plan that incorporates:
   - Environmental modification:
     ○ Improve the nutritional plane and basic husbandry.
     ○ Provide environmental enrichment where appropriate.
   - Behavioral modification techniques:
     ○ Focus on what you want the bird to do and reward the bird for that and/or engage in stimulating behavior that will accomplish that goal. Do not punish or deprive the bird.
     ○ Offer behavioral alternatives with emphasis in developing foraging behaviors for treats or food of increasing complexity, and training of basic skills.
   - Behavioral pharmacotherapy can be a useful component of treatment.
   - Whenever possible, consult with a behaviorist, preferably a member of the American College of Veterinary Behaviorists.
4. **Behavioral pharmacotherapy,** general principles:
   - These drugs may help the bird be more open to change, thereby reducing stress and increasing the chances of success.
   - Most behavioral drugs act by exerting effects on neurotransmitters (NT) in the central nervous system (CNS).
   - Serotonin (5-HT) affects mood, sleep patterns, and appetite; also plays a role in the suppression of impulses; low levels or an imbalance between serotonin and other hormones may be associated with maladaptive behaviors.
   - Norepinephrine (NE) plays an important role in attentiveness, sleeping, dreaming, and learning.
   - Gamma-aminobutyric acid (GABA) is a major inhibitory NT.
   - Behavioral drugs are classified based on their first clinical use in humans or on their structure and effects (tricyclics, selective serotonin reuptake inhibitors); major groups include anxiolytics, antipsychotics, and antidepressants, but their use may be more generalized outside of these broad areas.
   - A number of factors must be considered when selecting a psychotropic agent: the proposed mechanism of action, indications and contraindications, common side effects and the potential for other adverse effects, drug cost, and ease of administration; also consider the bird species, its age and underlying health, as well as reproductive status; see information that follows or consult a veterinary behavior text or a general formulary for more detailed information.

- Drugs commonly selected for:
  - Conditions of *fear, phobia, or anxiety* include benzodiazepines and buspirone; antidepressants may also be used for generalized anxiety and separation anxiety.
  - Obsessive-compulsive disorders such as stereotypical behaviors[a] include TCAs and SSRIs.
  - Stereotypy that involves self-injurious behavior include opioid antagonists (i.e., naltrexone), SSRIs, TCAs, and, in select cases, haloperidol.
  - Antipruritic effects include the TCAs; doxepin, followed by amitriptyline, have the most potent antihistaminic activity.[b]
  - Aggression, both hierarchical and anxiety-induced, are the SSRIs.
- Ancillary treatments may include opioid analgesics (Table 5-5), NSAIDs (Table 5-6), hormonal agents (Table 5-7), and/or essential fatty acid supplements when indicated.

5. **How much to give, how often, and for how long?**
   - Many of the doses in Table 5-10 are based on anecdotal experience or case reports; the few empirical studies referenced use small sample sizes.
   - Warn your client that, in many instances, dosing may be by trial and error; for instance, after giving an antidepressant for 4-8 weeks, it may be necessary to adjust the dose, or in some instances to change drugs.
   - Combination therapy can sometimes enhance drug effectiveness:
     - Benzodiazepines (BZDs) may be combined with antidepressants, but reduce the BZD dose to minimize the risk of CNS depression; this combination may be particularly helpful when psychotherapy is first started because it takes weeks for antidepressants to exert an effect.
     - Unless both dosages are decreased, avoid combining drugs that both increase serotonin levels since there is the risk of causing serotonin syndrome.[c]
   - Administer antidepressants for a minimum of 6-8 weeks.
   - Monitor blood work regularly.
   - When and if a beneficial result is achieved, it may be prudent to continue treatment for at least 2-6 months.
   - The process of weaning a bird off of medication may also require trial and error; one technique is to reduce the effective dose by 25% every 3 weeks; if signs relapse, return to the lowest effective dose; taper drug dosages over a minimum of 3 weeks.

6. **Client education**
   - Determine beforehand how you will document treatment response; identify target signs that can be monitored by the owner with respect to intensity, duration, and frequency.
   - Prepare clients for the possibility of trial and error dosing, possible side effects, the duration of treatment that may be necessary, and the length of time before onset of desired effects.
   - Extra-label drug use.

Characteristics	Anxiolytics			Antidepressants	
	Benzodiazepenes	Buspirone	Antipsychotics	Tricyclic Compounds (TCAs)	Selective Serotonin Reuptake Inhibitors (SSRIs)
Range of effects	Mild sedation,[d] to anxiolysis, to hypnosis as dose increases	Calming	Reduce motor activity	A variety of actions including potent antihistaminic activity and some sedation	A variety of actions including a mood-stabilizing effect
Specific examples	Diazepam Lorazepam Midazolam High potency: Alprazolam Clorazepate	—	Haloperidol	Amitriptyline Clomipramine Imipramine	Fluoxetine Paroxetine Sertraline
Disadvantages	Can interfere with learning and affect behavioral modification	Delayed onset of action (2-4 wk)	See below	Delayed onset of action (2-4 wk)	Delayed onset of action (3-6 wk)
Potential adverse effects	Sedation, ataxia,[d] paradoxical excitation; rare fatal idiopathic hepatic necrosis in cats given diazepam PO	Few to mild; confusion, nausea, anorexia	Extrapyramidal signs: tremors, dystonia, dyskinesia or akathisia; transient anorexia and regurgitation	Anticholinergic signs[e]	Uncommon and transient; anorexia most common[f] and serotonin syndrome is the most serious[c]
Contraindications and precautions	Liver or renal disease; aggression; consider potential for human abuse	Severe renal or hepatic disease	—	Discontinue slowly to prevent withdrawal responses; may lower seizure threshold in humans	—
Taste	Benign, although a bitter aftertaste has been described for diazepam	—	—	Lingering bitter taste	Odorless, tasteless tablets

[a]Stereotypies are repetitive behaviors such as circling or pacing, or in some instances, feather-destructive behavior.
[b]The antihistaminic activity of doxepin is 800 times that of diphenhydramine.
[c]Serotonin syndrome may cause muscle tremors, rigidity, agitation, hyperthermia, vocalization, hypertension or hypotension, tachycardia, seizures, coma, and death.
[d]Mild sedative effects create a risk of bird falling from perch; tolerance to sedation may develop over time.
[e]A variety of anticholinergic signs have been reported in mammals, including dry mouth, fatigue, variable degrees of sedation, constipation, tremor, hypotension, arrhythmias, weight gain, mydriasis, and vomiting; sedation and regurgitation are reported most commonly in birds.[497]
[f]Other possible adverse effects with SSRIs include diarrhea, increased agitation, irritability, insomnia, and in rare instances, vomiting.

REFERENCES

1. Aarons J. First aid and wound management in the ostrich. *Proc Annu Conf Assoc Avian Vet* 1995;201-208.
2. Aarons JE. Adverse effects of high environmental temperature on ostrich chicks. *Proc Annu Conf Assoc Avian Vet* 1996;153-158.
3. Aarons JE. Assessing the down bird. *Proc Annu Conf Assoc Avian Vet* 1997;175-179.
4. Abbas RZ, Iqbal Z, Khan MN, et al. Prophylactic efficacy of diclazuril in broilers experimentally infected with three field isolates of *Eimeria tenella*. *Intl J Ag Biol* 2009;11:606-610.
5. Abernathy DR, Arnold GJ, Azarnoff DL, et al., eds. *Mosby's Drug Consult*. St. Louis: Mosby; 2003.
6. Abou-Madi N. Avian anesthesia. *Vet Clin North Am Exot Anim Pract* 2001;4:147-167.
7. Abrams GA, Paul-Murphy J, Murphy CJ. Conjunctivitis in birds. *Vet Clin North Am Exot Anim Pract* 2002;5:287-309.
8. Abu J, Wünschmann A, Redig PT, Feeney D. Management of a cutaneous squamous cell carcinoma in an American flamingo (*Phoenicopterus ruber*). *J Avian Med Surg* 2009;23(1):44-48.
9. Acierno MJ, da Cunha A, Smith J, et al. Agreement between direct and indirect blood pressure measurements obtained from anesthetized Hispaniolan Amazon parrots. *J Am Vet Med Assoc* 2008;233:1587-1590.
10. Aguilar RF, Redig PT. Diagnosis and treatment of avian aspergillosis. In: Bonagura JD, ed. *Kirk's Current Veterinary Therapy XII: Small Animal Practice*. Philadelphia: WB Saunders Co; 1995:1294-1299.
11. Aguilar RF, Smith VE, Ogburn P, et al. Arrythmias associated with isoflurane anesthesia in bald eagles (*Haliaeetus leucocephalus*). *J Zoo Wildl Med* 1995;26:508-516.
12a. Alderton D. *A Birdkeeper's Guide to Pet Birds*. Morris Plains, NJ: Tetra Press; 1987.
12b. Alexander AB, Griffin L, Johnston MS. Radiation therapy of periorbital lymphoma in a blue and gold macaw (*Ara ararauna*). *J Avian Med Surg* 2017;31:39-46.
13. Allen DG, Pringle JK, Smith DA, et al., eds. *Handbook of Veterinary Drugs*. 2nd ed. Philadelphia: JB Lippincott Co; 1998:749-842.
14. Allen JL, Oosterhuis JE. Effect of tolazoline on xylazine-ketamine-induced anesthesia in turkey vultures. *J Am Vet Med Assoc* 1986;189:1011-1012.
15. Al-Sobayil FA, Ahmed AF, Al-Wabel NA, et al. The use of xylazine, ketamine, and isoflurane for induction and maintenance of anesthesia in ostriches (*Struthio camelus*). *J Avian Med Surg* 2009;23:101-107.
16. Al-Timimi F, Nolosco P, Al-Timimi B. Incidence and treatment of serratospiculosis in falcons from Saudi Arabia. *Vet Rec* 2009;165:408-409.
17. Ammersbach M, Beaufrère H, Gionet Rollick A, et al. Laboratory blood analysis in Strigiformes-Part II: plasma biochemistry reference intervals and agreement between the Abaxis Vetscan V2 and the Roche Cobas c501. *Vet Clin Pathol* 2015;44:128-140.
18a. Ammersbach M, Beaufrère H, Gionet Rollick A, Tully T. Laboratory blood analysis in Strigiformes—Part I: hematologic reference intervals and agreement between manual blood cell counting techniques. *Vet Clin Pathol* 2015;44:94-108.
18b. Anadón A, Martínez-Larrañaga MR, Díaz MJ, et al. Pharmacokinetic characteristics and tissue residues for marbofloxacin and its metabolite N-desmethyl-marbofloxacin in broiler chickens. *Am J Vet Res* 2002;63:927-933.
19. Anderson K, Garner MM, Reed HH, et al. Hemorrhagic diathesis in avian species following intramuscular administration of polysulfated glycosaminoglycan. *J Zoo Wildl Med* 2013;44(1):93-99.
20. Anderson NL, Johnson CK, Fender S, et al. Clinical signs and histopathologic findings associated with a newly recognized protozoal disease (*Trichomonas gallinae*) in free-ranging house finches (*Carpodacus mexicanus*). *J Zoo Wildl Med* 2010;41:249-254.
21. Andre J, Delverdier M. Primary bronchial carcinoma with osseous metastasis in an African grey parrot (*Psittacus erithacus*). *J Avian Med Surg* 1999;13(3):180-186.

22. Andrew SE, Clippinger TL, Brooks DE, Helmick KE. Penetrating keratoplasty for treatment of corneal protrusion in a great horned owl (*Bubo virginianus*). *Vet Ophthalmol* 2002;5(3): 201-205.
23. Angenvoort J, Fischer D, Fast C, et al. Limited efficacy of West Nile virus vaccines in large falcons (*Falco* spp.). *Vet Res* 2014;45:41.
24. Arabkhazaeli F, Madani SA, Ghavami S. Outbreak of an unusual tracheal mite, *Ptilonyssus morofskyi* (Acarina: Rhinonyssidae), in canaries (*Serinus canaria*) with concurrent infection with *Staphylococcus aureus* and *Macrorhabdus ornithogaster*. *J Avian Med Surg* 2016;30: 269-273.
25. Araghi M, Azizi S, Vesal N, et al. Evaluation of the sedative effects of diazepam, midazolam, and xylazine after intranasal administration in juvenile ostriches (*Struthio camelus*). *J Avian Med Surg* 2016;30:221-226.
26. Archawaranon M. Hematological investigations of captive Hill Mynah *Gracula religiosa* in Thailand. *Int J Poult Sci* 2005;4:679-682.
27. Asa C, Boutelle S. Contraception. In: Miller RE, Fowler ME, eds. *Fowler's Zoo and Wild Animal Medicine Current Therapy*. Vol 7: St. Louis: Elsevier; 2011:8-14.
28. Ashworth CD, Nelson DR. Antimicrobial potentiation of irrigation solutions containing tris-[hydroxymethyl] aminomethane-EDTA. *J Am Vet Med Assoc* 1990;197:1513-1514.
29. Atalan G, Uzun M, Demirkan I, et al. Effect of medetomidine-butorphanol-ketamine anaesthesia and atipamezole on heart and respiratory rate and cloacal temperature of domestic pigeons. *J Vet Med A Physiol Pathol Clin Med* 2002;49:281-285.
30. Axelson RD. *Caring for Your Pet Bird*. Toronto: Canaviax Publ Ltd; 1981.
31. Azizpour A, Hassani Y. Clinical evaluation of general anaesthesia in pigeons using a combination of ketamine and diazepam. *J S Afr Vet Assoc* 2012;83:12.
32. Baert K, de Backer P. Comparative pharmacokinetics of three non-steroidal anti-inflammatory drugs in five bird species. *Comp Biochem Physiol C Toxicol Pharmacol* 2003;134:25-33.
33. Baert K, Nackaerts J, de Backer P. Disposition of sodium salicylate, flunixin, and meloxicam after intravenous administration in ostriches (*Struthio camelus*). *J Avian Med Surg* 2002;16:123-128.
34. Baert L, Van Poucke S, Vermeersch H, et al. Pharmacokinetics and anthelmintic efficacy of febantel in the racing pigeon (*Columba livia*). *J Vet Pharmacol Therap* 1993;16:223-231.
35. Báez LA, Langston C, Givaruangsawat S, McLaughlin R. Evaluation of *in vitro* serial antibiotic elution from meropenem-impregnated polymethylmethacrylate beads after ethylene oxide gas and autoclave sterilization. *Vet Comp Orthop Traumatol* 2011;24(1):39-44.
36. Bailey J, Heard D, Schumacher J, et al. Midazolam, butorphanol, ketamine, and the clinically effective dose of isoflurane anesthesia in ostriches (*Struthio camelus*). *25th Annu Meet Am Coll Vet Anesthesiol* 2000;38.
37. Bailey T. Raptors: respiratory problems. In: Chitty J, Lierz M, eds. *BSAVA Manual of Raptors, Pigeons and Passerine Birds*. Gloucester, UK: BSAVA; 2008:223-233.
38. Bailey TA, Apo MM. Pharmaceutics commonly used in avian medicine. In: Samour J, ed. *Avian Medicine*. 3rd ed. Edinburgh: Mosby Elsevier; 2016:637-678.
39. Bailey TA, Apo MM. Pharmaceutics commonly used in avian medicine. In: Samour JH, ed. *Avian Medicine*. 2nd ed. Edinburgh: Mosby Elsevier; 2008:485-509.
40. Baillie JW. Alternative therapy ideas for feather picking. *Proc Annu Conf Assoc Avian Vet* 2001;191-196.
41. Baine K, Hendrix DVH, Kuhn SE, et al. The efficacy and safety of topical rocuronium bromide to induce bilateral mydriasis in Hispaniolan Amazon parrots (*Amazona ventralis*). *J Avian Med Surg* 2016;30(1):8-13.
42. Baine K, Jones MP, Cox S, et al. Pharmacokinetics of compounded intravenous and oral gabapentin in Hispaniolan Amazon parrots (*Amazona ventralis*). *J Avian Med Surg* 2015;29: 165-173.

43. Baine K, Jones MP, Cox S, Martín-Jiménez T. Pharmacokinetics of compounded intravenous and oral gabapentin in Hispaniolan Amazon parrots (*Amazona ventralis*). *J Avian Med Surg* 2015;29(3):165-173.
44. Barron HW, Roberts RE, Latimer KS, et al. Tolerance doses of cutaneous and mucosal tissues in ring-necked parakeets (*Psittacula krameri*) for external beam megavoltage radiation. *J Avian Med Surg* 2009;23(1):6-9.
45. Barsotti G, Briganti A, Spratte JR, et al. Bilateral mydriasis in common buzzards (*Buteo buteo*) and little owls (*Athene noctua*) induced by concurrent topical administration of rocuronium bromide. *Vet Ophthalmol* 2010;13(Suppl 1):35-40.
46. Barsotti G, Briganti A, Spratte JR, et al. Mydriatic effect of topically applied rocuronium bromide in tawny owls (*Strix aluco*): comparison between two protocols. *Vet Ophthalmol* 2010;13 (Suppl):9-13.
47. Barsotti G, Briganti A, Spratte JR, et al. Safety and efficacy of bilateral topical application of rocuronium bromide for mydriasis in European kestrels (*Falco tinnunculus*). *J Avian Med Surg* 2012;26(1):1-5.
48. Bartlett SL, Bailey R, Baitchman E. Diagnosis and management of diabetes mellitus in a Bali mynah (*Leucopsar rothschildi*). *J Avian Med Surg* 2016;30(2):146-151.
49. Bauck L. *A Practitioner's Guide to Avian Medicine*. American Animal Hospital Association: Lakewood, CO; 1993.
50. Bauck L, Brash M. Survey of diseases of the Lady Gouldian finch. *Proc Annu Conf Assoc Avian Vet* 1999;204-212.
51. Bauck L, Hoefer HL. Avian antimicrobial therapy. *Semin Avian Exot Pet Med* 1993;2:17-22.
52. Bauck L, Hillyer E, Hoefer H. Rhinitis: case reports. *Proc Annu Conf Assoc Avian Vet* 1992;134-139.
53. Beaufrère H. Nebulization in birds. In: Samour J, ed. *Avian Medicine*. 3rd ed. St. Louis, MO: Elsevier; 2016:208-209.
54. Beaufrère H. Parenteral fluid therapy. In: Samour J, ed. *Avian Medicine*. 3rd ed. St. Louis, MO: Elsevier; 2016:209-215.
55. Beaufrère H. *Personal observation.* 2017.
56. Beaufrère H, Guzman DS-M. Systemic diseases: disorders of the cardiovascular system. In: Samour J, ed. *Avian Medicine*. St. Louis: Elsevier; 2016:395-407.
57. Beaufrère H, Aertsens A, Fouquet J. Un cas d'insuffisance cardiaque congestive chez un perroquet gris. *L'Hebdo Vet* 2007;200:8-10.
58. Beaufrère H, Schilliger L, Pariaut R. Cardiovascular system. In: Mitchell M, Tully T, eds. *Current Therapy in Exotic Pet Practice*. St. Louis, MO: Elsevier; 2016:151-220.
59. Beaufrère H, Summa N, Le K. Respiratory system. In: Mitchell M, Tully T, eds. *Current Therapy in Exotic Pet Practice*. St. Louis, MO: Elsevier; 2016:76-150.
60. Beaufrère H, Holder KA, Bauer R, et al. Intermittent claudication-like syndrome secondary to atherosclerosis in a yellow-naped Amazon parrot (*Amazona ochrocephala auropalliata*). *J Avian Med Surg* 2011;25(4):266-276.
61. Beaufrère H, Laniesse D, Stickings P, et al. Generalized tetanus in a gyrfalcon (*Falco rusticolus*) with pododermatitis. *Avian Dis* 2016;60(4):850-855.
62. Beaufrère H, Nevarez J, Gaschen L, et al. Diagnosis of presumed acute ischemic stroke and associated seizure management in a Congo African grey parrot. *J Am Vet Med Assoc* 2011;239(1):122-128.
63. Beaufrère H, Nevarez J, Taylor WM, et al. Fluoroscopic study of the normal gastrointestinal motility and measurements in the Hispaniolan Amazon parrot (*Amazona ventralis*). *Vet Radiol Ultrasound* 2010;51(4):441-446.
64. Beaufrère H, Papich MG, Brandão J, et al. Plasma drug concentrations of orally administered rosuvastatin in Hispaniolan Amazon parrots (*Amazona ventralis*). *J Avian Med Surg* 2015;29 (1):18-24.

65. Beaufrère H, Pariaut R, Rodriguez D, et al. Comparison of transcoelomic, contrast transcoelomic, and transesophageal echocardiography in anesthetized red-tailed hawks (*Buteo jamaicensis*). *Am J Vet Res* 2012;73(10):1560-1568.
66. Beaufrère H, Rodriguez D, Pariaut R, et al. Estimation of intrathoracic arterial diameter by means of computed tomographic angiography in Hispaniolan Amazon parrots. *Am J Vet Res* 2011;72(2):210-218.
67. Beaufrère H, Pariaut R, Rodriguez D, Tully TN. Avian vascular imaging: a review. *J Avian Med Surg* 2010;24(3):174-184.
68. Bechert U, Christensen JM, Poppenga R, et al. Pharmacokinetics of orally administered terbinafine in African penguins (*Spheniscus demersus*) for potential treatment of aspergillosis. *J Zoo Wild Med* 2010;41:263-274.
69. Bechert U, Christensen JM, Poppenga R, et al. Pharmacokinetics of terbinafine after single oral dose administration in red-tailed hawks (*Buteo jamaicensis*). *J Avian Med Surg* 2010;24:122-230.
70. Beckwith-Cohen B, Horowitz I, Bdolah-Abram T, et al. Differences in ocular parameters between diurnal and nocturnal raptors. *Vet Ophthalmol* 2015;18(Suppl 1):98-105.
71. Beernaert LA, Baert K, Marin P, et al. Designing voriconazole treatment for racing pigeons: balancing between hepatic enzyme auto induction and toxicity. *Med Mycol* 2009;47:276-285.
72. Beernaert LA, Pasmans F, Baert K, et al. Designing a treatment protocol with voriconazole to eliminate *Aspergillus fumigatus* from experimentally inoculated pigeons. *Vet Microbiol* 2009;139:393-397.
73. Beernaert LA, Pasmans F, Van Waeyenberghe L, et al. Avian *Asperigillus fumigatus* strain resistant to both itraconazole and voriconazole. *Antimicrob Agents Chemother* 2009;53:2199-2201.
74. Bernard JB, Allen ME. Feeding captive piscivorous animals: nutritional aspects of fish as food. *Nutritional Advisory Group Handbook*. 1997;1-11.
75. Best R. Breeding problems. In: Beynon PH, Forbes NA, Lawton MPC, eds. *BSAVA Manual of Raptors, Pigeons and Waterfowl*. Ames: Iowa State University Press; 1996:202-215.
76. Beynon PH, Forbes NA, Harcourt-Brown NH. *Manual of Raptors, Pigeons and Waterfowl*. Ames: Iowa State University Press; 1996.
77. Beynon PH, Forbes NA, Lawton MPC. *Manual of Psittacine Birds*. Ames: Iowa State University Press; 1996.
78. Bicknese EJ. Review of avian sarcocystis. *Proc Annu Conf Assoc Avian Vet* 1993;52-58.
79. Bigby SE, Carter JE, Bauquier S, et al. Use of propofol for induction and maintenance of anesthesia in a king penguin (*Aptenodytes patagonicus*) undergoing magnetic resonance imaging. *J Avian Med Surg* 2016;30:237-242.
80. Bigham AS, Zamani Moghaddam AK. Finch (*Taeneopygia guttata*) sedation with intranasal administration of diazepam, midazolam or xylazine. *J Vet Pharmacol Ther* 2013;36:102-104.
81. Bird JE, Walser MM, Duke GE. Toxicity of gentamicin in red-tailed hawks (*Buteo jamaicensis*). *Am J Vet Res* 1983;44:1289-1293.
82. Bird JE, Miller KW, Larson AA, et al. Pharmacokinetics of gentamicin in birds of prey. *Am J Vet Res* 1983;44:1245-1247.
83. Bishop CR, Rorabaugh E. Evaluation of the safety and eficacy of selamectin in budgerigars with *Knemidokoptes* infection. *Proc Annu Conf Assoc Avian Vet* 2010;79-84.
84. Bishop CR, McCoy B, Peter B. Selamectin tolerance in *Taeniopygia guttata* with *Sternostoma tracheacolum*. *Proc Annu Conf Assoc Avian Vet* 2007;251-254.
85. Bishop Y, ed. *The Veterinary Formulary*. 5th ed. London: Pharmaceutical Press; 2001.
86. Bloomfield RB, Brooks D, Vulliet R. The pharmacokinetics of a single intramuscular dose of amikacin in red-tailed hawks (*Buteo jamaicensis*). *J Zoo Wildl Med* 1997;28:55-61.
87. Bonar CJ, Lewandowski AH. Use of a liposomal formulation of amphotericin B for treating wound aspergillosis in a goliath heron (*Ardea goliath*). *J Avian Med Surg* 2004;18:162-166.

88. Bonar CJ, Lewandowski AH, Schaul J. Suspected fenbendazole toxicosis in 2 vulture species (*Gyps africanus, Torgos tracheliotus*) and marabou storks (*Leptoptilos crumeniferus*). *J Avian Med Surg* 2003;17:16-19.
89. Boonstra JL, Cox SK, Martin-Jimenez T. Pharmacokintics of meloxicam after intramuscular and oral administration of a single dose to American flamingos (*Phoenicopterus ruber*). *Am J Vet Res* 2017;78:267-273.
90. Boothe DM. Antibacterial agents. *The Merck Veterinary Manual* 2015. Available at: www.merckvetmanual.com/pharmacology/antibacterial-agents. Accessed Dec 1, 2016.
91. Boothe DM. Antifungal agents. *The Merck Veterinary Manual* 2015. Available at: www.merckvetmanual.com/pharmacology/antifungal-agents. Accessed Dec 1, 2016.
92. Boothe DM. Drugs that modify animal behavior. In: Boothe DM, ed. *Small Animal Clinical Pharmacology and Therapeutics*. Philadelphia: WB Saunders; 2001:457-472.
93. Botman J, Dugdale A, Gabriel F, et al. Cardiorespiratory parameters in the awake pigeon and during anaesthesia with isoflurane. *Vet Anaesth Analg* 2016;43:63-71.
94. Botman J, Gabriel F, Dugdale AH, et al. Anaesthesia with sevoflurane in pigeons: minimal anaesthetic concentration (MAC) determination and investigation of cardiorespiratory variables at 1 MAC. *Vet Rec* 2016;178:560.
95. Bowles HL. Management with potassium bromide of seizures of undetermined origin in an umbrella cockatoo. *Exot DVM* 2003;4(5):7-8.
96. Bowles H, Lichtenberger M, Lennox A. Emergency and critical care of pet birds. *Vet Clin North Am Exot Anim Pract* 2007;10:345-394.
97. Bowman MR, Paré JA, Ziegler LE, et al. Effects of metoclopramide on the gastrointestinal tract motility of Hispaniolan parrots (*Amazona ventralis*). *Proc Annu Conf Am Assoc Zoo Vet* 2002;117-118.
98. Bowman MR, Waldoch J, Pittman JM, et al. Enrofloxacin plasma concentrations in sandhill cranes (*Grus canadensis*) after administration in drinking water: a preliminary study. *Proc Annu Conf Am Assoc Zoo Vet* 2002;389-390.
99. Brady S, Burgdorf A, Wack R. Treatment of pulmonary hypertension in a mealy Amazon parrot (*Amazona farinosa*) using sildenafil citrate. *J Avian Med Surg* 2016;30:368-373.
100. Brandão J, da Cunha AF, Pypendop B, et al. Cardiovascular tolerance of intravenous lidocaine in broiler chickens (*Gallus gallus domesticus*) anesthetized with isoflurane. *Vet Anaesth Analg* 2015;42:442-448.
101. Brandão J, Reynolds CA, Beaufrère H, et al. Cardiomyopathy in a Harris hawk (*Parabuteo unicinctus*). *J Am Vet Med Assoc* 2016;249(2):221-227.
102. Braun EJ. Comparative renal function in reptiles, birds, and mammals. *Semin Avian Exot Pet Med* 1998;7:62-71.
103. Brightsmith DJ, McDonald D, Matsafuji D, Bailey CA. Nutritional content of the diets of free-living scarlet macaw chicks in southeastern Peru. *J Avian Med Surg* 2010;24(1):9-23.
104. Brown CS. Wild bird rehabilitation for the practicing veterinarian. *Proc Annu Conf Assoc Avian Vet* 2003;207-219.
105. Bruch J von, Aufinger P, Jakoby JR. Untersuchungen zur pharmakokinetik und wirkung von intramuskulär, oral und über das trinkwasser verabreichtem sulfadimethoxine an gesunden und kokzidien-infizierten, adulten tauben (*Columba livia* Gmel., 1789, var. dom.). (Pharmacokinetics and efficacy of sulfadimethoxine in healthy and coccidia-infected adult pigeons.) *Vet Bull* 1986;56:7830.
106. Bueno MG, Lopez RP, de Menezes RM, et al. Identification of *Plasmodium relictum* causing mortality in penguins (*Spheniscus magellanicus*) from Sao Paulo Zoo, Brazil. *Vet Parasitol* 2010;173:123-127.
107. Bunting EM, Abou Madi N, Cox S, et al. Evaluation of oral itraconazole administration in captive Humboldt penquins (*Spheniscus humboldti*). *J Zoo Wildl Med* 2009;40:508-518.
108. Burke TJ. Antibiotic therapy in pet birds and reptiles. In: Weber AJ, Grey S, Townsend K, et al., eds. *Veterinary Pharmaceuticals and Biologicals*. 5th ed. Lenexa, KS: Veterinary Medicine Publishing Co; 1986.

109. Bush M, Locke D, Neal LA, et al. Gentamicin tissue concentration in various avian species following recommended dosage therapy. *Am J Vet Res* 1981;42:2114-2116.
110. Bush M, Locke D, Neal LA, et al. Pharmacokinetics of cephalothin and cephalexin in selected avian species. *Am J Vet Res* 1981;42:1014-1017.
111. Bush M, Neal LA, Custer RS. Preliminary pharmacokinetic studies of selected antibiotics in birds. *Proc Annu Conf Assoc Avian Vet* 1979;45-47.
112. Byrne RF, Davis C, Lister SA, et al. Prescribing for birds. In: Bishop Y, ed. *The Veterinary Formulary*. 5th ed. London: Pharmaceutical Press; 2001:43-56.
113. Cambre RC, Kenny D. Vaccination of zoo birds against avian botulism with mink botulism vaccine. *Proc Annu Conf Am Assoc Zoo Vet* 1993;383-385.
114. Campbell TW, Smith SA, Zimmerman KL. Hematology of waterfowl and raptors. In: Weiss DJ, Wardrop KJ, eds. *Schalm's Veterinary Hematology*. 6th ed. Ames: Blackwell Publishing; 2010:978-979.
115. Canny CJ, Ward DA, Patton S, et al. Microsporidian keratoconjunctivitis in a double yellow-headed Amazon parrot (*Amazona ochrocephala oratrix*). *J Avian Med Surg* 1999;13:279-286.
116. Carnarius M, Hafez HM, Henning A, et al. Clinical signs and diagnosis of thiamine deficiency in juvenile goshawks (*Accipiter gentilis*). *Vet Rec* 2008;163(7):215-217.
117. Carpenter JW. Cranes (Order Gruiformes). In: Fowler ME, ed. *Zoo and Wild Animal Medicine*. 2nd ed. Philadelphia: WB Saunders Co; 1986:315-326.
118. Carpenter JW. Infectious and parasitic diseases of cranes. In: Fowler ME, ed. *Zoo and Wild Animal Medicine: Current Therapy 3*. Philadelphia: WB Saunders Co; 1993:229-237.
119. Carpenter JW. Gruiformes (cranes, limpkins, rails, gallinules, coots, bustards). In: Fowler ME, Miller RE, eds. *Zoo and Wild Animal Medicine*. 5th ed. St. Louis: WB Saunders Co; 2003:171-180.
120. Carpenter JW. *Personal observation;* 2011.
121. Carpenter JW, Novilla MN, Hatfield JS. The safety and physiological effects of the anticoccidial drugs monensin and clazuril in sandhill cranes (*Grus canadensis*). *J Zoo Wildl Med* 1992;23:214-221.
122. Carpenter JW, Novilla MN, Hatfield JS. Efficacy of selected coccidiostats in sandhill cranes (*Grus canadensis*) following challenge. *J Zoo Wildl Med* 2005;36:391-400.
123. Carpenter JW, Hunter RP, Olsen JH, et al. Pharmacokinetics of marbofloxacin in blue and gold macaws (*Ara ararauna*). *Am J Vet Res* 2006;67:947-950.
124. Carpenter JW, Olsen JH, Randle-Port M, et al. Pharmacokinetics of azithromycin in the blue and gold macaw (*Ara ararauna*) after intravenous and oral administration. *J Zoo Wildl Med* 2005;36:606-609.
125. Carpenter JW, Tully Jr TN, Gehring R, et al. Single-dose pharmacokinetics of piperacillin/tazobactam in Hispaniolan Amazon parrots (*Amazona ventralis*). *J Avian Med Surg* 2017;31(2):95-101.
126. Carpenter NA. Anseriform and galliform therapeutics. *Vet Clin North Am Exot Anim Pract* 2000;3:1-17.
127. Carter RT, Murphy CJ, Stuhr CM, et al. Bilateral phacoemulsification and intraocular lens implantation in a great horned owl. *J Am Vet Med Assoc* 2007;230:559-561.
128. Ceulemans SM, Guzman DS, Olsen GH, et al. Evaluation of thermal antinociceptive effects after intramuscular administration of buprenorphine hydrochloride to American kestrels (*Falco sparverius*). *Am J Vet Res* 2014;75:705-710.
129. Chaleva EI, Vasileva IV, Savova MD. Absorption of lincomycin through the respiratory pathways and its influence on alveolar macrophages after aerosol administration to chickens. *Res Vet Sci* 1994;57:245-247.
130. Chan FT, Chang GR, Wang HC, et al. Anesthesia with isoflurane and sevoflurane in the crested serpent eagle (*Spilornis cheela hoya*): minimum anesthetic concentration, physiological effects, hematocrit, plasma chemistry and behavioral effects. *J Vet Med Sci* 2013;75:1591-1600.
131. Chang GJ, Davis BS, Stringfield C, et al. Prospective immunization of the endangered California condors (*Gymnogyps californianus*) protects this species from lethal West Nile virus infection. *Vaccine* 2007;25:2325-2330.

132. Chen LJ, Sun BH, Qu JP, et al. Avermectin induced inflammation damage in king pigeon brain. *Chemosphere* 2013;93:2528-2534.
133. Childs-Sanford SE, Rassnick KM, Alcaraz A. Carboplatin for treatment of a sertoli cell tumor in a mallard (*Anas platyrhynchos*). *Vet Comp Oncol* 2006;4(1):51-56.
134. Chitty J. Birds of prey. In: Meredith A, Redrobe S, eds. *BSAVA Manual of Exotic Pets*. Gloucester, GB: British Small Animal Veterinary Association; 2002:179-192.
135. Chitty J, Lierz M. Formulary. In: Chitty J, Lierz M, eds. *BSAVA Manual of Raptors, Pigeons and Passerine Birds*. Gloucester: British Small Animal Veterinary Association; 2008:384-390.
136. Clark CH, Thomas JE, Milton JL, et al. Plasma concentrations of chloramphenicol in birds. *Am J Vet Res* 1982;43:1949.
137. Clarke CR, Kocan AA, Webb AI, et al. Intravenous pharmacokinetics of penicillin G and antipyrine in ostriches and emus. *J Zoo Wildl Med* 2001;32:74-77.
138. Clubb SL. Therapeutics. In: Harrison GJ, Harrison LR, eds. *Clinical Avian Medicine and Surgery*. Philadelphia: WB Saunders Co; 1986:327-355.
139. Clubb SL. Birds. In: Johnston DE, ed. *The Bristol Veterinary Handbook of Antimicrobial Therapy*. 2nd ed. Veterinary Learning Systems Co: Trenton, NJ; 1987:188-199.
140. Clubb SL. Clinical management of psittacine birds affected with proventricular dilation disease. *Proc Annu Conf Assoc Avian Vet* 2006;85-90.
141. Clubb SL, Schubot RM, Joyner K, et al. Hematologic and serum biochemical reference intervals in juvenile eclectus parrots (*Eclectus roratus*). *J Assoc Avian Vet* 1990;4:218-225.
142. Clubb SL, Schubot RM, Joyner K, et al. Hematologic and serum biochemical reference intervals in juvenile cockatoos. *J Assoc Avian Vet* 1991;5:16-26.
143. Clubb SL, Schubot RM, Joyner K, et al. Hematologic and serum biochemical reference intervals in juvenile macaws (*Ara* sp. [sic.]). *J Assoc Avian Vet* 1991;5:154-162.
144. Clyde VL, Patton S. Diagnosis, treatment and control of common parasites in companion and aviary birds. *Semin Avian Exotic Pet Med* 1996;5:75-84.
145. Cockcroft PD, Jones AC, Harris JM. Antibacterial activity of ceftiofur-impregnated polymethylmethacrylate beads following manufacture, storage and sterilisation. *Vet Rec* 2003;152:21-22.
146. Cole GA, Paul-Murphy J, Krugner-Higby L, et al. Analgesic effects of intramuscular administration of meloxicam in Hispaniolan parrots (*Amazona ventralis*) with experimentally induced arthritis. *Am J Vet Res* 2009;70:1471-1476.
147. Coles BH. Appendix 1: An avian formulary. In: *Avian Medicine and Surgery*. 2nd ed. Oxford: Blackwell Science, Osney Mead; 1997:240-278.
148. Coles BH. Prescribing for exotic birds. In: Bishop Y, ed. *The Veterinary Formulary*. 5th ed. London: Pharmaceutical Press; 2001:99-105.
149a. Cooper JE. Appendix IX. Medicines and other agents used in treatment, including emergency anaesthesia kit and avian resuscitation protocol. In: Cooper JE, ed. *Birds of Prey: Health and Disease*. 3rd ed. Ames: Blackwell Publishing, Iowa State Press; 2002:271-277.
149b. Cooper RG. Bacterial, fungal and parasitic infections in the ostrich (*Struthio camelus* var. *domesticus*). *Anim Sci J* 2005;76:97-106.
150. Cornelissen H. Behavior, anatomy, feeding and medical problems of toucans in captivity. *Proc Euro Conf Avian Med Surg* 1993;446-453.
151. Cornelissen H, Ducatelle R, Roels S. Successful treatment of a channel-billed toucan (*Ramphastos vitellinus*) with iron storage disease by chelation therapy: sequential monitoring of the iron content of the liver during the treatment period by quantitative chemical and image analyses. *J Avian Med Surg* 1995;9:131-137.
152. Cornick JL. *Veterinary Anesthesia*. Woburn, MA: Butterworth-Heinemann; 2001;196-198.
153. Costantini V, Carraro C, Bucci FA, et al. Influence of a new slow-release GnRH analogue implant on reproduction in the budgerigar (*Melopsittacus undulatus*). *Anim Repro Sci* 2009;111:289-301.

154. Cowan ML, Martin GB, Monks DJ, et al. Inhibition of the reproductive system by deslorelin in male and female pigeons (*Columba livia*). *J Avian Med Surg* 2014;28:102-108.
155. Cray C. University of Miami Avian and Wildlife Laboratory avian reference ranges. University of Miami Web site. Available at: http://www.cpl.med.miami.edu/documents/avian_reference_ranges.pdf. Accessed June 15, 2017.
156. Crispin SM, Barnett KC. Ocular candidiasis in ornamental ducks. *Avian Pathol* 1978;7(1):49-59.
157. Cross G. Antiviral therapy. *Semin Avian Exot Pet Med* 1995;4:96-102.
158. Crosta L, Delli Carri AP. Oral treatment with clindamycin in racing pigeons. *Proc First Conf Euro Comm Assoc Avian Vet* 1991;293-296.
159. Cubas ZS. Medicine: Family Rhamphastidae (toucans). In: Fowler ME, Cubas ZS, eds. *Biology, Medicine, and Surgery of South American Wild Animals*. Ames: Iowa State University Press; 2001:188-199.
160. Cubas ZS. Toucans: husbandry and medicine. *Proc Annu Congr World Small Anim Vet Assoc*. Sao Paulo, Brazil; 2009. Avialable at: http://www.vin.com/proceedings/Proceedings.plx?CID=WSAVA2009&Category=8063&PID=53615&Print=1&O=Generic. Accessed Dec 12, 2010.
161. Curro TG. Evaluation of the isoflurane-sparing effects of butorphanol and flunixin in psittaciformes. *Proc Annu Conf Assoc Avian Vet* 1994;17-19.
162. Curro TG, Brunson DB, Paul-Murphy J. Determination of the ED_{50} of isoflurane and evaluation of the isoflurane-sparing effect of butorphanol in cockatoos (*Cacatua* spp.). *Vet Surg* 1994;23:429-433.
163. Cushing A, McClean M. Use of thiafentanil-medetomidine for the induction of anesthesia in emus (*Dromaius novaehollandiae*) within a wild animal park. *J Zoo Wildl Med* 2010;41:234-241.
164. Custer RS, Bush M, Carpenter JW. Pharmacokinetics of gentamicin in blood plasma of quail, pheasants, and cranes. *Am J Vet Res* 1979;40:892-895.
165. Cuthbert R, Parry-Jones J, Green RE, et al. NSAIDs and scavenging birds: potential impacts beyond Asia's critically endangered vultures. *Biol Lett* 2007;3:90-93.
166. Cutler DC, Shiomitsu K, Liu C-C, Nevarez JG. Comparison of calculated radiation delivery versus actual radiation delivery in military macaws (*Ara militaris*). *J Avian Med Surg* 2016;30(1):1-7.
167. da Cunha AF, Strain GM, Rademacher N, et al. Palpation- and ultrasound-guided brachial plexus blockade in Hispaniolan Amazon parrots (*Amazona ventralis*). *Vet Anaesth Analg* 2013;40:96-102.
168. Dahlhausen B, Aldred S, Colaizzi E. Resolution of clinical proventricular dilatation disease by cyclooxygenase 2 inhibition. *Proc Annu Conf Assoc Avian Vet* 2002;9-12.
169. Dahlhausen B, Lindstrom JG, Radabaugh CS. The use of terbinafine hydrochloride in the treatment of avian fungal disease. *Proc Annu Conf Assoc Avian Vet* 2000;35-39.
170. Davidson G. Veterinary pharmacy. In: Riviere JE, Papich MG, eds. *Veterinary Pharmacology and Therapeutics*. 9th ed. Hoboken, NJ: Wiley-Blackwell; 2009:1413.
171. Davies RR. Passerine birds: going light. In: Chitty J, Lierz M, eds. *BSAVA Manual of Raptors, Pigeons and Passerine Birds*. Gloucester: British Small Animal Veterinary Association; 2008:365-369.
172. Davis MR, Langan JN, Johnson YJ, et al. West Nile virus seroconversion in penguins after vaccination with a killed virus vaccine or a DNA vaccine. *J Zoo Wildl Med* 2008;39:582-589.
173. de Andrade JG, Lelis RT, Damatta RA, et al. Occurrence of nematodes and anthelmintic management of ostrich farms from different Brazilian states: *Libyostrongylus douglassii* dominates mixed infections. *Vet Parasitol* 2011;178:129-133.
174. De Francisco N, Ruiz Troya JD, Agüera EI. Lead and lead toxicity in domestic and free living birds. *Avian Pathol* 2003;32:3-13.

175. De Herdt P, Devriese LA, De Groote B, et al. Antibiotic treatment of *Streptococcus bovis* infections in pigeons. *Proc Euro Conf Avian Med Surg* 1993;297-304.
176. de Lucas JJ, Rodríguez C, Waxman S, et al. Pharmacokinetics of marbofloxacin after intravenous and intramuscular administration to ostriches. *Vet J* 2005;3:364-368.
177. de Matos R. Calcium metabolism in birds. *Vet Clin North Am Exot Anim Pract* 2008; 11(1):59-82.
178. de Souza LP, Lelis RT, Granja IR, et al. Efficacy of albendazole and moxidectin and resistance to ivermectin against *Libyostrongylus douglassii* and *Libyostrongylus dentatus* in ostriches. *Vet Parasitol* 2012;189:387-389.
179. De Voe RS, Trogdon M, Flammer K. Preliminary assessment of the effect of diet and L-carnitine supplementation on lipoma size and bodyweight in budgerigars (*Melopsittacus undulatus*). *J Avian Med Surg* 2004;18:12-18.
180. Degernes LA. Topics in emergency medicine: fluid therapy and parenteral nutrition. In: *Proc Avian Specialty Advanced Prog Small Mam and Rept Med Surg (Annu Conf Assoc Avian Vet)*; 1998:55-60.
181. Degernes LA, Crosier ML, Harrison LD, et al. Autologous, homologous, and heterologous red blood cell transfusions in cockatiels (*Nymphicus hollandicus*). *J Avian Med Surg* 1999; 13(1):2-9.
182. Degernes L, Davidson G, Flammer K, et al. Administration of total parenteral nutrition in pigeons. *Am J Vet Res* 1994;55:660-665.
183. Degernes LA, Fisher PE, Trogdon M, et al. Gastrointestinal scintigraphy in psittacines. *Proc Annu Conf Assoc Avian Vet* 1999;93-94.
184. Degernes LA, Harrison LD, Smith DW, et al. Autologous, homologous and heterologous red blood cell transfusions in conures of the genus *Aratinga*. *J Avian Med Surg* 1999; 13:10-14.
185. Delaski KM, Nelson S, Dronen NO, et al. Detection and management of air sac trematodes (*Szidatitrema* species) in captive multispecies avian exhibits. *J Avian Med Surg* 2015;29(4):345-353.
186. Delk K. Clinical management of seizures in avian patients. *J Exot Pet Med* 2012;21(2):132-139.
187. Denver MC, Tell LA, Galey FD. Comparison of two heavy metal chelators for treatment of lead toxicosis in cockatiels. *Am J Vet Res* 2000;61:935-940.
188. Desmarchelier M, Troncy E, Fitzgerald G, et al. Analgesic effects of meloxicam administration on postoperative orthopedic pain in domestic pigeons (*Columba livia*). *Am J Vet Res* 2012;73:361-367.
189. Dheeraj A, Seema A, Astha C. Effect of fipronil toxicity in haematological parameters in white leghorn cockerels. *Afri J Agricult Res* 2014;9:2759-2764.
190. Dijkstra B, Guzman DS, Gustavsen K, et al. Renal, gastrointestinal, and hemostatic effects of oral administration of meloxicam to Hispaniolan Amazon parrots (*Amazona ventralis*). *Am J Vet Res* 2015;76:308-317.
191. Dodwell GT. *The Complete Book of Canaries*. London: Merehurst Press; 1986.
192. Doneley B. Management of captive ratites. In: Harrison GJ, Lightfoot TL, eds. *Clinical Avian Medicine*. Vol II. Palm Beach: Spix Publishing; 2006:957-989.
193. Doneley B. The use of gabapentin to treat presumed neuralgia in a little corella (*Cacatua sanguinea*). *Proc Austral Assoc Avian Vet* 2007;169-172.
194. Doneley B. Formulary. In: Doneley B, ed. *Avian Medicine and Surgery in Practice: Companion and Aviary Birds*. London: Manson Publishing; 2011:285-320.
195. Doneley B. *Avian Medicine and Surgery in Practice: Companion and Aviary Birds*. 2nd ed. Boca Raton, FL: CRC Press; 2016.
196. Donnelly RF, Pascuet E, Ma C, et al. Stability of celecoxib oral suspension. *Canadian J Hosp Pharm* 2009;62:464-468.
197. Doolen M. Adriamycin® chemotherapy in a blue-front Amazon with osteosarcoma. *Proc Annu Conf Assoc Avian Vet* 1994;89-91.

198. Dorrestein GM. *Studies on Pharmacokinetics of Some Antibacterial Agents in Homing Pigeons (Columba livia)*. Thesis: Utrecht University; 1986.
199. Dorrestein GM. Formulation and (bio)availability problems of drug formulations in birds. *J Vet Pharmacol Therap* 1992;15:143-150.
200. Dorrestein GM. Antimicrobial drug use in companion birds. In: Prescott JF, Baggot JD, eds. *Antimicrobial Therapy in Veterinary Medicine*. 2nd ed. Ames: Iowa State University Press; 1993:491-506.
201. Dorrestein GM. Infectious diseases and their therapy in Passeriformes. In: *Antimicrobial Therapy in Caged Birds and Exotic Pets*. Trenton, NJ: Veterinary Learning Systems Co; 1995:11-27.
202. Dorrestein GM. Antimicrobial drug use in companion birds. In: Prescott JF, Baggot JD, Walker RD, eds. *Antimicrobial Therapy in Veterinary Medicine*. 3rd ed. Ames: Iowa State University Press; 2000:617-636.
203. Dorrestein GM. Passerine and softbill therapeutics. *Vet Clin North Am Exot Anim Pract* 2000;3:35-57.
204. Dorrestein GM, Kazemi SM, Eksik N. Comparative study of Synulox® and Augmentin® after intravenous, intramuscular and oral administration in collared doves (*Streptopelia decaocto*). In: Kösters J, et al, eds. *X. Tagung der Fachgruppe "Geflügelkrankheiten."* Giessen, Germany: Deutschen Veterinärmedizinischen Gesellschaft e.V; 1996:42-54.
205. Dorrestein GM, van Der Horst HHA, Cremers HJWM, et al. Quill mite (*Dermoglyphus passerinus*) infestation of canaries (*Serinus canaria*): diagnosis and treatment. *Avian Pathol* 1997;26:195-199.
206. Dorrestein GM, van Gogh H, Rinzema JD. Pharmacokinetic aspects of penicillins, aminoglycosides and chloramphenicol in birds compared to mammals: a review. *Vet Quart* 1984;6:216-224.
207. Dorrestein GM, Van Gogh H, Rinzema JD, et al. Comparative study of ampicillin and amoxicillin after intravenous, intramuscular and oral administration in homing pigeons (*Columba livia*). *Res Vet Sci* 1987;42:343-348.
208. d'Ovidio D, Noviello E, Adami C. Nerve stimulator-guided sciatic-femoral nerve block in raptors undergoing surgical treatment of pododermatitis. *Vet Anaesth Analg* 2015;42:449-453.
209. Dressen PJ, Wimsatt J, Burkhard MJ. The effects of isoflurane anesthesia on hematologic and plasma biochemical values of American kestrels (*Falco sparverius*). *J Avian Med Surg* 1999;173-179.
210. Dumonceaux G, Harrison GJ. Toxins. In: Ritchie BW, Harrison GJ, Harrison LR, eds. *Avian Medicine: Principles and Application*. Delray Beach, FL: Wingers Publishing; 1994:1030-1052.
211. Dyer DC, Van Alstine WG. Antibiotic aerosolization: tissue and plasma oxytetracycline concentrations in parakeets. *Avian Dis* 1987;31:677-679.
212. Edling TM. Anaesthesia and analgesia. In: Chitty J, Harcourt-Brown N, eds. *BSAVA Manual of Psittacine Birds*. Gloucester: British Small Animal Veterinary Association; 2005:87-96.
213. Efstathopoulos N, Giamarellos-Bourboulis E, Kanellakopoulou K, et al. Treatment of experimental osteomyelitis by methicillin resistant *Staphylococcus aureus* with bone cement system releasing grepafloxacin. *Injury* 2008;39:1384-1390.
214. Ehrlich PR, Dobkin DS, Wheye D. *The Birder's Handbook: A Field Guide to the Natural History of North American Birds*. New York: Simon & Schuster; 1988.
215. Elliston E, Perlman J. Meeting the protein requirements of adult hummingbirds in captivity. *J Wildl Rehab* 2002;25:14-19.
216. Emery LC, Cox SK, Souza MJ. Pharmacokinetics of nebulized terbinafine in Hispaniolan Amazon parrots (*Amazona ventralis*). *J Avian Med Surg* 2012;26(3):161-166.
217. Ensley PK, Janssen DL. A preliminary study comparing the pharmacokinetics of ampicillin given orally and intramuscularly to psittacines: Amazon parrots (*Amazona* spp.) and blue-naped parrots (*Tanygnathus lucionensis*). *J Zoo Anim Med* 1981;12:42-47.
218. Ernst S, Goggin JM, Biller DS, et al. Comparison of iohexol and barium sulfate as gastrointestinal contrast media in mid-sized psittacine birds. *J Avian Med Surg* 1998;12:16-20.

219. Escobar A, Thiesen R, Vitaliano SN, et al. Some cardiopulmonary effects of sevoflurane in crested caracara (*Caracara plancus*). *Vet Anaesth Analg* 2009;36:436-441.
220. Esperon F, Martin MP, Lopes F, et al. *Gongylonema* sp. infection in the scops owl (*Otus scops*). *Parasitol Int* 2013;62:502-504.
221. Esposito JF. Respiratory medicine. *Vet Clin North Am Exot Anim Pract* 2000;3:395-402.
222. Ethell MT, Bennett RA, Brown MP, et al. *In vitro* elution of gentamicin, amikacin and ceftiofur from polymethylmethacrylate and hydroxyapatite cement. *Vet Surg* 2000;29:375-382.
223. Eugenio CT. Amitriptyline HCl: clinical study for treatment of feather picking. *Proc Annu Conf Assoc Avian Vet* 2003;133-135.
224. Evans EE, Wade LL, Flammer K. Administration of doxycycline in drinking water for treatment of spiral bacterial infection in cockatiels. *J Am Vet Med Assoc* 2008;232:389-393.
225. Farca AM, Piromalli G, Maffei F, et al. Potentiating effect of EDTA-Tris on the activity of antibiotics against resistant bacteria associated with otitis, dermatitis and cystitis. *J Small Anim Pract* 1997;38:243-245.
226. Ferrell ST, Graham JE, Swaim SF. Avian wound healing and management. *Proc Annu Conf Assoc Avian Vet* 2002;337-347.
227. Ferrell ST, Marlar AB, Garner M, Lung NP. Intralesional cisplatin chemotherapy and topical cryotherapy for the control of choanal squamous cell carcinoma in an African penguin (*Spensiscus demersus*). *J Zoo Wildl Med* 2006;37(4):539-541.
228. Filippich LJ, O'Donoghue PJ. *Cochlosoma* infections in finches. *Aust Vet J* 1997;75:561-563.
229. Filippich LJ, Parker MG. Megabacteria and proventricular/ventricular disease in psittacines and passerines. *Proc Annu Conf Assoc Avian Vet* 1994;287-293.
230. Filippich LJ, Perry RA. Drug trials against megabacteria in budgerigars (*Melopsittacus undulatus*). *Aust Vet Pract* 1993;23:184-189.
231. Filippich LJ, Bucher AM, Charles BG. Platinum pharmacokinetics in sulphur-crested cockatoos (*Cacatua galerita*) following single-dose cisplatin infusion. *Aust Vet J* 2000;78:406-411.
232. Filippich LJ, Bucher AM, Charles BG, et al. Intravenous cisplatin administration in sulphur-crested cockatoos (*Cacatua galerita*): clinical and pathologic observations. *J Avian Med Surg* 2001;15:23-30.
233. Filippich LJ, Charles BG, Sutton RH, et al. Carboplatin administration in sulphur-crested cockatoos (*Cacatua galerita*): clinical observations. *J Avian Med Surg* 2005;19:92-97.
234. Fitzgerald B, Beaufrere H. Cardiology. In: Speer B, ed. *Current Therapy in Avian Medicine and Surgery*. St. Louis, MO: Elsevier; 2016:252-328.
235. Fitzgerald G, Cooper JE. Preliminary studies on the use of propofol in the domestic pigeon (*Columba livia*). *Vet Sci* 1990;49:334-338.
236. Flammer K. An overview of antifungal therapy in birds. *Proc Annu Conf Assoc Avian Vet* 1993;1-4.
237. Flammer K. A review of the pharmacology of antimicrobial drugs in birds. *Proc Avian/Exot Anim Med Symp* 1994;65-78.
238. Flammer K. Fluconazole in psittacine birds. *Proc Annu Conf Assoc Avian Vet* 1996;203-204.
239. Flammer K. Approach to the vomiting bird. In: *Proc 21st Annu Waltham®/OSU Symp*; 1997:19-21.
240. Flammer K. Common bacterial infections and antibiotic use in companion birds. *Antimicrobial Therapy in Exotics; Supplement to Comp Cont Edu Pract Vet* 1998;20(3A):34-48.
241. Flammer K. Doxycycline-medicated seed for treatment of chlamydiosis. *Proc Annu Conf Assoc Avian Vet* 2002;7-8.
242. Flammer K. Treatment of bacterial and mycotic diseases of the avian gastrointestinal tract. *Proc North Am Vet Conf* 2002;851-852.
243. Flammer K. Antifungal drug update. *Proc Annu Conf Assoc of Avian Vet* 2006;3.
244. Flammer K, Papich M. Assessment of plasma concentration and effects of injectable doxycycline in three psittacine species. *J Avian Med Surg* 2005;19:216-224.

245. Flammer K, Whitt-Smith D. Plasma concentrations of enrofloxacin psittacine birds offered water medicated with 200 mg/L of the injectable formulation of enrofloxacin. *J Avian Med Surg* 2002;16:286-290.
246. Flammer K, Aucoin DP, Whitt DA. Intramuscular and oral disposition of enrofloxacin in African grey parrots following single and multiple doses. *J Vet Pharmacol Therap* 1991; 41:359-366.
247. Flammer K, Whitt-Smith D, Papich M. Plasma concentrations of doxycycline in selected psittacine birds when administered in water for potential treatment of *Chlamydophila psittaci* infection. *J Avian Med Surg* 2001;15:276-282.
248. Flammer K, Aucoin DP, Whitt DA, et al. Plasma concentrations of enrofloxacin in African grey parrots treated with medicated water. *Avian Dis* 1990;34:228-234.
249. Flammer K, Aucoin DP, Whitt DA, et al. Potential use of long-acting injectable oxytetracycline for treatment of chlamydiosis in Goffin's cockatoos. *Avian Dis* 1990;34:1017-1022.
250. Flammer K, Clark CH, Drewes LA, et al. Adverse effects of gentamicin in scarlet macaws and galahs. *Am J Vet Res* 1990;51:404-407.
251. Flammer K, Massey JG, Roudybush T, et al. Assessment of plasma concentrations and potential adverse effects of doxycycline in cockatiels (*Nymphicus hollandicus*) fed a medicated pelleted diet. *J Avian Med Surg* 2013;27:187-193.
252. Flammer K, Nettifee-Osborne JA, Webb DJ, et al. Pharmacokinetics of voriconazole after oral administration of single and multiple doses in African grey parrots (*Psittacus erithacus timneh*). *Am J Vet Res* 2008;69:114-121.
253. Flinchum GB. Potential use of policosanol in the treatment of hyperlipidemia in pet birds. *Exot DVM* 2003;5:51-55.
254. Forbes N. The use of GNRH implants in the treatment of sexual derived behavioural abnormalities in birds. *Proc Eur Assoc Avian Vet* 2009;119-122.
255. Forbes NA. Birds of prey. In: Beynon PH, Cooper JE, eds. *BSAVA Manual of Exotic Pets*. Ames: Iowa State University Press; 1991:212-220.
256. Forbes NA. Raptors: parasitic diseases. In: Chitty J, Lierz M, eds. *BSAVA Manual of Raptors, Pigeons and Passerine Birds*. Gloucester: British Small Animal Veterinary Association; 2008:202-211.
257. Forbes NA, Richardson T. Husbandry and nutrition. In: Beynon PH, Forbes NA, Harcourt-Brown NH, eds. *BSAVA Manual of Raptors, Pigeons and Waterfowl*. Ames: Iowa State University Press; 1996:289-298.
258. Ford S, Chitty J, Jones MP. Raptor medicine master class. *Proc Annu Conf Assoc Avian Vet* 2009;143-162.
259. Fordham M, Rosenthal K, Durham A, et al. Intraocular osteosarcoma in an umbrella cockatoo (*Cacatua alba*). *Vet Ophthalmol* 2010;13(Suppl):103-108.
260. Forshaw JM, Cooper WT. *Parrots of the World*. 3rd ed. Lansdowne Editions: Melbourne; 1989.
261. Fourie T, Cromarty D, Duncan N, et al. The safety and pharmacokinetics of carprofen, flunixin and phenylbutazone in the Cape vulture (*Gyps coprotheres*) following oral exposure. *PLoS One* 2015;10.
262. Fowler ME. *Restraint and Handling of Wild and Domestic Animals*. 2nd ed. Ames: Iowa State University Press; 1995.
263. Fowler ME. *Restraint and Handling of Wild and Domestic Animals*. 3rd ed. Wiley-Blackwell: Ames; 2008.
264. France M. Chemotherapy treatment of lymphosarcoma in a Moluccan cockatoo. *Proc Annu Conf Assoc Avian Vet* 1993;15-19.
265. Frazier DL. Avian toxicology. In: Olsen GH, Orosz SE, eds. *Manual of Avian Medicine*. St. Louis: Mosby; 2000:228-263.
266. Freeman K, Hahn K, Adams W, et al. Radiation therapy for hemangiosarcoma in a budgerigar. *J Avian Med Surg* 1999;13(1):40-44.

267. Fudge AM. Laboratory reference ranges for selected avian, mammalian, and reptilian species. In: Fudge AM, ed. *Laboratory Medicine: Avian and Exotic Pets*. Philadelphia: WB Saunders Co; 2000:375-400.
268. Fudge AM, Joseph V. Disorders of avian leukocytes. In: Fudge AM, ed. *Laboratory Medicine: Avian and Exotic Pets*. Philadelphia: WB Saunders Co; 2000:19-25.
269. Fudge AM, Speer BL. Appendix 2: Normal clinical pathologic data. Hematology: laboratory reference ranges for selected species. In: Speer BL, ed. *Current Veterinary Therapy in Avian Medicine and Surgery*. St. Louis: Elsevier; 2016:825-856.
270. Gaggermeier B, Henke J, Schatzmann U. Investigations on analgesia in domestic pigeons (*C. livia*, Gmel., 1789, var. dom.) using buprenorphine and butorphanol. *Proc Eur Assoc Avian Vet* 2003;70-73.
271. Gaharan S, Gupta A, Boudreaux B, Beaufrère H. What is your diagnosis? Chronic lymphocytic leukemia. *J Avian Med Surg* 2012;26(1):45-48.
272. Galligan TH, Taggart MA, Cuthbert RJ, et al. Metabolism of aceclofenac in cattle to vulture-killing diclofenac. *Conserv Biol* 2016;30:1122-1127.
273. Gancz A. *Personal communication*; 2016.
274. Gancz A, Wellehan J, Boutette J, et al. Diabetes mellitus concurrent with hepatic haemosiderosis in two macaws (*Ara severa, Ara militaris*). *Avian Pathol* 2007;36:331-336.
275. Gancz AY, Lee S, Higginson G, et al. Horner's syndrome in an eastern screech owl (*Megascops asio*). *Vet Rec* 2006;159(10):320-322.
276. Gancz AY, Malka S, Sandmeyer L, et al. Horner's syndrome in a red-bellied parrot (*Poicephalus rufiventris*). *J Avian Med Surg* 2005;19(1):30-34.
277. García-Montijano M, Gonzáles F, Waxman S, et al. Pharmacokinetics of marbofloaxacin after oral administration to Eurasian buzzards (*Buteo buteo*). *J Avian Med Surg* 2003;17:185-190.
278. Garcia-Montijano M, Waxman S, de Lucas JJ, et al. The pharmacokinetic behaviour of marbofloxacin in Eurasian buzzards (*Buteo buteo*) after intraosseous administration. *Vet J* 2006;171:551-555.
279. Garcia-Montijano M, Waxman S, de Lucas JJ, et al. Disposition of marbofloxacin in vulture (*Gyps fulvus*) after intravenous administration of a single dose. *Res Vet Sci* 2010; epub.
280. Gaskins LA, Massey JG, Ziccardi MH. Effect of oral diazepam on feeding behavior and activity of Hawai'i' amakihi (*Hemignathus virens*). *Appl Anim Behav Sci* 2008;112:384-394.
281. Gibbons D, Morrissey C, Mineau P. A review of the direct and indirect effects of neonicotinoids and fipronil on vertebrate wildlife. *Environ Sci Pollution Res* 2015;22:103-118.
282. Giddings RF. Treatment of flukes in a toucan. *J Am Vet Med Assoc* 1988;193:1555-1556.
283. Gilbert CM, Filippich LJ, Charles BG. Doxorubicin pharmacokinetics following a single-dose infusion to sulphur-crested cockatoos (*Cacatua galerita*). *Aust Vet J* 2004;82(12):769-772.
284. Gilbert CM, Filippich LJ, McGeary RP, et al. Toxicokinetics of the active doxorubicin metabolite, doxorubicinol, in sulphur-crested cockatoos (*Cacatua galerita*). *Res Vet Sci* 2007;83(1):123-129.
285. Gill JH. Avian skin diseases. *Vet Clin North Am Exot Anim Pract* 2001;4:486.
286. Gozalo AS, Schwiebert RS, Lawson GW. Mortality associated with fenbendazole administration in pigeons (*Columba livia*). *J Am Assoc Lab Anim Sci* 2006;45:63-66.
287. Graham JE, Kollias-Baker C, Craigmill AL, et al. Pharmacokinetics of ketoprofen in Japanese quail (*Coturnix japonica*). *J Vet Pharmacol Ther* 2005;28:399-402.
288. Graham JE, Meola DM, Kini NR, et al. Comparison of the effects of glycerol, dimethyl sulfoxide, and hydroxyethyl starch solutions for cryopreservation of avian red blood cells. *Am J Vet Res* 2015;76(6):487-493.
289. Gray P, Gou J, Shivaprasad HL, et al. Use of antiviral drugs for treatment of avian bornavirus infection. *Proc Annu Conf Assoc Avian Vet* 2010;19.
290. Greenacre CB. Thyrogen for use in TSH testing of healthy and suspected hypothyroid parrots. *Proc Eur Assoc Avian Vet* 2009;125-126.

291. Greenacre CB, Olsen J, Wilson GH, et al. The use of synthetic TSH to evaluate the thyroid gland. *Proc Annu Conf Assoc Avian Vet* 2002;13.
292. Greenacre CB, Young DW, Behrend EN, et al. Validation of a novel high-sensitivity radioimmunoassay procedure for measurement of total thyroxine concentration in psittacine birds and snakes. *Am J Vet Res* 2001;62:1750-1754.
293. Greth A, Gerlach H, Gerbermann H, et al. Pharmacokinetics of doxycycline after parenteral administration in the houbara bustard (*Chlamydotis undulata*). *Avian Dis* 1993;37:31-36.
294. Grieves JL, Dick EJ, Schlabritz-Loutsevich NE, et al. Barbiturate euthanasia solution-induced tissue artifact in nonhuman primates. *J Med Primatol* 2008;37(3):154-161.
295. Grilo ML, Vanstreels RE, Wallace R, et al. Malaria in penguins—current perceptions. *Avian Pathol* 2016;45:393-407.
296. Grimm F, Serbest E. The therapy of osteomyelitis with clindamycin in patients suffering from fractures. *Proc VIII Tagung über Vogelkrankheiten, München* 1992;252-254.
297. Grizzle J, Hadley TL, Rotstein DS, et al. Effects of dietary milk thistle on blood parameters, liver pathology, and hepatobiliary scintigraphy in white carneaux pigeons (*Columba livia*) challenged with B1 aflatoxin. *J Avian Med Surg* 2009;23(2):114-124.
298. Gronwall R, Brown MP, Clubb S. Pharmacokinetics of amikacin in African gray parrots. *Am J Vet Res* 1989;50:250-252.
299. Gupta A, Tully TN, Beaufrère H, et al. What is your diagnosis? Bone marrow aspirate from a hyacinth macaw (*Anodorhynchus hyacinthinus*). *Vet Clin Pathol* 2011;40(4):565-566.
300. Gustavsen KA, Guzman DS, Knych HK, et al. Pharmacokinetics of buprenorphine hydrochloride following intramuscular and intravenous administration to American kestrels (*Falco sparverius*). *Am J Vet Res* 2014;75:711-715.
301. Guthrie AL, Gonzalez-Angulo C, Wigle WL, DeMaar TW. Radiation therapy of a malignant melanoma in a thick-billed parrot (*Rhynchopsitta pachyrhyncha*). *J Avian Med Surg* 2010;24(4):299-307.
302. Guzman DS, Beaufrère H, Kukanich B, et al. Pharmacokinetics of a single oral dose of pimobendan in Hispaniolan Amazon parrot (*Amazona ventralis*). *J Avian Med Surg* 2014;28(2):95-101.
303a. Guzman DS, Drazenovich TL, KuKanich B, et al. Evaluation of thermal antinociceptive effects and pharmacokinetics after intramuscular administration of butorphanol tartrate to American kestrels (*Falco sparverius*). *Am J Vet Res* 2014;75:11-18.
303b. Guzman DS, Drazenovich TL, Olsen GH, et al. Evaluation of thermal antinociceptive effects after intramuscular administration of hydromorphone hydrochloride to American kestrels (*Falco sparverius*). *Am J Vet Res* 2013;74:817-822.
303c. Guzman DS, Drazenovich TL, Olsen GH, et al. Evaluation of thermal antinociceptive effects after oral administration of tramadol hydrochloride to American kestrels (*Falco sparverius*). *Am J Vet Res* 2014;75(2):117-127.
304. Guzman DS, KuKanich B, Drazenovich TL, et al. Pharmacokinetics of hydromorphone hydrochloride after intravenous and intramuscular administration of a single dose to American kestrels (*Falco sparverius*). *Am J Vet Res* 2014;75:527-531.
305. Guzman DS-M, Diaz-Figueroa O, Tully Jr T, et al. Evaluating 21-day doxycycline and azithromycin treatments for experimental *Chlamydophila psittaci* infection in cockatiels (*Nymphicus hollandicus*). *J Avian Med Surg* 2010;24:35-45.
306. Guzman DS-M, Flammer K, Papich MG, et al. Pharmacokinetics of voriconazole after oral administration of single and multiple doses in Hispaniolan Amazon parrots (*Amazona ventralis*). *Am J Vet Res* 2010;71:460-467.
307. Hadley TL, Daniel GB, Rotstein DS, et al. Evaluation of hepatobiliary scintigraphy as an indicator of hepatic function in domestic pigeons (*Columba livia*) before and after exposure to ethylene glycol. *Vet Radiol Ultrasound* 48(2):155-162.
308. Halsema WB, Alberts H, de Bruijne JJ, et al. Collection and analysis of urine from racing pigeons (*Columba livia domestica*). *Avian Pathol* 1988;17:221-225.

309. Hamlin RL, Stalnaker PS. Basis for use of digoxin in small birds. *J Vet Pharmcol Therap* 1987;10:354-356.
310. Hammond EE, Guzman DS-M, Garner MM, et al. Long-term treatment of chronic lymphocytic leukemia in a green-winged macaw (*Ara chloroptera*). *J Avian Med Surg* 2010; 24(4):330-338.
311. Haneveld-v Laarhoven MA, Dorrestein GM. IME—sudden high mortality in canaries. *J Assoc Avian Vet* 1990;4:82.
312. Hannon DE, Swaim SF, Milton JL, et al. Full thickness mesh skin grafts in two great horned owls. *J Zoo Wildl Med* 1993;24:539-542.
313. Hanssen I, Grav HJ, Steen H. Vitamin C deficiency in growing willow ptarmigan (*Lagopus lagopus lagopus*). *J Nutr* 1979;109:2260-2276.
314. Hantash TM, Abu-Basha EA. Pharmacokinetics and bioavailability of a sulfadiazine/trimethoprim combination following intravenous, intramuscular, and oral administration in ostriches (*Struthio camelus*). *Proc Annu Conf Assoc Avian Vet* 2008;319-324.
315. Harcourt-Brown NH. Tendon repair in the pelvic limb of birds of prey: part II. Surgical techniques. In: *Raptor Biomedicine III*. Lake Worth, FL: Zoological Education Network; 2002: 217-231.
316. Harcourt-Brown N, Chitty J. Formulary. In: Harcourt-Brown N, Chitty J, eds. *BSAVA Manual of Psittacine Birds*. Gloucester: British Small Animal Veterinary Association; 2005:303-308.
317. Hardey J, Crick H, Wernham C, et al. *Raptors: A Field Guide to Survey and Monitoring*. Scottish Natural Heritage: Edinburgh; 2006.
318. Harlin RW. Pigeons. *Vet Clin North Am Small Anim Pract* 1994;24:157-173.
319. Harlin RW. Pigeons. *Proc Annu Conf Assoc Avian Vet* 1995;361-373.
320. Harlin RW. Pigeon therapeutics. *Vet Clin North Am Exot Anim Pract* 2000;3:19-34.
321. Harlin RW. Practical pigeon medicine. *Proc Annu Conf Assoc Avian Vet* 2006;249-262.
322. Harms CA, Hoskinson JJ, Bruyette DS, et al. Development of an experimental model of hypothyroidism in cockatiels (*Nymphicus hollandicus*). *Am J Vet Res* 1994;55:399-404.
323. Harper FDW. Poor performance and weight loss. In: Beynon PH, Forbes NA, Harcourt-Brown NH, eds. *BSAVA Manual of Raptors, Pigeons and Waterfowl*. Ames: Iowa State University Press; 1996:272-278.
324. Harrenstien LA, Tell LA, Vulliet R, et al. Disposition of enrofloxacin in red-tailed hawks (*Buteo jamaicensis*) and great horned owls (*Bubo virginianus*) after a single oral, intramuscular, or intravenous dose. *J Avian Med Surg* 2000;14:228-236.
325. Harris D. Therapeutic avian techniques. *Semin Avian Exot Pet Med* 1997;6:55-62.
326. Harrison GJ. What to do until a diagnosis is made. In: Harrison GJ, Harrison LR, eds. *Clinical Avian Medicine and Surgery*. Philadelphia: WB Saunders Co; 1986:356-361.
327. Harrison GJ, Harrison LR, eds. *Clinical Avian Medicine and Surgery*. Philadelphia: WB Saunders Co; 1986:662-663.
328. Harvey R. *Practical Incubation*. Payn Essex Printers Ltd, Sudbury: Suffolk, UK; 1990.
329. Harvey-Clark C, Gass CL. IME—Treating aspergillosis in hummingbirds. *J Assoc Avian Vet* 1993;7:216.
330. Hausmann JC, Mans C, Gosling A, et al. Bilateral uveitis and hyphema in a catalina macaw (*Ara ararauna × Ara macao*) with multicentric lymphoma. *J Avian Med Surg* 2016;30(2):172-178.
331. Hawk CT, Leary SL. *Formulary for Laboratory Animals*. 2nd ed. Ames: Iowa State University Press; 1999.
332a. Hawkey CM, Samour HJ. The value of clinical hematology in exotic birds. In: Jacobson ER, Kollias Jr GV, eds. *Exotic Animals*. New York: Churchill Livingstone; 1988:109-141.
332b. Hawkins MG. *Unpublished data;* 2016.
333. Hawkins MG, Barron H, Speer BL, et al. Birds. In: Carpenter JW, ed. *Exotic Animal Formulary*. 4th ed Elsevier Saunders: St. Louis, MO; 2013:183-437.
334. Hawkins MG, Malka S, Pascoe PJ, et al. Evaluation of the effects of dorsal versus lateral recumbency on the cardiopulmonary system during anesthesia with isoflurane in red-tailed hawks (*Buteo jamaicensis*). *Am J Vet Res* 2013;74:136-143.

335. Hawkins MG, Wright BD, Pascoe PJ, et al. Pharmacokinetics and anesthetic and cardiopulmonary effects of propofol in red-tailed hawks (*Buteo jamaicensis*) and great horned owls (*Bubo virginianus*). *Am J Vet Res* 2003;64:677-683.
336. Hayes B. British Columbia: deaths caused by barbiturate poisoning in bald eagles and other wildlife. *Can Vet J* 1988;29(2):173-174.
337. Heard D. Anesthesia and analgesia. In: Altman RB, Clubb SL, Dorrestein GM, et al. *Avian Medicine and Surgery*. Philadelphia: WB Saunders Co; 1997:807-827.
338. Heatley JJ, Gill H, Crandall L, et al. Enilconazole for treatment of raptor aspergillosis. *Proc Annu Conf Assoc Avian* 2007;287-288.
339. Heaton JT, Brauth SE. Effects of yohimbine as a reversing agent for ketamine-xylazine anesthesia in budgerigars. *Lab Anim Sci* 1992;42:54-56.
340. Heidenreich M. *Birds of Prey, Medicine and Management*. Blackwell Science Ltd: Malden, MA; 1997.
341. Helmer P. Psittacine sarcocystosis. *Proc Annu Conf Assoc Avian Vet* 2004;602.
342. Helmick KE, Boothe DM, Jensen JM. Disposition of single-dose intravenously administered amikacin in emus. *J Zoo Wildl Med* 1997;28:49-54.
343. Helmick KE, Boothe DM, Jensen JM. Disposition of single-dose intravenously administered enrofloxacin in emus. *J Zoo Wildl Med* 1997;28:43-48.
344. Hess L. Possible complications associated with topical corticosteroid use in birds. *Proc Annu Conf Assoc Avian Vet* 2001;29-32.
345. Hines R, Kolattukuty PE, Sharkey P. Pharmacological induction of molt and gonadal involution in birds. *Proc Annu Conf Assoc Avian Vet* 1993;127-134.
346. Hochleithner M. Reference values for selected psittacine species using a dry chemistry system. *J Assoc Avian Vet* 1989;3:207-209.
347. Hoefer H. IME—hepatic fibrosis and colchicine therapy. *J Assoc Avian Vet* 1991;5:193.
348. Hoefer HL. Antimicrobials in pet birds. In: Bonagura JD, ed. *Kirk's Current Veterinary Therapy XII: Small Animal Practice*. Philadelphia: WB Saunders Co; 1995:1278-1283.
349. Hoogesteijn AL, Raphael BL, Calle P, et al. Oral treatment of avian lead intoxication with meso-2,3-dimercaptosuccinic acid. *J Zoo Wildl Med* 2003;34:82-87.
350. Hooimeijer J. Coccidiosis in lorikeets infectious for budgerigar. *Proc Annu Conf Assoc Avian Vet* 1993;59-61.
351. Hoppes S, Flammer K, Hoersch K, et al. Disposition and analgesic effects of fentanyl in white cockatoos (*Cacatua alba*). *J Avian Med Surg* 2003;17:124-130.
352. Hoppes S, Heatley JJ, Guo JH, et al. Meloxicam treatment in cockatiels (*Nymphicus hollandicus*) infected with avian bornavirus. *J Exot Pet Med* 2013;22:275-279.
353. Hoppes S, Tizard I, Shivaprasad H, et al. Treatment of avian bornavirus-infected cockatiels (*Nymphicus hollandicus*) with oral meloxicam and cyclosporine. *Proc Annu Conf Assoc Avian Vet* 2012;27.
354. Hoppes S. Treatment of *Macrorhabdus ornithogaster* with sodium benzoate in budgerigars (*Melopsittacus undulatus*). *Proc Annu Conf Assoc Avian Vet* 2011;67.
355. Hornak S, Liptak T, Ledecky V, et al. A preliminary trial of the sedation induced by intranasal administration of midazolam alone or in combination with dexmedetomidine and reversal by atipamezole for a short-term immobilization in pigeons. *Vet Anaesth Analg* 2015;42:192-196.
356. Howard LL, Papendick R, Stalis IH, et al. Fenbendazole and albendazole toxicity in pigeons and doves. *J Avian Med Surg* 2002;16:203-210.
357. Hu J, McDougald LR. The efficacy of some drugs with known antiprotozoal activity against *Histomonas meleagridis* in chickens. *Vet Parasitol* 2004;121:233-238.
358. Huckabee JR. Raptor therapeutics. *Vet Clin North Am Exot Anim Pract* 2000;3:91-116.
359a. Hudelson KS, Hudelson PM. Endocrine considerations In: Harrison GJ, Lightfoot TL, eds. *Clinical Avian Medicine*. Palm Beach, FL: Spix Publishing; 2006:541-557.
359b. Hyatt MW, Georoff TA, Nollens HH, et al. Voriconazole toxicity in multiple penguin species. *J Wildl Med* 2015;46:880-888.

360. Iglauer F, Rasim R. Treatment of psychogenic feather picking in psittacine birds with a dopamine antagonist. *J Small Anim Pract* 1993;34:564-566.
361. Inghelbrecht S, Vermeersch H, Ronsmans S, et al. Pharmacokinetics and anti-trichomonal efficacy of a dimetridazole tablet and water-soluble powder in homing pigeons (*Columba livia*). *J Vet Pharmacol Therap* 1996;19:62-67.
362. Ingram K. Hummingbirds and miscellaneous orders. In: Fowler ME, ed. *Zoo and Wild Animal Medicine*. 2nd ed. Philadelphia: WB Saunders; 1986:447-456.
363. Isaza R, Budsberg SC, Sundlof SF, et al. Disposition of ciprofloxacin in red-tailed hawks following a single oral dose. *J Zoo Wildl Med* 1993;24:498-502.
364. Itoh N, Okada H. Pharmacokinetics and tolerability of chloramphenicol in budgerigars (*Melopsittacus undulatus*). *J Vet Med Sci* 1993;55:439-442.
365. Jaensch SM, Cullen L, Raidal SR. Assessment of liver function in galahs after partial hepatectomy: a comparison of plasma enzyme concentrations, serum bile acid levels, and galactose clearance tests. *J Avian Med Surg* 2000;14:164-171.
366. Jalanka HH. Medetomidine-ketamine and atipamezole: a reversible method for chemical restraint of birds. *Proc First Annu Conf Euro Comm Assoc Avian Vet* 1991;102-104.
367. Jalanka HH. New alpha two adrenoceptor agonists and antagonists. In: Fowler ME, ed. *Zoo and Wild Animal Medicine: Current Therapy*. 3rd ed. Philadelphia: WB Saunders Co; 1993:475-476.
368. Jamriska J, Lavilla LA, Thomasson A, et al. Treatment of atoxoplasmosis in the blue-crowned laughing thrush (*Dryonastes courtoisi*). *Avian Pathol* 2013;42:569-571.
369. Jankowski G, Nevarez J. Evaluation of a pediatric blood filter for whole blood transfusions in domestic chickens (*Gallus gallus*). *J Avian Med Surg* 2010;24(4):272-278.
370. Janovsky M, Ruf T, Wolfgang Z. Oral administration of tiletamine/zolazepam for the immobilization of the common buzzard (*Buteo buteo*). *J Raptor Res* 2002;36:188-193.
371. Jenkins JR. Avian critical care and emergency medicine. In: Altman RB, Clubb SL, Dorrestein GM, et al. *Avian Medicine and Surgery*. Philadelphia: WB Saunders Co; 1997:839-863.
372. Jenkins JR. Feather picking and self-mutilation in psittacine birds. *Vet Clin North Am Exot Anim Pract* 2001;4:663-667.
373. Jennings IB. Haematology. In: Beynon PH, Forbes NA, Harcourt-Brown NH, eds. *BSAVA Manual of Raptors, Pigeons and Waterfowl*. Ames: Iowa State University Press; 1996:68-78.
374. Jensen J, Westerman E. Amikacin pharmacokinetics in ostrich (*Struthio camelus*). *Proc Annu Conf Am Assoc Zoo Vet* 1990;238-242.
375. Jensen JM, Johnson JH, Weiner ST. *Husbandry & Medical Management of Ostriches, Emus & Rheas*. Wildlife and Exotic Animal TeleConsultants: College Station, TX; 1992.
376. Jeong MB, Kim YG, Yi NY, et al. Comparison of the rebound tonometer (TonoVet) with the applanation tonometer (TonoPen XL) in normal Eurasian eagle owls (*Bubo bubo*). *Vet Ophthalmol* 2007;10:376-379.
377. Johnson-Delaney CA, Harrison LR, eds. *Exotic Companion Medicine Handbook for Veterinarians*. Lake Worth, FL: Wingers Publishing; 1996.
378. Johnston MS, Ivey ES. Parathyroid and ultimobranchial glands: calcium metabolism in birds. *Semin Avian Exot Pet Med* 2002;11:84-93.
379. Jones MP, Arheart KL, Cray C. Reference intervals, longitudinal analyses, and index of individuality of commonly measured laboratory variables in captive bald eagles (*Haliaeetus leucocephalus*). *J Avian Med Surg* 2014;28:118-126.
380. Jones MP, Morandi F, Wall JS, et al. Distribution of 2-deoxy-2-fluoro-d-glucose in the coelom of healthy bald eagles (*Haliaeetus leucocephalus*). *Am J Vet Res* 2013;74(3):426-432.
381. Jones MP. Selected diseases of birds of prey. *Proc Annu Meet Am Board Vet Pract* 2001;31-39.
382. Jones MP. Selected infectious diseases of birds of prey. *J Exot Pet Med* 2006;15:5-17.
383. Jones MP, Orosz SE, Cox SK, et al. Pharmacokinetic disposition of itraconazole in red-tailed hawks (*Buteo jamaicensis*). *J Avian Med Surg* 2000;14:15-22.

384. Joseph V. Preventive health programs for falconry birds. *Proc Annu Conf Assoc Avian Vet* 1995;171-178.
385. Joseph V. Emergency care of raptors. *Vet Clin North Am Exot Anim Pract* 1998;1:77-98.
386. Joyner KL. Pediatric therapeutics. *Proc Annu Conf Assoc Avian Vet* 1991;188-199.
387. Joyner KL. Psittacine incubation and pediatrics. In: Fowler ME, ed. *Zoo and Wild Animal Medicine: Current Therapy*. 3rd ed. Philadelphia: WB Saunders; 1993:247-260.
388. Joyner PH, Jones MP, Ward D, et al. Induction and recovery characteristics and cardiopulmonary effects of sevoflurane and isoflurane in bald eagles. *Am J Vet Res* 2008;69:13-22.
389. Juarbe-Diaz SJ. Animal behavior case of the month. *J Am Vet Med Assoc* 2000;216:1562-1564.
390. Junge RE, Naeger LL, LeBeau MA, et al. Pharmacokinetics of intramuscular and nebulized ceftriaxone in chickens. *J Zoo Wildl Med* 1994;25:224-228.
391. Kahler J. Somatostatin treatment for diabetes mellitus in a sulfur breasted toucan. *Proc Annu Conf Assoc Avian Vet* 1994;269-273.
392. Kahler J. The use of gallium scanning in psittacine birds. *Proc Annu Conf Assoc Avian Vet* 2001;91-93.
393. Kamiloglu A, Atalan G, Kamiloglu NN. Comparison of intraosseous and intramuscular drug administration for induction of anaesthesia in domestic pigeons. *Res Vet Sci* 2008;85:171-175.
394. Kasper A. Rehabilitation of California towhees. *Proc Annu Conf Assoc Avian Vet* 1997;83-90.
395. Kearns KS. Paroxetine therapy for feather picking and self-mutilation in the waldrapp ibis (*Genonticus eremita*). *Proc Joint Conf Am Assoc Zoo Vet/Am Assoc Wildl Vet/Wildl Dis Assoc* 2004;254-255.
396. Keffen R. The ostrich: capture, care, accommodation, and transportation. In: McKenzie A, ed. *Capture and Care Manual*. Pretoria, South Africa: Wildlife Decision Services; 1993:634-652.
397. Keller D, Sanchez-Migallon Guzman D, Kukanich B, et al. Pharmacokinetics of nalbuphine hydrochloride after intravenous and intramuscular administration to Hispaniolan Amazon parrots (*Amazona ventralis*). *Am J Vet Res* 2011;72:741-745.
398. Keller KA, Beaufrère H, Brandao J, et al. Long-term management of ovarian neoplasia in two cockatiels (*Nymphicus hollandicus*). *J Avian Med Surg* 2013;27:44-52.
399. Keller KA, Beaufrère H, Brandão J, et al. Long-term management of ovarian neoplasia in two cockatiels (*Nymphicus hollandicus*). *J Avian Med Surg* 2013;27(1):44-52.
400. Kelly-Clarke WK, McBurney S, Forzan MJ, et al. Detection and characterization of a Trichomonas isolate from rehabilitated bald eagle (*Haliaeetus leucocephalus*). *J Zoo Wildl Med* 2013;44:1123-1126.
401. Kern T, Paul-Murphy J, Murphy C, et al. Disorders of the third eyelid in birds: 17 cases. *J Avian Med Surg* 1996;10(1):12-18.
402. Keymer I. Pigeons. In: Beynon P, Cooper J, eds. *BSAVA Manual of Exotic Pets*. Ames: Iowa State University Press; 1991:180-202.
403a. Kilburn JJ, Cox SK, Backues KA. Pharmacokinetics of ceftiofur crystalline free acids, a long-acting cephalosporin, in American flamingos (*Phoenicopterus ruber*). *J Zoo Wildl Med* 2016;47:457-462.
403b. Kilburn JJ, Cox SK, Kottyan J, et al. Pharmacokinetics of tramadol and its primary metabolite O-desmethyltramadol in African penguins (*Spheniscus demersus*). *J Zoo Wildl Med* 2014;45(1):93-99.
404. Kirchgessner MS, Tully TN, Nevarez J, et al. Magnesium therapy in a hypocalcemic African grey parrot (*Psittacus erithacus*). *J Avian Med Surg* 2012;26(1):17-21.
405. Kitulagodage M, Astheimer LB, Buttemer WA. Diacetone alcohol, a dispersant solvent, contributes to acute toxicity of a fipronil-based insecticide in a passerine bird. *Ecotoxicol Environ Saf* 2008;71:597-600.
406. Kitulagodage M, Buttemer WA, Astheimer LB. Adverse effects of fipronil on avian reproduction and development: maternal transfer of fipronil to eggs in zebra finch Taeniopygia guttata and in ovo exposure in chickens *Gallus domesticus*. *Ecotoxicology* 2011;20:653-660.

407. Kitulagodage M, Isanhart J, Buttemer WA, et al. Fipronil toxicity in northern bobwhite quail *Colinus virginianus*: reduced feeding behaviour and sulfone metabolite formation. *Chemosphere* 2011;83:524-530.
408. Klaphake E, Beazley-Keane SL, Jones M, et al. Multisite integumentary squamous cell carcinoma in an African grey parrot (*Psittacus erithacus erithacus*). *Vet Rec* 2006;158(17):593-596.
409. Klaphake E, Fecteau K, DeWit M, et al. Effects of leuprolide acetate on selected blood and fecal sex hormones in Hispaniolan Amazon parrots (*Amazona ventralis*). *J Avian Med Surg* 2009;23:253-262.
410. Klaphake E, Schumacher J, Greenacre C, et al. Comparative anesthetic and cardiopulmonary effects of pre- versus postoperative butorphanol administration in Hispaniolan Amazon parrots (*Amazona ventralis*) anesthetized with sevoflurane. *J Avian Med Surg* 2006;20:2-7.
411. Klein PN, Charmatz K, Langenberg J. The effect of flunixin meglumine (Banamine®) on the renal function in northern bobwhite (*Colinus virginianus*): an avian model. *Proc Annu Conf Am Assoc Zoo Vet* 1994;128-131.
412. Kleinschmidt LM, Hoppes SM, Heatley JJ, et al. Cyclosporine as a palliative treatment for proventricular dilatation disease in psittacines birds. *Proc Annu Conf Assoc Am Zoo Vet* 2015;47-48.
413. Koch J, Buss EG, Lobaugh B, et al. Blood pressure of chickens selected for leanness or obesity. *Poult Sci* 1983;62:904-907.
414. Koepff C. *The New Finch Handbook*. Barron's Educational Series: Woodbury, NY; 1983.
415. Kollias Jr GV, Palgut J, Rossi J, et al. The use of ketoconazole in birds: preliminary pharmacokinetics and clinical applications. *Proc Annu Conf Assoc Avian Vet* 1986;103.
416. Korbel R. Inhalation anaesthesia with isoflurane (Forene®) and sevoflurane (SEVOrane®) in domestic pigeons (*Columba livia*, Gmel., 1789, var. domestica). *Ger Vet Med Soc* 1998;209-217.
417. Korbel R. Avian ophthalmology—a practically orientated review on recent developments. *Proc Annu Assoc Avian Med* 2014;139-147.
418a. Korbel R. Avian ophthalmology: principles and application. *Proc Annu Conf Assoc Avian Vet: Exot Proc* 2016;173-180.
418b. Korbel RT. Disorders of the posterior eye segment in raptors—examination procedures and findings. In: Lumeij JT, Remple D, Redig PT, et al, eds. *Raptor Biomedicine III*. Lake Worth, FL: Zoological Education Network; 2000:179-194.
419. Korbel RT. Investigations into intraocular injection of recombinant tissue plasminogen activator (rTPA) for the treatment of trauma-induced intraocular hemorrhages in birds. *Proc Annu Conf Assoc Avian Vet* 2003;97.
420. Korbel RT. Avian ophthalmology: principles and application. *Proc Annu Conf Assoc Avian Vet* 2016;173-180.
421. Korbel RT, Goetz B. Investigations on topical anesthesia of the eye in racing pigeons (*Columba livia*) and common buzzards (*Buteo buteo*). *Proc Annu Conf Assoc Avian Vet* 2001;51-53.
422. Koutsos EA, Matson KD, Klasing KC. Nutrition of birds in the order Psittaciformes: a review. *J Avian Med Surg* 2001;15(4):257-275.
423. Koutsos EA, Tell LA, Woods LW, et al. Adult cockatiels (*Nymphicus hollandicus*) at maintenance are more sensitive to diets containing excess vitamin A than to vitamin A-deficient diets. *J Nutr* 2003;133:1898-1902.
424. Kozel CA, Kinney ME, Hanley CS, et al. Medical management of hypovitaminosis D with cholecalciferol and elastic therapeutic taping in red-legged seriema (*Cariama cristata*) chicks. *J Avian Med Surg* 2016;30(1):53-59.
425. Krautwald ME, Pieper K, Rullof R, et al. Further experiences with the use of Baytril in pet birds. *Proc Annu Conf Assoc Avian Vet* 1990;226-236.
426. Krautwald-Junghanns ME, Zebisch R, Schmidt V. Relevance and treatment of coccidiosis in domestic pigeons (*Columba livia forma domestica*) with particular emphasis on toltrazuril. *J Avian Med Surg* 2009;23:1-5.

427. Kreeger TJ, Degernes LA, Kreeger JS, et al. Immobilization of raptors with tiletamine and zolazepam (Telazol). In: Redig PT, Cooper JE, Remple DJ, et al. *Raptor Biomedicine*. Minneapolis: University of Minnesota Press; 1993:141-144.
428. Krinsley M. IME—use of DermCaps Liquid and hydroxyzine HCl for the treatment of feather picking. *J Assoc Avian Vet* 1993;7:221.
429. Kubiak M, Roach L, Eatwell K. The influence of a combined butorphanol and midazolam premedication on anesthesia in psittacid species. *J Avian Med Surg* 2016;30:317-323.
430. Kuhn SE, Jones MP, Hendrix DV, et al. Normal ocular parameters and characterization of ophthalmic lesions in a group of captive bald eagles (*Haliaeetus leucocephalus*). *J Avian Med Surg* 2013;27:90-98.
431. Kumar PS, Arivuchelvan A, Jagadeeswaran A, et al. Pharmacokinetics of enrofloxacin in emu (*Dromaius novaehollandiae*) birds after intravenous and oral bolus administration. *Proc Nat Acad Sci Indian Sec B-Bio Sci* 2015;85:845-851.
432a. Labelle AL, Whittington JK, Breaux CB, et al. Clinical utility of a complete diagnostic protocol for the ocular evaluation of free-living raptors. *Vet Ophthalmol* 2012;15:5-17.
432b. Lacasse C. Falconiformes (falcons, hawks, eagles, kites, harriers, buzzards, ospreys, caracaras, secretary birds, Old World and New World vultures). In: Miller RE, Fowler ME, eds. *Fowler's Wild Animal Medicine*. Vol 8. St. Louis, MO: Elsevier; 2015:127-142
433. Lacasse C, Gamble KC, Boothe DM. Pharmacokinetics of a single dose of intravenous and oral meloxicam in red-tailed hawks (*Buteo jamaicensis*) and great horned owls (*Bubo virginianus*). *J Avian Med Surg* 2013;27:204-210.
434. Lamberski N, Théon AP. Concurrent irradiation and intratumoral chemotherapy with cisplatin for treatment of a fibrosarcoma in a blue and gold macaw (*Ara ararauna*). *J Avian Med Surg* 2002;16(3):234-238.
435. Langan JN, Ramsay EC, Blackford JT, et al. Cardiopulmonary and sedative effects of intramuscular medetomidine-ketamine and intravenous propofol in ostriches (*Struthio camelus*). *J Avian Med Surg* 2000;14:2-7.
436. Langille BL, Jones DR. Central cardiovascular dynamics of ducks. *Am J Physiol* 1975;228:1856-1861.
437. Langlois I, Harvey RC, Jones MP, et al. Cardiopulmonary and anesthetic effects of isoflurane and propofol in Hispaniolan Amazon parrots. *J Avian Med Surg* 2003;17:4-10.
438. Laniesse D, Beaufrère H. Iron storage disease. In: Graham J, ed. *5-Minute Veterinary Consult: Avian*. Ames, IA: Wiley Blackwell; 2016:156-157.
439. Laniesse D, Beaufrère H, Smith D. Diabetes insipidus in a 4 year old Congo African grey parrot (*Psittacus erithacus erithacus*) concurrently infected with avian bornavirus. *Proc Annu Conf Assoc Avian Vet: Exot Proc* 2016;339.
440. Lawton MPC. Anaesthesia. In: Beynon PH, Forbes NA, Lawton MPC, eds. *BSAVA Manual of Psittacine Birds*. Ames: Iowa State University Press; 1996:49-55.
441. Lawton MPC. Anaesthesia. In: Beynon PH, Forbes NA, Harcourt-Brown NH, eds. *BSAVA Manual of Raptors, Pigeons and Waterfowl*. Ames: Iowa State University Press; 1996:79-88.
442. Leary S, Underwood W, Anthony R, et al. *AVMA Guidelines for the Euthanasia of Animals: 2013 Edition*. Schaumburg, IL: AVMA; 2013.
443. Legler M, Kothe R, Rautebschlein S, et al. Detection of psittacid herpesvirus 1 in Amazon parrots with cloacal papilloma [internal papillomatosis of parrots, IPP] in an aviary of different psittacine species. *Dtsch Tierarztl Wochenschr* 2008;115:461-470.
444. Lennox AM. Successful treatment of mycobacteriosis in three psittacine birds. *Proc Annu Conf Assoc Avian Vet* 2002;111-113.
445. Lennox AM. The use of Aldara™ (imiquimod) for the treatment of cloacal papillomatosis in psittacines. *Exot DVM* 2002;4:34-35.
446. Lennox AM. Mycobacteriosis in companion psittacine birds: a review. *J Avian Med Surg* 2007;21:181-187.
447. Lennox AM, VanDerHeyden N. Haloperidol for use in treatment of psittacine self-mutilation and feather plucking. *Proc Annu Conf Assoc Avian Vet* 1993;119-120.

448. Levi A, Perelman B, Waner T, et al. Haematological parameters of the otrich (*Struthio camelus*). *Avian Pathol* 1989;18:321-327.
449. Levy A, Perelman B, Waner T, et al. Reference blood chemical values in ostriches (*Struthio camelus*). *Am J Vet Res* 1989;50:1548-1550.
450. Lichtenberger M. Treatment of respiratory inhalant toxins in 4 psittacine birds. *Proc Annu Conf Assoc Avian Vet* 2003;39-43.
451. Lichtenberger M, Ko J. Critical care monitoring. *Vet Clin North Am Exot Anim Pract* 2007;10:317-344.
452. Lichtenberger M, Lennox A. Critical care. In: Speer B, ed. *Current Therapy in Avian Medicine and Surgery*. St. Louis, MO: Elsevier; 2016:582-588.
453. Lichtenberger M, Lennox A, Chavez W, et al. The use of butorphanol constant rate infusion in psittacines. *Proc Annu Conf Assoc Avian Vet/Assoc Exot Mam Vet* 2009;73.
454. Lichtenberger M, Orcutt C, Cray C, et al. Comparison of fluid types for resuscitation after acute blood loss in mallard ducks (*Anas platyrhynchos*). *J Vet Emerg Crit Care* 2009;19(5):467-472.
455. Lin HC, Todhunter PG, Power TA, et al. Use of xylazine, butorphanol, tiletamine-zolazepam, and isoflurane for induction and maintenance of anesthesia in ratites. *J Am Vet Med Assoc* 1997;210:244-248.
456. Lindemann DM, Carpenter JW, KuKanich B. Pharmacokinetics of a single dose of oral and subcutaneous meloxicam in Caribbean flamingos (*Phoenicopterus ruber ruber*). *J Avian Med Surg* 2016;30:14-22.
457. Lindemann DM, Eshar D, Nietfeld JC, et al. Suspected fenbendazole toxicity in an American white pelican (*Pelecanus erythrorhyncos*). *J Zoo Wildl Med* 2016;47:681-685.
458. Lindenstruth H, Frost JW. Enrofloxacin (Baytril)—an alternative for psittacosis prevention and therapy in imported psittacines. *DTW Dtsch Tierarztl Wochenschr* 1993;100:364-368.
459. Lloyd C, Hebel C, Padrtova R. Non-invasive indirect blood pressure measurements in Falconiformes. *Falco* 2007;30:20-21.
460. Locke D, Bush M. Tylosin aerosol therapy in quail and pigeons. *J Zoo Anim Med* 1984;15:67-72.
461. Locke D, Bush M, Carpenter JW. Pharmacokinetics and tissue concentrations of tylosin in selected avian species. *Am J Vet Res* 1982;43:1807-1810.
462. Loerzel SM, Smith PJ, Howe A, et al. Vecuronium bromide, phenylephrine and atropine combinations as mydriatics in juvenile double-crested cormorants (*Phalacrocorax auritus*). *Vet Ophthalmol* 2002;5:149-154.
463. Lohr JE, Haberkorn A. Efficacy of toltrazuril against natural infections with intestinal coccidia in aviary birds. *Praktische-Tierarzt* 1998;79:419-422.
464. Lopez-Antia A, Ortiz-Santaliestra ME, Camarero PR, et al. Assessing the risk of fipronil-treated seed ingestion and associated adverse effects in the red-legged partridge. *Environ Sci Technol* 2015;49:13649-13657.
465. Lothrop CD, Loomis MR, Olsen JH. Thyrotropin stimulation test for evaluation of thyroid function in psittacine birds. *J Am Vet Med Assoc* 1985;186:47-48.
466. Lothrop CD, Olsen JH, Loomis MR, et al. Evaluation of adrenal function in psittacine birds using ACTH. *J Am Vet Med Assoc* 1985;187:1113-1115.
467. Lovas EM, Johnston SD, Filippich LJ. Using a GnRH agonist to obtain an index of testosterone secretory capacity in the cockatiel (*Nymphicus hollandicus*) and sulphur-crested cockatoo (*Cacatua galerita*). *Aust Vet J* 2010;88:52-56.
468. Lowenstine L, Stasiak I. Update on iron overload in zoological species. In: Miller RE, Fowler ME, eds. *Fowler's Zoo and Wild Animal Medicine*. Vol 8. St. Louis, MO: Elsevier; 2015:674-681
469. Lublin A, Raz C, Weisman Y. Excretion of Baytril (enrofloxacin) in pigeon milk as an approach to treat squabs. *Israel J Vet Med* 1996;51:125-128.
470. Ludders JW, Mitchell GS, Rode J. Minimal anesthetic concentration and cardiopulmonary dose response of isoflurane in ducks. *Vet Surg* 1990;19:304-307.

471. Ludders JW, Rode J, Mitchell GS. Isoflurane anesthesia in sandhill cranes (*Grus canadensis*): minimal anesthetic concentration and cardiopulmonary dose-response during spontaneous and controlled breathing. *Anesth Analg* 1989;68:511-516.
472. Lumeij JT. Appendix: hematology and biochemistry—Columbiformes. In: Ritchie BW, Harrison GJ, Harrison LR, eds. *Avian Medicine: Principles and Application*. Lake Worth, FL: Wingers Publishing; 1994:1339-1340.
473. Lumeij JT. Psittacine antimicrobial therapy. In: *Antimicrobial Therapy in Caged Birds and Exotic Pets*. Trenton: Veterinary Learning Systems Co; 1995:38-48.
474. Lumeij JT, de Bruijne JJ. Blood chemistry reference values in racing pigeons (*Columba livia domestica*). *Avian Pathol* 1985;14:401-408.
475. Lumeij JT, Gorgevska D, Woestenborghs R. Plasma and tissue concentrations of itraconazole in racing pigeons (*Columba livia domestica*). *J Avian Med Surg* 1995;9:32-35.
476. Lumeij JT, Redig PT, Sprang EPM. Further studies on allopurinol induced hyperuricaemia and visceral gout in red-tailed hawks. *Avian Path* 1998;27:390-393.
477. Lupu C, Robins S. Comparison of treatment protocols for removing metallic foreign objects from the ventriculus of budgerigars (*Melopsittacus undulatus*). *J Avian Med Surg* 2009;23(3):186-193.
478. Lupu CA. Evaluation of side effects of tamoxifen in budgerigars. *J Avian Med Surg* 2000;14:237-242.
479. Machin KL, Caulkett NA. Evaluation of isoflurane and propofol anesthesia for intraabdominal transmitter placement in nesting female canvasback ducks. *J Wildl Dis* 2000;36:324-334.
480. Machin KL, Livingston A. Plasma bupivacaine levels in mallard ducks (*Anas platyrhynchos*) following a single subcutaneous dose. *Proc Annu Conf Am Assoc Zoo Vet/Am Assoc Wildl Vet/Assoc Rept Amph Vet/Nat Assoc Zoo Wildl Vet* 2001;159-163.
481. Machin KL, Tellier LA, Lair S, et al. Pharmacodynamics of flunixin and ketoprofen in mallard ducks (*Anas platyrhynchos*). *J Zoo Wildl Med* 2001;32:222-229.
482. MacLean RA, Beaufrère H. Gruiformes (cranes, limpkins, rails, gallinules, coots, bustards). In: Miller RE, Fowler ME, eds. *Fowler's Zoo and Wildlife Medicine*. Vol 8. St. Louis: Elsevier; 2015:155-163
483. Macwhirter P. Passeriformes. In: Ritchie RW, Harrison GJ, Harrison LR, eds. *Avian Medicine: Principles and Application*. Lake Worth, FL: Wingers Publishing; 1994:1172-1199.
484. Macwhirter P, Pyke D, Wayne J. Use of carboplatin in the treatment of renal adenocarcinoma in a budgerigar. *Exot DVM* 2002;4:11-12.
485. Mader JT, Calhoun J, Cobos J. *In vitro* evaluation of antibiotic diffusion from antibiotic-impregnated biodegradable beads and polymethylmethacrylate beads. *Antimicrob Agents Chemother* 1997;41:415-418.
486. Maier K, Olias P, Gruber AD, et al. Toltrazuril does not show an effect against pigeon protozoal encephalitis. *Parasitol Res* 2015;114:1603-1606.
487. Mainka SA, Dierenfeld ES, Cooper RM, et al. Circulating α-tocopherol following intramuscular or oral vitamin E administration in Swainson's hawks (*Buteo swainsonii*). *J Zoo Wildl Med* 1994;25:229-232.
488. Mama KR, Phillips LG, Pascoe PJ. Use of propofol for induction and maintenance of anesthesia in a barn owl (*Tyto alba*) undergoing tracheal resection. *J Zoo Wildl Med* 1996;27:397-401.
489. Mans C, Pilny A. Use of GnRH-agonists for medical management of reproductive disorders in birds. *Vet Clin North Am Exot Anim Pract* 2014;17:23-33.
490. Mans C, Guzman DS, Lahner LL, et al. Sedation and physiologic response to manual restraint after intranasal administration of midazolam in Hispaniolan Amazon parrots (*Amazona ventralis*). *J Avian Med Surg* 2012;26:130-139.
491. Mans C, Sanchez-Migallon Guzman D, Lahner LL, et al. Intranasal midazolam for conscious sedation in Hispaniolan Amazon parrots (*Amazona ventralis*). *Proc Annu Conf Am Assoc Zoo Vet* 2010;160.
492. Manucy T, Bennett R, Greenacre C, et al. Squamous cell carcinoma of the mandibular beak in a Buffon's macaw (*Ara ambigua*). *J Avian Med Surg* 1998;12(3):158-166.

493. Marshall KL, Craig LE, Jones MP, et al. Quantitative renal scintigraphy in domestic pigeons (*Columba livia domestica*) exposed to toxic doses of gentamicin. *Am J Vet Res* 2003;64:453-462.
494. Marshall R. Avian anthelmintics and antiprotozoals. *Semin Avian Exot Pet Med* 1993;2:33-41.
495. Martel-Arquette A, Mans C, Sladky K. Management of severe frostbite in a grey-headed parrot (*Poicephalus fuscicollis suahelicus*). *J Avian Med Surg* 2016;30(1):39-45.
496. Martin HD, Kollias GV. Evaluation of water deprivation and fluid therapy in pigeons. *J Zoo Wildl Med* 1989;20:173-177.
497. Martin KM. Psittacine behavioral pharmacotherapy. In: Leuscher AU, ed. *Manual of Parrot Behavior*. Ames: Blackwell Publishing; 2006:267-280.
498. Martinez R, Wobeser G. Immunization of ducks for type C botulism. *J Wildl Dis* 1999;35:710-715.
499. Marx D. Preventive health care with diagnostics. *AAV Today* 1988;2:92-94.
500. Marx KL, Roston MA. *The Exotic Animal Drug Compendium: An International Formulary*. Veterinary Learning Systems: Trenton; 1996.
501. Mashima TY, Ley DH, Stoskopf MK, et al. Evaluation of treatment of conjunctivitis associated with *Mycoplasma gallisepticum* in house finches (*Carpodacus mexicanus*). *J Avian Med Surg* 1997;11:20-24.
502. Massey JG, Work TM. Diclazuril therapy for clinical toxoplasmosis. *Proc Annu Conf Assoc Avian Vet* 2000;29-39.
503. Matthews NS. Anesthesia for big birds (ostriches and emus). *Proc North Am Vet Conf* 1993;705.
504. Mazet JAK, Newman SH, Gilardi KVK, et al. Advances in oiled bird emergency medicine and management. *J Avian Med Surg* 2002;16:146-149.
505. Mazor-Thomas JE, Mann PE, Karas AZ, et al. Pain-suppressed behaviors in the red-tailed hawk (*Buteo jamaicensis*). *Appl Anim Behav Sci* 2014;152:83-91.
506. McConnell HM, Morgan KJ, Sine A, et al. Using sea water for cleaning oil from seabird feathers. *Meth Ecol Evol* 2015;6(10):1235-1238.
507. McDonald SE. IME—injecting eggs with antibiotics. *J Assoc Avian Vet* 1989;1:9.
508. McDonald SE. IME—summary of medications for use in psittacine birds. *J Assoc Avian Vet* 1989;3:120-127.
509. McGill I, Feltrer Y, Jeffs C, et al. Isosporoid coccidiosis in translocated cirl buntings (*Emberiza cirlus*). *Vet Rec* 2010;167:656-660.
510. Mejia-Fava J, Divers SJ, Jimenez DA, et al. Diagnosis and treatment of proventricular nematodiasis in an umbrella cockatoo (*Cacatua alba*). *J Am Vet Med Assoc* 2013;242:1122-1126.
511. Mejia-Fava J, Holmes SP, Radlinsky M, et al. Use of a nitinol wire stent for management of severe tracheal stenosis in an eclectus parrot (*Eclectus roratus*). *J Avian Med Surg* 2015;29(3):238-249.
512. Menao MC, Bottino JA, Biasia I, et al. *Salmonella typhimurium* infection in hyacinth macaw (*Anodorhynchus hyacinthinus*). *Arquivos-do-Instituto-Biologico-Sao-Paulo* 2000;67:43-47.
513. Merryman JI, Buckles EL. The avian thyroid gland. *J Avian Med Surg* 1998;12:234-242.
514. Meteyer CU, Rideout BA, Gilbert M, et al. Pathology and proposed pathophysiology of diclofenac poisoning in free-living and experimentally exposed oriental white-backed vultures (*Gyps bengalensis*). *J Wildl Dis* 2005;41:707-716.
515. Midgley-DiGeronimo PM, Rinaldi M, da Cunha A, et al. Median toxic dose of intravenous bupivacaine in isoflurane-anesthetized Ross-708 broiler chickens. *Proc Annu Conf Assoc Avian Vet ExoticsCon* 2016;59.
516. Mikaelian I, Paillet I, Williams D. Comparative use of various mydriatic drugs in kestrels (*Falco tinnunculus*). *Am J Vet Res* 1994;55:270-272.
517. Millam JR. Leuprolide acetate can reversibly prevent egg laying in cockatiels. *Proc Annu Conf Assoc Avian Vet* 1993;46.
518. Millam JR, Finney HL. Leuprolide acetate can reversibly prevent egg laying in cockatiels (*Nymphicus hollandicus*). *Zoo Biol* 1994;13:149-155.

519. Miller EA, Welte SC. Caring for oiled birds. In: Fowler ME, Miller RE, eds. *Zoo and Wild Animal Medicine: Current Therapy 4*. Philadelphia: WB Saunders Co; 1998:300-309.
520. Mohan R. *Mycoplasma* in ratites. *Proc Annu Conf Assoc Avian Vet* 1993;294-296.
521. Molter CM, Court MH, Hazarika S, et al. Pharmacokinetics of parenteral and oral meloxicam in Hispaniolan parrots (*Amazona ventralis*). *Proc Annu Conf Assoc Avian Vet/Assoc Exot Mam Vet* 2009;317-318.
522. Monção-Silva R, Ofri R, Raposo AC, et al. Ophthalmic diagnostic tests in parrots (*Amazona amazonica*) and (*Amazona aestiva*). *J Exot Pet Med* 2016;25:186-193.
523. Montesinos A, Ardiaca M. Acid-base status in the avian patient using a portable point-of-care analyzer. *Vet Clin North Am Exot Anim Pract* 2013;16:47-69.
524a. Montesinos A, Ardiaca M, Gilabert JA, et al. Pharmacokinetics of meloxicam after intravenous, intramuscular and oral administration of a single dose to African grey parrots (Psittacus erithacus). *J Vet Pharmacol Ther* 2017;40:279-284.
524b. Montesinos A, Ardiaca M, Juan-Salles C, et al. Effects of meloxicam on hematologic and plasma biochemical analyte values and results of histologic examination of kidney biopsy specimens of African grey parrots (*Psittacus erithacus*). *J Avian Med Surg* 2015;29:1-8.
525. Moore DM, Rice RL. Exotic animal formulary. In: Holt KM, Boothe DM, Gaumnitz J, et al. *Veterinary Values*. 5th ed. Lenexa, KS: Veterinary Medicine Publishing Group; 1998:159-245.
526. Moore RP, Snowden KF, Phalen DN, et al. Diagnosis, treatment, and prevention of megabacteriosis in the budgerigar (*Melopsittacus undulatus*). *Proc Annu Conf Assoc Avian Vet* 2001;161-163.
527. Morgan K, Ziccardi M. Veterinary care of oiled birds. In: Samour J, ed. *Avian Medicine*. 3rd ed. St. Louis, MO: Elsevier; 2016:286-293.
528. Morishita TY. Clinical assessment of gallinaceous birds and waterfowl in backyard flocks. *Vet Clin North Am Exot Anim Pract* 1999;2:383-404.
529. Morrisey JK. Avian emergency medicine and critical care. In: Hoefer HL, ed. *Practical Avian Medicine: The Compendium Collection*. Trenton, NJ: Veterinary Learning Systems Co; 1997:53-57.
530. Morrisey JK, Hohenhaus AE, Rosenthal K, et al. Comparison of three media for the storage of avian whole blood. *Proc Annu Conf Am Assoc Zoo Vet* 1998;149-150.
531. Muir III WW, Hubbell JA, Bednarski RA, et al. Anesthetic procedures in exotic animals. In: Muir III WW, Hubbell JA, Bednarski RA, et al. *Handbook of Veterinary Anesthesia*. St. Louis: Elsevier Mosby; 2013:450-489.
532. Mukaratirwa S, Chimbwanda M, Matekwe N, et al. A comparison of the efficacy of doramectin, closantel and levamisole in the treatment of the "oriental eye fluke," *Philophthalmus gralli*, in commercially reared ostriches (*Struthio camelus*). *J S Afr Vet Assoc* 2008;79:101-103.
533. Mulcahy DM, Stoskopf MK, Esler D. Lack of isoflurane-sparing effect of butorphanol in field anesthesia of harlequin ducks (*Histrionicus histrionicus*). *Proc Annu Conf Am Assoc Zoo Vet/ Internat Assoc Aquatic Anim Med* 2000;532-533.
534. Muller MG, Kinne J, Schuster RK, et al. Outbreak of microsporidiosis caused by *Enterocytozoon bieneusi* in falcons. *Vet Parasitol* 2008;152:67-78.
535. Murase T, Ikeda T, Goto I, et al. Treatment of lead poisoning in wild geese. *J Am Vet Med Assoc* 1992;200:1726-1729.
536. Murphy CJ. Raptor ophthalmology. *Compend Contin Educ Pract Vet* 1987;9:241-260.
537. Murphy K, Wilson DA, Burton M, et al. Effectiveness of the GnRH agonist deslorelin as a tool to decrease levels of circulating testosterone in zebra finches. *Gen Comp Endocrinol* 2015;222:150-157.
538. Murray M, Tseng F. Diagnosis and treatment of secondary anticoagulant rodenticide toxicosis in a red-tailed hawk (*Buteo jamaicensis*). *J Avian Med Surg* 2008;22:41-46.
539. Mushi EZ, Binta MG, Isa JW. Biochemical composition of urine from farmed ostriches (Struthio camelus) in Botswana. *J South Afr Vet Assoc* 2001;72:46-48.
540. Musser JMB, Heatley JJ, Phalen DN. Pharmacokinetics after intravenous administration of flunixin meglumine in budgerigars (*Melopsittacus undulatus*) and Patagonian conures (*Cyanoliseus patagonus*). *J Am Vet Med Assoc* 2013;242:205-208.

541. Mutlow A, Forbes N. *Haemoproteus* in raptors: pathogenicity, treatment, and control. *Proc Annu Conf Assoc Avian Vet* 2000;157-163.
542. Naether CA. *Raising Pigeons and Doves*. New York: David McKay Co; 1979.
543. Naidoo V, Swan GE. Diclofenac toxicity in *Gyps* vulture is associated with decreased uric acid excretion and not renal portal vasoconstriction. *Comp Biochem Physiol C Toxicol Pharmacol* 2008;149:269-274.
544. Naidoo V, Venter L, Wolter K, et al. The toxicokinetics of ketoprofen in *Gyps coprotheres*: toxicity due to zero-order metabolism. *Arch Toxicol* 2010;84:761-766.
545. Naidoo V, Wolter K, Cromarty AD, et al. The pharmacokinetics of meloxicam in vultures. *J Vet Pharmacol Ther* 2008;31:128-134.
546. Naidoo V, Wolter K, Cromarty D, et al. Toxicity of non-steroidal anti-inflammatory drugs to *Gyps* vultures: a new threat from ketoprofen. *Biol Lett* 2010;6:339-341.
547. Napier JE, Hinrichs SH, Lampen F, et al. An outbreak of avian mycobacteriosis caused by *Mycobacterium intracellulare* in little blue penguins (*Eudyptula minor*). *J Zoo Wildl Med* 2009;40:680-686.
548. National Registration Authority for Agricultural and Veterinary Chemicals. Dimetridazole Scope Document. Canberra, Australia. 2002. Available at: http://www.apvma.gov.au/chemrev/dimetridazole_scope.pdf. Accessed June 16, 2017.
549. National Research Council. *Nutrient Requirements of Poultry*. Washington, DC: National Academy Press; 1994.
550. Nazifi S, Nabinejad A, Sepehrimanesh M, et al. Haematology and serum biochemistry of golden eagle (*Aquila chrysaetos*) in Iran. *Comp Clin Pathol* 2008;17:197-201.
551. Nemetz L. Deslorelin acetate long-term suppression of ovarian carcinoma in a cockatiel (*Nymphicus hollandicus*). *Proc Annu Conf Assoc Avian Vet* 2012;37-42.
552. Nemetz L, Broome M. Strontium-90 therapy for uropygial neoplasia. *Proc Annu Conf Assoc Avian Vet* 2004;15-20.
553. Nemetz LP, Lennox AM. Zosyn: a replacement for Pipracil in the avian patient. *Proc Annu Conf Assoc Avian Vet* 2004;11-13.
554. Neut D, van de Belt H, van Horn JR, et al. Residual gentamicin-release from antibiotic-loaded polymethylmethacrylate beads after 5 years of implantation. *Biomaterials* 2003;24:1829-1831.
555. Newell SM. Diagnosis and treatment of lymphocytic leukemia and malignant lymphoma in a Pekin duck (*Anas platyrhyncos domesticus*). *J Assoc Avian Vet* 1991;5:83-86.
556. Nguyen KQ, Hawkins MG, Taylor IT, et al. Stability and uniformity of extemporaneous preparations of voriconazole in two liquid suspension vehicles at two storage temperatures. *Am J Vet Res* 2009;7:908-914.
557. Nichols D, Wolff M, Phillips L, Montali R. Coagulopathy in pink-backed pelicans (*Pelecanus rufescens*) associated with hypervitaminosis E. *J Zoo Wildl Med* 1989;20(1):57-61.
558. Nolan PM, Duckworth RA, Hill GE, et al. Maintenance of a captive flock of house finches free of infection by *Mycoplasma gallisepticum*. *Avian Dis* 2000;44:948-952.
559. Norton TM. Medical protocols recommended by the US Bali mynah SSP. Available at: http://www.aazv.org/page/547/Bali-Mynah-Medical-Protocols.htm. Published 2001. Accessed June 16, 2017.
560. Norton TM, Greiner E, Latimer K. Medical protocols recommended by the U.S. bali mynah SSP. Available at: www.aazv.org/page/547/Bali-Mynah-Medical-Protocols.htm. Updated Sept 16, 2007. Accessed Feb 6, 2017.
561. Norton TM, Gaskin J, Kollias GV, et al. Efficacy of acyclovir against herpesvirus infection in Quaker parakeets. *Am J Vet Res* 1991;52:2007-2009.
562. Norton TM, Neiffer DL, Seibels B, et al. *Atoxoplasma medical protocols recommended by the passerine Atoxoplasma working group*. Available at: http://www.aazv.org/displaycommon.cfm?an=1&subarticlenbr=545; 2007. Accessed Jan 26, 2011.
563. Oaks J, Meteyer C. Nonsteroidal anti-inflammatory drugs in raptors. In: Miller RE, Fowler ME, eds. *Fowler's Zoo and Wild Animal Medicine: Current Therapy*. Vol 7. St. Louis: MO; 2012:349-355.

564. Oaks JL, Gilbert M, Virani MZ, et al. Diclofenac residues as the cause of vulture population decline in Pakistan. *Nature* 2004;427:630-633.
565. Okeson DM, Llizo SY, Miller CL, et al. Antibody response of five bird species after vaccination with a killed West Nile virus vaccine. *J Zoo Wildl Med* 2007;38:240-244.
566. Olsen GH, Carpenter JW, Langenberg JA. Medicine and surgery. In: Ellis DH, Gee GF, Mirande CM, eds. *Cranes: Their Biology, Husbandry, and Conservation*. Washington, DC: National Biological Service/International Crane Foundation; 1996:142-143.
567. Olsen GH, Turell MJ, Pagac BB. Efficacy of eastern equine encephalitis immunization in whooping cranes. *J Wildl Dis* 1997;33:312-315.
568. Olsen GH, Miller KJ, Docherty DE, et al. Pathogenicity of West Nile virus and response to vaccination in sandhill cranes (*Grus canadensis*) using a killed vaccine. *J Zoo Wildl Med* 2009;40:263-271.
569. Olsen GP, Russell KE, Dierenfeld E, et al. A comparison of four regimens for treatment of iron storage disease using the European starling (*Sturnus vulgaris*) as a model. *J Avian Med Surg* 2006;20:74-79.
570. Olsen GP, Russell KE, Dierenfeld E, et al. Impact of supplements on iron absorption from diets containing high and low iron concentrations in the European starling (*Sturnus vulgaris*). *J Avian Med Surg* 2009;20(2):67-73.
571. Onderka D, Doornenbal E. Mycotic dermatitis in ostriches. *Can Vet J* 1992;33:72-76.
572. Orosz SE, Frazier DL. Antifungal agents: a review of their pharmacology and therapeutic indications. *J Avian Med Surg* 1995;9:8-18.
573. Orosz SE, Schroeder EC, Frazier DL. Itraconazole: a new antifungal drug for birds. *Proc Annu Conf Assoc Avian Vet* 1994;13-19.
574. Orosz SE, Schroeder EC, Frazier DL. Pharmacokinetic properties of itraconazole in blue-fronted Amazon parrots (*Amazona aestiva aestiva*). *J Avian Med Surg* 1996;10:168-173.
575. Orosz SE, Jones MP, Cox SK, et al. Pharmacokinetics of amoxicillin plus clavulanic acid in blue-fronted Amazon parrots (*Amazona aestiva aestiva*). *J Avian Med Surg* 2000;14:107-112.
576. Orr KA, Fowler ME. Order Trochiliiformes (hummingbirds). In: Fowler ME, Cubas ZS, eds. *Biology, Medicine, and Surgery of South American Wild Animals*. Ames: Iowa State University Press; 2001:174-179.
577. Padilla LR, Miller RE, Flammer K. Doxycycline in drinking water for treatment of *Chlamydophila psittaci* in fruit doves. *Proc Annu Conf Am Assoc Zoo Vet* 2003;267-268.
578. Paesano F, Ceccherelli R, Briganti A. Partial intravenous anaesthesia (PIVA) with infusion of fentanyl and midazolam during orthopedic surgery in wild birds. *Intl Conf Avian Herp Exot Mam Med* 2015;332.
579. Paesano F, Ceccherelli R, Di Chiara G, et al. Clinical effects of alfaxalone based protocols in the yellow legged gull (*Larus michahellis*). *Intl Conf Avian Herp Exot Mam Med* 2015;334.
580. Page DC, Schmidt RE, English JH, et al. Antemortem diagnosis and treatment of sarcocystosis in two species of psittacines. *J Zoo Wildl Med* 1992;23:77-85.
581. Paley D, Herzenberg JE. Intramedullary infections treated with antibiotic cement rods: preliminary results in nine cases. *J Orthoped Trauma* 2002;16:723-729.
582. Papendick R, Stalis I, Harvey C, et al. Suspected fenbendazole toxicity in birds. *Proc Annu Conf Am Assoc Zoo Vet/Am Assoc Wildl Vet* 1998;144-146.
583. Park F. Vitamin A, toxicosis in a lorikeet flock. *Vet Clin North Am Exot Anim Pract* 2006;9(3):495-502.
584. Parrot TY, Cray C, Martin S. Daily dosing of voriconazole and correlation with serological testing. *Proc Annu Conf Assoc Avian Vet* 2010;69-70.
585. Paula VV, Fantoni DT, Otsuki DA, et al. Blood-gas and electrolyte values for Amazon parrots (*Amazona aestiva*). *Pesquisa Vet Brasil* 2008;28:108-112.
586. Paula VV, Otsuki DA, Auler Junior JO, et al. The effect of premedication with ketamine, alone or with diazepam, on anaesthesia with sevoflurane in parrots (*Amazona aestiva*). *BMC Vet Res* 2013;9:142.

587. Paul-Murphy J, Ludders JW. Avian analgesia. *Vet Clin North Am Exot Anim Pract* 2001;4: 35-45.
588. Paul-Murphy JR, Brunson DB, Miletic V. Analgesic effects of butorphanol and buprenorphine in conscious African grey parrots. *Am J Vet Res* 1999;60:1218-1221.
589. Paul-Murphy J, Hess JC, Fialkowski JP. Pharmacokinetic properties of a single intramuscular dose of buprenorphine in African grey parrots (*Psittacus erithacus erithacus*). *J Avian Med Surg* 2004;18:224-228.
590. Paul-Murphy J, Lowenstine L, Turrel J. Malignant lymphoreticular neoplasm in an African gray parrot. *J Am Vet Med Assoc* 1985;187(11):1216-1217.
591. Paul-Murphy J, Engilis A, Pascoe P, et al. Comparison of pentobarbital and thoracic (cardiac) compression to euthanize anesthetized sparrows (*Passer domesticus*) and starlings (*Sturnus vulgaris*). *Proc Annu Conf Assoc Avian Vet: Exot Proc* 2016;69-70.
592. Paul-Murphy JR, Sladky KK, Krugner-Higby LA, et al. Analgesic effects of carprofen and liposome-encapsulated butorphanol tartrate in Hispaniolan parrots (*Amazona ventralis*) with experimentally induced arthritis. *Am J Vet Res* 2009;70:1201-1210.
593. Pavez JC, Hawkins MG, Pascoe PJ, et al. Effect of fentanyl target-controlled infusions on isoflurane minimum anaesthetic concentration and cardiovascular function in red-tailed hawks (*Buteo jamaicensis*). *Vet Anaesth Analg* 2011;38:344-351.
594. Pedersoli WM, Ravis WR, Lee HS, et al. Pharmacokinetics of single doses of digoxin administered intravenously to ducks, roosters, and turkeys. *Am J Vet Res* 1990;51(11): 1751-1755.
595. Pees M, Krautwald-Junghanns M-E, Straub J. Evaluating and treating the cardiovascular system. In: Harrison GJ, Lightfoot TL, eds. *Clinical Avian Medicine*. Vol I. Palm Beach, FL: Spix Publishing; 2006:379-394.
596. Pees M, Kuhring K, Demiraij F, et al. Bioavailability and compatibility of enalapril in birds. *Proc Annu Conf Assoc Avian Vet* 2006;7-11.
597. Pees M, Schmidt V, Coles B, et al. Diagnosis and long-term therapy of right-sided heart failure in a yellow-crowned Amazon (*Amazona ochrocephala*). *Vet Rec* 2006;158:445-447.
598. Penguin Taxon Advisory Group. *Penguin (Spheniscidae) Care Manual*. Silver Springs: Association of Zoos and Aquariums; 2014.
599. Pereira ME, Werther K. Evaluation of the renal effects of flunixin meglumine, ketoprofen and meloxicam in budgerigars (*Melopsittacus undulatus*). *Vet Rec* 2007;160:844-846.
600. Perpinan D, Melero R. Suspected ivermectin toxicity in a Nanday parakeet (*Nandayus nenday*). *Proc Annu Conf Am Assoc Zoo Vet* 2003;298-299.
601. Peters TL, Fulton RM, Roberson KD, et al. Effect of antibiotics on *in vitro* and *in vivo* avian cartilage degradation. *Avian Dis* 2002;46:75-86.
602. Petritz OA, Guzman DS-M, Gustavsen K, et al. Evaluation of the mydriatic effects of topical administration of rocuronium bromide in Hispaniolan Amazon parrots (*Amazona ventralis*). *J Am Vet Med Assoc* 2016;248(1):67-71.
603. Petzinger C, Heatley JJ, Bailey CA, Bauer JE. Lipid metabolic dose response to dietary alpha-linolenic acid in monk parrot (*Myiopsitta monachus*). *Lipids* 2014;49(3):235-245.
604. Petzinger C, Larner C, Heatley JJ, et al. Conversion of α-linolenic acid to long-chain omega-3 fatty acid derivatives and alterations of HDL density subfractions and plasma lipids with dietary polyunsaturated fatty acids in Monk parrots (*Myiopsitta monachus*). *J Anim Physiol Anim Nutr (Berl)* 2014;98(2):262-270.
605. Phair KA, Larsen RS, Wack RF, et al. Determination of the minimum anesthetic concentration of sevoflurane in thick-billed parrots (*Rhynchopsitta pachyrhyncha*). *Am J Vet Res* 2012;73:1350-1355.
606. Phalen DN. Avian renal disorders. In: Fudge AM, ed. *Laboratory Medicine: Avian and Exotic Pets*. Philadelphia: WB Saunders Co; 2000:61-68.
607. Phalen DN. Common bacterial and fungal infectious diseases in pet birds. *Suppl Compend Contin Educ Pract Vet* 2003;25:43-48.

608. Phalen DN. Implications of viruses in clinical disorders. In: Harrison GJ, Lightfoot TL, eds. *Clinical Avian Medicine*. Vol II:Palm Beach: Spix Publishing; 2006:721-745.
609. Phalen DN. Preventive medicine and screening. In: Harrison GJ, Lightfoot TL, eds. *Clinical Avian Medicine*. Vol II:Palm Beach: Spix Publishing; 2006:573-585.
610. Phalen DN, Logan KS, Snowden KF. Encephalitozoon hellem infection as the cause of a unilateral chronic keratoconjunctivitis in an umbrella cockatoo (*Cacatua alba*). *Vet Ophthalmol* 2006;9:59-63.
611. Phalen DN, Hays HB, Filippich LJ, et al. Heart failure in a macaw with atherosclerosis of the aorta and brachiocephalic arteries. *J Am Vet Med Assoc* 1996;209:1435-1440.
612. Pignon C, Mayer J. Radiation therapy of uropygial gland carcinoma in psittacine species. *Proc Annu Conf Assoc Avian Vet* 2011;263.
613. Pikula J, Hajkova P, Bandouchova H, et al. Lead toxicosis of captive vultures: case description and responses to chelation therapy. *BMC Vet Res* 2013;9(1):11.
614. Plumb DC. *Plumb's Veterinary Drug Handbook*. 6th ed. Ames: Blackwell Publishing; 2008.
615. Plumb DC. *Plumb's Veterinary Drug Handbook*. 8th ed. Wiley-Blackwell: Ames, IA; 2015.
616. Poffers J, Lumeij JT, Redig PT. Investigations into the uricolytic properties of urate oxidase in a granivorous (*Columba livia domestica*) and in a carnivorous (*Buteo jamaicensis*) avian species. *Avian Pathol* 2002;31:573-579.
617. Poffers J, Lumeij JT, Timmermans-Sprang EPM, et al. Further studies on the use of allopurinol to reduce plasma uric acid concentrations in the red-tailed hawk (*Buteo jamaicensis*) hyperuricaemic model. *Avian Pathol* 2002;31:567-572.
618. Pollock CG, Schumacher J, Orosz SE, et al. Sedative effects of medetomidine in pigeons. *J Avian Med Surg* 2001;15:95-100.
619. Porter SL. Vehicular trauma in owls. *Proc Annu Conf Assoc Avian Vet* 1990;164-170.
620. Powers LV, Papich MG. Pharmacokinetics of orally administered phenobarbital in African grey parrots (*Psittacus erithacus erithacus*). *J Vet Pharmacol Ther* 2011;34(6):615-617.
621. Powers LV, Flammer K, Papich M. Preliminary investigation of doxycycline plasma concentrations in cockatiels (*Nymphicus hollandicus*) after administration by injection or in water or feed. *J Avian Med Surg* 2000;14:23-30.
622. Powers LV, Pokras M, Rio K, et al. Hematology and occurrence of hemoparasites in migrating sharp-shinned hawks (*Accipiter striatus*) during fall migration. *J Raptor Res* 1994;28:178-185.
623. Prather JF. Rapid and reliable sedation induced by diazepam and antagonized by flumazenil in zebra finches (*Taeniopygia guttata*). *J Avian Med Surg* 2012;26:76-84.
624. Product insert.
625. Proenca LM, Mayer J, Schnellbacher R, et al. Antemortem diagnosis and successful treatment of pulmonary candidiasis in a sun conure (*Aratinga solstitialis*). *J Avian Med Surg* 2014;28:316-321.
626. Prus SE, Clubb SL, Flammer K. Doxycycline plasma concentrations in macaws fed a medicated corn diet. *Avian Dis* 1992;36:480-483.
627. Quandt JE, Greenacre CB. Sevoflurane anesthesia in psittacines. *J Zoo Wildl Med* 1999;30:308-309.
628. Quesenberry KE, Hillyer EV. Supportive care and emergency therapy. In: Ritchie BW, Harrison GJ, Harrison LR, eds. *Avian Medicine: Principles and Application*. Lake Worth, FL: Wingers Publishing; 1994:382-416.
629. Quintavalla F, Zucca P. Birds of prey: blood chemistry profile for peregrine falcons (*Falco peregrinus*) and eagle owls (*Bubo bubo*) in a raptor centre in north Italy. *Proc Euro Conf Assoc Avian Vet* 1993;544-551.
630. Raath JP, Quandt SKF, Malan JH. Ostrich (*Struthio camelus*) immobilization using carfentanil and xylazine and reversal with yohimbine and naltrexone. *J South Afr Vet Assoc* 1992;63:138-140.
631. Raghav R, Middleton R, Ahamad R, et al. Analysis of arterial and venous blood gases in healthy gyrfalcons (*Falco rusticolus*) under anesthesia. *J Avian Med Surg* 2015;29:290-297.

632. Raghav R, Taylor M, Guincho M, Smith D. Potassium chloride as a euthanasia agent in psittacine birds: clinical aspects and consequences for histopathologic assessment. *Can Vet J* 2011;52(3):303-306.
633. Ramer JC, Paul-Murphy J, Brunson D, et al. Effects of mydriatic agents in cockatoos, African gray parrots, and blue-fronted Amazon parrots. *J Am Vet Med Assoc* 1996;208:227-230.
634. Ramos JR, Howard RD, Pleasant RS, et al. Elution of metronidazole and gentamicin from polymethylmethacrylate beads. *Vet Surg* 2003;32(3):251-261.
635. Ramsay E, Bos J, McFadden C. Use of intratumoral cisplatin and orthovoltage radiotherapy in treatment of a fibrosarcoma in a macaw. *J Assoc Avian Vet* 1993;7(2):87-90.
636. Ramsay EC, Grindlinger H. Use of clomipramine in the treatment of obsessive behavior in psittacine birds. *J Assoc Avian Vet* 1994;8:9.
637. Ramsay EC, Vulliet R. Pharmacokinetic properties of gentamicin and amikacin in the cockatiel. *Avian Dis* 1993;37:628-634.
638. Ramsay EC, Drew ML, Johnson B. Trichomoniasis in a flock of budgerigars. *Proc Annu Conf Assoc Avian Vet* 1990;309-311.
639. Randolph K. Equine encephalitis virus in ratites. *Proc Annu Conf Assoc Avian Vet* 1995;249-252.
640. Rathinam T, Chapman HD. Sensitivity of isolates of *Eimeria* from turkey flocks to the anticoccidial drugs amprolium, clopidol, diclazuril, and monensin. *Avian Dis* 2009;53:405-408.
641. Ratzlaff K, Papich MG, Flammer K. Plasma concentrations of fluconazole after a single oral dose and administration in drinking water in cockatiels (*Nymphicus hollandicus*). *J Avian Med Surg* 2011;25:23-31.
642. Ravich M, Cray C, Hess L, et al. Lipid panel reference intervals for Amazon parrots (*Amazona* species). *J Avian Med Surg* 2014;28:209-215.
643. Redig P. *Medical Management of Birds of Prey: A Collection of Notes on Selected Topics.* The Raptor Center: St. Paul; 1993.
644. Redig P. Infectious diseases; fungal diseases. In: Samour J, ed. *Avian Medicine.* London: Harcourt Publishers; 2000:275-291.
645. Redig P. Aspergillosis. In: Samour J, ed. *Avian Medicine.* 3rd ed. St. Louis, MO: Elsevier; 2016:460-472.
646. Redig PT. Fluid therapy and acid-base balance in the critically ill avian patient. *Proc Annu Conf Assoc Avian Vet* 1984;59-73.
647. Redig PT. Treatment protocol for bumblefoot types 1 and 2. *AAV Today* 1987;1:207-208.
648. Redig PT. Avian emergencies. In: Beynon PH, Forbes NA, Harcourt-Brown NH, eds. *BSAVA Manual of Raptors, Pigeons and Waterfowl.* Ames: Iowa State University Press; 1996:30-41.
649. Redig PT. Nursing avian patients. In: Beynon PH, Forbes NA, Harcourt-Brown NH, eds. *Manual of Raptors, Pigeons and Waterfowl.* Ames: Iowa State University Press; 1996:42-46.
650. Redig PT. Falconiformes (vultures, hawks, falcons, secretary bird). In: Fowler ME, Miller RE, eds. *Zoo and Wild Animal Medicine.* 5th ed. Philadelphia: WB Saunders Co; 2005:150-161.
651. Redig P, Arent L. Raptor toxicology. *Vet Clin North Am Exot Anim Pract* 2008;11:261-282.
652. Redig PT, Cruz-Martinez L. Raptors. In: Tully TN, Dorrestein GM, Jones AK, eds. *Avian Medicine.* Edinburgh: Saunders Elsevier; 2009:209-242.
653. Redig PT, Duke GE. Intravenously administered ketamine HCl and diazepam for anesthesia of raptors. *J Am Vet Med Assoc* 1976;169:886-888.
654. Redig PT, Ponder J. Raptors: practical information every avian practitioner can use. *Proc Annu Conf Assoc Avian Vet* 2010;171-180.
655. Redig PT, Talbot B, Guarnera T. Avian malaria. *Proc Annu Conf Assoc Avian Vet* 1993;173-181.
656. Reidarson TH, McBain JF, Denton D. The use of medroxyprogesterone acetate to induce molting in chinstrap penguins. *J Zoo Wildl Med* 1999;30:278-280.

657. Reiss AE, Badcock NR. Itraconazole levels in serum, skin and feathers of Gouldian finches (*Chloebia gouldiae*) following in-seed medication. *Proc Joint Conf Am Assoc Zoo Vet/Am Assoc Wildl Vet* 1998;142-143.
658. Reither NP. Medetomidine and atipamezole in avian practice. *Proc Euro Conf Avian Med Surg* 1993;43-48.
659. Remple JD. Intracellular hematozoa of raptors: a review and update. *J Avian Med Surg* 2004;18:75-88.
660. Remple JD, Forbes NA. Antibiotic-impregnated polymethyl methacrylate beads in the treatment of bumblefoot in raptors. In: *Raptor Biomedicine III*. Lake Worth. FL: Zoological Education Network; 2002:255-263.
661. Reuter A, Muller K, Arndt G, et al. Reference intervals for intraocular pressure measured by rebound tonometry in ten raptor species and factors affecting the intraocular pressure. *J Avian Med Surg* 2011;25:165-172.
662. Riedesel D. Respiratory pharmacology. In: Hsu W, ed. *Handbook of Veterinary Pharmacology*. Ames, IA: Wiley-Blackwell; 2008:221-233.
663. Riggs SM, Hawkins MG, Craigmill AL, et al. Pharmacokinetics of butorphanol tartrate in red-tailed hawks (*Buteo jamaicensis*) and great horned owls (*Bubo virginianus*). *Am J Vet Res* 2008;69:596-603.
664. Ritchie BW. *Avian Viruses: Function and Control*. Lake Worth, FL: Wingers Publishing; 1995.
665. Ritchie BW. Diagnosing and preventing common viral infections in companion birds. In: *Proc 21st Annu Waltham/OSU Symp*; 1997:7-13.
666. Ritchie BW, Harrison GJ. Formulary. In: Ritchie BW, Harrison GJ, Harrison LR, eds. *Avian Medicine: Principles and Application*. Lake Worth, FL: Wingers Publishing; 1994:457-478.
667. Ritchie BW, Harrison GJ. Formulary. In: Ritchie BW, Harrison GJ, Harrison LR, eds. *Avian Medicine: Principles and Application*. Abridged ed. Lake Worth, FL: Wingers Publishing; 1997:227-253.
668. Ritchie BW, Harrison GJ, Harrison LR. Hematology and biochemistry. In: Ritchie BW, Harrison GJ, Harrison LR, eds. *Avian Medicine: Principles and Application*. Lake Worth, FL: Wingers Publishing; 1994:1331-1347.
669. Ritchie BW, Latimer KS, Leonard J, et al. Safety, immunogenicity and efficacy of an inactivated avian polyomavirus vaccine. *Am J Vet Res* 1998;59:143-148.
670. Ritchie BW, Vaughn SB, St. Leger J, et al. Use of an inactivated virus vaccine to control polyomavirus outbreaks in nine flocks of psittacine birds. *J Am Vet Med Assoc* 1998;212:685-690.
671. Rivera S, McClearen J, Reavill DR. Suspected fenbendazole toxicity in pigeons (*Columba livia*). *Proc Annu Conf Assoc Avian Vet* 2000;207-209.
672. Robbe D, Todisco G, Giammarino A, et al. Use of a synthetic GnRH analog to induce reproductive activity in canaries (*Serinus canaria*). *J Avian Med Surg* 2008;22:123-126.
673. Rivera S, McClearen JR, Reavill DR. Treatment of nonepitheliotropic cutaneous B-cell lymphoma in an umbrella cockatoo (*Cacatua alba*). *J Avian Med Surg* 2009;23:294-302.
674. Robbins PK, Tell LA, Needham ML, et al. Pharmacokinetics of piperacillin after intramuscular injection in red-tailed hawks and great horned owls. *J Zoo Wildl Med* 2000;31:47-51.
675. Roberts MF. *Pigeons*. Jersey City: TFH Publications; 1962.
676. Romagnano A. Examination and preventive medicine protocols in psittacines. *Vet Clin North Am Exot Anim Pract* 1999;2(333):352-355.
677. Romagnano A, Shiroma JT, Heard DJ, et al. Magnetic resonance imaging of the brain and coelomic cavity of the domestic pigeon (*Columba livia domestica*). *Vet Radiol Ultrasound* 1996;37(6):431-440.
678. Rosenthal KL, Johnston M. Hypothyroidism in a red-lored Amazon (*Amazona autumnalis*). *Proc Annu Conf Assoc Avian Vet* 2003;33-36.
679. Rosenthal K, Stamoulis M. Diagnosis of congestive heart failure in an Indian Hill mynah bird (*Gracula religiosa*). *J Assoc Avian Vet* 1993;7:27-30.

680. Rosenthal K, Duda L, Ivey ES, et al. A report of photodynamic therapy for squamous cell carcinoma in a cockatiel. *Proc Annu Conf Assoc Avian Vet* 2001;175-176.
681. Rosskopf WJ, Woerpel RW. Practical avian therapeutics with dosages of commonly used medications. *Proc Basics Avian Med (Sydney, Australia)* 1996;75-81.
682. Rouffaer LO, Adriaensen C, De Boeck C, et al. Racing pigeons: a reservoir for nitro-imidazole-resistant *Trichomonas gallinae*. *J Parasitol* 2014;100:360-363.
683. Rundfeldt C, Wyska E, Steckel H, et al. A model for treating avian aspergillosis: serum and lung tissue kinetics for Japanese quail (*Coturnix japonica*) following single and multiple aerosol exposures of a nanoparticulate itraconazole suspension. *Med Mycol* 2013;51(8):800-810.
684. Rupiper DJ. Diseases that affect race performance of homing pigeons. Part 1: Husbandry, diagnostic strategies, and viral diseases. *J Avian Med Surg* 1998;12:70-77.
685. Rupiper DJ. *Personal communication*. 2004.
686. Rupiper DJ, Ehrenberg M. Introduction to pigeon practice. *Proc Annu Conf Assoc Avian Vet* 1994;203-211.
687. Rupiper DJ, Ehrenberg M. Practical pigeon medicine. *Proc Annu Conf Assoc Avian Vet* 1997;479-497.
688. Rupley AE. Respiratory bacterial, fungal and parasitic diseases. In: *Proc Avian Specialty Advanced Prog Small Mam Rept Med Surg (Annu Conf Assoc Avian Vet)*; 1997:23-44.
689. Rupley AE. Critical care of pet birds. *Vet Clin North Am Exot Anim Pract* 1998;1:11-41.
690. Russell RE, Franson JC. Causes of mortality in eagles submitted to the National Wildlife Health Center 1975-2013. *Wildl Soc Bull* 2014;38(4):697-704.
691. Sabrautzki S. The course of gentamicin concentrations in serum and tissues of pigeons. *Inaugural dissertation Tierarztliche Fakultat der Ludwig-Maximilians-Universitat Munchen Vet Bull* 1983;54:5915.
692. Sacre B, Oppenheim Y, Steinberg H, et al. Presumptive histiocytic sarcoma in a great horned owl. *J Zoo Wildl Med* 1992;23:113-121.
693. Sadar MJ, Hawkins MG, Drazenovich T, et al. Pharmacokinetic-pharmacodynamic integration of an extended-release ceftiofur formulation administered to red-tailed hawks (*Buteo jamaicensis*). *Proc Annu Conf Assoc Avian Vet* 2014;11.
694. Sadar MJ, Sanchez-Migallon Guzman D, Mete A, et al. Mange caused by a novel Micnemidocoptes mite in a golden eagle (*Aquila chrysaetos*). *J Avian Med Surg* 2015;29:231-237.
695. Sadegh AB. Comparison of intranasal administration of xylazine, diazepam, and midazolam in budgerigars (*Melopsittacus undulatus*): clinical evaluation. *J Zoo Wildl Med* 2013;44:241-244.
696. Saggese MD, Tizard I, Phalen DN. Efficacy of multi-drug therapy with azithromycin, rifampin, and ethambutol for the treatment of ring-necked doves (*Streptopelia risoria*) naturally infected with avian mycobacteriosis. *Proc Annu Conf Assoc Avian Vet* 2007;27-29.
697. Samour J. Pharmaceutics commonly used in avian medicine. In: Samour J, ed. *Avian Medicine*. Philadelphia: Mosby; 2000:388-418.
698. Samour J. Management of raptors. In: Harrison GJ, Lightfoot TL, eds. *Clinical Avian Medicine*. Vol II. Palm Beach: Spix Publishing; 2006:948-954.
699. Samour J. Toxicology. In: Samour J, ed. *Avian Medicine*. 3rd ed. St. Louis, MO: Elsevier; 2016:275-286.
700. Samour JH, Naldo J. Serratospiculiasis in captive falcons in the Middle East: a review. *J Avian Med Surg* 2001;15:2-9.
701. Samour JH, Naldo J. Diagnosis and therapeutic management of lead toxicosis in falcons in Saudi Arabia. *J Avian Med Surg* 2002;16:16-20.
702. Samour JH, Naldo J. Diagnosis and therapeutic manangement of trichomoniasis in falcons in Saudi Arabia. *J Avian Med Surg* 2003;17:135-143.
703. Samour JH, Irwin-Davies J, Faraj E. Chemical immobilisation in ostriches using etorphine hydrochloride. *Vet Rec* 1990;127:575-576.
704. Samour JH, Naldo JL, John SK. Therapeutic management of *Babesia shortii* infection in a peregrine falcon (*Falco peregrinus*). *J Avian Med Surg* 2005;19:294-296.

705. Samour JH, Jones DM, Knight JA, et al. Comparative studies of the use of some injectable anesthetic agents in birds. *Vet Rec* 1984;115:6-11.
706. Sanchez-Migallon Guzman D. Advances in avian clinical therapeutics. *J Exot Pet Med* 2014; 23(1):6-20.
707. Sanchez-Migallon Guzman D, Flammer K, Paul-Murphy J, et al. Pharmacokinetics of butorphanol after oral, intravenous and intramuscular administration in Hispaniolan Amazon parrots (*Amazona ventralis*). *J Avian Med Surg* 2011;25:185-191.
708. Sanchez-Migallon Guzman D, Houck E, Beaufrère H, et al. Evaluation of the thermal antinociceptive effects of hydromorphone hydrochloride in cockatiels (*Nymphicus hollandicus*). In: *Proc 35th Annul Conf Assoc Avian Vet*; 2014:23.
709. Sanchez-Migallon Guzman D, Knych H, Olsen G, et al. Evaluation of the thermal antinociceptive effects and pharmacokinetics of a sustained-release buprenorphine formulation in American kestrels (*Falco sparverius*). In: *Proc 36th Annu Conf Assoc Avian Vet ExoticsCon*; 2015:13.
710a. Sanchez-Migallon Guzman D, Kukanich B, Keuler NS, et al. Antinociceptive effects of nalbuphine hydrochloride in Hispaniolan Amazon parrots (*Amazona ventralis*). *Am J Vet Res* 2011;72:736-740.
710b. Sanchez-Migallon Guzman D, Souza MJ, Braun JM, et al. Antinociceptive effects after oral administration of tramadol hydrochloride in Hispaniolan Amazon parrots (Amazona ventralis). *Am J Vet Res* 2012;73(8):1148-1152.
711. Sandmeier P. Evaluation of medetomidine for short-term immobilization of domestic pigeons (*Columba livia*) and Amazon parrots (*Amazona* species). *J Avian Med Surg* 2000;14:8-14.
712. Sandmeier P, Clauss M, Donati OF, et al. Use of deferiprone for the treatment of hepatic iron storage disease in three hornbills. *J Am Vet Med Assoc* 2012;240(1):75-81.
713. Santangelo B, Ferrari D, Di Martino I, et al. Dexmedetomidine chemical restraint in two raptor species undergoing inhalation anaesthesia. *Vet Res Commun* 2009;33:S209-S211.
714a. Scaglione FE, Cannizzo FT, Chiappino L, et al. *Plasmodium* spp. in a captive raptor collection of a safaripark in northwest Italy. *Res Vet Sci* 2016;104:123-125.
714b. Schäffer DP, Raposo AC, Libório FA, et al. Intranasal administration of midazolam in blue-and-yellow macaws (Ara araruana): evaluation of sedative effects. *Vet Anaesth Analg* 2016;43 (4):459-460.
715. Schink B, Korbel RT. Investigations on pharmacokinetics and pharmacodynamics of cefovecin in domestic pigeons. *Proc Annu Conf Assoc Avian Vet* 2010;301-302.
716. Schmidt V, Demiraj F, Di Somma A, et al. Plasma concentrations of voriconazole in falcons. *Vet Rec* 2007;161:265-268.
717. Schnellbacher R, Beaufrère H, Arnold RD, et al. Pharmacokinetics of levetiracetam in healthy Hispaniolan Amazon parrots (*Amazona ventralis*) after oral administration of a single dose. *J Avian Med Surg* 2014;28(3):193-200.
718. Schnellbacher RW, da Cunha AF, Beaufrère H, et al. Effects of dopamine and dobutamine on isoflurane-induced hypotension in Hispaniolan Amazon parrots (*Amazona ventralis*). *Am J Vet Res* 2012;73(7):952-958.
719. Schobert E. Telazol® use in wild and exotic animals. *Vet Med* 1987;(Oct):1080-1088.
720. Schoemaker N, Schottert M, Mesu S, et al. Distribution of nebulized fluorescein-labeled propylene glycol or saline in pigeons. In: *Proc ExoticsCon(San Antonio, TX)*; 2015:3-4.
721. Schroeder EC, Frazier DL, Morris PJ, et al. Pharmacokinetics of ticarcillin and amikacin in blue-fronted Amazon parrots (*Amazona aestiva aestiva*). *J Avian Med Surg* 1997;11: 260-267.
722. Schuetz S, Krautwald-Junghanns ME, Lutz F, et al. Pharmacokinetic and clinical studies of the carbapenem antibiotic, meropenem, in birds. *Proc Annu Conf Assoc Avian Vet* 2001; 183-190.
723. Schumacher J, Citino SB, Hernandez K, et al. Cardiopulmonary and anesthetic effects of propofol in wild turkeys. *Am J Vet Res* 1997;58:1014-1017.

724. Scope A, Filip T, Gabler C, et al. The influence of stress from transport and handling on hematologic and clinical chemistry blood parameters of racing pigeons (*Columba livia domestica*). *Avian Dis* 2002;46:224-229.
725. Scott DE. Successful treatment of aspergillosis with voriconazole in a red-tailed hawk (*Buteo jamaicensis*). *Proc Annu Conf Assoc Avian Vet* 2011;53-57.
726. Sedacca CD, Campbell TW, Bright JM, et al. Chronic cor pulmonale secondary to pulmonary atherosclerosis in an African grey parrot. *J Am Vet Med Assoc* 2009;234(8):1055-1059.
727. Seibels B, Lamberski N, Gregory CR, et al. Effective use of tea to limit dietary iron available to starlings (*Sturnus vulgaris*). *J Zoo Wildl Med* 2003;34:314-316.
728. Seibert LM. Animal behavior case of the month. A cockatiel was examined because of repetitive chewing of the third digit of the right foot. *J Am Vet Med Assoc* 2004;224(9):1433-1435.
729. Seibert LM, Tobias K, Sequin B. Understanding behavior: husbandry considerations for better behavioral health in psittacine species. *Compend Contin Educ Vet* 2007;29:303-306.
730. Seibert LM, Crowell-Davis SL, Wilson GH, et al. Placebo-controlled clomipramine trial for the treatment of feather picking disorder in cockatoos. *J Am Anim Hosp Assoc* 2004;40:261-269.
731. Sellers C. *Personal communication;* 2003.
732. Seok SH, Jeong DH, Hong IH, et al. Cardiorespiratory dose-response relationship of isoflurane in cinereous vulture (*Aegypius monachus*) during spontaneous ventilation. *J Vet Med Sci* 2017;79(1):160-165.
733. Sharma AK, Saini M, Singh SD, et al. Diclofenac is toxic to the Steppe eagle (*Aquila nipalensis*): widening the diversity of raptors threatened by NSAID misuse in South Asia. *Bird Conserv Intl* 2014;24:282-286.
734. Shaver SL, Robinson NG, Wright BD, et al. A multimodal approach to management of suspected neuropathic pain in a prairie falcon (*Falco mexicanus*). *J Avian Med Surg* 2009;23:209-213.
735. Shlosberg A. Treatment of monocrotophos-poisoned birds of prey with pralidoxime iodide. *J Am Vet Med Assoc* 1976;169(9):989-990.
736. Shlosberg A, Egyed MN, Eilat A, et al. Efficacy of pralidoxime iodide and obidoxime dichloride as antidotes in diazinon-poisoned goslings. *Avian Dis* 1976;20(1):162-166.
737. Sibley DA. *The Sibley Guide to Birds.* New York: Knopf; 2000.
738. Siddalls M, Currier TA, Pang J, et al. Infestation of research zebra finch colony with 2 novel mite species. *Comp Med* 2015;65:51-53.
739. Siegal-Willot JL, Carpenter JW, Glaser AL. Lack of detectable antibody response in greater flamingos (*Phoeniopterus ruber ruber*) after vaccination against West Nile virus with a killed equine vaccine. *J Avian Med Surg* 2006;20:89-93.
740. Silveira LF, Hofling E, Moro MEG, et al. Order Tinamiformes (tinamous). In: Fowler ME, Cubas ZS, eds. *Biology, Medicine, and Surgery of South American Wild Animals.* Ames: Iowa State University Press; 2001:72-80.
741. Simone-Freilicher E. Use of isoxsuprine for treatment of clinical signs associated with presumptive atherosclerosis in a yellow-naped Amazon parrot (*Amazona ochrocephala auropalliata*). *J Avian Med Surg* 2007;21:215-219.
742. Simone-Freilicher E. Recurrent smoke-induced respiratory infections in a ruby blue-headed pionus parrot (*Pionus menstruus rubrigularis*). *J Avian Med Surg* 2008;22(2):138-145.
743. Simpson BS, Papich MG. Pharmacologic management in veterinary behavioral medicine. *Vet Clin North Am Small Anim Pract* 2003;33:365-404.
744. Sinclair KM, Church ME, Farver TB, et al. Effects of meloxicam on hematologic and plasma biochemical analysis variables and results of histologic examination of tissue specimens of Japanese quail (*Coturnix japonica*). *Am J Vet Res* 2012;73:1720-1727.
745. Siperstein LJ. Use of neurontin (gabapentin) to treat leg twitching/foot mutilation in a Senegal parrot. *Proc Annu Conf Assoc Avian Vet/Assoc Exot Mam Vet* 2007;335.
746. Sladky KK, Krugner-Higby L, Meek-Walker E, et al. Serum concentrations and analgesic effects of liposome-encapsulated and standard butorphanol tartrate in parrots. *Am J Vet Res* 2006;67:775-781.

747. Smith JA. Passeriformes (songbirds, perching birds). In: Miller RE, Fowler ME, eds. *Fowler's Zoo and Wildlife Medicine*. Vol 8. St. Louis: Elsevier; 2015:236-246
748. Smith JA, Tully TN, Cornick JL. Determination of isoflurane minimum anesthetic concentration in emus. *Proc Annu Conf Assoc Avian Vet* 1997;181-182.
749. Smith SA. Diagnosis and treatment of helminths in birds of prey. In: Redig PT, Cooper JE, Remple JD, et al., eds. *Raptor Biomedicine*. Minneapolis: University of Minnesota Press; 1993:21-27.
750. Smith SA. Parasites of birds of prey: their diagnosis and treatment. *Semin Avian Exot Pet Med* 1996;5:97-105.
751. Snowden K, Phalen DN. *Encephalitozoon* infection in birds. *Semin Avian Exot Pet Med*. 2004;13:94-99.
752. Snyder SB, Richard MJ. Treatment of avian tuberculosis in a whooping crane (*Grus americana*). *Proc Annu Conf Am Assoc Zoo Vet* 1994;167-170.
753. Soenens J, Vermeersch H, Baert K, et al. Pharmacokinetics and efficacy of amoxycillin in the treatment of an experimental *Streptococcus bovis* infection in racing pigeons (*Columba livia*). *Vet J* 1998;156:59-65.
754. Souza M, Wall J, Stuckey A, et al. Static and dynamic (18) FDG-PET in normal Hispaniolan Amazon parrots (*Amazona ventralis*). *Vet Radiol Ultrasound* 2011;52(3):340-344.
755a. Souza MJ, Cox SK. Tramadol use in zoological medicine. *Vet Clin North Am Exot Anim Pract* 2011;14:117-130.
755b. Souza MJ, Gerhardt L, Cox S. Pharmacokinetics of repeated oral administration of tramadol hydrochloride in Hispaniolan Amazon parrots (*Amazona ventralis*). *Am J Vet Res* 2013;74(7): 957-962.
756. Souza MJ, Martin-Jimenez T, Jones MP, et al. Pharmacokinetics of intravenous and oral tramadol in the bald eagle (*Haliaeetus leucocephalus*). *J Avian Med Surg* 2009;23:247-252.
757. Souza MJ, Martin-Jimenez T, Jones MP, et al. Pharmacokinetics of oral tramadol in red-tailed hawks (*Buteo jamaicensis*). *J Vet Pharmacol Ther* 2010;34:86-88.
758. Sreter T, Szell Z, Varga I. Anticryptosporidial prophylactic efficacy of enrofloxacin and paromomycin in chickens. *J Parasitol* 2002;88:209-211.
759. Stadler C, Carpenter JW. Parasites of backyard game birds. *Semin Avian Exot Pet Med* 1996;5:85-96.
760. Stalis IH, Rideout BA, Allen JL, et al. Possible albendazole toxicity in birds. *Proc Joint Conf Am Assoc Zoo Vet/Wildl Dis Assoc/Am Assoc Wildl Vet* 1995;190-191.
761. Stanford M. Use of Doxirobe Gel®. *Exot DVM* 2002;4:11.
762. Stanford M. Interferon treatment of circovirus infection in grey parrots (*Psittacus erithacus*). *Vet Rec* 2004;154:435-436.
763. Stanford M. Significance of cholesterol assays in the investigation of hepatic lipidosis and atherosclerosis in psittacine birds. *Exot DVM* 2005;7(3):28-34.
764. Stanford M. Clinical pathology of hypocalcaemia in adult grey parrots (*Psittacus erithacus*). *Vet Rec* 2007;161:456-457.
765. Starkey SR, Morrisey JK, Hickam JD, et al. Extrapyramidal side effects in a blue and gold macaw (*Ara ararauna*) treated with haloperidol and clomipramine. *J Avian Med Surg* 2008;22:234-239.
766. Starkey SR, Wood C, de Matos R, et al. Central diabetes insipidus in an African grey parrot. *J Am Vet Med Assoc* 2010;237:415-419.
767. Steinhort LA. Avian fluid therapy. *J Avian Med Surg* 1999;13:83-91.
768. Steinhort LA. Diagnosis and treatment of common diseases of finches. In: Bongaura JD, ed. *Kirk's Current Veterinary Therapy XIII*. Philadelphia: WB Saunders Co; 2000:1119-1123.
769. Stetter MD, Sheppard C, Cook RA. Itraconazole-impregnated synthetic grit for sustained release dosing in avian species. *Proc Annu Conf Am Assoc Zoo Vet* 1996;181-185.
770. Stewart JS. IME—restraint and anesthesia of ratites. *J Assoc Avian Vet* 1990;4:90.
771. Stiles J, Buyukmihci NC, Farver TB. Tonometry of normal eyes in raptors. *Am J Vet Res* 1994;55:477-479.

772. Stone EG. Preliminary evaluation of hetastarch for the management of hypoproteinemia and hypovolemia. *Proc Annu Conf Assoc Avian Vet* 1994;197-199.
773. Storey ES, Carboni DA, Kearney MT, et al. Use of phenol red thread tests to evaluate tear production in clinically normal Amazon parrots and comparison with Schirmer tear test findings. *J Am Vet Med Assoc* 2009;235:1181-1187.
774. Straub J, Zenker I. First experience with hormonal treatment of sertoli cell tumors in budgerigars (*Melopsittacus undulatus*) with absorbable, extended-release GnRH chips (Suprelorelin®). In: *Proc 1st Intl Conf Avian Herpetol Exot Mam Med*; 2013:299-300.
775. Straub J, Forbes NA, Pees M, et al. Pulsed-wave Doppler-derived velocity of diastolic ventricular inflow and systolic aortic outflow in raptors. *Vet Rec* 2004;154:145-147.
776. Straub J, Pees M, Enders F, et al. Pericardiocentesis and the use of enalapril in a Fischer's lovebird (*Agapornis fischeri*). *Vet Rec* 2003;152:24-26.
777. Stringer EM, De Voe RS, Loomis MR. Suspected anaphylaxis to leuprolide acetate depot in two elf owls (*Micrathene whitneyi*). *J Zoo Wildl Med* 2011;42:166-168.
778. Stunkard JA. *Diagnostics, Treatment and Husbandry of Pet Birds*. Edgewater, MD: Stunkard Publ Co; 1984.
779. Suarez DL. Appetite stimulation in raptors. In: Redig PT, Cooper JE, Remple DJ, et al., eds. *Raptor Biomedicine*. Minneapolis: University of Minnesota Press; 1993:225-228.
780. Suedmeyer W, Henry C, McCaw D, Boucher M. Attempted photodynamic therapy against patagial squamous cell carcinoma in an African rose-ringed parakeet (*Psittacula kremeri*). *J Zoo Wildl Med* 2007;38(4):597-600.
781. Suedmeyer WK. IME—use of Adequan in articular diseases of avian species. *J Assoc Avian Vet* 1993;7:105.
782. Suedmeyer WK, Haynes N, Roberts D. Clinical management of endoventricular mycoses in a group of African finches. *Proc Annu Conf Assoc Avian Vet* 1997;225-227.
783. Suedmeyer WK, McCaw D, Turnquist S. Attempted photodynamic therapy of squamous cell carcinoma in the casque of a great hornbill (*Buceros bicornis*). *J Avian Med Surg* 2001;15(1):44-49.
784. Summa NM, Sanchez-Migallon Guzman D, Wils-Plotz EL, et al. Evaluation of the effects of a 4.7-mg deslorelin acetate implant on egg laying in cockatiels (*Nymphicus hollandicus*). *Am J Vet Res* 2017;78:745-751.
785. Summa NM, Sanchez-Migallon Guzman D, Larrat S, et al. Evaluation of high dosages of oral meloxicam in American kestrels (*Falco sparverius*). *J Avian Med Surg* 2017;31(2):108-116.
786. Swan GE, Cuthbert R, Quevedo M, et al. Toxicity of diclofenac to *Gyps* vultures. *Biol Lett* 2006;2:279-282.
787. Swarup D, Patra RC, Prakash V, et al. Safety of meloxicam to critically endangered *Gyps* vultures and other scavenging birds in India. *Anim Cons* 2007;10:192-198.
788a. Swinnerton KJ, Greenwood AG, Chapman RE, et al. The incidence of the parasitic disease trichomoniasis and its treatment in reintroduced and wild pink pigeons *Columba mayeri*. *Ibis* 2005;147:772-782.
788b. Swisher SD, Phillips KL, Tobias JR, et al. External beam radiation therapy of squamous cell carcinoma in the beak of an African grey parrot (*Psittacus timneh*). *J Avian Med Surg* 2016;30:250-256.
789. Sykes IV J. Piciformes (honeyguides, barbets, woodpeckers, toucans). In: Miller RE, Fowler ME, eds. *Fowler's Zoo and Wild Animal Medicine*. Vol 8. St. Louis, MO: Elsevier; 2015:230-235.
790. Tarello W. Serratospiculosis in falcons from Kuwait: incidence, pathogenicity and treatment with melarsomine and ivermectin. *Parasite* 2006;13:59-63.
791. Tarello W. Clinical signs and response to primaquine in falcons with *Haemoproteus tinnunculi* infection. *Vet Rec* 2007;161:204-206.
792. Tarello W. Efficacy of ivermectin (Ivomec) against intestinal capillariosis in falcons. *Parasite* 2008;15:171-174.

793. Tavernier P, Saggese M, Van Wettere A, et al. Malaria in an eastern screech owl (*Megascops asio*). *Avian Dis* 2005;9:433-435.
794. Teare JA, Schwark WS, Shin SJ, et al. Pharmacokinetics of a long-acting oxytetracycline preparation in ring-necked pheasants, great horned owls and Amazon parrots. *Am J Vet Res* 1985;46:2639-2643.
795. Tell L, Harrenstien L, Wetzlich S, et al. Pharmacokinetics of ceftiofur sodium in exotic and domestic avian species. *J Vet Pharmacol Therap* 1998;21:85-91.
796. Tell LA, Stephens K, Teague SV, Pinkerton KE, Raabe OG. Study of nebulization delivery of aerosolized fluorescent microspheres to the avian respiratory tract. *Avian Dis* 2012; 56(2):381-386.
797. Tengelsen LA, Bowen RA, Royals MA, et al. Response to and efficacy of vaccination against eastern equine encephalomyelitis virus in emus. *J Am Vet Med Assoc* 2001;218:1469-1473.
798. Ter Beest J, McClean M, Cushing A, et al. Efficacy of thiofentanil-dexmedetomidine-Telazol for greater rhea (*Rhea americana*) immobilizations. *Proc Joint Conf Am Assoc Zoo Vet/Am Assoc Wildl Vet* 2010;202.
799. Ter Beest J, McClean M, Cushing A, et al. Thiofentanil-dexmedetomidine-telazol anesthesia in greater rheas (*Rhea americana*). *J Zoo Wildl Med* 2012;43:802-807.
800. Todisco G, Paoletti B, Giammarino A, et al. Comparing therapeutic efficacy between ivermectin, selamectin, and moxidectin in canaries during natural infection with *Dermanyssus gallinae*. *Ann N Y Acad Sci* 2008;1149:365-367.
801. Tschopp R, Bailey T, Di Somma A, et al. Urinalysis as a noninvasive health screening procedure in Falconidae. *J Avian Med Surg* 2007;21:8-12.
802. Tseng FS. Considerations in care for birds affected by oil spills. *Semin Avian Exot Pet Med* 1999;8:21-31.
803. Tsourvakas S, Alexandropoulos C, Karatzios C, et al. Elution of ciprofloxacin from acrylic bone cement and fibrin clot: an *in vitro* study. *Acta Orthop Belg* 2009;75(4):537-542.
804. Tudor DC. *Pigeon Health and Disease*. Ames: Iowa State University Press; 1991.
805. Tully T, Shane S, Kearney M. Evaluation of two *Lactobacillus acidophilus* formulations as dietary supplements in neonatal cockatiels (*Nymphicus hollandicus*). *J Avian Med Surg* 1998;12 (1):25-29.
806. Tully TN. Therapeutics. In: Tully TN, Shane SM, eds. *Ratite Management, Medicine, and Surgery*. Malabar, FL: Krieger Publishing Co; 1996:155-163.
807. Tully TN. Formulary. In: Altman RB, Clubb SL, Dorrestein GM, et al. *Avian Medicine and Surgery*. Philadelphia: WB Saunders Co; 1997:671-688.
808. Tully TN. Psittacine therapeutics. *Vet Clin North Am Exot Anim Pract* 2000;3:59-90.
809. Tully TN. *Personal communication*. 2003.
810. Tully Jr TN. Birds. In: Mitchell MA, Tully Jr TN, eds. *Manual of Exotic Pet Practice*. St. Louis: Saunders/Elsevier; 2009:250-298.
811. Ueblacker SN. Trichomoniasis in American kestrels (*Falco sparverius*) and Eastern screech-owls (*Otus asio*). In: Lumeij JT, Remple JD, Redig PT, et al. *Raptor Biomedicine III*. Lake Worth, FL: Zoological Education Network; 2000:59-63.
812. Uzun M, Onder F, Atalan G, et al. Effects of xylazine, medetomidine, detomidine, and diazepam on sedation, heart and respiratory rates, and cloacal temperature in rock partridges (*Alectoris graeca*). *J Zoo Wildl Med* 2006;37:135-140.
813. Vaden SL, Cullen JM, Riviere JE. Pharmacokinetics of cyclosporine in woodchucks and Pekin ducks. *J Vet Pharmacol Ther* 1995;18(1):30-33.
814. Valverde A, Honeyman VL, Dyson DH, et al. Determination of a sedative dose and influence of midazolam on cardiopulmonary function in Canada geese. *Am J Vet Res* 1990;51:1071-1074.
815. Van Alstine WG, Dyer DC. Antibiotic aerosolization: tissue and plasma oxytetracycline concentrations in turkey poults. *Avian Dis* 1985;29:430-436.
816. Van Cutsem J. Antifungal activity of enilconazole on experimental aspergillosis in chickens. *Avian Dis* 1983;27(1):36-42.

817. van Zeeland Y, Bastiaansen P, Kooistra H, Schoemaker N. Diagnosis and treatment of Cushing's syndrome in a senegal parrot. In: *Proc Exot Conf* (San Antonio, TX); 2015:119.
818. van Zeeland Y, Friedman S, Bergman L. Behavior. In: Speer B, ed. *Current Therapy in Avian Medicine and Surgery*. St. Louis, MO: Elsevier; 2016:177-251.
819. van Zeeland Y, Schoemaker N, Lumeij J. Syncopes associated with second degree atrioventricular block in a cockatoo. *Proc Annu Conf Assoc Avian Vet* 2010;345-346.
820. van Zeeland YRA, Schoemaker NJ, Haritova A, et al. Pharmacokinetics of paroxetine, a selective serotonin reuptake inhibitor, in grey parrots (*Psittacus erithacus erithacus*): influence of pharmaceutical formulation and length of dosing. *J Vet Pharmacol Ther* 2013; 36(1):51-58.
821. VanDerHeyden N. Update on avian mycobacteriosis. *Proc Annu Conf Assoc Avian Vet* 1994;53-61.
822. VanDerHeyden N. New strategies in the treatment of avian mycobacteriosis. *Semin Avian Exot Pet Med* 1997;6:25-33.
823. Vanhaecke E, De Backer P, Remon JP, et al. Pharmacokinetics and bioavailability of erythromycin in pigeons (*Columba livia*). *J Vet Pharmacol Ther* 1990;13:356-360.
824. Van Heerden J, Keffen R. Preliminary investigation into the immobilizing of ostriches. *J South Afr Vet Assoc* 1991;62:114-117.
825. Van Sant F, Stewart GR. Ponazuril used as a treatment for suspected *Cryptosporidium* infection in 2 hybrid falcons. *Proc Annu Conf Assoc Avian Vet* 2009;368-371.
826. Vanstreels RE, Kolesnikovas CK, Sandri S, et al. Outbreak of avian malaria associated to multiple species of *Plasmodium* in magellanic penguins undergoing rehabilitation in southern Brazil. *PLoS One* 2014;9.
827a. Vercruysse J. Efficacy of toltrazuril and clazuril against experimental infections with *Eimeria labbeana* and *E. columbarum* in racing pigeons. *Avian Dis* 1990;34:73-79.
827b. Vergneau-Grosset C, Polley T, Holt DC, et al. Hematologic, plasma biochemical, and lipid panel reference intervals in orange-winged Amazon parrots (*Amazona amazonica*). *J Avian Med Surg* 2016;30:335-344.
828. Verwoerd D. Aerosol use of a novel disinfectant as part of an integrated approach to preventing and treating aspergillosis in falcons in the UAE. *Falco* 2002;17:15-18.
829. Vesal N, Eskandari MH. Sedative effects of midazolam and xylazine with or without ketamine and detomidine alone following intranasal administration in ring-necked parakeets. *J Am Vet Med Assoc* 2006;228:383-388.
830. Vesal N, Zare P. Clinical evaluation of intranasal benzodiazepines, alpha-agonists and their antagonists in canaries. *Vet Anaesth Analg* 2006;33:143-148.
831. Villaverde-Morcillo S, Benito J, Garcia-Sanchez R, et al. Comparison of isoflurane and alfaxalone (Alfaxan) for the induction of anesthesia in flamingos (*Phoenicopterus roseus*) undergoing orthopedic surgery. *J Zoo Wildl Med* 2014;45:361-366.
832. Viner TC, Hamlin BC, McClure PJ, Yates BC. Integrating the forensic sciences in wildlife case investigations: a case report of pentobarbital and phenytoin toxicosis in a bald eagle (*Haliaeeetus leucocephalus*). *Vet Pathol* 2016;53(5):1103-1106.
833. Vink-Nooteboom M, Lumeij JT, Wolvekamp WT. Radiography and image-intensified fluoroscopy of barium passage through the gastrointestinal tract in six healthy Amazon parrots (*Amazona aestiva*). *Vet Radiol Ultrasound* 2003;44:43-48.
834. Visser M, Boothe D. Population pharmacokinetics of levetiracetam and zonisamide in the African grey parrot (*Psittacus erithacus*). In: *Proc Exot Conf (San Antonio, TX)*; 2015:7-10.
835. Visser M, Ragsdale MM, Boothe DM. Pharmacokinetics of amitriptyline HCl and its metabolites in healthy African grey parrots (*Psittacus erithacus*) and cockatoos (*Cacatua species*). *J Avian Med Surg* 2015;29(4):275-281.
836. Vriends MM. *Simon & Schuster's Guide to Pet Birds*. New York: Simon & Schuster; 1984.
837. Wagner CH, Hochleitner M, Rausch W-D. Ketoconazole plasma levels in buzzards. *Proc First Conf Euro Comm Assoc Avian Vet* 1991;333-340.

838. Wallace RS. Spheniciformes (penguins). In: Miller RE, Fowler ME, eds. *Fowler's Zoo and Wild Animal Medicine*. Vol 8. St. Louis, MO: Elsevier; 2015:82-88.
839. Wallace RS. Spheniciformes (penguins). In: Miller RE, Fowler ME, eds. *Fowler's Zoo and Wild Animal Medicine*. Vol 8. St. Louis, MO: Elsevier; 2015:82-88.
840. Weber MA, Terrell SP, Neiffer DL, et al. Bone marrow hypoplasia and intestinal crypt cell necrosis associated with fenbendazole administration in five painted storks. *J Am Vet Med Assoc* 2002;221:417-419.
841. Wellehan J. Frostbite in birds: pathophysiology and treatment. *Comp Contin Educ Pract Vet* 2003;25(10):776-781.
842. Wellehan JFX, Zens MS, Calsamiglia M, et al. Diagnosis and treatment of conjunctivitis in house finches associated with mycoplasmosis in Minnesota. *J Wildl Dis* 2001;37(2):245-251.
843. Welsh RD, Nieman RW, Vanhooser SL, et al. Bacterial infections in ratites. *Vet Med* 1997;92:992-998.
844. Westerhof I, Pellicaan C. Effects of different application routes of glucocorticoids on the pituitary-adrenocortical axis in pigeons (*Columba livia domestica*). *J Avian Med Surg* 1995;9(3):175-181.
845. Weston HS. The successful treatment of sarcocystosis in two keas (*Nestor nobilis*) at the Franklin Park Zoo. *Proc Annu Conf Am Assoc Zoo Vet* 1996;186-191.
846. Wheler C. Avian anesthetics, analgesics, tranquilizers. *Semin Avian Exot Pet Med* 1993;2:7-12.
847. Whitehead MC, Hoppes SM, Perkins PL, et al. The use of alfaxalone in Quaker parrots (*Myiopsitta monachus*). *Proc Annu Conf Assoc Avian Vet ExoticsCon* 2016;55.
848. Whiteside DP, Barker IK, Conlon PD, et al. Pharmacokinetic disposition of the oral iron chelator deferiprone in the domestic pigeon (*Columba livia*). *J Avian Med Surg* 2007;21(2):121-129.
849. Whiteside DP, Barker IK, Mehren KG, et al. Clinical evaluation of the oral iron chelator deferiprone for the potential treatment of iron overload in bird species. *J Zoo Wildl Med* 2004;35(1):40-49.
850. Wickstrom ML. Antiseptics and disinfectants. *The Merck Veterinary Manual* 2015; Available at: www.merckvetmanual.com/pharmacology/antiseptics-and-disinfectants. Accessed Dec 1, 2016.
851. Willette M, Ponder J, Cruz-Martinez L, et al. Management of select bacterial and parasitic conditions of raptors. *Vet Clin North Am Exot Anim Pract* 2009;12:491-517.
852. Williams DL, Cooper JE. Horner's syndrome in an African spotted eagle owl (*Bubo africanus*). *Vet Rec* 1994;134(3):64-66.
853. Williams M, Smith PJ, Loerzel SM, et al. Evaluation of the efficacy of vecuronium bromide as a mydriatic in several different species of aquatic birds. *Proc Annu Conf Assoc Avian Vet* 1996;113-117.
854. Williams SM, Fulton RM, Render JA, et al. Ocular and encephalic toxoplasmosis in canaries. *Avian Dis* 2001;45:262-267.
855. Wills S, Pinard C, Nykamp S, et al. Ophthalmic reference values and lesions in two captive populations of northern owls: great grey owls (*Strix nebulosa*) and snowy owls (*Bubo scandiacus*). *J Zoo Wildl Med* 2016;47:244-255.
856. Wilson GH, Greenacre CB, Howerth EW, et al. Ascaridosis in a group of psittacine birds. *J Avian Med Surg* 1999;13:32-39.
857. Wilson GH, Hernandez-Divers S, Budsberg SC, et al. Pharmacokinetics and use of meloxicam in psittacine birds. *Proc Annu Conf Assoc Avian Vet* 2004;7-9.
858. Wilson RC, Zenoble RD, Horton Jr CR, et al. Single dose digoxin pharmacokinetics in the Quaker conure (*Myiopsitta monachus*). *J Zoo Wildl Med* 1989;20:432-434.
859. Wismer T. Advancements in diagnosis and management of toxicologic problems. In: Speer B, ed. *Current Therapy in Avian Medicine and Surgery*. St. Louis, MO: Elsevier; 2016:589-599.
860. Wlaź P, Knaga S, Kasperek K, et al. Activity and safety of inhaled itraconazole nanosuspension in a model pulmonary *Aspergillus fumigatus* infection in inoculated young quails. *Mycopathologia* 2015;180(1-2):35-42.

861. Woods LW, Higgins RJ, Joseph VJ, et al. Ronidazole toxicosis in 3 society finches (*Lonchura striata*). *Vet Pathol* 2010;47:231-235.
862. Woolcock PR. Duck hepatitis virus type I: studies with inactivated vaccines in breeder ducks. *Avian Pathol* 1991;20:509-522.
863. Yadav S, Srivastav AK. Influence of calcitonin administration on ultimobranchial and parathyroid glands of pigeon, *Columba livia*. *Microsc Res Tech* 2009;72:380-384.
864. Yaw TJ, Zaffarano BA, Gall A, et al. Pharmacokinetic properties of a single administration of oral gabapentin in the great horned owl (*Bubo virginianus*). *J Zoo Wildl Med* 2015;46(3):547-552.
865. Zantop D. Medetomidine in birds. *Exot DVM* 1999;1:34.
866. Zantop DW. Treatment of bile duct carcinoma in birds with carboplatin. *Exot DVM* 2000;2:76-78.
867. Zantop DW. Using leuprolide acetate to manage common avian reproductive problems. *Exot DVM* 2000;2:70.
868. Zehnder A, Graham J, Reavill D, McLaughlin A. Neoplastic diseases in avian species. In: Speer B, ed. *Current Therapy in Avian Medicine and Surgery*. St. Louis, MO: Elsevier; 2016:107-141.
869. Zehnder AM, Hawkins MG, Pascoe PJ, et al. Evaluation of indirect blood pressure monitoring in awake and anesthetized red-tailed hawks (*Buteo jamaicensis*): effects of cuff size, cuff placement, and monitoring equipment. *Vet Anaesth Analg* 2009;36:464-479.
870. Zenker W, Janovsky M, Kurzwell J, et al. Immobilisation of the Eurasian buzzard (*Buteo buteo*) with oral tiletamine/zolazepam. In: Lumeij JT, Remple JD, Redig PT, et al., eds. *Raptor Biomedicine III*. Lake Worth, FL: Zoological Education Network; 2002:295-300.
871. Zenoble RD, Kempppainen RJ, Young DW, et al. Endocrine responses of healthy parrots to ACTH and thyroid stimulating hormone. *J Am Vet Med Assoc* 1985;187:1116-1118.
872. Zoller G, Chassang L, Loos P, et al. Evaluation of dexmedetomidine-alfaxalone-butorphanol and dexmedetomidine-ketamine-butorphanol anesthesia in domestic doves (*Streptotelia risoria*). *Proc Annu Assoc Avian Vet ExoticsCon* 2016;49.
873. Zollinger TJ, Gamble KC, Alvarado TP, et al. Rhabdomyolysis, steatitis, and coagulopathy in East African white pelicans (*Pelecanus onocrotalus*) and pink-backed pelicans (*Pelecanus rufescens*). *Proc Annu Conf Am Assoc Zoo Vet* 2002;111-113.
874. Zollinger TJ, Hoover JP, Payton ME, et al. Clinicopathologic, gross necropsy, and histologic findings after intramuscular injection of carprofen in a pigeon (*Columba livia*) model. *J Avian Med Surg* 2011;25:173-184.
875. Zordan MA, Papich MG, Pich AA, et al. Population pharmacokinetics of a single dose of meloxicam after oral and intramuscular administration to captive lesser flamingos (*Phoeniconaias minor*). *Am J Vet Res* 2016;77:1311-1318.
876. Zuba JR, Singleton C, Papendick R. Avian chlamydiosis and doxycycline toxicity in a flock of free-contact rainbow lorikeets (*Trichoglossus haematodus haematodus*): considerations, concerns, and quandaries. *Proc Annu Conf Am Assoc Zoo Vet* 2002;105-107.
877. Zwijnenberg RJG, Vulto AG, Van Miert AS, et al. Evaluation of antibiotics for racing pigeons (*Columba livia* var. *domestica*) available in the Netherlands. *J Vet Pharmacol Therap* 1992;15:364-378.

Chapter 6 Backyard Poultry and Waterfowl

Cheryl B. Greenacre | G. Lynne Luna | Teresa Y. Morishita

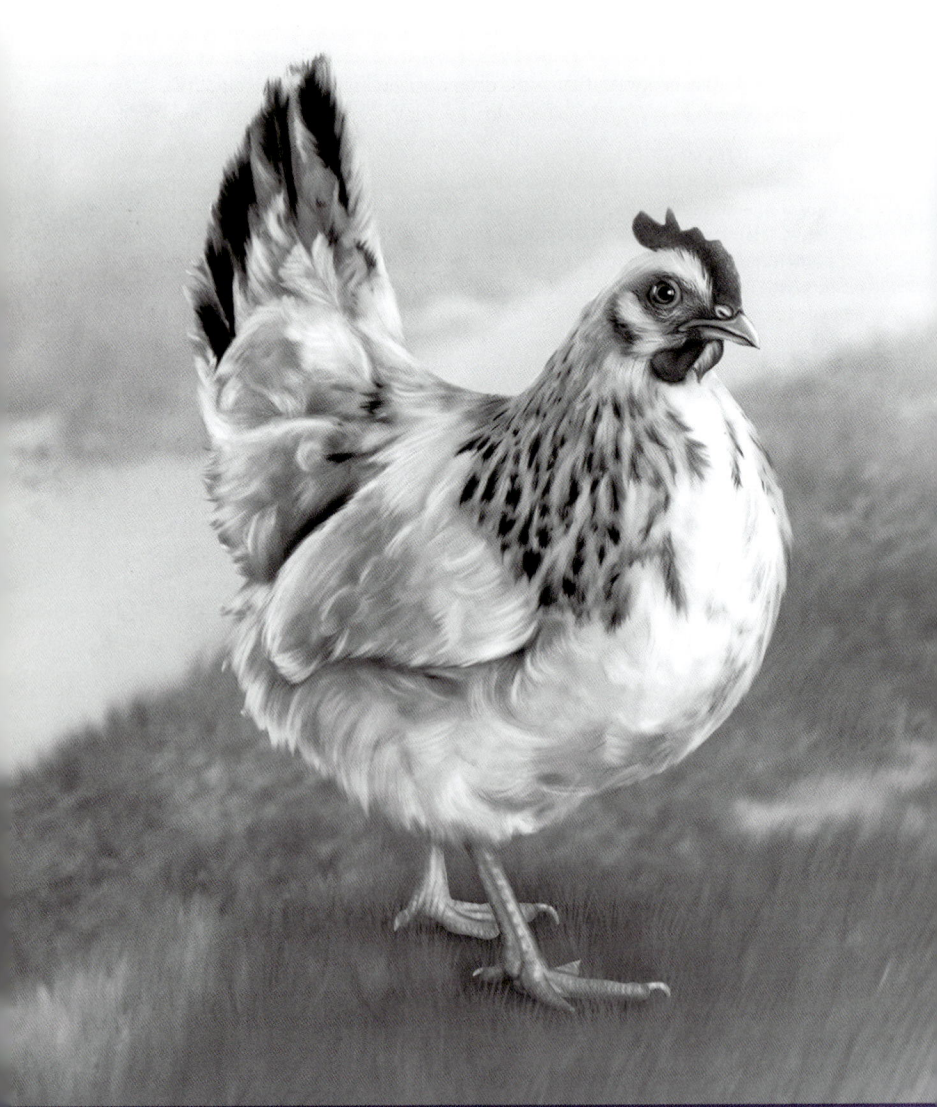

Note: Many poultry species are considered food-producing animal *species,* and as such, these species are regulated by the U.S. Food and Drug Administration (FDA).[166] Even if the individual animal of any of these species is never used for food, it is still regulated by the FDA. The FDA prohibits the use of certain drugs, with no allowable extra-label drug use, in any food-producing animal species. These prohibited drugs are clearly identified in the tables, and the doses are provided in case they are needed for a similar but non-food-producing animal species (e.g., Attwater's prairie chicken), and listings should in no way be misconstrued as an endorsement of using FDA-prohibited drugs in any food-producing animal species. Please refer to the appropriate tables at the end of this chapter regarding the definitions of prohibited drugs, extra-label drugs, labeled drugs, and drugs needing a Veterinary Feed Directive prior to choosing a drug and dose. Please refer to the Food Animal Residue Avoidance Databank at www.farad.org and other sources listed in Table 6.25 for meat and egg withdrawal times. Please be aware that most drug dosages are listed in standard international units (SI), such as mg/kg, but some dosages may be in conventional units, such as mg/lb, mg/gallon, or grams/ton to match the dose on the label.

TABLE 6-1 Antimicrobial Agents Used in Backyard Poultry and Waterfowl.[a–c]

Agent	Dosage	Species/Comments
Amikacin	10 mg/kg SC, IM q8h × 14 days[85]	Ring-necked pheasants/PD; renal toxicosis appeared at 11 days; uric acid levels abnormal up to 7 days after cessation
	20 mg/kg IM q8h[45]	Chickens/PD
	5.3 mg/kg IV RLP once[137b]	Chickens/pododermatitis; regional limb perfusion (RLP) into medial metatarsal vein with a tourniquet placed proximal to hock joint for 15 min[137b]
Amoxicillin/clavulanate (Clavamox, Zoetis)	125 mg/kg PO q8h[173]	Poultry
	500 mg/L drinking water[179]	Chickens/PD
Amoxicillin trihydrate	15 mg/kg/day PO × 3 days[48]	Chickens, turkeys
	20 mg/kg PO[92]	Chickens, turkeys/no frequency listed
	15 mg/kg body weight in drinking water × 3-5 days[123]	Chickens not laying eggs for human consumption[123]
	15-20 mg/kg body weight in drinking water × 3-5 days[123]	Turkeys not laying eggs for human consumption[123]
	20 mg/kg body weight in drinking water × 3 consecutive days[123]	Ducks not laying eggs for human consumption[123]
	330 mg/L drinking water, provide on alternate days × 3 treatments[27]	Waterfowl
	1 g/3 L of drinking water, provide on alternate days × 3 treatments[16]	Waterfowl

Continued

TABLE 6-1 Antimicrobial Agents Used in Backyard Poultry and Waterfowl. (cont'd)

Agent	Dosage	Species/Comments
Ampicillin trihydrate	55-110 mg/kg IM q8-12h[69]	Poultry
	170 mg/L drinking water[16,69]	Game birds
	250 mg/8 oz of drinking water[16]	Galliformes
	1000 mg/L drinking water[16,69]	Galliformes/flock use
Apramycin (Apralan, Elanco)	—	Therapeutic levels not achieved in Japanese quail at 50 mg/kg IV;[87] not available in the United States
	250-500 mg/L drinking water[16,69]	Game birds, poultry/primarily used against *Salmonella* spp.
Bacitracin methylene disalicylate (Solu-Tracin 200, Solu-Tracin 50, BMD Soluble 50%, Zoetis)	100-400 mg/gal drinking water[30a]	Chickens, turkeys
	220 mg/L[27]	Quail/*Clostridium perfringens*; prepare daily
	400 mg/gal drinking water[30a]	Poultry
	55-220 mg/kg feed[69]	Quail
	4-200 g/ton feed[30a]	Chickens, turkeys
Bacitracin methylene disalicylate (BMD 60, BMD 50 Granular A, BMD 30 Granular A, BMD 30 BMD 50, Zoetis)	4-50 g/ton feed[165]	Pheasant, turkeys (growing)/no use class stated or implied; increased rate of weight gain and improved feed efficiency
	5-20 g/ton feed[165]	Quail (not over 5 wk)/increased rate of weight gain and improved feed efficiency
	10-25 g/ton feed[165]	Chicken/layers, first 7 mo of production; aid in increased egg production and improved feed efficiency; feed continuously as the sole ration for the first 7 mo of egg production
	40-50 g/ton feed[165]	Chickens (broilers, replacements)/increased rate of gain and improved feed efficiency; no limitations[165]
	50 g/ton feed[165]	Prevention of necrotic enteritis; feed as sole ration
	100-200 g/ton feed × 5-7 days[165]	Aid in control of necrotic enteritis; feed as sole ration; start at first signs of disease; vary dose based on severity
	200 g/ton feed[165]	Quail (growing)/prevention of ulcerative enteritis; feed continuously as the sole ration
	200 g/ton feed[165]	Turkeys (growing)/aid in the control of transmissible enteritis

TABLE 6-1 Antimicrobial Agents Used in Backyard Poultry and Waterfowl. (cont'd)

Agent	Dosage	Species/Comments
Bacitracin methylene disalicylate (Pennitracin MD 50G, Zoetis)	4-50 g/ton of feed[165]	Chickens (broiler, replacement), turkeys (growing), pheasants (growing)/administer continuously throughout feeding period for increased rate of weight gain and improved feed efficiency
	5-20 g/ton of feed[165]	Quail (growing)/administer continuously through 5 wk of age for increased rate of weight gain and improved feed efficiency
Bacitracin zinc (Baciferm 10, 25, 50, 40, Zoetis)	4-50 g/ton feed[30a,165]	Chickens, turkeys, pheasants (growing)/for increased rate of weight gain and improved feed efficiency
	5-20 g/ton of feed[165]	Quail (growing)/for increased rate of weight gain and improved feed efficiency; feed to starting quail through 5 wk of age[165]
	10-25 g/ton of feed[165]	Chickens (laying)/for improved feed efficiency and increased egg production
Cefazolin	22-110 mg/kg IM q8-12h[69]	Poultry/restricted drug[b]
Cefovecin (Convenia, Zoetis)	10 mg/kg SC, IM, IV q1h[162a]	Chickens/PK; not recommended for use in birds due to short half-life Poultry/restricted drug[b]
Cefquinome	5 mg/kg IM q24h[178]	Ducks/no effect PO Poultry/restricted drug[b]
Ceftiofur (Naxcel, Zoetis)	0.08-0.2 mg SC once[30a,166]	Chickens (1- to 3-day-old chicks)/as a single SC injection in the neck for the control of early mortality associated with *Escherichia coli* organisms; restricted drug[b]
	0.17-0.5 mg SC once[30a,166]	Turkeys (1- to 3-day-old poults)/as a single SC injection in the neck for the control of early mortality associated with *E. coli* organisms;[165,166] restricted drug[b]
	0.16 mg/chick SC q24h[156]	Chickens (chicks)/PK; treatment of early mortality associated with *E. coli* Poultry/restricted drug[b]
	0.17-0.5 mg/poult SC q24h[156]	Turkeys, poultry/restricted drug[b]
	2-4 mg/kg SC q24h[31]	Ducks, poultry/restricted drug[b]
	2.8-5.8 mg/kg SC q24h[156]	Turkeys (poults)/PK; treatment of early mortality associated with *E. coli* Poultry/restricted drug[b]
	10 mg/kg IM q72h[69]	Guinea fowl/PD Poultry/restricted drug[b]

Continued

TABLE 6-1 Antimicrobial Agents Used in Backyard Poultry and Waterfowl. (cont'd)

Agent	Dosage	Species/Comments
Ceftriaxone	100 mg/kg IM q4h[80]	Chickens/PK; not approved for food animal products in the United States Poultry/restricted drug[b]
Cephalexin	35-50 mg/kg IM q2-3h[69]	Quail, ducks/PD Poultry/restricted drug[b]
	55-110 mg/kg PO q12h[69]	Poultry/*Mycoplasma, Haemophilus;* restricted drug[b]
Cephalothin	100 mg/kg IM q2-3h[16,69]	Quail, ducks/PD; not approved for food animal products in the United States Poultry/restricted drug[b]
Chloramphenicol palmitate (oral suspension)	50 mg/kg PO q6-12h[69]	Galliformes (turkeys), chickens[9] Poultry/restricted drug[c]
Chloramphenicol succinate	22 mg/kg IM, IV q3h[41a]	Ducks/PD Poultry/restricted drug[c]
	50 mg/kg IM q24h[32]	Peafowl Poultry/restricted drug[c]
	50 mg/kg IM, IV q6-12h[32]	Chickens, turkeys, geese (PK), ducks Poultry/restricted drug[c]
	79 mg/kg IM q12h[32]	Turkeys/PK Poultry/restricted drug[c]
Chlortetracycline bisulfate (Aureomycin Soluble Powder, Zoetis)	25 mg/lb body weight in drinking water[166]	Turkeys/control of complicating bacterial organisms associated with bluecomb (transmissible enteritis, coronaviral enteritis); prepare fresh solution daily as a sole source of chlortetracycline; do not slaughter animals for food within 24 hours of treatment; do not use for more than 14 days[166]
	40-120 mg/L drinking water[69]	Galliformes (game birds)
	100-400 mg/gal drinking water[30a]	Turkeys
	100-1000 mg/gal drinking water[30a]	Chickens
	200-400 mg/gal drinking water[166]	Chickens/control of infectious synovitis caused by *Mycoplasma synoviae;* prepare fresh solution daily as sole source of chlortetracycline; do not slaughter animals for food within 24 hr of treatment; do not use for more than 14 days; do not use in laying chickens[166]

TABLE 6-1	Antimicrobial Agents Used in Backyard Poultry and Waterfowl. (cont'd)	
Agent	Dosage	Species/Comments
Chlortetracycline bisulfate (Aureomycin Soluble Powder, Zoetis) (cont'd)	400 mg/gal drinking water[166]	Turkeys (growing)/control of infectious synovitis caused by *Mycoplasma synoviae*; prepare fresh solution daily as sole source of chlortetracycline; do not slaughter animals for food within 24 hr of treatment; do not use for more than 14 days[166]
	400-800 mg/gal drinking water[166]	Chickens/control of chronic respiratory disease (CRD) and air sac infections caused by *Mycoplasma gallisepticum* and *E. coli*; prepare fresh solution daily as sole source of chlortetracycline; do not slaughter animals for food within 24 hr of treatment; do not use for more than 14 days; do not use in laying chickens[166]
	1000 mg/gal drinking water[166]	Chickens/control of mortality due to fowl cholera caused by *Pasteurella multocida*; prepare fresh solution daily as sole source of chlortetracycline; do not slaughter animals for food within 24 hr of treatment; do not use for more than 14 days; do not use in laying chickens[166]
	1000 ppm (18.2 g/kg) in feed for 45 days[16]	Waterfowl
	2500 mg/kg feed[180] and 2500 mg/L drinking water[30a,180]	Chickens, turkeys/PD; simultaneous medication of feed and water required to reach therapeutic level
Chlortetracycline (Aureomycin granular, Zoetis)	25 mg/lb body weight q24h × 7-14 days[165]	Turkeys/control of complicating bacterial organisms associated with bluecomb
	10-50 g/ton of feed[165]	Chickens, turkeys (growing)/increase rate of weight gain, feed efficiency
	100-200 g/ton of feed × 7-14 days[165]	Chickens/control of infectious synovitis caused by *Mycoplasma synoviae*
	200 g/ton of feed × 7-14 days[165]	Turkeys/control of infectious synovitis caused by *Mycoplasma synoviae*
	200-400 g/ton of feed × 7-14 days[165]	Chickens/control of CRD and air sac infection caused by *Mycoplasma gallisepticum* and *E. coli*

Continued

TABLE 6-1 Antimicrobial Agents Used in Backyard Poultry and Waterfowl. (cont'd)

Agent	Dosage	Species/Comments
Chlortetracycline (Aureomycin granular, Zoetis) (cont'd)	200-400 g/ton of feed not more than 21 days[165]	Ducks/control and treatment of fowl cholera caused by *Pasteurella multocida*; feed in complete ration to provide from 16-62 mg/kg of body weight per day depending on age and severity of disease[165]
	400 g/ton of feed × 7-14 days[165]	Turkeys/control of *Hexamita meleagridis* Turkeys (poults not over 4 wk of age)/reduction of mortality due to paratyphoid caused by *Salmonella typhimurium*
	500 g/ton of feed × 5 days[165]	Chickens/reduce mortality due to *E. coli* infections
Chlortetracycline (ChlorMax, Aureomycin granular, Zoetis)	200-600 mg/kg feed[69]	Galliformes
	300-400 mg/kg feed[27]	Waterfowl/colibacillosis, *Chlamydia*, *Salmonella*
	1000 mg/kg feed[69]	Waterfowl
	10-400 g/ton feed[30a]	Turkeys
	10-500 g/ton feed[30a]	Chickens
Ciprofloxacin	2 mg/kg IV[121]	Chicks/no toxic effects observed; prohibited drug[c]
	5 mg/kg/day PO × 5 days[55]	Chickens/PD; prohibited drug[c]
	10-20 mg/kg PO q12h[46]	Chickens/prohibited drug[c]
Clindamycin	100 mg/kg PO q24h × 3-5 days[69]	Quail/*Clostridium*
Danofloxacin mesylate (A180, Zoetis)	5 mg/kg PO, IM, IV[46,152]	Chickens/PD; higher therapeutic efficacy of water medication for enrofloxacin compared to danofloxacin can be expected when given at 5 mg/kg;[84] prohibited drug[c]
	50 mg/L in drinking water × 3 days[113,152]	Chicks/*Mycoplasma*; prohibited drug[c]
Doxycycline (Vibramycin, Zoetis)	8-25 mg/kg PO q12h[27]	Waterfowl
	20 mg/kg/day PO × 3 days[177]	Chickens
	25-50 mg/kg/day PO[173]	Poultry
	35 mg/kg/day PO × 7 days max[173]	Poultry
	50 mg/kg PO q12h × 3-5 days[16,69]	Waterfowl/45 days for chlamydiosis
	100 mg/L drinking water[51]	Chickens/PD
	265-525 mg/L drinking water[69]	Poultry/*Mycoplasma*, *Haemophilus*; can use in combination with tylosin
	250-300 mg/kg seed[69]	Waterfowl

CHAPTER 6 Backyard Poultry and Waterfowl

TABLE 6-1 Antimicrobial Agents Used in Backyard Poultry and Waterfowl. (cont'd)

Agent	Dosage	Species/Comments
Enrofloxacin	—	IM formulation has an extremely alkaline pH and should not be given repeatedly; best to avoid IV use in birds; fluoroquinolones may be used in PMMA beads with success;[43] prohibited drug[c]
	5 mg/kg/day PO × 5 days[55]	Chickens/PD; accumulates in eggs; prohibited drug[c]
	10 mg/kg PO q12h × 4 days[10,12]	Chickens/PK; high efficacy for intestinal salmonellosis; prohibited drug[c]
	10-15 mg/kg PO, IM q12h × 5-7 days[16]	Waterfowl/prohibited drug[c]
	50 mg/kg via nebulization × 4 hr (day 1, AM), then 25 mg/kg × 4 hr/day × 4 days[164]	Muscovy, Pekin ducklings/ *Riemerella* (*Pasteurella*); prohibited drug[c]
	26 mg/L drinking water[27]	Galliformes/prohibited drug[c]
	50 mg/L drinking water[71,81]	Chickens, turkeys/PK; prohibited drug[c]
	50-100 mg/L drinking water[69]	Game birds/prohibited drug[c]
	200-800 mg/L drinking water[69]	Chickens/no detected effect on cartilage in day-old chicks;[69] prohibited drug[c]
Erythromycin	25.5 mg/kg PO q24h × 5 days[111]	Chickens/*Mycoplasma* spp.; do not use in hens laying eggs for human consumption
	55-110 mg/kg PO q12h[69]	Poultry/*Mycoplasma*, *Haemophilus*
	102 mg/L drinking water[42]	Chicks/PD
	92.5-185 g/ton feed[30a]	Chickens, turkeys/do not use high dose level (185 g/ton) in layers
Erythromycin phosphate (Gallimycin, Cross VetPharm Group)	500 mg/gal drinking water × 5-7 days[165]	Chickens (broilers, replacements)/ aid control of chronic respiratory disease (5 days) and aid control of infectious coryza due to *Haemophilus gallinarum;* do not use in replacement pullets over 16 wk of age; do not use in chickens producing eggs for human consumption; solutions older than 3 days should not be used[165]

Continued

TABLE 6-1 Antimicrobial Agents Used in Backyard Poultry and Waterfowl. (cont'd)

Agent	Dosage	Species/Comments
Erythromycin thiocyanate (Gallimycin, Cross VetPharm Group)	25.5 mg/kg PO q24h × 5 days[111]	Chickens/*Mycoplasma* spp.; do not use in hens laying eggs for human consumption
	4.6-18.5 g/ton feed[165]	Chickens/growth promotion and feed efficiency
	9.25-18.5 g/ton of feed[165]	Turkeys (not over 12 wk of age)/ growth promotion and feed efficiency
	18.5 g/ton of feed[165]	Chickens (laying)/aids in increasing egg production; no limitations are included in the CFR for this species when using this product in this amount
	92.5 g/ton feed[165]	Chickens, turkeys/aid in the prevention of chronic respiratory disease during periods of stress (2 days before and 3-6 days after stress); aid in the prevention of infectious coryza (7-14 days); withdraw 24 hr before slaughter
	92.5-185 g/ton feed[30a]	Chickens, turkeys/do not use high dose level (185 g/ton) in layers
	185 g/ton feed × 5-8 days[165]	Chickens, turkeys/aid in the prevention and reduction of lesions and in lowering severity of chronic respiratory disease; do not use in birds producing eggs for food purposes; withdraw 48 hr before slaughter
Furazolidone (NF180, Hess and Clark)	220-440 mg/kg feed[27]	Waterfowl/*Salmonella* Poultry/prohibited drug[c,54,166]
Gentamicin sulfate (Garasol, Intervet)	0.2 mg SC[30a]	Chickens/35-day meat withdrawal time; Turkeys/65-day meat withdrawal time
	5 mg/kg IM q8h[35,69]	Pheasants/PK
	10 mg/kg IM q6h[35,69]	Quail/PK
Lincomycin HCl (Lincocin, Upjohn)	64 mg/gal drinking water[30a]	Chickens
	2 g/L drinking water × 5-7 days[16]	Waterfowl
Lincomycin hydrochloride monohydrate (Lincomix, Zoetis)	2 g/L drinking water × 5-7 days[69]	Waterfowl/*Pasteurella*, *Mycoplasma tenosynovitis*
	2 g/ton feed[30a]	Chickens
	2-4 g/ton of feed[165]	Chickens (broilers)

TABLE 6-1 Antimicrobial Agents Used in Backyard Poultry and Waterfowl. (cont'd)

Agent	Dosage	Species/Comments
Lincomycin/spectinomycin (LS-50 Water Soluble, Upjohn; Linco-Spectin 100 Soluble Powder, Upjohn)	2.5-5 mg/chick IM once[63]	Chickens (chicks)/PD; may prevent *E. coli* and *Staphylococcus aureus* infections; injectable form not available in the United States
	528 mg/L drinking water for first 5 days of life[64]	Turkey poults/PD; *Mycoplasma* airsacculitis
	750 mg/L drinking water × 3-7 days[16,27]	Waterfowl/*Mycoplasma* synovitis, sinusitis
Lincomycin hydrochloride monohydrate/spectinomycin sulfate tetrahydrate (LS 50 Water Soluble Powder, Zoetis)	2 g/gal drinking water first 5-7 days of age[165]	Chicken (up to 7 days old)/aid in control of airsacculitis
	750 mg/L drinking water × 3-7 days[27]	Waterfowl
Marbofloxacin (Zeniquin, Zoetis)	2 mg/kg PO q24h[11]	Chickens (broilers)/PD; prohibited drug[c,54,166]
	3-12 mg/kg PO q24h[66]	Turkeys/PK; prohibited drug[c,54,166]
Metronidazole	—	Poultry/prohibited drug[c,54,166]
Miporamicin	100 mg/kg feed × 5 days[69,151]	Poultry/macrolide; under development; make preparation fresh daily
Neomycin	80-264 mg/L drinking water[27]	Waterfowl
	126 mg/L drinking water[69]	Galliformes
	70-220 mg/kg feed × 14-21 days[27,69]	Waterfowl, galliformes/*Clostridium*, necrotizing enteritis
Neomycin sulfate (Neomycin 325 Soluble Powder, Zoetis)	10 mg/lb (22 mg/kg) body weight per day in drinking water × 2-5 days[166]	Turkeys (growing)/for the control of mortality associated with *E. coli*[166]
Nitrofuran	26 mg/L drinking water × 5-7 days[27]	Galliformes/prohibited drug[c,167]
	50-200 mg/kg feed × 5-7 days[27]	Galliformes/*Clostridium*, *Salmonella*; prohibited drug[c,167]
Nitrofurazone	—	Poultry/prohibited drug[c,167]
Norfloxacin (Noroxin, Merck; Vetriflox 20% Oral Solution, Lavet)	8 mg/kg PO q24h[12]	Chickens/PD; prohibited drug[c,167]
	10 mg/kg PO q24h[16,86]	Chickens, geese/PD; prohibited drug[c,167]
	10 mg/kg PO q6-8h[16,86]	Turkeys/PD; prohibited drug[c,167]
	15 mg/kg in water over 2-4 hr[139]	Turkeys/PD; once-per-day pulse dosing was more efficacious than continuous dosing in the water; prohibited drug[c,167]
	20-40 mg/kg PO q24h × 5 days[96]	Chickens/prohibited drug[c,167]
	100 mg/L drinking water × 5 days[139]	Chickens/PD; prohibited drug[c,167]
	175 mg/L drinking water × 5 days[138]	Chickens/prohibited drug[c,167]

Continued

TABLE 6-1 Antimicrobial Agents Used in Backyard Poultry and Waterfowl. (cont'd)

Agent	Dosage	Species/Comments
Novobiocin sodium	15-30 mg/kg PO q24h[151]	Poultry/effective against some gram-positive cocci
	220-385 mg/kg feed[69]	Poultry, waterfowl
Novobiocin (Albamix Feed Medication, Zoetis)	4-5 mg/lb body weight/day in feed[166]	Turkeys/aid in the treatment of breast blisters associated with susceptible staphylococcal infections[166]
	5-8 mg/lb body weight/day in feed[166]	Turkeys/aid in the control of recurring outbreaks of fowl cholera caused by susceptible strains of *Pasteurella multocida* following initial treatment with 7-8 mg/lb body weight/day[166]
	6-7 mg/lb body weight/day in feed × 5-7 days[166]	Chickens/aid in the treatment of breast blisters associated with susceptible staphylococcal infections; administer as sole ration feed that contains not less than 200 g/ton of feed; not for laying chickens[166]
	10-14 mg/lb body weight/day in feed × 5-7 days[166]	Chickens/treatment of susceptible staphylococcal infections; administer as sole ration in feed that contains not less than 350 g/ton of feed; not for laying chickens[166]
Oleandomycin	—	Macrolide; not available in the United States
Orbifloxacin (Orbax, Intervet)	15-20 mg/kg PO q24h[70]	Japanese quail/PK[70] Poultry/prohibited drug[c,168]
Ormetoprim-sulfadimethoxine (Primor, Zoetis)	200-800 mg/kg feed[27]	Waterfowl/colibacillosis
Oxytetracycline	5 mg/kg SC, IM q12-24h[20]	Chickens (chicks)/PD
	23 mg/kg IV q6-8h[155]	Pheasants/PK
	43 mg/kg IM q24h[155]	Pheasants/PD
	200 mg/kg IM q24h[69]	Waterfowl/*Pasteurella*
	2500 mg/L drinking water and 2500 mg/kg feed[69,180]	Chickens (PD), turkeys (PD), waterfowl/simultaneous medication of feed and water required to reach therapeutic level
Oxytetracycline (Liquamycin injectable, Terramycin Soluble Powder, Zoetis)		Chickens (broilers, breeders), turkeys/*Mycoplasma gallisepticum*, *Mycoplasma synoviae*, *E. coli*, and *Pasteurella multocida*; treatment must be discontinued at least 5 days prior to slaughter; do not administer to laying hens unless the eggs are used for hatching only; in light turkey breeds, no more than 55 mg/kg of body weight is administered; treatment not to exceed a total of 4 consecutive days[165]

TABLE 6-1	Antimicrobial Agents Used in Backyard Poultry and Waterfowl. (cont'd)	
Agent	Dosage	Species/Comments
Oxytetracycline (Liquamycin injectable, Terramycin Soluble Powder, Zoetis) (cont'd)	6.25 mg/chick or poult/day SC diluted 1 part drug to 3 parts sterile water[165]	Chickens, turkeys (1 day to 2 wk of age)
	12.5 mg/pullet or poult/day SC diluted 1 part drug to 3 parts sterile water[165]	Chickens, turkeys (2-4 wk of age)
	25 mg/chicken/day SC[165]	Chickens (4-8 wk of age)
	50 mg/chicken or poult/day SC[165]	Chickens (8 wk of age), turkeys (4-6 wk of age)
	100 mg/chicken or poult/day SC[165]	Chickens (adult), turkeys (6-12 wk of age)
	200 mg/poult/day SC undiluted[165]	Turkeys (12 wk of age and older)
	50-100 mg injected into swollen sinus; may be repeated in 5-7 days[165]	Turkeys/infectious sinusitis; treat concurrently with SC doses described above
Oxytetracycline (Terramycin Soluble Powder, Zoetis)	25 mg/lb body weight × 7-14 days[166]	Turkeys (growing)
	200-400 mg/gal drinking water × 7-14 days[166]	Turkeys (not laying eggs for human consumption)
	200-800 mg/gal drinking water × 7-14 days[166]	Chickens
	37 g/15 L drinking water × 5-7 days[16]	Waterfowl/pasteurellosis and other sensitive bacterial infections
Penicillin	50,000 U/kg IM[27]	Waterfowl/*Erysipelas*, new duck disease
Penicillin G (Penicillin G Potassium, Zoetis)	1,500,000 U/gal drinking water × 5 days[166]	Turkeys/not laying eggs for human consumption
Penicillin procaine	100 mg/kg IM q24-48h[73]	Turkeys/PD
Sarafloxacin (Saraflox, Abbott)	10 mg/kg PO q8h[16]	Chickens/prohibited drug[c,168]
	20-40 mg/L drinking water × 5 days[16]	Chickens/colibacillosis; prohibited drug[c,168]
	30-50 mg/L drinking water × 5 days[16]	Turkeys/colibacillosis; prohibited drug[c,168]
Spectinomycin	0.5 g/gal drinking water[166]	Chickens (floor-raised broilers)/use first 3 days of life × 3 days; 1 day following each vaccination[166]
	1 g/gal drinking water[166]	Chickens (broilers)/use first 3-5 days of life[166]
	2 g/gal drinking water[166]	Chickens (growing)/use first 3 days of life × 3 days; use 1 day following each vaccination[166]
Streptomycin	22-33 mg/kg PO[165]	Chickens/not laying eggs for human consumption
	25-50 mg/kg IM q24h[16]	Chickens/PD
	0.6-0.9 g/gal drinking water for up to 5 days[165]	Chickens/not laying eggs for human consumption

Continued

TABLE 6-1 Antimicrobial Agents Used in Backyard Poultry and Waterfowl. (cont'd)

Agent	Dosage	Species/Comments
Sulfachloropyridazine/trimethoprim (Cosumix Plus, Ciba)	400 mg/kg feed[16]	Geese
Sulfadimethoxine	0.938 g/gal (0.025%) × 6 days[166]	Turkeys (meat)/fowl cholera; do not administer to turkeys over 24 wk of age; withdraw 5 days prior to slaughter[165]
	1.875 g/gal (0.05%) × 6 days[166]	Chickens (broilers and replacements)/fowl cholera and infectious coryza; do not administer to chickens over 16 wk of age; withdraw 5 days prior to slaughter[166]
Sulfamethazine (SMZ, Cross VetPharm Group)	128-187 mg/kg body weight/day in drinking water[165]	Chickens/not laying eggs for human consumption[165]
	110 to 273 mg/kg body weight/day in drinking water[166]	Turkeys/not laying eggs for human consumption[166]
Sulfaquinoxaline (Sulquin 6-50, Zoetis; Sul-Q-Nox, S. Q., Huvepharma)	0.04% in drinking water × 2-3 days[166]	Chickens, turkeys/acute fowl cholera due to *P. multocida*; fowl typhoid due to *Salmonella gallinarum*
	250-500 mg/kg feed[27]	Waterfowl/avian cholera, new duck disease
Tetracycline	40-200 mg/L drinking water[27]	Game birds
	100-600 mg/kg feed[27,69]	Game birds
Tiamulin (Denagard; Elanco)	12.5 mg/kg PO q24h × 3 days[75]	Poultry/intestinal spirochetosis; adverse effects, including death, if administered with ionophores
	30 mg/kg PO q24h × 7 days[69]	Poultry (adults)
	60 mg/kg PO q24h × 7 days[69]	Poultry (chicks)
	225-250 mg/L drinking water × 3-7 days[69]	Poultry
	1000 mg/L water[69]	Poultry eggs/dip
	300-400 mg/kg feed × 7 days[69]	Game birds
Tiamulin/chlortetracycline (Tetramutin, Elanco)	1-1.5 mg/kg feed × 7 days[149]	Chickens/*Mycoplasma; Brachyspira*-related diseases; may be used with salinomycin at low doses of 60 mg/kg without signs of incompatibility[69]
Tilmicosin (Micotil 300 Injection, Provitil-powder and Pulmotil AC-liquid, Elanco)	30 mg/kg PO q24h[2]	Poultry/PK; not labeled for use in poultry[69]
	100-500 mg/L drinking water × 5 days[79,82]	Poultry chicks/*Mycoplasma*

TABLE 6-1 Antimicrobial Agents Used in Backyard Poultry and Waterfowl. (cont'd)

Agent	Dosage	Species/Comments
Tobramycin	2.5-5 mg/kg IM, IV q12h[69]	Pheasants
Trimethoprim/sulfadiazine	107 mg/L drinking water[69]	Galliformes
Trimethoprim/sulfamethoxazole	20-50 mg/kg PO q12h[173]	Ducks
	50 mg/kg PO q12h[173]	Chickens
	400 mg/kg feed[69]	Geese
Tylosin (Tylan, Elanco)	6.6-11 mg/kg SC[69]	Galliformes
	10-40 mg/kg IM q6-8h[69]	Poultry
	20-30 mg/kg IM q8h × 3-7 days[16,69]	Waterfowl/*Mycoplasma*
	25 mg/kg IM q6h[94]	Quail/PK
	851-1419 mg/gal (225-375 ppm) in drinking water × 5 days[166]	Chickens/control mortality caused by necrotic enteritis[166]
	2000 mg/gal (528 ppm) in drinking water × 1-5 days[166]	Chickens (broiler and replacement chicks)/chronic respiratory disease[166]
	2000 mg/gal (528 ppm) in drinking water × 2-5 days[166]	Turkeys/infectious sinusitis associated with *Mycoplasma gallisepticum*[166]
	500 mg/L drinking water × 3-28 days[69,79,152]	Galliformes, waterfowl/*Mycoplasma*
	2.5 g/5 L drinking water × 3 days[16]	Waterfowl
	2000 mg/L drinking water[69]	Poultry/*Mycoplasma*, *Haemophilus*
	200 mg/kg feed[69]	Galliformes
	100 mg/10 mL saline nasal flush × 10 days[16]	Waterfowl/*Mycoplasma*
Virginiamycin (Stafac, Phibro)	22 mg/kg feed[151]	Poultry
	5-20 g/ton feed[165]	Chickens (broilers)
	10-20 g/ton feed[165]	Turkeys (growing)

[a]Many poultry species are considered food-producing animal *species*, and as such, these species are regulated by the U.S. Food and Drug Administration (FDA).[166] Even if the individual animals of any of these species are never used for food, they are still regulated by the FDA. The FDA prohibits the use of certain drugs, with no allowable extra-label drug use, in any food-producing animal species. These prohibited drugs are clearly identified in the tables, and the doses are provided in case they are needed for a similar but non-food-producing animal species (e.g., Attwater's prairie chicken), and listings should in no way be misconstrued as an endorsement of using FDA-prohibited drugs in any food-producing animal species. Please refer to the appropriate tables at the end of this chapter regarding the definitions of prohibited drugs, extra-label drugs, labeled drugs, and drugs needing a Veterinary Feed Directive prior to choosing a drug and dose. Please refer to the Food Animal Residue Avoidance Databank at www.farad.org and other sources listed in Table 6.25 for meat and egg withdrawal times.[54]

[b]The FDA restricts the extra-label use of the cephalosporin class of antibiotics, except for cephapirin, in food-producing animal species, such as chickens and turkeys.[54,166,169]

[c]The FDA prohibits the use of chloramphenicol, clenbuterol, diethylstilbestrol (DES), fluoroquinolone-class antibiotics, glycopeptides (all agents, including vancomycin), medicated feeds, nitroimidazoles (all agents, including dimetridazole, ipronidazole, metronidazole, and others), and nitrofurans (all agents, including furazolidone, nitrofurazone, and others), with no allowable extra-label drug use, in any food-producing animal species.[54,166]

TABLE 6-2 Antifungal Agents Used in Backyard Poultry and Waterfowl.[a]

Agent	Dosage	Species/Comments
Copper sulfate ("bluestone")	Dissolve 0.5 lb copper sulfate and 0.5 cup vinegar in 1 gal of water for a "stock" solution; dispense stock solution at the rate of 1 oz per gal for the final drinking solution;[114] alternate method of preparing the solution: dissolve 1 oz copper sulfate and 1 Tbs of vinegar in 15 gal water[114]	Poultry/mycosis (thrush) in the crop; "follow-up" treatment after flushing crop with Epsom salt solution[114]
Epsom salts	1 tsp Epsom salt in 1 oz water to flush crop[114]	Chicken/mycotic ingluvitis; individual dose
	1 lb Epsom salt per 5 gal water × 1 day[114]	Poultry/to flush digestive system of toxins
	1 lb Epsom salt per 15 lb feed[114]	Poultry/laxative or flush prior to copper sulfate treatment; give the Epsom salt feed mixture as the sole feed source for a 1-day period
Fluconazole	100 mg/kg PO q24h[69]	Chickens/avian gastric yeast
Flucytosine (Ancobon, Roche)	60 mg/kg PO q12h[69]	Galliformes, swans/birds >500 g; syringeal aspergilloma
	150 mg/kg PO q12h[69]	Galliformes, swans/birds <500 g; syringeal aspergilloma
Itraconazole	—	Study using SC controlled-release gel formulation in ducks showed unacceptable tissue and plasma levels of the drug[160]
	5 mg/kg PO q24h[69]	Galliformes, swans/aspergillosis
	5-10 mg/kg PO q12h[69]	Waterfowl
	10 mg/kg PO q24h × 7-10 days[16]	Waterfowl/prophylactic dose
	10 mg/kg PO q12h 4-6 wk[16]	Waterfowl/therapeutic dose
	16% itraconazole-impregnated PMMA fed as grit stones in 1-g pieces[148]	Indian peafowl/PD; therapeutic levels achieved in 2 days and decreased over 7 days
Ketoconazole	12.5 mg/kg PO q24h × 30 days[69]	Swans/candidiasis
Nystatin	300,000 U/kg PO q12h × 7-14 days[16,69]	Waterfowl
Parconazole (Parcomyc, Janssen-Cilag)	30-60 mg/kg feed[69]	Guinea fowl/candidiasis; prophylaxis; not available in the United States
Voriconazole	10 mg/kg PO, IV q12h[22]	Chickens/PK
	40 mg/kg PO q24h[159]	Quail/PD

[a]Many poultry species are considered food-producing animal *species*, and as such, these species are regulated by the U.S. Food and Drug Administration (FDA).[166] Even if the individual animals of any of these species are never used for food, they are still regulated by the FDA. The FDA prohibits the use of certain drugs, with no allowable extra-label drug use, in any food-producing animal species. These prohibited drugs are clearly identified in the tables, and the doses are provided in case they are needed for a similar but non-food-producing animal species (e.g., Attwater's prairie chicken), and listings should in no way be misconstrued as an endorsement of using FDA-prohibited drugs in any food-producing animal species. Please refer to the appropriate tables at the end of this chapter regarding the definitions of prohibited drugs, extra-label drugs, labeled drugs, and drugs needing a Veterinary Feed Directive prior to choosing a drug and dose. Please refer to the Food Animal Residue Avoidance Databank at www.farad.org and other sources listed in Table 6.25 for meat and egg withdrawal times.

TABLE 6-3 Antiviral and Immunomodulating Agents Used in Backyard Poultry and Waterfowl.[a]

Note: The U.S. Food and Drug Administration (FDA) restricts the extra-label use of adamantane and neuraminidase inhibitors in all poultry, including ducks, because of the potential resistance production against avian influenza.[54,166]

Agent	Dosage	Species/Comments
Acyclovir	10 mg/kg IM q24h × 5-14 days starting 3 days post-exposure[69]	Chickens/Marek's disease
Famciclovir	25 mg/kg PO q12h[16,69,163]	Ducklings/PD; duck hepatitis; toxic effects were not reported
Levamisole	1.25-2.5 mg/kg PO, SC[69]	Poultry
Penciclovir (Denavir, Novartis)	10 mg/kg IP q24h × 12-24 wk[91]	Ducks/PD; herpesviruses; duck hepatitis B virus; viral levels were significantly reduced; no toxic effects observed; dissolve in 2 mL of 1% DMSO

[a]Many poultry species are considered food-producing animal *species*, and as such, these species are regulated by the U.S. Food and Drug Administration (FDA).[166] Even if the individual animals of any of these species are never used for food, they are still regulated by the FDA. The FDA prohibits the use of certain drugs, with no allowable extra-label drug use, in any food-producing animal species. These prohibited drugs are clearly identified in the tables, and the doses are provided in case they are needed for a similar but non-food-producing animal species (e.g., Attwater's prairie chicken), and listings should in no way be misconstrued as an endorsement of using FDA-prohibited drugs in any food-producing animal species. Please refer to the appropriate tables at the end of this chapter regarding the definitions of prohibited drugs, extra-label drugs, labeled drugs, and drugs needing a Veterinary Feed Directive prior to choosing a drug and dose. Please refer to the Food Animal Residue Avoidance Databank at www.farad.org and other sources listed in Table 6.25 for meat and egg withdrawal times.

TABLE 6-4 Antiparasitic Agents Used in Backyard Poultry and Waterfowl.[a,b]

Agent	Dosage	Species/Comments
Albendazole (11.36%) (Valbazen, Zoetis)	10 mg/kg PO once[34]	Poultry/PK
	47 mg/kg PO once, then repeat in 4 wk[69]	Chickens/lower ascarid *Heterakis* fecal counts than nontreated
Amprolium	13-26 mg/kg PO[62]	Chickens/PK, PD; bioavailability almost 4 times greater in fasted birds
	575 mg/L drinking water[27]	Poultry/using a 9.6% solution
	¼ tsp/L drinking water × 3-5 days[69]	Poultry/20% soluble powder
	115-235 mg/kg feed[69]	Poultry, pheasants/coccidia; *Sarcocystis*; lower dose is prophylactic; higher dose is therapeutic
	125 mg/kg feed[137a]	Turkeys/31 of 33 *Eimeria* isolates were resistant
Carbaryl 5% (Sevin Dust, Bayer)	—	No longer approved for use in poultry
Chloroquine phosphate	5 mg/kg PO q24h or in feed[69]	Game birds/generally used with primaquine for *Plasmodium*, *Haemoproteus*, and *Leucocytozoon*; overdose can result in death[16]
	2000 mg/L drinking water q24h × 14 days[69]	Game birds/juice covers bitter taste of drug

Continued

TABLE 6-4 Antiparasitic Agents Used in Backyard Poultry and Waterfowl. (cont'd)

Agent	Dosage	Species/Comments
Clazuril (Appertex, Janssen)	3 mg/kg PO once, or × 5 days[57]	Chickens/PK; drug detected in eggs after multiple dosing
	5-10 mg/kg PO q72h × 3 treatments[16,69]	Waterfowl/coccidiosis
	5-10 mg/kg PO q24h × 3 days, off 2 days, on 3 days[69]	Poultry
Clopidol	0.0125%-0.025% in feed (113.5 or 227 g/ton feed)[30a]	Turkeys/leucocytozoonosis prevention
	0.0125%-0.025% in feed[30a]	Chickens (broilers and layer replacements)/coccidiosis prevention; do not feed to chickens over 16 wk of age
	125 mg/kg feed[137a]	Turkeys/16 of 33 *Eimeria* isolates showed partial to complete resistance
	125-250 mg/kg feed[69]	Game birds/coccidiosis, *Leucocytozoon, Plasmodium*
Clorsulon (Curatrem, Merial)	20 mg/kg PO q14d × 3 treatments[69]	Waterfowl/trematodes, cestodes
	20 mg/kg PO 3 ×/wk × 14 days[69]	Waterfowl/trematodes, cestodes
Cypermethrin (5%) (Max Con, Y-Tex)	60-120 mg/chicken topically over dorsal neck[4a]	Chickens/effective against *Triatoma infestans*
Decoquinate (Deccox, Alpharma)	20-40 mg/kg feed[61,151]	Chickens/*Eimeria;* very effective in isolates studied
Diatomaceous earth (kitchen/food grade)	2% in feed, feed continuously[106]	Chickens/lowers numbers of *Heterakis* and *Capillaria*
Diclazuril (Clinicox 0.5%, Huvepharma AD; DiClosol 1%, Pharmaswede)	—	Benzene-acetonitrile anticoccidial; some *Eimeria* resistance in poultry documented recently;[1a,137a] rotation suggested for long-term prevention
	5 mg/L drinking water × 6 days[69]	Chickens/reduced oocyst viability and virulence
	5-10 mg/L drinking water × 2 days[44]	Chickens/effective in preventing disease and reducing total oocysts, lesions, and mortality in infected birds with mixed *Eimeria* infections
	0.5-1 mg/kg feed[29,44]	Chickens, turkeys/coccidia
	1 mg/kg feed[137a]	Turkeys/21 of 33 *Eimeria* isolates were partially or completely resistant
Dimetrida-zole[b] (Emtryl 40% powder, Rhone Merieux)	200-400 mg/L drinking water × 5 days[69]	Game birds/*Trichomonas, Giardia, Hexamita, Spironucleus, Histomonas;* low therapeutic index; highly toxic to geese, and ducks;[69] not available in many countries (United States, European Union) because of human health risks; Canada has banned use in food-producing animals;[124] prohibited drug[b]

TABLE 6-4 Antiparasitic Agents Used in Backyard Poultry and Waterfowl. (cont'd)

Agent	Dosage	Species/Comments
Dimetrida-zoleb (Emtryl 40% powder, Rhone Merieux) (cont'd)	800 mg/L drinking water[69]	Poultry, game birds/prohibited drug[b]
	185-187.5 mg/kg feed[69]	Poultry, game birds/prohibited drug[b]
	200-400 mg/kg feed[69]	Chickens/highly effective against *Histomonas*; prohibited drug[b]
Dinitolmide (Zoamix, Alpharma)	40-187 mg/kg feed[69]	Chickens, turkeys/coccidia
Fenbendazole (Safeguard, Ralston Purina; Panacur, Intervet)	—	Anthelmintic effective against cestodes, nematodes, trematodes, *Giardia*, acanthocephalans; can cause feather abnormalities if administered during molting[16]
	1.5-3.9 mg/kg PO q24h × 3 days[16,153]	Chickens/PK, PD; *Capillaria*
	5-15 mg/kg q24h × 5 days[16]	Waterfowl
	10-50 mg/kg PO once; repeat in 10 days[106]	Chickens/*Ascaris* spp.
	10-50 mg/kg PO q24h × 5 days[106]	Chickens/*Capillaria* and other nematodes
	12 mg/kg PO[69]	Partridges, pheasants/*Syngamus, Heterakis, Ascaridia*
	20 mg/kg PO once[16,69]	Waterfowl,[16] pheasants/cestodes, nematodes, acanthocephalans; reduced *Heterakis* and *Eimeria* in pheasants
	20-100 mg/kg PO once[106]	Chickens/nematodes other than *Capillaria*
	125 mg/L of drinking water × 5 days[106]	Chickens/nematodes other than *Capillaria*
	53 mg/kg in feed × 5-7 days[69]	Game birds/nematodes, trematodes
	79 mg/kg feed (75 ppm) × 3 days[d,114]	Chickens, quail
	80 mg/kg feed[153]	Chickens/PK, PD; *Capillaria*
	375 mg/kg feed × 1 day[c,114]	Chickens/*Capillaria, Heterakis, Ascaridia, Syngamus* Bobwhites (280-g size)/will treat about 1000 birds[114]
	14.5 g/ton feed (16 ppm) × 6 days[106]	Turkeys (growing)/*Ascaridia dissimilis* and *Heterakis gallinarium*
Flubendazole (Flutelmium 7.5%, Janssen-Cilag)	30 mg/kg feed × 7 days[16]	Poultry
	60 mg/kg feed × 7-14 days[16,69]	Partridges, pheasants
Halofuginone	—	Not available in the United States
	1.3-2.72 mg/kg feed[27]	Turkeys/coccidia; not approved for birds intended for food
	2.7 mg/kg feed[27]	Chickens/coccidia, *Plasmodium*

Continued

TABLE 6-4 Antiparasitic Agents Used in Backyard Poultry and Waterfowl. (cont'd)

Agent	Dosage	Species/Comments
Hygromycin B (Hygromix 8, Elanco)	—	Aminoglycoside antibiotic used as anthelmintic feed additive
	8-12 g/ton feed[106]	Chickens/*Ascaridia, Heterakis, Capillaria*
	9-13 mg/kg feed[69]	Game birds/ascarids, cecal worms; some efficacy against *Capillaria*
	18-26 mg/kg feed × 2 mo[69]	Game birds/cecal worms
Ivermectin	—	Most nematodes, acanthocephalans, leeches, most ectoparasites (including *Knemidokoptes, Dermanyssus*); can dilute with water or saline for immediate use; dilute with propylene glycol for extended use
	0.2 mg/kg PO, SC, IM once, can repeat in 10-14 days[16,69]	Guinea fowl, waterfowl
Lasalocid (Avatec, Alpharma)	67-125 mg/kg feed continuously[69,151]	Game birds, chickens/coccidia
Levamisole	—	Nematodes; immunostimulant; low therapeutic index (toxic reactions, deaths reported); do not use in debilitated birds;[16] IM administration may cause severe toxicity[69]
	13 g/25 gal drinking water × 1 day; can repeat in 5-7 days[f,114]	Poultry/*Capillaria, Heterakis,* and *Ascaridia*; solution contains 0.5 g of levamisole per 3.8 L of water[114]
	52 g/100 gal drinking water × 1 day; can repeat in 5-7 days[e,114]	Poultry/*Capillaria, Heterakis,* and *Ascaridia*; solution contains 0.5 g of levamisole per 3.8 L of water[114]
	52 g/3 L water stock solution that is then added at 30 mL stock solution/3.8 L drinking water × 1 day; can repeat in 5-7 days[114]	Poultry/*Capillaria, Heterakis,* and *Ascaridia*; solution contains 0.5 g of levamisole per 3.8 L of water[114]
	20-25 mg/kg SC[69]	Game birds
	20-50 mg/kg PO, SC once[16]	Waterfowl
	25-30 mg/kg[106]	Chicken/*Ascaridia dissimilis, H. gallinarium, Capillaria obsingnata*
	40 mg/kg PO once[47,69]	Chickens/PK; *Capillaria*; significantly higher bioavailability, volume of distribution, and total body clearance in laying hens[47]
	265-525 mg/L drinking water × 1 day, repeat in 7-14 days[69]	Game birds, poultry
Maduramicin ammonium (Cygro, Alpharma)	5-6 mg/kg feed[69]	Chickens, turkeys/coccidia; not available in the United States

TABLE 6-4 Antiparasitic Agents Used in Backyard Poultry and Waterfowl. (cont'd)

Agent	Dosage	Species/Comments
Mebendazole (Telmin Suspension, Telmintic Powder, Schering-Plough)		Broad-spectrum ovicidal antihelmintic; primarily used for *Capillaria*[16]
	5-15 mg/kg PO q24h × 2 days[16,69]	Waterfowl/nematodes
	1.2 mg/kg feed × 14 days[69]	Waterfowl/nematodes
Metronidazole[b]	—	Antiprotozoal, including alimentary tract protozoa (especially flagellates such as *Giardia, Histomonas, Spironucleus, Trichomonas*); prohibited drug[54,166]
	25 mg/kg PO q12h × 10 days[27]	Turkeys/*Trichomonas*; prohibited drug[166]
	30 mg/kg PO q12h[36]	Poultry/PK, PD; prohibited drug[166]
	50 mg/kg PO[27]	Waterfowl/flagellates; prohibited drug[166]
	110 mg/kg PO q12h[69]	Poultry/*Histomonas*; prohibited drug[166]
	400 mg/L drinking water × 5-15 days[69]	Game birds, passerines/protozoal sinusitis; prohibited drug[166]
	200-400 mg/kg feed[69]	Chickens/highly effective against *Histomonas* but reduced weight gains at higher dosage; prohibited drug[166]
Milbemycin oxime (Interceptor, Novartis)	2 mg/kg PO, repeat in 28 days[69]	Galliformes/nematodes
Monensin (Coban 45, Elanco)	—	Ionophore antibiotic anticoccidial feed additive; keep away from horses (toxic)
	53-94 mg/kg feed × 10 wk[29,69]	Turkeys
	73 mg/kg feed × 10 wk[27]	Quail
	94 mg/kg feed[69]	Quail, cranes/coccidia (including disseminated visceral coccidiosis)
	94-108 mg/kg feed × 8 wk[69]	Chickens
	99.2 mg/kg feed[137a]	Turkeys/23 of 33 *Eimeria* isolates were resistant
Narasin (Monteban 45, Elanco)	20-80 mg/kg feed[151]	Chickens/prophylactic coccidiostat; toxic to turkeys
Nicarbazin (Nicarb 25%, Merck AgVet)	20-125 mg/kg feed[151]	Chickens/prophylactic coccidiostat
Oregano essential oil (Orego-Stim 5% Meriden AnimalHealth Ltd)	500 ppm in feed[116]	Chickens (growing)/PD; coccidiostat; lower oocysts per gram of feces and displayed lower coccidiosis lesion scores in upper and middle regions of intestine than controls[116]
Phenylarsonic acid (Merck European Laboratories)	22-45 mg/kg[27]	Chickens, turkeys/*Histomonas* prevention; not recommended or approved for game birds; not available in the United States

Continued

TABLE 6-4 Antiparasitic Agents Used in Backyard Poultry and Waterfowl. (cont'd)

Agent	Dosage	Species/Comments
Piperazine (Wazine, Fleming Laboratories)	—	Ascarids, oxyurids; less efficacious than fenbendazole; resistance is widespread[106]
	45-200 mg/kg PO once[69]	Waterfowl/*Tetrameres, Capillaria*
	50 mg/bird PO[106]	Chickens (<6 wk old)
	50-100 mg/kg PO once[69]	Chickens
	100 mg/bird PO[106]	Chickens (≥6 wk old), turkeys (<12 wk old)
	100-400 mg/bird PO[69]	Turkeys
	100-500 mg/kg PO once, repeat in 10-14 days[69]	Game birds
	200 mg/bird PO[106]	Turkeys (≥12 wk old)
	1000 mg/L drinking water; repeat in 10-14 days[16]	Gallinaceous birds/should be completely consumed within a few hours because only relatively high concentrations of the drug eliminate worms[106]
	1000-2000 mg/L drinking water × 1-2 days[69]	Game birds
	1600-2600 mg/L drinking water[27]	Waterfowl/*Tetrameres, Capillaria*
Praziquantel	5-10 mg/kg PO, SC q24h × 14 days[27,69]	Waterfowl/trematodes
	8.5 mg/kg IM[69]	Chickens/cestodes, trematodes[16,69]
	10 mg/kg PO[69]	Chickens
	10 mg/kg PO, SC q24h × 14 days[16]	Waterfowl/trematodes
	10-20 mg/kg PO, repeat in 10 days[16,69]	Waterfowl/cestodes, trematodes[69]
	10-20 mg/kg SC, repeat in 10 days[69]	Waterfowl/cestodes
	11 mg/kg SC once[69]	Chickens
Primaquine	—	Game birds/hematozoa (i.e., *Plasmodium, Haemoproteus, Leucocytozoon*); use in conjunction with chloroquine; dosage based on amount of active base rather than total tablet weight
	0.03 mg/kg PO q24h × 3 days[69]	Game birds
Pyrimethamine (Fansidar, Roche)	0.25-0.5 mg/kg PO q12h × 30 days[69]	Waterfowl/*Sarcocystis, Toxoplasma*
	0.5 mg/kg PO q12h × 30 days[69]	Waterfowl/*Sarcocystis*
	0.25-0.5 mg/kg PO q12h × 30 days[16]	Waterfowl
	1 mg/kg feed[69]	Game birds
Pyrimethamine/ sulfaquinoxaline (Microquinox, C-Vet Livestock Products)	60 mg/L drinking water, 3 days on, 2 days off, 3 days on[16]	Waterfowl/coccidiosis
Robenidine HCl (Bio-Cox, Alpharma)	33 mg/kg feed[69]	Chickens

TABLE 6-4 Antiparasitic Agents Used in Backyard Poultry and Waterfowl. (cont'd)

Agent	Dosage	Species/Comments
Sulfadiazine/trimethoprim (DiTrim, Zoetis)	60 mg/kg PO q12h × 3 days[16]	Waterfowl/coccidiosis
Sulfadimethoxine (12.5%)	250 mg/L drinking water × 5 days[69]	Turkeys (meat)/coccidiosis
	500 mg/L drinking water × 6 days[69]	Chickens (broilers and replacements)/coccidiosis
	0.938 g/gal (0.025%) × 6 days[166]	Turkeys (meat)/coccidiosis
	1.875 g/gal (0.05%) × 6 days[166]	Chickens (broilers and replacements)/coccidiosis
Sulfadimethoxine/ormetoprim (Rofenaid, Hoffmann-La Roche)	10 mg/kg feed[69]	Game birds/coccidiosis, *Leucocytozoon, Sarcocystis*
	320-525 mg/L drinking water[69]	Poultry
Sulfamethazine (Sulmet, Boehringer-Ingelheim)	125-185 mg/kg PO q24h × 2 days, then 64-94 mg/kg × 4 days[69]	Chickens
Sulfaquinoxaline (Sulquin 6-50, Solvay)	0.04% in drinking water × 2-3 days, off 3 days, then use 0.025% × 2 days (repeat 0.025% × 2 days if needed)[166]	Chickens/coccidiosis caused by *Eimeria tenella, E. necatrix, E. acervulina, E. maxima,* and *E. brunetti*; do not change litter unless absolutely necessary; do not give flushing mashes; medicated chickens must actually consume enough medicated water to provide a recommended dosage of approximately 22-99 mg/kg/day depending on the age, class of animal, ambient temperature, and other factors; do not give to chickens within 10 days of slaughter for food; do not medicate chickens producing eggs for human consumption; make fresh drinking water daily[166]
	0.025% in drinking water × 2 days, off 3 days, give 2 days, off 3 days and on 2 days more; repeat if necessary[166]	Turkeys/coccidiosis caused by *Eimeria meleagrimitis* and *E. adenoides*;[166] must consume enough medicated water to provide approximately 77-121 mg/kg/day depending on age, class of animal, ambient temperature; do not give to turkeys within 10 days of slaughter for food; do not use in turkeys producing eggs for human consumption
	250 mg/L drinking water × 6 days, off 2 days, on 6 days[69]	Turkeys
	400 mg/L (1.4 mL/L) drinking water × 6 days, off 2 days, on 6 days[69]	Chickens
	225 mg/kg feed continuously[69]	Turkeys
	450 mg/kg feed continuously[69]	Chickens

Continued

TABLE 6-4 Antiparasitic Agents Used in Backyard Poultry and Waterfowl. (cont'd)

Agent	Dosage	Species/Comments
Thiabendazole	—	Nematodes, acanthocephalans; generally less efficacious than fenbendazole; may be toxic to diving ducks[16]
	425 mg/kg feed × 14 days[69]	Pheasants
Tinidazole (Fasigyn, Pfizer)	200-400 mg/kg feed[69]	Giardia, Trichomonas, Entamoeba Chickens/Histomonas; depressed weight gain on higher dosage
Toltrazuril (Baycox, Bayer)	—	Coccidiocidal;[69] efficacious for refractory coccidiosis; 2.5% solution is very alkaline and should not be gavaged directly into the crop[69]
	12.5 mg/L drinking water × 2 days[69]	Waterfowl
	25 mg/L drinking water × 2 days[44]	Chickens/effective in preventing disease and reducing total oocysts, lesions, and mortality in infected birds with mixed Eimeria infections
	25 mg/L drinking water × 2 days, repeat in 5 days[69]	Geese
Trimethoprim/sulfachlorpyridazine (1:5 ratio; Cosumix Plus, Novartis)	400 mg/kg feed[69]	Geese
Trimethoprim/sulfadiazine	60 mg/kg PO, SC q12h × 3 days, off 2 days, on 3 days[16]	Waterfowl/coccidiosis
Trimethoprim/sulfamethoxazole	320-525 mg/L drinking water[16,69]	Poultry/coccidiosis

[a]Many poultry species are considered food-producing animal *species,* and as such, these species are regulated by the U.S. Food and Drug Administration (FDA).[166] Even if the individual animals of any of these species are never used for food, they are still regulated by the FDA. The FDA prohibits the use of certain drugs, with no allowable extra-label drug use, in any food-producing animal species. These prohibited drugs are clearly identified in the tables, and the doses are provided in case they are needed for a similar but non-food-producing animal species (e.g., Attwater's prairie chicken), and listings should in no way be misconstrued as an endorsement of using FDA-prohibited drugs in any food-producing animal species. Please refer to the appropriate tables at the end of this chapter regarding the definitions of prohibited drugs, extra-label drugs, labeled drugs, and drugs needing a Veterinary Feed Directive prior to choosing a drug and dose. Please refer to the Food Animal Residue Avoidance Databank at www.farad.org and other sources listed in Table 6.25 for meat and egg withdrawal times.
[b]The FDA prohibits the use of chloramphenicol, clenbuterol, diethylstilbestrol (DES), fluoroquinolone class antibiotics, glycopeptides (all agents, including vancomycin), medicated feeds, nitroimidazoles (all agents, including dimetridazole, ipronidazole, metronidazole, and others), and nitrofurans (all agents, including furazolidone, nitrofurazone, and others), with no allowable extra-label drug use, in any food-producing animal species.[54,166]
[c]375 mg/kg feed × 1 day is equivalent to 1 oz of 10% Safeguard or 10% Panacur per 15-20 lb feed.[114]
[d]79 mg/kg feed × 3 days is equivalent to 1.2 oz of 10% Safeguard or 10% Panacur in 100 lb feed or a 4-oz packet of Worm-A-Rest Litter Pack (Ralston Purina) in 50 lb feed or a 5-lb bag of Worm-A-Rest Mix Pack in 495 lb feed.[114]
[e]Dissolve a 52-g (1.84-oz) packet of Tramisol Cattle and Sheep Wormer per 100 gal of drinking water.[114]
[f]Dissolve a 13-g (0.46-oz) packet of Tramisol Sheep Drench Powder per 25 gal of drinking water.[114]

TABLE 6-5 Chemical Restraint/Anesthetic/Analgesic Agents Used in Backyard Poultry and Waterfowl.[a-c]

Agent	Dosage	Species/Comments
Alphachloralose (Fisher Scientific)	30 mg/kg PO once[18]	Canada geese/immobilization of nuisance geese; prepare suspension in corn oil, inject into individual bread baits, and hand-toss to target individuals; onset approximately 60 min, duration up to 24 hr; low therapeutic index in chickens suggests only marginally safe in domestic species or for field applications where dosage difficult to control[95]
	250-430 mg/cup of bait[27,69]	Waterfowl (including Canada geese)/immobilization
Alphaxalone/alphadolone (Saffan, Schering-Plough)	36 mg/kg IP[69]	Waterfowl/immobilization; relatively low therapeutic index
Atipamezole (Antisedan, Zoetis)	—	α_2 adrenergic antagonist; 1:1 volume reversal of dexmedetomidine and medetomidine is general rule; although the same effects would be expected as with medetomidine (no longer available but can be compounded), there are no data available on the efficacy of this volume of atipamezole reversal of dexmedetomidine in birds
	2.5-5 × medetomidine dose IM, IV[69,100]	Geese/righting reflex regained 2-10 min after administration; for reversal of dexmedetomidine and medetomidine (no longer commercially available but can be compounded)
	0.18-0.28 mg/kg IV[99]	Mallard ducks
	0.25-0.38 mg/kg IM[100]	Mallard ducks
	1.3-1.6 mg/kg IV[69]	Chickens
Atropine sulfate	0.1 mg/kg IM, IV q3-4h[16]	Waterfowl
Bupivacaine HCl	1.94 mg/kg IV[112]	Chickens/TD_{50}; dose with 50% probability of a clinically significant change in blood pressure in isoflurane-anesthetized chickens
	2 mg/kg infused SC[103]	Mallard ducks/PD; high plasma levels at 6 and 12 hr post-administration, so delayed toxicity is possible
	2-8 mg/kg perineurally[21]	Mallard ducks/variable effectiveness for brachial plexus nerve block
	2-10 mg/kg infused into incision site[69]	Eider ducks/high bupivacaine dose toxicity or cumulative toxicity of bupivacaine and ketoprofen may have occurred
	3 mg/0.3 mL saline injected intraarticular[69]	Chickens/arthritis
	5 mg/kg (with 10 μg/kg epinephrine) perineurally[69]	Chickens/unsuccessful brachial plexus nerve block
	50:50 mixture with dimethyl sulfoxide topically[69]	Chickens/topical anesthesia; applied to amputated beaks

Continued

TABLE 6-5 Chemical Restraint/Anesthetic/Analgesic Agents Used in Backyard Poultry and Waterfowl. (cont'd)

Agent	Dosage	Species/Comments
Buprenorphine HCl	0.05-1 mg/kg intraarticular[56a]	Chickens/PD; no significant antinociceptive effects
Butorphanol tartrate	0.5-2 mg/kg IM[118]	Harlequin ducks/no isoflurane-sparing effects detected when administered 15 min prior to induction;[118] 4 mg/kg IM caused severe adverse cardiopulmonary effects in Guinea fowl[50]
	2 mg/kg IM q8-12h[173]	Chicken/as part of bimodal pain therapy with PO carprofen
Butorphanol (B)/midazolam (Mi)	(B) 1 mg/kg + (Mi) 1 mg/kg[69]	Chickens/adequate sedation for lateral recumbency
Detomidine (Dormosedan, Zoetis)	0.3 mg/kg IM[69,171]	Chickens, rock partridges/marked sedation; significant decrease in HR and RR, decrease in cloacal temperature, and prolonged recoveries (260 ± 17.6 min) in partridges
Diazepam	0.5-1 mg/kg IM, IV q8-12h[16]	Waterfowl/sedation; anticonvulsant; IM administration may cause severe muscle irritation, and absorption may be delayed
	6 mg/kg IM[171]	Rock partridges/decrease in cloacal temperature; prolonged recoveries (149 ± 8.3 min)
Fentanyl citrate	0.5-1 mg/kg intraarticular[56a]	Chickens/PD; no effect on pain behavior
	5 mg/kg transdermal (intrascapular skin)[174]	Guinea fowl/PK; plasma concentrations greater than those reported to be analgesic for dogs for at least 7 days; no longer available in the United States
	25 μg/h patch for 72 hr[41b]	Chickens/PK; wide variability; placed over plucked skin on dorsum; reached human therapeutic levels by 2-4 hr post-application[41b]
Flumazenil	0.018-0.028 mg/kg IV[99]	Mallard ducks
	0.05 mg/kg intranasally[69,100]	Mallard ducks
	0.1 mg/kg IM[39]	Quail/PD; reversed midazolam in 1.4-1.8 min
Isoflurane	1.3%[97,98]	Ducks/minimum anesthetic concentration
	1.15%[108]	Chickens/minimum anesthetic concentration
	1.1% ± 0.1%[49]	Chickens/minimum anesthetic concentration
Ketamine HCl	15-25 mg/kg IM, IV[69]	Waterfowl/seldom used as sole agent because of poor muscle relaxation and prolonged (up to 3 hr), violent recovery;[69] may produce excitation or convulsions in golden pheasants;[69] may fail to produce general anesthesia in some species, including waterfowl[69]
	20-50 mg/kg SC, IM, IV[69]	Waterfowl/restraint 30-60 min; smaller species require a higher dose; large birds tend to recover more slowly

CHAPTER 6 Backyard Poultry and Waterfowl

TABLE 6-5 Chemical Restraint/Anesthetic/Analgesic Agents Used in Backyard Poultry and Waterfowl. (cont'd)

Agent	Dosage	Species/Comments
Ketamine (K)/diazepam (D)	(K) 10-40 mg/kg IV + (D) 1-1.5 mg/kg IM, IV[69]	Waterfowl/induction or surgical anesthesia; rapid bolus may produce apnea, arrhythmia, and increased risk of death
	(K) 75 mg/kg IM + (D) 2.5 mg/kg IV[69]	Chickens/diazepam given 10 min after ketamine; pain reflexes elicited at all times; recovery in 90-100 min
	(K) 75 mg/kg IM + (D) 2.5 mg/kg IV[107]	White leghorn cockerels/diazepam administered 5 min before ketamine for typhlectomy; smooth induction/recovery, some limb contracture, hypothermia, hypoxia, hypercapnia
Ketamine (K)/ medetomidine (Me)	(K) 1.5-2 mg/kg + (Me) 60-85 µg/kg IM, IV[69]	Waterfowl/sedation; medetomidine no longer available but can be compounded; see dexmedetomidine[69]
	(K) 5-10 mg/kg + (Me) 100-200 µg/kg IM, IV[69]	Geese
Ketamine (K)/ medetomidine (Me)/ midazolam (Mi)	(K) 10 mg/kg + (Me) 50 µg/kg + (Mi) 2 mg/kg IV[99,100]	Mallard ducks/PD; medetomidine not currently available but can be compounded; anesthesia of 30-min duration; reverse with atipamezole, flumazenil intranasally; regimen considered unsafe due to acidosis, bradypnea, apnea, and in 1/12 birds, death[100]
Ketamine (K)/ midazolam (Mi)	(K) 50 mg/kg IV + (Mi) 2 mg/kg IM[107]	Chickens (white leghorn cockerels)/midazolam administered 5 min before ketamine for typhlectomy; hypoxia, hypercapnia, torticollis, dyspnea, salivation noted; prolonged recovery (92-105 min)
Ketamine (K)/xylazine (X)	(K) 10 mg/kg + (X) 2 mg/kg IV[107]	Chickens (white leghorn cockerels)/for typhlectomy; smooth induction/recovery; optimal to excellent surgical anesthesia
	(K) 20 mg/kg + (X) 1 mg/kg IV[69,98]	Pekin ducks/bradypnea, acidemia, hypoxemia, moderate hyperthermia
	(K) 25 mg/kg + (X) 1 mg/kg IM[154]	Guinea fowl/lateral recumbency 1-6 min; adequate anesthesia; arousal in 1.4 ± 0.7 min after yohimbine administration
Ketamine (K)/xylazine (X)/diazepam (D)	(K) 25 mg/kg + (X) 3 mg/kg + (D) 4 mg/kg IM[117]	Roosters/use with caution; significant decreases in HR, RR, cloacal temperatures; prolonged recoveries (up to 4 hr)
Ketamine (K)/xylazine (X)/midazolam (Mi)	(K) 15 mg/kg + (X) 2.5 mg/kg + (Mi) 0.3 mg/kg IM[3]	Guinea fowl/midazolam improved anesthetic quality
Lidocaine	2.5 mg/kg IV (give over 20 sec)[37]	Chickens/PK; under isoflurane anesthesia
	15 mg/kg (with 3.8 µg/kg epinephrine) perineurally[21]	Mallard ducks/variable effectiveness for brachial plexus nerve block
	20 mg/kg (with 10 µg/kg epinephrine) perineurally[69]	Chickens/unsuccessful brachial plexus nerve block

Continued

TABLE 6-5 Chemical Restraint/Anesthetic/Analgesic Agents Used in Backyard Poultry and Waterfowl. (cont'd)

Agent	Dosage	Species/Comments
Medetomidine	250-350 µg/kg PO[69]	Chickens/sedation; 60 µg given to male birds, 40 µg given to female birds; average time of sedation was 6 min; not commercially available but can be compounded
Methohexital sodium (Brevital, JHP Pharmaceuticals)	4-8 mg/kg IV[69]	Poultry
	5-10 mg/kg IV[69]	Ducks
Metomidate HCl (Hypnodil, Janssen)	4 g/cup of bait (usually corn)[69]	Turkeys (wild)
Midazolam HCl	2 mg/kg IM[69]	Canada geese/sedation for 15-20 min
	2-6 mg/kg IM[39]	Quail/PD; mild to heavy sedation
	4-6 mg/kg IM[69]	Waterfowl
	5 mg/kg IV[33]	Turkeys, chickens, ring-necked pheasants, bobwhites/PK; rapid absorption, $t_{1/2}=0.42$, 1.45, 1.90, and 9.71 hr for turkeys, chickens, bobwhites, and pheasants, respectively
Morphine sulfate	1-3 mg/kg intraarticular[56a]	Chickens/PD; no analgesic effect for arthritis noted; early work in chickens demonstrated confusing clinical dosage results[69]
	2.5-3 mg/kg SC, IM q4h[69]	Galliformes/analgesia
	2 mg/kg IV[145]	Chickens/PK; plasma concentrations greater than MEC for humans for 2 hr
	10-20 mg/kg IM[52]	Japanese quail/PD; exhibited antinociceptive effects on foot withdrawal and pressure tests; no effect on locomotion, eating, or drinking at these doses
Propofol	5 mg/kg IV (induction); 0.5 mg/kg/min IV (maintenance)[143]	Wild turkeys/PD; anesthesia; intubation, ventilation, and supplemental oxygen strongly recommended[69,143]
	6-14 mg/kg (induction); boluses prn[69]	Eider ducks/anesthesia with inhalant, bupivacaine, ketoprofen; significant mortality but high-dose bupivacaine toxicity or cumulative bupivacaine/ketoprofen toxicity may have occurred
	8 mg/kg IV (induction); 0.85 mg/kg/min IV (maintenance)[119]	Swans (mute)/PD
	8-10 mg/kg IV (induction); 1-4 mg/kg IV boluses prn (maintenance)[99,100,102]	Mallard ducks, canvasback ducks/PD; anesthesia
	15 mg/kg IV (induction); 0.8 mg/kg/min IV (maintenance)[101]	Canvasback ducks/PD; some excitement during induction; 2 deaths; significant reduction in ventilation

TABLE 6-5 Chemical Restraint/Anesthetic/Analgesic Agents Used in Backyard Poultry and Waterfowl. (cont'd)

Agent	Dosage	Species/Comments
Ropivacaine (Ropi 0.75%, Cristália Chemical & Pharmaceutical)	7.5 mg/kg perineurally[26]	Chickens/15 min to effect for brachial plexus nerve block; approximately 110 min anesthesia; no toxic effects noted at this dose
Sevoflurane	2.21 ± 0.32%[122]	Chickens/PD; minimum anesthetic concentration; dose-dependent hypotension noted
Tiletamine/zolazepam (Telazol, Zoetis)	4-25 mg/kg IM[69]	Waterfowl/sedation; dose generally decreases as body weight increases in waterfowl
	6.6 mg/kg IM[69]	Swans
	9-30 mg/kg IM[69]	Wood partridges/restraint
Tramadol HCl	7.5 mg/kg PO[19]	Peafowl/PK; only 2/6 birds reached human tramadol analgesic concentrations; 5/6 maintained O-desmethyl-tramadol (M1) concentrations above human analgesic concentrations for 10-12 hr and 3/6 for 24 hr; analgesia not evaluated
Xylazine	1 mg/kg IV[98]	Pekin ducks
	1-20 mg/kg IM, IV[27]	Waterfowl/sedation
	10 mg/kg IM[171]	Rock partridges/good sedation; significant decrease in respiratory rate; decrease in cloacal temperature; prolonged recoveries (205 ± 22.2 min)
Yohimbine HCl (Yobine, Lloyd)	—	α_2 adrenergic antagonist; excitement and mortality observed at doses >1 mg/kg[69]
	0.1-0.2 mg/kg IV[27,69]	Waterfowl
	1 mg/kg IV[154]	Guinea fowl/excitement and mortality observed in birds at doses >1 mg/kg[69]

[a]The anesthetic agents of choice in most avian species are the inhalant agents isoflurane and sevoflurane.
[b]All opiod agonists and agonist antagonists may cause respiratory depression; profound bradypnea may occur with potent opioid agonists.
[c]Many poultry species are considered food-producing animal *species,* and as such, these species are regulated by the U.S. Food and Drug Administration (FDA).[166] Even if the individual animals of any of these species are never used for food, they are still regulated by the FDA. The FDA prohibits the use of certain drugs, with no allowable extra-label drug use, in any food-producing animal species. These prohibited drugs are clearly identified in the tables, and the doses are provided in case they are needed for a similar but non-food-producing animal species (e.g., Attwater's prairie chicken), and listings should in no way be misconstrued as an endorsement of using FDA-prohibited drugs in any food-producing animal species. Please refer to the appropriate tables at the end of this chapter regarding the definitions of prohibited drugs, extra-label drugs, labeled drugs, and drugs needing a Veterinary Feed Directive prior to choosing a drug and dose. Please refer to the Food Animal Residue Avoidance Databank at www.farad.org and other sources listed in Table 6.25 for meat and egg withdrawal times.

TABLE 6-6 Nonsteroidal Antiinflammatory Agents Used in Backyard Poultry and Waterfowl.[a,b]

Agent	Dosage	Species/Comments
Acetaminophen	10 mg/kg IM q24h × 7 days[76]	Chicken/no adverse clinical signs, normal serum creatinine and uric acid, no gross or histopathologic changes in kidneys observed
Aspirin (acetylsalicylic acid)	25 mg/kg IV[14,15]	Chickens, ducks, turkeys
	50 mg/kg PO[134a]	Chickens, turkeys/PK; mean residue time 7 hr and 4.5 hr, respectively;[134a] chickens/400 mg/kg PO × 14 days led to decreased weight gain and ventricular ulceration[133,134a]
	50 mg/kg IV[134a]	Chickens, turkeys/PK; mean residue time 6 hr and 3.3 hr, respectively
	100-200 mg/kg IM[74]	Chickens/partially reduced arthritic behaviors after 1 hr
	Dissolve five (5-grain) aspirin tablets in 1 gal of water (=324 mg/gal of drinking water)[114]	Poultry/offer solution free choice to obtain a dosage rate of about 55 mg/kg body weight/day[114]
Carprofen	1 mg/kg SC[110]	Chickens/improved locomotion for at least 90 min post-injection
	5-8 mg/kg PO q12h[173]	Chickens
	15-25 mg/kg SC[25]	Chickens/PD; therapeutically effective treatment of induced articular pain at 6 hr
	30 mg/kg IM[74]	Chickens/PD; arthritis painful behaviors reduced 1 hr post-treatment only with this high dose
	40 mg/kg body weight provided in feed[38]	Chickens/analgesia; dosage required to reach similar mammalian therapeutic plasma concentrations (8.3 μg/mL), but much lower plasma concentrations (0.28 μg/mL) provided some analgesia
Diclofenac	—	Chickens/toxic at dose of 2.5 mg/kg IM q24h × 7 days; severe clinical signs of renal toxicity and high mortality with increased serum creatinine and uric acid concentrations[76]
Flunixin meglumine	—	Potential nephrotoxicity; histologic glomerular changes were demonstrated in bobwhite quail given doses as low as 0.1 mg/kg (severity of lesions was directly correlated to dose);[83] IM administration caused muscle necrosis in mallard ducks[105]
	1.1 mg/kg IV[14]	Chickens, ducks, turkeys, and chickens had long half-life, but ostrich $t_{1/2}$ = 10 min
	3 mg/kg IM[74]	Chickens/PD; arthritis behaviors reduced 1 hr after treatment
	5 mg/kg IM[105]	Mallard ducks/PD; reduced thromboxane activity for 12 hr; muscle necrosis at injection site

TABLE 6-6	Nonsteroidal Antiinflammatory Agents Used in Backyard Poultry and Waterfowl. (cont'd)	
Agent	Dosage	Species/Comments
Flunixin meglumine (cont'd)	5 mg/kg IV[176]	Chickens/PK; $t_{1/2} = 3$ hr
	1.3 mg/kg IV RLP once[137b]	Chickens/pododermatitis; regional limb perfusion (RLP) into medial metatarsal vein with a tourniquet placed proximal to hock joint for 15 min[137b]
Ketoprofen	1 mg/kg IM q24h × 1-10 days[14-16,69]	Waterfowl/arthritis
	2 mg/kg PO, SC, IM, IV[59,60]	Japanese quail/PK, PD; poor bioavailability and rapid clearance after PO or IM administration
	2-5 mg/kg PO, IM, IV q12-24h[69]	Eider ducks/high mortality in male ducks may be due to high bupivacaine dose or cumulative toxicity of bupivacaine and ketoprofen
	3 mg/kg IM q24h × 5 days[115]	Chickens/no adverse clinical signs; normal creatinine, uric acid, ALT, AST
	5 mg/kg IM q12h[104,105]	Mallard ducks/PD; inhibited thromboxane for approximately 12 hr
	5-10 mg/kg IM, IV[27,69]	Waterfowl
	12 mg/kg IM[74]	Chickens/reduced arthritic pain behaviors for 12 hr
Meloxicam	0.5 mg/kg IV[14,15]	Chickens, ducks, turkeys/PK; variable distribution
	1 mg/kg PO, IM q12h[173]	Chicken
	1 mg/kg PO once[146]	Chickens/PK; $t_{1/2} = 2.8$ hr; drug detected in egg white up to 4 days and egg yolk up to 8 days after dosing
	1-1.5 mg/kg PO q12-24h[173]	Chicken
	2 mg/kg IM q12h × 14 days[144]	Japanese quail/PD; unremarkable histologic and minimal biochemical changes
	3-5 mg/kg SC[25]	Chickens/PD; therapeutically effective treatment of induced articular pain at 6 hr
Tepoxalin	30 mg/kg PO, IV[40]	Chickens/PK; rapidly metabolized, $t_{1/2} = 2.8$ hr and 1 hr, respectively[40]

[a]Nonsteroidal antiinflammatory agents may potentially cause gastrointestinal upset and hemorrhage as well as adverse renal effects ranging from fluid retention to renal failure.

[b]Many poultry species are considered food-producing animal *species*, and as such, these species are regulated by the U.S. Food and Drug Administration (FDA).[166] Even if the individual animals of any of these species are never used for food, they are still regulated by the FDA. The FDA prohibits the use of certain drugs, with no allowable extra-label drug use, in any food-producing animal species. These prohibited drugs are clearly identified in the tables, and the doses are provided in case they are needed for a similar but non-food-producing animal species (e.g., Attwater's prairie chicken), and listings should in no way be misconstrued as an endorsement of using FDA-prohibited drugs in any food-producing animal species. Please refer to the appropriate tables at the end of this chapter regarding the definitions of prohibited drugs, extra-label drugs, labeled drugs, and drugs needing a Veterinary Feed Directive prior to choosing a drug and dose. Please refer to the Food Animal Residue Avoidance Databank at www.farad.org and other sources listed in Table 6.25 for meat and egg withdrawal times.

TABLE 6-7 Hormones and Steroids Used in Backyard Poultry and Waterfowl.[a]

Agent	Dosage	Species/Comments
Estradiol benzoate	1 mg/kg IM q24h × 12 days[72]	Mallard ducks/induces molt
Levonorgestrel depot form (Levonorgestrel, Sigma Chemical)	40 mg/kg SC[53,157]	Japanese quail, turkeys/halts egg laying but may cause ovostasis if already in oviduct; repeat in 60 days in turkeys
Levothyroxine (l-thyroxine)	200-400 µg/bird PO q24h × 14 days[150]	Chickens/induces molt
Oxytocin	3-5 U/kg IM, may repeat q30min[69]	Waterfowl
Prostaglandin E_2 (dinoprostone) (Prepidil Gel, Upjohn)	0.02-0.1 mg/kg applied topically to the uterovaginal sphincter[69]	Waterfowl/dystocia; relaxes uterovaginal sphincter; lower dosage may be effective; freeze into aliquots
Prostaglandin $F_{2\alpha}$ (Dinoprost tromethamine) (Lutalyse, Upjohn)	0.02-0.1 mg/kg IM, intracloacal once[16]	Waterfowl/dystocia
Tamoxifen citrate	40 mg/kg IM[72,147]	Galliformes, ducks/induces molt

[a]Many poultry species are considered food-producing animal *species,* and as such, these species are regulated by the U.S. Food and Drug Administration (FDA).[166] Even if the individual animals of any of these species are never used for food, they are still regulated by the FDA. The FDA prohibits the use of certain drugs, with no allowable extra-label drug use, in any food-producing animal species. These prohibited drugs are clearly identified in the tables, and the doses are provided in case they are needed for a similar but non-food-producing animal species (e.g., Attwater's prairie chicken), and listings should in no way be misconstrued as an endorsement of using FDA-prohibited drugs in any food-producing animal species. Please refer to the appropriate tables at the end of this chapter regarding the definitions of prohibited drugs, extra-label drugs, labeled drugs, and drugs needing a Veterinary Feed Directive prior to choosing a drug and dose. Please refer to the Food Animal Residue Avoidance Databank at www.farad.org and other sources listed in Table 6.25 for meat and egg withdrawal times.[54]

TABLE 6-8 Nebulization Agents Used in Backyard Poultry and Waterfowl.[a,b]

Agent	Dosage	Species/Comments
Ceftriaxone	40 mg/mL sterile water[69,80]	Poultry/PD; prohibited drug[54,166]
	40 mg/mL sterile water and DMSO[80]	Poultry/PD; 1 g ceftriaxone in 10 mL sterile water, plus 15 mL DMSO; prohibited drug[54,166]
	200 mg/mL sterile water and DMSO[80]	Poultry/PD; 4 g ceftriaxone in 10 mL sterile water, plus 10 mL DMSO; prohibited drug[54,166]
Lincomycin	250 mg aerosolized drug/m^3 chamber × 15-30 min[28]	Chickens/PD; antibiotic; therapeutic concentrations in blood, lungs, and trachea for up to 24 hr

TABLE 6-8 Nebulization Agents Used in Backyard Poultry and Waterfowl. (cont'd)

Agent	Dosage	Species/Comments
Oxytetracycline	1 g/m^3 of air using a DeVilbiss ultrasonic nebulizer, or 0.075 g/m^3 of air using a Fogmaster fogger[172]	Turkey poults
Tylosin	20 mg/mL DMSO or distilled water × 1 hr[93,94]	Quail/PD

[a]Many poultry species are considered food-producing animal *species*, and as such, these species are regulated by the U.S. Food and Drug Administration (FDA).[166] Even if the individual animals of any of these species are never used for food, they are still regulated by the FDA. The FDA prohibits the use of certain drugs, with no allowable extra-label drug use, in any food-producing animal species. These prohibited drugs are clearly identified in the tables, and the doses are provided in case they are needed for a similar but non-food-producing animal species (e.g., Attwater's prairie chicken), and listings should in no way be misconstrued as an endorsement of using FDA-prohibited drugs in any food-producing animal species. Please refer to the appropriate tables at the end of this chapter regarding the definitions of prohibited drugs, extra-label drugs, labeled drugs, and drugs needing a Veterinary Feed Directive prior to choosing a drug and dose. Please refer to the Food Animal Residue Avoidance Databank at www.farad.org and other sources listed in Table 6.25 for meat and egg withdrawal times.
[b]Nebulization is an adjunctive therapy indicated for rhinitis, sinusitis, tracheitis, pneumonia, airsacculitis, and syringeal aspergilloma, where there is air movement occurring in the patient's disease state; optimal particle size for deposition in the trachea is 2-10 μm; optimal particle size for peripheral airways is 0.5-5 μm; treatments of 30-45 min repeated q4-12h are recommended; caution: do not overhydrate airways.[69]

TABLE 6-9 Agents Used in the Treatment of Toxicologic Conditions of Backyard Poultry and Waterfowl.[a]

Agent	Dosage	Species/Comments
Atropine sulfate	0.1 mg/kg IM, IV q3-4h[16,69]	Waterfowl/acetylcholinesterase toxicosis
Botulinum type C antitoxin (100 U/mL) (National Wildlife Health Center)	1 mL IP[69,109]	Waterfowl/not commercially available; produced for experimental use in migratory birds[69]
Calcium EDTA (edetate calcium disodium)	10-40 mg/kg IM, IV q12h × 5-10 days[16]	Waterfowl
	25-50 mg/kg IV q12h[69]	Geese
Deferiprone (Ferriprox, Apotex)	50 mg/kg PO q12h × 30 days[69,175]	Chickens/PK; iron chelation; may produce rust-colored urates; supplemental zinc may be indicated;[69] an orphan drug in the United States
Magnesium sulfate (Epsom salts)	500-1000 mg/kg PO q24h × 1-3 days[16,69]	Waterfowl/cathartic used in lead toxicosis to encourage passage of heavy-metal particles[16]
Melatonin	10 mg/kg in feed[128]	Chickens/aflatoxin exposure; liver and kidney damage greatly reduced in chicks administered aflatoxin and melatonin concurrently for 21 days[128]
Penicillamine (Cuprimine, Merck)	30-55 mg/kg PO q12h × 7-14 days[69]	Waterfowl
	55 mg/kg PO q12h × 7-14 days[16]	Waterfowl

Continued

TABLE 6-9 Agents Used in the Treatment of Toxicologic Conditions of Backyard Poultry and Waterfowl. (cont'd)

Agent	Dosage	Species/Comments
Pralidoxime mesylate (2-PAM) (Protopam, Wyeth-Ayerst)	10-100 mg/kg IM q24-48h or repeat once after 6 hr[69]	Waterfowl
	100 mg/kg IM, repeat once after 6 hr[16]	Waterfowl

[a]Many poultry species are considered food-producing animal *species,* and as such, these species are regulated by the U.S. Food and Drug Administration (FDA).[166] Even if the individual animals of any of these species are never used for food, they are still regulated by the FDA. The FDA prohibits the use of certain drugs, with no allowable extra-label drug use, in any food-producing animal species. These prohibited drugs are clearly identified in the tables, and the doses are provided in case they are needed for a similar but non-food-producing animal species (e.g., Attwater's prairie chicken), and listings should in no way be misconstrued as an endorsement of using FDA-prohibited drugs in any food-producing animal species. Please refer to the appropriate tables at the end of this chapter regarding the definitions of prohibited drugs, extra-label drugs, labeled drugs, and drugs needing a Veterinary Feed Directive prior to choosing a drug and dose. Please refer to the Food Animal Residue Avoidance Databank at www.farad.org and other sources listed in Table 6.25 for meat and egg withdrawal times.

TABLE 6-10 Nutritional/Mineral Support Used in Backyard Poultry and Waterfowl.

Nutritional and mineral support are uncommon in poultry fed commercially prepared diets that are formulated for their particular physiologic state. To determine if you have a potential nutrient deficiency, at least 5% of your flock should display deficiency signs.[132]

Agent	Dosage	Species/Comments
Biotin	150 mg/ton[89]	Poultry/biotin deficiency
Calcium	—	Recommended dietary levels
	4-8 mg/kg feed (0.4%-0.8%)[125]	Growing Muscovy ducks
	8 mg/kg feed (0.8%)[125]	Growing Japanese quail
	8-10 mg/kg feed (0.8%-1%)[125]	Growing chickens
	18.8-32.5 mg/kg feed (1.88%-3.25%)[125]	Laying chickens/3.25% recommended for hens that lay eggs daily
	22.5 mg/kg feed (2.25%)[125]	Laying turkeys
Folic acid	50-100 μg IM[13]	Poultry chicks/treatment of deficiency; anemia improved in 4 days
	1 mg/kg of feed[89]	Poultry/folic acid deficiency
Iron dextran	10 mg/kg IM, repeat in 7-10 days prn[16,69]	Waterfowl/iron deficiency anemia
Niacin	30 mg/kg of feed[89]	Chickens/niacin deficiency
	55-70 mg/kg of feed[89]	Poultry/niacin deficiency

TABLE 6-10 Nutritional/Mineral Support Used in Backyard Poultry and Waterfowl. (cont'd)

Agent	Dosage	Species/Comments
Pantothenic acid	12 mg/kg of feed[89]	Poultry/pantothenic acid deficiency
	2 mg (calcium pantothenate) +0.5 mg riboflavin in 50 gal (190 L) water × 2-3 day[89]	Poultry/pantothenic acid deficiency
Riboflavin	10 mg/kg of feed[89]	Poultry/riboflavin deficiency
Thiamine	4 mg/kg of feed[89]	
Vitamin B_{12}	Up to 20 mcg/g of feed × 1-2 wk	Poultry/vitamin B_{12} deficiency
Vitamin C (ascorbic acid)	150 mg/kg PO q24h[65]	Willow ptarmigan chicks/PD; supplemental daily requirements over 265-mg/kg diet
Vitamin D3	11-30 min of direct sunlight/day[69]	Chickens/sufficient for endogenous synthesis of vitamin D
Vitamin E/γ-linolenic acid (2%), linoleic acid (71%) (Derm Caps, DVM Pharmaceuticals)	4000 mg linolenic acid/kg feed[120]	Japanese quail/PD; reduces essential fatty acid deficient hepatic lipidosis
Vitamin K_1 (phytonadione)	0.1 mg/kg feed[77]	Turkeys/PD; as effective as 1-2 mg/kg in reducing plasma prothrombin time
Vitamin K_1 (menadione)	1-4 mg/ton of feed[89]	Poultry/for vitamin K deficiency, double the dose

TABLE 6-11 Ophthalmologic Agents Used in Backyard Poultry and Waterfowl.[a]

Agent	Dosage	Species/Comments
Amphotericin B	125 μg/5 mL sterile water subconjunctival[69]	Ducks (ornamental)/candidiasis of third eyelid
Amphotericin B ointment (4%) (formulated)	Topical q24h[69]	Ducks (ornamental)/candidiasis of third eyelid; administered in conjunction with systemic antifungal therapy
Ivermectin	0.005-0.05 mg topical q24h × 10 days[161]	Chicken/PD; conjunctival oxyspirurid (nematode) infection; no adverse effects were seen with topical use

[a]Variable amounts of skeletal muscle are present in the avian iris, giving birds voluntary control over pupil dilation. In many avian patients, the pupils are best dilated by restraining the animal in a dark room.

TABLE 6-12 Oncologic Agents Used in Backyard Poultry and Waterfowl.[a]

Agent	Dosage	Species/Comments
Chlorambucil (Leukeran, GlaxoSmithKline)	1 mg/bird PO 2×/wk[126]	Pekin ducks/lymphocytic leukemia or lymphosarcoma; responded to treatment initially, but was euthanatized 1 mo after presentation because of respiratory distress and hemorrhages
Prednisone	1 mg/kg PO q12h[126]	Ducks/lymphoma; lymphocytic leukemia
Vincristine sulfate	0.5 mg/m2 IV, then 0.75 mg/m² q7d × 3 treatments[126]	Ducks/lymphoma; lymphocytic leukemia

[a]Many poultry species are considered food-producing animal *species*, and as such, these species are regulated by the U.S. Food and Drug Administration (FDA).[166] Even the individual animals of any of these species are never used for food, they are still regulated by the FDA. The FDA prohibits the use of certain drugs, with no allowable extra-label drug use, in any food-producing animal species. These prohibited drugs are clearly identified in the tables, and the doses are provided in case they are needed for a similar but non-food-producing animal species (e.g., Attwater's prairie chicken), and listings should in no way be misconstrued as an endorsement of using FDA-prohibited drugs in any food-producing animal species. Please refer to the appropriate tables at the end of this chapter regarding the definitions of prohibited drugs, extra-label drugs, labeled drugs, and drugs needing a Veterinary Feed Directive prior to choosing a drug and dose. Please refer to the Food Animal Residue Avoidance Databank at http://www.farad.org and other sources listed in Table 6.25 for meat and egg withdrawal times.[54]

TABLE 6-13 Euthanasia Agents Used in Backyard Poultry and Waterfowl.[a]

Agent	Dosage	Comments
Argon	90% Argon with 2% residual oxygen[8,136a]	Chickens/little to no aversion;[8,136a] conditionally acceptable method of euthanasia by the American Veterinary Medical Association (AVMA) if used[8]
Carbon dioxide (CO_2)	—	Chickens/renders the bird unconscious prior to death; unconscious motor activity such as flapping of wings may damage tissues for necropsy and may be disconcerting to the observer;[8] conditionally acceptable method of euthanasia by AVMA if used properly[8]
	>40%[8]-70%[140]	Chickens
Carbon monoxide (CO)	Minimum 6% concentration in a closed container[8,140]	Causes rapid unconsciousness; inexpensive;[69] conditionally acceptable method of euthanasia by AVMA if used properly[8]
Inhalant anesthetics (ex., isoflurane, sevoflurane)	Saturated cotton ball in closed container or face mask;[130a,140] high concentrations (5% or more) using vaporizer are preferred[8]	Rapid induction; wing flapping and vocalizing may occur, less tissue damage compared with other methods;[88,135] conditionally acceptable by AVMA as a sole method of euthanasia if high concentrations used and safety considerations to personnel followed;[8] can also be used to render birds unconscious prior to other methods of euthanasia[8,127]
Nitrogen	100% gas exposure[8]	Conditionally acceptable method of euthanasia by AVMA if used properly

TABLE 6-13 Euthanasia Agents Used in Backyard Poultry and Waterfowl. (cont'd)

Agent	Dosage	Comments
Pentobarbital sodium	0.2-1 mL/kg IV[8]	Acceptable method by AVMA to give IV either conscious or unconscious (under anesthesia); conditionally acceptable method to give intraosseous or intracoelomically only if unconscious or under anesthesia; unacceptable to administer IM due to the low pH, which causes pain;[8,129] birds may react unpredictably with IV administration[8]
Potassium chloride	1-2 mmol/kg IV[8,17]	Conditionally acceptable method by AVMA to give IV only if unconscious or under anesthesia[8]

[a]The 2013 AVMA Guidelines for Euthanasia state that methods regarded as "Acceptable with Conditions" are equivalent to "Acceptable" methods of euthanasia.[8] The AVMA acceptable method is administering a pentobarbital euthanasia solution IV in either an awake or unconscious bird. The AVMA conditionally acceptable methods include inhalant anesthetic overdose, argon, nitrogen, CO, CO_2, cervical dislocation, decapitation, KCl, gunshot, and exsanguination as long as the conditions are met.[8]

TABLE 6-14 Miscellaneous Agents Used in Backyard Poultry and Waterfowl.

Agent	Dosage	Species/Comments
9,10 Anthraquinone (Flight Control, Environmental Biocontrol)	12.6 mL/L water, sprayed q7d on dry, grassy areas where geese frequent[69]	Nuisance Canada geese/deterrent if ingested; birds become nauseated and subsequently avoid the area that contains an ultraviolet dye readily detected by the avian eye
Digoxin	0.0035 mg/kg IV q24h[69]	Turkeys
	0.0049 mg/kg IV q12h[69]	Poultry
	0.01 mg/kg PO q24h × 6 wk[69]	Chickens/ascites syndrome; reduced ascites; no apparent toxicity
	0.019 mg/kg IV q12h[69]	Pekin ducks
Doxapram	10 mg/kg IV once[16]	Waterfowl
Hemoglobin glutamer-200 (Oxyglobin, OPK Biotech)	—	Currently not available in the United States
	5 mL/kg IV[90]	Mallard ducks/PD
	15 mL/kg IV[69]	Chickens/PD; hemoglobin levels fell to near zero by 50 min post-administration
Methocarbamol	32.5 mg/kg PO q12h[69]	Swans/capture myopathy
	50 mg/kg IV (slow bolus)[69]	Swans/muscle relaxation; capture myopathy; may be given q12h for muscle relaxation
Metoclopramide	2 mg/kg IM, IV q8-12h[69]	Waterfowl/crop stasis; ileus
Nicarbazin (OvoControl, Innolytics)	Formulated pellets provided at baiting stations	Waterfowl/egg-hatch control; inhibits sperm receptor sites on the vitelline membrane to prevent fertilization of eggs; check federal and state permit requirements prior to use
Polysulfated glycosaminoglycan (PSGAG) (Adequan, Luitpold)	5 mg/kg IM q7d[69]	Pekin ducks/degenerative joint disease
	10 mg/kg IM, intraarticular q7d × 3 mo[69]	Pheasants/noninfectious or traumatic joint dysfunction; 250 mg/mL for intraarticular use; 500 mg/mL for IM use

TABLE 6-15 Hematologic and Serum Biochemical Values of Selected Galliformes.

Measurement	Chicken (Gallus gallus)[78]	Quail (Coturnix spp.)[a,78,142]	Ring-Necked Pheasant (Phasianus colchicus)[141,181]	Turkey (Meleagris gallopavo)[78]
Hematology				
PCV (%)	23-55	30-45	—	30-46
RBC ($10^6/\mu L$)	1.3-4.5	4-5.2	1.2-3.5	1.7-3.7
Hgb (g/dL)	7-18.6	10.7-14.3	8-11.2	8.8-13.4
MCV (fL)	100-139	60-100	—	112-168
MCH (pg)	25-48	23-35	—	32-49.3
MCHC (g/dL)	20-34	28-39	—	23-35
WBC ($10^3/\mu L$)	9-32	12.5-24.6	18-39	16-25.5
Heterophils (%)	15-50	25-50	12-30	29-52
Lymphocytes (%)	29-84	50-70	63-83	35-48
Monocytes (%)	0.1-7	0.5-3.8	2-9	3-10
Eosinophils (%)	0-16	0-15	0	0-5
Basophils (%)	0-8	0-1.5	0-3	1-9
H:L ratio	0.2-1.7	0.4-1	0.14-0.48	0.6-1.5
Chemistries				
ALT (U/L)	—	6.5-9.6	—	—
AST (U/L)	—	402-422	—	—
Calcium (mg/dL)	13.2-23.7	—	—	11.7-38.7
Cholesterol (mg/dL)	86-211	—	—	81-129
Creatinine (mg/dL)	0.9-1.8	0.01-0.08	—	0.8-0.9
GGT (U/L)	—	1.7-1.9	—	—
Glucose (mg/dL)	227-300	259-312	—	275-425
Phosphorus (mg/dL)	6.2-7.9	—	—	5.4-7.1
Potassium (mEq/L)	3-7.3	1.4	—	6-6.4
Protein, total (g/dL)	3.3-5.5	3.4-3.6	4.5-5.1	4.9-7.6
Albumin (g/dL)	1.3-2.8	1.3-1.5	2.6-2.7	3-5.9
Globulin (g/dL)	1.5-4.1	—	1.9-2.1	1.7-1.9
Sodium (mEq/L)	131-171	180	—	149-155
Uric acid (mg/dL)	2.5-8.1	5.4-5.5	5.6-6	3.4-5.2

[a]Except for phosphorus, protein (total), and sodium, biochemistry values are reported in 16-wk-old Japanese quail.

TABLE 6-16 Hematologic and Serum Biochemical Values of Selected Anseriformes (Waterfowl).

Measurement	Canada Goose (*Branta canadensis*)[24,78]	Mallard Duck (*Anas platyrhynchos*)[181]	Wood Duck (*Aix sponsa*)[24]
Hematology			
PCV (%)	38-58	39-49	46 ± 3
RBC (10^6/μL)	1.6-2.7	2-3.8	2.8 ± 0.2
Hgb (g/dL)	12.7-19.1	7.4-15.6	15 ± 1
MCV (fL)	145-210	148-200	164 ± 14
MCH (pg)	53.7-70	—	—
MCHC (g/dL)	28-32	29-32	33 ± 4
WBC (10^3/μL)	13-21.8	23.4-24.8	25.6 ± 5.7
Heterophils (%)	39	26-38	—
Lymphocytes (%)	46	54-63	—
Monocytes (%)	6	1-4	—
Eosinophils (%)	2	0.2-0.4	—
Basophils (%)	7	0-4	—
H:L ratio	0.5-0.9	0.4-2	0.4-0.7
Chemistries			
ALP (U/L)	72 ± 43	—	160-780
ALT (U/L)	43 ± 11	—	19-48
AST (U/L)	75 ± 17	—	45-123
Bile acid (μmol/L)			
RIA	—	—	22-60
Colorimetric	—	—	—
Calcium (mg/dL)	10.2 ± 0.7	—	7.6-10.4
Chloride (mEq/L)	105 ± 4	—	101-113
Cholesterol (mg/dL)	172 ± 28	—	—
CK (U/L)	—	—	110-480
Creatinine (mg/dL)	0.8 ± 0.3	—	0.3-0.4
GGT (U/L)	2 ± 3	—	0-2.9
Glucose (mg/dL)	210 ± 31	—	232-269
LDH (U/L)	301 ± 80	—	30-205
Phosphorus (mg/dL)	2.8 ± 0.9	—	1.8-4.1
Potassium (mEq/L)	3.4 ± 0.6	—	3.9-4.7
Protein, total (g/dL)	4.8 ± 0.7	—	2.1-3.3
Albumin (g/dL)	2.1 ± 0.2	—	1.5-2.1
Globulin (g/dL)	2.8 ± 0.6	—	0.6-1.2
A:G ratio	0.76 ± 0.13	—	1.5-3.6
Sodium (mEq/L)	142 ± 4	—	141-149
Uric acid (mg/dL)	8.3 ± 2.3	—	2.5-12.9

TABLE 6-17 Biologic and Physiologic Values of Selected Galliformes.[67,68,78]

Species	Incubation Period (days)	Fledgling Age (days)	Weaning Age (days) Parent-Raised	Weaning Age (days) Hand-Reared	Sexual Maturity	Lifespan in Captivity (Maximum) (years)	Body Weight (g)
Galliformes							
Bobwhite quail	—	—	Precocial	—	—	6	—
Peafowl	—	12	Precocial	—	—	20	—
Pheasant, ring-necked	22-24	—	Precocial	—	1 yr	10-18	1150

TABLE 6-18 Biologic and Physiologic Values of Selected Anseriformes (Waterfowl) Species.[69]

Species	Clutch Size	Incubation Period (days)	Fledgling (days)	Sexual Maturity (yr)	Longevity (yr)	Weight (kg) Male	Weight (kg) Female	Respiratory Rate (breaths per minute)	Heart Rate (beats per minute)
Bar-headed goose	4-6	27	—	2	15-20	2-3	2-3	13-40	80-150
Canada goose	4-10	25-30	40-73	—	—	—	—	—	—
Common eider	3-6	25-30	65-75	1	10-15	2.25	2.12	30-95	180-230
European goldeneye	9-11	27-32	—	1	10-15	0.99-1.16	0.7-0.8	30-95	180-230
European wigeon	7-11	23-25	—	1	10-15	0.7	0.64	30-95	180-230
Hawaiian goose	3-5	29	—	2	15-20	2.2	1.9	13-40	80-150
Mallard[a]	8-12	23-29	42-60	1	10-15	1.26	1.1	30-95	180-230
Mandarin duck	9-12	28-30	—	1	10-15	0.44-0.55	0.44-0.55	30-95	180-230
Muscovy duck	8-15	35	—	1	10-15	2-4	1.1-1.5	30-95	180-230
Mute swan	4-8	35-40	—	5	25-30	12.2	8.9	13-40	80-150
Pink-footed goose	3-5	26-27	—	2	15-20	2.6	2.35	13-40	80-150
Red-breasted goose	3-7	23-25	—	2	15-20	1.3-1.6	1.15	13-40	80-150
Tufted duck	6-14	23-25	—	1	10-15	1.1	1.05	30-95	180-230

[a]Except for the Muscovy, all breeds of domestic duck are descended from the mallard (*Anas platyrhynchos*).

TABLE 6-19 Selected Nutritional Recommendations for Wild Bird Rehabilitation.[69]

Waterfowl
- Offer domestic waterfowl, mallard ducks, and Canada geese cracked corn, scratch grains, leafy greens, and nonmedicated waterfowl or poultry diet.
- Swans, particularly trumpeter swans, may refuse to eat for 3 or more days; place the swan in an isolated area, with a slurry of food and fresh greens; do not disturb unless absolutely necessary.
- Offer water in a dish or bucket deep enough to allow the bird to submerge its entire neck before its bill touches the bottom of the container.
- Do not use galvanized metal containers because the zinc may leach into food and water.
- For ducklings, goslings, and cygnets, offer nonmedicated waterfowl or chick starter in shallow dishes and scattered on the floor of the enclosure.
- Tiny pieces of bright fruit, like strawberries, or small, live mealworms may stimulate self-feeding in a hospital setting.

TABLE 6-20 Veterinary Feed Directive (VFD) Order Information.[6,7]

- Note: A VFD is used for drugs given in the food or water of food animals that are given *exactly* per label instructions in regard to dose, concentration, frequency, duration, and so forth and is *not* for extra-label drug use. A VFD is valid up to 6 mo.
- For your convenience, a Veterinary Feed Directive Order fillable form and detailed information can be found on the American Veterinary Medical Association's Web site at www.avma.org/KB/Resources/Pages/VFDInstructions.aspx.[7]
- According to the U.S. Food and Drug Administration (FDA), a valid VFD Order is needed for any feed additive given to a food animal and must be associated with a Valid Client Patient Relationship (VCPR), and it must contain the following:[6]
  - Veterinarian information (name, address, phone) with signature
  - Client information (name, address, phone)
  - Name of the drug, drug concentration, indications for use, and duration of use
  - Dose, withdrawal time
  - Where animals are located (premises) and type (species) and number of animals
  - Date issued, expiration date, indication for use
  - Specified verbiage: "Use of feed containing this VFD drug in a manner other than as directed on the labeling (extra-label use) is not permitted"

TABLE 6-21 Partial List of Antimicrobials Transitioning From Over-the-Counter (OTC) to Veterinary Feed Directive (VFD) Status (as of January 2016).[169]

- Chlortetracycline (CTC)
- Chlortetracycline/sulfamethazine
- Chlortetracycline/sulfamethazine/penicillin
- Hygromycin B
- Lincomycin
- Oxytetracycline
- Oxytetracycline/neomycin
- Penicillin/sulfadimethoxine/ormetoprim
- Tylosin
- Tylosin/sulfamethazine
- Virginiamycin

Note: Apramycin, erythromycin, neomycin (alone), oleandomycin, sulfamerazine, and sulfaquinoxaline are also approved for use in feed and are expected to transition to VFD status but are not marketed at this time. If they return to the market after January 1, 2017, they will require a VFD.

TABLE 6-22 Serologic Tests for Poultry.[23,170]

Test	Test Type[a]	Sample Needed
Avian adenovirus	FA	Tissues
Avian encephalomyelitis	ELISA	Serum
Avian encephalomyelitis	PCR	Tissues
Avian hemorrhagic enteritis	ELISA	Serum
Avian influenza	AGID	Serum
Avian influenza	AGID (egg yolk)	Egg
Avian influenza	ELISA	Serum
Avian influenza	FA	Serum
Avian influenza	PCR	Tissues
Avian influenza	H5 and H7 Typing	Nasal swab
Avian influenza screen	PCR	Tissues, nasal swab, cloacal swab
Avian pneumovirus	PCR	Tissues, tracheal swab, cloacal swab
Avian pneumovirus—type C	PCR	Liver, spleen, heart, kidney, nasal swab
Avian reovirus	ELISA	Serum
Bordetella avium	ELISA	Serum
Chicken profile testing	—	Serum
Chlamydia psittaci	Culture	Affected tissues (heart, liver, spleen, feces)
Chlamydia psittaci	FA	Affected tissues (heart, liver, spleen)
Chlamydia spp.	PCR	Affected tissues
Day-old monitoring	Pathology	1-day-old poultry
Eastern equine encephalitis (EEE) Virus	RT-PCR	Brain tissues, blood
Erysipelothrix spp.	Culture	Affected tissues (kidney, heart, liver, spleen, lung, joint swab, skin)
Exotic Newcastle disease	PCR	Tissues, nasal swab, cloacal swab
Fungal culture	Culture	Affected tissues, poultry litter
Infectious bronchitis virus	ELISA	Serum
Infectious bronchitis virus	PCR	Lung, trachea, kidney swab
Infectious bursal disease virus	ELISA	Serum
Infectious bursal disease virus	PCR	Spleen, bursa
Infectious laryngotracheitis virus	PCR	Trachea, lung
Influenza virus—type A	AGID	Serum
Influenza virus—type A	FA	Affected tissues
Influenza virus—type A screen	PCR	Swabs, tissues
Lead	—	Whole blood
Mycoplasma gallisepticum	ELISA	Serum
Mycoplasma gallisepticum	HI	Serum
Mycoplasma gallisepticum	PCR	Tissues (swab)
Mycoplasma gallisepticum	SPT	Serum
Mycoplasma iowae	PCR	Tissues
Mycoplasma meleagridis	ELISA	Serum

Continued

TABLE 6-22 Serologic Tests for Poultry. (cont'd)

Test	Test Type	Sample Needed
Mycoplasma meleagridis	HI	Serum
Mycoplasma meleagridis	PCR	Tissues
Mycoplasma meleagridis	SPT	Serum
Mycoplasma spp.	Culture	Affected tissues (lung, tracheal wash, nasal swab, joint swab, air sac)
Mycoplasma spp.	PCR	Choanal swab
Mycoplasma synoviae	ELISA	Serum
Mycoplasma synoviae	HI	Serum
Mycoplasma synoviae	PCR	Tissue
Mycotoxin screen (aflatoxin B_1, zearalenone, ochratoxin D, vomitoxin)	—	Stomach contents, feed
Newcastle disease virus (paramyxovirus—type 1)	HI	Serum
Newcastle disease virus screen	PCR	Tissues, swabs
Ornithobacterium rhinotracheale	Culture	Affected tissues (lung, tracheal wash, nasal swab, air sac swab)
Ornithobacterium rhinotracheale	SPT	Serum
Paramyxovirus—type 2	HI	Serum
Paramyxovirus—type 3	HI	Serum
Paramyxovirus—type 7	HI	Serum
Pasteurella multocida	ELISA	Serum
Salmonella enteritidis—phage typing[b]	—	—
Salmonella enteritidis—rapid test	Culture	Pool 50 eggs
Salmonella enteritidis—serotyping confirmation[b]	—	—
Salmonella enteritidis—egg culture BAM method[b]	—	Egg
Salmonella pullorum	MAT	Serum
Salmonella pullorum	SPT	Serum
Salmonella pullorum	STT	Serum
Salmonella pullorum or Salmonella enteritidis	Culture	Tissues
Salmonella spp.	Culture	Affected tissues, feces, feed, water, swabs
Salmonella spp.	Environmental culture	Environmental
Salmonella typhimurium	MAT	Serum
Salmonella typhimurium	STT	Serum
Turkey profile	—	Serum
West Nile virus	PCR	Brain, blood

[a] AGID, Agar gel immunodiffusion; ELISA, enzyme linked immunosorbent assay; FA, fluorescent antibody; FDA, Food and Drug Administration; HI, hemagglutinin inhibition; MAT, modified agglutination test; PCR, polymerase chain reaction; RT-PCR, reverse transcriptase polymerase chain reaction; SPT, skin puncture test; STT, standard tube test.

[b] Following a positive test for Salmonella enteritidis, state and federal authorities are contacted, and additional testing will be performed by those agencies to further an epidemiologic investigation.

TABLE 6-23 Definitions of the Various Designations of Drugs in Food-Producing Animals According to the U.S. Food and Drug Administration (FDA) as They Pertain to Poultry.[5,166]

Designation	Definition	Example
Prohibited, group 1	Drugs with no allowable extra-label uses in any food-producing animal species[166,168]	Chloramphenicol, clenbuterol, diethylstilbestrol (DES), fluoroquinolone-class antibiotics, glycopeptides (all agents, including vancomycin), medicated feeds, nitroimidazoles (all agents, including dimetridazole, ipronidazole, metronidazole, and others), nitrofurans (all agents, including furazolidone, nitrofurazone, and others)
Prohibited, group 2	Drugs with restricted extra-label uses in food-producing animal species[166]	Adamantane and neuraminidase inhibitors (in all poultry, including ducks), cephalosporin-class of antibiotics except cephapirin (in all classes of chickens and turkeys), gentian violet (prohibited from use in food or feed of food-producing animals), and indexed drugs (some exceptions for minor use species); extra-label drug use (ELDU) restrictions apply to all production classes of major food animal species (no ELDU for purpose of disease prevention; no ELDU that involves unapproved dose, treatment duration, frequency, or administration route; and agent must be approved for that species and production class); ELDU restrictions *do not apply* to minor-use food animal species
Extra-label drug use (ELDU)		Use in another species: trimethoprim sulfamethoxazole directly orally to a duck
		Use for a different indication: erythromycin administered as per label instructions but for pododermatitis rather than chronic respiratory disease
		Use at a different dose or frequency: administering spectinomycin for more than the first 3 days of life
		Use via a different route of administration: erythromycin directly orally, not in food or drinking water
		Contact www.farad.org for information regarding potential meat and egg withdrawal
Labeled drug	Used exactly as written on the label, including the species, duration, dose, concentration, frequency, route, and indication	Erythromycin (erythromycin thiocyanate, Gallimycin, Cross VetPharm Group Ltd.): 185 g/ton of feed, to aid in the prevention and reduction of lesions and in lowering severity of chronic respiratory disease; feed for 5 to 8 days; do not use in birds producing eggs for food purposes; withdraw 48 hr before slaughter

TABLE 6-24 Water and Feed Consumption Rates for Backyard Poultry.

Estimated water consumption rates per 100 birds based on age and use. Estimated feed consumption rates for chickens based on weight of food eaten per day expressed as a percentage of body weight.[158]

Use (Age)	Weight (kg)	Water per 100 birds (L)	Feed Expressed as %BW
Hens (non-laying)	—	19	—
Hens (laying)	—	19-28	—
Chickens (4 wk)	—	7.6	—
Chickens (8 wk)	—	15.5	—
Chickens (12 wk)	—	21	—
—	0.23	—	14
—	0.45	—	11.4
—	0.68	—	9.7
—	1.59	—	6.7
—	2.5	—	5.0

TABLE 6-25 Sources of Information on Meat and Egg Withdrawal for Backyard Poultry and Waterfowl.

These sources of information are provided rather than quoting meat and egg withdrawal times because of frequently changing regulations. The status of any medication should be checked prior to administration.[54]

Source	Comments
www.farad.org[54]	Provides information on labeled drug meat and egg withdrawal times as well as an interactive section (VetGram) to ask about estimated meat and egg withdrawal times on extra-label drugs
www.animaldrugsatfda.fda.gov/adafda/views/#/home/previewsearch[165]	Food and Drug Administration website listing all animal drug products approved for safety and effectiveness (a.k.a. the "Green Book"); updated monthly
"Pharmacokinetics of Veterinary Drugs in Laying Hens and Residues in Eggs; a Review of the Literature"[58]	Extensive review article on meat and egg withdrawal for many labeled and extra-labeled drugs
Poultry Medications Formulary, www.poultrymeds.cvpservice.com/catindex/main[131]	A continually updated resource on meat and egg withdrawal times for labeled drugs

TABLE 6-26 Values Reported for Selected Ophthalmic Diagnostic Tests in Avian Species.

Species	Intraocular Pressure (mmHg) by Rebound Tonometry	Phenol Red Thread Test (mm/15 sec $\pm$ STD)
Helmeted guinea fowl, 15-40 mo old[136b]	9.1 ± 0.9	-16.5 ± 1.3
Chicken, 3 wk old[134b]	17.5 ± 0.1	

TABLE 6-27 Selected Vaccines Used in Backyard Poultry.

Disease	Vaccine	Route[a]	Age Administered	Comments
Avian encephalomyelitis	Attenuated	DW	8 wk	Chickens/vaccinate layer/breeder flocks to prevent vertical transmission; may be given in DW up to 4 wk prior to start of production[130b]
	Attenuated	WW	9-15 wk	Chickens/vaccinate breeders to prevent vertical transmission[1b,4b,130b]
Coccidiosis	Live attenuated	PO	1 day+	Chickens, turkeys/controversial results; to use properly, must allow chick access to its own feces to develop cell-mediated immunity by re-exposure to the attenuated strain; for the same reason, do not concurrently treat with anticoccidial drugs; mainly used in breeders or heavily infected flocks[4b,56b,130b]
Fowl cholera	Live attenuated	WW, PO	6 wk	Chickens/not typically given to backyard poultry[4b,30b]
Fowl cholera bacterin		SC	8 and 12 wk	Chickens/killed preparation; may require 2 injections; not typically used in backyard flocks[130b]
Fowl pox	Live vaccine of chick embryo origin	WW	>4 wk	Chickens/used in backyard flocks if there has been a previous problem with this disease; if given <6 wk of age, will not ensure lasting immunity, so repeat at 12-16 wk of age;[162b] not typically given to backyard flocks unless there is a past history of the disease; control mosquitos and reduce stress with good management practices[130b]
			2-3 mo	Turkeys/WW vaccine can cause vaccine reaction on head, so use "thigh-stick" route[4b]
	Tissue culture origin	WW	1 day+	Chickens/can be used in chicks as young as 1 day of age[130b]
	Pigeon pox	WW	—	Chickens/mild vaccine that can be used at any age[130b]
Hemorrhagic enteritis	Live attenuated	—	4-5 wk	Turkeys/reduces clinical signs of disease[4b,130b]
Infectious laryngotracheitis		—	6 wk	Chickens/do not develop permanent immunity until at least 6 wk of age; not typically given to backyard flocks unless there is a past history of the disease[130a]

Continued

TABLE 6-27	Selected Vaccines Used in Backyard Poultry. (cont'd)			
Disease	Vaccine	Route	Age Administered	Comments
Marek's disease	HVT[b] serotype 3	SC, OV	1 day or in ovo	Chickens/typically given at hatchery; most common Marek's vaccine used in backyard flocks[130b]
	Serotype 2	—	1 day	Chickens/naturally avirulent isolates[130b]
	Rispens	—	1 day	Chickens/nononcogenic strains of serotype[130b]
Newcastle's disease	Type B	IN, DW, or spray	1 day, 14 days, and 6 wk	Chickens/usually given in combination with IBV vaccine; common to monitor response to vaccine by HI or ELISA testing; not typically given to backyard flocks[130b]
	Type B	IN, DW, or spray	3 wk	Turkeys/followed by LaSota strain vaccine at 8 wk[130b]
	LaSota	IN, DW, or spray	16-18 wk, q60d during production	Laying chickens/usually administered as a combination vaccine with IBV; can develop upper respiratory vaccine reaction; not typically given to backyard flocks[130b]
Newcastle disease and infectious bronchitis combination		DW, IO, IN	10, 35, and 84 days	Chickens/not typically given to backyard flocks due to varying strains of IBV and morbidity from live IBV vaccine; in layer/breeder flocks, repeat at 3-mo intervals[130b]

[a]*DW*, Drinking water; *IN*, intranasal; *IO*, intraocular; *OV*, in ovo; *PO*, per os; *SC*, subcutaneous; *WW*, wing web (chickens).
[b]*HVT*, Turkey herpesvirus vaccine.

REFERENCES

1a. Abbas RZ, Iqbal Z, Khan MN, et al. Prophylactic efficacy of diclazuril in broilers experimentally infected with three field isolates of *Eimeria tenella*. *Intl J Ag Biol* 2009;11:606-610.
1b. Abdul-Aziz T. Overview of avian encephalomyelitis. *Merck Veterinary Manual*. Available at: http://www.merckvetmanual.com/poultry. Accessed May 19, 2017.
2. Abu-Basha EA, Idkaidek NM, Al-Shunnaq AF. Pharmacokinetics of tilmicosin (Provitil powder and Pulmotil liquid AC) oral formulations in chickens. *Vet Res Com* 2007;31:477-485.
3. Ajadi RA, Kasali OB, Makinde AF, et al. Effects of midazolam on ketamine-xylazine anesthesia in guinea fowl (*Numida meleagris galeata*). *J Avian Med Surg* 2009;23:199-204.
4a. Amelotti I, Catala SS, Gorla DE. Response of *Triatoma infestans* to pour-on cypermethrin applied to chickens under laboratory conditions. *Mem Inst Oswaldo Cruz* 2009;104:481-485.
4b. American Poultry Association. The Poultry Site. Available at: http://www.thepoultrysite.com/diseaseinfo. Accessed May 19, 2017.
5. American Veterinary Medical Association. ELDU and AMDUCA FAQs. Available at: http://www.avma.org/KB/Resources/FAQs/Pages/ELDU-and-AMDUCA-FAQs.aspx. Accessed Feb 4, 2017.
6. American Veterinary Medical Association. AVMA Instructions for Completing a Veterinary Feed Directive (VFD) Order. Available at: http://www.avma.org/KB/Resources/Pages/VFDInstructions.aspx. Accessed Feb 16, 2017.

7. American Veterinary Medical Association. Regulatory Brief: Veterinary Feed Directive. Available at: http://www.avma.org/Advocacy/National/Federal/Pages/FDA-Veterinary-Feed-Directive.aspx. 2017. Accessed Feb 16, 2017.
8. American Veterinary Medical Association Panel on Euthanasia. AVMA Guidelines on Euthanasia: 2013 Edition. www.avma.org/kb/policies/documents/euthanasia.pdf. 2013. Accessed Feb 16, 2017.
9. Anadón A, Bringas P, Martinez-Larrañaga MR, et al. Bioavailability, pharmacokinetics and residues of chloramphenicol in the chicken. *J Vet Pharmacol Therap* 1994;17:52-58.
10. Anadón A, Martinez-Larrañaga MR, Diaz MJ, et al. Pharmacokinetics and residues of enrofloxacin in chickens. *Am J Vet Res* 1995;56:501-506.
11. Anadón A, Martínez-Larrañaga MR, Díaz MJ, et al. Pharmacokinetic characteristics and tissue residues for marbofloxacin and its metabolite N-desmethyl-marbofloxacin in broiler chickens. *Am J Vet Res* 2002;63:927-933.
12. Anadón A, Martinez-Larrañaga MR, Velez C, et al. Pharmacokinetics and residues of enrofloxacin in chickens. *Am J Vet Res* 1992;53:2084-2089.
13. Austic RE, Scott ML. Nutritional diseases. In: Calnek BW, ed. *Diseases of Poultry*. 10th ed. Ames: Iowa State University Press; 1997:47-73.
14. Baert K, de Backer P. Disposition of sodium salicylate, flunixin, and meloxicam after intravenous administration in broiler chickens. *J Vet Pharmacol Therap* 2002;25:449-453.
15. Baert K, de Backer P. Comparative pharmacokinetics of three non-steroidal anti-inflammatory drugs in five bird species. *Comp Biochem Physiol C Toxicol Pharmacol* 2003;134:25-33.
16. Bailey TA, Apo MM. Pharmaceutical products commonly used in avian medicine. In: Samour JH, ed. *Avian Medicine*. 3rd ed. Edinburgh: Mosby Elsevier; 2016:637-678.
17. Beaver BV, Reed W, Leary S, et al. Report of the AVMA panel on euthanasia. *J Am Vet Med Assoc* 2001;218:669-696.
18. Belant JL, Seamans TW. Comparison of three formulations of alpha-chloralose for immobilization of Canada geese. *J Wildl Dis* 1997;33:606-610.
19. Black PA, Cox SK, Macek M, et al. Pharmacokinetics of tramadol hydrochloride and its metabolite O-desmethyltramadol in peafowl (*Pavo cristatus*). *J Zoo Wildl Med* 2010;41:671-676.
20. Black WD. A study of the pharmacodynamics of oxytetracycline in the chicken. *Poult Sci* 1977;56:1430-1434.
21. Brenner DJ, Larsen RS, Dickinson PJ, et al. Development of an avian brachial plexus nerve block technique for perioperative analgesia in mallard ducks (*Anas platyrhynchos*). *J Avian Med Surg* 2010;24:24-34.
22. Burhenne J, Haefeli WE, Hess M, et al. Pharmacokinetics, tissue concentrations, and safety of the antifungal agent voriconazole in chickens. *J Avian Med Surg* 2008;22:199-220.
23. California and Health and Food Safety Laboratory. Lab Test and Fees. cahfs.ucdavis.edu/test_fees/index.cfm. Accessed May 8, 2017.
24. Campbell TW, Smith SA, Zimmerman KL. Hematology of waterfowl and raptors. In: Weiss DJ, Wardrop KJ, eds. *Schalm's Veterinary Hematology*. 6th ed. Ames: Blackwell Publishing; 2010:978-979.
25. Caplen G, Baker L, Hothersall B, et al. Thermal nociception as a measure of non-steroidal anti-inflammatory drug effectiveness in broiler chickens with articular pain. *Vet J* 2013;198:616-619.
26. Cardozo LB, Almeida RM, Fiuza LC, et al. Brachial plexus blockade in chickens with 0.75% ropivacaine. *Vet Anaesth Analg* 2009;36:396-400.
27. Carpenter NA. Anseriform and galliform therapeutics. *Vet Clin North Am Exot Anim Pract* 2000;3:1-17.
28. Chaleva EI, Vasileva IV, Savova MD. Absorption of lincomycin through the respiratory pathways and its influence on alveolar macrophages after aerosol administration to chickens. *Res Vet Sci* 1994;57:245-247.

29. Chapman HD, Matsler PL, Chapman ME. Control of coccidiosis in turkeys with diclazuril and monensin: effects upon performance and development of immunity to *Eimeria* species. *Avian Dis* 2004;48:631-634.
30a. Charlton BR. Poultry use guide. In: Charlton BR, ed. *Avian Disease Manual*. 6th ed. Athens, GA: American Association of Avian Pathologists; 2006:227-231.
30b. Christensen JP. Overview of fowl cholera. *Merck Veterinary Manual*. Available at: http://www.merckvetmanual.com/poultry. Accessed May 19, 2017.
31. Chung HS, Jung WC, Kim DH, et al. Ceftiofur distribution in plasma and tissues following subcutaneously administration in ducks. *J Vet Med Sci* 2007;69:1081-1085.
32. Clark CH, Thomas JE, Milton JL, et al. Plasma concentrations of chloramphenicol in birds. *Am J Vet Res* 1982;43:1949.
33. Cortright KA, Wetzlich SE, Craigmill AL. Plasma pharmacokinetics of midazolam in chickens, turkeys, pheasants and bobwhite quail. *J Vet Pharmacol Ther* 2007;30:429-436.
34. Csikó GY, Banhidi GY, Semjén G, et al. Metabolism and pharmacokinetics of albendazole after oral administration to chickens. *J Vet Pharmacol Therap* 1996;19:322-325.
35. Custer RS, Bush M, Carpenter JW. Pharmacokinetics of gentamicin in blood plasma of quail, pheasants, and cranes. *Am J Vet Res* 1979;40:892-895.
36. Cybulski W, Larsson P, Tjälve H, et al. Disposition of metronidazole in hens (*Gallus gallus*) and quails (*Coturnix coturnix japonica*): pharmacokinetics and whole-body autoradiography. *J Vet Pharmacol Therap* 1996;19:352-358.
37. Da Cunha AF, Messenger KM, Stout RW, et al. Pharmacokinetics of lidocaine and its active metabolite monoethylglycinexylidide after a single intravenous administration in chickens (Gallus domesticus) anesthetized with isoflurane. *J Vet Pharmacol Ther* 2012;35:604-607.
38. Danbury TC, Weeks CA, Chambers JP, et al. Self-selection of the analgesic drug carprofen by lame broiler chickens. *Vet Rec* 2000;146:307-311.
39. Day TK, Roge CK. Evaluation of sedation in quail induced by use of midazolam and reversed by use of flumazenil. *J Am Vet Med Assoc* 1996;209:969-971.
40. De Boever S, Neirinckx E, Baert K, et al. Pharmacokinetics of tepoxalin and its active metabolite in broiler chickens. *J Vet Pharmacol Ther* 2009;32:97-100.
41a. Dein FJ, Monard DF, Kowalczyk DF. Pharmacokinetics of chloramphenicol in Chinese spot-billed ducks. *J Vet Pharmacol Therap* 1980;3:161-168.
41b. Delaski KM, Gehring R, Heffron BT, et al. Plasma concentrations of fentanyl achieved with transdermal application in chickens. *J Avian Med and Surg* 2017;31:6-15.
42. Devriese L, Dutta G. Effects of erythromycin inactivating *Lactobacillus* crop flora on blood levels. *J Vet Pharmacol Therap* 1984;7:49-53.
43. Efstathopoulos N, Giamarellos-Bourboulis E, Kanellakopoulou K, et al. Treatment of experimental osteomyelitis by methicillin resistant *Staphylococcus aureus* with bone cement system releasing grepafloxacin. *Injury* 2008;39:1384-1390.
44. El-Banna HA, El-Bahy MM, El-Zorba HY, et al. Anticoccidial efficacy of drinking water soluble diclazuril on experimental and field coccidiosis in broiler chickens. *J Vet Med A Physiol Pathol Clin Med* 2005;52:287-291.
45. El-Gammal AA, Ravis WR, Krista LM, et al. Pharmacokinetics and intramuscular bioavailability of amikacin in chickens following single and multiple dosing. *J Vet Pharmacol Therap* 1992;15:133-142.
46. El-Gendi AY. el-Banna HA, Abo Norag M, et al. Disposition kinetics of danofloxacin and ciprofloxacin in broiler chickens. *Dtsch Tierarztl Wochenschr* 2001;429-434.
47. El-Kholy H, Kemppainen B, Ravis W, et al. Pharmacokinetics of levamisole in broiler breeder chickens. *J Vet Pharm Therap* 2006;29:49-53.
48. Elviss NC, Williams LK, Jørgensen F, et al. Amoxicillin therapy of poultry flocks: effect upon the selection of amoxicillin-resistant commensal *Campylobacter* spp. *J Antimicrob Chemother* 2009;64:702-711.
49. Escobar A, da Rocha RW, Pypendop BH, et al. Effects of methadone on the minimum anesthetic concentration of isoflurane, and its effects on heart rate, blood pressure and

ventilation during isoflurane anesthesia in hens (*Gallus gallus domesticus*). *PLoS One* 2016;28 (11):1-12.
50. Escobar A, Valadao CA, Brosnan RJ, et al. Cardiopulmonary effects of butorphanol in sevoflurane-anesthetized guinea fowl (*Numida meleagris*). *Vet Anesth Anal* 2014;41:284-289.
51. Espigol C, Artigas C, Palmada J, et al. Serum levels of doxycycline during water treatment in poultry. *J Vet Pharmacol Therap* 1997;20:192-193.
52. Evrard HC, Balthazart J. The assessment of nociceptive and non-nociceptive skin sensitivity in the Japanese quail (*Coturnix japonica*). *J Neurosci Methods* 2002;116:135-146.
53. Fontenot DK, Terrell SP, Neiffer DL, et al. Clinical trial of a depot form of levonorgestrel in domestic turkeys. *Proc Annu Conf Assoc Avian Vet* 2002;43.
54. Food Animal Residue Avoidance Databank (FARAD). Available at http://www.farad.org. Accessed May 18, 2017.
55. García-Ovando H, Chiostri E, Ugnia L, et al. HPLC residues of enrofloxacin and ciprofloxacin in eggs of laying hens. *J Vet Pharmacol Therap* 1997;20:204.
56a. Gentle MJ, Hocking PM, Bernard R, et al. Evaluation of intraarticular opioid analgesia for the relief of articular pain in the domestic fowl. *Pharmacol Biochem Behav* 1999;63:339-343.
56b. Gerhold R. Parasitic diseases. In: Greenacre CB, Morishita TY, eds. *Backyard Poultry Medicine and Surgery: A Guide for Veterinary Practitioners.* Ames: Wiley; 2015:297-320.
57. Giorgi M, Soldani G. Pharmacokinetic study of clazuril (Appertex) in eggs and plasma from laying hens after single or multiple treatments, using a new HPLC method for detection. *Br Poult Sci* 2008;49:609-618.
58. Goetting V, Lee KA, Tell LA. Pharmacokinetics of veterinary drugs in laying hens and residues in eggs; a review of the literature. *J Vet Pharmacol Therap* 2011;34:521-556.
59. Graham JE, Tell LA, Kollias-Baker C, et al. Pharmacokinetics of ketoprofen in adult Japanese quail (*Coturnix japonica*). *Proc Annu Conf Assoc Avian Vet* 2001;19-21.
60. Graham JE, Tell LA, Kollias-Baker C, et al. Preliminary investigation into the pharmacodynamics of ketoprofen in quail. *Proc Annu Conf Assoc Avian Vet* 2002;75-76.
61. Guo FC, Suo X, Zhang GZ, et al. Efficacy of decoquinate against drug sensitive laboratory strains of *Eimeria tenella* and field isolates of *Eimeria* spp. in broiler chickens in China. *Vet Parasitol* 2007;147:239-245.
62. Hamamoto K, Koike R, Machida Y. Bioavailability of amprolium in fasting and nonfasting chickens after intravenous and oral administration. *J Vet Pharmacol Ther* 2000;23:9-14.
63. Hamdy AH, Kratzer DD, Paxton LM, et al. Effect of a single injection of lincomycin, spectinomycin, and linco-spectin on early chick mortality caused by *E. coli* and *S. aureus*. *Avian Dis* 1979;24:164-173.
64. Hamdy AH, Saif YM, Kasson CW. Efficacy of lincomycin-spectinomycin water medication on *Mycoplasma meleagridis* airsacculitis in commercially reared turkey poults. *Avian Dis* 1982;26:227-233.
65. Hanssen I, Grav HJ, Steen H. Vitamin C deficiency in growing willow ptarmigan (*Lagopus lagopus lagopus*). *J Nutr* 1979;109:2260-2276.
66. Haritova AM, Rusenova NV, Parvanov PR, et al. Integration on pharmacokinetic and pharmacodynamic indices of marbofloxacin in turkeys. *Antimicrob Agents Chemother* 2006;50:3779-3785.
67. Harrison GJ, Harrison LR, eds. In: *Clinical Avian Medicine and Surgery*. Philadelphia: WB Saunders Co; 1986:662-663.
68. Harvey R. *Practical Incubation*. Payn Essex Printers Ltd, Sudbury: Suffolk, UK; 1990.
69. Hawkins MG, Barron HW, Speer BL, et al. Birds. In: Carpenter JW, ed. 4th ed. St. Louis: Elsevier; 2013:183-437. Exotic Animal Formulary.
70. Hawkins MG, Taylor IT, Byrne BA, et al. The pharmacokinetics and pharmacodynamics of orbifloxacin in Japanese quail (*Coturnix coturnix japonica*). *Proc Annu Conf Assoc Avian Vet* 2010;25.
71. Heinen E, DeJong A, Scheer M. Antimicrobial activity of fluoroquinolones in serum and tissues in turkeys. *J Vet Pharmacol Therap* 1997;20(Suppl 1):196-197.

72. Hines R, Kolattukuty PE, Sharkey P. Pharmacological induction of molt and gonadal involution in birds. *Proc Annu Conf Assoc Avian Vet* 1993;127-134.
73. Hirsh DC, Knox SJ, Conzelman Jr GM, et al. Pharmacokinetics of penicillin-G in the turkey. *Am J Vet Res* 1978;39:1219-1221.
74. Hocking PM, Robertson GW, Gentle MJ. Effects of non-steroidal anti-inflammatory drugs on pain-related behaviour in a model of articular pain in the domestic fowl. *Res Vet Sci* 2005;78:69-75.
75. Islam KM, Klein U, Burch DG. The activity and compatibility of the antibiotic tiamulin with other drugs in poultry medicine—a review. *Poult Sci* 200;88:2353-2359.
76. Jayakumar K, Mohan K, Swamy HD, et al. Study of nephrotoxic potential of acetaminophen in birds. *Toxicol Int* 2010;17:86-89.
77. Jin S, Sell JL. Dietary vitamin K_1 requirements and comparison of biopotency of different vitamin K sources for young turkeys. *Poult Sci* 2001;80:615-620.
78. Johnson-Delaney CA, Harrison LR, eds. *Exotic Companion Medicine Handbook for Veterinarians*. Lake Worth, FL: Wingers Publishing; 1996.
79. Jordan FTW, Horrocks BK. The minimum inhibitory concentration of tilmicosin and tylosin for *Mycoplasma gallisepticum* and *Mycoplasma synoviae* and a comparison of their efficacy in the control of *Mycoplasma gallisepticum* infection in chickens. *Avian Dis* 1997;41:802-807.
80. Junge RE, Naeger LL, LeBeau MA, et al. Pharmacokinetics of intramuscular and nebulized ceftriaxone in chickens. *J Zoo Wildl Med* 1994;25:224-228.
81. Keitzmann M, Knoll U, Glünder G. Pharmacokinetics of enrofloxacin and danofloxacin in broiler chickens. *J Vet Pharmacol Therap* 1997;20(Suppl 1):202.
82. Kempf I, Reeve-Johnson L, Gesbert F, et al. Efficacy of tilmicosin in the control of experimental *Mycoplasma gallisepticum* infection in chickens. *Avian Dis* 1997;41:802-807.
83. Klein PN, Charmatz K, Langenberg J. The effect of flunixin meglumine (Banamine®) on the renal function in northern bobwhite (*Colinus virginianus*): an avian model. *Proc Annu Conf Am Assoc Zoo Vet* 1994;128-131.
84. Knoll U, Glunder G, Kietzmann M. Compare study of the plasma pharmacokinetics and tissue concentrations of danofloxacin and enrofloxacin in broiler chickens. *J Vet Pharmacol Ther* 1999;22:239-246.
85. Kollias GV, Zgola MM, Weinkle TK, et al. Amikacin sulfate pharmacokinetics in ring-necked pheasants (*Phasianus colchicus*): age and route dependent effects. *Proc Annu Conf Am Assoc Zoo Vet* 1996;178-180.
86. Laczay P, Semjén G, Nagy G, et al. Comparative studies on the pharmacokinetics of norfloxacin in chickens, turkeys, and geese after a single oral administration. *J Vet Pharmacol Therap* 1998;21:161-164.
87. Lashev LD, Mihailov R. Pharmacokinetics of apramycin in Japanese quail. *J Vet Pharmacol Therap* 1994;17:394-395.
88. Latimer KS, Rakich PM. Necropsy examination. In: Ritchie BW, Harrison GJ, Harrison LR, eds. *Avian Medicine: Principles and Application*. Lake Worth: Wingers Publishing Inc; 1994:355-379.
89. Leeson S. Vitamin deficiencies in poultry. *Merck Veterinary Manual*. Available at: http://www.merckvetmanual.com/poultry/nutrition-and-management-poultry/vitamin-deficiencies-in-poultry#v3347924. Accessed May 8, 2017.
90. Lichtenberger M, Chavez W, Cray C, et al. Mortality and response to fluid resuscitation after acute blood loss in mallard ducks. *Proc Annu Conf Assoc Avian Vet* 2003;7-10.
91. Lin E, Luscombe C, Colledge G, et al. Long-term therapy with the guanine nucleoside analog penciclovir controls chronic duck hepatitis B virus infection in vivo. *Antimicrob Agents Chemother* 1998;42:2132-2137.
92. Lister S, Houghton-Wallace J. Backyard poultry 2. Veterinary care and disease control. *In Pract* 2012;34:214-225.
93. Locke D, Bush M. Tylosin aerosol therapy in quail and pigeons. *J Zoo Anim Med* 1984;15:67-72.

94. Locke D, Bush M, Carpenter JW. Pharmacokinetics and tissue concentrations of tylosin in selected avian species. *Am J Vet Res* 1982;43:1807-1810.
95. Loibl MF, Clutton RE, Marx BD, et al. Alpha-chloralose as a capture and restraint agent of birds: therapeutic index determination in the chicken. *J Wildl Dis* 1988;24:684-687.
96. Lublin Z, Mechani S, Malkinson M, et al. Efficacy of norfloxacin nicotinate treatment of broiler breeders against *Haemophilus paragallinarum*. *Avian Dis* 1993;37:673-679.
97. Ludders JW, Mitchell GS, Rode J. Minimal anesthetic concentration and cardiopulmonary dose response of isoflurane in ducks. *Vet Surg* 1990;19:304-307.
98. Ludders JW, Rode J, Mitchell GS, et al. Effects of ketamine, xylazine, and a combination of ketamine and xylazine in Pekin ducks. *Am J Vet Res* 1989;50:245-249.
99. Machin KL, Caulkett NA. Cardiopulmonary effects of propofol and a medetomidine-midazolam-ketamine combination in mallard ducks. *Am J Vet Res* 1998;59:598-602.
100. Machin KL, Caulkett NA. Investigation of injectable anesthetic agents in mallard ducks (*Anas platyrhynchos*): a descriptive study. *J Avian Med Surg* 1998;12:255-262.
101. Machin KL, Caulkett NA. Cardiopulmonary effects of propofol infusion in canvasback ducks (*Aythya valisineria*). *J Avian Med Surg* 1999;13:167-172.
102. Machin KL, Caulkett NA. Evaluation of isoflurane and propofol anesthesia for intraabdominal transmitter placement in nesting female canvasback ducks. *J Wildl Dis* 2000;36:324-334.
103. Machin KL, Livingston A. Plasma bupivacaine levels in mallard ducks (*Anas platyrhynchos*) following a single subcutaneous dose. *Proc Annu Conf Am Assoc Zoo Vet/Am Assoc Wildl Vet/Assoc Rept Amph Vet/Nat Assoc Zoo Wildl Vet* 2001;159-163.
104. Machin KL, Livingston A. Assessment of the analgesic effects of ketoprofen in ducks anesthetized with isoflurane. *Am J Vet Res* 2002;63:821-826.
105. Machin KL, Tellier LA, Lair S, et al. Pharmacodynamics of flunixin and ketoprofen in mallard ducks (*Anas platyrhynchos*). *J Zoo Wildl Med* 2001;32:222-229.
106. Macklin KS. Overview of helminthiasis in poultry. *Merck Veterinary Manual*. Available at: http://www.merckvetmanual.com/poultry/helminthiasis/overview-of-helminthiasis-in-poultry. Accessed May 18, 2017.
107. Maiti SK, Tiwary R, Vasan P, et al. Xylazine, diazepam and midazolam premedicated ketamine anaesthesia in white Leghorn cockerels for typhlectomy. *J S Afr Vet Assoc* 2006;77:12-18.
108. Martin-Jurado O, Vogt R, Kutter APN, et al. Effect of inhalation of isoflurane at end-tidal concentrations greater than, equal to, and less than the minimum anesthetic concentration on the bispectral index in chickens. *Am J Vet Res* 2008;69:1254-1261.
109. Martinez R, Wobeser G. Immunization of ducks for type C botulism. *J Wildl Dis* 1999;35:710-715.
110. McGeown D, Danbury TC, Waterman-Pearson AE, et al. Effect of carprofen on lameness in broiler chickens. *Vet Rec* 1999;144:668-671.
111. Meredith A. Chickens as patients. *Proc Assoc Avian Vet (AC) and Unusual/Exot Pets*. Available at: http://www.vin.com/members/cms/project/defaultadv1.aspx?id=6422183&pid=11392. 2013. Accessed May 18, 2017.
112. Midgley-DiGeronimo PM, Rinaldi M, da Cunha A, et al. Median toxic dose of intravenous bupivacaine in isoflurane-anesthetized Ross-708 broiler chickens. *Proc Annu Conf Assoc Avian Vet/ExoticsCon* 2016;59.
113. Migaki TT, Avakian AP, Barnes HJ, et al. Efficacy of danofloxacin and tylosin in the control of mycoplasmosis in chicks infected with tylosin-susceptible or tylosin-resistant field isolates of *Mycoplasma gallisepticum*. *Avian Dis* 1993;37:508-514.
114. Mississippi State University Extension. Solutions and treatments. Available at: http://www.extension.msstate.edu/content/solutions-and-treatments. Accessed Feb 13, 2017.
115. Mohan K, Jayakumar K, Narayanaswamy HD, et al. An initial safety assessment of hepatotoxic and nephrotoxic potential of intramuscular ketoprofen at single repetitive dose level in broiler chickens. *Poult Sci* 2012;91:1308-1314.
116. Mohiti-Asli M, Ghanaatparast-Rashti M. Dietary oregano essential oil alleviates experimentally induced coccidiosis in broilers. *Prev Vet Med*. 2015;120:195-202.

117. Mostachio GQ, de-Oliveira LD, Carciofi AC. The effects of anesthesia with a combination of intramuscular xylazine-diazepam-ketamine on heart rate, respiratory rate and cloacal temperature in roosters. *Vet Anaesth Analg* 2008;35:232-236.
118. Mulcahy DM, Stoskopf MK, Esler D. Lack of isoflurane-sparing effect of butorphanol in field anesthesia of harlequin ducks (*Histrionicus histrionicus*). *Proc Annu Conf Am Assoc Zoo Vet/ Int Assoc Aquatic Anim Med* 2000;532-533.
119. Muller K, Holzapfel J, Brunnberg L. Total intravenous anaesthesia by boluses or by continuous rate infusion of propofol in mute swans (*Cygnus olor*). *Vet Anaesth Analg* 2011;38:286-291.
120. Murai A, Furuse M, Okumura J-I. Involvement of (n-6) essential fatty acids and prostaglandins in liver lipid accumulation in Japanese quail. *Am J Vet Res* 1996;57:342-345.
121. Naccari F, Salpietro DC, DeSarro A, et al. Tolerance and pharmacokinetics of ciprofloxacin in the chick. Preliminary experience in subjects of pediatric age with urinary tract infections. *Res Commun Mol Pathol Pharmacol* 1998;99:187-192.
122. Naganobu K, Fujisawa Y, Ohde H, et al. Determination of the minimum anesthetic concentration and cardiovascular dose response for sevoflurane in chickens during controlled ventilation. *Vet Surg* 2000;29:102-105.
123. National Office for Animal Health (NOAH). Antibiotics for Animals. Available at: http://www.noah.co.uk/medicine-topics/antibiotics-for-animals. Accessed Feb 13, 2017.
124. National Registration Authority for Agricultural and Veterinary Chemicals. *Dimetridazole Scope Document*. 2012. Available at: http://apvma.gov.au/sites/default/files/publication/15036-dimetridazole-final-report.pdf. Accessed July 18, 2017.
125. National Research Council. *Nutrient Requirements of Poultry*. Washington, DC: National Academy Press; 1994.
126. Newell SM. Diagnosis and treatment of lymphocytic leukemia and malignant lymphoma in a Pekin duck (*Anas platyrhyncos domesticus*). *J Assoc Avian Vet* 1991;5:83-86.
127. Orosz S. Birds. In: American Association of Zoo Veterinarians (AAZV). *Guidelines for Euthanasia of Nondomestic Animals*. Yulee: AAZV, 2006:46-49.
128. Ozen H, Karaman M, Ciğremiş Y, et al. Effectiveness of melatonin on aflatoxicosis in chicks. *Res Vet Sci* 2009;86:485-489.
129. Paul-Murphy J, Koch VW, Briscoe JA, et al. Advancements in the management of the welfare of avian species. In: Speer BL, ed. *Current Therapy in Avian Medicine and Surgery*. St. Louis: Elsevier; 2016:669-718.
130a. Porter SL. Euthanasia techniques for wildlife. *Proc North Am Vet Conf* 1994;925.
130b. Morishita TY, Porter RE. Gastrointestinal and hepatic diseases. In: Greenacre CB, Morishita TY, eds. *Backyard Poultry Medicine and Surgery: A Guide for Veterinary Practitioners*. Ames: Wiley; 2015:297-320.
131. *Poultry Medications Formulary*. North American Compendiums. Available at: http://www.poultrymeds.cvpservice.com/catindex/main. Accessed Feb 16, 2017.
132. Poultry Site. Available at http://www.thepoultrysite.org. Accessed Feb 16, 2017.
133. Poźniak B, Świtała M, Jaworski K, et al. Comparative pharmacokinetics of acetylsalicylic acid and sodium salicylate in chickens and turkeys. *Br Poult Sci* 2013;54:538-544.
134a. Poźniak B, Switała M, Bobrek K, et al. Adverse effects associated with high-dose acetylsalicylic acid and sodium salicylate treatment in broilers. *Br Poult Sci* 2012;53:777-783.
134b. Prashar A, Guggenheim JA, Erichsen JT, et al. Measurement of intraocular pressure (IOP) in chickens using a rebound tonometer: quantitative evaluation of variance due to position inaccuracies. *Exp Eye Res* 2007;85:563-571.
135. Rae M. Necropsy. In: Palm Beach: Spix Publishing; 2006:661–678. Lightfoot TL, Harrison GJ, eds. Clinical Avian Medicine; Vol 2.
136a. Raj ABM, Gregory NG, Wotton SB. Changes in the somatosensory evoked potentials and spontaneous electroencephalogram of hens during stunning in argon-induced anoxia. *Br Vet J* 1991;147:322-330.

136b. Rajaei SM, Ansari Mood M, Sohail Ghazanfari Hashemi S. Measurement of tear production and intraocular pressure in healthy captive helmeted guinea fowl (*Numida meleagris*). *J Avian Med Surg* 2016;30:324-328.
137a. Rathinam T, Chapman HD. Sensitivity of isolates of *Eimeria* from turkey flocks to the anticoccidial drugs amprolium, clopidol, diclazuril, and monensin. *Avian Dis* 2009;53:405-408.
137b. Ratliff CM, Zaffarano BA. Therapeutic use of regional limb perfusion in a chicken. *J Avian Med Surg* 2017;31:29-32.
138. Rolinski Z, Kowalski C, Wlaz P. Distribution and elimination of norfloxacin from broiler chicken tissues and eggs. *J Vet Pharmacol Therap* 1997;20:200-201.
139. Sarkozy G, Semjen G, Laczay P, et al. Treatment of experimentally induced *Pasteurella multocida* in broilers and turkeys: comparative studies of different oral treatment regimens. *J Vet Med B Infect Dis Vet Public Health* 2002;49:130-134.
140. Schaeffer DO. Avian euthanasia. *Proc Annu Conf Assoc Avian Vet* 1996;287-288.
141. Schmidt EMS, Paulillo AC, Dittrich RL, et al. Serum biochemical parameters in the ring-necked pheasant (*Phasianus colchius*) on breeding season. *Int J Poult Sci* 2007;6:673-674.
142. Scholtz N, Halle I, Flachowsky G, et al. Serum chemistry reference values in adult Japanese quail (*Coturnix coturnix japonica*) including sex-related differences. *Poult Sci* 2009;88:1186-1190.
143. Schumacher J, Citino SB, Hernandez K, et al. Cardiopulmonary and anesthetic effects of propofol in wild turkeys. *Am J Vet Res* 1997;58:1014-1017.
144. Sinclair K, Paul-Murphy J, Church M, et al. Renal physiologic and histopathologic effects of meloxicam in Japanese quail (*Coturnix japonica*). *Proc Annu Conf Assoc Avian Vet/Assoc Exotic Mam Vet* 2010;287-288.
145. Singh PM, Johnson C, Gartrell B, et al. Pharmacokinetics of morphine after intravenous administration in broiler chickens. *J Vet Pharmacol Ther* 2010;33:515-518.
146. Souza MJ, White MS, Gordon KI, et al. Pharmacokinetics and egg residues after oral meloxicam use in poultry. *Proc Annu Conf Assoc Avian Vet/ExoticsCon* 2016;43.
147. Stake PE. Tamoxifen induced forced-rest/molt in laying hens. *Poult Sci* 1979;58:1111.
148. Stetter MD, Sheppard C, Cook RA. Itraconazole-impregnated synthetic grit for sustained release dosing in avian species. *Proc Annu Conf Am Assoc Zoo Vet* 1996;181-185.
149. Stipkovits L, Burch DGS, Salyi G, et al. Study to test the compatibility of Tetramutin® given in feed at different levels with salinomycin (60 ppm) in chickens. *J Vet Pharmacol Therap* 1997;20:191-192.
150. Szelenyi Z, Peczely P. Thyroxine induced moult in domestic hen. *Acta Physiol Hung* 1988;72:143-149.
151. Tanner AC. Antimicrobial drug use in poultry. In: Prescott J, Baggot J, eds. *Antimicrobial Therapy in Veterinary Medicine*. 3rd ed. Ames: Iowa State University Press; 2000:637-655.
152. Tanner AC, Avakian AP, Barnes HJ, et al. A comparison of danofloxacin and tylosin in the control of induced *Mycoplasma gallisepticum* infection in broiler chicks. *Avian Dis* 1993;37:515-522.
153. Taylor SM, Kenny J, Houston A, et al. Efficacy, pharmacokinetics and effect on egg-laying and hatchability of two dose rates of in-feed fenbendazole for the treatment of *Capillaria* species infections in chickens. *Vet Rec* 1993;133:519-521.
154. Teare JA. Antagonism of xylazine hydrochloride-ketamine hydrochloride immobilization in guinea fowl (*Numidia meleagris*) by yohimbine hydrochloride. *J Wildl Dis* 1987;23:301-305.
155. Teare JA, Schwark WS, Shin SJ, et al. Pharmacokinetics of a long-acting oxytetracycline preparation in ring-necked pheasants, great horned owls and Amazon parrots. *Am J Vet Res* 1985;46:2639-2643.
156. Tell L, Harrenstien L, Wetzlich S, et al. Pharmacokinetics of ceftiofur sodium in exotic and domestic avian species. *J Vet Pharmacol Therap* 1998;21:85-91.

157. Tell L, Shukla A, Munson L, et al. A comparison of the effects of slow release, injectable levonorgestrel and depot medroxyprogesterone acetate on egg production in Japanese quail (*Coturnix coturnix japonica*). *J Avian Med Surg* 1999;13:23-31.
158. Tell LA. Regulatory considerations for medicine use in poultry. In: Greenacre CB, Morishita TY, eds. *Backyard Poultry Medicine and Surgery: A Guide for Veterinary Practitioners*. Ames: Wiley; 2015:297-320.
159. Tell LA, Clemons KV, Kline Y, et al. Efficacy of voriconazole in Japanese quail (*Coturnix japonica*) experimentally infected with Aspergillus fumigatus. *Med Mycol* 2010;48:234-244.
160. Tell LA, Craigmill AL, Clemons KV, et al. Studies on itraconazole delivery and pharmacokinetics in mallard ducks (*Anas platyrhynchos*). *J Vet Pharmacol Therap* 2005;28:267-274.
161. Thomas-Baker B, Dew RD, Patton S. Ivermectin treatment of ocular nematodiasis in birds. *J Am Vet Med Assoc* 1986;189:1113.
162a. Thuesen LR, Bertelsen MF, Brimer L, et al. Selected pharmacokinetic parameters for cefovecin in hens and green iguanas. *J Vet Pharmacol Ther* 2009;32:613-617.
162b. Tripathy DN. Fowl pox in chickens and turkeys. *Merck Veterinary Manual*. Available at: http://www.merckvetmanual.com/poultry. Accessed May 19, 2017.
163. Tsiquaye KN, Slomka MJ, Maung M. Oral famciclovir against duck hepatitis B virus replication in hepatic and nonhepatic tissues of ducklings infected in ovo. *J Med Virol* 1994;42:306-310.
164. Turbahn A, De Jäckel SC, Greuel E, et al. Dose response study of enrofloxacin against *Riemerella anatipestifer* septicaemia in Muscovy and Pekin ducklings. *Avian Pathol* 1997;26:791-802.
165. U.S. Food and Drug Administration. Animal Drugs. Available at: https://animaldrugsatfda.fda.gov/adafda/views/#/home/previewsearch. Accessed May 18, 2017.
166. U.S. Food and Drug Administration. Extralabel Use and Microbials. Available at: http://www.fda.gov/AnimalVeterinary/SafetyHealth/AntimicrobialResistance/ucm421527.htm. Accessed Feb 16, 2017.
167. U.S. Food and Drug Administration. FDA Prohibits Nitrofuran Drug Used in Food-Producing Animal. Available at: http://www.fda.gov/cvm/index/updates/nitroup.htm. 2002. Accessed Feb 16, 2017.
168. U.S. Food and Drug Administration. Reminder—Extra-Label Use of Fluoroquinolones Prohibited. Available at: http://www.fda.gov/cvm/index/updates/noeluflq.htm. 2002. Accessed Feb 16, 2017.
169. U.S. Food and Drug Administration. Drugs Transitioning from Over-the-Counter (OTC) to Veterinary Feed Directive (VFD) Status. Available at: http://www.fda.gov/AnimalVeterinary/DevelopmentApprovalProcess/ucm482107.htm. 2016. Accessed Feb 13, 2017.
170. University of Connecticut Cooperative Extension, College of Agriculture and Natural Resources. *Poultry Diseases and Medications for Small Flocks*. Available at: http://web.uconn.edu/poultry/poultrypages/diseasefactsheet.html#deficiencies. Accessed Feb 13, 2017.
171. Uzun M, Onder F, Atalan G, et al. Effects of xylazine, medetomidine, detomidine, and diazepam on sedation, heart and respiratory rates, and cloacal temperature in rock partridges (*Alectoris graeca*). *J Zoo Wildl Med* 2006;37:135-140.
172. Van Alstine WG, Dyer DC. Antibiotic aerosolization: tissue and plasma oxytetracycline concentrations in turkey poults. *Avian Dis* 1985;29:430-436.
173. Veterinary Information Network (VIN). Message Boards. Available at: http://www.vin.com. Accessed May 17, 2017.
174. Waugh L, Kynch H, Cole G, et al. Pharmacokinetic evaluation of a long-acting fentanyl solution after transdermal administration in helmeted guinea fowl (*Numida meleagridis*). *J Zoo Wildl Med* 2016;47:468-473.
175. Whiteside DP, Barker IK, Conlon PD, et al. Pharmacokinetic disposition of the oral iron chelator deferiprone in the white leghorn chicken. *J Avian Med Surg* 2007;21:110-120.
176. Yang F, Li GH, Meng XB, et al. Pharmacokinetic interactions of flunixin meglumine and doxycycline in broiler chickens. *J Vet Pharmacol Ther* 2013;36:85-88.

177. Yang F, Si HB, Wang YQ, et al. Pharmacokinetics of doxycycline in laying hens after intravenous and oral administration. *Br Poult Sci* 2016;57:576-580.
178. Yuan L, Sun J, Wang R, et al. Pharmacokinetics and bioavailability of cefquinome in healthy ducks. *Am J Vet Res* 2011;72:122-126.
179. Ziv G, Shem-Tov M, Glickman A, et al. Concentrations of amoxycillin and clavulanic acid in the serum of broilers during continuous and pulse-dosing of the drinking water. *J Vet Pharmacol Therap* 1997;20(Suppl 1):183-184.
180. Ziv G, Shem-Tov M, Glickman A, et al. Serum oxytetracycline and chlortetracycline concentrations in broilers and turkeys treated with high doses of the drugs via the feed and water. *J Vet Pharmacol Therap* 1997;20(Suppl 1):190-191.
181. Zuchowska E. Some blood parameters in zoo birds. *Proc Euro Conf Avian Med Surg* 1993;493-506.

Chapter 7 Sugar Gliders

David M. Brust | *Christoph Mans*

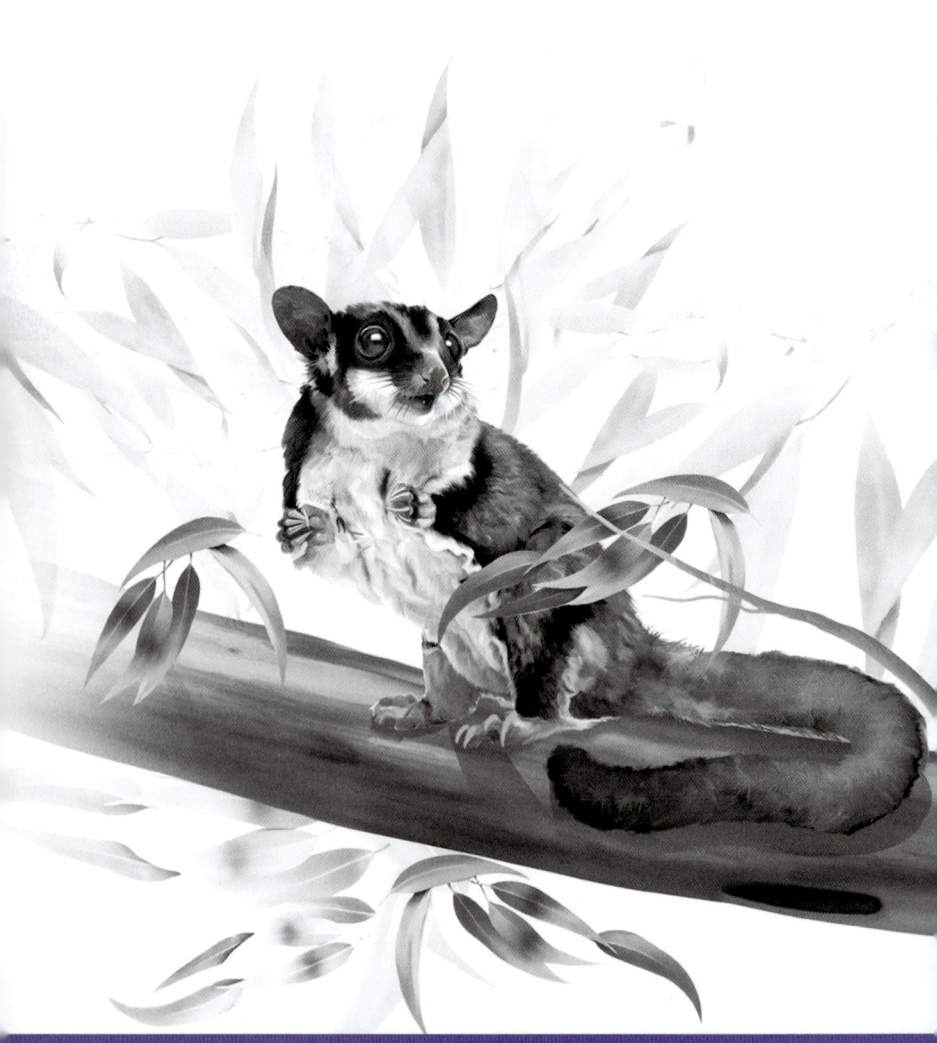

CHAPTER 7 Sugar Gliders

TABLE 7-1 Antimicrobial and Antifungal Agents Used in Sugar Gliders.

Agent	Dosage	Comments
Amikacin sulfate	3 mg/kg IM, SC q12h[19] 10 mg/kg IM, SC q12h × 5 days[21]	Severe Gram-negative infections
Amoxicillin	30 mg/kg PO, SC q12-24h[18,19,21]	
Amoxicillin/clavulanic acid	12.5 mg/kg PO, SC divided q12h[18,19,21]	
Cefovecin sodium (Convenia, Zoetis)	—	Not recommended due to high interspecies variability in PD
Cephalexin	30 mg/kg PO, SC divided q12h[19,21,24]	
Chloramphenicol	50 mg/kg PO q12h[18]	
Ciprofloxacin	10 mg/kg PO q12h[19]	
Clindamycin	5.5-10 mg/kg PO q12h[18]	
Enrofloxacin	2.5-5 mg/kg PO, SC IM q12-24h[21] 5 mg/kg PO, SC, IM q12h[25]	Tissue necrosis may occur when administered parenterally; dilute for SC injection
Gentamicin	1.5-2.5 mg/kg SC, IM q12h[18,21] 2 mg/kg SC, IM divided q12-24h[19]	Not recommend due to nephrotoxicity; use amikacin instead
Griseofulvin	20 mg/kg PO q24h × 30-60 days[21]	Dermatophytes; fungistatic
Itraconazole	5-10 mg/kg PO q12-24h[19] 5-10 mg/kg PO q24h[18]	
Lincomycin	30 mg/kg PO, SC, IM q24h[18,21]	Dose can be divided q12h
Marbofloxacin	2-5 mg/kg PO, SC, IM q24h[18]	
Metronidazole	25 mg/kg PO q12-24h × 7-10 days[19,21] 80 mg/kg PO q24h[18]	CNS toxicity possible at high doses or if underlying hepatic disorder; compound at 5 mg/mL in tutti-frutti flavor[3]
Nystatin	2000 U/kg PO q12h[3] 5000 U/kg PO q8h[21]	Candidiasis
Penicillin	22,000-25,000 U/kg SC, IM q12-24h[18,19,21]	
Trimethoprim/sulfamethoxazole	10-20 mg/kg PO q12-24h[21] 15 mg/kg PO q12h[19] 50 mg/kg PO q24h[25]	

TABLE 7-2 Antiparasitic Agents Used in Sugar Gliders.

Agent	Dosage	Comments
Carbaryl powder (5%)	Topical[19,21]	Ectoparasites; use sparingly; can be used in nest boxes
Fenbendazole	20-50 mg/kg PO q24h × 3 days, repeat in 14 days[18,19,21]	Roundworms, hookworms, whipworms; cestodes; lower end of dosage range may be preferable

Continued

TABLE 7-2 — Antiparasitic Agents Used in Sugar Gliders. (cont'd)

Agent	Dosage	Comments
Ivermectin	0.2 mg/kg SC, repeat in 10-14 days[19,21]	Roundworms, hookworms, whipworms; mites
	0.2-0.4 mg/kg PO, SC, repeat at 14 and 28 days[18]	Mites, nematodes
Levamisole	10 mg/kg PO[21]	
Metronidazole	25 mg/kg PO q12h[19]	Intestinal protozoa; compound at 5 mg/mL in tutti-frutti flavor[3]
	25 mg/kg/day PO, repeat in 14 days[7]	
	80 mg/kg PO q24h[18]	CNS toxicity possible at high doses or if underlying hepatic disorder
Piperazine	50 mg/kg PO q24h[18]	GI nematodes; safe in pregnant animals
	100 mg/kg PO[7]	
Praziquantel	5-10 mg/kg PO, SC, repeat in 10-14 days[23]	Cestodes, trematodes
Pyrethrin powder	Topical[7]	Ectoparasites; use products safe for kittens
Selamectin (Revolution, Zoetis)	6-18 mg/kg topically, repeat in 30 days[3,19]	Ectoparasites

TABLE 7-3 — Chemical Restraint/Anesthetic Agents Used in Sugar Gliders.

Agent	Dosage	Comments
Acepromazine	—	See butorphanol, ketamine for combinations
Atropine	0.01-0.02 mg/kg SC, IM[18,19]	
	0.02-0.04 mg/kg SC, IM, IV[7]	
Bupivacaine	1-2 mg/kg (local infiltrate)[18]	Local anesthesia
Buprenorphine	—	Buprenorphine combination follows
Buprenorphine (Bu)/ midazolam (Mi)/ meloxicam (Mel)	(Bu) 0.01 mg/kg + (Mi) 0.1 mg/kg + (Mel) 0.2 mg/kg IM[22]	Give preemptively for the reduction of postsurgical self-mutilation
Butorphanol (Torbugesic, Fort Dodge)	—	Butorphanol combination follows
Butorphanol (B) + acepromazine (A)	(B) 1.7 mg/kg + (A) 1.7 mg/kg PO[5]	Postoperative sedation and analgesia to prevent self-trauma to incision site
Dexmedetomidine (Dexdomitor, Pfizer)	—	α-2 agonist that is the active optical enantiomer of racemic compound medetomidine; ½ the dose of medetomidine should be administered; limited data on safety or efficacy available
Diazepam	0.5-2 mg/kg PO, IM, SC[7,19]	Sedative, anticonvulsant; avoid parenteral injection if possible (use midazolam instead)

TABLE 7-3 Chemical Restraint/Anesthetic Agents Used in Sugar Gliders. (cont'd)

Agent	Dosage	Comments
Glycopyrrolate	0.01-0.02 mg/kg SC, IM, IV[19]	Controls salivation during sedation
Isoflurane	5% induction; 1%-3% maintenance[19,21]	Anesthetic of choice
Ketamine	—	Ketamine combinations follow
	20 mg/kg IM[19]	
	30-50 mg/kg IM[21]	
Ketamine (K)/ acepromazine (A)	(K) 10 mg/kg + (A) 1 mg/kg SC[19]	Postoperative sedation and analgesia to prevent self-trauma to incision site
	(K) 30 mg/kg + (A) 2 mg/kg SC, IM[21]	For immobilization
Ketamine (K)/ medetomidine (Me)	(K) 2-3 mg/kg + (Me) 0.05-0.1 mg/kg SC, IM[19,21]	For immobilization (see medetomidine)
Ketamine (K)/ midazolam (Mi)	(K) 10-20 mg/kg + (Mi) 0.35-0.5 mg/kg SC, IM[19,21]	
Ketamine (K)/ Xylazine (X)	(K) 10-25 mg/kg + (X) 5 mg/kg SC, IM[21]	
Lidocaine	<4 mg/kg local infiltration or topical[18]	Local anesthesia; dilute to avoid toxicity from accidental overdosing
Medetomidine	—	No longer commercially available, but can be obtained through various compounding services; see dexmedetomidine; see ketamine for combination
Midazolam	—	See buprenorphine, ketamine for combinations
	0.1-0.5 mg/kg IM, SC, intranasal[5,18,19,21,26]	Anxiolytic; anticonvulsant, preanesthetic; sedation
Sevoflurane	1%-5% to effect[19]	Anesthesia
Tiletamine/zolazepam	—	Do not use; has caused neurological syndromes and death in squirrel gliders at 10 mg/kg[19]
Xylazine	—	See ketamine for combination
Yohimbine	0.2 mg/kg SC, IM[19]	Reversal of xylazine

TABLE 7-4 Analgesic Agents Used in Sugar Gliders.

Agent	Dosage	Comments
Buprenorphine	0.01-0.03 mg/kg PO, SC, IM q8-12h[4,19]	
	0.05 mg/kg IM[15]	
Butorphanol	0.1-0.5 mg/kg SC, IM q6-8h[19,21]	
Meloxicam	0.2 mg/kg PO, SC q24h[19]	Nonsteroidal antiinflammatory
	0.1-0.2 mg/kg PO, SC q12-24h[7]	
	0.5 mg/kg PO q24h[15]	

TABLE 7-5 Miscellaneous Agents Used in Sugar Gliders.

Agent	Dosage	Comments
Calcitonin	50-100 U/kg[21] SC	Nutritional osteodystrophy; ensure serum calcium levels are normal prior to use; salmon origin
Calcium glubionate	150 mg/kg PO q24h[4,21]	Nutritional osteodystrophy; calcium deficiency
Calcium gluconate	100 mg/kg SC q12h × 3-5 days; dilute in saline to 10 mg/mL[4]	Nutritional osteodystrophy; calcium deficiency
Cisapride	0.25 mg/kg q8-24h PO, SC[4,21]	Gastrointestinal prokinetic
Dexamethasone	0.1-0.6 mg/kg SC, IM, IV[19]	Antiinflammatory; allergies
	0.2 mg/kg SC, IM, IV q12-24h[21]	
	0.5-2 mg/kg SC, IM, IV[12]	Shock
Doxapram	2 mg/kg SC, IM, IV[19]	Respiratory stimulant; can also place under tongue
Enalapril	0.22-0.44 mg/kg PO q24h[16,19,21]	Vasodilator for the treatment of heart failure and hypertension; can compound at 1 mg/mL in tutti-frutti flavor[16]
	0.5 mg/kg PO q24h[18]	
Epinephrine	0.003 mg/kg IV[16,19]	Stimulates heart; antagonizes effects of histamine; raises blood sugar
Fluoxetine (Prozac, Eli Lilly)	1-5 mg/kg PO q8h[14]	Self-mutilation; use liquid form
	2-5 mg/kg PO q12h[13]	
Furosemide	1-4 mg/kg PO, SC, IM q8h[18]	Diuretic
	1-5 mg/kg PO, SC, IM q6-12h[4,7,19]	
L-carnitine	100 mg/kg PO q12h[21]	
Maropitant citrate (Cerenia, Zoetis)	0.2 mg/kg SC q24h[5]	Dilute 1:20 with sterile water; cannot store diluted drug
Metoclopramide	0.05-0.1 mg/kg PO, SC, IM q6-12h prn[21]	Gastrointestinal prokinetic
Pimobendan	0.3-0.5 mg/kg PO q12h[18]	Positive inotropic and vasodilatory effect; administration with food may reduce bioavailability
Prednisolone	0.1-0.2 mg/kg PO, SC, IM q24h[18,19,21]	Antiinflammatory
	0.2 mg/kg PO q12h[17]	
Vitamin A	500-5000 U/kg IM[19]	
Vitamin B complex	0.01-0.2 mL/kg SC, IM[19,21]	Use small animal formulation; dilute; stings on injection
	10 U/kg PO, SCa[3]	Neurological conditions
Vitamin E	10 U/kg SC[3]	
	25-100 U/animal/day[21]	
Vitamin K	2 mg/kg SC q24-72h[19]	

TABLE 7-6 Hematologic and Serum Biochemical Values of Sugar Gliders.[a]

Measurement	Sugar Gliders: A Complete Veterinary Care Guide[3,b]	International Species Information System[8]	Merck Veterinary Manual[7]
Hematology			
PCV (%)	51-54 (62)	43 ± 4 (24)	45-53
RBC ($10^6/\mu L$)	8.31-8.83 (53)	7.8 ± 0.9 (20)	5.1-7.2
Hgb (g/dL)	15.8-16.9 (53)	15.4 ± 1.6 (21)	13-15
MCH (pg)	18.8-19.4 (53)	19.9 ± 1.3 (20)	18.2-20.6
MCHC (g/dL)	30.6-31 (53)	35.1 ± 2 (21)	30-33
MCV (fL)	60-68 (54)	56.8 ± 5.4 (20)	—
WBC ($10^3/\mu L$)	5.49-9.31 (62)	7.7 ± 5.5 (23)	5-12.2
Neutrophils ($10^3/\mu L$)	1.46-2.2 (61)	1.2 ± 1 (23)	1.5-3
Lymphocytes ($10^3/\mu L$)	3.69-7.16 (62)	6.2 ± 5.1 (23)	2.8-9.2
Monocytes ($10^3/\mu L$)	0.11-0.17 (45)	0.19 ± 0.17 (18)	0.06-0.2
Eosinophils ($10^3/\mu L$)	0.09-0.28 (10)	0.18 ± 0.24 (16)	0.02-0.14
Basophils ($10^3/\mu L$)	0.03-0.06 (8)	0.04 (1)	0
NRBC/100 WBC	—	2 ± 1 (7)	—
Platelets ($10^3/\mu L$)	292-400 (53)	728 ± 176 (3)	—
Chemistries			
ALP (U/L)	89-115 (75)	231 ± 93 (7)	—
ALT (U/L)	97-137 (81)	67 ± 38 (16)	50-106
AST (U/L)	54-100 (38)	70 ± 65 (17)	46-179
Bilirubin, total (mg/dL)	0.12-0.7 (72)	0.3 ± 0.2 (15)	—
Calcium (mg/dL)	8.5-8.9 (97)	7.4 ± 2.9 (7)	6.9-8.4
Chloride (mEq/L)	106-109 (94)	105 ± 3 (5)	—
Cholesterol (mg/dL)	112-124 (78)	159 ± 49 (6)	—
CPK (U/L)	1081-1637 (47)	639 ± 477 (5)	210-589
Creatinine (mg/dL)	0.5-0.6 (100)	0.7 ± 0.3 (8)	0.2-0.5
Glucose (mg/dL)	153-172 (85)	135 ± 75 (17)	130-183
LDH (U/L)	—	246 ± 33 (3)	—
Phosphorus (mg/dL)	4.4-6.1 (62)	6.7 ± 2.0 (6)	3.8-4.4
Potassium (mEq/L)	4.6-5.5 (93)	3.3 ± 0.7 (5)	3.3-5.9
Protein, total (g/dL)	6.7-7 (92)	6.0 ± 0.6 (15)	5.6-6.9
Albumin (g/dL)	3.1-4.6 (99)	3.8 ± 0.7 (8)	3-3.5
Globulin (g/dL)	2.9-3.1 (92)	2.3 ± 0.8 (7)	2.2-3.6
Sodium (mEq/L)	139-143 (92)	142 ± 4 (5)	135-145
Urea nitrogen (mg/dL)	15-18 (100)	19 ± 11 (16)	—

[a]Sample size is presented in parentheses.
[b]Values shown are the 95% reference intervals after outliers were removed; blood was collected from the cranial vena cava; glucose levels were measured immediately after collection.

TABLE 7-7 Biologic and Physiologic Values of Sugar Gliders.[2,3,8,24]

Parameter	Normal Values
Average life span (wild)	
Male	4-5 years
Female	5-7 years
Maximum reported life span	
Captivity	15 years
Wild	9 years
Colony size (wild)	7 (avg) (1 dominant male, 2 subordinate males, 4 adult females)
Colony size (captivity)	Minimum 2 (more is better)
Adult weight	Male, 100-160 g
	Female, 80-135 g
Body length	16-21 cm (avg 17 cm)
Tail length	16.5-21 cm (avg 19 cm)
Heart rate	200-300 beats/min
Respiratory rate	16-40 breaths/min
Cloacal temperature	36.2°C ± 0.4°C (97.2°F ± 0.7°F)
Torpor cloacal temperature	≤15°C (59°F)
Thermoneutral zone	27-31°C (81-88°F)
Basal metabolic rate	2.54 (weight in kg)$^{0.75}$
Estrus cycle	
Type	Seasonally polyestrus
Length	29 days
Gestation period	15-17 days
Litter size	1-4 (usually 2)
Birth weight	0.2 g
Pouch emergence	50-74 days (usually 60 days)
Weaning age	85-120 days (usually 100 days)
Dispersal from nest	7-10 months
Sexual maturity	Male, 12-14 months; female 8-12 months

TABLE 7-8 Urinalysis Values of Sugar Gliders.[3]

Measurement	Avg	Reference Interval[a,b]
Specific gravity	1.030	1.020-1.040 (103)
pH	6.2	6-6.3 (98)
Protein (mg/dL)	12	9.5-14.6 (82)

[a]Values shown are the 95% reference intervals after outliers were removed; analysis performed using IDEXX Vetlab UA™.
[b]Sample size is presented in parentheses.

TABLE 7-9 Growth and Development of Sugar Gliders.[2,4,6]

Stage 1: In Pouch

Age (days)	Weight (g)	Head (mm)	Leg (mm)	Key Developmental Characteristics
1	0.2	—	—	Mouth and forelimbs most developed feature
20	0.8	11	6	Ears free from head; papillae of mystacial vibrissae (whiskers) visible
30	1.6	14	9	—
35	2	—	—	Mystacial vibrissae erupt; ears pigmented
40	3.2	17	12	Start to pigment on shoulders; eye slits present
50	6.2	20	16	Typical detachment from teat and emergence from pouch at 50-60 days

Stage 2: Out of Pouch (OOP)[a,b]

Age (weeks)	Weight (g)	Key Developmental Characteristics
1	8-18	Dorsal stripe developing; little to no fur; slick tail; closed eyes
2	12-22	Eyes open at approximately 17-21 days; fur lengthens
3	17-29	Very fine fur, except abdominal area; tail still slick; eyes still closed
4	18-35	Fur becoming more prominent; tail beginning to fluff; weaning begins
5	19-39	Complete fur coverage; light fur on abdominal area; tail continues to fill out
6	20-45	Tail fully fluffed out; abdominal area fully furred; mostly weaned
7	21-60	Very active at night; eating mainly solid foods
8	23-75	Fully self-sufficient and weaned

[a]On a practical level, estimating an exact out of pouch (OOP) date is often problematic because of the nocturnal nature of the animal and protectiveness of parents; joeys often exhibit wide weight differentials at the same age; the most reliable method for estimating age is to visually assess key distinguishing characteristics of their physical development, especially the abdominal area and tail.[3]
[b]Once joey is observed out of pouch, age is typically measured in weeks.[1]

TABLE 7-10 Dietary Components for Sugar Gliders in Captivity.[3]

Common presentations	Obesity, malnutrition, and osteodystrophy often caused by nutritional inconsistencies of homemade diets and excessive sweet and fatty items
Daily consumption	15%-20% of body weight
Pelleted kibble	Nutritionally-balanced, commercial sugar glider kibble (Glide-R-Chow™ [www.sugarbears.com], NutriMax™ [www.vetspride.com]), VitaSmart Sugar Glider Formula & Vita Prima™ Sunscription Exotics Sugar Glider Formula (www.vitakraftsunseed.com)
Fresh fruits and vegetables	Apples, apricots, bananas, berries, corn, grapes, green beans, kiwifruit, mangos, melons, oranges, papaya, peas, sweet potatoes, squash, and watermelon
Supplement	Calcium-based multivitamin supplement formulated specifically for sugar gliders (Glide-A-Mins™ [www.sugarbears.com], VitaMax™ [www.vetspride.com])
Treats[a]	Must be strictly controlled; applesauce, yogurt, and limited invertebrates such as mealworms, grasshoppers, moths, fly pupae, and crickets

Continued

TABLE 7-10　Dietary Components for Sugar Gliders in Captivity. (cont'd)

Bottled or filtered water	Refresh drip water bottle daily; introduction of weighted container such as small ashtray may also be necessary for young joeys
Blossoms and branches	*Eucalyptus, Banksia, Leptospermum, Grevillea, Acacia, Melaleuca, Callistemum,* and *Hakea*

[a]Sugar gliders will preferentially eat sweet/fatty items to excess and to the exclusion of more nutritious foods, so they should not be presented with too wide a selection of foods.

TABLE 7-11　Suggested Sugar Glider Diets.[3,11]

Diet 1[3]

75%: Nutritionally balanced, commercial sugar glider kibble: 1-2 oz (28-56 g)/day/animal; available free choice in cage at all times (Glide-R-Chow™ [www.sugarbears.com], NutriMax™ [www.vetspride.com])

25%: Fresh fruits and vegetables: approximately ⅛ of an apple, or the equivalent in mixed fruits/vegetables per animal per day; introduce each evening and remove leftovers in morning; apples, apricots, bananas, berries, corn, grapes, green beans, kiwifruit, mangos, melons, oranges, paw paw (papaya), peas, sweet potatoes, squash, and watermelon

Calcium-based multivitamin supplement: Sprinkle lightly on fruits/vegetables every other day; can also be mixed into applesauce or fruit baby food and hand-fed daily to promote bonding (Glide-A-Mins™ [www.sugarbears.com], VitaMax™ [www.vetspride.com])

Treats: Not to exceed 5% of daily diet; introduce gradually and individually, checking for diarrhea; treat items must be strictly controlled and may include fruits, applesauce, yogurt, and invertebrates such as mealworms, grasshoppers, moths, fly pupae, and crickets

Diet 2[a-c,9]

50%: Leadbeater's mixture (150 mL warm water; 150 mL honey; 1 shelled, hard-boiled egg; 25 g high protein baby cereal; 1 tsp vitamin/mineral supplement)

- Mix warm water and honey
- In separate container, blend egg until homogenized
- Gradually add honey/water, then vitamin powder, then baby cereal, and blend after each addition until smooth
- Keep refrigerated until served

50%: Insectivore/omnivore diet (e.g., Mazuri Brand, Purina Mills, St. Louis, MO; Reliable Protein Products, Palm Desert, CA; ZuPreem, Mission, KS)

Diet 3[d,9]

- Apple: 3 g; banana/corn: 3 g; grapes/kiwifruit: 3 g; orange with skin: 4 g; pear: 2 g; rockmelon/melon/paw paw (payaya): 2 g
- Sweet potato: 3 g
- Dog kibble: 1.5 g
- Fly pupae: 1 tsp
- Leadbeater's mix (see Diet 2): 2 tsp
- Day-old chick (1 day/week)
- Large insects or mealworms (when available)

[a]Insects can be added to this diet to help prevent dental problems.
[b]Feed fresh portions in evening; chop items together to reduce only favorite foods being selected; can offer treats (meats, diced fruits with multiple vitamin/mineral powder, bee pollen, worms, and crickets or other gut-loaded insects) at approximately 5% of daily intake.
[c]Pelleted sugar glider food (e.g., Marion Zoological, Plymouth, MN) might be preferable to other dry omnivore diets.
[d]Recipe feeds two animals; without native foods (e.g., North America), add calcium carbonate to this diet.

CHAPTER 7 Sugar Gliders

TABLE 7-12 Feed Estimates for Hand-Rearing Sugar Gliders.[a-d,6]

Age (days)	Feed (mL/day)	Wombaroo Possum Milk Replacer
20	0.7	Formula "<0.8"
30	1.1	Formula "<0.8"
40	1.8	Formula "<0.8"
50	3	Formula "<0.8"
51-53	4 (3 mL ["<0.8"]+1 mL [">0.8"])	Transition from Formula "<0.8" to Formula ">0.8"
54-56	4 (2 mL ["<0.8"]+2 mL [">0.8"])	Transition from Formula "<0.8" to Formula ">0.8"
57-59	4 (1 mL ["<0.8"]+3 mL [">0.8"])	Transition from Formula "<0.8" to Formula ">0.8"
60	3	Formula ">0.8"
70	4	Formula ">0.8"
80	6	Formula ">0.8"
90	7	Formula ">0.8"
100	8	Formula ">0.8"

[a]Using Table 7.9, estimate the age of the sugar glider using developmental characteristics and weight measurements. Feed the volume listed according to the estimated age of the sugar glider. In emaciated joeys, the head and leg measurement is a more accurate method to determine age than the animal's weight.
[b]Note that marsupial milk changes in composition and energy as the joey develops. Therefore, there are two formulas of Wombaroo Possum Milk Replacer that are used for hand-rearing sugar gliders. Formula "<0.8" is for younger joeys; Formula ">0.8" is for gliders out of the pouch. When a joey has fully emerged from the pouch, it then uses Formula ">0.8" entirely.
[c]Wombaroo Possum Milk Replacer "<0.8" and ">0.8" is available in the United States from the Exotic Nutrition Co, Newport News, VA; (866) 988-0301; exoticdiet@cox.net or from Perfect Pets Inc., Belleville, MI; (800) 366-8794; www.wombaroo.com.
[d]For hand-rearing procedures, refer to Barnes[1] and Ness and Booth.[20]

REFERENCES

1. Barnes M. Sugar gliders. In: Gage LJ, ed. *Hand-Rearing Wild and Domestic Mammals*. Ames: Iowa State Press; 2002:55-62.
2. Booth RJ. General husbandry and medical care of sugar gliders. In: Bonagura JD, ed. *Kirk's Current Veterinary Therapy XIII: Small Animal Practice*. Philadelphia: WB Saunders; 2000:1157-1163.
3. Brust DM. *Sugar Gliders: A Complete Veterinary Care Guide*. Sugarland: Veterinary Interactive Publications; 2009.
4. Brust DM. What every veterinarian needs to know about sugar gliders. *Exotic DVM* 2009;11:32-41.
5. Brust DM. Personal observation. 2016.
6. Donneley B. Hand-rearing orphan marsupials. *Exotic DVM* 2002;4:79-82.
7. Hess L. Sugar gliders. In: Aiello SE, ed. *The Merck Veterinary Manual*. 11th ed. Kenilworth, NJ: Merck & Co; 2015:2035-2043.
8. Species 360 (formerly International Species Information System [ISIS]). Bloomington, MN, 2002. Available at: www.species360.org/. Accessed March 6, 2017.
9. Johnson-Delaney C. Feeding sugar gliders. *Exotic DVM* 1998;1:4.
10. Johnson-Delaney C. Marsupial nutrition and physiology. *Exotic DVM* 2002;4:75-77.
11. Johnson-Delaney CA. Marsupials. In: Johnson-Delaney CA, ed. *Exotic Companion Medicine Handbook*. West Palm Beach: Zoological Education Network; 2000.
12. Johnson-Delaney CA. Therapeutics of companion exotic marsupials. *Vet Clin North Am Exot Anim Pract* 2000;3:173-181.

13. Johnson-Delaney CA. Practical marsupial medicine. *Annu Conf Assoc Exot Mam Vet* 2006;51-60.
14. Johnson-Delaney CA. Marsupials. In: Meredith A, Johnson-Delaney CA, eds. *BSAVA Manual of Exotic Pets*. 5th ed. Gloucester: British Small Animal Veterinary Association; 2010:103-126.
15. Keller KA, Nevarez JG, Rodriguez D, et al. Diagnosis and treatment of anaplastic mammary carcinoma in a sugar glider (*Petaurus breviceps*). *J Exot Pet Med* 2014;23:277-282.
16. Lennox AM. Emergency and critical care procedures in sugar gliders (*Petaurus breviceps*), African hedgehogs (*Atelerix albiventris*), and prairie dogs (*Cynomys* spp.). *Vet Clin North Am Exot Anim Pract* 2007;10:533-555.
17. Lindemann DM, Carpenter JW, DeBey BM, et al. Concurrent adrenocortical carcinoma and hepatocellular carcinoma with hemosiderosis in a sugar glider (*Petaurus breviceps*). *J Exot Pet Med* 2016;25:144-149.
18. Meredith A. *BSAVA Small Animal Formulary. Part B: Exotic Pets*. 9th ed. Gloucester: British Small Animal Veterinary Association; 2015.
19. Morrisey JK, Carpenter JW. Formulary. In: Quesenberry KE, Carpenter JW, eds. *Ferrets, Rabbits, and Rodents: Clinical Medicine and Surgery*. 3rd ed. St. Louis: Saunders/Elsevier; 2012:566-575.
20. Ness RD, Booth RJ. Sugar gliders. In: Quesenberry KE, Carpenter JW, eds. *Ferrets, Rabbits, and Rodents: Clinical Medicine and Surgery*. 2nd ed. St. Louis: Saunders/Elsevier; 2004:330-338.
21. Ness RD, Johnson-Delaney C. Sugar gliders. In: Quesenberry KE, Carpenter JW, eds. *Ferrets, Rabbits, and Rodents: Clinical Medicine and Surgery*. 3rd ed. St. Louis: Saunders/Elsevier; 2012:393-410.
22. Pye GW. Personal communication. 2010.
23. Pye GW. Personal communication. 2016.
24. Pye GW, Carpenter JW. A Guide to medicine and surgery in sugar gliders. *Vet Med* 1999;94:891-905.
25. Pye GW, Carpenter JW. Sugar Gliders. *Exotic Animal Formulary*. 3rd ed. St. Louis: Saunders/Elsevier; 2005:347-360.
26. Rivas AE, Pye GW, Papendick R. Dermal hemangiosarcoma in a sugar glider (*Petaurus breviceps*). *J Exot Pet Med* 2014;23:384-388.

Chapter 8 **Hedgehogs**

Peter J. Helmer | *James W. Carpenter*

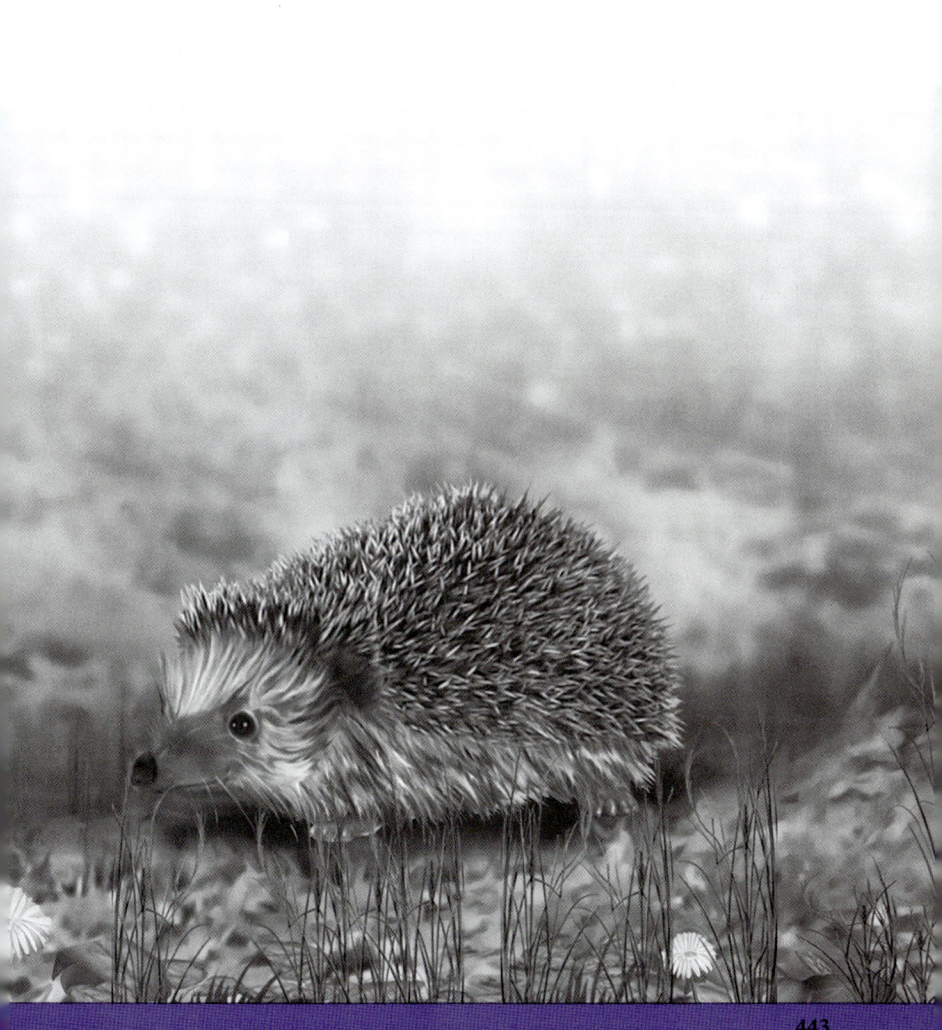

TABLE 8-1 Antimicrobial Agents Used in Hedgehogs.

Agent	Dosage	Comments
Amikacin	2.5-5 mg/kg IM q8-12 h[36]	Make sure animal is hydrated; do not use in animals with renal disease[44]
	1 mg per 4 g powder[35]	Polymethylmethacrylate (PMMA) beads
Amoxicillin	15 mg/kg PO, SC, IM q12h[19a,54]	Palatable to most hedgehogs[13]
Amoxicillin/clavulanic acid (Clavamox, Pfizer)	12.5 mg/kg PO q12h[40,56]	Palatable to most hedgehogs[13]
Ampicillin	10 mg/kg IM q12h[19a,23,54]	Not recommended or use with caution[27]
Ceftiofur sodium	20 mg/kg SC q12-24h[36]	
	1 g per 20 mL powder[35]	Polymethylmethacrylate (PMMA) beads
Cephalexin	25 mg/kg PO q8h[36]	May make stools loose[27]
Chloramphenicol	30 mg/kg IM q12h[19a,23]	Acute salmonellosis; potentially toxic to humans—have dosage giver avoid contact with medication[44]
	30-50 mg/kg PO, SC, IM, IV q12h[54]	
	50 mg/kg PO, SC, IM q12h[18,19a,23]	
Chlorhexidine	Topical[54] q8-12h[27]	Bacterial dermatitis; traumatic skin lesions; wound treatments; soaking (e.g., appendages); use properly diluted
Chlorhexidine shampoo	2%-3% shampoo[36]	Bacterial, mycotic dermatitis
Chlortetracycline	5-20 mg/kg PO q12h[40]	
Ciprofloxacin	5-20 mg/kg PO q12h[40]	
Clarithromycin	5.5 mg/kg PO q12h[40]	
Clindamycin	5.5-10 mg/kg PO q12h[36,56]	Anaerobes; dental disease
Doxycycline	2.5-10 mg/kg PO, SC, IM q12h[40]	Concentration of active drug declines rapidly after 7 days in compounded formulation[43]
Enrofloxacin	2.5-5 mg/kg PO, IM q12h[51]	Avoid IM administration
	5-10 mg/kg PO, SC, IM q12h[18,54]	Dilute if administering SC; avoid IM administration[51]
Erythromycin	10 mg/kg PO, IM q12h[19a,23]	Penicillin-resistant Gram-positive cocci; *Mycoplasma*; *Pasteurella*; *Bordetella*
Gentamicin	2 mg/kg SC, IM q8h[18]	Rarely indicated; best to avoid; nephrotoxic
Gentamicin ophthalmic drops	Topical to cornea or conjunctiva[36] q8h[27]	Corneal abrasions or conjunctivitis; use as in dog or cat
Metronidazole	20 mg/kg PO q12h[36,40]	Anaerobes
Mupirocin (2%) (Muricin, Dechra)	Topical to cutaneous lesions q12-24h prn[36]	Bacterial dermatitis or traumatic skin lesions
Neomycin, polymyxin B, bacitracin ophthalmic ointment	Topical to cornea or conjunctiva[36] q8-12h[27]	Corneal abrasions or conjunctivitis; use as in dog or cat

TABLE 8-1 Antimicrobial Agents Used in Hedgehogs. (cont'd)

Agent	Dosage	Comments
Neomycin, thiabendazole, dexamethasone solution (Tresaderm, Merial)	Topical to cutaneous lesions or ear canal q12h prn[36]	Bacterial, mycotic dermatitis; otitis externa; antiinflammatory
Nystatin, neomycin, thiostrepton, triamcinolone cream (Panalog, Fort Dodge)	Topical to cutaneous lesions q12-24h prn[36]	Bacterial, mycotic dermatitis; antiinflammatory
Orbifloxacin (Orbax suspension, Intervet)	10-20 mg/kg PO q12-24h[16]	
Oxytetracycline	25-50 mg/kg PO q24h × 5-7 days[11,13,36]	*Bordetella*; may be administered in food
Oxytetracycline ophthalmic ointment (Terramycin, Pfizer)	Topical to cornea or conjunctiva[36] q8-12h[27]	Corneal abrasions or conjunctivitis; use as in dog or cat
Penicillin G	40,000 U/kg SC, IM q24h[19a,40]	
Piperacillin	10 mg/kg SC q8-12h[36]	
Spiramycin	15 mg/kg PO × 8 days[19a]	Gingivitis; frequency not listed; not available in the United States
Sulfadimethoxine	2-20 mg/kg PO, SC, IM q24h[18,19a]	May have slight nephrotoxicity[27]
Trimethoprim/sulfa	30 mg/kg PO, SC, IM q12h[18,51]	Respiratory infections; trimethoprim/sulfamethoxazole is available in injectable form
Tylosin	10 mg/kg PO, SC q12h[23]	*Mycoplasma*; *Clostridium*; do not administer IM (causes muscle necrosis)

TABLE 8-2 Antifungal Agents Used in Hedgehogs.

Agent	Dosage	Comments
Chlorhexidine	2%-3% shampoo[36]	Dermatophytosis
Enilconazole (Imaverol, Janssen)	Topical q24h[56] 100 mg/mL water topically q4d[42]	Dermatophytosis; dilute 1:50 Dermatophytosis
Griseofulvin (microsize)	—	Skin and deep mycoses; long-term therapy
	25 mg/kg PO q12h[19a]	
	50 mg/kg PO q24h[19a,54] × 14-21 days[38]	
Itraconazole	5-10 mg/kg PO q12-24h[36]	Systemic mycoses
	10 mg/kg PO q12h[6]	European hedgehogs/dermatophytosis
	10 mg/kg PO q24h[12]	Cutaneous paecilomycosis
Ketoconazole	10 mg/kg PO q24h × 6-8 wk[19a,54]	Mycoses; use long term
Lime sulfur	Topical[17]	Dermatophytosis
Nystatin	30,000 U/kg PO q8-24h[36]	Yeast infections
Terbinafine	100 mg/kg PO q12h[6]	European hedgehogs/dermatophytosis

TABLE 8-3 Antiparasitic Agents Used in Hedgehogs.

Agent	Dosage	Comments
Amitraz (Mitaban, Pfizer)	0.3% topical q7d × 2-3 treatments[34,36]	Mites (*Caparinia, Chorioptes*, etc.); may dilute; use with caution
Fenbendazole	10-15 mg/kg PO q14d × 2-3 treatments[54]	Nematodes
	10-30 mg/kg PO q24h × 5 days[23]	Nematodes (i.e., *Crenosoma, Capillaria*)
	25 mg/kg PO q10d[36]	Nematodes
Fipronil spray (Frontline, Merial)	Topical, repeat in 10 days[27,33]	Mites; apply 1 spray over dorsum
Flea products (feline)	Topical[17]	Use sparingly
Imidacloprid	½ puppy/kitten dose topical q30d[13]	Fleas; apply to quilled areas behind head
Imidacloprid 10% + moxidectin 1%	0.1 mL/kg[28]	*Caparinia*
Ivermectin	0.2 mg/kg PO, SC q14d × 3 treatments[54]	Mites (*Caparinia*, etc.); nematodes; a pyrethrin-based shampoo q7d × several treatments is often needed concurrently for full response
	0.2 mg/kg SC q21d[9b]	*Caparinia* mites
	0.2-0.4 mg/kg PO, SC q10-14d × 3-5 treatments[20,40]	Ectoparasites
	0.5 mg/kg PO, SC q14d × 3 treatments[7]	Mites; resistance to the lower doses of ivermectin has been noted
	<1 mg/kg[27] PO, SC	For resistant *Chorioptes*
Levamisole (1%)	10 mg/kg SC,[11] repeat q48h; repeat prn q14d[19a]	Nematodes, including lungworms
Lufenuron	½ puppy/kitten dose PO q30d[13]	Fleas
Mebendazole	15 mg/kg PO, repeat q14d[27]	Nematodes; do not use in animals with hepatic disease
	25 mg/animal <500 g q12h; 50 mg/animal >500 g q24h PO × 5 days, repeat q14-21[27]	*Capillaria, Crenosoma, Brachylaernus, Hymenolepsis, Physaloptera*
Metronidazole	25 mg/kg PO q12h × 5 days[17,54]	Intestinal protozoa
Moxidectin (Cydectin, Bayer)	0.3 mg/kg SC q10d[42]	Notoedric mange
Permethrin (1%)	Topical[55]	Mites; apply once via fine mist; change bedding
Praziquantel	7 mg/kg PO, SC, repeat q14d[17,54]	Cestodes, trematodes
Selamectin (Revolution, Pfizer)	6 mg/kg topically[3]	Ectoparasites; higher dose may be required
	6-18 mg/kg topically q30d × 2 treatments[22]	External mites
Sulfadimethoxine	2-20 mg/kg PO,[19a] SC, IM[23] q24h × 2-5 days, off 5 days, on 2-5 days[19a]	Coccidia
	10 mg/kg PO q24h × 5-7 days[36]	Coccidia
Sulfadimidine	100-200 mg/kg SC q24h × 3 days[11]	Coccidia
Toltrazuril	10 mg/kg PO q24h × 2 treatments then repeated q7d × 3 wk[21]	Coccidia (*Eimeria*)

CHAPTER 8 Hedgehogs

TABLE 8-4 Chemical Restraint/Anesthetic Agents Used in Hedgehogs.

Agent	Dosage	Comments
Acepromazine	0.1-1 mg/kg PO, SC, IM[13]	Sedative; hypotension may occur when used alone; atropine pretreatment may alleviate this effect
Atipamezole (Antisedan, Zoetis)	0.3-0.5 mg/kg IM[56] 1 mg/kg SC, IM, IV, IP[4,27]	Reversal of medetomidine and dexmedetomidine
Atropine	0.01-0.05 mg/kg SC, IM[21,40]	Preanesthetic to decrease hypersalivation
Buprenorphine	—	See midazolam for combination
Butorphanol	—	See midazolam for combination
Dexmedetomidine (Dexdomitor, Zoetis)	0.02 mg/kg IM[32]	Avoid use in ill or debilitated animals; reversible with atipamezole
Diazepam	—	Diazepam combination follows
	0.5-2 mg/kg IM[51]	Mild sedation; may be given with ketamine for anesthesia; seizures; midazolam preferred for IM use
Diazepam (D)/ ketamine (K)	(D) 0.5-2 mg/kg + (K) 5-20 mg/kg IM[7]	Anesthesia; do not use in neck area where there is brown fat;[23] midazolam preferred for IM use
Enflurane	To effect[40]	Anesthesia; not commonly used; isoflurane or sevoflurane preferred
Fentanyl	—	See medetomidine for combination
Isoflurane	3%-5% induction[54]	Anesthetic of choice; generally occurs in an induction chamber or mask
	0.5%-3% maintenance[53,54]	By mask or endotracheal tube
Ketamine	—	See diazepam and medetomidine for combinations; combinations follow
	5-20 mg/kg IM[51]	Sedation; anesthesia; do not use in neck area where there is brown fat;[23] may use in combination with midazolam (or less preferably diazepam) or an α_2 agonist; recovery may be prolonged and/or rough
Ketamine (K)/ medetomidine (M)	(K) 5 mg/kg + (M) 0.1 mg/kg IM[40,56]	Anesthesia; (M) reverse with atipamezole (0.3-0.5 mg/kg IM); see medetomidine[a]
Ketamine (K)/ midazolam (Mi)	(K) 3-10 mg/kg + (Mi) 0.5-1 mg/kg IM[32]	
Medetomidine	—	Medetomidine[a] combination follows; not commercially available, but can be obtained through select compounding pharmacies; recommend equal volume of dexmedetomidine, but no reports of safety or efficacy available
	0.05-0.1 mg/kg IM[36,56]	Light sedation; reverse with atipamezole (0.3-0.5 mg/kg IM)
	0.2 mg/kg SC, IM[5]	Heavy sedation; reverse with atipamezole (0.3-0.5 mg/kg IM)
Medetomidine (M)/ ketamine (K)/ fentanyl (F)	(M) 0.2 mg/kg + (K) 2 mg/kg + (F) 0.1 mg/kg SC[4]	Anesthesia; good muscle relaxation; (M) reversed with atipamezole (1 mg/kg IM) and (F) reversed with naloxone (0.16 mg/kg IM); see medetomidine[a]

Continued

TABLE 8-4 Chemical Restraint/Anesthetic Agents Used in Hedgehogs. (cont'd)

Agent	Dosage	Comments
Midazolam	—	Midazolam combinations follow; it is the preferred benzodiazepine for IM use
	0.25-0.5 mg/kg IM[31]	Preanesthetic
	0.5-1.0 mg/kg IM[32]	
Midazolam (Mi)/ buprenorphine (Bup)	(Mi) 0.25-0.5 mg/kg + (Bup) 0.03 mg/kg IM[31]	Painful or stressful procedures
Midazolam (Mi)/ butorphanol (But)	(Mi) 0.25-0.5 mg/kg + (But) 0.4 mg/kg IM[31]	Stressful procedures; also see butorphanol comments in Table 8.5
	(Mi) 0.5-1 mg/kg + (But) 0.2-0.5 mg/kg IM[32]	
Naloxone	0.1-0.16 mg/kg SC, IM q6-8h[4,27]	Reversal of fentanyl
Sevoflurane	To effect[40]	Anesthesia; may provide more rapid induction and plane changes than isoflurane
Tiletamine/ zolazepam (Telazol, Zoetis)	1-5 mg/kg IM[54]	Sedation; anesthesia; recovery may be prolonged and/or rough; rarely indicated because gas anesthesia is preferred
Xylazine	0.5-1 mg/kg IM[51]	Anesthesia; may be given with ketamine; rarely indicated because gas anesthesia is preferred
Yohimbine	0.5-1 mg/kg IM[40]	Reversal of xylazine

^aDexmedetomidine (0.5 mg/mL) is an α-2 agonist that is the active optical enantiomer of racemic compound medetomidine; ½ the dose of medetomidine (1 mg/mL) but same volume; although the same effects would be expected as with medetomidine (not commercially available, but can be obtained through various compounding services), there is no data on the efficacy and safety of dexmedetomidine in hedgehogs, and, to date, it appears to have been seldom used clinically in this species; the effects of the v/v use of the two drugs may not be equivalent, so the dose of dexmedetomidine may need to be adjusted based on clinical response.

TABLE 8-5 Analgesic Agents Used in Hedgehogs.

Agent	Dosage	Comments
Buprenorphine	0.01 mg/kg SC, IM q6-8h[11,53,56]	Analgesia; higher dose will likely be required
	0.01-0.5 mg/kg SC, IM q8-12h[24]	Analgesia
Butorphanol	0.05 mg/kg q8h SC prn[23]	Analgesia; when compared with other opiate analgesics, this drug appears to be less useful in small animals for treating moderate to severe pain and has to be dosed more frequently
	0.05-0.1 mg/kg SC, IM q8-12h[24]	Analgesia
	0.2-0.4 mg/kg SC, IM q6-8h[53,54]	Analgesia

TABLE 8-5   Analgesic Agents Used in Hedgehogs. (cont'd)

Agent	Dosage	Comments
Carprofen	1 mg/kg PO, SC q12-24h[27]	Nonsteroidal, antiinflammatory
Dexamethasone	0.1-1.5 mg/kg IM[19a]	Glucocorticoid; inflammation; allergies
Flunixin meglumine	0.3 mg/kg SC q24h[24]	Nonsteroidal, antiinflammatory; arthritis; chronic inflammation; higher dose may be required
Hydromorphone	0.1 mg/kg SC[49]	Preoperative analgesia
Meloxicam	0.08 mg/kg PO q24h[49] 0.2 mg/kg PO, SC q24h[26,27,57]	Nonsteroidal, antiinflammatory
Methylprednisolone	1-2 mg/kg SC[36]	Glucocorticoid; antiinflammatory
Naloxone	0.1-0.16 mg/kg SC, IM q6-8h[4,27]	Reversal of fentanyl
Prednisolone	2.5 mg/kg PO, SC, IM q12h prn[19a,40]	Glucocorticoid; allergies
Tramadol	2-4 mg/kg PO q12h	Synthetic μ-receptor opiate-like agonist
Triamcinolone	0.2 mg/kg SC, IM[13]	Glucocorticoid; antiinflammatory; no frequency given

TABLE 8-6   Miscellaneous Agents Used in Hedgehogs.

Agent	Dosage	Comments
Acyclovir	40-100 mg/kg PO q24h[21]	Herpes simplex infection
Aluminum hydroxide	100 mg/kg PO with each syringe feeding[45]	Renal failure; hyperphosphatemia
Atropine	0.05-0.2 mg/kg SC[13]	Bradycardia
Bupivicaine	1.1 mg/kg diluted with saline 1:12[49]	Surgical site infiltration
Calcium gluconate (10%)	50 mg/kg IM[36]	Hypocalcemia
Calcium gluconate (23%)	100-150 mg/kg IV[31]	
Carnivore Care (Oxbow)	2-3 mL PO[26] Mix 1:1 with Critical Care Fine Grind[1] (Oxbow)	Gavage feed; may require slight sedation
Cimetidine	10 mg/kg PO q8h[36]	Treatment of gastric ulcers
Doxapram	2-10 mg/kg IV, IP[13,31]	Respiratory stimulant; use with caution as use may increase CNS oxygen demand[44]
Emeraid Carnivore (Lafeber)	3 mL/100 g BW q6h	Mix 1:1 with Emeraid Omnivore per label

Continued

TABLE 8-6 Miscellaneous Agents Used in Hedgehogs. (cont'd)

Agent	Dosage	Comments
Enalapril	0.5 mg/kg PO q24h[36]	Vasodilator; heart failure
Epinephrine	0.003 mg/kg IV[31]	Cardiac arrest
Erythropoietin (Epogen, Amgen)	100 U/kg SC q48-72h[36]	Chronic anemia
Famotidine	1 mg/kg SC q24h[45]	Prevention or treatment of gastric ulcers
Furosemide	2.5-5 mg/kg PO, SC, IM q8h[40,56]	Edema; diuretic
	2-4 mg/kg PO, SC q8h[15]	Congestive heart failure
Glycopyrrolate	0.01-0.02 mg/kg SC[13]	Bradycardia
Hetastarch	5 mL/kg IV[31]	Give over 5-10 min
Hyaluronidase	100-150 U/L[36]	Add to SC fluids; may facilitate fluid absorption
Iron dextran	25 mg/kg IM[56]	Anemia
Lactated Ringer's solution (LRS)	—	Fluid replacement; dehydration; shock
	1-15 mL/kg IV[31]	
	25 mL/kg SC q12h[57]	
	50-100 mL/kg/day[26]	
Lactobacilli	2.5 mL/kg q24h[19a]	May aid in restoring gastrointestinal flora
Lactulose	0.3 mL/kg PO q8-12h[36]	Hepatic disease; constipation[27]
Lysine	250-500 mg/kg PO q24h[21]	Herpes simplex
Metoclopramide	0.2-0.5 mg/kg PO, SC[36]	Regurgitation; antiemetic; GI motility enhancer[27]
Milk thistle (Silybum marianum)	4-15 mg/kg PO q12h[21]	Hepatoprotectant
Pimobendan	0.3 mg/kg PO q12h[15]	Congestive heart failure
Sucralfate	10 mg/kg PO q8-12h[40]	Gastrointestinal ulcers
Theophylline	10 mg/kg PO, IM q12h[36]	Bronchodilator
Trilostane	2 mg/kg PO q24h[21]	Hyperadrenocorticism
Vitamin A	400 U/kg IM q24h × 10 days[19a]	Skin disorders; excessive quill loss
Vitamin B complex	1 mL/kg SC, IM once[23,40]	CNS signs; paralysis of unknown origin; anorexia; use small animal formulation
Vitamin C	50-200 mg/kg PO, SC q24h[19a]	Deficiency; infections; gingivitis
	1 g ascorbic acid/L drinking water[19a]	Change daily; not recommended; alternative routes of supplementation preferred; use oral pills or powder[27]

TABLE 8-7 Hematologic and Serum Biochemical Values of Hedgehogs.

Measurement	Reference Range[19]	Reference Range[41]
Hematology		
PCV (%)	36 ± 7 (22-64)	42.0 ± 0.9 (33.5-47.0)
RBC ($10^6/\mu L$)	6 ± 2 (3-16)	5.0 ± 0.1 (4.3-6.0)
Hgb (g/dL)	12 ± 2.8 (7-21.1)	13.1 ± 0.3 (10.7-14.9)
MCV (fL)	67 ± 9 (41-94)	87.8 ± 1.8 (76.3-99.8)
MCH (pg)	22 ± 4 (11-31)	27.1 ± 0.7 (22.5-31.4)
MCHC (g/dL)	34 ± 5 (17-48)	30.9 ± 0.5 (27.7-35.2)
Platelets ($10^3/\mu L$)	226 ± 108 (60-347)	Not reported
WBC ($10^3/\mu L$)	11 ± 6 (3-43)	15.0 ± 0.7 (11.5-21.7)
Neutrophils ($10^3/\mu L$)	5.1 ± 5.2 (0.6-37.4)	9.5 ± 0.5 (6.1-14.6)
Lymphocytes ($10^3/\mu L$)	4 ± 2.2 (0.9-13.1)	5.2 ± 0.4 (3.3-8.9)
Monocytes ($10^3/\mu L$)	0.3 ± 0.3 (0-1.6)	0.2 ± 0.1 (0-0.8)
Eosinophils ($10^3/\mu L$)	1.2 ± 0.9 (0-5.1)	0.2 ± 0 (0-0.3)
Basophils ($10^3/\mu L$)	0.4 ± 0.3 (0-1.5)	0.1 ± 0 (0-0.2)
Chemistries		
ALP (U/L)	51 ± 21 (8-92)	22.4 ± 1.0 (18.2-25.5)
ALT (U/L)	53 ± 24 (16-134)	22.8 ± 1.4 (15.2-28.8)
Amylase (U/L)	510 ± 170 (244-858)	Not reported
AST (U/L)	34 ± 22 (8-137)	33.5 ± 3.5 (19.0-65.6)
Bilirubin, total (mg/dL)	0.3 ± 0.3 (0-1.3)	Not reported
BUN (mg/dL)	27 ± 9 (13-54)	47.1 ± 2.3 (34.3-57.3)
Calcium (mg/dL)	8.8 ± 1.4 (5.2-11.3)	9.7 ± 0.3 (8.6-11.4)
Chloride (mEq/L)	109 ± 10 (92-128)	Not reported
Cholesterol (mg/dL)	131 ± 25 (86-189)	132.5 ± 5.3 (100-150)
Creatine kinase (U/L)	863 ± 413 (333-1964)	Not reported
Creatinine (mg/dL)	0.4 ± 0.2 (0-0.8)	0.7 ± 0.1 (0.5-1.0)
GGT (U/L)	4 ± 1 (0-12)	Not reported
Glucose (mg/dL)	89 ± 30	86.1 ± 4.7 (60-125)
LDH (U/L)	441 ± 258 (57-820)	Not reported
Phosphorus (mg/dL)	5.3 ± 1.9 (2.4-12)	Not reported
Potassium (mEq/L)	4.9 ± 1 (3.2-7.2)	Not reported
Protein, total (g/dL)	5.8 ± 0.7 (4-7.7)	6.0 ± 0.2 (4.6-6.9)
Albumin (g/dL)	2.9 ± 0.4 (1.8-4.2)	3.4 ± 0.2 (2.7-3.9)
Globulin (g/dL)	2.7 ± 0.5 (1.6-3.9)	2.6 ± 0.2 (1.9-3.6)
Sodium (mEq/L)	141 ± 9 (120-165)	Not reported
Triglycerides (mg/dL)	38 ± 22 (10-96)	37.8 ± 2.3 (30.8-46.2)

TABLE 8-8 Biological and Physiological Values of Hedgehogs.[1,13,16,20,29,39,47,52,54,60]

Parameter	Biological and Physiological Values
Weight	Male, 400-600 g
	Female, 300-400 g
Life span	Avg 4-6 years, may live 8 years
Temperature, rectal	95.7-98.6°F (35.4-37°C)
Preferred environmental temperature	75-85°F (24-29°C)
	Temperatures <60°F (16°C) induce torpor state
Adult dental formula	2 (I3/2:C1/1:P3/2:M3/3) = 36; variations have been noted
Gastrointestinal system	Simple stomach; no cecum; transit time 12-16 hours
Heart rate	180-280 beats/min
Respiratory rate	25-50 breaths/min
Age at sexual maturity	Male, 6-8 months
	Female, 2-6 months
Reproductive life span	Male, throughout life
	Female, 2-3 years
Gestation	34-37 days
Milk composition	Protein, 16 g/100 g; carbohydrate, trace; fat, 25.5 g/100 g
Litter size	Avg 3-4 (range 1-7)
Birth weight	10-18 g
Eyes open	14-18 days
Deciduous teeth eruption	Begins on day 18; all deciduous teeth erupt by 9 weeks
Permanent teeth eruption	Begins at 7-9 weeks
Age at weaning	4-6 weeks (start eating solids at 3 weeks)
Endotracheal tube size	14 g over-the-needle IV catheter to 2.0 mm
Esophagostomy tube size	8 Fr

TABLE 8-9 Suggested Diets for Hedgehogs.[9b,20,23,27,47,51]

The exact nutritional requirements of hedgehogs are unknown. Diets for captive animals have been developed taking into consideration their omnivorous nature, simple gastrointestinal tract, ability to digest chitin, poor digestibility of cellulose, propensity toward obesity, and lack of reports of specific nutritional problems (with the exception of lactose intolerance).

Hedgehogs in captivity will thrive on a base diet composed of approximately 30%-50% protein (dry matter basis) and 10%-20% fat. Because scientific studies regarding hedgehog nutritional needs are lacking, commercial diets appear to be the most balanced diet that a pet owner can offer. If a commercial hedgehog food is not used, a premium commercial feline (adults may use "lite" adult cat foods), ferret, or insectivore diets may be used. Dry foods may be advantageous to help with dental health as periodontal disease is fairly common in hedgehogs. It is inappropriate to use these commercial diets as a sole nutrition source. Supplement with small portions of cooked egg, pinky mice, vegetable and meat jarred human baby foods, gut-loaded crickets and mealworms,[a] chopped vegetables, and fruits. Dairy products, such as cottage cheese and milk, should be avoided, however, because of reports of lactose intolerance.

TABLE 8-9 Suggested Diets for Hedgehogs. (cont'd)

In general, pets should not be fed ad libitum as obesity is very common. Approximately 1-2 Tbs of food daily is a reasonable starting point for adults, with growing animals and reproductively active females being fed the usual diet ad libitum, and calcium-rich foods should be supplemented. Young or pregnant/lactating hedgehogs can also use kitten or ferret formulations. Hedgehogs are generally nocturnal eaters. Fresh water should be provided ad libitum in a shallow dish; animals can also learn to drink from sipper bottles.

In addition to the main diet, 1-2 tsp of varied moist foods (e.g., canned cat or dog food, cooked meat or egg, low-fat cottage cheese) and approximately ½ tsp of fruit (e.g., banana, grape, apple, pear, berries) or vegetables (e.g., beans, cooked carrots, squash, peas, tomatoes, leafy greens) should also be provided daily.[b] One key to balanced nutrition is to provide variety. Acceptable treats include mealworms, earthworms, waxworms, crickets, and cat treats; these may be hidden in the bedding to promote foraging behavior as environmental enrichment.

---

[a]Mealworms are high calorie, low calcium and should be limited to 6-10 smaller mealworms 2-3 times a week; 1-2 crickets (more if hedgehog is pregnant or lactating) can be fed insectivore diet plus some of the fruit/vegetable mixture for a minimum of 3 days after purchase before being fed to the hedgehog; other types of commercially available insects can also be fed. Insects can be dusted with a calcium supplement before feeding to hedgehogs.

[b]An alternative fruit/vegetable mix: chop together ½ tsp diced leafy dark greens (spinach, kale, leaf lettuce), ¼ tsp diced carrot, ¼ tsp diced apple, ¼ tsp diced banana, ¼ tsp diced grape or raisin, ¼ tsp vitamin/mineral powder (Vionate or crushed feline vitamin tab).

TABLE 8-10 Hand-Rearing Orphaned Hedgehogs.[20,31,47,52]

1. Leave neonates with the mother if possible for the first 24-72 hours for colostrum ingestion.
2. In cases of lactation failure or abandonment by the female, fostering the pups to another dam with similarly aged pups is generally successful.
3. Feed a canine milk replacer with added lactase (Lactaid, McNeil Nutritionals) using a 1-cc syringe with a catheter tip or an eye dropper.
4. Neonates should be fed as much as they will consume every 2-4 hours for about 3 weeks, then the time between feedings can be gradually lengthened; the newborns should gain 1-2 g/day during the first week, about 3-4 g/day during the second week, 4-5 g/day during the third and fourth weeks, and 7-9 g/day until they are 60 days old; at 4-6 weeks, parent- or hand-raised young should be weaned by offering canned dog or cat food, minced beef, or freshly molted mealworms; hand-rearing hedgehogs is often associated with high mortality.
5. The ambient temperature should be maintained at 90-95°F (32-35°C) for the first few weeks.
6. Manual stimulation is required for defecation and should be performed after each meal by massaging the ventrum and perineal area with a cloth or swab moistened in warm water.

TABLE 8-11 Common Injection and Venipuncture Sites in Hedgehogs.[16,25,26,37]

Injection Sites	Comments
Subcutaneous	5-10 mL/site; flank at junction of furred skin and spined mantle; SC under mantle requires 1.5- to 3-inch needle
Intramuscular	0.5 mL/site; anterior thigh, triceps; may require sedation; orbicularis up to 1 mL/site
Intravenous	Lateral saphenous, jugular
Intraperitoneal	5-10 mL; requires sedation for access; caudal right abdominal quadrant; useful for fluid administration
Intraosseous	0.5-1 mL slow bolus; requires anesthesia for tibial placement; rarely used

TABLE 8-11   Common Injection and Venipuncture Sites in Hedgehogs. (cont'd)

Venipuncture Sites	Comments
Saphenous	0.5-1 mL; requires sedation; common site for catheterization with 24g-26g catheter
Jugular	0.5-1 mL; requires sedation; easier in thin animals; not visible or palpable; blind stick
Cephalic	Requires sedation; common site for catheterization with 24g-26g catheter
Cranial vena cava	Requires sedation; risk of cardiac puncture

TABLE 8-12   Preventive Medicine in Hedgehogs.[25]

- Prevent obesity; have owners weigh hedgies at least monthly
- Dental prophylaxis—routine brushing, scaling
- Nails need periodic trimming
- Annual (or semi-annual) physical examination, including fecal flotation and direct smear
- No routine vaccines recommended
- Prevent chilling; provide heated environment with dry bedding
- Microchip for personal identification

TABLE 8-13   Common Differential Diagnoses Based on Physical Examination Findings.[2,10,13,14,16,21,22,27,30,46,59]

- Ataxia: brain neoplasia, herpes simplex infection, intervertebral disk disease, wobbly hedgehog syndrome
- Cutaneous/subcutaneous masses: cutaneous hemangiosarcoma, mammary neoplasia, mast cell tumor, thyroid tumor
- Dermatitis/quill loss: bacterial pyoderma, fungal dermatophytosis, mange (*Caparinia*, *Chorioptes*, *Notoedres*)
- Dyspnea: cardiomyopathy, mitral valve disease, bacterial pneumonia, pulmonary metastases
- Gastroenteritis: bacterial (*Salmonella*), lymphosarcoma, parasitic
- Hematuria: bacterial cystitis, endometrial polyps, endometrial sarcoma, uterine spindle cell tumor
- Oral cavity masses: odontogenic fibroma, spindle cell carcinoma, squamous cell carcinoma

TABLE 8-14   Confirmed Zoonotic Diseases Carried by Hedgehogs.[48,50,58]

- Bacterial: *Salmonella* spp., *Yersinia pseudotuberculosis*, *Mycobacterium marinum*
- Viral: Herpesvirus, including human herpes simplex
- Mycotic: *Trychophyton metagrophytes* var. erinacei, *Microsporum* spp.

TABLE 8-15   Common Vocalizations in Hedgehogs.[13]

Snorting/huffing; hissing/grunting	Aggressive or warning sounds produced by sharp vibrating exhalations through the nostrils; generally made when the animal is disturbed, when it encounters another animal, or when it is in the process of rolling up
Screaming	Severe distress call given when the animal is in distress or pain
Twittering/whistling	High-pitched sounds of neonates; whistling stimulates contact by the dam
Clucking	High-pitched contact call of the dam to neonates; also made by courting males
Snuffling	Made as hedgehogs search for food
Inaudible sounds	Hedgehogs can make and hear sounds in the 40- to 90-kHz range, above the range of human hearing

TABLE 8-16 Cardiac Measurements in Hedgehogs.[a,8]

Radiographic Measurements[b]	Mean ± SD (Range)
AB/CD	1.38 ± 0.11 (1.24-1.59)
AB/H	0.88 ± 0.07 (0.74-1.01)
AB/R5-7	1.89 ± 0.29 (1.55-2.73)
CD/H	0.63 ± 0.04 (0.58-0.7)
VHS	8.16 ± 0.48 (7.25-8.75)
L/W	1.4 ± 0.11 (1.16-1.55)
L/C	1.64 ± 0.25 (1.38-2.13)
W/T	0.6 ± 0.03 (0.55-0.66)
W/C	1.17 ± 0.17 (1-1.45)
Echocardiographic Measurements[c]	**Mean ± SD (Range)**
IVSd (cm)	0.15 ± 0.01 (0.13-0.17)
IVSs (cm)	0.22 ± 0.02 (0.19-0.24)
LVIDd (cm)	0.74 ± 0.05 (0.67-0.84)
LVIDs (cm)	0.58 ± 0.03 (0.54-0.65)
LVFWd (cm)	0.16 ± 0.01 (0.14-0.18)
LVFWs (cm)	0.23 ± 0.02 (0.19-0.27)
FS (%)	21.45 ± 2.5 (17.4-26.8)
EPSS (cm)	0.11 ± 0.02 (0.09-0.14)
AO (cm)	0.36 ± 0.02 (0.31-0.4)
LA (cm)	0.56 ± 0.04 (0.51-0.62)
LA/AO (cm)	1.55 ± 0.16 (1.37-1.92)
LVOT Vmax (m/sec)	0.489 ± 0.108 (0.296-0.662)
RVOT Vmax (m/sec)	0.335 ± 0.094 (0.236-0.512)
R-wave amplitude (mV)	0.22 ± 0.11 (0.08-0.5)
QRS duration (sec)	0.03 ± 0 (0.03-0.03)
Mean electrical axis	−10 ± 13 (−28 to 8)
Heart rate (beats/min)	200 ± 48 (100-260)

[a] $n=13$; 5 male, 8 female; age range 6 mo-5 yr, 7 <1 yr, 6 >1 yr.
[b] *AB*, apicobasilar length of heart; *CD*, maximum width of heart perpendicular to AB; *H*, vertical depth of thorax from ventral border of spine to dorsal border of sternum at level of tracheal birfurcation; *R5-7*, distance from 5th rib cranial edge to 7th rib caudal edge; *VHS*, vertebral heart score; *L*, heart length; *W*, maximum width perpendicular to L; *C*, length of clavicle; *T*, thoracic width at level of 6th rib articulation with vertebral column.
[c] *IVSd*, interventricular septal thickness in diastole; *IVSs*, interventricular septal thickness in systole; *LVIDd*, left ventricular internal diameter in diastole; *LVIDs*, left ventricular internal diameter in systole; *LVFWd*, left ventricular free wall thickness in diastole; *LVFWs*, left ventricular free wall thickness in systole; *FS*, fractional shortening; *EPSS*, E-point-to-septal separation length; *AO*, aortic diameter in diastole; *LA*, left atrium internal dimension; *LVOT*, maximum velocity of left ventricular outflow; *RVOT*, maximum velocity of right ventricular outflow.

REFERENCES

1. Adamovicz L, Bullen L, Saker K, et al. Use of an esophagostomy tube for management of traumatic subtotal glossectomy in an African pygmy hedgehog (*Atelerix albiventris*). *J Exot Pet Med* 2016;25:231-236.
2. Allison N, Chang TC, Steele KE, et al. Fatal herpes simplex infection in a pygmy African hedgehog (*Atelerix albiventris*). *J Comp Pathol* 2002;126:76-78.
3. Applegate J. Ectoparasite control in small mammals. http://lafeber.com/vet/ectoparasite-control-in-small-mammals; 2016.
4. Arnemo JM, Soli NE. Chemical immobilization of free-ranging European hedgehogs (*Erinaceus europaeus*). *J Zoo Wildl Med* 1995;26:246-251.
5. Barbiers R. Insectivora (hedgehogs, tenrecs, shrews, moles) and Dermoptera (flying lemurs). In: Fowler ME, Miller RE, eds. *Zoo and Wild Animal Medicine*. 5th ed. Philadelphia: WB Saunders Co; 2003:304-315.
6. Baxton S, Nelson H. Comparison of two systemic antifungal agents, itraconazole and terbinafine, for the treatment of dermatophytosis in European hedgehogs (*Erinaceus europaeus*). *Vet Dermatol* 2016;27:500-e133.
7. Bennett RA. Husbandry and medicine of hedgehogs. *Proc Exotic Sm Mam Med Mgt (Annu Conf Assoc Avian Vet)* 2000;109-114.
8. Black PA, Marshall C, Seyfried AW, et al. Cardiac assessment of African hedgehogs (*Atelerix albiventris*). *J Zoo Wildl Med* 2011;42:49-53.
9. Dierenfeld ES. Feeding behavior and nutrition of the African pygmy hedgehog (*Atelerix albiventris*). *Vet Clin North Am Exot Anim Pract* 2009;12:335-337.
10. Demkowska-Kutrzepa M, Tomczuk K, Studzinska M, et al. *Caparinia tripilis* in African hedgehog (*Atelerix albiventris*). *Vet Dermatol* 2015;26:73-75.
11. Done LB, Deem SL, Fiorello CV. Surgical and medical management of a uterine spindle cell tumor in an African hedgehog (*Atelerix albiventris*). *J Zoo Wildl Med* 2007;38:601-603.
12. Gregory MW, Stocker L. Hedgehogs. In: Beynon PH, Cooper JE, eds. *BSAVA Manual of Exotic Pets*. Gloucestershire: British Small Animal Veterinary Association; 1991:63-68.
13. Han JI, Na KJ. Cutaneous paecilomycosis caused by *Paecilomyces variotii* in an African pygmy hedgehog (*Atelerix albiventris*). *J Exot Pet Med* 2010;19:309-312.
14. Heatley JJ. Hedgehogs. In: Mitchell MA, Tully Jr TN, eds. *Manual of Exotic Pet Practice*. St. Louis: Saunders/Elsevier; 2009:433-455.
15. Heatley JJ, Mauldin GE, Cho DY. A review of neoplasia in the captive African hedgehog (*Atelerix albiventris*). *Semin Avian Exot Pet Med* 2005;14:182-192.
16. Hedley J, Benato L, Fraga G, et al. Congestive heart failure due to endocardiosis of the mitral valves in an African pygmy hedgehog. *J Exot Pet Med* 2013;22:212-217.
17. Helmer PJ. Personal observation. 2016.
18. Hoefer HL. Hedgehogs. *Vet Clin North Am Small Anim Pract* 1994;24:113-120.
19. Hoefer HL. Clinical approach to the African hedgehog. *Proc North Am Vet Conf* 1999;836-838.
19a. Hoppes S. Common diseases of hedgehogs. *Southwest Vet Symp* 2016.
20. International Species Information System. Apple Valley, MN. 2002.
21. Isenbügel E, Baumgartner RA. Diseases of the hedgehog. In: Fowler ME, ed. *Zoo and Wild Animal Medicine: Current Therapy*. 3rd ed. Philadelphia: WB Saunders Co; 1993:294-302.
22. Ivey E, Carpenter JW. African hedgehogs. In: Quesenberry KE, Carpenter JW, eds. *Ferrets, Rabbits, and Rodents: Clinical Medicine and Surgery*. 3rd ed. Philadelphia: Saunders/Elsevier; 2012:411-427.
23. Jepson L. Hedgehogs. In: Jepson L. *Exotic Animal Medicine: A Quick Reference Guide*. 2nd ed. St. Louis: Elsevier; 2016:198-230.
24. Johnson D. Diagnosing and treating African pygmy hedgehogs. *Proc Atlantic Coast Vet Conf* 2004.
25. Johnson-Delaney CA. *Exotic Companion Medicine Handbook for Veterinarians*. Lake Worth, FL: Wingers Publishing; 1996.

26. Johnson-Delaney CA. Other small mammals. In: Meredith A, Redrobe S, eds. *BSAVA Manual of Exotic Pets*. 4th ed. Quedgeley: British Small Animal Veterinary Association; 2002:102-115.
27. Johnson-Delaney CA. Hedgehogs. In: Johnson-Delaney CA, ed. *Exotic Companion Medicine Handbook for Veterinarians*. Lake Worth, FL: Zoological Education Network; 2005.
28. Johnson-Delaney CA. Common procedures in hedgehogs, prairie dogs, exotic rodents, and companion marsupials. *Vet Clin North Am Exot Anim Pract* 2006;9:415-435.
29. Johnson-Delaney CA. What veterinarians need to know about hedgehogs. *Exot DVM* 2007;9:38-44.
30. Kim KR, Ahn KS, Oh DS, et al. Efficacy of a combination of 10% imidacloprid and 1% moxidectin against *Caparinia tripilis* in African pygmy hedgehog (*Atelerix albiventris*). *Parasit Vectors* 2012;5:158.
31. Landes E, Zentek J, Wolf P, et al. Investigations on the composition of milk and development of sucklings in hedgehogs. *Kleintierpraxis* 1997;42:647-658.
32. LaRue MK, Flesner BK, Higbie CT. Treatment of a thyroid tumor in an African pygmy hedgehog (*Atelerix albiventris*). *J Exot Pet Med* 2016;25:226-230.
33. Lennox AM. Emergency and critical care procedures in sugar gliders (*Petaurus breviceps*), African hedgehogs (*Atelerix albiventris*), and prairie dogs (*Cynomys* spp.). *Vet Clin North Am Exot Anim Pract* 2007;10:533-555.
34. Lennox AM. Safe sedation and immobilization of unusual exotic species encountered in practice. *J Exot Pet Med* 2014;23:363-368.
35. Leonatti SR. *Ornithonyssus bacoti* mite infestation in an African pygmy hedgehog. *Exot DVM* 2007;9:3-4.
36. Letcher JD. Amitraz as a treatment for acariasis in African hedgehogs (*Atelerix albiventris*). *J Zoo Anim Med* 1988;19:24-29.
37. Levine BS. Review of antibiotic-impregnated polymethylmethacrylate beads in avian and exotic pets. *Exot DVM* 2003;5:11.
38. Lightfoot TL. Therapeutics of African pygmy hedgehogs and prairie dogs. *Vet Clin North Am Exot Anim Pract* 2000;3:155-172.
39. Longley L. Anaesthesia of other small mammals. In: Longley L, ed. *Anaesthesia of Exotic Pets*. Philadelphia: Saunders/Elsevier; 2008:96-102.
40. Marshall KL. Fungal diseases in small mammals: therapeutic trends and zoonotic considerations. *Vet Clin North Am Exot Anim Pract* 2003;6:415-427.
41. Morgan KR, Berg BM. Body temperature regulation and energy metabolism in pygmy hedgehogs. *Am Zool* 1997;37:150A.
42. Morrisey JK, Carpenter JW. Formulary. In: Quesenberry KE, Carpenter JW, eds. *Ferrets, Rabbits, and Rodents: Clinical Medicine and Surgery*. 3rd ed. St. Louis: Saunders/Elsevier; 2012:566-575.
43. Okorie-Kanu CO, Onoja RL, Achegbulu EE, et al. Normal haematological and serum biochemistry values of African hedgehog (*Atelerix albiventris*). *Comp Clin Pathol* 2015;24:127-132.
44. Pantchev N, Hofmann T. Notoedric mange caused by *Notoedres cati* in a pet African pygmy hedgehog (*Atelerix albiventris*). *Vet Rec* 2006;158:59-60.
45. Papich MG, Davidson GS, Fortier LA. Doxycycline concentration over time after storage in a compounded veterinary preparation. *J Am Vet Med Assoc* 2013;242:1674-1678.
46. Plumb DC. *Plumb's Veterinary Drug Handbook*. 8th ed. Ames: Wiley-Blackwell; 2015.
47. Powers LV. Subcutaneous implantable catheter for fluid administration in an African pygmy hedgehog. *Exot DVM* 2002;4.5:16-17.
48. Raymond JT, Aguilar R, Dunker F, et al. Intervertebral disc disease in African hedgehogs (*Atelerix albiventris*): four cases. *J Exot Pet Med* 2009;18:220-223.
49. Reeve N. *Hedgehogs*. London: T & AD Poyser Ltd; 1994.
50. Rhee DY, Kim MS, Chang SE, et al. A case of tinea manuum caused by *Trichophyton mentagrophytes* var. erinacei: the first isolation in Korea. *Mycoses* 52:287-290.

51. Rhody JL, Schiller CA. Spinal osteosarcoma in a hedgehog with pedal self-mutilation. *Vet Clin North Am Exot Anim Pract* 2006;9:625-631.
52. Riley PY, Chomel BB. Hedgehog zoonoses. *Emerg Infect Dis* 2005;11:1-5.
53. Smith AJ. Husbandry and medicine of African hedgehogs (*Atelerix albiventris*). *J Small Exotic Anim Med* 1992;2:21-28.
54. Smith AJ. Neonatology of the hedgehog (*Atelerix albiventris*). *J Small Exot Anim Med* 1995;3:15-18.
55. Smith AJ. Medical management of hedgehogs. *Proc 21st Annu Waltham/OSU Symp* 1997;57-61.
56. Smith AJ. General husbandry and medical care of hedgehogs. In: Bonagura JD, ed. *Kirk's Current Veterinary Therapy XIII: Small Animal Practice*. Philadelphia: WB Saunders Co; 2000:1128-1133.
57. Staley EC, Staley EE, Behr MJ. Use of permethrin as a miticide in the African hedgehog (*Atelerix albiventris*). *Vet Hum Toxicol* 1994;36:138.
58. Stocker L. *Medication for Use in the Treatment of Hedgehogs*. Marshcliff: Ayelsbury; 1992.
59. Vuolo S, Whittington JK. Dystocia secondary to a perianal fetal hernia in an African hedgehog. *Exot DVM* 2008;10.3:10-12.
60. Weishaupt J, Kolb-Maurer A, Lempert S, et al. A different kind of hedgehog pathway: tinea manus due to *Trichophyton erinacei* transmitted by an African pygmy hedgehog (*Atelerix albiventris*). *Mycoses* 2014;57:125-127.
61. Wozniak A, Janeczek M, Janus I, et al. Surgical resection of peripheral odontogenic fibromas in African pygmy hedgehogs (*Atelerix albiventris*): a case study. *BMC Vet Res* 2015;11:145.
62. Wrobel D, Brown SA. *The Hedgehog: An Owner's Guide to a Happy, Healthy Pet*. New York: Howell Book House; 1997.

Chapter 9 Rodents

Jörg Mayer | Christoph Mans

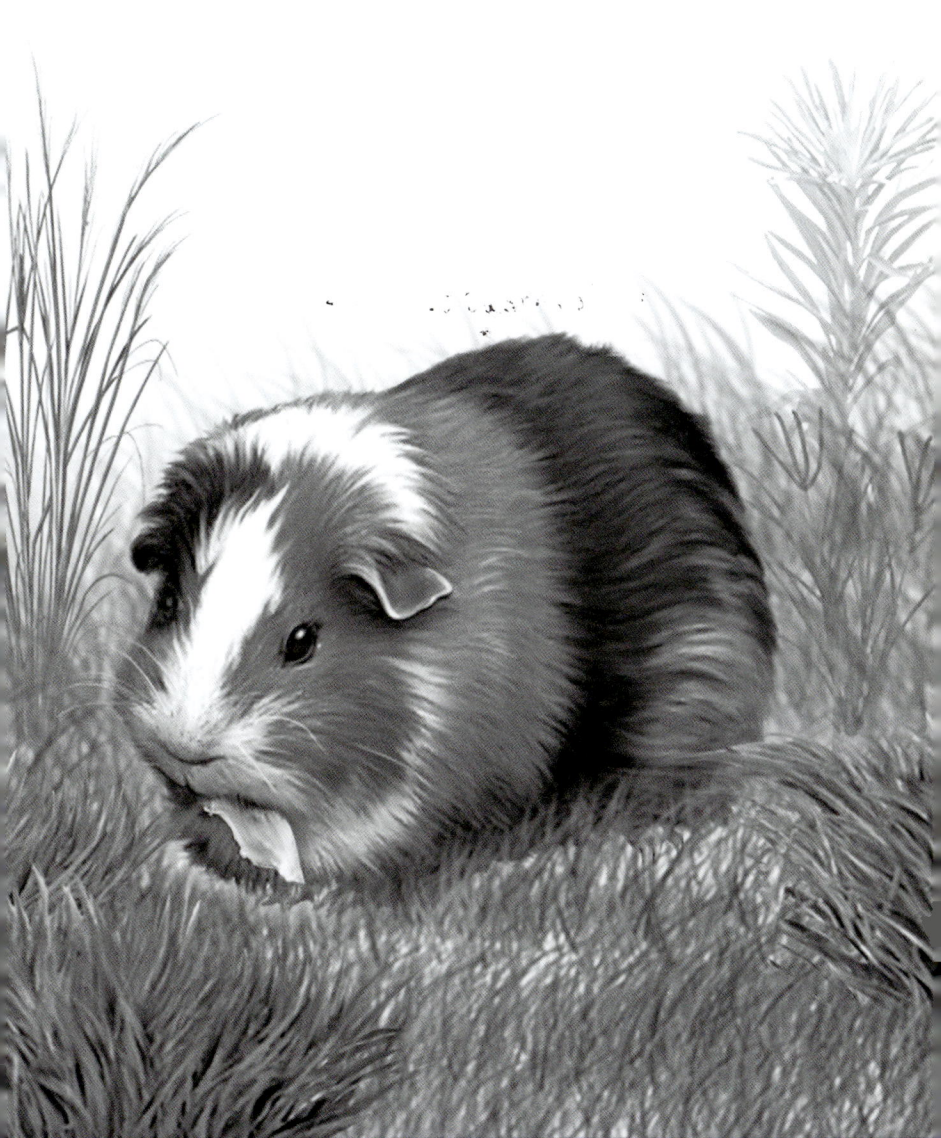

TABLE 9-1 Antimicrobial and Antifungal Agents Used in Rodents.[a]

Agent	Dosage	Comments
Amikacin	5-15 mg/kg SC, IM, IV q8-12h[84]	All species/also administer fluid therapy
	15 mg/kg IM q12h[79]	Guinea pigs/high peak dosing regimen as efficacious as divided regimen
	16 mg/kg SC, IM, IV divided q8-24h[90]	All species/also administer fluid therapy
Amoxicillin	—	Do not use orally in hamsters, guinea pigs, chinchillas; may cause enterocolitis[2]
	25 mg/kg PO q12h[82]	Rats
	10-15 mg/kg PO q12h[113]	Rats
	100-150 mg/kg IM, SC[84]	Rats, mice
	0.25 mg/mL drinking water for 7 days[73]	Mice/only effective against highly susceptible bacteria; plasma levels reached <300 ng/mL[73]
Amoxicillin/clavulanic acid	20 mg/kg PO q12h[90]	Mice, rats
Amphotericin B	0.11 mg/kg SC q24h[84,90]	Mice/use with caution; may cause renal toxicity
	0.43 mg/kg PO q24h[84,90]	Mice/candidiasis
	1.25-2.5 mg/kg SC q24h[84]	Guinea pigs/cryptococcosis
Ampicillin	—	Do not use orally in hamsters, guinea pigs, chinchillas; may cause enterocolitis[2]
	6-30 mg/kg PO q8h[84]	Gerbils
	20-100 mg/kg PO, SC, IM q8h[84]	Gerbils
	20-250 mg/kg PO q12h[113]	Rats
	25 mg/kg SC, IM q12h[84]	Rats, mice
	50-200 mg/kg PO q12h[84]	Rats, mice
Azithromycin	15-30 mg/kg PO q24h[31,90]	Most species, including guinea pigs, chinchillas, hamsters
	30 mg/kg PO q24h[8,20]	Chinchillas
	50 mg/kg PO q12h for 14 days[84]	Rats, mice
Captan powder	1 tsp/2 cups dust[49]	Chinchillas/fungicide to prevent spread of dermatophytes between cagemates; add to dust box
Cephalexin	15 mg/kg SC, IM q12h[33]	Rats, mice
	15 mg/kg SC q12h[33]	Guinea pigs
	20 mg/kg PO q8h[113]	Rats
	25 mg/kg IM q12-24h[84,113]	Guinea pigs
	25 mg/kg SC q24h[90]	Hamsters, gerbils
	60 mg/kg PO q12h[90]	Mice
Chloramphenicol	30-50 mg/kg PO q8-12h[31,90]	Most species
	200 mg/kg PO q12h[84]	Mice
	0.5 mg/mL drinking water[84]	Mice
	0.83 mg/mL drinking water[84]	Gerbils
	1 mg/mL drinking water[84]	Guinea pigs

TABLE 9-1 Antimicrobial and Antifungal Agents Used in Rodents. (cont'd)

Agent	Dosage	Comments
Chlortetracycline	10 mg/kg SC, IM q12h[90]	Rats
	20 mg/kg PO, SC, IM q12h[90]	Hamsters, gerbils
	25 mg/kg PO, SC, IM q12h[90]	Mice
	50 mg/kg PO q12h[90]	Chinchillas
Ciprofloxacin	5-25 mg/kg PO q12-24h[84,90]	Chinchillas, guinea pigs/may cause arthropathies in young of any species
	10 mg/kg PO q12h[84]	Rats, mice
	10-20 mg/kg PO q12h[84]	Hamster
Clarithromycin	15 mg/kg PO q12h[7]	Chinchillas
Clindamycin	7.5 mg/kg SC q12h[90]	Most species/can cause diarrhea; do not give orally; avoid or use with caution in chinchillas and guinea pigs; excellent bone penetration
Doxycycline	2.5-5 mg/kg PO q12h[90]	All species/pneumonia; may give in combination with enrofloxacin; do not use in young and pregnant animals
	70-100 mg/kg SC, IM q7d[90]	Mice, rats/use long-acting formulation
	0.05 mg/mL drinking water for 7 days[73]	Mice/failed to achieve effective plasma concentrations.
Enilconazole	Dip in a 0.2% (1:50) solution q7d[2,84]	Dermatophytosis
	0.2% solution topical q3-4d[31]	All species/dermatophytosis
Enrofloxacin	—	Very high doses may cause arthropathies in young if given for a prolonged time; limit SC, IM injections; SC injections can be diluted in NaCl or lactated Ringer's solution
	5-20 mg/kg PO, SC, IM q12-24h[2,84,90]	Most species/may combine with doxycycline for chronic respiratory infections in rats
	10 mg/kg SC q12h[33]	Most species
	0.25 mg/mL drinking water × 7 days[73]	Mice/failed to achieve effective plasma concentrations; remains stable for 7 days
Enrofloxacin (E)/ doxycycline (D)	10 mg/kg (E) + 5 mg/kg (D) PO q12h[83]	Rats/chronic respiratory infection
Erythromycin	—	Do not use orally in chinchillas, guinea pigs; use with caution in hamsters and gerbils[90]
	10 mg/kg PO q24h[113]	Rats, chronic respiratory disease
	20 mg/kg PO q12h[84,90]	Mice, rats, hamsters
	0.13 mg/mL drinking water[84]	Hamsters/outbreaks of proliferative ileitis; use with caution: can cause enterotoxemia; equivalent to 500 mg/gal drinking water
Gentamicin	—	Use cautiously; nephrotoxic; ensure adequate hydration; can be used topically in nostrils for upper respiratory tract infections; consider use of amikacin instead
	2-5 mg/kg SC, IM q24h[84]	All species
	4-24 mg/kg SC, IM q12h[2]	All species
	20 mg/kg SC q24h[2]	Rats

Continued

TABLE 9-1 Antimicrobial and Antifungal Agents Used in Rodents. (cont'd)

Agent	Dosage	Comments
Griseofulvin	—	Dermatophytosis; do not use in pregnant animals; can cause diarrhea, leukopenia, anorexia
	15-50 mg/kg PO q24h × 14-28 days[90]	Guinea pigs
	25 mg/kg PO q24h[90]	Most species
Itraconazole	2.5-10 mg/kg PO q24h[84,90]	Most species, in guinea pigs less effective than terbinafine for treatment of dermatophytosis[85]
	5 mg/kg PO q24h[31]	Guinea pigs/dermatophytosis; consider pulse therapy, 7 days on/off until culture negative[31]
	50-150 mg/kg PO q24h[84,90]	Mice/blastomycosis
Ketoconazole	10-40 mg/kg PO q24h × 14 days[90]	All species/systemic mycoses; candidiasis
Lime sulfur dip	Dip q7d × 4 treatments[90]	All species/dermatophytosis; dilute 1:40 with water
Marbofloxacin	2-5 mg/kg PO, SC, IM q24h[84]	All species/do not give during lactation, pregnancy, or while growing; injectable can be given orally
	4 mg/kg PO, SC q24h[90]	
Metronidazole	—	Use with caution in chinchillas; objectionable taste may result in reduced food consumption
	10-20 mg/kg PO q12h[90]	Most species
	10-40 mg/kg PO q24h[90]	Mice, rats
	20-60 mg/kg PO q8-12h[2]	Prairie dogs
	2.5 mg/mL drinking water × 5 day[14]	Mice
Neomycin	—	No absorption following oral administration, therefore not effective against systemic infections; extremely nephrotoxic following parenteral administration
	15 mg/kg PO q12h[84]	Chinchillas, guinea pigs
	25 mg/kg PO q12h[84]	Mice, rats, hamsters
	0.5 mg/mL drinking water[84]	Hamsters
	2 mg/mL drinking water[33]	Mice, rats
	2.6 mg/mL drinking water[84]	Mice, rats, gerbils
Nystatin	60,000-90,000 U/kg PO q12h × 7-10 days[84]	Gastrointestinal mycoses; not absorbed from gastrointestinal tract
Oxytetracycline	5 mg/kg IM q12h, or 10-20 mg/kg PO q8h[84]	Guinea pigs
	15 mg/kg IM q12h, or 50 mg/kg PO q12h[84]	Chinchillas
	10 mg/kg PO q8h[14]	Gerbils
	10-20 mg/kg PO q8h[84]	Mice, rats/Tyzzer's disease (mice); *Mycoplasma pneumonia* (rats)
	20-25 mg/kg IM q8-12h[84]	Hamsters, gerbils
	100 mg/kg SC q24h[104]	All species
	0.25-1 mg/mL drinking water[14]	Hamsters, mice, rats, gerbils

TABLE 9-1 Antimicrobial and Antifungal Agents Used in Rodents. (cont'd)

Agent	Dosage	Comments
Oxytetracycline (cont'd)	200 mg/L drinking water for 30 days[113]	Rats/prophylactic treatment
	400 mg/L drinking water for 10 days[113]	Rats/curative treatment
	3 g/L drinking water[104]	Chinchillas, guinea pigs
Penicillin G	22,000 U/kg SC, IM q24h[90]	Rats
Penicillin G (benzathine and procaine)	22,000 U/kg SC, IM q24h[84,90]	Most species
	50,000 U/kg SC q3-5d[69,72]	Chinchillas, guinea pigs, degus
Sulfonamide/ trimethoprim combinations	15-30 mg/kg PO, SC, IM 12-24h[84,90]	Most species
	25 mg/kg PO q12h[113]	Rats
	50-100 mg/kg PO, SC q24h[84]	Gerbils, rats, mice
	0.8 mg/mL drinking water[73]	Mice/failed to achieve effective plasma concentrations; remains stable for 7 days
Terbinafine	10-30 mg/kg PO q24h × 4-6 wk[90]	Most species/antifungal
	20 mg/kg PO q24h[85]	Guinea pigs/PD; dermatophytosis; more effective than itraconazole
Tetracycline	10 mg/kg PO q8-12h[90]	Guinea pigs, chinchillas/use with caution[90]
	10 mg/kg PO, SC q24h[31]	Guinea pigs
	20 mg/kg PO q12h[2]	Most species
	20 mg/kg PO, IM q24h[2]	Gerbils
	30 mg/kg PO q6h[2]	Hamsters
	0.2-0.5 mg/mL drinking water for 7-10 mL days[113]	Rats
	0.4 mg/mL drinking water[2]	Hamsters
	0.6 mg/mL drinking water[2]	Mice
	0.7 mg/mL drinking water[2]	Guinea pigs/toxicity reported[73]
	0.1%-0.5% feed × 14 days[2]	Rats
Trimethoprim/ sulfonamides	—	See Sulfonamide/trimethoprim combinations
Tylosin	2-10 mg/kg PO, SC q12h[90]	Hamsters, gerbils/use with caution
	10 mg/kg PO, SC q12h[84,90,115]	Chinchillas, guinea pigs, mice, rats/toxicity reported in guinea pigs
	10 mg/kg PO q24h × 5 days[113]	Rats
	0.5 mg/mL (500 mg/L) drinking water[15]	Gerbils, hamsters, mice, rats/PD in rats;[18] toxicity in hamsters reported[3]
Vancomycin	20 mg/kg PO q24h[46]	Tyzzer's disease

[a]Oral antibiotic treatment can result in enteritis and antibiotic-associated clostridial enterotoxemia, especially when antibiotics with a primary Gram-positive spectrum are given. Chinchillas, guinea pigs, and hamsters are most susceptible. Also, direct toxicity due to streptomycin and dihydrostreptomycin occurs in gerbils, guinea pigs, hamsters, and mice. Procaine, included in some penicillin preparations, can be toxic to mice. Guinea pigs and chinchillas are highly susceptible to the ototoxic effects of chloramphenicol and aminoglycosides at dosages above those recommended clinically. Antibiotics implicated in antibiotic-associated clostridial enterotoxemia following oral administration include:[49,97]

- Chinchillas: penicillins (including ampicillin, amoxicillin), bacitracin, cephalosporins, clindamycin, erythromycin, lincomycin.
- Guinea pigs: penicillins (including ampicillin, amoxicillin), cefazolin, clindamycin, erythromycin, lincomycin, dihydrostreptomycin, streptomycin, bacitracin, chlortetracycline, oxytetracycline, tetracycline, tylosin.
- Hamsters: penicillins (including ampicillin, amoxicillin), bacitracin, cephalosporins, clindamycin, erythromycin, lincomycin, vancomycin, dihydrostreptomycin, streptomycin, tylosin.

TABLE 9-2 Antiparasitic Agents Used in Rodents.

Agent	Dosage	Comments
Albendazole	5 mg/kg PO q12h[10]	Guinea pigs
	25 mg/kg PO q12h × 2 days[90]	Chinchillas/giardiasis
Amitraz	1.4 mL/L (0.007%) topical q7-14d × 3 treatments[2,84,90]	Gerbils, hamsters/demodecosis; apply with cottonball, brush; use with caution; not recommended in young
	0.3% solution topically q7-14d × 3-6 treatments[84,90]	Guinea pigs/mites
	1.4 mL/L topical, repeat q14d[113]	Rats
Carbaryl powder (5%)	Topical q7d × 3 treatments[90]	Guinea pigs/ectoparasites
Dimetridazole	20-50 mg/kg PO q24h × 7 days[10]	Guinea pigs/*Trichomonas, Giardia*
	1.2-10 mg/mL drinking water for 5 days[99]	Mice/trichomoniasis, but not effective; use metronidazole or tinidazole instead[99]
	500 mg/L drinking water[10,103]	Degus, hamsters/*Trichomonas, Giardia*
	1 g/L drinking water for 40 days[10]	Chinchillas, degus, chipmunks, squirrels/*Giardia*
	4 g/L drinking water for 7 days[10,113]	Rats, mice/*Giardia, Hexamita*
Doramectin	0.2-0.5 mg/kg SC q7-14d for 2-3 treatments[10]	Most species
Emodepside/ praziquantel (Profender, Bayer)	0.07-0.7 mL/kg topical[81]	Mice/PD; nematodes; cestodes; contains 21.4 mg/mL of emodepside and 85.9 mg/mL of praziquantel
Fenbendazole	20 mg/kg PO q24h for 5 days[10,113]	Rats, guinea pigs
	20-50 mg/kg PO q24h × 5 days[2,84,90]	All species/giardiasis; a lower dose is generally preferred; higher end for giardiasis only[84]
	25-150 ppm in feed for 5 days[113]	Mice/*Oxyurids*
	50 ppm in feed for 5 days[113]	Mice/*Hymenolepis dimunata*
	300 ppm in feed for 5 days[113]	Mice/*Rodentolepis nana*
Fipronil	7.5 mg/kg topically q30-60d[84]	Most species/fleas, ticks, and lice
	1-2 spray pumps topical, repeat 1-2 × q7-10d[31]	Guinea pigs
Imidacloprid	20 mg/kg topically q30d[84,90]	Most species/flea control
Imidacloprid 10%/ moxidectin 1% (Advocate, Bayer)	0.1 mL/animal[52]	Guinea pigs/ectoparasites (i.e., fleas, biting lice, mites)
Ivermectin	0.2-0.4 mg/kg PO, SC q7-14d[90]	Most species/ectoparasites; preferred dosage appears to be 0.4 mg/kg q7d (higher doses have also been reported); for *Demodex*, use q7d
	0.2-0.5 mg/kg SC, PO q7-14d[84]	Most species
	0.3 mg/kg PO q24h[111]	Hamsters/PD; demodicosis
	0.4 mg/kg SC q7d[11]	Hamsters/notoedric mites
	0.4 mg/kg SC, repeat q14d[27]	Guinea pigs/PD; *Trixacarus caviae*

TABLE 9-2 Antiparasitic Agents Used in Rodents. (cont'd)

Agent	Dosage	Comments
Ivermectin (cont'd)	Spray animals or topical drops[9]	Mice/clinical trial for mite control;[9] use 1% ivermectin diluted 1:100 with 1:1 propylene glycol:water (0.1 mg/mL); sprayed onto mice or topical behind ear
	8 mg/L drinking water × 4 days/wk × 5 wk[60]	Mice/pinworms
	25 mg/L drinking water × 4 days/wk × 5 wk[60]	Rats/pinworms
	48 mg/L drinking water × 3 days[34]	Rats/pinworms, *Giardia*, *Hymenolepis*
Levimasol	25 mg/kg SC[10]	Guinea pigs
Lime sulfur dip	Dip q7d × 6 wk[90]	All species/ectoparasites; dilute 1:40 with water
Mebendazole	20 mg/kg PO[10]	Guinea pigs
	40 mg/kg PO q7d × 21 days[2]	Mice, rats/pinworms
	50-60 mg/kg PO q12h × 5 days[10]	Chinchillas, degus, chipmunks
Metronidazole	10-20 mg/kg PO q12h, or 40 mg/kg q24h[84]	Guinea pigs, chinchillas/use with caution in chinchillas; objectionable taste may result in reduced food intake
	20-40 mg/kg PO q24h[84]	Rats, mice, gerbils, hamsters
	20-50 mg/kg PO q8h[90]	Gerbils, hamsters
	25 mg/kg PO q12h[10]	Guinea pigs, chinchillas
	50-60 mg/kg PO q12h for 5 days[113]	Rats
	2.5 mg/mL drinking water × 5 days[2,10,99]	Rats, mice/trichomoniasis
Moxidectin	—	See Imidacloprid
Niclosamid	100 mg/kg PO 2 × q7d[10]	Guinea pigs/*Hymenolepis* spp.
Nitenpyram (Capstar, Novartis)	1 mg/kg PO once[84]	Most species/fleas, flystrike; safe in pregnant animals[84]
Permethrin	0.25% dust in cage[74]	All species/ectoparasites
Piperazine adipate	500 mg/kg PO q24h[90]	Chinchillas
	3-5 mg/mL drinking water × 7 days, off 7 days, on 7 days[90]	Hamsters, gerbils
	4-7 mg/mL drinking water × 3-10 days[90]	Guinea pigs, mice, rats
Piperazine citrate	100 mg/kg PO q24h × 2 days[90]	Chinchillas
	4-5 mg/mL drinking water × 7 days, off 7 days, on 7 days[84]	Rats, mice
	4-7 g/L drinking water[10]	Guinea pigs
	10 mg/mL drinking water × 7 days, off 7 days, on 7 days[84,90]	Guinea pigs, hamsters
Ponazuril	30 mg/kg PO q48h × 2 treatments[38]	Prairie dogs/*Eimeria*

Continued

TABLE 9-2 Antiparasitic Agents Used in Rodents. (cont'd)

Agent	Dosage	Comments
Praziquantel	5-10 mg/kg PO, SC q10d × 2 treatments[31]	Guinea pigs
	6-10 mg/kg PO, SC, repeat in 10 days[31,90]	All species/cestodes, trematodes
	30 mg/kg PO q14d × 3 treatments[84]	Gerbils, mice, rats
	140 ppm in feed for 7 days[2]	Mice
Pyrantel pamoate	50 mg/kg PO[84,90]	Most species/gastrointestinal nematodes
Pyrethrin powder	Topical 3×/wk[90]	Gerbils, hamsters, mice, rats/ectoparasites
	Topical q7d × 3 treatments[90]	Chinchillas, guinea pigs/ectoparasites
Pyrethrin shampoo (0.05%)	Shampoo q7d × 4 treatments[90]	Hamsters, gerbils, mice, rats/fleas
Ronidazole	400 mg/L drinking water[10,113]	Rats, mice, gerbils
Selamectin	15 mg/kg topically once[27]	Guinea pigs/PD; *Trixacarus caviae*
	15-30 mg/kg topically q21-28d × 2 treatments (q14d for *Demodex*)[29,31]	Most species/use 30 mg/kg for *Sarcoptes*
Sulfadimethoxine	15-100 mg/kg PO q24h × 3 days, 5 days break, then treat for 3 more days[10]	Guinea pigs
	25-50 mg/kg PO q24h × 10 days[90]	Most species
	50 mg/kg PO once, then 25 mg/kg q24h × 10-20 days	All species/coccidiosis
Sulfamerazine	1 mg/mL drinking water[90]	Most species/coccidiosis
	1.5 mg/L drinking water for 10 days[10]	Chinchillas, degus, chipmunks, squirrels/coccidia
Sulfamethazine	1 mg/mL drinking water × 4 days, then 4 days off, repeat for 3 more treatments[10]	Chinchillas, degus, chipmunks, squirrels/coccidia
	1-5 mg/mL drinking water[2]	All species/coccidiosis
Sulfamethoxypyrazine	25 mg/kg PO q24h × 3-5 days[10]	Guinea pigs
Sulfaquinoxaline	1 mg/mL drinking water × 14-21 days[2,90]	All species/coccidiosis
Thiabendazole	50-100 mg/kg PO q24h × 5 days[90]	Most species/ascaridiasis
	100-200 mg/kg PO q24h × 5 days[10]	Guinea pigs
Tinidazole	50-100 mg/kg PO[69]	Prairie dogs/*Giardia*
	2.5 g/L drinking water[10,99]	Rats, mice, gerbils
Toltrazuril (Baycox, Bayer)	10 mg/kg PO q24h × 3 days, off 3-5 days, on 3 days[30,103,113]	Most species/drug of choice for coccidiosis; 2.5% solution has very low pH; needs to be diluted with equal parts water and propylene glycol (1:1:1);[106] 5% solution does not need to be diluted
	10-20 mg/kg PO q24h for 3 days, 5 days break, then give for 3 more days[113]	Hamsters/coccidiosis
	25 mg/L drinking water[10]	Most species

TABLE 9-3 Chemical Restraint/Anesthetic Agents Used in Rodents.

Agent	Dosage	Comments
Acepromazine	—	See ketamine for combinations
	0.5-1 mg/kg IM[90,114]	Most species
	0.5-2.5 mg/kg IM, SC, PO[84]	Rats
	0.5-5 mg/kg IM, SC, PO[84]	Guinea pigs, hamsters, mice/higher doses should only be given PO
Alfaxalone	—	Licensed for IV administration; can be administered IM, SC, IP, but high doses needed, resulting in large volumes
	2-5 mg/kg IV[65]	Rats/anesthesia; mean duration <15 min
	5-10 mg/kg SC, IM administration[94]	Chinchillas, not effective[94]
	20 mg/kg IP[65]	Rats/anesthesia, 20-60 min; no induction in 30% of animals
	40 mg/kg IM, IP[84]	Guinea pigs
	80 mg/kg IP[108]	Mice/surgical anesthesia for ~60 min
	100 mg/kg SC, IP[48]	Mice/anesthesia
Alfaxalone (A)/ butorphanol (B)	(A) 5 mg/kg + (B) 0.5 mg/kg IM[94]	Chinchillas/short-term inconsistent anesthesia (<20 min); significant postanesthetic reduction in food intake and fecal output[94]
Alfaxalone (A)/ medetomidine (Me)/ butorphanol (B)	(A) 40-80 mg/kg + (Me) 0.3 mg/kg + (B) 5 mg/kg SC[48]	Mice/anesthesia; surgical anesthesia for 35-85 min dependent on alfaxalone dose; not effective after IP administration
Alfaxalone (A)/ xylazine (X)	(A) 80 mg/kg + (X) 10 mg/kg IP[108]	Mice/surgical anesthesia for 80 ± 18 min
Atipamezole (Antisedan, Pfizer)[a]	5 × the administered medetomidine dose, or 10 × the administered dexmedetomidine dose SC, IM[84]	Dexmedetomidine/medetomidine reversal
	1 mg/kg SC[90]	All species
Atropine	0.04-0.4 mg/kg SC, IM[90]	Gerbils, hamsters, mice, rats/rats possess serum atropinesterase
	0.05-0.2 mg/kg SC, IM, IV[90]	Chinchillas, guinea pigs
	0.1-0.2 mg/kg SC, IM[84]	Chinchillas, guinea pigs
Bupivacaine	0.5 mg/kg[3]	Guinea pigs/nerve blocks
	1 mg/kg + 0.1 mg/kg morphine (preservative free) epidural[84]	Limit volume to 0.33 mL/kg
	1-2 mg/kg local nerve block[84]	Guinea pig, rats
	1.6 mg/kg epidural[84]	Anesthesia to level of L4
	2.3 mg/kg epidural[84]	Anesthesia to level of T11-13
Dexmedetomidine (Dexdomitor, Orion)	—	α_2-agonist similar to medetomidine; see ketamine for combination
Diazepam	—	See fentanyl/fluanisone and ketamine for combinations
	0.5-5 mg/kg IM[84]	Guinea pigs
	2.5-5 mg/kg IM[84]	Chinchillas, hamsters, gerbils, rats, mice

Continued

TABLE 9-3 Chemical Restraint/Anesthetic Agents Used in Rodents. (cont'd)

Agent	Dosage	Comments
Fentanyl/fluanisone (Hypnorm, Janssen)	—	Anesthesia
	0.2-0.6 mL/kg IM, IP[74]	Mice, rats
	0.5-1 mL/kg IM[84]	Guinea pigs
Flumazenil	0.1 mg/kg SC[46]	Chinchillas/midazolam reversal
Glycopyrrolate	0.01-0.02 mg/kg SC[50]	All species/excess oral or respiratory mucus
Isoflurane	2%-5% induction, then 0.25%-4% maintenance[74,84]	All species/inhalant anesthetic of choice
Ketamine	—	Avoid use alone, due to high doses needed; ketamine combinations follow
	20-40 mg/kg IM[74]	Chinchillas, hamsters/light sedation; heavy sedation at higher doses in hamsters
	22 mg/kg IM[74]	Mice, rats/light sedation; heavy sedation at 44 mg/kg in mice and 25-40 mg/kg in rats
	22-44 mg/kg IM[74]	Guinea pigs/light sedation; heavy sedation at higher doses
	40-60 mg/kg IM[74]	Gerbils/light sedation; heavy sedation at higher doses (marked individual variation)
Ketamine (K)/ acepromazine (A)	(K) 40 mg/kg + (A) 0.5 mg/kg IM[89]	Chinchillas/anesthesia; prolonged recovery
	(K) 50-150 mg/kg + (A) 2.5-5 mg/kg IM[88]	Mice, rats/lower end of doses preferred
Ketamine (K)/ dexmedetomidine (De)	(K) 2-4 mg/kg + (Me) 0.025 mg/kg IM[84]	Most species/sedation
	(K) 3-5 mg/kg + (De) 0.05 mg/kg SC, IM[84]	Guinea pigs/short anesthesia
	(K) 4 mg/kg + (De) 0.015 mg/kg[24,35]	Chinchillas/surgical anesthesia; provide supplemental oxygen; reverse with atipamezole[35]
	(K) 75 mg/kg + (De) 0.5 mg/kg IP[74]	Mice, rats
Ketamine (K)/ diazepam (D)	(K) 20-30 mg/kg + (D) 1-2 mg/kg IM[74]	Guinea pigs/anesthesia
	(K) 20-40 mg/kg + (D) 1-2 mg/kg IM[49]	Chinchillas/anesthesia
Ketamine (K)/ medetomidine (Me)	(K) 2-4 mg/kg + (Me) 0.05 mg/kg IM[84]	Most species/sedation
	(K) 3-5 mg/kg + (Me) 0.1 mg/kg SC, IM[84]	Guinea pigs/short anesthesia
	(K) 4-5 mg/kg + (Me) 0.03 mg/kg[69]	Chinchillas/anesthesia; provide supplemental oxygen; reverse with atipamezole
	(K) 5 mg/kg + (Me) 0.06 mg/kg IM[46]	Chinchillas/anesthesia
	(K) 5-10 mg/kg + (Me) 0.02-0.04 mg/kg IM[51]	Degus/anesthesia; supplement with isoflurane if needed
	(K) 20 mg/kg + (Me) 0.1 mg/kg + buprenorphine 0.03 mg/kg IM[3]	Guinea pigs/premedication
	(K) 40 mg/kg + (Me) 0.5 mg/kg IM, IP[31,74]	Guinea pigs/20-30 min duration of anesthesia
	(K) 40-75 mg/kg + (Me) 1 mg/kg IP[22]	Mice/anesthesia; minor procedures; use the higher dose of ketamine in females; (Me) reversal is atipamezole

TABLE 9-3 Chemical Restraint/Anesthetic Agents Used in Rodents. (cont'd)

Agent	Dosage	Comments
Ketamine (K)/ medetomidine (Me) (cont'd)	(K) 75-90 mg/kg + (Me) 0.5 mg/kg IM, IP[74,90]	Rats, gerbils/surgical anesthesia 20-30 min duration
	(K) 100 or 200 mg/kg + (Me) 0.25 mg/kg IP, SC[25,58]	Hamsters (Syrian)/anesthesia
Ketamine (K)/ midazolam (M)	(K) 5-10 mg/kg + (M) 0.5-1 mg/kg IM[90]	Chinchillas, guinea pigs, prairie dogs
	(K) 40 mg/kg + (M) 1-2 mg/kg IM, SC, IP[31]	Rats/anesthesia
Ketamine (K)/ midazolam (M)/ butorphanol (B)	(K) 5-10 mg/kg + (M) 0.2-0.4 mg/kg + (B) 0.3-0.5 mg/kg IM[51]	Degus/anesthesia; supplement with isoflurane if needed
Ketamine (K)/ xylazine (X)	(K) 20-40 mg/kg + (X) 2 mg/kg IM[41]	Guinea pigs/light anesthesia
	(K) 40 mg/kg + (X) 2 mg/kg IM[46]	Chinchillas/anesthesia
	(K) 50 mg/kg + (X) 2 mg/kg IP[41]	Gerbils/anesthesia
	(K) 60 mg/kg + (X) 6 mg/kg IP[56]	Mice/anesthesia; <40 min
	(K) 80 mg/kg + (X) 5 mg/kg IM, IP[41]	Hamsters/anesthesia
	(K) 80 mg/kg + (X) 8 mg/kg IP[56]	Mice/anesthesia; <30 min
	(K) 100 mg/kg + (X) 5 mg/kg IM, IP[29]	Rats/anesthesia
Medetomidine	—	See ketamine for combinations
	0.1 mg/kg SC[74]	Hamsters/light to moderate sedation
	0.1-0.2 mg/kg SC[74]	Gerbils/light to moderate sedation
	0.15 mg/kg IM[12,31]	Rats, guinea pigs/sedation
	0.15-0.25 mg/kg IM[42]	Rats/sedation
	0.2-0.3 mg/kg SC[31]	Hamsters/sedation
Medetomidine (Me)/ butorphanol (B)	(Me) 0.1 mg/kg + (B) 2 mg/kg IM[12]	Rats/sedation
Midazolam	—	See ketamine for combination
	0.4-2 mg/kg IM[114]	Guinea pigs, chinchillas
	1-2 mg/kg IM[74]	All species/preanesthetic
	2-3 mg/kg IM[114]	Rats, mice, gerbils
Midazolam (M)/ butorphanol (B)	(M) 0.2-0.8 mg/kg + (B) 0.3-0.5 mg/kg IM[51]	Degus/sedation
Midazolam (M)/ medetomidine (Me)/ butorphanol (B)	(M) 1 mg/kg + (Me) 0.05 mg/kg + (B) 2 mg/kg IP[12]	Rats/sedation; completely reversible
	(M) 2 mg/kg + (Me) 0.15 mg/kg + (B) 2.5 mg/kg IP[59]	Rats/anesthesia; completely reversible
	(M) 4 mg/kg + (Me) 0.3 mg/kg + (B) 5 mg/kg IP[48,56]	Mice/anesthesia; <60 min; completely reversible
Midazolam (M)/ medetomidine (Me)/ fentanyl (F)	(M) 1 mg/kg + (Me) 0.05 mg/kg + (F) 0.02 mg/kg IM[46]	Chinchillas/anesthesia, completely reversible with flumazenil (0.1 mg/kg) + atipamezole (0.5 mg/kg) + naloxone (0.05 mg/kg) SC[46]
	(M) 2 mg/kg + (Me) 0.15 mg/kg + (F) 0.005 mg/kg IM[4]	Rats/anesthesia, completely reversible with flumazenil (0.2 mg/kg) + atipamezole (0.75 mg/kg) + naloxone (0.12 mg/kg)

Continued

TABLE 9-3 — Chemical Restraint/Anesthetic Agents Used in Rodents. (cont'd)

Agent	Dosage	Comments
Midazolam (M)/ medetomidine (Me)/ fentanyl (F) (cont'd)	(M) 2 mg/kg + (Me) 0.2 mg/kg + (F) 0.025-0.05 mg/kg IM[31]	Guinea pigs/anesthesia; completely reversible with flumazenil (0.1 mg/kg) + atipamezole (1 mg/kg) + naloxone (0.03 mg/kg)[31]
	(M) 3.3 mg/kg + (Me) 0.33 mg/kg + (F) 0.033 mg/kg SC[31]	Hamsters/anesthesia; completely reversible
Naloxone	0.01-0.1 mg/kg SC, IP[46,74,84]	All species/opioid reversal
	0.02 mg/kg/h IV[84]	Constant rate infusion (CRI)
Pentobarbital	—	Anesthesia; not recommended; marginal analgesia; autonomic depression; euthanasia dose is 150 mg/kg[84]
	30-45 mg/kg IP[41]	Guinea pigs, chinchillas, rats
	50 mg/kg IP[56]	Mice/anesthesia, <45 min; no surgical anesthesia achieved
	50-90 mg/kg IP[41]	Gerbils, hamsters, mice
Propofol	—	Anesthesia; induction
	3-5 mg/kg IV[90]	Guinea pigs, chinchillas, prairie dogs
	7.5-10 mg/kg IV[74,84]	Rats
Sevoflurane	To effect[90]	Most species
Tiletamine/ zolazepam (Telazol, Fort Dodge)	20-40 mg/kg IM[74]	Chinchillas, rats/anesthesia
	30 mg/kg IM IP[31]	Hamsters
	50-80 mg/kg IM[88]	Mice, rats
Tiletamine/ zolazepam (T)/ xylazine (X)	(T) 20 mg/kg + (X) 10 mg/kg IP[74]	Gerbils/anesthesia
	(T) 30 mg/kg + (X) 10 mg/kg IM, IP[41]	Hamsters/anesthesia
Xylazine	—	See ketamine, tiletamine/zolazepam for combinations
	5-10 mg/kg SC, IM, IP[88]	Most species/may cause muscle necrosis when given IM
Yohimbine	0.5-1 mg/kg IV, IP[41]	All species/xylazine reversal

TABLE 9-4 — Analgesic Agents Used in Rodents.

Agent	Dosage	Comments
Acetaminophen	100 mg/kg PO[86]	Rats/PD
	200 mg/kg PO[33]	Mice, rats
	1-2 mg/mL drinking water[50]	All species
Acetylsalicylic acid	50-150 mg/kg PO q4-8h[84]	All species
	87 mg/kg PO[33]	Guinea pigs
	100 mg/kg PO[33,37]	Rats
	120 mg/kg PO q4h[33]	Mice

TABLE 9-4 Analgesic Agents Used in Rodents. (cont'd)

Agent	Dosage	Comments
Buprenorphine	0.01-0.05 mg/kg IM, SC q6-12h[29,84]	Gerbils, hamsters
	0.01-0.05 mg/kg SC, IV q8-12h[33]	Rats
	0.05 mg/kg SC q8-12h[31,33]	Guinea pigs, chinchillas
	0.05 mg/kg q12h SC, IM[107]	Rats/PD; PK
	0.05-0.1 SC q12h[33]	Mice
	0.1 mg/kg SC q12h[57]	Mice/PD; not sufficient analgesia following laparotomy
	0.1-0.25 mg/kg PO q8-12h[33]	Rats
	0.1-0.4 mg/kg PO[87,100]	Rats
	0.2 mg/kg SC q4-6h[71]	Chinchillas/PD
	0.2 mg/kg q5h oral transmucosal[102]	Guinea pigs/PK
	0.2 mg/kg IV q7h[102]	Guinea pigs/PK
	0.5 mg/kg SC q8h[31]	Hamsters
Buprenorphine, extended release (Animalgesics for Mice and Rats, Animalgesic Labs)	0.65 mg/kg SC q48h[54]	Rats/PD
Buprenorphine, sustained release (Buprenorphine SR, Zoopharm)	—	Injections site lesions have been reported
	0.3-1.2 mg/kg SC q48-72h[21]	Rats/PD
	0.6 mg/kg SC q72h[57]	Mice/PD; sufficient post-laparotomy analgesia
	1.2 mg/kg SC q72-96h[54,107]	Rats/PD; PK
	1.2 mg/kg SC q72h[16]	Prairie dogs/PK
	1.5 mg/kg SC q48h[44]	Mice/PD
	2.2 mg/kg SC q24-48h[53]	Mice/PD; PK
Butorphanol	0.2-2 mg/kg q2-4h[6,90]	Most species
	1-2 mg/kg SC q4h[33]	Guinea pigs, rats, mice
	1-5 mg/kg SC q4h[29,84,90]	Gerbils, rats, mice, hamsters
Carprofen	—	Nonsteroidal antiinflammatory; high end of dosage reflects total daily dose; can be divided
	2-5 mg/kg PO, SC, IM, IV total daily dose give q12-24h[84]	All species
	4 mg/kg SC q12-24h[87]	Guinea pigs, chinchillas
	5 mg/kg SC[29,33]	Rats, mice, gerbils
	5-10 mg/kg PO[67,114]	Rats, mice, gerbils
	5-15 mg/kg SC[100,101]	Rats/PD
Celecoxib	10-20 mg/kg PO[86]	Rats/PD
Clonidine	0.25-0.5 mg/kg PO[37]	Mice
Codeine	40 mg/kg SC[80]	Rats/PD

Continued

TABLE 9-4 Analgesic Agents Used in Rodents. (cont'd)

Agent	Dosage	Comments
Diclofenac	2.1 mg/kg PO[33]	Guinea pigs
	8 mg/kg PO[33]	Mice
	10 mg/kg PO[33]	Rats
Dipyrone	—	See metamizole
Duloxetine	10 mg/kg IP[55]	Mice/PD
	30 mg/kg PO q24h[55]	Mice/PD
Fentanyl	0.025-0.6 mg/kg SC[37]	Mice
	0.16 mg/kg SC[80]	Rats/PD
Flunixin meglumine	—	Nonsteroidal antiinflammatory; do not use in dehydrated animals
	2.5 mg/kg SC[87]	Most species
	2.5-5 mg/kg SC q12-24h[33]	Most species
Gabapentin	10-30 mg/kg PO[55]	Mice/PD
	30 mg/kg PO q8h[84]	Rats
	50 mg/kg PO q24h[84]	Hamsters
Hydrocodone	10-40 mg/kg SC[80]	Rats/PD
Hydromorphone	0.4 mg/kg SC <q2h[110]	Rats/PD
	2 mg/kg SC <q4h[70]	Chinchillas/PD
Ibuprofen	10 mg/kg PO q4h[33]	Guinea pigs
	15 mg/kg PO[33]	Rats
	30 mg/kg IP[91]	Rats/PD
	30 mg/kg PO[33]	Mice
	40 mg/kg PO[43]	Mice/PD study
Indomethacin	8 mg/kg PO[33]	Guinea pigs
Ketoprofen	1-3 mg/kg SC, IM q12-24h[84,90]	Chinchillas, guinea pigs, prairie dogs/in prairie dogs, doses of 3-5 mg/kg have been used
	5 mg/kg SC[33]	Rats, mice
	5-15 mg/kg SC[101]	Rats/PD
Meloxicam	0.1-0.3 mg/kg PO, SC q24h[33,87]	Guinea pigs
	≥0.5 mg/kg PO, SC q24h[90]	Chinchillas, guinea pigs, hamsters, gerbils
	1 mg/kg PO, SC[33,87]	Rats
	1-2 mg/kg PO q12-24h[6,84]	Rats
	1-5 mg/kg PO, SC q24h[90]	Mice
	5 mg/kg PO, SC[33]	Mice
Meloxicam, sustained release (Meloxicam SR, Zoopharm Fort Collins, CO)	4 mg/kg SC q72h[16]	Prairie dogs/PK
	4 mg/kg SC q96h[107]	Rats/PD
Meperidine	10-20 mg/kg SC, IM q2-3h[33]	Guinea pigs, mice, rats
Metamizole	20-50 mg/kg PO, SC q6-12h[29,30]	Most species

TABLE 9-4 Analgesic Agents Used in Rodents. (cont'd)

Agent	Dosage	Comments
Methadone	0.5-3 mg/kg SC[26]	Rats/PD
	1-2 mg/kg SC, IM[6]	Mice
	1-4 mg/kg SC, IM[6]	Rats
	5-10 mg/kg IP[1]	Rats/PD
Morphine	1-3 mg/kg SC[55]	Mice/PD
	2-5 mg/kg SC, IM q4h[6,33,90]	Most species, guinea pigs
	2.5 mg/kg SC q2-4h[33,84]	Rats, mice, hamsters
Nalbuphine	1-2 mg/kg IM q3h[33]	Guinea pigs, rats
	2-4 mg/kg IM q4h[33]	Mice
Oxycodone	10-40 mg/kg SC[80]	Rats/PD
Oxymorphone	0.2-0.5 mg/kg SC, IM q4h[33,87]	Guinea pigs, rats, mice
Pentazocine	5-10 mg/kg SC q2-4h[84]	Gerbils, guinea pigs, hamsters, mice, rats
	5-10 mg/kg SC q3-4h[33]	Rats, mice
Pethidine	10-20 mg/kg SC, IM q2-3h[33,84]	Most species
Piroxicam	3.4-20 mg/kg PO[84]	Mice
Tolfenamic acid	2 mg/kg SC q24h[84]	Guinea pigs
	4 mg/kg PO, SC q24h for 3 doses max[29,30]	Most species
Tramadol	—	Oral route unlikely to be effective
	5 mg/kg SC, IP[6,33]	Rats/mice
	10-20 mg/kg PO, SC q8-12h[84]	Rats
	10-40 mg/kg SC q12h[84]	Mice
	10-40 mg/kg SC[70]	Chinchillas/PD; no analgesic effects; side effects at >40 mg/kg; single-dose study

TABLE 9-5 Cardiovascular Agents Used in Rodents.

Agent	Dosage	Comments
Atenolol	0.2-2 mg/kg PO q24h[52]	Most species/beta-blocker; hypertension and tachyarrhythmias
	2-10 mg/kg IV, IP q24h[84]	Mice
Atropine	0.05-0.5 mg/kg SC, IM[2,52]	All species/preanesthetic, cardiac problems
	0.1-0.2 mg/kg SC IM[84]	Guinea pigs, chinchillas
	Up to 10 mg/kg IM, SC, IV q20min[41,84]	All species/organophosphate toxicity
Benazepril	0.05–0.1 mg/kg PO q24h[52,84]	Most species/ACE inhibitor; heart failure, hypertension, and chronic renal failure
	0.125-0.25 mg/kg PO q24h[29,30]	

Continued

TABLE 9-5 Cardiovascular Agents Used in Rodents. (cont'd)

Agent	Dosage	Comments
Carvedilol	1-11 mg/kg PO q24h[84]	Hamsters/beta-blocker
	2-30 mg/kg PO q24h[84]	Rats/beta-blocker
Digoxin	0.005-0.01 mg/kg PO q12-24h[29-31]	Most species
	0.05-0.1 mg/kg PO q12-24h[74,84]	Hamsters/dilated cardiomyopathy
Diltiazem	0.5-1 mg/kg PO q12-24h[31,52]	Most species/Ca channel blocker; hypertension and hypertrophic cardiomyopathy
Dopamine	0.08 mg/kg IV prn[64]	Guinea pigs/hypotension, especially anesthetic related
Enalapril	0.5-1 mg/kg PO q24h[30,31]	ACE inhibitor; heart failure
Epinephrine (adrenaline)	0.003-0.1 mg/kg IV prn[31]	Guinea pigs/cardiac arrest
	0.01 mg/kg IV[84]	Most species
	0.1 mg/kg IV[90]	Most species
Etilefrine	0.5-1 mg/kg PO q6-8h[30]	Sympathomimetic
Furosemide	1-4 mg/kg SC, IM q4-6h, or 5-10 mg/kg SC, IM q12h[84]	Most species
	1-5 mg/kg PO, SC, IM q12-24h[29,30]	Most species/congestive heart failure
Glyceryl trinitrate ointment (2%)	3 mm strip applied to inner pinna q6-12h[52,84]	Most species/congestive heart failure
Glycopyrrolate	0.01-0.02 mg/kg SC, IM, IV[84]	Most species/anticholinergic agent used for bradycardia; premedication
Imidapril hydrochloride	0.125-0.25 mg/kg PO q24h[30]	ACE inhibitor
Lidocaine	1-2 mg/kg IV, or 2-4 mg/kg IT[52]	Most species/arrhythmias
Metildigoxin	0.005-0.01 mg/kg PO q24h[30]	Dilative cardiomyopathy, tachycardic arrhythmia
Pimobendan	0.2-0.4 mg/kg PO q12h[74]	Most species/inodilator for treating heart failure
	0.25 mg/kg PO q12h[29,30]	Most species
Propentofyllin	10-25 mg/kg PO q12-24h[29,30]	Ischemia; phosphodiesterase inhibitor
Taurine	100 mg/kg PO q12h × 8 wk[52]	Most species/cardiomyopathy
Verapamil	0.25-0.5 mg/kg SC q12h[84]	Hamsters/calcium channel blocker

TABLE 9-6 Emergency Drugs Used in Rodents.

Agent	Dosage	Comments
Atropine	0.05-0.1 mg/kg SC[29,30]	All species/bradycardia; some rats possess serum atropinase
	0.1-0.2 mg/kg SC, IM[84]	Chinchillas, guinea pigs
	Up to 10 mg/kg IM, SC, IV q20min[41,84]	All species/organophosphate toxicity

TABLE 9-6 Emergency Drugs Used in Rodents. (cont'd)

Agent	Dosage	Comments
Calcium gluconate	100 mg/kg IM, IP once[31,74]	Guinea pigs/dystocia; follow with 1 U oxytocin (see Table 8.7)
	100 mg/kg IM, IP once[84]	Chinchillas/hypocalcemic tetany; eclampsia
Charcoal (activated)	0.5-5 g/kg PO prn[84]	Acute poisoning with organophosphates and other pesticides
Dexamethasone	—	All species/antiinflammatory
	0.5-2 mg/kg SC, IM, IV[90]	
	0.6 mg/kg IM, IV[2,84]	Guinea pigs/pregnancy toxemia
	4-5 mg/kg SC, IM, IP, IV[74]	Shock
Diazepam	0.5-5 mg/kg IM, IV, IP[84]	All/treatment of seizures, sedation
Diphenhydramine	—	Antihistamine; anaphylaxis
	1-2 mg/kg PO, SC q12h[90]	All species
	1-5 mg/kg SC prn[84,90]	Guinea pigs
Dopamine	0.08 mg/kg IV[64]	Guinea pigs/hypotension
Doxapram	—	Respiratory stimulant
	2-5 mg/kg IV, IP, SC[31,84]	Guinea pigs
	5-10 mg/kg IV, IP[30,84]	Most species
Ephedrine	1 mg/kg IV[84]	Guinea pigs/antihistamine; stimulant
Epinephrine (adrenalin)	0.003-0.1 mg/kg IV prn[31]	Guinea pigs/cardiac arrest
	0.01 mg/kg IV[84]	Most species
	0.1 mg/kg IV[90]	Most species
Furosemide	—	Diuretic for edema, pulmonary congestion, ascites
	1-4 mg/kg SC, IM q4-6h, or 5-10 mg/kg SC, IM q12h[84]	Most species
	1-5 mg/kg PO, SC, IM q12-24h[29,30]	Most species/congestive heart failure
Glycopyrrolate	0.01-0.02 mg/kg SC, IM, IV[84]	Most species/anticholinergic agent used for bradycardia; premedication
Hetastarch	1-10 mL/kg IV[84]	Rats/hypotension, shock
	3 mL/kg IV, IO[66]	Shock; administer with hypertonic saline (3 mL/kg) over 10 min
Lactated Ringer's solution	10-25 mL/kg IV, IO[96]	Most species/give slowly over 5-10 min (if unsuccessful, administer IP)
Mannitol	0.3 g/kg/h IV[30]	Reduction of intracranial pressure, acute glaucoma, oliguric renal failure
Prednisolone	10-20 mg/kg IV, IM, IP once[30]	Most species/shock
Saline, hypertonic (7.2%-7.5%)	3 mL/kg IV, IO slow over 10 min[66]	Shock; administer with hetastarch (3 mL/kg) over 10 min

TABLE 9-7 Miscellaneous Agents Used in Rodents.

Agent	Dosage	Comments
Acetylcysteine	3 mg/kg PO, SC q12h[29,30]	Mucolytic
	2% solution nebulization over 30-60 min prn[84]	Injectable form can be used for nebulization; dilute in 0.9% NaCl
Aglepristone	10 mg/kg IM, SC on days 1, 2, and 8[84]	Guinea pigs/progesterone antagonist for treatment of pyometra/metritis, pregnancy termination
	10 mg/kg SC q24h for 2 doses[29]	Rats, hamsters, gerbils/pyometra
	10-20 mg/kg SC q12h for 2 doses, repeat after 8 days[31]	Hamsters/pyometra
Aluminum hydroxide	20-40 mg/animal PO prn[84]	Guinea pigs/hyperphosphatemia caused by renal failure
Aminophylline	10 mg/kg PO q12-24h[93]	Rats
	50 mg/kg PO, SC[84,90]	Guinea pigs
Aminotriptyline	5-20 mg/kg PO q24h[84]	Rats/antidepressant; chronic antianxiety treatment
Asparaginase (L-asparaginase)	400 IU/kg SC q7d[31]	Guinea pigs/lymphoma
	10,000 IU/m² SC, IM q21d[84]	Guinea pigs/lymphoma
Atropine (1%)/ phenylephrine (10%)	Topical to eyes[41]	All species/mydriasis for non-albino eyes
Barium sulfate (1000 mg/mL)	5-10 mL/kg PO[29,30]	Most species/contrast studies; might need to be diluted with water (1:1)
Bromhexine	0.5 mg/kg PO q12-24h[29,30]	Bronchial secretolytic
	0.5-1 mg/kg PO q12-24h[31]	Guinea pigs
Cabergoline	10-50 µg/kg PO q12-24h[84]	Rats/pituitary adenoma
	0.6 mg/kg PO q72h[76]	
	12.5-15 µg/kg PO q24h × 4-6 days[29,30]	Most species/pseudopregnancy
Calcium EDTA	25-30 mg/kg SC q6-12h, 5 days on, 5 day off cycle[84]	Lead or zinc intoxication; treat until blood levels within normal range at end of off period
	30 mg/kg SC q12h[49,90]	All species/lead chelation
Carbimazole	1-2 mg/kg PO q24h[30,78]	Guinea pigs/hyperthyroidism
Charcoal (activated)	1 g/kg PO[29]	Most species/use only in cases of toxicity (not with general diarrhea)
Chlorpheniramine maleate	0.6 mg/kg PO q24h[2,84]	Guinea pigs/antihistamine
Cholestyramine	1 g/animal mixed with water PO q24h[84]	Guinea pigs/gastrointestinal clostridial overgrowth; decreases toxin absorption
Cimetidine	5-10 mg/kg PO, SC, IM, IV q6-12h[84]	All species/H_2-blocker; gastric, duodenal ulceration; esophagitis, gastroesophageal reflux
Cisapride	0.1-0.5 mg/kg PO q8-12h[31]	All species/may enhance gastrointestinal motility; not commercially available in the United States; must be compounded
	0.1-1 mg/kg PO q8-12h[84]	Chinchillas, guinea pigs

TABLE 9-7 Miscellaneous Agents Used in Rodents. (cont'd)

Agent	Dosage	Comments
Clomipramine	16-32 mg/kg PO q12h[84]	Rats
Cyclophosphamide	300 mg/kg IP q24h[64]	Guinea pigs/antineoplastic
	300 mg/m² IP q24h[84]	
Cyclosporine	10 mg/kg PO q24h[84]	Rats
Cyproheptadine	0.5 mg/kg PO q12h[84]	Guinea pigs, chinchillas/appetite stimulation
Deslorelin acetate	4.7 mg implant/animal SC[62,105]	Guinea pigs/suppression of estrus; ovarian cysts (not effective against serous cysts)
	4.7 mg implant/animal SC[5,19,40,109]	Rats/anti-gonadal effects, for at least 12 mo[5,19]
Dexamethasone	—	Antiinflammatory
	0.5-2 mg/kg PO, SC, then decreasing dose q12h × 3-14 days[41]	All species
	0.6 mg/kg IV, IM, SC q24h[84]	Guinea pigs/pregnancy toxemia
Diazoxide	25 mg/kg PO q12h[47]	Guinea pigs/insulinoma
Diphenhydramine	—	Antihistamine; anaphylaxis
	1-2 mg/kg PO, SC q12h[90]	Chinchillas, hamsters, mice, rats
	1-5 mg/kg SC prn[84]	Guinea pigs
Diphenylhydantoin	25-50 mg/kg q12h[52]	Most species/seizures
Dorzolamide	1 drop of 1% solution q12h[84]	Rats/glaucoma
Ephedrine	1 mg/kg PO, IV prn[64,84]	Guinea pigs/antihistamine; anaphylaxis
Famotidine	0.4-0.5 mg/kg PO, SC, q24h[84]	Guinea pigs, chinchillas
Fluoxetine	1-1.5 mg/kg PO q24h[84]	Rats
	5-10 mg/kg PO q24h[52]	Most species/for behavioral problems (i.e., fur chewing)
Furosemide	1-4 mg/kg SC, IM q4-6h, or 5-10 mg/kg SC, IM q12h[84]	Most species
	1-5 mg/kg PO, SC, IM q12-24h[29,30]	Most species/congestive heart failure
GnRH (e.g., gonadorelin)	20 µg/animal IM once[39]	Guinea pigs/follicular ovarian cysts, short-acting formulations
	25 µg/animal q14d × 2 treatments[75]	Guinea pigs/follicular ovarian cysts
Heparin	5 mg/kg IV prn[64]	Guinea pigs/disseminated intravascular coagulation
Human chorionic gonadotropin (hCG)	100 U/kg SC q10-14d × 3 injections[30]	Guinea pigs/follicular ovarian cysts
	100 U/kg SC q7d for 3 injections[84]	Guinea pigs/follicular ovarian cysts
Insulin	1 U/kg SC q12h[84]	Chinchillas
	1-3 U/kg q12-24h SC[30]	Guinea pigs, chinchillas, degus/starting dose is 1 U/kg[30]
	1-2 U/animal SC q12h[84]	Guinea pigs

Continued

TABLE 9-7 Miscellaneous Agents Used in Rodents. (cont'd)

Agent	Dosage	Comments
Insulin (cont'd)	1-3 U/animal SC q12h[84]	Rats
	2 U/animal SC[84]	Hamsters, gerbils
Iodine, I-131 (radioactive)	1 mCi/animal SC once[78]	Guinea pigs/hyperthyroidism
Kaolin pectin	0.2 mL PO q6-8h[2]	Guinea pigs/antidiarrheal
	1-2 mL/kg PO q2-6h[84]	
Lactulose	0.5 mL/kg PO q12h[84]	Most species/constipation, hepatic disorders
	2 mL/kg PO prn[29,30]	Most species/constipation
Leuprolide acetate depot (Lupron Depot, TAP Pharmaceuticals)	0.2-0.3 mg/kg IM q28d[92]	Guinea pigs/follicular ovarian cysts
Levetiracetam	20 mg/kg PO q8h[84]	Prairie dogs/seizures
Levothyroxine	5 µg/kg PO q12h[84]	Most species/hypothyroidism
	10-20 µg/kg PO q24h[30]	Guinea pigs/hypothyroidism
Loperamide	0.1 mg/kg PO q8h[41,84]	All species/diarrhea; limit use to avoid gastrointestinal stasis
Magnesium hydroxide	4 mg/kg PO[52] prn	Prevention of calcium oxalate uroliths
Methimazole	0.5-2 mg/kg PO q24h[78]	Guinea pigs/hyperthyroidism
	1-3 mg/kg PO q8-24h[63]	Guinea pigs/hyperthyroidism
Metoclopramide	0.2-1 mg/kg PO, SC, IM q12h[90]	Most species
	0.5-1 mg/kg PO, SC q6-12h[84]	Guinea pigs/antiemetic and upper gastrointestinal prokinetic
	1-5 mg/kg q8-12h SC, PO[29,30]	
Metyrapone	8 mg/animal PO q24h × 4 wk[31,52]	Hamsters/hyperadrenocorticism
Milk thistle (*Silybum marianum*)	4-15 mg/kg PO q8-12h[52]	Most species/hepatic disorders
Mitotane	5 mg/animal PO q24h × 4 wk[52]	Hamsters/hyperadrenocorticism
Oxytocin	0.2-3 U/kg SC, IM, IV[84]	All species/delayed parturition if unobstructed
	1 U/kg SC, IM[29,30]	All species
	1-2 U/animal IM[2]	Guinea pigs/uterine contraction; milk letdown
	6.25 U/kg SC[2]	Mice/milk letdown
Pentosan polysulphate	3 mg/kg SC q5-7d for 4 doses[84]	Guinea pigs/osteoarthritis, idiopathic cystitis
Phenobarbital	5-20 mg/kg PO, IV, IP[90]	Guinea pigs/antiseizure medication; sedative
	5-25 mg/kg IV, IP q12-24h[84]	Guinea pigs, gerbils/seizures
Phenoxybenzamine	0.25 mg/kg PO q12h[69]	Guinea pigs/urolithiasis
Potassium citrate	10-30 mg/kg PO q12h[90]	Guinea pigs

TABLE 9-7 Miscellaneous Agents Used in Rodents. (cont'd)

Agent	Dosage	Comments
Prednisolone	1-2 mg/kg PO, SC q12-24h[30,31]	Guinea pigs
Prednisone	0.5-2.2 mg/kg PO, SC, IM[90]	All species
Pseudoephedrine	1.2 mg/animal PO q12h[98]	Chinchillas/nasal and sinus decongestant
Ranitidine	5 mg/kg PO q12h[84]	Guinea pigs, chinchillas
S-Adenosylmethionine (SAMe)	20-100 mg/kg PO q24h[84]	Most species
Sildenafil citrate	5 mg/kg PO q24h[61]	Rats
Silymarin	50-200 mg/kg/day PO[17]	Rats
Sucralfate	25-50 mg/kg PO q6-8h[84]	Most species/oral, esophageal, gastric, and duodenal ulcers
	25-100 mg/kg PO q8-12h[90]	Most species/oral, esophageal, gastric, and duodenal ulcers
Terbutaline	5 mg/kg every PO q12h[84,95]	Most species
Theophylline	2-3 mg/kg PO q8-12h[29,30]	Most species
	4-10 mg/kg PO q8-12h[31]	Guinea pigs
	10-20 mg/kg PO q8-12h[84]	Rats, prairie dogs
Thiamazol	102 mg/kg PO q24h[30]	Most species/hyperthyroidism
Thiamine	1 mg/kg feed[52]	Most species/thiamine deficiency
Thyroid stimulating hormone (TSH); human recombinant	100 μg/animal IM[77]	Guinea pigs/thyroid function testing
Toremifene	12 mg/kg PO q24h[52]	Rats/pituitary hyperplasia/adenoma
Trilostane	2-4 mg/kg PO q24h[84]	Hyperadrenocorticism
Vitamin A	50-500 U/kg IM[84]	Guinea pigs, hamsters
	2000 U/animal[52]	Chinchillas/hypovitaminosis A
	2 μg vitamin A palmitate/g feed[84]	Hamsters
	10 mg β-carotene/kg of feed[84]	Guinea pigs
Vitamin B complex (small animal)	0.02-0.2 mL/kg SC, IM[84]	All species/B_1 (100 mg/mL), B_2 (2 mg/mL), B_{12} (0.1 mg/mL)
Vitamin C (ascorbic acid)	10-30 mg/kg PO, SC, IM[84]	Guinea pigs/maintenance
	50-100 mg/kg SC, PO[31]	Guinea pigs/treatment of deficiency
	100-200 mg/kg PO q24h[84]	Guinea pigs/hypovitaminosis C
	0.2-0.4 mg/mL drinking water[84]	Guinea pigs/prevents deficiency; change daily
Vitamin D	200-400 U/kg SC, IM[74]	All species
Vitamin E	50 mg/kg PO q24h[31]	Guinea pigs
Vitamin K_1	1-5 mg/kg SC q12-24h[29,30]	Most species
	1-10 mg/kg IM q24h × 4-6 days[41]	All species/warfarin poisoning; menadiols not used in acute cases

TABLE 9-8 Common and Scientific Names of Pet Rodents.[31]

Common Name	Other Common Names	Scientific Name
Chinchilla	Long-tailed chinchilla	Chinchilla lanigera
Chipmunk	Siberian chipmunk; Korean chipmunk	Eutamias sibericus
Degu	Common degu	Octodon degus
Gerbil	Mongolian gerbil; Mongolian jird, clawed jird	Meriones unguiculatus
Guinea pig	Cavy, cuy	Cavia porcellus
Hamster, Chinese	Striped hamster	Cricetulus griseus
Hamster, dwarf	Russian dwarf hamster, Siberian dwarf hamster, Djungarian hamster	Phodopus sungorus
	Campbell dwarf hamster	Phodopus campbelli
	Roborowski dwarf hamster	Phodopus roborovskii
Hamster, golden	Syrian hamster	Mesocricetus auratus
Mouse	Common mouse	Mus musculus
Prairie dog	Black-tailed prairie dog	Cynomys ludovicianus
Rat	Brown rat, Norway rat	Rattus norvegicus

Measurement	Mouse	Rat	Gerbil	Hamster	Guinea Pig	Chinchilla	Prairie Dog
PCV (%)	35-40	35-45	35-45	45-50	35-45	27-54	36-54
RBC (10^6/μL)	7-11	7-10	7-8	7-8	4-7	5.6-8.4	5.9-9.4
Hgb (g/dL)	10-20	12-18	14-16	16.6-18.6	11-17	11.8-14.6	12.7-19.6
WBC (10^3/μL)	4-12	5-23	7.5-10.9	7-10	7-14	5.4-15.6	1.9-10.1
Neutrophils (%)	5-40	10-50	22	18-40	20-60	39-54	43-87
Lymphocytes (%)	30-90	50-70	75	56-80	30-80	45-60	8-54
Monocytes (%)	0-10	0-10	0-4	2	2-20	0-5	0-12
Eosinophils (%)	0-5	0-5	0-3	0-1	0-5	0-5	0-10
Basophils (%)	0-1	0-1	0-1	0-1	0-1	0-1	0-2
ALT (U/L)	26-77	20-92	—	22-128	10-25	10-35	26-91
ALP (U/L)	45-222	16-96	—	99-186	—	6-72	25-64
AST (U/L)	54-269	—	—	28-122	—	96	16-53
Bilirubin, total (mg/dL)	0.1-0.9	0.2-0.6	0.2-0.6	0.1-0.9	0.3-0.9	0.6-1.3	0.1-0.3
BUN (mg/dL)	17-28	15-21	17-27	12-26	9-32	17-45	21-44
Calcium (mg/dL)	3.2-8	5.3-13	3.7-6.2	5.3-12	7.8-10.5	5.6-12.1	8.3-10.8
Chloride (mEq/L)	82-114	—	—	—	98-115	108-129	—
Cholesterol (mg/dL)	26-82	40-130	90-150	55-181	20-43	50-302	—
Creatinine (mg/dL)	0.3-1	0.2-0.8	0.6-1.4	0.4-1	0.6-2.2	0.4-1.3	0.8-2.3
Glucose (mg/dL)	62-175	50-135	50-135	37-198	60-125	109-193	120-209
Phosphorus (mg/dL)	6-10.4	5.8-8.2	3.7-7	3-9.9	5.3	4-8	3.6-10
Potassium (mEq/L)	5.1-10.4	5.9	3.3-6.3	3.9-5.5	6.8-8.9	3.3-5.7	4-5.7
Protein, total (g/dL)	3.5-7.2	5.6-7.6	4.3-12.5	5.2-7	4.6-6.2	3.8-5.6	5.8-8.1
Albumin (g/dL)	2.5-4.8	3.8-4.8	1.8-5.5	3.5-4.9	2.1-3.9	2.3-4.1	2.4-3.9
Globulin (g/dL)	0.6	1.8-3	1.2-6	2.7-4.2	1.7-2.6	0.9-2.2	3.4-4.2
Sodium (mEq/L)	112-193	135-155	141-172	128-144	146-152	142-166	144-175
Triglycerides (mg/dL)	—	26-145	—	72-227	0-145	—	—

TABLE 9-10 Biologic and Physiologic Data of Rodents.[30,31,74]

Species	Life Span	Avg wt (g) (male/female)	Temperature °C (°F)	Heart Rate (beats/min)	Respiratory (breaths/min)
Chinchilla	10-20	450-600/550-800	34.9-37.9 (94.8-100.2)	200-240	40-80
Degu	5-7	170-350	37-39 (98.6-102.2)	240-390	80-150
Gerbil	3-4	65-130/70-100	37-39 (98.6-102.2)	260-450	70-130
Guinea pig	4-6	900-1500/700-1000	37.5-39.5 (99.5-103.1)	230-380	40-120
Hamster, Chinese	1.5-3	30-45/30-45	—	—	—
Hamster, golden	2-3	80-150/90-160	37-39 (98.6-102.2)	250-500	50-135
Hamster, Russian dwarf and Campbell	2-3	19-45/19-36	37-39 (98.6-102.2)	200-560	90-120
Hamster, Roborowski dwarf	1.5-2	20-28/18-23	37-39 (98.6-102.2)	200-560	90-120
Mouse	1.5-3	20-40/18-35	36-38 (96.8-100.4)	300-800	70-220
Prairie dog	8-10	1000-2200/500-1500	35.4-39.1 (95.7-102.3)	150-320	30-60
Rat	1.5-3	350-500/250-350	37.5-39.5 (98.6-103.1)	250-450	70-120

TABLE 9-11 Blood Volumes of Rodents with Safe-Bleeding Volume Recommendations.[92]

Species	Blood Volume (Average)	Safe Venipuncture Volume
Gerbil	67 mL/kg	0.3 mL/animal
Guinea pig	75 mL/kg	7.7 mL/kg
Hamster	78 mL/kg	5.5 mL/kg
Mouse	79 mL/kg	7.7 mL/kg
Rat	64 mL/kg	5.5 mL/kg

TABLE 9-12 Urinalysis Reference Values of Rodents.[a,23,28,29,32,52,74]

Measurement	Chinchilla	Gerbil	Guinea Pig	Hamster	Mouse	Prairie Dog	Rat
Specific gravity	1.014->1.060	1.006-1.080	1.005-1.050	1.014-1.060	1.034-1.058	1.005-1.059	1.022-1.050
pH	≥8.5	6.2-8.2	8.4±0.3	6.9-9	7.3-8.5	8-8.5	7.3-8.5
Protein[b] (mg/dL)	Present[b] (6–87)	Present[b]	Present[b]	Present[b]	Present[b]	Present[b] (6-124)	Present[b]
Crystals	Common, amorphous crystals predominant	—	Amorphous crystals predominant	—	—	Rare, amorphous	—
Parasites	—	—	Cysts of *Klossiella cobaye* might be seen	—	—	—	*Trichosomoides crassicauda* (bladder threadworm), larvated ova in urine

[a]Values should be considered as guides; values are likely to vary between groups of animals according to such variables as strain, age, sex, fasting, and methodology.
[b]Proteinuria is a normal feature in most rodent species, and dip stick protein levels do not correlate with actual urinary protein levels in most species, in particular in the presence of alkaline urine.

TABLE 9-13 Reproductive Data for Rodents.[13,31,41,74]

Species	Estrus Cycle Length (days)	Gestation (days)	Litter Size	Birth Weight (g)	Age Eyes Open (days)	Weaning Age (days)	Breeding Life	Separate Adults Before Birth
Chinchilla	30-50	105-115	1-4	30-50	birth	36-48	—	—
Degu	18-21	87-93	1-10	10-20	2-3	35-42	—	—
Gerbil	4-6	24-26	1-12	2.5-3.5	16-20	21-28	15-20 months	No (mate for life)
Guinea pig	15-19	59-72	2-5	60-100	birth	21-28	3-4 years	No
Hamster	4-5	15-22	4-12	2	14-16	20-28	11-18 months	Yes
Mouse	4-5	19-21	10-12	0.5-1.5	10-14	21-28	12-18 months	No
Prairie dog	14-21	33-38	1-10	15	14	37-51	—	—
Rat	4-5	19-23	6-12	5-6	12-17	17-21	14 months	No

TABLE 9-14 Determining the Sex of Mature Rodents.[74]

Male	Female
• Anogenital distance is longer in the male • Manipulate prepuce to protrude penis • Palpate for testicles either in a scrotal sac (if present) or subcutaneous in inguinal region • Males have only two external openings in the inguinal area: 　○ Anus 　○ Urethral orifice at tip of penis • In very fat males, there may be a depression between the penis and anus; this depression can be obliterated by manipulating the skin in that area	• Anogenital distance is shorter in the female • Look for three external openings in the inguinal area: 　○ Anus (most caudal opening) 　○ Vaginal orifice (middle opening)—look carefully 　○ Urethral orifice at tip of urethral papilla (most cranial opening) • The urethral papilla is located outside the vagina (unlike most other mammals) • In very fat females or young females, the vaginal orifice may be either hidden by folds of skin (the former) or sealed (latter); gentle manipulation of the skin in this area will divulge the orifice

TABLE 9-15 Nutritional Data for Rodents.[31,74]

	Consumption (per 100 g BW/day)		Nutritional Recommendations			
Species	Food (g)	Water (mL)	Minimum Fiber (%)	Carbo-hydrates (%)	Fat (%)	Protein (%)
Chinchilla	3-6	—	16-18	—	2-4	14-16
Gerbil	5-8	4-7	—	—	2-4	16-22
Guinea pig	6	10	16-18	16	—	18-30
Hamster	8-12	8-10	—	8	3-5	15-25
Mouse	12-18	15	—	45-55	5-25	16-20
Prairie dog	2.3-4.1	—	—	—	—	—
Rat	5-6	≥10-12	—	—	5-25	12-27

TABLE 9-16 Zoonotic Diseases in Rodents.[74]

Species	Potential Zoonotic Disease
Chinchilla	*Giardia duodenalis; Listeria monocytogenes*
	Lymphocytic choriomeningitis (LCM); rare
	Dermatophytes (*Trichophyton mentagrophytes, Microsporum canis, M. gypseum*)
Gerbil	Salmonellosis; rare
	Hymenolepis nana; rare
Guinea pig	Allergies (cutaneous and respiratory) to dander and urinary proteins
	Bordetella, salmonellosis, *Yersinia pseudotuberculosis, Streptococcus*; rare
	Dermatophyte (*Trichophyton mentagrophytes*)
	Sarcoptic mites (*Trixacarus caviae, Sarcoptes scabei*)

Continued

TABLE 9-16 Zoonotic Diseases in Rodents. (cont'd)

Species	Potential Zoonotic Disease
Hamster	Salmonellosis, *Acinetobacter*
	Lymphocytic choriomeningitis (LCM); rare
	Dermatophytes (*Trichophyton mentagrophytes, Microsporum* spp.)
	Hymenolepis nana
Mouse	Allergies (cutaneous and respiratory) to dander and urinary proteins
	Salmonellosis; rare
	Lymphocytic choriomeningitis (LCM); rare
Prairie dog	*Clostridium piliforme, Pasteurella multocida,* salmonellosis, *Yersinia pseudotuberculosis, Y. pestis, Y. enterocolitica*
	Hantavirus (wild-caught), rabies virus (wild-caught)
	Dermatophytes (*Trichophyton mentagrophytes, Microsporum gypseum*)
	Various ectoparasites (mites, fleas, lice)
Rat	Allergies (cutaneous and respiratory) to dander and urinary proteins
	Leptospirosis, salmonellosis, cestodiasis, streptococcal infection
	Seoul virus (hantavirus; hemorrhagic fever with renal syndrome), sylvatic plague (vector: rat fleas), St. Louis encephalitis (vector: *Liponyssus sylviarum*), rat bite fever (*Streptobacillus moniliformis*)

TABLE 9-17 Disease Testing in Rodents.[21]

Laboratory	Test
Animal Health Diagnostic Center College of Veterinary Medicine Cornell University, 240 Farrier Rd, Ithaca, NY 14853, USA 607-253-3900 www.diagcenter.vet.cornell.edu Email: diagcenter@cornell.edu	Serum neutralization and direct fluorescence for canine distemper virus, *Giardia* and *Cryptosporidium* antigen ELISA, fungal serology
Avian Biotech International 1336 Timberlane Road Tallahassee, FL 32312, USA 800-514-9672 Email: contact@avianbiotech.com www.avianbiotech.com	PCR for *Mycobacterium, Candida, Cryptosporidium, Giardia, Salmonella*
Avian Biotech International UK PO Box 107 Truro Cornwall, TR1 2YR, England 011-44-1872-262737 Email: contact@avianbiotech.co.uk www.avianbiotech.co.uk	PCR for *Mycobacterium, Candida, Cryptosporidium, Giardia, Salmonella*
BioReliance Ltd. Todd Campus Glasgow, G20 0XA, Scotland 44 (0)141 946 9999	Rodent and rabbit serology, rodent PCR
Charles River Laboratories International, Inc. 251 Ballardvale Street Wilmington, MA 01887, USA 877-274-8371 (US and Canada) 800 3195 3430 (International) www.criver.com/products-services/basic-research/health-monitoring-diagnostic-services	Serology and PCR for rodents

TABLE 9-17 Disease Testing in Rodents. (cont'd)

Laboratory	Test
IDEXX BioResearch 4011 Discovery Drive Columbia, MO 65201, USA 573-499-5700 800-669-0825 www.idexxbioresearch.com.animal-health-monitoring	PCR testing for rodents and serology for rodents and rabbits
Laboratory Animal Diagnostic Services (LADS) BioReliance Corporation 14920 Broschart Road Rockville, MD 20850, USA 301-738-1000 800-533-5372	Rodent and rabbit serology, rodent PCR
Taconic Anmed One Hudson City Centre, Hudson, NY 12534, USA 888-822-6642 www.taconic.com Email: custserv@taconic.com European Customer Services Email: TaconicEurope@taconic.com	Serology for rodents and rabbits
University of Georgia 110 Riverbend Rd, Riverbend North Athens, GA 30602, USA 706-542-5812 www.vet.uga.edu/IDL/	PCR for *Salmonella* and *Pasteurella*, serology for *Pasteurella*, Aleutian disease virus ELISA
University of Miami–Comparative Pathology 1120 NW 14th Street CRB Building Miami, FL 33136, USA 800-596-7390 www.cpl.med.miami.edu Email: compathlab@med.miami.edu	Serology for rodents, *Giardia* and *Cryptosporidium* antigen ELISA
Zoologix Inc 9811 Owensmouth Avenue, Suite 4 Chatsworth, CA 91311, USA 818-717-8880 www.zoologix.com Email: info@zoologix.com	Extensive list of avian, primate, wildlife, and rodent PCR tests

TABLE 9-18 Endocrine Values in Rodents.[36,52]

Test	Guinea Pig	Syrian Hamster	Mouse	Rat
Free plasma cortisol (µg/dL)	0.6-5.8	0.5-1	—	—
Salivary cortisol[a] (ng/mL)	Baseline: 6.6 ± 3.4	—	—	—
	Post-ACTH stim: 157 ± 53	—	—	—
Total serum T_4 (µg/dL)	2.26-5.82[36]	3.6	3.08-4.74	3.4-6.22
Free T_4 (ng/dL)	1.26-2.03	—	—	1.17-2.8
Total T_3 (ng/dL)	39-44	45.45	84.42-110.39	—
Free T_3 (ng/dL)	0.221-0.26	—	52-77.9	110-1038 (pg/dL)

[a]For ACTH stimulation test, inject 20 U ACTH IM; repeat sample 4 hr postinjection.

TABLE 9-19 Echocardiographic Measurements in Rodents.[18,45,68,74,116]

Parameters	Chinchilla	Guinea Pig[a]	Hamster[a]	Mouse[a]	Rat[a]
Left ventricular internal diameter in diastole (mm)	4.3-7.5	6.49-7.21	3.7-4.5	3.48-3.66	5.93-6.43
Left ventricular internal diameter in systole (mm)	1.8-4.0	4.18-4.52	1.9-2.7	2.26-2.42	4.08-4.42
Thickness of left ventricular free wall in diastole (mm)	1.8-3.1	1.44-2.06	0.9-1.1	0.41-0.43	1.12-1.7
Thickness of left ventricular free wall in systole (mm)	—	1.91-2.61	—	0.86-0.92	2.02-2.7
Thickness of interventricular septum in diastole (mm)	1.6-2.5	1.88-2.68	0.9-1.1	0.42-0.44	1.06-1.36
Thickness of interventricular septum in systole (mm)	—	2.22-3.38	—	0.89-0.93	1.4-1.9
Left atrial diameter (mm)	4.3-5.9	4.61-5.29	—	—	—
Aortic diameter (mm)	3.6-4.9	4.4-4.9	—	—	—

[a]Measurements obtained in anesthetized animals.

TABLE 9-20 Electrocardiographic Measurements in Rodents.[45,112]

Parameters	Guinea Pig	Prairie Dog, Black-Tailed
P-wave duration (sec)	0.015-0.035	0.02-0.03
P-wave amplitude (mV)	0.01	0.01-0.06
PR interval (sec)	0.048-0.06	0.04-0.06
QRS duration (sec)	0.008-0.046	0.02
QRS wave amplitude (mV)	1.1-1.9	0.1-1.15
QT interval (sec)	0.106-0.144	0.1-0.14
T-wave amplitude (mV)	0.062	
Mean electrical axis (degrees)	120 to 180	−15 to +120

REFERENCES

1. Abreu M, Aguado D, Benito J, et al. Reduction of the sevoflurane minimum alveolar concentration induced by methadone, tramadol, butorphanol and morphine in rats. *Lab Anim* 2012;46:200-206.
2. Adamcak A, Otten B. Rodent therapeutics. *Vet Clin North Am Exot Anim Pract* 2000;3:221-237, viii.
3. Aguiar J, Mogridge G, Hall J. Femoral fracture repair and sciatic and femoral nerve blocks in a guinea pig. *J Small Anim Pract* 2014;55:635-639.
4. Albrecht M, Henke J, Tacke S, et al. Effects of isoflurane, ketamine-xylazine and a combination of medetomidine, midazolam and fentanyl on physiological variables continuously measured by telemetry in Wistar rats. *BMC Vet Res* 2014;10:1.
5. Alkis I, Cetin Y, Sendag S, et al. Long term suppression of oestrus and prevention of pregnancy by deslorelin implant in rats. *Bull Vet Inst Pulawy* 2011;55:237-240.

6. Allweiler SI. How to improve anesthesia and analgesia in small mammals. *Vet Clin North Am Exot Anim Pract* 2016;19:361-377.
7. Alper CM, Doyle WJ, Seroky JT, et al. Efficacy of clarithromycin treatment of acute otitis media caused by infection with penicillin-susceptible, -intermediate, and -resistant *Streptococcus pneumoniae* in the chinchilla. *Antimicrob Agents Chemother* 1996;40:1889-1892.
8. Babl FE, Pelton SI, Li Z. Experimental acute otitis media due to nontypeable *Haemophilus influenzae*: comparison of high and low azithromycin doses with placebo. *Antimicrob Agents Chemother* 2002;46:2194-2199.
9. Baumans V, Havenaar R, van Herck H, et al. The effectiveness of Ivomec and Neguvon in the control of murine mites. *Lab Anim* 1988;22:243-245.
10. Beck W, Pantchev N. *Praktische Parasitologie bei Heimtieren*. Schluetersche Verlagsgesellschaft: Hannover; 2006.
11. Beco L, Petite A, Olivry T. Comparison of subcutaneous ivermectin and oral moxidectin for the treatment of notoedric acariasis in hamsters. *Vet Rec* 2001;149:324-327.
12. Bellini L, Banzato T, Contiero B, et al. Evaluation of three medetomidine-based protocols for chemical restraint and sedation for non-painful procedures in companion rats (*Rattus norvegicus*). *Vet J* 2014;200:456-458.
13. Bishop CR. Reproductive medicine of rabbits and rodents. *Vet Clin North Am Exot Anim Pract* 2002;5:507-535.
14. Burgmann P, Percy DH. Antimicrobial drug use in rodents and rabbits. In: Prescott JF, Baggot JD, eds. *Antimicrobial Therapy in Veterinary Medicine*. 2nd ed. Ames, IA: Iowa State University Press; 1993:524-541.
15. Carter KK, Hietala S, Brooks DL, et al. Tylosin concentrations in rat serum and lung tissue after administration in drinking water. *Lab Anim Sci* 1987;37:468-470.
16. Cary CD, Lukovsky-Akhsanov NL, Gallardo-Romero NF, et al. Pharmacokinetic profiles of meloxicam and sustained-release buprenorphine in prairie dogs (Cynomys ludovicianus). *J Am Assoc Lab Anim Sci* 2017; in press.
17. Cavaretta M. Therapeutic review: milk thistle. *J Exot Pet Med* 2015;24:470-472.
18. Çetin N, Çetin E, Toker M. Echocardiographic variables in healthy guinea pigs anaesthetized with ketamine–xylazine. *Lab Anim* 2005;39:100-106.
19. Cetin Y, Alkis I, Sendag S, et al. Long-term effect of deslorelin implant on ovarian pre-antral follicles and uterine histology in female rats. In: Rodriguez-Martinez H, ed. *Reproduction in Domestic Animals*: 2013:195-199. United Kingdom: Blackwell Publishing Inc. 482013.
20. Chan KH, Swarts JD, Doyle WJ, et al. Efficacy of a new macrolide (azithromycin) for acute otitis media in the chinchilla model. *Arch Otolaryngol Head Neck Surg* 1988;114:1266-1269.
21. Chum HH, Jampachairsri K, McKeon GP, et al. Antinociceptive effects of sustained-release buprenorphine in a model of incisional pain in rats (*Rattus norvegicus*). *J Am Assoc Lab Anim Sci* 2014;53:193-197.
22. Cruz JI, Loste JM, Burzaco OH. Observations on the use of medetomidine/ketamine and its reversal with atipamezole for chemical restraint in the mouse. *Lab Anim* 1998;32:18-22.
23. Doss GA, Mans C, Houseright RA, et al. Urinalysis in chinchillas (*Chinchilla lanigera*). *J Am Vet Med Assoc* 2016;248:901-907.
24. Doss GA, Mans C, Stepien RL. Echocardiographic effects of dexmedetomidine-ketamine in chinchillas (*Chinchilla lanigera*). *Lab Anim* 2016;51:89-92.
25. Erhardt W, Wohlrab S, Kilic N, et al. Comparison of the anaesthesia combinations racemic-ketamine/medetomidine and S-ketamine/medetomidine in Syrian golden hamsters (*Mesocricetus auratus*). *Vet Anaesth Analg* 2001;28:212-213.
26. Erichsen HK, Hao J-X, Xu X-J, et al. Comparative actions of the opioid analgesics morphine, methadone and codeine in rat models of peripheral and central neuropathic pain. *Pain* 2005;116:347-358.
27. Eshar D, Bdolah-Abram T. Comparison of efficacy, safety, and convenience of selamectin versus ivermectin for treatment of *Trixacarus caviae* mange in pet guinea pigs (*Cavia porcellus*). *J Am Vet Med Assoc* 2012;241:1056-1058.

28. Eshar D, Pohlman LM, Harkin KR. Urine properties of captive black-tailed prairie dogs (*Cynomys ludovicianus*). *J Exot Pet Med* 2016;25:213-219.
29. Ewringmann A, Gloeckner B. *Leitsymptome bei Hamster, Ratte, Maus und Rennmaus*. 2nd ed. Stuttgart: Enke; 2014.
30. Ewringmann A, Gloeckner B. *Leitsymptome bei Meerschweinchen, Chinchilla und Degu*. 2nd ed. Stuttgart: Enke; 2012.
31. Fehr M, Sassenburg L, Zwart P. *Krankheiten der Heimtiere*. 8th ed. Schluetersche Verlagsgesellschaft: Hannover; 2015.
32. Fisher PG. Exotic mammal renal disease: diagnosis and treatment. *Vet Clin North Am Exotic Anim Pract* 2006;9:69-96.
33. Flecknell PA. Analgesia and post-operative care. In: *Laboratory Animal Anaesthesia*. 4th. Boston: Academic Press; 2016:141-192.
34. Foletto VR, Vanz F, Gazarini L, et al. Efficacy and security of ivermectin given orally to rats naturally infected with *Syphacia* spp., *Giardia* spp. and *Hymenolepis nana*. *Lab Anim* 2015;49:196-200.
35. Fox L, Snyder LB, Mans C. Comparison of dexmedetomidine-ketamine with isoflurane for anesthesia of chinchillas (*Chinchilla lanigera*). *J Am Assoc Lab Anim Sci* 2016;55:312-316.
36. Fredholm DV, Cagle LA, Johnston MS. Evaluation of precision and establishment of reference ranges for plasma thyroxine using a point-of-care analyzer in healthy guinea pigs (*Cavia porcellus*). *J Exot Pet Med* 21:87-93.
37. Gaertner DJ, Hallman TM, Hankenson FC, et al. Anesthesia and analgesia for laboratory rodents. In: Brown MJ, Danneman PJ, Karas AZ, eds. *Anesthesia and Analgesia in Laboratory Animals*. 2nd ed. San Diego: Academic Press; 2008:239-297.
38. Gardhouse S, Eshar D. Diagnosis and successful treatment of *Eimeria* infection in a group of zoo-kept black-tailed prairie dogs (*Cynomys ludovicianus*). *J Zoo Wildl Med* 2015;46:367-369.
39. Goebel T, Erwingmann A. *Heimtierkrankheiten: Kleinsaeuger, Amphibien, Reptilien*. Stuttgart: UTB Publishing; 2005.
40. Grosset C, Peters S, Peron F, et al. Contraceptive effect and potential side-effects of deslorelin acetate implants in rats (*Rattus norvegicus*): preliminary observations. *Can J Vet Res* 2012;76:209-214.
41. Harkness JE. *A Practitioner's Guide to Domestic Rodents*. American Animal Hospital Association: Lakewood, CO; 1993.
42. Hauptman K, Jekl V, Knotek Z. Use of medetomidine for sedation in the laboratory rat (*Rattus norvegicus*). *Acta Veterinaria Brno* 2003;72:583-591.
43. Hayes KE, Raucci Jr JA, Gades NM, et al. An evaluation of analgesic regimens for abdominal surgery in mice. *J Am Assoc Lab Anim Sci* 2000;39:18-23.
44. Healy JR, Tonkin JL, Kamarec SR, et al. Evaluation of an improved sustained-release buprenorphine formulation for use in mice. *Am J Vet Res* 2014;75:619-625.
45. Heatley JJ. Cardiovascular anatomy, physiology, and disease of rodents and small exotic mammals. *Vet Clin North Am Exot Anim Pract* 2009;12:99-113.
46. Henke J, Baumgartner C, Roltgen I, et al. Anaesthesia with midazolam/medetomidine/fentanyl in chinchillas (*Chinchilla lanigera*) compared to anaesthesia with xylazine/ketamine and medetomidine/ketamine. *J Vet Med A Physiol Pathol Clin Med* 2004;51:259-264.
47. Hess LR, Ravich ML, Reavill DR. Diagnosis and treatment of an insulinoma in a guinea pig (*Cavia porcellus*). *J Am Vet Med Assoc* 2013;242:522-526.
48. Higuchi S, Yamada R, Hashimoto A, et al. Evaluation of a combination of alfaxalone with medetomidine and butorphanol for inducing surgical anesthesia in laboratory mice. *Jpn J Vet Res* 2016;64:131-139.
49. Hoefer HL. Chinchillas. *Vet Clin North Am Small Anim Pract* 1994;24:103-111.
50. Huerkamp M. Anesthesia and postoperative management of rabbits and pocket pets. In: Current Veterinary Therapy XII Small Animal Practice; 1995:1322-1327.
51. Jekl V. *Personal observation*: 2016.

52. Jepson L. *Exotic Animal Medicine: A Quick Reference Guide.* Philadelphia: Saunders/Elsevier; 2009.
53. Jirkof P, Tourvieille A, Cinelli P, et al. Buprenorphine for pain relief in mice: repeated injections vs sustained-release depot formulation. *Lab Anim* 2015;49:177-187.
54. Johnson RA. Voluntary running-wheel activity, arterial blood gases, and thermal antinociception in rats after 3 buprenorphine formulations. *J Am Assoc Lab Anim Sci* 2016;55:306-311.
55. Jones CK, Peters SC, Shannon HE. Efficacy of duloxetine, a potent and balanced serotonergic and noradrenergic reuptake inhibitor, in inflammatory and acute pain models in rodents. *J Pharmacol Exp Therapeut* 2005;312:726-732.
56. Kawai S, Takagi Y, Kaneko S, et al. Effect of three types of mixed anesthetic agents alternate to ketamine in mice. *Exp Anim* 2011;60:481-487.
57. Kendall LV, Wegenast DJ, Smith BJ, et al. Efficacy of sustained-release buprenorphine in an experimental laparotomy model in female mice. *J Am Assoc Lab Anim Sci* 2016;55:66-73.
58. Kilic N, Henke J, Erhardt W. Ketamine/medetomidine-anaesthesia in the hamster: a clinical comparison between the subcutaneous and intraperitoneal way of application. *Tierärztliche Praxis Kleintiere* 2004;32:384-388.
59. Kirihara Y, Takechi M, Kurosaki K, et al. Effects of an anesthetic mixture of medetomidine, midazolam, and butorphanol in rats—strain difference and antagonism by atipamezole. *Exp Anim* 2016;65:27-36.
60. Klement P, Augustine JM, Delaney KH, et al. An oral ivermectin regimen that eradicates pinworms (*Syphacia* spp.) in laboratory rats and mice. *Lab Anim Sci* 1996;46:286-290.
61. Knafo ES. Sildenafil citrate as a pulmonary protectant in chronic murine *Mycoplasma pulmonis* infection. *Proc Annu Assoc Exot Mam Vet* 2014;6.
62. Kohutova S, Jekl V, Knotek Z, et al. The effect of deslorelin acetate on the oestrous cycle of female guinea pigs. *Veterinarni Medicina* 2015;60:155-160.
63. Kunzel F, Hierlmeier B, Christian M, et al. Hyperthyroidism in four guinea pigs: clinical manifestations, diagnosis, and treatment. *J Small Anim Pract* 2013;54:667-671.
64. Laird KL, Swindle MM, Flecknell PA. *Handbook of Rodent and Rabbit Medicine.* New York: Pergamon; 1996.
65. Lau C, Ranasinghe MG, Shiels I, et al. Plasma pharmacokinetics of alfaxalone after a single intraperitoneal or intravenous injection of Alfaxan (R) in rats. *J Vet Pharmacol Ther* 2013;36:516-520.
66. Lichtenberger M, Lennox AM. Critical care of the exotic companion mammal (with a focus on herbivorous species): the first twenty-four hours. *J Exot Pet Med* 2012;21:284-292.
67. Liles JH, Flecknell PA. A comparison of the effects of buprenorphine, carprofen and flunixin following laparotomy in rats. *J Vet Pharmacol Ther* 1994;17:284-290.
68. Linde A, Summerfield NJ, Johnston MS, et al. Echocardiography in the chinchilla. *J Vet Intern Med* 2004;18:772-774.
69. Mans C. *Personal observation;* 2016.
70. Mans C, Evenson E. Analgesic efficacy and safety of hydromorphone and tramadol in chinchillas (*Chinchilla lanigera*). In: *Proc 2nd Exoticscon Conf*; 2016:409.
71. Mans C, Fox L, Sladky KK. Efficacy and safety of buprenorphine in chinchillas. In: *Proc 2nd ICARE Conf (Paris)*; 2015:458.
72. Mans C, Jekl V. Anatomy and disorders of the oral cavity of chinchillas and degus. *Vet Clin North Am Exot Anim Pract* 2016;19:843-869.
73. Marx JO, Vudathala D, Murphy L, et al. Antibiotic administration in the drinking water of mice. *J Am Assoc Lab Anim Sci* 2014;53:301-306.
74. Mayer J. Rodents. In: Carpenter JW, ed. *Exotic Animal Formulary.* 4th ed. St. Louis: Saunders/Elsevier; 2012:476-516.
75. Mayer J. The use of GnRH to treat cystic ovaries in a guinea pig. *Exotic DVM* 2003;3:36.
76. Mayer J, Sato A, Kiupel M, et al. Extralabel use of cabergoline in the treatment of a pituitary adenoma in a rat. *J Am Vet Med Assoc* 2011;239:656-660.

77. Mayer J, Wagner R, Mitchell MA, et al. Use of recombinant human thyroid-stimulating hormone for evaluation of thyroid function in guinea pigs (*Cavia porcellus*). *J Am Vet Med Assoc* 2013;242:346-349.
78. Mayer J, Wagner R, Taeymans O. Advanced diagnostic approaches and current management of thyroid pathologies in guinea pigs. *Vet Clin North Am Exot Anim Pract* 2010;13:509-523.
79. McClure JT, Rosin E. Comparison of amikacin dosing regimens in neutropenic guinea pigs with *Escherichia coli* infection. *Am J Vet Res* 1998;59:750-755.
80. Meert TF, Vermeirsch HA. A preclinical comparison between different opioids: antinociceptive versus adverse effects. *Pharmacol Biochem Behav* 2005;80:309-326.
81. Mehlhorn H, Schmahl G, Frese M, et al. Effects of a combination of emodepside and praziquantel on parasites of reptiles and rodents. *Parasitol Res* 2005;97(Suppl 1):S65-S69.
82. Melo ME, Silva CA, de Souza Gomes WD, et al. Immediate tooth replantation in rats: effect of systemic antibiotic therapy with amoxicillin and tetracycline. *Clin Oral Investig* 2016;20:523-532.
83. *Merck Veterinary Manual*. 11th ed. Kenilworth, New Jersey: Merck & Co; 2016.
84. Meredith A. *BSAVA Small Animal Formulary: Part B: Exotic Pets*. Quedgeley, Glouchester, UK: British Small Animal Veterinary Association; 2015.
85. Mieth H, Leitner I, Meingassner JG. The efficacy of orally applied terbinafine, itraconazole and fluconazole in models of experimental trichophytoses. *J Med Vet Mycol* 1994;32:181-188.
86. Millecamps M, Jourdan D, Leger S, et al. Circadian pattern of spontaneous behavior in monarthritic rats: a novel global approach to evaluation of chronic pain and treatment effectiveness. *Arthrit Rheumat* 2005;52:3470-3478.
87. Miller AL, Richardson CA. Rodent analgesia. *Vet Clin North Am Exot Anim Pract* 2011;14:81-92.
88. Mitchell MA, Tully TN. *Manual of Exotic Pet Practice*. Saunders/Elsevier: St. Louis, MO; 2009.
89. Morgan RJ, Eddy LB, Solie TN, et al. Ketamine-acepromazine as an anaesthetic agent for chinchillas (*Chinchilla laniger*). *Lab Anim* 1981;15:281-283.
90. Morrisey JK, Carpenter JW. Formulary. In: Quesenberry KE, Carpenter JW, eds. *Ferrets, Rabbits, and Rodents: Clinical Medicine and Surgery*. 3rd ed. St. Louis: Saunders/Elsevier; 2012:566-575.
91. Munro G. Pharmacological assessment of the rat formalin test utilizing the clinically used analgesic drugs gabapentin, lamotrigine, morphine, duloxetine, tramadol and ibuprofen: influence of low and high formalin concentrations. *Euro J Pharmacol* 2009;605:95-102.
92. Ness RD. Rodents. In: Carpenter JW, ed. *Exotic Animal Formulary*. 3rd ed. St. Louis: Saunders/Elsevier; 2005:375-408.
93. Oglesbee BL. *Blackwell's Five Minute Veterinary Consult: Small Mammals*. 2nd ed. Wiley-Blackwell: Chichester, West Sussex; 2011.
94. Parkinsin L, Mans C. Anesthetic and post-anesthetic effects of alfaxalone-butorphanol compared with dexmedetomidine-ketamine in chinchillas (Chinchilla lanigera). *J Am Assoc Lab Anim Sci* 2017: in press.
95. Petersen NT. Therapeutic review: terbutaline. *J Exot Pet Med* 2012;21:260-263.
96. Plunkett SJ. *Emergency Procedures for the Small Animal Veterinarian*. 3rd ed. London: Elsevier; 2013.
97. Quesenberry KE. Guinea pigs. *Vet Clin North Am Small Anim Pract* 1994;24:67-87.
98. Richardson VCG. *Diseases of Small Domestic Rodents*. Malden: Blackwell Scientific Publications; 1997.
99. Roach PD, Wallis PM, Olson ME. The use of metronidazole, tinidazole and dimetridazole in eliminating trichomonads from laboratory mice. *Lab Anim* 1988;22:361-364.
100. Roughan JV, Flecknell PA. Behaviour-based assessment of the duration of laparotomy-induced abdominal pain and the analgesic effects of carprofen and buprenorphine in rats. *Behav Pharmacol* 2004;15:461-472.

101. Roughan JV, Flecknell PA. Behavioural effects of laparotomy and analgesic effects of ketoprofen and carprofen in rats. *Pain* 2001;90:65-74.
102. Sadar M, Knych H, Drazenovich T, et al. Pharmacokinetics of buprenorphine in the guinea pig (*Cavia porcellus*): intravenous and oral transmucosal administration. *Annu Assoc Exot Mam Vet Conf* 2014.
103. Degu Sassenburg L. In: Fehr M, Sassenburg L, Zwart P, eds. *Krankheiten der Heimtiere* Hannover: Schluetersche Verlagsgesellschaft 2015;239-270.
104. Schoeb TR. Respiratory diseases of rodents. *Vet Clin North Am Exot Anim Pract* 2000;3:481-496.
105. Schuetzenhofer G, Goericke-Pesch S, Wehrend A. Effects of deslorelin implants on ovarian cysts in guinea pigs. *Schweizer Archiv für Tierheilkunde* 2011;153:416-417.
106. Schweigart G. *Arzneimittelanwendung bei Nagetieren und Kanninchen*. 2nd ed. Berlin: Veterinärmedizinischer Fachverlag; 2009.
107. Seymour TL, Adams SC, Felt SA, et al. Postoperative analgesia due to sustained-release buprenorphine, sustained-release meloxicam, and carprofen gel in a model of incisional pain in rats (*Rattus norvegicus*). *J Am Assoc Lab Anim Sci* 2016;55:300-305.
108. Siriarchavatana P, Ayers JD, Kendall LV. Anesthetic activity of alfaxalone compared with ketamine in mice. *J Am Assoc Lab Anim Sci* 2016;55:426-430.
109. Smith A, Asa C, Edwards B, et al. Predominant suppression of FSHβ-immunoreactivity after long-term treatment of intact and castrate adult male rats with the GnRH agonist deslorelin. *J Neuroendocrinol* 2012;24:737-747.
110. Smith LJ, Valenzuela JR, Krugner-Higby LA, et al. A single dose of liposome-encapsulated hydromorphone provides extended analgesia in a rat model of neuropathic pain. *Comp Med* 2006;56:487-492.
111. Tani K, Iwanaga T, Sonoda K, et al. Ivermectin treatment of demodicosis in 56 hamsters. *J Vet Med Sci* 2001;63:1245-1247.
112. Thomason JD, Eshar D, Zimmer Coyle C, et al. The static electrocardiogram in clinically healthy, anesthetized, zoo-kept black-tailed prairie dogs (*Cynomys ludovicianus*). *J Vet Cardiol* 2015;17:293-297.
113. Visser C, Wijnbergen A, Bleich A. Maeuse und Ratten. In: Fehr M, Sassenburg L, Zwart P, eds. *Krankheiten der Heimtiere*. Hannover: Schluetersche Verlagsgesellschaft; 2015:129-182.
114. Wenger S. Anesthesia and analgesia in rabbits and rodents. *J Exot Pet Med* 2012;21:7-16.
115. Wyre NR. Rats, chronic respiratory disease. In: Mayer J, Donnelly TM, eds. *Clinical Veterinary Advisor: Birds and Exotic Pets*. St. Louis: WB Saunders; 2013:242-252.
116. Yang X-P, Liu Y-H, Rhaleb N-E, et al. Echocardiographic assessment of cardiac function in conscious and anesthetized mice. *Am J Physiol-Heart Circulat Physiol* 1999;277:H1967-H1974.

Chapter 10 Rabbits

Peter Fisher | Jennifer Graham

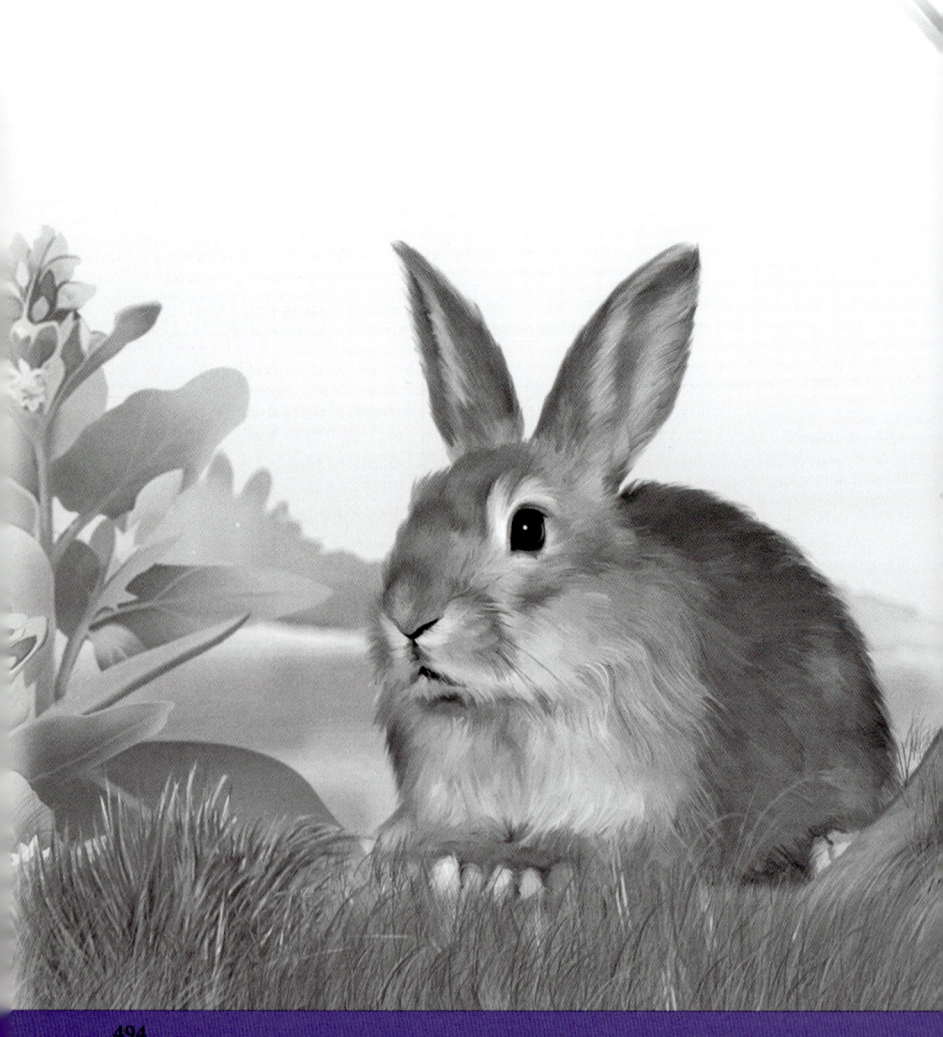

TABLE 10-1 Antimicrobial Agents Used in Rabbits.[a]

Agent	Dosage	Comments
Amikacin	5-10 mg/kg SC, IM, IV divided q8-24h[41]	
	8-16 mg/kg SC, IM, IV q24h[112]	Increased efficacy and decreased toxicity when given once daily; for IV use, dilute in 4 mL/kg saline and give over 20 min
	1.25 g/20 g methylmethacrylate[41]	Place in bone after surgical debridement of jaw abscess
Azithromycin	4-5 mg/kg IM q48h × 7 days[19]	Effective against syphilis
	15-30 mg/kg PO q24h × 15 days[41]	PD; pulmonary infections
Cefazolin	2 g/20 g methylmethacrylate[41]	Place in bone after surgical debridement of jaw abscess
Cefotaxime	50 mg/kg IM q8h[41]	Pneumococcal endocarditis
Ceftazidime	50 mg/kg IM, IV q3h[1]	PK
	100 mg/kg IM q12h[41]	
Ceftiofur	2 g/20 g methylmethacrylate[41]	Place in bone after surgical debridement of jaw abscess
Ceftriaxone	40 mg/kg IM q12h × 2-3 days[41]	Effective against syphilis, pneumococcal endocarditis
	71 mg/kg IV q24h[28]	Pneumococcal pneumonia
Cephalexin	—	Oral cephalosporins are not recommended[41]
	15 mg/kg SC q12h[41]	Parenteral form not available in the United States; not generally recommended
Cephalothin	12.5 mg/kg IM q6h × 6 days[41]	Cephalosporins are generally not recommended;[112] not available in the United States
	2 g/20 g methylmethacrylate[41]	Place in bone after surgical debridement of jaw abscess
Chloramphenicol	—	The use of chloramphenicol in food-producing animals is prohibited in the United States
	25 mg/kg PO q8-12h[41]	
	30-50 mg/kg SC, IM, IV q8-24h[41,112]	
	55 mg/kg PO q12h × 4 wk[41]	Effective against syphilis
Chlortetracycline	50 mg/kg PO q24h[41]	
Ciprofloxacin[b]	—	May cause arthropathies in young animals[126]
	5-20 mg/kg PO q12h[41]	Suspension in water is stable for 14 days
	1 drop topical q8-12h[53]	Nasal pasteurellosis; maintains therapeutic levels in tear film for at least 6hr after application (tears drain into nasal sinus)
Difloxacin[b] (Dicural, Fort Dodge)	5 mg/kg IM, IV q24h[3]	PK; dose appropriate for E. coli infections
Doxycycline	2.5 mg/kg PO q12h[20]	
	4 mg/kg PO q24h[41]	

Continued

TABLE 10-1 Antimicrobial Agents Used in Rabbits. (cont'd)

Agent	Dosage	Comments
Enrofloxacin[b]	—	May cause arthropathies in young dogs, but similar effects using standard dosages in rabbits have not been reported; SC and IM injections may cause muscle necrosis or sterile abscesses; dilute before giving parenterally[41]
	5 mg/kg IM, IV q12-24h[36]	Angora rabbits/PK
	5 mg/kg PO, SC, IM, IV q12h[15,16,41]	PK;[15,16] clinical trial for pasteurellosis, × 14 days[41]
	5-20 mg/kg PO, IM q12h × 14-30 days[41]	Pasteurellosis
	200 mg/L drinking water × 14 days[41]	
Florfenicol	—	In the United States, use of related drug chloramphenicol is prohibited in food-producing animals
	25 mg/kg IM, IV q6h[74]	PK
	30 mg/kg PO, IV q8h[2]	PK
Furazolidone	5 mg/kg PO q24h × 14 days[41]	The FDA has prohibited extra-label use in food animals
	5.5 g/L drinking water[41]	
	50 mg/kg feed[41]	
Gentamicin	—	Seldom indicated; use with caution
	4 mg/kg SC, IM q24h[41]	
	5-8 mg/kg SC, IM, IV q8-24h[41]	Decreased toxicity when given once daily; for IV use, dilute in 4 mL/kg saline and give over 20 min
	1 g/20 g methylmethacrylate[41]	Place in bone after surgical debridement of jaw abscess
Marbofloxacin[b]	—	Lowest MIC of nine antibiotics tested against bacteria responsible for upper respiratory infections[120]
	2 mg/kg SC, IM, IV q24h[4,92]	PK; study during *Pasteurella* infection[4]
	5 mg/kg PO q24h × 10 days[22]	PK
Metronidazole	5 mg/kg IV q12h[112]	Administer slowly
	20 mg/kg PO q12h × 3-5 days[112]	
	40 mg/kg PO q24h × 3 days[41]	
Minocycline	6 mg/kg IV q8h[100]	PK
Moxifloxacin[b]	5 mg/kg PO, IM q24h × 10 days[39]	PK; susceptible infections (some bacteria may require higher doses)
	40 mg/kg IV q12h × 2 doses, then q24h[104]	Bacterial meningitis
Netilmicin (Netromycin, Schering)	6-8 mg/kg SC, IM, IV q24h[41]	For IV use, dilute and give over 20 min
	7 mg/kg IV q12h[122]	PK; induced renal tubular necrosis in 50% of animals

TABLE 10-1   Antimicrobial Agents Used in Rabbits. (cont'd)

Agent	Dosage	Comments
Ofloxacinb (Ocuflox, Allergan)	20 mg/kg SC q8h[91]	Urogenital, skin, respiratory infections
Orbifloxacin[b]	20 mg/kg PO q24h × 7-21 days[138]	PK
Oxytetracycline	15 mg/kg IM q8h[84]	PK; anorexia and diarrhea at 30 mg/kg IM q8h; tissue irritation can occur
	25 mg/kg SC q24h[41]	
	50 mg/kg PO q12h[41]	
	1 mg/mL drinking water[41]	
Penicillin G	—	Do not give any form of penicillin orally to rabbits
Benzathine form	42,000-60,000 U/kg IM q48h[41]	Benzathine penicillin achieves lower serum levels than other forms and is effective against only highly susceptible organisms
	42,000-84,000 U/kg SC q7d × 3 wk[41]	
Procaine form	40,000 U/kg IM q24h × 5-7 days[41]	Rabbit syphilis
	42,000-84,000 U/kg SC, IM q24h[41]	
	60,000 U/kg IM q8h[139]	PK
Benzylpenicillin	60,000 U/kg IM q12h[64]	PK
Rifampin (R)/azithromycin (A)	(R) 40 mg/kg PO q12h + (A) 50 mg/kg PO q24h[41]	*Staphylococcus* osteomyelitis
Rifampin (R)/clarithromycin (C)	(R) 40 mg/kg + (C) 80 mg/kg PO q12h[41]	*Staphylococcus* osteomyelitis
Silver sulfadiazine cream (Silvadene, Marion)	Topical q24h[41]	Does not cause diarrhea if ingested
Spectinomycin	1 g/L drinking water × 7 days[112]	May cause diarrhea in weanling rabbits
Sulfadimethoxine	10-15 mg/kg PO q12h[112]	
Sulfamethazine	1 mg/mL drinking water[41]	
	5-10 g/kg feed[41]	
Sulfaquinoxaline	1 mg/mL drinking water[41]	
	0.6 g/kg feed[41]	
Tetracycline	50-100 mg/kg PO q8-12h[112]	
	250-1000 mg/L drinking water[41]	Therapeutic levels not achieved even at 800-1600 mg/L;[108] 250 mg/L not effective in clinical trial for pasteurellosis[41]
Tilmicosin (Micotil, Elanco)	12.5 mg/kg PO q24h × 7 days[48]	PK
	25 mg/kg SC once[41]	Pasteurellosis; use cautiously: at least one rabbit death and several human deaths have been reported;[20] has been associated with anemia and leukopenia

Continued

TABLE 10-1	Antimicrobial Agents Used in Rabbits. (cont'd)	
Agent	**Dosage**	**Comments**
Tobramycin	1 g/20 g methylmethacrylate[41]	Place in bone after surgical debridement of jaw abscess
	10% in calcium sulfate pellets[99]	Biodegradable implants for treatment of osteomyelitis
Trimethoprim/sulfa	15 mg/kg PO q12h[41]	
	30 mg/kg PO, SC, IM q12h[41,112]	May cause tissue necrosis when given SC[112]
	15-30 mg/kg PO q12-24h[112]	
	30-48 mg/kg SC q12h[112]	
Tylosin	10 mg/kg PO, SC, IM q12-24h[112]	
Vancomycin	50 mg/kg IV q8h[100]	PD
	10 mg vancomycin and 50 mg DL-lactide-co-glycolide copolymer[41]	Osteomyelitis; effective locally for 56 days

[a]There is a potential for antibiotic-induced enterotoxemia following administration of some antimicrobial agents (see Table 10.15). Appetite and fecal character must be monitored closely during and following therapy.
[b]The use of fluoroquinolones in food-producing animals is strictly prohibited in the United States. Do not use these drugs in rabbits that may be consumed by humans.

TABLE 10-2	Antifungal Agents Used in Rabbits.[a]	
Agent	**Dosage**	**Comments**
Albaconazole	5 mg/kg PO q24h[98]	Cryptococcal meningitis
	50 mg/kg PO q24h[18]	Disseminated *Scedosporium prolificans*
Amphotericin B	—	Severe fungal infections; use in combination with fluconazole;[41] potentially nephrotoxic and hepatotoxic
Desoxycholate form	1 mg/kg IV q24h[41,112,121]	
Liposomal form	5 mg/kg IV q24h[110]	Invasive aspergillosis
Clotrimazole (Lotrimin, Bayer)	Topical[41]	Localized dermatophytosis
Fluconazole	5 mg/kg PO q24h[98]	Cryptococcal meningitis
	25-43 mg/kg IV (slow) q12h[87,112]	Systemic fungal disease
	38 mg/kg PO q12h[8]	*Aspergillus* keratitis
	80 mg/kg PO q24h × 21 days[41]	Coccidioidal meningitis; controlled but did not cure

TABLE 10-2 Antifungal Agents Used in Rabbits. (cont'd)

Agent	Dosage	Comments
Griseofulvin	12.5-25 mg/kg PO q12-24h × 30-45 days[41]	Advanced cases of dermatophytosis; decrease dose by 50% if using ultra-microsize form (Gris-PEG, Allergan Herbert), which has better absorption
	15-25 mg/kg PO q24h, or divided q12h × 30 days[58]	At high doses may cause bone marrow suppression and panleukopenia
Itraconazole	5-10 mg/kg PO q24h × 30 days[38,58]	Dermatophytosis
	20-40 mg/kg PO q24h[41]	*Aspergillus* pneumonia
	40 mg/kg PO q24h[107]	Invasive aspergillosis
Ketoconazole	10-40 mg/kg PO q24h × 14 days[38,41]	Dermatophytosis
Lime sulfur (2%-3%)	Topical q5-7d × 4 wk[41]	Dermatophytosis; use with caution
	Topical 1:32 dilution with water 2×/wk[58]	
Micafungin	0.25-2 mg/kg IV q24h[110]	Systemic candidiasis
Miconazole (Conofite, Merck)	Topical q24h × 14-28 days[41]	Localized dermatophytosis
Miconazole/chlorhexidine shampoo	Bathe once daily[65]	Dermatophytosis
Nystatin	20 mg/kg PO q12h × 10 days[41]	*Cyniclomyces guttulatus* yeast overgrowth
Posaconazole	6 mg/kg PO q24h[109]	*Aspergillus* pneumonia
	20 mg/kg PO q24h[41]	*Aspergillus* pneumonia
Terbinafine	—	Best used as part of combination therapy; little activity when used as a single agent[41,73]
	10 mg/kg PO q24h[58]	Dermatophytosis
	100 mg/kg PO q12h × 21 days[41]	Less effective than fluconazole for coccidioidal meningitis
	100 mg/kg PO q12-24h[41]	
	100 mg/kg PO q24h in combination with amphotericin B 0.4 mg/kg IV q24h[73]	Invasive aspergillosis
Voriconazole	—	The short terminal elimination half-life of less than 1 hr in the rabbit indicates that the efficacy of voriconazole is less than optimal in this species;[117] however, voriconazole is effective as a topical antifungal ophthalmic preparation in the rabbit (see Table 10.6)

[a]Antifungal protocols using amphotericin B administered intravenously or itraconazole, fluconazole, or ketoconazole administered orally alone or in combination for deep mycotic infections have been based on those used successfully in the dog and may be adequate treatment options in the rabbit; however, this hypothesis requires confirmation and validation.[14] Certain antifungal protocols have not caused death in rabbit models, even when given for extended periods.[18,41,107,109,110,121]

TABLE 10-3 Antiparasitic Agents Used in Rabbits.

Agent	Dosage	Comments
Albendazole	7.5-20 mg/kg PO q24h[41] × 3-14 days[41,112]	Potential treatment for encephalitozoonosis; use cautiously, deaths have been reported[52]
Amprolium (9.6%)	0.5 mL/pint drinking water × 10 days[112]	Coccidiosis
	0.625 mL/pint drinking water × 21 days[41]	
Carbaryl powder 5%	Topically q7d[41]	Ectoparasites; use sparingly
Cyromazine 6% (Rearguard, Novartis)	Topically q6-10wk[41]	Preventative for myiasis
Decoquinate (Deccox, Rhone-Poulenc)	62.5 ppm in feed[41]	Coccidiosis
Diclazuril	4 mg/kg SC[106]	
	1 ppm in feed[41,135]	PD; intestinal and hepatic coccidiosis
Doramectin	0.2 mg/kg IM once[68,112]	*Psoroptes* mites
	0.3 mg/kg SC[50]	PD
Emodepside 2.1%/ praziquantel 8.6% (Profender, Bayer)	0.14 mL/kg topically once[41]	*Trichostrongylus colubriformis*
Eprinomectin	0.2-0.3 mg/kg SC once[105]	*Psoroptes* mites
	2 mg/kg topically once[140]	*Psoroptes* mites
Febantel/pyrantel pamoate/ praziquantel (Drontal Plus, Bayer)	½ tablet/5 kg PO once[41]	Use tablet for puppies and small dogs (2-25 lb); effective against nematodes and cestodes
Fenbendazole	—	On rare occasions, anemia and arteritis have been reported[52]
	5 mg/kg PO[41]	
	5-20 mg/kg PO q24h × 5 days; repeat in 14 days[41]	Nematodes; use 20 mg/kg for *Passalurus ambiguous*
	20 mg/kg PO q24h × 7 days before and 2 days after mixing rabbits[130]	Preventive against encephalitozoonosis
	20 mg/kg PO q24h × 28 days[112,130]	Treatment for encephalitozoonosis; failed to clear all parasites
	50 ppm in feed × 2-6 wk[41]	
Fipronil (Frontline, Merial)	Contraindicated[41]	Can cause neurologic disease and death
Imidacloprid (Advantage, Bayer)	10-16 mg/kg topically once[41,61]	Flea adulticide; use single 0.4 mL dose, 10% solution
Imidacloprid (I) 10%/ moxidectin (M) 1% (Advantage Multi for Cats, Bayer)	10 mg/kg (I) + 1 mg/kg (M) topically q4wk × 3 treatments[41]	*Psoroptes* mites
Imidacloprid 8.8%/ permethrin 44% (Advantix, Bayer)	11-16.6 mg/kg topically once[12]	*Leporacarus gibbus* (rabbit fur mite)

TABLE 10-3 Antiparasitic Agents Used in Rabbits. (cont'd)

Agent	Dosage	Comments
Ivermectin	—	Ectoparasites
	0.1-0.2 mg/kg SC, repeat in 14 days[41]	Ear mites, clinical trial
	0.2-0.44 mg/kg PO, SC q8-14d[112]	*Psoroptes* (ear mites)
	0.3-0.4 mg/kg SC, repeat in 14 days[112]	*Sarcoptes scabiei* (sarcoptic mange); *Notoedres cati*
	0.4 mg/kg SC q80h × 3 doses[69]	Sarcoptic mange
Lasalocid	120 ppm in feed[41]	Coccidiosis
Lime sulfur (2%-3%)	1-2 dips/wk × 28 days[41]	Ectoparasites; young animals
	Dip q7d × 4-6 wk[41,112]	
Lufenuron (Program, Novartis)	30 mg/kg PO q30d[112]	Flea larvicide
Metronidazole	20 mg/kg PO q12h[41]	Antiprotozoal agent
Monensin (CoBan 60, Elanco)	0.002%-0.004% in feed[41]	Coccidiosis
Moxidectin	0.2 mg/kg PO, repeat in 10 days[112,136]	Psoroptic mange
	0.3 mg/kg SC[50]	PD
Oxibendazole	30 mg/kg PO q24h × 7-14 days, then 15 mg/kg PO q24h for 30-60 days[112]	Encephalitozoonosis; no highly effective treatment has been identified; bone marrow suppression has been reported with the use of benzimidazoles, so an intratreatment CBC is recommended[52]
Piperazine	100 mg/kg PO q24h × 2 days[41]	Use with citrate formulation
	200 mg/kg PO, repeat in 14-21 days[112]	Use with citrate formulation
	200-500 mg/kg PO × 2 days[112]	Adults; use with adipate formulation
	750 mg/kg PO × 2 days[41]	Juveniles; wash perianal area
	2-5 mg/mL drinking water × 7 days[41]	
Praziquantel	5-10 mg/kg PO, SC, IM, repeat in 10 days[112]	Cestodes, trematodes
Pyrantel pamoate	5-10 mg/kg PO, SC, IM, repeat in 10 days[41]	
	5-10 mg/kg PO, repeat in 14-21 days[112]	
Pyrethrins	Topically as directed for puppies/kittens q7d[41]	Flea control
Selamectin (Revolution, Zoetis)	12 mg/kg topically at base of neck once[72]	Cheyletiellosis
	20 mg/kg topically q7d[21]	PK/flea infestation; further studies are needed to assess long-term safety in rabbits at this dose following repeated application[21]

Continued

TABLE 10-3 Antiparasitic Agents Used in Rabbits. (cont'd)

Agent	Dosage	Comments
Selamectin (Revolution, Zoetis) (cont'd)	30 mg (8-14 mg/kg) topically q30 days × 2 doses[37,76]	Sarcoptic mange
	30 mg (6-18 mg/kg) topically once[76,96]	*Psoroptes*
Sulfadimethoxine	50 mg/kg PO once, then 25 mg/kg q24h × 10-20 days[41]	Coccidiosis
Sulfadimethoxine/ ormetoprim (Rofenaid 40, Roche)	62.5-250 ppm in feed[41]	Coccidiosis
Sulfadimidene	100-233 mg/L drinking water[41]	Coccidiosis
Sulfamerazine	100 mg/kg PO[41]	Coccidiosis
	0.05%-0.15% in drinking water[41]	
Sulfamethazine	100 mg/kg PO q24h[41]	Coccidiosis
	0.77 g/L drinking water[41]	
	0.5%-1% in feed[41]	
Sulfamethoxine	50 mg/kg PO once, then 25 mg/kg PO q24h × 10-20 days[41]	Coccidiosis
Sulfaquinoxaline	0.02%-0.05% in drinking water[41]	Coccidiosis; prevention
	0.025%-0.1% in drinking water[112]	Alternating 2 wk periods for 4-8 wk during weaning
	0.1%-0.15% in drinking water[41]	Coccidiosis; treatment
	1 mg/mL in drinking water[41]	
	0.025%-0.03% in feed × 4-6 wk[112]	During weaning
	125-250 ppm in feed[41]	
Thiabendazole	25-50 mg/kg PO[41]	
	50-100 mg/kg PO q24h × 5 days[112]	
	0.1% in feed × 3 mo[41]	
Toltrazuril	2.5-5 mg/kg PO[115]	Intestinal coccidiosis
	10 mg/kg PO[60,71]	PK;[41] coccidiosis due to *Eimeria tenella*[41]
	25 ppm in drinking water (or 25 mg/kg PO) q24h × 2 days, repeat after 5 days[41]	Coccidiosis
	50 ppm in drinking water[17]	Hepatic coccidiosis due to *Eimeria stiedae*

TABLE 10-4 Chemical Restraint/Sedative/Anesthetic/Analgesic Agents Used in Rabbits.[a,b]

Agent	Dosage	Comments
Acepromazine	—	See butorphanol, ketamine, ketamine/xylazine for combinations
	0.25-1 mg/kg IM[41]	Preanesthetic; sedative; tranquilizer
	1-5 mg/kg SC, IM[41]	Preanesthetic; lower end of dose range is preferred
Acetaminophen (Tylenol, McNeil)	—	Short-term use only; use with caution as associated with liver failure[88]
	200-500 mg/kg PO[41]	Analgesia
	1-2 mg/mL drinking water[41]	
Acetaminophen/codeine (120 mg/12 mg per 5 mL)	1 mL elixir/100 mL drinking water[41]	Analgesia
Acetylsalicylic acid (aspirin)	5-20 mg/kg PO q24h[112]	Antiinflammatory; for low grade analgesia
	10-100 mg/kg PO q8-12h[41]	
	100 mg/kg PO q8-24h[25,41]	
	100 mg/kg PO q48h[41]	
Alfaxalone (Alfaxan, Jurox)	—	Neurosteroid anesthetic; IV dose dependent respiratory depression; no analgesic properties
	0.5-1 mg/kg IM[85]	For additional sedation when combined with midazolam, an opioid, and ketamine[85]
	1 mg/kg IV slowly to effect[85]	Anesthetic induction when used in conjunction with preanesthetic sedatives (i.e., midazolam 0.5 mg/kg, hydromorphone 0.1 mg/kg, ketamine 7 mg/kg, and dexmedetomidine 0.005 mg/kg combined in single syringe and given IM)[85]
	2-3 mg/kg IV[55]	Anesthetic induction; give slow to effect
	4 mg/kg IV[111]	Dilute with 5% dextrose and give over 1 min for smooth induction that allows intubation
	4-6 mg/kg IM[62]	Deep sedation; longer duration of action with higher dose
Atipamezole (Antisedan, Orion)	Give same volume SC, IV, IP as medetomidine or dexmedetomidine (5 × medetomidine or 10 × dexmedetomidine dose in mg)[41]	Dexmedetomidine and medetomidine[c] reversal[41]
	0.25 mg/kg IV[112]	
	0.5 mg/kg SC, IM[112]	
	1 mg/kg SC, IM, IV[41]	
Atracurium	0.1 mg/kg IV[41]	Paralysis for intraophthalmic surgery; requires assisted ventilation

Continued

TABLE 10-4 Chemical Restraint/Sedative/Anesthetic/Analgesic Agents Used in Rabbits. (cont'd)

Agent	Dosage	Comments
Atropine	—	Many rabbits possess serum atropinase, hence very high doses are often administered; glycopyrrolate often preferred
	0.1-0.5 mg/kg SC, IM[41]	
	0.1-3 mg/kg SC[41]	
	0.8-1 mg/kg IM[41]	
	10 mg/kg SC q20min[41,112]	To treat organophosphate toxicity
Bupivicaine 0.125%, 0.5%	—	Local and regional anesthetic techniques; concentrations of 0.125% or less produce a good sensory block with least motor effect; epidural anesthesia; dilute with preservative-free saline only; total volume should not exceed 0.33 mL/kg[56]
	1 mg/kg[20]	Injectable epidural; use 0.125% preparation[56]
	2 mg/kg[84]	
Buprenorphine	—	Partial agonist that exerts significant actions at the mu opioid receptor; duration of analgesia may be dose dependent; may cause respiratory depression;[10] see midazolam for combination
	0.01-0.05 mg/kg SC, IM, IV q6-12h[25,41]	Analgesia
	0.012 mg/kg[20,56]	Epidural anesthesia; dilute with preservative-free saline only; total volume should not exceed 0.33 mL/kg[56]
	0.02-0.1 mg/kg SC, IM, IV[41,83]	Preanesthetic
	0.06 mg/kg IV q8h[125]	Analgesia
Buprenorphine SR-LAB (1 mg/mL, ZooPharm)	0.12 mg/kg SC[32]	Compounded formulation of sustained-release buprenorphine
Butorphanol	—	See ketamine/xylazine and midazolam for combinations; mixed agonist/antagonist with low intrinsic activity at the mu receptor and strong agonist activity at kappa and sigma receptors; duration of analgesia may be dose dependent; use lower doses IV
	0.1-0.5 mg/kg SC, IM, IV q4h[25,41]	Analgesia
	0.3-0.5 mg/kg SC, IM, IV q2-4h[123]	
	0.1-1 mg/kg SC, IM, IV q4-6h[41]	
Butorphanol (B)/acepromazine (A)	(A) 0.5 mg/kg + (B) 0.5 mg/kg SC, IM[43]	

TABLE 10-4 Chemical Restraint/Sedative/Anesthetic/Analgesic Agents Used in Rabbits. (cont'd)

Agent	Dosage	Comments
Carprofen	—	Nonsteroidal antiinflammatory; chronic osteoarthritis or degenerative joint disease
	1-2.2 mg/kg PO q12h[25]	
	1-5 mg/kg PO q12-24h[41]	
	2-4 mg/kg PO q12-24h[10]	
	2-4 mg/kg SC q24h[25,41]	
	4 mg/kg SC, IM q24h[10,41]	
Dexmedetomidine (Dexdomitor, Orion)	—	See ketamine/fentanyl and midazolam/hydromorphone/ketamine for combinations; α_2 agonist similar to medetomidine; reverse with atipamezole
	0.005 mg/kg IM[79]	Preanesthetic when combined with ketamine
	0.035-0.05 mg/kg IM[79]	Induction/maintenance when combined with ketamine
Diazepam	—	Benzodiazepine sedative; IV route preferred; see ketamine for combination
	0.5-2 mg/kg IM, IV[41,67,112]	For sedation
	1 mg/kg intracavernous[33]	Seizures; alternative to IV route
	1-3 mg/kg IM[41]	Preanesthetic; tranquilizer
	1-5 mg/kg IM, IV[25,41]	Preanesthetic; tranquilizer
Etomidate	1-2 mg/kg [79,80,83]	Give slow to effect for anesthetic induction; short-acting induction agent; good choice with cardiac patients
Fentanyl	—	Mu opioid agonist; analgesia; see ketamine/dexmedetomidine and medetomidine/midazolam for combinations
	0.0074 mg/kg IV[25,41]	
Fentanyl patch	½ patch/medium-sized rabbit (3 kg) × 3 days[41]	Postoperative analgesia; do not cut patch; cover portion not in use
	25 µg/h patch/3 kg rabbit × 3 days[45]	Note: rapid hair regrowth decreases plasma concentrations
	12.5 µg/h patch/3/ kg rabbit × 3 days[25]	Do not cut patches; may cause drowsiness when initially applied
Fentanyl/fluanisone (Hypnorm, Janssen)	0.2-0.3 mL/kg[41]	Premedication; analgesia; sedation
	0.25 mL/kg SC[41]	
Flumazenil	0.01-0.1 mg/kg IM, IV[41]	Reversal for benzodiazepines
Flunixin meglumine	—	Analgesia; nonsteroidal antiinflammatory[41]
	0.3-2 mg/kg PO, IM, IV q12-24h[41]	Use for no more than 3 days

Continued

TABLE 10-4 Chemical Restraint/Sedative/Anesthetic/Analgesic Agents Used in Rabbits. (cont'd)

Agent	Dosage	Comments
Flunixin meglumine (cont'd)	1.1 mg/kg SC, IM q12h[41] 1-2 mg/kg SC q12-24h[41]	
Gabapentin	—	Neuropathic pain analgesic; indicated for adjunctive treatment of chronic or neurogenic pain in dogs and cats at 3 mg/kg PO q24h and for ancillary therapy of refractory seizures in dogs at 10-30 mg/kg PO q8h[112]
	3-5 mg/kg PO q12-24h[41]	
	25 mg/kg SC[75]	Dose used to approximate plasma concentrations in humans
Glycopyrrolate	—	Anticholinergic; premedication to prevent salivation and bradycardia
	0.01-0.02 mg/kg SC[41] 0.01-0.1 mg/kg SC, IM[41] 0.02 mg/kg IV, IO, intratracheally[57]	
Hydromorphone	—	Opioid analgesic; mainly a mu agonist with less affinity for delta receptors
	0.05-0.2 mg/kg SC, IM q6-8h[20] 0.1-0.2 mg/kg SC, IM, IV q6-8h[66]	
Ibuprofen	—	Analgesia; nonsteroidal antiinflammatory; may have gastrointestinal side effects
	2-7.5 mg/kg PO q4h[41] 7.5 mg/kg PO q6-8 h41	
Isoflurane	3%-5% induction, 1.5%-1.75% maintenance[41]	MAC = 2.05%;[41] prior use of a sedative or injectable induction agent(s) is recommended, as use of preanesthetic agent or combinations will lower the MAC of inhalants
	3%-5% induction, 2%-3% maintenance[41]	
Ketamine	—	NMDA receptor antagonist; should be administered in combination with other agents; combinations to follow
	1-10 mg/kg IM[80] 5-50 mg/kg SC, IM[41] 7-10 mg/kg IM[79,81]	Preanesthetic; add to midazolam/opioid combination if additional sedation required[81]
	15 mg/kg IV[41] 15-20 mg/kg IV[41]	
	20-50 mg/kg IM[41]	60 min of sedation
	20 mg/kg IM[79]	Anesthetic induction, maintenance

TABLE 10-4 Chemical Restraint/Sedative/Anesthetic/Analgesic Agents Used in Rabbits. (cont'd)

Agent	Dosage	Comments
Ketamine (K)/acepromazine (A)	(K) 25-40 mg/kg + (A) 0.25-1 mg/kg IM, IV[41]	Anesthesia
	(K) 40 mg/kg + (A) 0.5-1 mg/kg IM[41]	Anesthesia
Ketamine (K)/dexmedetomidine (D)/fentanyl (F)	(D) 0.02 mg/kg + (K) 5 mg/kg + (F) 0.01 mg/kg IM[119]	May result in mild respiratory depression, respiratory acidosis and hypoxemia; supplemental oxygen recommended
Ketamine (K)/diazepam (D)	(K) 10 mg/kg + (D) 0.5 mg/kg IV[41]	Anesthesia; follow with isoflurane
	(K) 15 mg/kg + (D) 0.3 mg/kg IM[41]	Anesthesia; follow with isoflurane
	(K) 20-40 mg/kg + (D) 1-5 mg/kg IM[41]	Anesthesia; follow with inhalant as needed
	(K) 30-40 mg/kg + (D) 2-5 mg/kg IM[41]	Surgical anesthesia; lower end of dose range for (D) is preferred; less preferable than aforementioned (K)/(D) combinations
Ketamine (K)/medetomidine (Me)[c]	(K) 5 mg/kg + (Me) 0.35 mg/kg IM, IV[41]	Surgical anesthesia
	(K) 15 mg/kg + (Me) 0.25 mg/kg SC,[41] IM[54]	Anesthetic induction; laryngospasm common
Ketamine (K)/midazolam (Mi)	(K) 15 mg/kg IM + (Mi) 3 mg/kg IM[54]	Anesthetic induction
	(K) 25 mg/kg + (Mi) 2-5 mg/kg IM[41]	May be preferable to use (Mi) at <2 mg/kg
Ketamine (K)/xylazine (X)	—	Anesthesia; may result in bradycardia; less preferable than (K)/(D) with isoflurane combinations; seldom indicated
	(K) 10 mg/kg + (X) 3 mg/kg IV[41]	
	(K) 30-40 mg/kg + (X) 3-5 mg/kg IM[41]	
Ketamine (K)/xylazine (X)/acepromazine (A)	(K) 35 mg/kg + (X) 5 mg/kg + (A) 0.75 mg/kg IM[41]	Anesthesia; may result in bradycardia; less preferable than (K)/(D) with isoflurane combinations; seldom indicated
Ketamine (K)/xylazine (X)/butorphanol (B)	(K) 35 mg/kg + (X) 5 mg/kg + (B) 0.1 mg/kg IM[41]	Anesthesia; may result in bradycardia; less preferable than (K)/(D) with isoflurane combinations; seldom indicated
Ketamine (K)/midazolam (Mi)/hydromorphone (H)/dexmedetomidine (D)	(K) 7 mg/kg + (Mi) 0.5 mg/kg + (H) 0.1 mg/kg + (D) 0.005 mg/kg IM[85]	Preanesthetic
Ketoprofen	—	Nonsteroidal antiinflammatory
	1 mg/kg IM q12-24h[41]	Musculoskeletal pain; nonsteroidal antiinflammatory
	1-3 mg/kg IM q12-24h[41]	
	3 mg/kg SC, IM q24h[25,41]	Estimated duration of action 12-24 hr[44]

Continued

TABLE 10-4 Chemical Restraint/Sedative/Anesthetic/Analgesic Agents Used in Rabbits. (cont'd)

Agent	Dosage	Comments
Ketoprofen 2.5% topical gel (Menarini, France)	Apply topically (visceral) q6-12 h[7]	Musculoskeletal pain
Lidocaine (2% injectable)	—	Amide local anesthetic; local, regional, topical, and epidural anesthesia; also see Table 5
	1 mg/kg[78]	
	2-3 mg/kg[83]	
1.5%	0.4 mL/kg epidural[41]	Epidural anesthesia
10%	Topical to glottis[41]	Facilitates intubation
Lidocaine 2.5%/prilocaine 2.5% (Emla cream)	Topical to skin	Facilitates IV catheter placement
Maropitant citrate (Cerenia, Zoetis)	2 mg/kg SC q24h × 3-5 days[24]	Neurokinin (NK1) receptor antagonist; gastrointestinal (visceral) and arthritic pain; can be administered long term q48h or 3 × weekly as needed[24]
Medetomidine	—	Medetomidine is no longer commercially available in the United States, although it may be obtained from select compounding services
	0.1-0.25 mg/kg IM[41]	
Medetomidine (Me)^c/fentanyl (F)/midazolam (Mi)	(Me) 0.2 mg/kg + (F) 0.02 mg/kg + (Mi) 1 mg/kg IM[41]	Anesthesia; endotracheal intubation and supplemental oxygen are required
Medetomidine (Me)^c/propofol (P)	(Me) 0.35 mg/kg IM + (P) 3 mg/kg IV[41]	Surgical anesthesia; note high medetomidine dose[41]
Meloxicam	—	Nonsteroidal antiinflammatory; analgesia; antipyretic; used for osteoarthritis and postoperative pain; palatable PO form
	0.2 mg/kg SC, IM q24h[41]	
	0.2-0.5 mg/kg PO, SC, IM q24h[25]	
	0.3 mg/kg PO q24h × 10 days[23]	PK; a higher dose (≥0.5 mg/kg)[20] may be required, but efficacy and safety studies have not been performed[22]
	0.3 mg/kg PO q24h[41]	
	0.3-1.5 mg/kg PO q24h × 5 days[133]	PK; the higher dose was based on a limited sample size, but efficacy and safety studies have not been performed
	1 mg/kg PO q24h[46]	PK; dose required to achieve plasma levels associated with analgesia in other species; clinical efficacy was not evaluated

TABLE 10-4 Chemical Restraint/Sedative/Anesthetic/Analgesic Agents Used in Rabbits. (cont'd)

Agent	Dosage	Comments
Meloxicam (cont'd)	1 mg/kg PO q24h × 29 days[30]	PK; safety studies indicated may be safe for long-term use in rabbits
Midazolam	—	Benzodiazepine sedative; may reverse with flumazenil; more potent, shorter action than diazepam; water soluble; rapidly absorbed and less painful than diazepam when given IM; combinations to follow
	0.25-0.5 mg/kg IM[57]	When combined with an opioid
	0.5-2 mg/kg IM, IV, IP[25,41,57]	Preanesthetic; tranquilizer
	1-2 mg/kg IM, IV, IP[41]	Preanesthetic; tranquilizer
Midazolam (Mi)/buprenorphine (Bpr)	(Mi) 0.5 mg/kg + (Bpr) 0.01-0.05 mg/kg SC, IM[57]	Add ketamine (1-10 mg/kg) for additional sedation
Midazolam (Mi)/butorphanol (B)	(Mi) 0.5 mg/kg + (B) 0.2-0.4 mg/kg SC, IM[57]	Add ketamine (1-10 mg/kg) for additional sedation and analgesia
	(Mi) 0.5-1 mg/kg + (B) 0.25-0.5 mg/kg IM[90]	Add ketamine 5-10 mg/kg IM for additional sedation and analgesia
Midazolam (Mi)/oxymorphone (O)	(Mi) 0.5 mg/kg + (O) 0.05-0.2 mg/kg SC, IM[57]	Add ketamine (1-10 mg/kg) for additional sedation
Morphine	—	Analgesic; mu receptor agonist; decreases GI transit time[29]
	0.1 mg/kg[20,56]	Epidural anesthesia; dilute with preservative-free saline only; total volume should not exceed 0.33 mL/kg[56]
	0.5-2.0 mg/kg SC, IM q2-4h[20]	Analgesia
	2-5 mg/kg SC, IM q2-4h[25,41]	
	10 mg/kg IM[29]	Decreased GI transit time and affected stomach and cecum motility[29]
Naloxone	0.01-0.1 mg/kg IM, IV[25,41]	Narcotic reversal; note that analgesic effects are also reversed; avoid use following painful procedure as sudden awareness of pain may predispose to breath-holding, increased catecholamine release, and fatal arrhythmias;[41] mu opioid agonist
Oxymorphone	0.05-0.2 mg/kg SC, IM q8-12h[41]	Analgesia
	0.1-0.3 mg/kg SC, IM, IV q3-4h[10,112]	
Pentazocine (Talwin-V, Upjohn)	5-10 mg/kg IM, IV q2-4h[41]	Analgesia
Pentobarbital	20-45 mg/kg IV, IP[41]	Marginal analgesia; autonomic depression; not recommended

Continued

TABLE 10-4 Chemical Restraint/Sedative/Anesthetic/Analgesic Agents Used in Rabbits. (cont'd)

Agent	Dosage	Comments
Piroxicam	0.2 mg/kg PO q8h[41]	Analgesia; nonsteroidal antiinflammatory
Propofol	—	Intravenous nonbarbiturate anesthetic; slow IV; lower dose after pre-med, higher dose when used alone; see medetomidine for combination
	2-3 mg/kg IV[41]	Induction after premedication; maintain with approximately 1 mg/kg IV q15min
	3-6 mg/kg IV[41]	
	5-14 mg/kg slow IV (20 mg/kg/min)[41,112]	To effect
	6-8 mg/kg IV induction, followed by 0.8-1 mg/kg/min CRI[118]	Anesthetic induction and maintenance; premedicated with dexmedetomidine (20 µg/kg IM), ketamine (5 mg/kg IM), fentanyl (10 µg/kg IM)[118]
	7.5-15 mg/kg IV[26]	
	12.5 mg/kg IV, IO followed by 1 mg/kg/min CRI[93]	Anesthetic induction and maintenance
	16 ± 5 mg/kg IV[6]	Anesthetic induction
Sevoflurane	To effect[6]	Anesthesia; MAC = 3.7%[41]
	6%-8% induction, 1%-3% maintenance	Prior use of a sedative or injectable induction agent is recommended, as use of preanesthetic combinations will lower the MAC of inhalants
Thiamylal	15-25 mg/kg IV to effect[41]	
Thiopental	15-30 mg/kg IV to effect[41]	
Tiletamine/zolazepam (Telazol, Zoetis, Fort Dodge)	3 mg/kg IM[41]	Sedation prior to gas anesthetic; tiletamine causes severe renal tubular necrosis at 32 mg/kg and mild nephrosis at 7.5 mg/kg;[41] not generally recommended for use in rabbits
Tramadol	—	Pharmacokinetic data reported to be variable, data on clinical efficacy lacking[10]
	4.4 mg/kg IV[34]	Did not result in isoflurane-sparing effects[34]
	5 mg/kg SC, IV q8h[25]	
	5-15 mg/kg PO q8-12h[25]	
	10 mg/kg PO q12-24h[10]	Recommendation based on personal experience and anecdotal reports
	11 mg/kg PO[127]	PK; did not achieve adequate plasma concentrations for analgesia based on human levels

TABLE 10-4 Chemical Restraint/Sedative/Anesthetic/Analgesic Agents Used in Rabbits. (cont'd)

Agent	Dosage	Comments
Xylazine	—	See ketamine for combinations
	1-5 mg/kg SC, IM[41]	Preanesthetic; tranquilizer; lower end of dose range preferred; seldom indicated
Yohimbine	0.2-1 mg/kg IM, IV[41]	Alpha$_2$-adrenergic antagonist; xylazine reversal

[a]See Table 10-5 for Constant Rate Infusion (CRI) protocols.
[b]Drugs and doses chosen dependent on individual patient requirements and health status, procedure planned, and level of sedation desired. Combination of drugs mixed in one syringe unless otherwise indicated. Atipamezole may be used to reverse dexmedetomidine or medetomidine, flumazenil may be used to reverse midazolam, and naloxone may be used to reverse opioids.
[c]Medetomidine is no longer commercially available in the United States although it may be obtained from select compounding services.

TABLE 10-5 Constant Rate Infusion (CRI) Protocols Used in Rabbits.[a]

Agent(s)	Loading Dose IV	CRI Rate IV Per Hour Unless Noted
Butorphanol	0.2-0.4 mg/kg[56]	0.1-0.2 mg/kg[112]
		0.2-0.4 mg/kg[56]
Fentanyl	5-10 µg/kg[56]	10-30 µg/kg[56]
		30-100 µg/kg/min[41]
Ketamine	2-5 mg/kg[56]	0.3-1.2 mg/kg[56]
Ketamine (K)/ butorphanol (B)	(K) 0.4-0.5 mg/kg + (B) 0.02-0.06 mg/kg[81]	(K) 0.6 mg/kg (0.4-1) + (B) 0.1-0.2 mg/kg[81]
Ketamine (K)/ butorphanol (B)	(K) 0.4-0.5 mg/kg + (B) 0.02-0.06 mg/kg[82]	(K) 0.4-1 mg/kg + (B) 0.1-0.2 mg/kg[82]
Ketamine (K)/ fentanyl (F)	(K) 0.4-0.5 mg/kg + (F) 0.005 mg/kg[81]	(K) 0.6 mg/kg (0.4-1) + (F) 0.005-0.02 mg/kg[81]
Ketamine (K)/ hydromorphone (H)	(K) 0.4-0.5 mg/kg + (H) 0.05 mg/kg[81]	(K) 0.6 mg/kg (0.4-1) + (H) 0.025-0.05 mg/kg[81]
Ketamine (K)/ hydromorphone (H)	(K) 0.4-0.5 mg/kg + (H) 0.05 mg/kg[82]	(K) 0.4-1 mg/kg + (H) 0.025-0.05 mg/kg[82]
Lidocaine	2 mg/kg[124]	50 or 100 µg/kg/min;[124] both CRI doses decreased the isoflurane MAC[124]

[a]Surgical fluid rate is 10 mL/kg/h IV.[81]

TABLE 10-6 Ophthalmologic Agents Used in Rabbits.

Agent	Dosage	Comments
Amphotericin B (liposomal form) (A)/moxifloxacin (Mo)	(A) 10 µg in 0.05 mL + (Mo) 100 µg in 0.05 mL intravitreally[31]	(Mo) strongly augments efficacy of (A)
Atropine 1%	Topical to eyes q12h prn[41]	Mydriasis; systemic effects are possible; may be ineffective in rabbits with pigmented irides or those that produce atropinase[141]

Continued

TABLE 10-6 Ophthalmologic Agents Used in Rabbits. (cont'd)

Agent	Dosage	Comments
Atropine 1%/phenylephrine 10%	Topical to eyes[41]	Mydriasis for non-albino eyes
Azithromycin 1% (Azasite, Akorn)	Topical to eyes q12h × 2 days, then q24h × 5 days[5]	Bacterial conjunctivitis
Besifloxacin 0.6% (Besivance, Bausch & Lomb)	Topical to eyes q12h[113]	Fluoroquinolone; bacterial conjunctivitis/endophthalmitis;[102] minimal systemic absorption
Betaxolol 0.5% (Betoptic, Alcon)	Topical to eyes q12h[70]	Glaucoma; effectively decreases intraocular pressure in rabbits
Ciprofloxacin 0.3% (Ciloxan, Alcon)	Topical to eyes q8-12h[41] 2 drops topical q1h for 7-14 hr [41]	Susceptible infections Ocular penetration injuries; good penetration into aqueous and vitreous humor
Cyclosporine A 0.05% (Restasis, Allergan)	Topical to eyes q12h[131]	Dry eye due to autoimmune dacryoadenitis
Cyclosprine A 0.2% (Optimmune, Schering-Plough)	Topical to eyes q12h[132]	Shown to increase tear production in rabbits; may inhibit recurrence of precorneal membranous occlusion postoperatively[49]
Dichlorophenamide (Daranide, Merck)	1-2 mg/kg PO q24h[41]	Glaucoma
Diclofenac sodium 0.1%	Topical to eyes[137] Topical to eyes q12h[89]	Nonsteroidal antiinflammatory Blepharitis[141]
Dorzolamide 2% (Trusopt, Merck)	Topical to eyes q8-12h[41,89]	Glaucoma
Doxycycline monohydrate	2.5 mg/kg PO q12h[89]	*Encephalitozoon cuniculi*-induced glaucoma
Fluconazole	37.5 mg/kg PO q12h[8]	*Aspergillus* keratitis
Flurbiprofen sodium 0.03%	Topical to eyes[41]	Nonsteroidal antiinflammatory; blepharitis[141]
Fusidic acid (Fucithalmic, Leo)	Topical to eyes q12-24h[41]	Bacterial conjunctivitis
Gatifloxacin 0.3% (Zymar, Allergan)	Topical to eyes q8h[113]	Bacterial conjunctivitis
Gentamicin (Tiacil, Virbac)	Topical to eyes q8h[41]	Bacterial conjunctivitis
Ketorolac tromethamine 0.1%	Topical to eyes[137]	Nonsteroidal antiinflammatory; blepharitis[141]
Marbofloxacin (Marbocyl FD, Vetoquinol)	4 mg/kg IV[116]	Penetration of marbofloxacin into the aqueous and vitreous humor after IV administration was significantly enhanced by intraocular inflammation
Methylsulfonylmethane (MSM) ophthalmic 15% (Alcon)	Topical to eyes q12h[89]	*Encephalitozoon cuniculi*-induced glaucoma
Metipranolol 0.1%/pilocarpine 2%	Topical to eyes q8-12h[41]	Glaucoma

TABLE 10-6 Ophthalmologic Agents Used in Rabbits. (cont'd)

Agent	Dosage	Comments
Moxifloxacin 0.5% (Vigamox, Alcon)	Topical to eyes q6h[95,102]	Bacterial conjunctivitis; good aqueous concentration with both oral and ophthalmic administration; oral better for vitreous concentration[47]
Micafungin 0.1%	0.5 mL subconjunctivally q24h × 3 wk[59]	*Candida* keratitis
Neomycin/bacitracin/polymyxin B	Topical to eyes q6h[41]	Susceptible infections; corneal ulceration
Penicillin G	40,000 U/kg SC q7d × 3 treatments[49]	*Treponema cuniculi*-induced blepharitis
Phenylephrine 10%	—	See atropine for combination
	Topical to eyes[41]	Mydriasis
Prednisolone acetate 1%	Topical to eyes q6-12h[41]	Inflammation of eyes; rabbits are a corticosteroid-sensitive species; use with extreme caution
	Topical to eyes q12h[89]	*Encephalitozoon cuniculi*-induced glaucoma
Terbinafine 1% ointment	Topical q6h × 8 wk[13,112]	Keratomycosis; compounded
Timolol 0.5% (Timoptic, Merck)	Topical to eyes q12h[70]	Glaucoma
Tobramycin 0.3%	Topical to eyes q6h[13]	Bacterial ulcerative keratitis
Tropicamide 1%	Topical to eyes[41]	Mydriasis
Trovafloxacin 0.5%	Topical to eyes[9]	Broad-spectrum; safe for intravitreal injection up to 25 μg
Vancomycin 0.3%, 1%	Topical to eyes q2h for 10 hr each day × 5 days[35]	Commercially available product not available in the United States; compounded from injectable form of vancomycin; used to treat methicillin-resistant *Staphylococcus aureus*
Voriconazole	Topical to eyes q12h[128]	Fungal keratitis; compounded to a 1% voriconazole solution[112]

TABLE 10-7 Miscellaneous Agents Used in Rabbits.

Agent	Dosage	Comments
Activated charcoal (1 g/5 mL water)	1 g/kg PO q4-6h[63,103]	May reduce intestinal absorption of toxins
Aluminum hydroxide	30-60 mg/kg PO q8-12h[41]	Phosphorus-binder; hyperphosphatemia due to renal failure
Barium	10-14 mL/kg PO[41]	Gastrointestinal contrast studies
Benazepril	0.25-0.5 mg/kg PO q24h[41]	Vasodilator; potentially less nephrotoxic than enalapril
Blood transfusion (whole blood)	10-20 mL/kg given no faster than 22 mL/kg/h[41]	Cross-matching advised, especially for repeated transfusions

Continued

TABLE 10-7 Miscellaneous Agents Used in Rabbits. (cont'd)

Agent	Dosage	Comments
Calcium EDTA (edetate calcium disodium) (Calcium Disodium Versenate, 3 M)	13-27 mg/kg SC, IV[41] 27 mg/kg SC q6-12h prn[41]	Chelation therapy Lead toxicosis; diluted to <10 mg/mL with 0.45% NaCl/2.5% dextrose
Cellulose powder (Unifiber, Niche)	½-1 tsp/feeding[41]	Nonsoluble fiber source for rabbits on liquid enteral diets; will pass through small diameter feeding tubes
Chlorpheniramine maleate	0.2-0.4 mg/kg PO q12h[41]	Antihistamine
Cholestyramine (Questran Light, Squibb)	2 g/animal PO q24h × 18-21 days[41]	Ion exchange resin for toxin absorption following inappropriate antibiotic administration; use for treating enterotoxemia; gavage with 20 mL water; may result in constipation
Chondroitin sulfate (Cosequin, Nutramax)	Used empirically at feline dose[134]	Arthritis; nutraceutical
Cimetidine	5-10 mg/kg PO, SC, IM, IV q6-12h[65,112]	Gastric and duodenal ulcers
Cisapride	0.5 mg/kg PO q8-12h[112]	Enhances gastrointestinal motility; must be compounded in United States
Cyclizine	8 mg/rabbit PO q12h[41]	Vertigo associated with torticollis
Cyproheptadine	1-4 mg/rabbit PO q12-24h[51]	Possible appetite stimulant
Dexamethasone	—	Corticosteroids are seldom indicated in rabbits; rabbits are a corticosteroid-sensitive species;[41] use with extreme caution and consider concurrent administration of a gastroprotective agent
	0.2-0.6 mg/kg SC, IM, IV[41]	Antiinflammatory
	0.5-2 mg/kg PO, SC, then taper dose q12h × 3-14 days[41]	
	2 mg/kg IM, IV[41]	Shock; effectiveness is controversial
Digoxin	0.005-0.01 mg/kg PO q12-24h[41]	Congestive heart failure; atrial fibrillation
Diltiazem	0.5-1 mg/kg PO q12-24h[41]	Calcium channel blocker for hypertrophic cardiomyopathy
Diphenhydramine	2 mg/kg PO, SC q8-12h[41,112]	Torticollis, antihistamine
Doxapram	2-5 mg/kg SC, IV q15min[41]	Respiratory stimulant
Enalapril	0.1-0.5 mg/kg PO q24-48h[65]	Beware of hypotensive side effects
Epinephrine	0.2-0.4 mg/kg IM, IV, intratracheally[112]	Cardiac arrest
Epoetin alpha, recombinant (Epogen, Amgen)	50-150 U/kg SC q2-3d[112]	Biosynthetic form of erythropoietin; treatment of anemia; use until PCV is normal, then q7d for at least 4 wk
Famotidine	0.5-1 mg/kg PO, SC, IV q12-24h[40,112]	H_2-receptor antagonist used to reduce GI acid production
Fecal transfaunation	Mix fresh cecotrophs with warm saline, strain through gauze, and administer by gavage[41]	Dysbiosis; placement of E-collar on donor facilitates collection of sample
Ferrous sulfate	4-6 mg/kg PO q24h[41]	Iron deficiency anemia

TABLE 10-7 Miscellaneous Agents Used in Rabbits. (cont'd)

Agent	Dosage	Comments
Furosemide	—	Loop diuretic
	0.3-2 mg/kg SC, IM, IV[41] prn	
	1-4 mg/kg SC, IM, IV q4-6h[112]	Pulmonary edema
	2-5 mg/kg PO, SC, IM, IV q12h[112] prn	Congestive heart failure
Hetastarch (Hespan, DuPont)	5 mL/kg IV given over 5-10 min; repeat if necessary[41]	Volume expansion in hypoproteinemic patients; may be of benefit in endotoxemia
	20 mL/kg IV[101]	
Human chorionic gonadotropin (hCG)	20-25 U/animal IV[41]	Ovulation
Hydroxyzine	2 mg/kg PO q8-12h[41]	Antihistamine; antipruritic
Iron dextran	4-6 mg/kg IM once[41]	Iron deficiency anemia (treatment or prevention)
Lactated Ringer's solution or other appropriate fluid of choice	60-90 mL/kg × 1 hr[41]	Treatment for shock
	100-150 mL/kg/day CRI or divided SC q6-12h[41]	Maintenance fluid support
Lactobacilli	—	May aid in treatment of enteritis;[41] efficacy not determined
	Administer PO during antibiotic treatment period, then 5-7 days beyond cessation[41]	Give 2 hr before or 2 hr after antibiotic treatment
Levetiracetam (Keppra, UCB)	20 mg/kg PO q8h[11]	Anticonvulsant; dosage not established in rabbits, but PD are similar to those in dogs
Lidocaine	1-2 mg/kg IV (bolus)[41]	Cardiac arrhythmia
	2-4 mg/kg intratracheally[41]	Cardiac arrhythmia
Loperamide	0.1 mg/kg PO q8h × 3 days, then q24h × 2 days[112]	Enteropathies (nonspecific diarrhea); give in 1 mL water
Maropitant citrate (Cerenia, Zoetis)	2 mg/kg SC q24h × 3-5 days, then q48h or 3 × weekly if needed[24]	May be helpful in arthritis or inflammatory conditions; reduces visceral pain
Meclizine	2-12 mg/kg PO q24h[112]	Reduces disorientation and rolling with torticollis (for prevention of motion sickness in small animals)
	12.5-25 mg/kg PO q8-12h[41]	
Metoclopramide	0.2-0.5 mg/kg PO, SC q6-8 h[41]	Stimulates gastrointestinal motility
	0.2-1 mg/kg PO, IM, SC q6-24h[112]	
	0.5 mg/kg PO, SC q4-12 h[41]	
Mirtazapine	0.3-0.5 mg/kg PO q24h[114]	Appetite stimulant; dosage not established in rabbits; cat dose given here
Nandrolone (Deca-Durabolin, Organon)	2 mg/kg SC, IM[41]	Anabolic steroid; appetite stimulant; adjunct to treatment for anemia, especially in chronic renal failure

Continued

TABLE 10-7 Miscellaneous Agents Used in Rabbits. (cont'd)

Agent	Dosage	Comments
Omeprazole	20 mg/kg SC q12h[77]	Proton pump inhibitor used as a gastroprotective agent
Oxytocin	0.1-3 U/kg SC, IM[41]	Use in delayed, but unobstructed, parturition; agalactia
Pimobendan	0.1-0.3 mg/kg PO q12-24h[41]	Phosphodiesterase inhibitor; increases cardiac contractility with dilated cardiomyopathy or mitral valve disease
Polysulfated glycosaminoglycan (Adequan, Luitpold)	2.2 mg/kg SC, IM q3d × 21-28 days, then q14d[112]	Noninfectious, traumatic, or degenerative joint disease
Potassium citrate	33 mg/kg q8h[41]	Urinary calculi; may decrease calcium-based stone formation
Prednisolone	—	See dexamethasone; rarely indicated
	0.25-0.5 mg/kg PO q12h × 3 days, then q24h × 3 days, then q48h[41]	Treatment of nonresponsive torticollis, when negative for pasteurellosis; give antibiotics concurrently
	0.5-2 mg/kg PO q12h[112]	
Prednisone	—	See dexamethasone; rarely indicated
	0.5-2 mg/kg PO[41,112]	Antiinflammatory
Prochlorperazine	0.2-0.5 mg/kg PO q8h[41]	Torticollis; doses as high as 30 mg/kg q8h are used to treat labyrinthine disorders in humans
Ranitidine	2 mg/kg IV q24h[41] 2-5 mg/kg PO q12h[112]	Gastric ulceration (often in inappetant rabbits)
Sevelamer	Dosage not established in animals	Human dosage is 2-4 capsules PO q8h;[112] phosphorus binder for hyperphosphatemia associated with chronic renal failure; consider monitoring coagulation parameters, as vitamin K absorption may be affected; drug is not absorbed systemically so toxicity is unlikely
Silymarin (milk thistle)	4-15 mg/kg PO q8-12h[65] 20-50 mg/kg PO q24h[112]	Nutraceutical used as an adjunctive treatment for liver disease; hepatoprotectant; dosage not established for rabbits; suggested dose for small animals
Simethicone	65-130 mg/animal PO q1h × 2-3 treatments[41]	May reduce abdominal discomfort associated with excess gas
Sodium bicarbonate	2 mEq/kg IV, IP[41]	Ketoacidosis (pregnancy toxemia); dose is approximate
Stanozolol	0.5-2 mg PO once[112]	Stimulates appetite following surgery or illness; may be available from compounding pharmacy
Succimer (DMSA)	1050 mg/m^2 PO × 1 wk, then 700 mg/m^2 × 2 wk[142]	Lead toxicity
Sucralfate	25 mg/kg PO q8-12h[41]	Gastrointestinal ulcers; may interfere with other orally administered drugs

TABLE 10-7   Miscellaneous Agents Used in Rabbits. (cont'd)

Agent	Dosage	Comments
Sulfasalazine	⅛-¼ crushed 500 mg tablet/animal q8-24 h[41]	May reduce inflammation of intestinal mucosa
Verapamil	2.5-25 µg/kg/h IP[129]	Postoperative administration decreases adhesion formation
	8-16 mg/kg PO plus 0.5-2 mg/kg SC q24h[112]	Slow-channel calcium blocking agent
Vitamin A	500-1000 U/kg IM[41]	
Vitamin B complex	0.02-0.4 mL/rabbit SC, IM q24h[51]	Possible appetite stimulant; vitamin B deficiency
Vitamin C (ascorbic acid)	100 mg/kg PO q12h[112]	Nutritional supplement
Vitamin K	1-10 mg/kg IM prn[41]	Select bleeding disorders and toxicities

TABLE 10-8   Hematologic and Serum Biochemical Values of Rabbits.[41]

Measurement	Normal Values
Hematology	
PCV (%)	30-50
Hgb (g/dL)	8-17.5
RBC (10^6/µL)	4-8
MCV (fL)	58-75
MCH (pg)	17.5-23.5
MCHC (g/dL)	29-37
Reticulocytes (%)	2-4
Platelets (10^3/µL)	290-650
WBC (10^3/µL)	5-12
Heterophils (neutrophils) (%)	35-55
Lymphocytes (%)	25-60
Monocytes (%)	2-10
Eosinophils (%)	0-5
Basophils (%)	2-8
Chemistries	
ALP (U/L)	4-70
ALT (U/L)	14-80
Amylase (U/L)	200-500
AST (U/L)	14-113
Bicarbonate (mEq/L)	16.2-31.8
Bile acids (µmol/L)	<40
Bilirubin, total (mg/dL)	0-0.75

Continued

TABLE 10-8 Hematologic and Serum Biochemical Values of Rabbits. (cont'd)

Measurement	Normal Values
Calcium (mg/dL)	8-14.8
Chloride (mEq/L)	92-112
Cholesterol (mg/dL)	12-116
Creatinine (mg/dL)	0.5-2.6
Glucose (mg/dL)	75-150
LDH (U/L)	34-129
Lipids, total (mg/dL)	280-350
Phosphorus (mg/dL)	2.3-6.9
Potassium (mEq/L)	3.5-7
Protein, total (g/dL)	5.4-7.5
Albumin (g/dL)	2.5-5
Globulin (g/dL)	1.5-3.5
Sodium (mEq/L)	138-155
Triglycerides (mg/dL)	124-156
T_3 (ng/dL)	130-430
T_4 (μg/dL)	1.7-2.4
Urea nitrogen (mg/dL)	15-50
Vitamin A, plasma (μg/mL)	30-80
Vitamin E, plasma (μg/mL)	>1
Vitamin D_3 (pmol/L)	20-45 (free-range, outdoors)

TABLE 10-9 Rabbit Blood Glucose and Sodium Levels as Prognostic Indicators.[65]

Physiologic State	Blood Glucose (mg/dL)	Sodium (mEq/L)	Osmolarity[a] (mOsm/L)	Tonicity[a] (mOsm/L)
Normal	76-148	136-147	284-312	278-302
Stress (e.g., handling)	144-180	—	—	—
Severe disease (e.g., enterotoxemia, mucoid enteropathy, GI obstruction)	360-540	<129 carries a 2.3 times mortality risk	—	—
Diabetes mellitus	540-601	—	—	—

[a]Osmolarity and tonicity may be used to differentiate true hyponatremia from pseudohyponatremia (may occur with hyperlipidemia, severe liver disease, or congestive heart failure).

Calculated tonicity:

$\text{Ton (mOsm/L)} = 2 \times \text{Na (mEq/L)} + \text{glucose (mg/dL)}/18$

Calculated osmolarity:

$P_{osm} \text{ (mOsm/L)} = 2 \times \text{Na (mEq/L)} + \text{glucose (mg/dL)}/18 + \text{BUN (mg/dL)}/2.8$

TABLE 10-10 Biologic and Physiologic Data of Rabbits.[41]

Parameter	Normal Values
Adult body weight, male (buck)	1.5-5 kg
Adult body weight, female (doe)	1.5-6 kg
Birth weight	30-80 g
Respiratory rate	30-60 breaths/min
Tidal volume	4-6 mL/kg
Heart rate	130-325 beats/min
Rectal temperature	38.5-40°C (101.3-104°F)
Life span	5-6 years (up to 15 years)
Food consumption	50 g/kg/day
Water consumption	100 mL/kg/day
Gastrointestinal transit time	4-5 hours
Breeding onset, male	6-10 months
Breeding onset, female	4-9 months
Breeding life of female	4 months to 3.75 years
Reproductive cycle	Induced ovulation
Gestation period	29-35 days
Litter size	4-10
Weaning age	4-6 weeks
Dental formula	I2/1 C0/0 P3/2 M3/3

TABLE 10-11 Urinalysis Values in Rabbits.[41]

Measurement	Normal Values
Urine volume	
Large breeds	20-350 mL/kg/day
Average breeds	130 mL/kg/day
Specific gravity	1.003-1.051
pH	7.7-9.6
Crystals	Ammonium magnesium phosphate, calcium carbonate monohydrate, anhydrous calcium carbonate
Casts, epithelial cells, or bacteria	Absent to rare
Leukocytes or erythrocytes	Occasional
Albumin	Occasional in young rabbits
Protein:creatinine ratio	0.11-0.47
Protein (g/L, reference assay)	0.57-10.66
Protein (Multistix dipsticks)	Negative to +++

TABLE 10-12 Cerebrospinal Fluid Values in Rabbits.[41]

Measurement	Normal Values
Leukocyte count	≤4 cells/μL (1-97 cells/μL in *E. cuniculi* positive rabbits)
Alkaline phosphatase	5 U/dL
Calcium	5.4 mEq/L
Carbon dioxide	41.2-48.5 mL%
Chloride	127 mEq/L
Cholesterol	33 mg/dL
Creatinine	17 mg/dL
Glucose	75 mg/dL
Lactic acid	1.4-4 mg/dL
Magnesium	2.2 mEq/L
Nitrogen, nonprotein	5.6-16.8 mg/dL
Phosphate	2.3 mEq/L
Potassium	3 mEq/L
Protein, total	13-59 mg/dL (31-154 mg/dL in *E. cuniculi* positive rabbits)
Sodium	149 mEq/L
Urea nitrogen	20 mg/dL

TABLE 10-13 Electrocardiographic (ECG) and Echocardiographic Values in Rabbits.[41]

ECG Parameter	Normal Values
Heart rate	198-330 beats/min[a]
Measurements (lead II)	
P wave	
Duration (width)	0.01-0.05 sec
Amplitude (height)	0.04-0.12 mv
P-R interval	
Duration	0.04-0.08 sec
QRS complex	
Duration	0.02-0.06 sec
R-wave amplitude	0.03-0.039 mv
Q-T interval	
Duration	0.08-0.16 sec
T wave	
Amplitude	0.05-0.17 mv
Electrical axis (frontal plane)	−43 to +80 degrees
Thickness of interventricular septum in diastole	0.143-0.310 cm
Thickness of interventricular septum in systole	0.217-0.403 cm
Left ventricular internal diameter in diastole	1.187-1.906 cm

TABLE 10-13 Electrocardiographic (ECG) and Echocardiographic Values in Rabbits. (cont'd)

ECG Parameter	Normal Values
Left ventricular internal diameter in systole	0.783-1.353 cm
Thickness of left ventricular free wall in diastole	0.16-0.28 cm
Thickness of left ventricular free wall in systole	0.243-0.455 cm
Fractional shortening	22.6%-36.83%
Ejection fraction	49.07%-70%
Aortic diameter	0.673-0.980 cm
Left atrial appendage diameter	0.753-1.200 cm
Left atrial appendage diameter:aortic diameter	0.94-1.54
Mitral valve E-point–to–septal separation interval	0.120-0.233 cm
Doppler heart rate	115-234 beats/min
Maximal aortic outflow velocity	0.56-1.06 m/sec
Maximal pulmonary artery outflow velocity	0.34-0.84 m/sec
Maximal mitral E-wave velocity	0.41-0.83 m/sec
Maximal mitral A-wave velocity	0.19-0.44 m/sec
Maximal mitral E-wave velocity:A-wave velocity	1.34-3.55

[a]Lower values may be expected in acclimated rabbits.

TABLE 10-14 Determining the Sex of Mature Rabbits.[41]

Male	Female
• Protrude penis by manipulating skin of prepuce • Palpate for testicles • Anogenital distance is longer	• There is a common orifice for both the vagina and urethra (like dogs and cats) • No structure like a "penis" can be protruded from the urogenital orifice • Anogenital distance is shorter

TABLE 10-15 Drugs Reported to Be Toxic in Rabbits.[a]

Drug	Comments
Amoxicillin[41]	Enteritis; enterotoxemia
Amoxicillin/clavulanic acid[41]	Enteritis; enterotoxemia
Ampicillin[41]	Enteritis; enterotoxemia, high risk especially if given orally
Benzimidazoles (fenbendazole, oxibendazole, albendazole)[52]	Bone marrow suppression reported; recommend intratreatment CBC to r/o anemia, leukopenia, thrombocytopenia
Cephalosporins[41]	Enteritis; enterotoxemia if given orally
Clindamycin[41]	Enteritis; enterotoxemia, high risk
Erythromycin[41]	Enteritis; enterotoxemia
Fipronil[41]	Can cause neurologic disease and death

Continued

TABLE 10-15 Drugs Reported to Be Toxic in Rabbits. (cont'd)

Drug	Comments
Lincomycin[41]	Enteritis; enterotoxemia, high risk
Penicillin[112]	Enteritis; enterotoxemia if given orally
Procaine[41]	May be fatal at doses of 0.4 mg/kg
Tiletamine[41]	Nephrotoxic

[a]There have also been some reports of antibiotic-related colitis in rabbits given penicillin/streptomycin, trimethoprim/sulfamethoxazole, tetracycline, and gentamicin.

TABLE 10-16 Treatments Used in the Management of Rabbit Gastrointestinal Syndrome (RGIS).[a]

Agent	Dosage	Comments
Buprenorphine	0.01-0.05 mg/kg SC, IV, IP q6-12h[41]	Analgesia
Butorphanol	0.1-0.5 mg/kg SC, IM, IV q4h[41]	Analgesia
Cisapride	0.5 mg/kg PO q8-12h[112]	Enhances gastrointestinal motility; compounded in United States
Cyproheptadine HCl	1-4 mg/rabbit PO q12-24h[51]	Possible appetite stimulant
Enrofloxacin	5 mg/kg PO, SC, IM, IV q12h[15,16,41]	Suspected primary bacterial enteritis (rare in rabbits)
Famotidine	0.5-1 mg/kg PO, SC, IV q12-24h[40,111]	H2-receptor antagonist used to reduce GI acid production
Fluid therapy	Weight (kg) × % dehydration × 1000 mL = fluid deficit divided into SC boluses or divided IV per hr over 12-24 hr[51]	Add deficit to maintenance requirement of 3-4 mL/kg/h
	60-90 mL/kg × 1 hr	Shock therapy
	100-150 mL/kg/day constant rate infusion or divided SC q6-12h	Maintenance fluid support
Herbivore critical care diet	Follow manufacturer's instructions	Syringe feeding; use fine grind for nasogastric tubes
Hydromorphone	0.05-0.2 mg/kg SC, IM, IV q6-8h[20]	Analgesia
Lidocaine	2 mg/kg IV loading dose given over 5 minutes followed by 60-100 μg/kg/min[124]	CRI for severe, refractory cases of RGIS
	100 μg/kg/min × 2 days[125]	Better surgical and postoperative outcome than buprenorphine
Maropitant citrate (Cerenia, Zoetis)	2 mg/kg SC q24h × 3-5 days; then q48h or 3 × weekly if needed[24]	May be helpful in inflammatory conditions; reduces visceral pain
Meloxicam	0.3-1 mg/kg PO q24h[23,133]	NSAID; use only if well hydrated with normal renal parameters
Metoclopramide	0.2-0.5 mg/kg PO, SC q6-8h[41]	Stimulates gastrointestinal motility
	0.01-0.09 mg/kg/h IV[112]	CRI
Metronidazole	20 mg/kg PO q12h for 3-5 days[112]	For suspected clostridial overgrowth and enterotoxemia
	5 mg/kg slow IV q12h[112]	

TABLE 10-16 Treatments Used in the Management of Rabbit Gastrointestinal Syndrome (RGIS). (cont'd)

Agent	Dosage	Comments
Midazolam	0.25-0.5 mg/kg IM, IV[57]	Antianxiety; may also stimulate appetite
Ranitidine	2 mg/kg IV q24h[41] 2-5 mg/kg PO q12h[112]	Gastric ulceration (often in inappetant rabbits)
Simethicone	65-130 mg/animal PO q1h × 2-3 treatments[41]	May reduce abdominal discomfort associated with excess gas
Thermal support	Provide thermal support if body temperature <99°F[51]	Avoid overheating
Trimebutine	1.5 mg/kg PO, IV[86]	Enhance GI motility; not available in the United States; oral available in Canada
Vitamin B Complex	0.02-0.4 mL/rabbit SC, IM q24h[51]	Possible appetite stimulant

[a]Concurrent to treatment, it is important to correct the cause (e.g., boredom, stress, excessive shedding, inadequate dietary roughage, nutritional deficiency or imbalance, disease, toxin, obesity). Surgical intervention is no longer considered the primary treatment option and is rarely indicated except in cases of complete obstruction.

TABLE 10-17 Bronchoalveolar Lavage (BAL) in Rabbits.[a,41]

BAL Parameter	Results and Comments
Volume	40%-76% recovery = 1.2-2.3 mL
Leukocyte count	200-700 cells/µL, predominantly macrophages
Heterophils	0-28 cells/µL (0%-5%)
Lymphocytes	15-98 cells/µL (4%-30%)
Macrophages	180-602 cells/µL (69%-94%)
Eosinophils	0-60 cells/µL (0%-12%)

[a]Bronchoscopic bronchoalveolar lavage in New Zealand white rabbits was performed with 3 mL of sterile saline into both left bronchus and right bronchus.

TABLE 10-18 Clinical Signs and Behavioral Changes Used in the Assessment of Pain in Rabbits.[a]

Clinical Signs	Behavioral Changes
Change of body posture; tensing of abdominal muscles, pressing abdomen onto ground	Decreased grooming activity; piloerection; unkempt and ruffled fur coat
Change of body posture; tucking of abdomen, hunched body; abdominal splinting on palpation	Decreased interest in food or cessation of food intake
Eyelids squinted; lack of focus; orbit may be retracted or bulging	Decreased frequency and duration of exploring/searching
Muzzle and nares contracture; increased intensity associated with level of pain	Decreased frequency and duration of movement or response to stimuli
Increased teeth grinding (bruxism)	Decreased conspecific interaction
Ears pinned back, held close to head	Irritable or aggressive temperament

Continued

TABLE 10-18 Clinical Signs and Behavioral Changes Used in the Assessment of Pain in Rabbits. (cont'd)

Clinical Signs	Behavioral Changes
Increased heart rate; increased frequency and depth of respirations	Stiff gait, lameness, staggering; difficulty finding comfortable resting position
Decreased body weight over time	Decreased fecal output or decreased size of fecal pellets

[a]Modified from Fisher (2010).[42]

TABLE 10-19 Percentage of Antibiotic Susceptibility Results for the Most Common Bacteria Isolated From Nasal Cultures of 121 Rabbits With Signs of Upper Respiratory Disease.[120]

	Bacteria[a]			
	Pateurella multocida (N=106)	Bordetella bronchiseptica (N=99)	Pseudomonas spp. (N=41)	Staphylococcus spp. (N=27)
Antibiotic	S I R	S I R	S I R	S I R
Cephalexin	100 0 0	2.0 0 98.0	2.4 2.4 95.2	88.9 0 11.1
Danofloxacin	100 0 0	43.4 40.4 16.2	65.9 22.0 12.1	77.8 18.5 3.7
Doxycycline	97.2 2.8 0	88.9 2.0 9.1	56.1 7.3 36.6	74.1 3.7 22.2
Enrofloxacin	100 0 0	71.7 15.2 13.1	58.5 22.0 19.5	81.5 14.8 3.7
Gentamicin	99.1 0.9 0	96 1.0 3.0	75.6 4.9 19.5	85.2 0 14.8
Marbofloxacin	100 0 0	88.9 6.1 5.0	87.8 4.9 7.3	96.3 0 3.7
Oxytetracycline	97.2 0 2.8	86.9 2.0 11.1	63.4 9.8 26.8	74.1 0 25.9
Trimethoprim-sulfamethoxazole	93.4 5.7 0.9	81.8 1.0 17.2	24.4 19.5 56.1	92.6 3.7 3.7

[a]S, sensitivity; I, intermediate; R, resistant.

TABLE 10-20 Sensitivity and Specificity Calculators for IgM and IgG Titers and CRP Levels Relative to the Diagnosis of Suspected Encephalitozoon cuniculi Infections in Pet Rabbits.[a,27]

IgM ≥ 1:64	IgG ≥ 1:512	CRP > 38 mg/L	Sensitivity (%)	Specificity (%)	Positive Predictive Value (%)	Negative Predictive Value (%)
+	ND	ND	69	75	88	48
ND	+	ND	62	78	88	44
ND	ND	+	40	89	90	38
+	+	ND	58	89	92	41
+	ND	+	27	100	100	34
ND	+	+	22	97	95	32
+	+	+	20	100	100	32

[a]CRP, C-Reactive Protein; ND, results of analyte not included in analysis.

REFERENCES

1. Abd El-Aty AM, Goudah A, Abo El-Sooud K. Pharmacokinetics, intramuscular bioavailability and tissue residue profiles of ceftazidime in a rabbit model. *Dtsch Tierarztl Wochenschr* 2001;108:168-171.
2. Abd El-Aty AM, Goudah A, Abo El-Sooud K, et al. Pharmacokinetics and bioavailability of florfenicol following intravenous, intramuscular, and oral administration in rabbits. *Vet Res Commun* 2004;28:515-524.
3. Abd El-Aty AM, Goudah A, Ismail M, et al. Disposition kinetics of difloxacin in rabbits after intravenous and intramuscular injection of Dicural. *Vet Res Commun* 2005;29:297-304.
4. Abo-El-Sooud K, Goudah A. Influence of *Pasteurella multocida* infection on the pharmacokinetic behavior of marbofloxacin after intravenous and intramuscular administrations in rabbits. *J Vet Pharmacol Ther* 2009;33:63-68.
5. Akpek EK, Vittitow J, Verhoeven RS, et al. Ocular surface distribution and pharmacokinetics of a novel ophthalmic 1% azithromycin formulation. *J Ocul Pharmacol Ther* 2009;25:433-440.
6. Allweiler S, Leach MC, Flecknell PA. The use of propofol and sevoflurane for surgical anaesthesia in New Zealand white rabbits. *Lab Anim* 2010;44:113-117.
7. Audeval-Gerard C, Nivet C, el Amrani A, et al. Pharmacokinetics of ketoprofen in rabbits after single topical application. *Eur J Drug Metab Pharmacokinet* 2000;25:227-230.
8. Avunduk AM, Beuerman RW, Warnel ED, et al. Comparison of efficacy of topical and oral fluconazole treatment in experimental *Aspergillus* keratitis. *Curr Eye Res* 2003;26:113-117.
9. Barequet IS, Denton P, Osterhout GJ, et al. Treatment of experimental bacterial keratitis with topical trovafloxacin. *Arch ophthalmol* 2004;122:65-69.
10. Barter LS. Rabbit analgesia. *Vet Clin North Am Exot Anim Pract* 2011;14:93-104.
11. Benedetti M, Coupez R, Whomsley R, et al. Comparative pharmacokinetics and metabolism of levetiracetam, a new anti-epileptic agent, in mouse, rat, rabbit, and dog. *Xenobiotic* 2004;34:281-300.
12. Birke L, Molina P, Baker D, et al. Comparison of selamectin and imidacloprid plus permethrin in eliminating *Leporacarus gibbus* infestation in laboratory rabbits. *J Am Assoc Lab Anim Sci* 2009;48:757-762.
13. Bourguet A, Guyonnet A, Donzel E, et al. Keratomycosis in a pet rabbit (*Oryctolagus cuniculus*) treated with topical 1% terbinafine ointment. *Vet Ophthalmol* 2015;6:1-6.
14. Brandao J, Woods S, Fowlkes N, et al. Disseminated histoplasmosis (*Histoplasma capsulatum*) in a pet rabbit: case report and review of the literature. *J Vet Diagn Invest* 2014;26:158-162.
15. Broome RL, Brooks DL, Babish JG, et al. Pharmacokinetic properties of enrofloxacin in rabbits. *Am J Vet Res* 1991;52:1835-1841.
16. Cabanes A, Arboix M, Anton JMG, et al. Pharmacokinetics of enrofloxacin after intravenous and intramuscular injection in rabbits. *Am J Vet Res* 1992;53:2090-2093.
17. Cam Y, Atasever A, Eraslan G, et al. Experimental infection in rabbits and the effect of treatment with toltrazuril and ivermectin. *Exper Parasitol* 2008;119:164-172.
18. Capilla J, Yustes C, Mayayo E, et al. Efficacy of albaconazole (UR-9825) in treatment of disseminated *Scedosporium prolificans* infection in rabbits. *Antimicrob Agents Chemother* 2003;47:1948-1951.
19. Carceles CM, Fernandez-Varon E, Marin P, et al. Tissue disposition of azithromycin after intravenous and intramuscular administration to rabbits. *Vet J* 2007;174:154-159.
20. Carpenter JW, Hawkins MG. *Personal communication*; 2016.
21. Carpenter JW, Dryden M, KuKanich B. Pharmacokinetics, efficacy, and adverse effects of selamectin following topical administration in flea-infested rabbits. *Am J Vet Res* 2012;73:562-566.
22. Carpenter JW, Pollock CG, Koch DE, et al. Single- and multiple-dose pharmacokinetics of marbofloxacin after oral administration to rabbits. *Am J Vet Res* 2009;70:522-526.
23. Carpenter JW, Pollock CG, Koch DE, et al. Single- and multiple-dose pharmacokinetics of meloxicam after oral administration to the rabbit (*Oryctolagus cuniculus*). *J Zoo Wildl Med* 2009;40:601-606.

24. Chen S. *Personal communication;* 2016.
25. Chitty J. Formulary. In: Harcourt-Brown F, Chitty J, eds. *BSAVA Manual of Rabbit Surgery, Dentistry and Imaging.* Gloucestershire: BSAVA Press; 2013:430-431.
26. Cocksholt ID, Douglas EJ, Plummer GF, et al. The pharmacokinetics of propofol in laboratory animals. *Xenobiotica* 1992;22:369-375.
27. Cray C, McKenny S, Perritt E, et al. Utility of IgM titers with IgG and C-reactive protein quantitation in the diagnosis of suspected *Encephalitozoon cuniculi* infection in rabbits. *J Exot Pet Med* 2015;24:356-360.
28. Croisier-Bertin D, Piroth L, Charles PE, et al. Ceftaroline versus ceftriaxone in a highly penicillin-resistant pneumococcal pneumonia rabbit model using simulated human dosing. *Antimicrob Agents Chemother* 2011;55:3557-3563.
29. Deflers H, Bolen G, Gandar F, et al. Proc Assoc Exot Mam Vet Conf: Influence of morphine on the rabbit gastrointestinal tract; 2014.
30. Delk KW, Carpenter JW, Kukanich B, et al. Pharmacokinetics of meloxicam administered orally to rabbits (*Oryctolagus cuniculis*) for 29 days. *Am J Vet Res* 2014;75:195-199.
31. Deren YT, Ozdek S, Kalkanci A, et al. Comparison of antifungal efficacies of moxifloxacin, liposomal amphotericin B, and combination treatment in experimental *Candida albicans* endophthalmitis in rabbits. *Can J Microbiol* 2010;56:1-7.
32. DiVencenti L, Meirelles LAD, Westcott RA. Safety and clinical effectiveness of a compounded sustained-release formulation of buprenorphine for postoperative analgesia in New Zealand white rabbits. *J Am Vet Med Assoc* 2016;248:795-801.
33. Dundaroz R, DeGim T, Sizlan A, et al. Intracavernous application of diazepam: an alternative route of the seizure treatment—an experimental study in rabbits. *Pediatr Int* 2002;44:163-167.
34. Egger CM, Souza MJ, Greenacre CB, et al. Effect of intravenous administration of tramadol hydrochloride on the minimum alveolar concentration of isoflurane in rabbits. *Am J Vet Res* 2009;70:945-949.
35. Eguchi H, Shiota H, Oguro S, et al. The inhibitory effect of vancomycin ointment on the manifestation of MRSA keratitis in rabbits. *J Infect Chemother* 2009;15:279-283.
36. Elmas M, Uney K, Yazar E, et al. Pharmacokinetics of enrofloxacin following intravenous and intramuscular administration in Angora rabbits. *Res Vet Sci* 2007;82:242-245.
37. Farmaki R, Koutinas AF, Papazahariadou MG, et al. Effectiveness of a selamectin spot-on formulation in rabbits with sarcoptic mange. *Vet Rec* 2009;164:431-432.
38. Fehr M. Zoonotic potential of dermatophytosis in small mammals. *J Exot Pet Med* 2015;24:308-316.
39. Fernandez-Varon E, Bovaira MJ, Espuny A, et al. Pharmacokinetic-pharmacodynamic integration of moxifloxacin in rabbits after intravenous, intramuscular and oral administration. *J Vet Pharmacol Ther* 2005;28:343-348.
40. Fiorello CV. *Personal communication;* 2011.
41. Fiorello CV, Divers SJ. Rabbits. In: Carpenter JW, ed. *Exotic Animal Formulary.* 4th ed. St. Louis: Elsevier; 2013:518-559.
42. Fisher P. Standards of care in the 21st century: the rabbit. *J Exot Pet Med* 2010;19:22-35.
43. Flecknell P. Anaesthesia and perioperative care. In: Meridith A, Flecknell P, eds. *BSAVA Manual of Rabbit Medicine and Surgery.* 2nd ed. Gloucestershire: BSAVA Press; 2006:154-165.
44. Flecknell P. Analgesia and perioperative care. *Proc World Vet Conf* 2008; accessed via Veterinary Information Network.
45. Foley P, Henderson A, Bissonette E, et al. Evaluation of fentanyl transdermal patches in rabbits: blood concentrations and physiologic response. *Comp Med* 2001;51:239-244.
46. Fredholm DV, Carpenter JW, KuKanich B, et al. Pharmacokinetics of meloxicam in rabbits after oral administration of single and multiple doses. *Am J Vet Res* 2013;74:636-641.
47. Fukuda M, Shibata N, Osada H, et al. Vitreous and aqueous penetration of orally and topically administered moxifloxacin. *Ophthalmic Res* 2011;46:113-117.
48. Gallina G, Lucatello L, Drigo I, et al. Kinetics and intrapulmonary disposition of tilmicosin after single and repeated oral bolus administrations to rabbits. *Vet Res Commun* 2010;34:S69-S72.

49. Gelatt KN. Exotic animal ophthalmology. In: Gelatt KN, ed. *Essentials of Veterinary Ophthalmology*. Oxford: Blackwell; 2005:413-438.
50. Gokbulut C, Biligili A, Kart A, et al. Plasma dispositions of ivermectin, doramectin and moxidectin following subcutaneous administration in rabbits. *Lab Anim* 2010;44:138-142.
51. Graham JE. *Personal observation*; 2016.
52. Graham JE, Garner MM, Reavill DR. Benzimidazole toxicosis in rabbits: 13 cases (2003-2011). *J Exot Pet Med* 2014;23:188-195.
53. Green LC, Callegan MC, Engel LS, et al. Pharmacokinetics of topically applied ciprofloxacin in rabbit tears. *Jpn J Ophthalmol* 1996;40:123-126.
54. Grint NJ, Murison PJ. A comparison of ketamine-midazolam and ketamine-medetomidine combinations for induction of anaesthesia in rabbits. *Vet Anaesth Analg* 2008;35:113-121.
55. Grint NJ, Smith HE, Senior JM. Clinical evaluation of alfaxalone in cyclodextrin for the induction of anaesthesia in rabbits. *Vet Rec* 2008;163:395-396.
56. Hawkins MG. Advances in exotic mammal clinical therapeutics. *J Exot Pet Med* 2014;23:39-49.
57. Hernandez-Divers SJ, Lennox AM. Sedation and anesthesia in exotic companion mammals. *Proc Annu Conf Assoc of Avian Vet* 2009;287-298.
58. Hess L, Tater K. Rabbits: dermatologic diseases. In: Quesenberry KE, Carpenter JW, eds. *Ferrets, Rabbits and Rodents: Clinical Medicine and Surgery*. 3rd ed. St. Louis: Saunders/Elsevier; 2012:232-244.
59. Hiraoka T, Kaji Y, Wakabayashi T, et al. Comparison of micafungin and fluconazole for experimental *Candida* keratitis in rabbits. *Cornea* 2007;26:336-342.
60. Hu L, Liu C, Shang C, et al. Pharmacokinetics and improved bioavailability of toltrazuril after oral administration to rabbits. *J Vet Pharmacol Ther* 2010;33:503-506.
61. Hutchinson MJ, Jacobs DE, Bell GD, et al. Evaluation of imidacloprid for the treatment and prevention of cat flea (*Ctenocephalides felis felis*) infestations on rabbits. *Vet Rec* 2001;148:695-696.
62. Huynh M, Poumeyrol S, Pignon C, et al. Intramuscular administration of alfaxalone for sedation in rabbits. *Vet Rec* 2015;176:255-260.
63. Idid S, Lee C. Effects of Fuller's Earth and activated charcoal on oral absorption of paraquat in rabbits. *Clin Exp Pharmacol Physiol* 1996;23:679-681.
64. Jekl V, Hauptman A, Minarikova A, et al. Pharmacokinetic study of benzylpenicillin potassium after intramuscular administration in rabbits. *Vet Rec* 2016;179:18 Epub May 2016.
65. Jepson L. Rabbits. In: Jepson L, ed. *Exotic Animal Medicine, A Quick Reference Guide*. 2nd ed. St. Louis: Elsevier; 2016:42-87.
66. Johnston MS. Clinical approaches to analgesia in ferrets and rabbits. *J Exot Pet Med* 2005;14:229-235.
67. Kaiser-Klingler S. Exotic animal anesthesia for the small animal practice. *Proc West Vet Conf* 2009; accessed via Veterinary Information Network.
68. Kanbur M, Atalay O, Ica A, et al. The curative and antioxidative efficiency of doramectin and doramectin + vitamin AD_3E treatment on *Psoroptes cuniculi* infestation in rabbits. *Res Vet Sci* 2008;85:291-293.
69. Kaya D, Inceboz T, Kolatan E, et al. Comparison of efficacy of ivermectin and doramectin against mange mite (*Sarcoptes scabiei*) in naturally infested rabbits in Turkey. *Vet Ital* 2010;46:51-56.
70. Kiel JW, Patel P. Effects of timolol and betaxolol on choroidal blood flow in the rabbit. *Exp Eye Res* 1998;67:501-507.
71. Kim MS, Lim JH, Hwang YH, et al. Plasma disposition of toltrazuril and its metabolites, toltrazuril sulfoxide and toltrazuril sulfone, in rabbits after oral administration. *Vet Parasitol* 2010;169:51-56.
72. Kim SH, Lee JY, Jun HK, et al. Efficacy of selamectin in the treatment of cheyletiellosis in pet rabbits. *Vet Dermatol* 2008;19:26-27.

73. Kirkpatrick WR, Vallor AC, McAtee RK, et al. Combination therapy with terbinafine and amphotericin B in a rabbit model of experimental invasive aspergillosis. *Antimicrob Agents Chemother* 2005;49:4751-4753.
74. Koc F, Ozturk M, Kadioglu Y, et al. Pharmacokinetics of florfenicol after intravenous and intramuscular administration in New Zealand white rabbits. *Res Vet Sci* 2009;87:102-105.
75. Kozer E, Levicheck Z, Hoshino N, et al. The effect of amitriptyline, gabapentin, and carbamazepine on morphine-induced hypercarbia in rabbits. *Anesth Analg* 2008;107:1216-1222.
76. Kurtdede A, Karaer Z, Acar A, et al. Use of selamectin for the treatment of psoroptic and sarcoptic mite infestation in rabbits. *Vet Dermatol* 2007;18:18-22.
77. Lee M, Kallal S, Feldman M. Omeprazole prevents indomethacin-induced gastric ulcers in rabbits. *Aliment Pharmacol Ther* 1996;10:571-576.
78. Lennox AM. Clinical technique: small exotic companion mammal dentistry-anesthetic considerations. *J Exot Pet Med* 2008;17:102-106.
79. Lennox AM. Protocols and tips for anesthesia and analgesia for rabbit and rodent dentistry and orofacial surgery. *Proc Assoc Exot Mam Vet Con* 2012;77-78.
80. Lennox AM. Sedation and local anesthesia as an alternative to general anaesthesia in exotic companion mammals. *Proc Brit Small Anim Vet Cong* 2013.
81. Lennox AM. Sedation, anesthesia and analgesia in the critical exotic surgery patient. *Proc Internat Vet Emer Crit Care Symp* 2013.
82. Lennox AM. The use of constant rate infusion analgesia in exotic companion mammals. *Proc Assoc Exot Mam Vet Conf* 2013.
83. Lennox AM. Anesthesia and analgesia for dentistry of rabbits and rodents. *Proc Am Board Vet Pract Conf* 2014.
84. Lennox AM. Anesthesia and analgesia for critical exotic companion mammals. *Proc Internat Vet Emer Crit Care Symp* 2015.
85. Lennox AM. Introducing alfaxalone into exotic companion mammal practice. *Proc Assoc Exot Med Vet Conf* 2015;321-323.
86. Lennox AM. *Personal communication*; 2016.
87. Louie A, Liu QF, Drusano GL, et al. Pharmacokinetic studies of fluconazole in rabbits characterizing doses which achieve peak levels in serum and area under the concentration-time curve values which mimic those of high-dose fluconazole in humans. *Antimicrob Agents Chemother* 1998;42:1512-1514.
88. Maciejewska-Paszek I, Pawlowska-Góral K, Kostrzewski M, et al. The influence of small doses of paracetamol on rabbit liver. *Exp Toxicol Pathol* 2007;59:139-141.
89. Maguire R, Gallinato MJ. Novel treatment of *Encephalitozoon cuniculi*-induced glaucoma in a rabbit. *Proc Assoc Exot Mam Vet Conf* 2011;125.
90. Mans C. *Personal communication*; 2016.
91. Marangos MN, Zhu Z, Nicolau DP, et al. Disposition of ofloxacin in female New Zealand white rabbits. *J Vet Pharmacol Ther* 1997;20:17-20.
92. Marín P, Álamo LF, Escudero E, et al. Pharmacokinetics of marbofloxacin in rabbit after intravenous, intramuscular, and subcutaneous administration. *Res Vet Sci* 2013;94:698-700.
93. Mazaheri-Khameneh R, Sarrafzadeh-Rezaei F, Asri-Rezaei S, et al. Comparison of time to loss of consciousness and maintenance of anesthesia following intraosseous and intravenous administration of propofol in rabbits. *J Am Vet Med Assoc* 2012;241:73-80.
94. McElroy DE, Ravis WR, Clark CH. Pharmacokinetics of oxytetracycline hydrochloride in rabbits. *Am J Vet Res* 1987;48:1261-1263.
95. McGee DH, Holt WF, Kastner PR, et al. Safety of moxifloxacin as shown in animal and in vitro studies. *Surv Ophthalmol* 2005;50:S46-S54.
96. McTier TL, Hair JA, Walstrom DJ, et al. Efficacy and safety of topical administration of selamectin for treatment of ear mite infestation in rabbits. *J Am Vet Med Assoc* 2003;223:322-324.
97. Mercier P, Morel-Saives A, Verdelhan S, et al. Tolerance of decoquinate in the rabbit. *Proc 8th World Rabbit Congr* 2004; 597-600.

98. Miller JL, Schell WA, Wills EA, et al. In vitro and in vivo efficacies of the new triazole albaconazole against *Cryptococcus neoformans*. *Antimicrob Agents Chemother* 2004;48:384-387.
99. Nelson CL, McLaren SG, Skinner RA, et al. The treatment of experimental osteomyelitis by surgical debridement and the implantation of calcium sulfate tobramycin pellets. *J Orthop Res* 2002;20:643-647.
100. Nicolau DP, Freeman CD, Nightingale CH, et al. Pharmacokinetics of minocycline and vancomycin in rabbits. *Lab Anim Sci* 1993;43:222-225.
101. Nielson VG, Sidhartha T, Brix AE, et al. Hextend® (hetastarch solution) decreases multiple organ injury and xanthine oxidase release after hepatoenteric ischemia-reperfusion in rabbits. *Crit Care Med* 1997;25:1565-1574.
102. Norcross EW, Sanders ME, Moore Q, et al. Comparative efficacy of besifloxacin and other fluoroquinolones in a prophylaxis model of penicillin-resistant *Streptococcus pneumoniae* rabbit endophthalmitis. *J Ocul Pharmacol Ther* 2010;26:237-243.
103. Ofoefule SI, Onuoha LC, Okonta MJ, et al. Effect of activated charcoal on isoniazid absorption in rabbits. *Boll Chim Farm* 2001;140:183-186.
104. Ostergaard C, Sorensen TK, Knudsen JD, et al. Evaluation of moxifloxacin, a new 8-methoxyquinolone, for treatment of meningitis caused by a penicillin-resistant pneumococcus in rabbits. *Antimicrob Agents Chemother* 1998;42:1706-1712.
105. Pan B, Wang M, Xu F, et al. Efficacy of an injectable formulation of eprinomectin against *Psoroptes cuniculi*, the ear mange mite in rabbits. *Vet Parasitol* 2006;137:386-390.
106. Pan BL, Zhang YF, Suo X, et al. Effect of subcutaneously administered diclazuril on the output of *Eimeria* species oocysts by experimentally infected rabbits. *Vet Rec* 2008;162:153-155.
107. Patterson TF, Fothergill AW, Rinaldi MG. Efficacy of itraconazole solution in a rabbit model of invasive aspergillosis. *Antimicrob Agents Chemother* 1993;37:2307-2310.
108. Percy DH, Black WD. Pharmacokinetics of tetracycline in the domestic rabbit following intravenous or oral administration. *Can J Vet Res* 1988;52:5-11.
109. Petraitiene R, Petraitis V, Groll AH, et al. Antifungal activity and pharmacokinetics of posaconazole (SCH 56592) in treatment and prevention of experimental invasive pulmonary aspergillosis: correlation with galactomannan antigenemia. *Antimicrob Agents Chemother* 2001;45:857-869.
110. Petraitis V, Petraitiene R, Groll AH, et al. Comparative antifungal activities and plasma pharmacokinetics of micafungin (FK463) against disseminated candidiasis and invasive pulmonary aspergillosis in persistently neutropenic rabbits. *Antimicrob Agents Chemother* 2002;46:1857-1869.
111. Pignon C. *Personal communication*; 2016.
112. Plumb DC. *Plumb's Veterinary Drug Handbook*. 8th ed. Ames: Wiley Blackwell Publishing: 2015.
113. Proksch JW, Ward KW. Ocular pharmacokinetics/pharmacodynamics of besifloxacin, moxifloxacin, and gatifloxacin following topical administration to pigmented rabbits. *J Ocul Pharmacol Ther* 2010;26:449-458.
114. Quimby JM, Gustafson DL, Samber BJ, et al. Studies on the pharmacokinetics and pharmacodynamics of mirtazapine in healthy young cats. *J Vet Pharmacol Ther* 2011;34:388-396.
115. Redrobe S, Gakos G, Elliot SC, et al. Comparison of toltrazuril and sulphadimethoxine in the treatment of intestinal coccidiosis in pet rabbits. *Vet Rec* 2010;167:287-290.
116. Regnier A, Schneider M, Concordet D, et al. Intraocular pharmacokinetics of intravenously administered marbofloxacin in rabbits with experimentally induced acute endophthalmitis. *Am J Vet Res* 2008;69:410-415.
117. Roffey SJ, Cole S, Comby P, et al. The disposition of voriconazole in mouse, rat, rabbit, guinea pig, dog, and human. *Drug Metab Dispos* 2003;31:731-741.
118. Rota S, Briganti A, Portela DA, et al. Anesthesia and recovery time in rabbits (*Oryctolagus cuniculus*) premedicated with dexmedetomidine, ketamine and fentanyl and maintained with an infusion of propofol. *Proc Assoc Exot Mam Vet Conf* 2012;3.

119. Rota S, Briganti I, Tayari A, et al. Effect of dexmedetomidine-fentanyl-ketamine anesthesia on arterial gas analysis in rabbits (*Oryctolagus cuniculus*). *Proc Assoc Exot Mam Vet* 2013.
120. Rougier S, Galland D, Boucher S, et al. Epidemiology and susceptibility of pathogenic bacteria responsible for upper respiratory tract infections in pet rabbits. *Vet Microbiol* 2006;115:192-198.
121. Sanati H, Ramos C, Bayer A, et al. Combination therapy with amphotericin B and fluconazole against invasive candidiasis in neutropenic-mouse and infective-endocarditis rabbit models. *Antimicrob Agents Chemother* 1997;41:1345-1348.
122. Santos M, Arévalo M, Colino CI, et al. Study on pharmacokinetics and nephrotoxicity of netilmicin in rabbits using a new dosage regimen. *Methods Find Exp Clin Pharmacol* 1997;19:53-59.
123. Schnellbacher R. Butorphanol *J Exot Pet Med* 2010;19:192-195.
124. Schnellbacher RW, Carpenter JW, Mason DE, et al. Effects of lidocaine administration via continuous rate infusion on the minimum alveolar concentration of isoflurane in New Zealand white rabbits (*Oryctolagus cuniculus*). *Am J Vet Res* 2013;74:1377-1384.
125. Schnellbacher R, Divers S, Maglaras C, et al. Intravenous lidocaine and buprenorphine on postoperative pain and gastrointestinal motility in New Zealand white rabbits following ovariohysterectomy. *Am J Vet Res*. In press.
126. Sharpnack DD, Mastin JP, Childress CP, et al. Quinolone arthropathy in juvenile New Zealand white rabbits. *Lab Anim Sci* 1994;44:436-442.
127. Souza MJ, Greenacre CB, Cox SK. Pharmacokinetics of orally administered tramadol in domestic rabbits (*Oryctolagus cuniculus*). *Am J Vet Res* 2008;69:979-982.
128. Sponsel W, Chen N, Dang D, et al. Topical voriconazole as a novel treatment for fungal keratitis. *Antimicrob Agents Chemother* 2006;50:262-268.
129. Steinleitner A, Lambert H, Kazensky C, et al. Reduction of primary postoperative adhesion formation under calcium channel blockade in the rabbit. *J Surg Res* 1990;48:42-45.
130. Suter C, Muller-Doblies UU, Hatt JM, et al. Prevention and treatment of *Encephalitozoon cuniculi* infection in rabbits with fenbendazole. *Vet Rec* 2001;148:478-480.
131. Thomas P, Samant D, Zhu Z, et al. Long-term topical cyclosporine treatment improves tear production and reduces keratoconjunctivitis in rabbits with induced autoimmune dacryoadenitis. *J Ocul Pharmacol Ther* 2009;25:285-291.
132. Toshida H, Nakayasu K, Kanai A. Effect of cyclosporine A eyedrops on tear secretion in the rabbit. *Jpn J Ophthalmol* 1998;42:168-173.
133. Turner P, Chen H, Taylor W. Pharmacokinetics of meloxicam in rabbits after single and repeat oral dosing. *Comp Med* 2006;56:63-67.
134. Uebelhart D, Thonar EJ, Zhang JW, et al. Protective effect of exogenous chondroitin 4,6-sulfate in the acute degradation of articular cartilage in the rabbit. *Osteoarthr Cartilage* 1998;6:6-13.
135. Vanparijs O, Hermans L, van der Flaes L, et al. Efficacy of diclazuril in the prevention and cure of intestinal and hepatic coccidiosis in rabbits. *Vet Parasitol* 1989;32:109-117.
136. Wagner R, Wendlberger U. Field efficacy of moxidectin in dogs and rabbits naturally infested with *Sarcoptes* spp., *Demodex* spp., and *Psoroptes* spp. mites. *Vet Parasitol* 2000;93:149-158.
137. Waterbury L, Flach A. Comparison of ketorolac tromethamine, diclofenac sodium, and loteprednol etabonate in an animal model of ocular inflammation. *J Ocul Pharmacol Ther* 2006;22:155-159.
138. Watson MK, Wittenburg LA, Bui CT, et al. Pharmacokinetics and bioavailability of orbifloxacin oral suspension in New Zealand white rabbits (*Oryctolagus cuniculus*). *Am J Vet Res* 2015;76:946-951.
139. Welch WD, Lu YS, Bawdon RE. Pharmacokinetics of penicillin-G in serum and nasal washings of *Pasteurella multocida*-free and -infected rabbits. *Lab Anim Sci* 1987;37:65-68.

140. Wen H, Pan B, Wang F, et al. The effect of self-licking behavior on pharmacokinetics of eprinomectin and clinical efficacy against *Psoroptes cuniculi* in topically administered rabbits. *Parasitol Res* 2010;106:607-613.
141. Williams DL. Common features of exotic animal ophthalmology. In: Williams DL, ed. *Ophthalmology in Exotic Pets*. Oxford: Wiley-Blackwell; 2012:9-14.
142. Yu GY, Yan CH, Yu XG, et al. Effects of chelation therapy with succimer in young rabbits of moderate lead poisoning. *Zhonghua Yu Fang Yi Xue Za Zhi* 2009;43:8-13.

Chapter 11 Ferrets

James K. Morrisey | *Matthew S. Johnston*

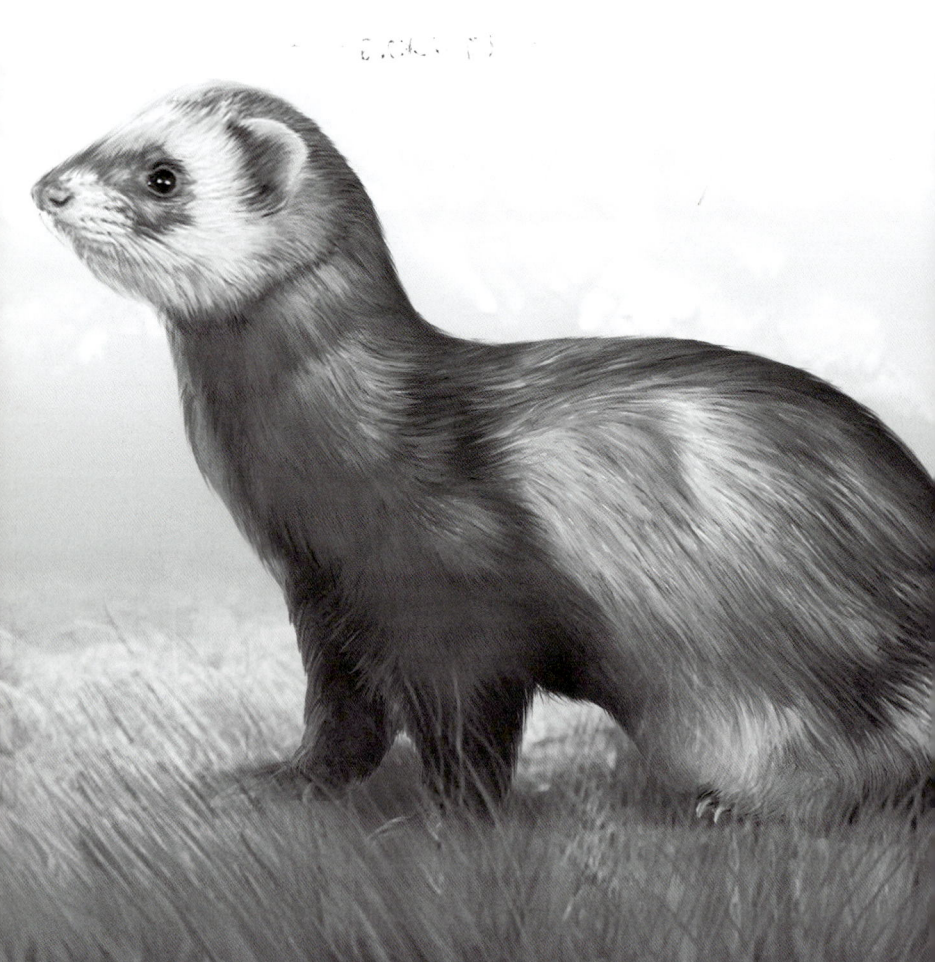

TABLE 11-1 Antimicrobial and Antifungal Agents Used in Ferrets.

Agent	Dosage	Comments
Amikacin	8-16 mg/kg SC, IM, IV divided q8-24h[53]	Potentially ototoxic and nephrotoxic
	10-15 mg/kg SC, IM q12h[52]	
Amoxicillin	20 mg/kg PO, SC q12h[52]	
	30 mg/kg PO q8h × 21 days[16]	*Helicobacter*; can use with metronidazole and bismuth subsalicylate
Amoxicillin/clavulanic acid (Clavamox, Zoetis)	13-25 mg/kg PO q8-12h[52]	
	18.75 mg per jill PO q12h[15]	For treatment of *E. coli* induced mastitis
Amphotericin B	0.15 mg/kg IV 3×/wk × 2-4 mon[25]	Treatment of cryptococcosis
	0.25-1 mg/kg IV q24h or q48h until total dose of 7-25 mg has been given[25]	
	0.4-0.8 mg/kg IV q7d[52]	Blastomycosis; monitor for azotemia; total dose 7-25 mg
Ampicillin	5-30 mg/kg SC, IM, IV q8-12h[51,52]	
Azithromycin	5 mg/kg PO q24h[60]	
Cefadroxil	15-20 mg/kg PO q12h[52]	
Cefovecin (Convenia, Zoetis)	8 mg/kg SC q2-3d[49]	Second generation parenteral cephalosporin; long-acting antibiotic
Cephalexin	15-30 mg/kg PO q8-12h[53]	
Cephaloridine	10-25 mg/kg SC, IM q24h × 5-7 days[53]	Dermatitis
Chloramphenicol	25-50 mg/kg PO, SC, IM, IV q12h[53]	14-day minimum for proliferative bowel disease
	50 mg/kg SC, IM q12h[15]	For treatment of mastitis
Ciprofloxacin	10-30 mg/kg PO q24h[53]	Mix 500 mg tablet in 10 mL water (50 mg/mL); flavor for improved acceptance
Clarithromycin	12.5 mg/kg PO q8-12h × 14 days[44]	*Helicobacter*; use with ranitidine bismuth citrate
	50 mg/kg PO q24h or divided q12h × 14 days[51]	*Helicobacter*; use with omeprazole (or ranitidine) and metronidazole
Clindamycin	5.5-10 mg/kg PO q12h[53]	Anaerobic infections; bone and dental disease
	12.5 mg/kg PO q12h[53]	Toxoplasmosis
Cloxacillin	10 mg/kg PO, IM, IV q6h[65]	
Doxycycline	10 mg/kg PO q12h[37]	May help with ferret systemic coronavirus infection
Enrofloxacin (Baytril, Bayer)	5 mg/kg PO, IM q12h[15]	For treatment of mastitis
	5-10 mg/kg PO, SC, IM q12h[53]	IM for short term (generally 1 injection); injectable form can be given PO in palatable liquid; liquid for PO can also be compounded
	10-20 mg/kg PO, SC, IM q12-24h[52]	
Erythromycin	10 mg/kg PO q6h[52]	
	220 g/ton feed[53]	Controlling *Campylobacter* diarrhea in large groups

Continued

TABLE 11-1 Antimicrobial and Antifungal Agents Used in Ferrets. (cont'd)

Agent	Dosage	Comments
Fluconazole	50 mg/kg PO q12h[53]	
Gentamicin	2 mg/kg PO q12h × 10-14 days[21]	Parenteral form can be given PO; proliferative colitis that is nonresponsive to chloramphenicol[12,21]
	2-5 mg/kg SC, IM, IV q12-24h[52]	If given IV, dilute with saline and administer over 20 min
Griseofulvin	25 mg/kg PO q12-24h[53]	Refractory dermatomycosis; use with lime-sulfur dips q7d
Itraconazole	1.5 mg/kg PO q24h[41]	Invasive nasal cryptococcosis
	10 mg/kg PO q12h[20]	Histoplasmosis
	10-20 mg/kg PO q24h[67]	Cryptococcosis
	25-33 mg/kg PO q24h[25,72]	
Ketoconazole	10-50 mg/kg PO q12-24h[39]	
Lime sulfur	Dip q7d[52]	Dermatomycosis; see griseofulvin
Lincomycin	11 mg/kg PO q8h[53]	
Metronidazole	15-20 mg/kg PO q12h[52]	Anaerobic infections; can use with amoxicillin and bismuth subsalicylate for *Helicobacter*
Neomycin	10-20 mg/kg PO q6h[52]	Potential nephrotoxicity and neuromuscular blockage
Netilmicin (Netromycin, Schering)	6-8 mg/kg SC, IM, IV q24h[53]	Severe staphylococcal infections
Nitazoxanide (Alinia, Romark Laboratories)	5 mg/kg PO q12h[25]	Treatment of cryptosporidiosis
Oxytetracycline	20 mg/kg PO q8h[52]	
Penicillin G (sodium or potassium)	20,000 U/kg IM q12h[39] 40,000 U/kg SC, IM q24h[52]	
Pentamidine isethionate	3-4 mg/kg SC q48h[25]	*Pneumocystis* pneumonia
Pyremethamine	0.5 mg/kg PO q12h[25]	Combine with trimethoprim sulfa (30 mg/kg PO q12h) and folic acid (3-5 mg/kg PO q24h) for treatment of toxoplasmosis
Sulfadimethoxine	25 mg/kg PO, SC, IM q24h[53] 30-50 mg/kg PO q12-24h[52]	
Sulfamethazine	1-5 mg/mL drinking water[52]	
Sulfasoxazole	50 mg/kg PO q8h[53]	
Sulfathalidine	Mix in food at dose of 1 g/day/kg body weight[12]	Opioid useful for management of *Salmonella* and to reduce shedding in colonies
Tetracycline	20-25 mg/kg PO q8-12h[52]	
Trimethoprim/sulfa	5 mg/kg PO q24h[15]	Pyelonephritis
	15 mg/kg IV q12h[8]	
	15-30 mg/kg PO, SC q12h[52]	Dosage amount of combined drugs
Tylosin (Tylan, Elanco)	5-10 mg/kg PO, SC, IM, IV q12h[51,52]	

TABLE 11-2 Antiparasitic Agents Used in Ferrets.

Agent	Dosage	Comments
Amitraz (Mitaban, Upjohn)	0.0125% topical solution q7d × 3 treatments, then 0.0375% q7d × 3 treatments[52]	Demodecosis secondary to other illness
	0.03% topical solution to affected area q7d × 3-6 treatments[53]	Demodecosis; use full concentration
Amprolium	19 mg/kg PO q24h[52]	Coccidiosis
	100 mg/kg PO in food or water for 7 days[25]	*Isospora*
Carbaryl powder (5%)	Topical q7d × 3-6 treatments[52]	Ectoparasites
Decoquinate	0.5 mg/kg PO for at least 2 wk[60]	Coccidiosis; larger groups of ferrets
Fenbendazole	20 mg/kg PO q24h × 5 days[52]	
	50 mg/kg PO q24h × 30 days[52]	*Mesocestoides* infection
Fipronil (Frontline, Merial)	1 pump of spray or 1/5-1/2 of cat pipette topical q60d[52]	Flea adulticide
	0.2-0.4 mL topically q30d[52]	
Imidacloprid (Advantage, Bayer)	10 mg/kg topically[36]	Flea treatment; PD
	0.1-0.4 mL topically q30d[39,52]	Flea adulticide; use small cat/kitten vial
Imidacloprid/moxidectin (Advantage Multi, Bayer)	1.9-3.3 µg/kg topically q30d[60]	Heartworm prevention
Ivermectin	0.02 mg/kg PO, SC q30d[69]	Heartworm prevention
	0.05 mg/kg PO q30d until negative testing[69]	Recommended treatment for heartworms; give prednisolone (1 mg/kg/day) concurrently
	0.05-0.3 mg/kg PO q24h for 1 mo after negative skin scraping[6]	Demodecosis
	0.2-0.5 mg/kg SC q14d × 3 treatments[52]	Sarcoptic mange
	0.4 mg/kg PO, SC, repeat in 14-28 days[52]	Ear mites, ticks
	0.5-1 mg/kg in ears, repeat in 14 days[52]	Ear mites; half dose in each ear; treat cats and dogs in house concurrently
Lime sulfur	Dip 1:40 dilution q7d × 6 wk[21]	Demodectic mange
Lufenuron (Program, Novartis)	10 mg/kg SC[25]	Flea larvicide
	30 mg/kg PO in food[25]	
	30-45 mg/kg PO q30d[52]	
Mebendazole	50 mg/kg PO q12h × 2 days[25]	Nematodes
Melarsomine dihydrochloride (Immiticide, Merial)	2.5 mg/kg IM once, repeat in 30 days with 2 treatments 24 hr apart[52]	Heartworm adulticide; less commonly used; use prednisone (1 mg/kg q24h × 4 mo) following treatment
Metronidazole	15-20 mg/kg PO q12h × 14 days[52]	Gastrointestinal protozoa
Milbemycin oxime (Interceptor, Novartis)	1.15-2.33 mg/kg PO q30d[52]	Heartworm preventive
Moxidectin	0.17 mg SC once[60]	Heartworm adulticide
Paromomycin	165 mg/kg PO q12h × 5 days[60]	Cryptosporidiosis; possible treatment; use with caution, severe renal disease possible

Continued

TABLE 11-2 Antiparasitic Agents Used in Ferrets. (cont'd)

Agent	Dosage	Comments
Piperazine citrate	50-100 mg/kg PO q14d[53]	Intestinal nematodes
Praziquantel (Droncit, Bayer)	5-10 mg/kg PO, SC, repeat in 10[53]-14d[52]	Cestodes
	25 mg/kg PO × 3 days[60]	Trematodes
Pyrantel pamoate	4.4 mg/kg PO, repeat in 14 days[52]	
Pyrethrins	Topical q7d prn[52]	Fleas; use products safe for puppies and kittens
Pyrimethamine	0.5 mg/kg PO q12h[25]	Toxoplasmosis; antiprotozoal
Selamectin (Revolution, Zoetis)	6-18 mg/kg topically[51-53,60]	Ectoparasites (fleas, lice, most mites except *Demodex*)
	15 mg topically q30d[14]	Ear mites, fleas; PD
	45 mg/ferret topically[50]	Ear mites; although this dose has been reported in a PD study, it appears that lower (safer?) doses (see previous) are also quite effective
Sulfadimethoxine	20-50 mg/kg PO q24h[7]	Coccidia
	50 mg/kg PO, then 25 mg/kg q24h × 9 days[52]	
	0.5 mL/kg of a 12.5% solution mixed into drinking water[56]	For treatment of enteric coccidiosis in a large group of ferrets
Thiabendazole/dex-amethasone/neomycin (Tresaderm, Merial)	2 drops in each ear q24h × 7 days, off 7 days, on 7 days[55]	Ear mites

TABLE 11-3 Chemical Restraint/Anesthetic Agents Used in Ferrets.

Agent	Dosage	Comments
Acepromazine	—	See ketamine for combination
	0.1-0.25 mg/kg SC, IM[52]	Preanesthetic; light sedation
	0.1-0.5 mg/kg SC, IM[33]	Rapid onset of sedation if given IM; doses above 0.2 mg/kg are associated with prolonged recovery times and hypothermia
	0.2-0.5 mg/kg SC, IM[52]	Tranquilization
Alfaxalone (Alfaxan, Jurox)	5 mg/kg IV[18]	Anesthetic induction; PD
	5-15 mg/kg IM[28]	Sedative
Atipamezole (Antisedan, Zoetis)	0.4 mg/kg IM[53]	Dexmedetomidine and medetomidine reversal; give same volume SC, IV, IP as medetomidine or dexmedetomidine (5 × medetomidine or 10 × dexmedetomidine dose in mg)
	1 mg/kg SC, IV, IP[52]	
Atropine	0.04-0.05 mg/kg SC, IM, IV[52]	Preanesthetic; bradycardia; hypersalivation
Bupivacaine	1 mg/kg epidurally[52]	Epidural anesthesia; analgesia
	1-1.5 mg/kg SC infiltrate[27]	Local anesthesia; lasts several hours

TABLE 11-3 Chemical Restraint/Anesthetic Agents Used in Ferrets. (cont'd)

Agent	Dosage	Comments
Butorphanol	Loading dose 0.05-0.2 mg/kg; maintenance 0.1-0.4 mg/kg/hr[21]	Constant-rate infusion (CRI) for perioperative analgesia; see ketamine, midazolam, and tiletamine/zolazepam for combinations
Dexmedetomidine (Dexdomitor, Zoetis)	0.04-0.1 mg/kg IM[49]	α_2 agonist similar to medetomidine; not commonly used because of bradycardia and other side effects
Diazepam	—	See ketamine for combinations; drug is slowly and incompletely absorbed following IM administration
	0.5 mg/kg PO, IM, IV q6-8 h[59]	Smooth muscle relaxation in urethral obstruction cases
	0.5-1.5 mg/kg/h constant-rate infusion[3]	Seizure control
	1 mg/animal IV[52]	Seizure control; 1-2 boluses
	2 mg/kg SC, IM[25]	Tranquilization; seizure control
Enflurane	2% maintenance[52]	Anesthesia
Etomidate	1 mg/kg IV[27]	Induction and intubation of critically ill animal
Fentanyl citrate/fluanisone (Hypnorm, Janssen)	0.3 mg/kg IM[52]	Anesthesia; not available in the United States
Fentanyl/droperidol (Innovar-Vet, Schering Plough)	0.15 mL/kg IM[52]	Minor surgical procedures; deep sedation
Glycopyrrolate	0.01 mg/kg IM[52]	Preanesthetic; bradycardia; hypersalivation
Isoflurane	To effect[32]	Inhalant anesthesia
Ketamine	—	Ketamine combinations follow
	10-20 mg/kg IM[52]	Tranquilization; induction
	30-60 mg/kg IM[52]	Anesthesia; when used alone, high doses cause poor muscle relaxation, rough recoveries, and convulsions; not recommended as a sole agent
Ketamine (K)/acepromazine (A)	(K) 20-35 mg/kg + (A) 0.2-0.35 mg/kg SC, IM[52]	Anesthesia
Ketamine (K)/diazepam (D)	(K) 10-20 mg/kg + (D) 1-2 mg/kg IM[52]	Anesthesia; poor analgesia[61]
	0.1 mL/kg IV[52]	Induction; will allow intubation with premedication; use equal volumes of (K) at 100 mg/mL and (D) at 5 mg/mL
Ketamine (K)/dexmedetomidine (D)	(K) 5 mg/kg IM + (D) 0.03 mg/kg IM[52]	Medetomidine no longer commercially available; dexmedetomidine at half the dose of medetomidine may be effective
Ketamine (K)/medetomidine (M) or dexmedetomidine (D)/butorphanol (B)	(K) 5 mg/kg + (M) 0.08 mg/kg or (D)	Medetomidine no longer commercially available; induction or total injectable

Continued

TABLE 11-3 Chemical Restraint/Anesthetic Agents Used in Ferrets. (cont'd)

Agent	Dosage	Comments
	0.04 mg/kg + (B) 0.2 mg/kg IM[32]	anesthesia; allows for intubation; 60-80 min of surgical plane of anesthesia
Ketamine (K)/midazolam (M)	(K) 5-10 mg/kg + (M) 0.25-0.5 mg/kg IV[51]	
	0.1 mL/kg IV[52]	Induction; use equal volumes of (K) at 100 mg/mL and (M) at 5 mg/mL
Ketamine (K)/xylazine (X)	(K) 10-25 mg/kg + (X) 1-2 mg/kg IM[52]	Anesthesia; avoid in sick animals;[39] may result in cardiac arrhythmias[61]
Lidocaine	1-2 mg/kg total SC[27]	Local anesthesia; use 1%-2% solution; lasts 15-30 min
	0.5-1.0 mg/kg IV q12h[52]	
Midazolam (Versed, Roche)	—	See ketamine for combination; can be reversed with flumazenil at same volume
	0.25-0.3 mg/kg SC, IM[25]	Mild sedation; premedication
	0.25-0.5 mg/kg SC, IM, IV[53]	
Midazolam (M)/butorphanol (B)	(M) 0.2 mg/kg + (B) 0.2 mg/kg IM[10,58]	Good sedation; premedication for minor procedures (i.e., ultrasonography, endoscopy, etc.); if needed, can follow with gas anesthesia or IV propofol; can reverse midazolam with flumazenil
Naloxone (Narcan, Dupont)	0.01-0.03 mg/kg IM, IV[52]	Reversal of opioids; up to 1 mg/kg may be used
	0.04 mg/kg SC, IM, IV[52]	
Propofol	1-3 mg/kg IV[32]	Induction when premedicants are used; bradypnea or apnea and hypoxia common; intubation and oxygen insufflation is recommended
	2-10 mg/kg IV[25]	Induction
Sevoflurane	To effect[51]	Inhalant anesthesia
Tiletamine/zolazepam (Telazol, Fort Dodge)	—	Tiletamine/zolazepam combinations follow
	12-22 mg/kg IM[52]	Minor surgical procedures at 22 mg/kg; recovery may be prolonged at higher doses; poor muscle relaxation; rarely indicated
Tiletamine/zolazepam (T)/xylazine (X)	3 mg/kg (T) + 3 mg/kg (X) IM[34]	Small injection volume; rapid and smooth induction; allows for endotracheal intubation
Tiletamine/zolazepam (T)/xylazine (X)/butorphanol (B)	1.5 mg/kg (T) + 1.5 mg/kg (X) + 0.2 mg/kg (B)[34]	Small injection volume; rapid and smooth induction; allows for endotracheal intubation; analgesia; profound cardiorespiratory depression necessitates oxygen insufflation
Tiletamine/zolazepam (T)/dexmedetomidine (D)/butorphanol (B)	0.03 mL/kg IM of prepared solution (see comment)[32]	Telazol powder is reconstituted with 2.5 mL of dexmedetomidine and 2.5 mL of butorphanol (10 mg/mL) to form final volume of 5 mL

TABLE 11-3 Chemical Restraint/Anesthetic Agents Used in Ferrets. (cont'd)

Agent	Dosage	Comments
Xylazine	—	See ketamine and tiletamine/zolazepam for combinations
	0.1-0.5 mg/kg SC, IM[53]	Tranquilization; may cause hypotension, bradycardia, and arrhythmias; use with care in sick animals
	2 mg/kg IM[33]	Rapid immobilization within 3-5 minutes; associated with arrhythmias, hypotension, bradycardia
Yohimbine (Yobine, Lloyd)	0.2-0.5 mg/kg IV[52] 0.5-1 mg/kg IM[52,53]	Xylazine reversal

TABLE 11-4 Analgesic Agents Used in Ferrets.

Agent	Dosage	Comments
Acetylsalicylic acid (aspirin)	0.5-22 mg/kg PO q8-24h[52]	Analgesia; antiinflammatory; antipyretic; cannot be compounded as molecule is unstable in aqueous solution
Amantadine	3-5 mg/kg PO[49]	May potentiate other analgesics via NMDA antagonist action
Bupivicaine	1-2 mg/kg SC[32]	
Buprenorphine	12 µg/kg epidurally[21]	Epidural analgesia/anesthesia
	0.04 mg/kg IM q4-6h[29]	PK
	0.01-0.05 mg/kg oral transmucosal, SC, IM, IV q6-12h[32,52]	Analgesia
Butorphanol	—	See ketamine, midazolam, and tiletamine/zolazepam (see Table 11-3) for anesthetic combinations
	0.05-0.5 mg/kg SC, IM q8-12h[32,52]	Analgesia; lower end of dose may be too low for clinical effect; higher end of dose range may cause profound sedation
	0.3 mg/kg SC q2-4h[29]	PK
Carprofen (Rimadyl, Zoetis)	1-5 mg/kg PO q12-24h[21,52]	Nonsteroidal antiinflammatory; use caution in animals with gastritis or enteritis
	4 mg/kg SC[32]	
Fentanyl citrate	1.25-5 µg/kg/h IV via constant-rate infusion[21,49]	Postoperative analgesia
	10-30 µg/kg/h IV via constant-rate infusion[21,49]	Perioperative analgesia; administer after loading dose of 5-10 µg/kg IV

Continued

TABLE 11-4 Analgesic Agents Used in Ferrets. (cont'd)

Agent	Dosage	Comments
Flunixin meglumine (Banamine, Schering)	0.3-2 mg/kg IV, PO, SC q12-24h[52,53] 2.5 mg IM q12h[14]	Nonsteroidal antiinflammatory; use caution in animals with gastritis or enteritis; use caution in using drug more than 5 days continuously; mix injectable form with palatable syrup for PO
Gabapentin	3-5 mg/kg PO q8-24h[52]	Neurotropic pain; may cause sedation at higher doses
Hydromorphone	0.1 mg/kg SC q1-2h[29] 0.1-0.2 mg/kg SC, IM, IV[39]	Opioid; PK
Ibuprofen	1 mg/kg PO q12-24h[51]	Nonsteroidal antiinflammatory
Ketamine	0.1-0.4 mg/kg/h IV via constant-rate infusion[21] 0.3-1.2 mg/kg/h IV via constant-rate infusion[21]	Postoperative analgesia Perioperative analgesia; administer after 2-5 mg/kg IV loading dose
Ketoprofen (Ketofen, Fort Dodge)	1-3 mg/kg PO, SC, IM q24h[53]	Nonsteroidal antiinflammatory; use caution with gastritis or enteritis or if using >5 days
Meloxicam	0.1-0.3 mg/kg PO, SC, IM q24h[24,25,27]	Nonsteroidal antiinflammatory; monitor liver and kidney values
Meperidine (Demerol, Winthrop-Breon)	5-10 mg/kg SC, IM, IV q2-4h[25]	Analgesia
Morphine	0.1 mg/kg epidurally[21] 0.2-5 mg/kg SC, IM q2-6h[52]	Analgesia SC administration of 1 mg/kg associated with emesis, excitability, and ptyalism[39]
Nalbuphine (Nubain, Endo Labs)	0.5-1.5 mg/kg IM, IV q2-3h[25]	Analgesia
Oxymorphone	0.05-0.2 mg/kg SC, IM, IV q8-12 h[27,52]	Analgesia
Pentazocine (Talwin, Sanofi Winthrop)	5-10 mg/kg IM q4h[52]	Analgesia
Tramadol	5-10 mg/kg PO q12-24[25]	Analgesia; synergistic with NSAIDs

TABLE 11-5 Cardiopulmonary Agents Used in Ferrets.

Agent	Dosage	Comments
Aminophylline	4-6.6 mg/kg PO, IM, IV q12h[52]	Bronchodilator
Amlodipine (Norvasc, Pfizer)	0.2-0.4 mg/kg PO q12h[28]	Vasodilator
Atenolol (Tenormin, ICI)	3.125-6.25 mg/kg PO q24h[35,52] 6.25 mg/animal PO q24h[52]	β-adrenergic blocker for hypertrophic cardiomyopathy
Atropine	0.02-0.04 mg/kg SC, IM[52] 0.1 mg/kg intratracheal[52]	Bradycardia

TABLE 11-5 Cardiopulmonary Agents Used in Ferrets. (cont'd)

Agent	Dosage	Comments
Benazepril	0.25-0.5 mg/kg PO q24h[35,68]	Vasodilator; less nephrotoxic than enalapril
Captopril (Capoten, Squibb)	⅛ of 12.5 mg tablet/animal PO q48h[52]	Vasodilator; starting dose, gradually increase to q12-24h; can cause lethargy
Digoxin (Cardoxin, Evsco)	0.005-0.01 mg/kg PO q12-24h[52]	Positive inotrope for dilated cardiomyopathy; monitor serum levels
Diltiazem (Cardizem, Marion Merrill Dow)	1.5-7.5 mg/kg PO q12h[35,52]	Calcium channel blocker for hypertrophic cardiomyopathy
Dobutamine	0.01 mL/animal IV prn[28]	Hypotension
Doxapram	1-2 mg/kg IV[52] 5-11 mg/kg IV[52]	Respiratory stimulant
Enalapril (Enacard, Merck)	0.25-0.5 mg/kg PO q24-48h[35,52]	Vasodilator for dilated cardiomyopathy; do not use with concurrent renal disease
Epinephrine	0.02 mg/kg SC, IM, IV, intratracheal[43]	Cardiac arrest; anaphylactic reactions (including vaccine reactions)
	0.2 mg/kg IV, intracardiac, IO[25]	
	0.2-0.4 mg/kg diluted in 0.9% NaCl[25] intratracheal	Administer during cardiopulmonary arrest
Furosemide	1-4 mg/kg PO, SC, IM, IV q8-12h[52]	Diuretic; use high dose in fulminant heart failure
	2-3 mg/kg IM, IV q8-12h followed by 1-2 mg/kg PO q12h for long-term management[69]	Emergency management of fulminant heart failure
Hyperimmune serum	1 mL/animal IV once[57]	Use serum from a healthy, appropriately vaccinated ferret for treatment of canine distemper virus infection
Isoproterenol	20-25 μg/animal SC, IM q4-6h[69] 40-50 μg/animal PO q4-6h[69]	Positive chronotrope to increase ventricular rate in third-degree AV block
Metaproterenol	0.25-1 mg/kg PO q12h[69]	Positive chronotrope to increase ventricular rate in third-degree AV block
Nitroglycerin (2%) ointment (Nitrol, Savage)	1/16-⅛ inch/animal q12-24h[52]	Vasodilator for cardiomyopathy; apply to shaved inner thigh or pinna
Pimobendan	0.25-1.25 mg/kg PO q12h[25] 0.5 mg/kg PO q12h[69] 0.625-1.25 mg/kg PO q12h[39]	Phosphodiesterase inhibitor; increases cardiac contractility with dilated cardiomyopathy or mitral valve disease
Propranolol (Inderal, Wyeth-Ayerst)	0.2-1 mg/kg PO q8-12h[52] 2 mg/kg PO, SC q12h[52]	β-blocker for hypertrophic cardiomyopathy; may cause lethargy, loss of appetite
Pseudophedrine	5 mg/kg PO q8h[69]	Positive chronotrope to increase ventricular rate in third-degree AV block
Terbutaline	2.5-5 mg/kg PO q12-24h[27]	Bronchodilator
Theophylline	4.25 mg/kg PO q8-12h[12]	Bronchodilator; use elixir

TABLE 11-6 Adrenal Gland Disease Agents Used in Ferrets.

Agent	Dosage	Comments
Anastrazole (Arimidex, Astrazeneca Pharmaceuticals)	0.1 mg/kg PO q24h[52]	Estrogen inhibitor; precursor hormones blocked by inhibition of aromatase enzyme; use until signs resolve, then 7 days on, 7 days off, etc.; pregnant owners should avoid handling agent
Bicalutamide (Casodex, Astrazeneca Pharmaceuticals)	5 mg/kg PO q24h[52]	Testosterone inhibitor; competitively inhibits androgen by binding to receptors in target tissues; use until clinical signs resolve, then 7 days on, 7 days off, etc.; pregnant owners should avoid handling agent
Deoxycorticosterone pivalate (DOCP)	2 mg/kg IM q21d[52]	Treatment of adrenal insufficiency following bilateral adrenalectomy
Deslorelin (Suprelorin, Virbac Animal Health)	—	Long-acting GnRH analog that may suppress LH and FSH; used to control signs of adrenal disease; given as a subcutaneous implant approximately once yearly; now available in the United States
	2.7 mg implant SC[38]	Alternative to spay/neuter; the 2.7 mg implant is not available in the United States
	3 mg or 4.7 mg SC[38,71]	The 3 mg implant is not available in the United States
	4.7 mg implant SC[25]	Treatment of adrenal disease; lasts 10-18 months
	9.4 mg implant SC[25]	Treatment of adrenal disease; lasts 16-48 months; not available in the United States
Finasteride (Proscar, Merck)	5 mg/kg PO q24h[52]	Inhibits conversion of testosterone to active form of dihydrotestosterone; also used in treatment of prostatic enlargement
Flutamide (Eulexin, Schering)	5-10 mg/kg PO q12-24h[11,52,63]	Androgen inhibitor; reduces enlarged periurethral prostate tissue; lifetime treatment; associated with mammary tumors
Leuprolide acetate (Lupron, AbbVie)	—	Long-acting GnRH analog that may cause an initial stimulation, then suppression of LH and FSH; palliative treatment of adrenal disease (will not resolve tumor); administer q28d until clinical signs regress, then treatment interval can be up to 6-8 wk; lifetime treatment; higher dosage may shrink prostate within 12-48 hr which may improve urine flow in cases of urethral obstruction; must be prepared in aliquots and frozen (although the effects of freezing on drug efficacy are questionable) until used; very expensive
	1 mg IM q60-75d[11] 3 month depot	Adrenal disease
Lupron, Depot 30 day (TAP)	100-150 µg/kg IM q4-8wk[1,70] 250 µg/kg IM q4-8wk[26]	
Lupron, Depot 4 month (TAP)	250 µg/kg IM[59] 2 mg/kg SC, IM q16wk[52]	
Melatonin	0.5-1 mg/animal PO q24h[61] prn	Symptomatic treatment of hyperadrenocorticism; may not affect tumor growth
	5.4 mg implant SC[52]	Should last 6-12 mo

TABLE 11-6 Adrenal Gland Disease Agents Used in Ferrets. (cont'd)

Agent	Dosage	Comments
Mitotane (o,p'-DDD) (Lysodren, Bristol-Myers)	—	Hyperadrenocorticism; variable results and not a reliable alternative to adrenalectomy or other drugs mentioned above; results have been largely unsatisfactory and, therefore, use is not recommended
Trilostane (Vetoryl, Dechra)	2 mg/kg PO q12h[52]	May be useful for treating pituitary-dependent hyperadrenocorticism or adrenal dependent hyperadrenocorticism; reduces synthesis of adrenal androgens

TABLE 11-7 Miscellaneous Agents Used in Ferrets.[a]

Agent	Dosage	Comments
Activated charcoal	1-3 g/kg PO[52]	Orally administered adsorbent for gastrointestinal tract toxins/drug overdoses
Amantadine (Symmetrel, Endo Labs)	6 mg/kg as aerosol q12h[5,25,52]	Influenza; experimental antiviral
Apomorphine	0.7 mg/kg SC[52]	Emetic
	5 mg/kg SC[52]	Emetic; may cause excitation
Atropine	5-10 mg/kg SC, IM[52]	Organophosphate toxicity
Azathioprine (Imuran, GlaxoSmithKline)	0.9 mg/kg PO q24-72h[9]	Immunosuppressive agent; may use in chronic hepatitis
Barium (30%)	8-13 mL/kg PO[52]	Gastrointestinal contrast study
Barium (60%)	17 mL/kg PO[66]	Followed 30 minutes later by 42 mL/kg of air for a double contrast gastrointestinal study
Bismuth subcitrate, colloidal	6 mg/kg PO q12h[52]	In combination with enrofloxacin at 4.25 mg/kg q12h for *Helicobacter*
Bismuth subsalicylate (Pepto-Bismol, Procter & Gamble)	0.25-1 mL/kg PO q4-8h[52]	Gastrointestinal ulcers; may help prevent *Helicobacter* colonization
	17.5 mg/kg PO q8-12h[52]	
Bleomycin (Blenoxane, BristolMyersSquibb)	10 U/m² SC[52]	Treatment of squamous cell carcinoma
Budesonide (Entocort, Astrazeneca)	Up to 1 mg/ferret PO q24h[49]	Novel steroid may have use as single agent treatment for inflammatory bowel disease
Cabergoline	5 µg/kg PO q24h × 5 days[27]	Pseudopregnancy
Calcium EDTA	20-30 mg/kg SC q12h[62]	Treatment of heavy metal toxicosis
Chitosan	0.5 mg/kg on food q12h[49]	Intestinal phosphorus and uremic toxin absorbent; cellulose-like biopolymer from exoskeletons of marine invertebrates
Chlorambucil (Leukeran, Glaxo)	1 mg/kg PO[4]	Antineoplastic; in chemotherapy protocols for lymphoma[a]
	20 mg/m² PO[52]	

Continued

TABLE 11-7 Miscellaneous Agents Used in Ferrets. (cont'd)

Agent	Dosage	Comments
Chlorpheniramine (Chlor-Trimeton, Squibb)	1-2 mg/kg PO q8-12h[52]	Antihistamine; control sneezing and coughing when they interfere with eating or sleeping
Cimetidine (Tagamet, SmithKline)	5-10 mg/kg PO, SC, IM q8h[52] 10 mg/kg PO, IV q8h[25]	H_2 blocker; inhibits acid secretion; gastrointestinal ulcers; unpalatable; give IV (slow)
Ciproheptadine (Periactin, Merck)	0.5 mg/kg PO q12h[49]	Appetite stimulation
Cisapride (Propulsid, Janssen)	0.5 mg/kg PO q8-12h[52]	Antiemetic; motility enhancer; not currently available in the United States; must be compounded
Cobalamin	25 µg/kg SC q7d × 6 wk, then q14d × 6 wk, then q30d[24]	Chronic diarrhea; with cobalamin malabsorption
Cyclophosphamide	10 mg/kg PO, SC[52] 200 mg/m² PO, SC[4] 250 mg/m² PO q4-5wk[47]	Antineoplastic; use at higher dose for salvage treatment of lymphoma[a] Part of a noninvasive protocol for treatment of lymphoma[a]
Cyclosporine	4-6 mg/kg PO q12h[42]	Pure red cell aplasia
Cytarabine (Cytosar-U, Zoetis)	300 mg/m² q8wk[47]	Part of a noninvasive protocol for treatment of lymphoma[a]
Dexamethasone	0.5 mg/kg SC, IM, IV[52] 1 mg/kg IM[52]	 Post-adrenalectomy; follow with prednisone
Dexamethasone sodium phosphate	1-2 mg/kg IV[3] 2 mg/kg IM, IV[19] 4-8 mg/kg IM, IV[52]	Cerebral edema therapy Anaphylactic reaction to vaccine Shock therapy
Dextrose 50%	0.25-2 mL IV[40] 1.25%-5% IV[40]	Bolus for hypoglycemia; give to effect Infusion for hypoglycemic or inappetant animal
Diazoxide (Proglycem, Medical Market Specialties)	5-30 mg/kg PO q12h[45,52] 10 mg/kg PO q24h or divided q8-12h[52]	Insulinoma; insulin-blocker; can cause hypertension, lethargy, depression, nausea
Diphenhydramine	0.5-2 mg/kg PO, IM, IV q8-12h[43,52]	Antihistamine; controls sneezing and coughing when they interfere with eating or sleeping; give at high dose IM prevaccination when previous reaction occurred or for treatment of vaccine reaction
Doxapram	1-2 mg/kg IV[52] 2-5 mg/kg IV[53]	Respiratory stimulant
Doxorubicin	1 mg/kg IV q21d × 4 treatments[4]	Antineoplastic agent; lymphoma;[a] salvage treatment
Epinephrine	0.02 mg/kg SC, IM, IV, IT[52]	Severe vaccine reaction; cardiac arrest
Epoetin alfa (Epogen, Amgen)	50-150 U/kg PO, IM q48h[52]	Stimulates erythropoiesis; after desired PCV is reached, administer q7d for maintenance

TABLE 11-7 Miscellaneous Agents Used in Ferrets. (cont'd)

Agent	Dosage	Comments
Famotidine (Pepcid, Merck)	0.25-0.5 mg/kg PO, SC, IV q24h[52] 2.5 mg PO, SC, IV q24h[25]	Inhibits acid secretion; gastrointestinal ulcers
Fludrocortisone (Florinef, SquibbMark)	0.05-0.1 mg/kg PO q24h or divided q12h[52]	Mineralocorticoid replacement after adrenal gland removal
Flunixin meglumine (Banamine, Schering)	1 mg/kg SC, IM[52]	Prevention of prostaglandin-mediated hypotension of endotoxemia
	2.5 mg/animal SC, IM q12h prn[14]	Reduce inflammation in mastitis
Flurbiprofen sodium	1-2 drops q12-24h[25]	Ophthalmic inflammation
Gadolinium-diethylenetriamine pentaacetic acid (Gl-DPTA) (Omniscan, GE Healthcare)	0.2 mL/kg[3]	MRI contrast agent for neurological studies
Glucagon	15 ng/kg/min IV constant-rate infusion[8]	Emergency management of hypoglycemia secondary to insulinoma
Glutamine	—	Amino acid; L form available OTC as a nutritional supplement; improves immune system, digestive health, and enhances muscle production
	0.5 g/kg PO divided daily[49]	Enterocyte supplementation with starvation
Gonadotropin-releasing hormone (GnRH) (Cystorelin, Sanofi)	20 μg/animal IM[14]	Termination of estrus after day 10 of estrus; repeat in 2 wk prn
Hairball laxative, feline	1-2 mL/animal PO q48h[52]	Trichobezoar prophylaxis
Heparin	100 U/animal (0.45-1.35 kg) SC q24h × 21 days[35]	May be used in some heartworm treatments
	200 U/kg SC, IM q12h × 5 days[52]	Decreases thromboembolism; start day prior to some heartworm adulticide treatments
Human chorionic gonadotropin (hCG) (Pregnyl, Organon)	—	Use 10 or more days after onset of estrus to induce ovulation and prevent hyperestrogenemia; repeat in 1-2 wk prn
	50-100 U/animal IM[14]	
	200-1000 U/animal IM[52]	
Hydrocortisone sodium succinate	25-40 mg/kg IV[52]	Shock
Hydrogen peroxide (3%)	2.2 mL/kg PO[52]	Emetic
Hydroxyzine (Atarax, Roerig)	2 mg/kg PO q8h[52]	Antihistamine; pruritus; may cause drowsiness
Insulin, glargine	0.5 U SC q12h[23]	
Insulin, NPH	0.1 U/animal SC q12h[52]	
	0.5-1 U/kg (or to effect) SC[49]	Diabetes mellitus; diabetic ketoacidosis; monitor blood glucose

Continued

TABLE 11-7 Miscellaneous Agents Used in Ferrets. (cont'd)

Agent	Dosage	Comments
Insulin, ultralente	0.1 U/animal SC q24h[52]	Diabetes mellitus; monitor blood glucose
Interferon-α	107 units IV or intranasal q24h for several days[31]	Adjunctive therapy for influenza
Iohexol	0.25-0.5 mL injected epidurally at the L5-L6 intervertebral disc space/kg[3]	Myelography
	10 mL/kg PO[52]	Gastrointestinal contrast study; can dilute 1:1 with water
	2.3 mL/kg IV[66]	Excretory urography
Ipecac (7%)	2.2-6.6 mL/animal PO[52]	Emetic
Iron dextran	10 mg/animal IM once[49]	Iron deficiency anemia; hemorrhage
Isotretinoin	2 mg/kg PO q24h[4]	Cutaneous epitheliotropic lymphoma
Kaolin/pectin	1-2 mL/kg PO q2-6h prn[52]	Gastrointestinal protectant
Lactulose syrup (Cephulac, Merrill Dow)	0.15-0.75 mL/kg PO q12h[52]	Absorption of blood ammonia in hepatic disease; may cause soft stools at higher dose
	150-175 mg/kg PO q8-12h[25]	
L-asparaginase	400 U/kg SC, IM[4]	Antineoplastic
	10,000 U/m² SC q7d × 3 treatments[47]	Part of a noninvasive chemotherapy protocol
Levothyroxine	50-100 µg/animal q12h[72]	Hypothyroidism
Loperamide	0.2 mg/kg PO q12h[52]	Antidiarrheal
Mannitol	0.5-1 g/kg IV[3]	Give over 20 min
Methotrexate	0.5 mg/kg IV[4]	Antineoplastic
	0.8 mg/kg IM[47]	Part of noninvasive protocol for treatment of lymphoma[a]
Metoclopramide	0.2-1 mg/kg PO, SC, IM q6-8h[53]	Antiemetic; motility enhancer
Milk thistle (*Silybum marianum*)	4-15 mg/kg PO q8-12h[25]	Hepatoprotective
Misoprostol (Cytotech, Searle)	1-5 µg/kg PO q8h[52]	Gastric ulcers
Nandrolone decanoate	1-5 mg/kg IM q7d[52]	Anabolic steroid
Nutri-Cal (EVSCO)	1-3 mL/animal PO q6-8h[52]	Nutritional supplement
Octreotide (Sandostatin, Novartis)	1-2 µg/kg SC q8-12h[49]	Somatostatin analogue; potential treatment for insulinomas
Omeprazole (Prilosec, Astra Merck)	0.7 mg/kg PO q24h[17]	Proton-pump inhibitor; decreases gastric secretion of HCl
	4 mg/kg PO q24h[25]	*Helicobacter*; use with clarithromycin and metronidazole
Ondansetron	1 mg/kg PO q12-24h[49]	Antiemetic
Oseltamivir phosphate (Tamiflu, Genentech)	5-10 mg/kg PO q12h × 10 days[31]	Antiviral for influenza treatment
Oxytocin	0.2-3 U/kg SC, IM[52]	Expels retained fetuses; stimulates lactation
Penicillamine	10 mg/kg PO q24h[25]	Copper toxicity

TABLE 11-7   Miscellaneous Agents Used in Ferrets. (cont'd)

Agent	Dosage	Comments
Pentoxifylline (Pentoxil, Upsher-Smith)	20 mg/kg PO q12h[37]	Improves perfusion to hypoperfused tissue by increasing deformability of erythrocytes; supportive treatment for ferret systemic coronavirus
Pet-Tinic (SmithKline)	0.2 mL/kg PO q24h[52]	Nutritional/iron supplement for anemia
Phenobarbital	1-2 mg/kg PO q8-12h[39,52]	Seizure control
	2-10 mg/kg/h IV constant-rate infusion[3]	Seizure control if diazepam is not effective
Phenoxybenzamine (Dibenzyline, SmithKline Beecham)	3.75-7.5 mg/animal PO q24-72h[59]	α-Adrenergic antagonist; smooth muscle relaxation for urethral obstruction; potential gastrointestinal or cardiovascular side effects
Polyprenol (Vetimmune, Sass & Sass)	3 mg/kg PO 3×/wk[37]	Antioxidant and immunostimulant; supportive treatment for ferret systemic coronavirus
Potassium bromide	—	Seizure control
	22-30 mg/kg q24h PO[3]	Dose if used with phenobarbitol
	70-80 mg/kg q24h PO[3]	Dose if used alone
Prazosin (Minipress, Zoetis)	0.05-0.1 mg/kg PO q8h[59]	α-Adrenergic antagonist; smooth muscle relaxation for urethral obstruction; potential for gastrointestinal and cardiovascular side effects
Prednisone	0.25 mg/kg PO q12h × 5 days, then 0.1 mg/kg q12h × 10 days[52]	Postoperative adrenalectomy; after initial dose of dexamethasone
	0.25-1 mg/kg PO divided q12h[52]	Insulinoma; gradually increase to 4 mg/kg/day prn; up to 2 mg/kg/day when given with diazoxide
	0.5 mg/kg PO q12h × 7-10 days, then q24h × 7-10 days, then q48h × 7-10 days[52]	Postoperative adrenalectomy
	1 mg/kg PO q24h × 7-14 days[52]	Use following heartworm adulticide treatment; thromboembolism
	1.25-2.5 mg/kg PO q24h[52]	Eosinophilic gastroenteritis; treat until clinical signs abate; gradually decrease to q48h
	1.5 mg/kg PO q24h × 7 days, then taper to 0.8 mg/kg PO q24h[46]	Management of eosinophilic gastroenteritis
	2 mg/kg PO q24h[52]	Palliative therapy for lymphosarcoma[a] or chronic inflammatory bowel disease; taper dose as able
Procarbazine	50 mg/m² PO q24h × 14 days[4]	Part of a noninvasive protocol for treatment of lymphoma[a]
Proligestone	50 mg SC[59]	Induce ovulation when jill has been in estrus for 10 days; not available in the United States

Continued

TABLE 11-7 Miscellaneous Agents Used in Ferrets. (cont'd)

Agent	Dosage	Comments
Prostaglandin F_2-α (Lutalyse, Upjohn)	0.1-0.5 mg/animal IM prn[7]	Metritis; expels necrotic debris
	0.5 mg/animal IM[7]	Can induce delivery on day 41 if only one kit; follow with 6 U oxytocin 1-4 hr later
Pyridostigmine (Mestinon, Valeant)	1 mg/kg PO q8h[13]	Oral cholinesterase inhibitor for potential treatment of myasthenia gravis
	1 mg/kg PO q8-12h[2]	Myasthenia gravis; overdose possible with long-term use
Ranitidine bismuth citrate (Pylorid, Glaxo Wellcome)	24 mg/kg PO q8h[44]	*Helicobacter*; use in combination with clarithromycin; not available in the United States
Ranitidine HCl (Zantac, Glaxo Wellcome)	3.5 mg/kg PO q12h[25,66]	Inhibits acid secretion; gastrointestinal ulcers
S-adenosylmethionine (SAMe) (Vetri-SAMe, Vetriscience Labs)	20-100 mg/kg PO q24h[49]	Adjunctive treatment for liver disease; hepatoprotectant; improves synthesis of glutathione and other compounds important for liver function
Saw palmetto	0.15 mL/animal PO q12h[52]	Homeopathic remedy used for dysuria associated with prostatic enlargement
Stanozolol (Winstrol, Upjohn)	0.5 mg/kg PO, SC q12h[52]	Anemia; anabolic steroid; use with caution in hepatic disease
Sucralfate (Carafate, Hoechst Marion Roussel)	25-125 mg/kg PO q8-12h[52]	Gastrointestinal ulcers; give before meals; requires acidic pH
Sulfasalazine	62.5-125 mg PO q8-24h[49]	Management of colitis
Theophylline elixir	4.25 mg/kg PO q8-12h[52]	Bronchodilator
Thyroid-stimulating hormone (TSH)	1 U IV[30]	Blood for T_4 measurement taken 120 min later
Thyroxine	0.2-0.4 mg/kg q12h[52]	Hypothyroidism; adjust and taper as needed
Trientine (Syprine, Valeant)	10 mg/kg PO q12h[25]	Chelating agent used for copper toxicosis
Ursodiol (Actigall, Ciba)	15 mg/kg PO q12h[9]	Treatment of chronic hepatopathies
Vincristine	0.12-0.2 mg/kg IV[4]	
	0.75 mg/m^2 IV[4]	Minimal myelosuppression
Vitamin A (retinol palmitate)	50,000 U IM q24h × 2 treatments[62]	Reduced mortality secondary to canine distemper virus infection
Vitamin B complex	1-2 mg/kg IM prn[52]	Dose based on thiamine content
Vitamin C	50-100 mg/kg PO q12h[25]	Adjunct therapy for lymphoma
Vitamin K	2.5 mg/kg SC, then 1-2.5 mg/kg PO divided q8-12h × 5-7 days[49]	First generation rodenticide toxicity (e.g., warfarin class)
	5 mg/kg SC, then 2.5 mg/kg PO divided q8-12h × 3 wk[49]	Second generation rodenticide toxicity (e.g., brodifacoum class)
	2.5-5 mg/kg SC, then 2.5 mg/kg PO divided q8-12h × 3-4 wk[49]	Inandione or unknown anticoagulant toxicity

TABLE 11-7 Miscellaneous Agents Used in Ferrets. (cont'd)

Agent	Dosage	Comments
Yeast, brewer's	⅛-¼ tsp PO q12h[52]	Source of chromium to stabilize glucose and insulin for animals with insulinomas
Zanamivir (Relenza, GlaxoSmithKline)	12.5 mg/kg intranasal only[5] 0.3-1 mg/kg via inhalation q12h[31]	Antiviral for influenza treatment; greater effect if used with amantadine

[a]See Table 11-13 for chemotherapy protocols for lymphoma.

TABLE 11-8 Hematologic and Biochemical Values of Ferrets.[22,43,52]

Measurements	Female	Male
Hematology[a]		
PCV (%)	34.6-55	33.6-61
RBC ($10^6/\mu L$)	6.77-9.76	7.1-13.2
Hgb (g/dL)	11.9-17.4	12-18.5
MCV (fL)	44.4-53.7	42.6-52.5
MCH (pg)	16.4-19.4	13.7-19.7
MCHC (g/dL)	33.2-42.2	30.3-34.9
WBC ($10^3/\mu L$)	2.5-18.2	4.4-19.1
Neutrophils (%)	12-84	11-82
Band cells (%)	0-4.2	0-2.2
Lymphocytes (%)	12-95	12-73
Monocytes (%)	1-8	0-9
Eosinophils (%)	0-9	0-8.5
Basophils (%)	0-2.9	0-2.7
Platelets ($10^3/\mu L$)	264-910	297-730
Reticulocytes (%)	2-14	1-12
Biochemistries		
ALP (U/L)	3-62	11-120
ALT (U/L)	54-280	54-289
AST (U/L)	40-120	28-248
Bilirubin, total (mg/dL)	0-1	0-0.1
Bile acids (μmol/L)	0.0-28.9	0.0-28.9
BUN (mg/dL)	10-45	11-42
Calcium (mg/dL)	8-10.2	8.3-11.8
Carbon dioxide (mEq/L)	16.5-27.8	12.2-28
Chloride (mEq/L)	112-124	102-126
Cholesterol (mg/dL)	122-296	64-221
Creatinine (mg/dL)	0.2-1	0.2-1
GGT (U/L)	0-5	0-5

Continued

TABLE 11-8 Hematologic and Biochemical Values of Ferrets. (cont'd)

Measurements	Female	Male
Glucose (mg/dL)	85-207	62.5-198
LDH (U/L)	—	241-752
Lipase (U/L)	—	0-200
Phosphorus (mg/dL)	4.2-10.1	4-8.7
Potassium (mEq/L)	4.2-7.7	4.1-7.3
Protein, total (g/dL)	5.1-7.2	5.3-7.4
Albumin (g/dL)	3.2-4.1	2.8-4.2
Globulin (g/dL)	2.2-3.2	2-4
Albumin:globulin	1-1.6	0.8-2.1
Sodium (mEq/L)	142-156	137-162
Triglycerides (mg/dL)	—	10-32

[a]Several of these hematology values were obtained from ferrets under isoflurane anesthesia. This can artificially lower red cell indices and may be responsible for the wide ranges in some values.

TABLE 11-9 Protein Electrophoresis Values for Ferrets.[48]

Parameter	Normal Values
Total protein (g/dL)	5.6-7.2
Albumin (g/dL)	3.3-4.1
Alpha$_1$ globulins (g/dL)	0.33-0.56
Alpha$_2$ globulins (g/dL)	0.36-0.60
Beta globulins (g/dL)	0.83-1.2
Gamma globulins (g/dL)	0.3-0.8
A/G	1.3-2.1

TABLE 11-10 Biologic and Physiologic Data of Ferrets.[43,52,64]

Parameter	Normal Values
Adult body weight, male	1-2 kg
Adult body weight, female	0.65-0.95 kg
Birth weight	6-12 g
Weight at 7 days	30 g average
Weight at 14 days	60-70 g
Sexual maturity	6-12 mo (usually 1st spring after birth)
Reproductive cycle	Induced ovulator
Gestation period	42 ± 2 days
Litter size	1-18 (average 8, primiparous jill 10)
Weaning age	6-8 wk
Eyes open	34 days

TABLE 11-10 Biologic and Physiologic Data of Ferrets. (cont'd)

Parameter	Normal Values
Hearing	32 days
Life span	5-9 yr (average in United States)
Food consumption	43 g/kg/day
Water consumption	75-100 mL/day
Gastrointestinal transit time	3-4 hr
Enteral feeding requirements	2000-3000 kcal/kg/day
Dental formula	2(I 3/3 C 1/1 P 3/3 M 1/2) = 34
Deciduous teeth erupt	20-28 days
Permanent teeth erupt	50-74 days
Canines erupt	50 days
Molars erupt (first to fourth)	53-74 days
Heart rate	200-400 beats/min
Mean systolic blood pressure	133-161 mmHg
Respiratory rate	33-36 breaths/min
Rectal temperature	37.8-40°C (100-104°F)
Blood volume	60-80 mL (5%-7% body weight)
Intraocular pressure	22.8 ± 5.5 mmHg
Endotracheal tube size	2-4 mm ID
Prothrombin time (PT)	8-16.5 sec
Partial thromboplastin time (PTT)	16-25 sec

TABLE 11-11 Urinalysis Values of Ferrets.[52]

Parameter	Male	Female
Volume (mL/24 hr)	26 (8-48)	28 (8-140)
Sodium (mmol/24 hr)	1.9 (0.4-6.7)	1.5 (0.2-5.6)
Potassium (mmol/24 hr)	2.9 (1-9.6)	2.1 (0.9-5.4)
Chloride (mmol/24 hr)	2.4 (0.7-8.5)	1.9 (0.3-7.8)
pH	6.5-7.5[a]	6.5-7.5[a]
Protein (mg/dL)	7-33	0-32
Exogenous creatinine clearance (mL/min/kg)[b]	—	3.32 ± 2.16
Insulin clearance (mL/min/kg)	—	3.02 ± 1.78
Specific gravity	1.040-1.052	—

[a]Urine pH can vary according to diet; normal urine pH in ferrets on a high-quality, meat-based diet is approximately 6.
[b]Endogenous creatinine clearance (mL/min/kg) = 2.5 ± 0.93.

TABLE 11-12 Proposed Schedule of Vaccinations and Routine Prophylactic Care for Ferrets.[43,52]

Age	Recommendation
4-6 wk	CDV[a] vaccination if dam is unvaccinated
6-8 wk	CDV[a,b] vaccination if dam was vaccinated; physical examination; fecal examination
10-11 wk	CDV[a-c] vaccination; physical examination; fecal examination
12-14 wk	CDV[a-c] vaccination; rabies vaccination;[d] physical examination; fecal examination (optional)
4-8 mo	Spay/castrate; fecal examination; remove musk glands (optional); start heartworm and flea prevention (endemic areas)
1 yr	CDV[a,e] booster; rabies booster;[d] physical examination; dental prophylaxis and fecal examination if indicated; CBC; heartworm and flea prevention
2 yr	CDV[a,e,f] booster; rabies booster;[d] physical examination; dental prophylaxis and fecal examination if indicated; CBC; heartworm and flea prevention
3 yr and older (every 6 mo)	CDV[a,e,f] booster (annual); rabies booster[d] (annual); physical examination; dental prophylaxis and fecal examination if indicated; CBC; serum chemistries, including fasting blood glucose; heartworm and flea prevention

[a]CDV, canine distemper vaccine; Purevax (Merial) is the only CDV approved for use in ferrets; if Purevax is unavailable, other vaccines which have been used include Novibac DPv (Merck) and Recombitek (Merial).
[b]Purevax is recommended to be administered at 8 wk, then every 3 wk for 3 doses.
[c]Vaccinations are generally administered at 2-3 wk intervals until the ferret is 12-14 wk of age.
[d]Only a killed virus vaccine (Imrab 3, Rhône Merieux) should be used. Vaccines should be separated by several days to reduce vaccine reactions.
[e]In previously unvaccinated adults, an initial series of two vaccinations given 14-28 days apart should be given.
[f]Rabies and distemper titers are under evaluation and may alter the revaccination schedule of older animals.

TABLE 11-13 Chemotherapy Protocols for Lymphoma in Ferrets.[a]

		Protocol I[47,52]	
Week	Day	Agent	Dosage
1	1	Prednisone	1-2 mg/kg PO q12h and continued throughout therapy
	1	Vincristine	0.025 mg/kg IV
	3	Cyclophosphamide	10 mg/kg PO, SC
2	8	Vincristine	0.025 mg/kg IV
3	15	Vincristine	0.025 mg/kg IV
4	22	Vincristine	0.025 mg/kg IV
	24	Cyclophosphamide	10 mg/kg PO, SC
7	46	Cyclophosphamide	10 mg/kg PO, SC
9	63	Prednisone	Gradually decrease dose to 0 over the next 4 wk

TABLE 11-13 Chemotherapy Protocols for Lymphoma in Ferrets. (cont'd)

Protocol II[b,52]		
Week	Agent	Dosage
1	Vincristine	0.025 mg/kg IV
	L-asparaginase	400 U/kg IP
	Prednisone	1 mg/kg PO q24h and continued throughout therapy
2	Cyclophosphamide	10 mg/kg SC
3	Doxorubicin	1 mg/kg IV
4-6	As weeks 1-3 above, but discontinue L-asparaginase	—
8	Vincristine	0.025 mg/kg IV
10	Cyclophosphamide	10 mg/kg SC
12	Vincristine	0.025 mg/kg IV
14	Methotrexate	0.5 mg/kg IV

Protocol III[47]		
Week	Agent	Dosage
1	L-asparaginase	10,000 U/m^2 SC
	Cytoxin	250 mg/m^2 PO, SC (in 50 mL/kg of NaCl SC)
	Prednisone	2 mg/kg PO daily for 7 days, then q48h throughout therapy
2	L-asparaginase	10,000 U/m^2 SC
	Perform CBC[c]	
3	L-asparaginase	10,000 U/m^2 SC
	Cytosar	300 mg/m^2 SC × 2 days (dilute 100 mg with 1 mL H$_2$O)
4	Perform CBC[c]	
5	Cytoxin	250 mg/m^2 PO, SC (in 50 mL/kg of NaCl SC)
7	Methotrexate Perform CBC[c]	0.8 mg/kg IM
8	Perform CBC[c]	
9	Cytoxin	250 mg/m^2 PO, SC (in 50 mL/kg of NaCl SC)
11	Cytosar	300 mg/m^2 SC × 2 days (dilute 100 mg with 1 mL H$_2$O)
	Leukeran	1 tablet/animal PO or ½ tablet/animal PO × 2 days
12	Perform CBC[c]	
13	Cytoxin	250 mg/m^2 PO, SC (in 50 mL/kg of NaCl SC)
15	Procarbazine	50 mg/m^2 PO q24h × 14 days
16	Perform CBC[c]	
17	Perform CBC[c]	
18	Cytoxin	250 mg/m^2 PO, SC (in 50 mL/kg of NaCl SC)
20	Cytosar	300 mg/m^2 SC × 2 days (dilute 100 mg with 1 mL H$_2$O)
	Leukeran	1 tablet/animal PO or ½ tablet/animal PO × 2 days
23	Cytoxin	250 mg/m^2 PO, SC (in 50 mL/kg of NaCl SC)
26	Procarbazine	50 mg/m^2 PO q24h × 14 days
27	Perform CBC[c] and chemistry panel	If not in remission, continue weeks 20-26 for 3 cycles

Continued

TABLE 11-13 Chemotherapy Protocols for Lymphoma in Ferrets. (cont'd)

	Protocol IV[4]	
Week	Agent	Dosage
3 days	L-asparaginase	400 U/kg SC (premedicate with diphenhydramine)
1	Vincristine	0.12 mg/kg IV
	Prednisone	1 mg/kg PO q24h continue throughout therapy
	Cyclophosphamide	10 mg/kg PO
2	Vincristine	0.12 mg/kg IV
3	Vincristine	0.12 mg/kg IV
4	Vincristine	0.12 mg/kg IV
	Cyclophosphamide	10 mg/kg PO
7, 10, 13, etc.	Vincristine	0.12 mg/kg IV
	Cyclophosphamide	10 mg/kg PO
		Continue therapy every 3 wk for 1 yr, then decrease to every 4-6 wk
Rescue treatment	Doxorubicin	1-2 mg/kg IV (over 20 min)

[a]CBC should be checked weekly during therapy; after therapy is discontinued, continue to monitor CBC and do physical examination at 3-mo intervals.
[b]Protocol is continued in sequence biweekly after week 14, making the therapy protocol less intensive.
[c]If CBC shows severe myelosuppression, reduce dosage by 25% for all subsequent treatments of the previously used myelosuppressive drug.

TABLE 11-14 Conversion of Body Weight (kg) to Body Surface Area (m^2).[47]

Body Weight (kg)	Body Surface Area (m^2)
0.5	0.063
0.6	0.071
0.7	0.079
0.8	0.086
0.9	0.093
1.0	0.100
1.1	0.107
1.2	0.113
1.3	0.119
1.4	0.125
1.5	0.131
1.6	0.137
1.7	0.142
1.8	0.148
1.9	0.153
2.0	0.159
2.1	0.164
2.2	0.169
2.3	0.174
2.4	0.179
2.5	0.184

REFERENCES

1. Antinoff N. Neoplasia in ferrets. In: Bonagura JD, ed. *Kirk's Current Veterinary Therapy XIII: Small Animal Practice*. Philadelphia: WB Saunders Co; 2000:1149-1152.
2. Antinoff N. Diagnosis and successful treatment of myasthenia gravis in a ferret. *ExoticsCon*. 2015;367.
3. Antinoff N, Giovanella CJ. Musculoskeletal and neurologic diseases. In: Quesenberry KE, Carpenter JW, eds. *Ferrets, Rabbits, and Rodents: Clinical Medicine and Surgery*. 3rd ed. St. Louis: Saunders/Elsevier; 2012:132-140.
4. Antinoff N, Hahn K. Ferret oncology. *Vet Clin North Am Exot Anim Pract*. 2004;7:579-626.
5. Barron HW, Rosenthal KL. Respiratory diseases. In: Quesenberry KE, Carpenter JW, eds. *Ferrets, Rabbits, and Rodents: Clinical Medicine and Surgery*. 3rd ed. St. Louis: Saunders/Elsevier; 2012:78-85.
6. Beaufrère H, Neta M, Smith DA. Demodectic mange associated with lymphoma in a ferret. *J Exot Pet Med*. 2009;18:57-61.
7. Bell JA. Periparturient and neonatal diseases. In: Quesenberry KE, Carpenter JW, eds. *Ferrets, Rabbits, and Rodents: Clinical Medicine and Surgery*. 2nd ed. St. Louis: WB Saunders Co; 2004:50-57.
8. Bennett KR, Gaunt MC, Parker DL. Constant rate infusion of glucagon as an emergency treatment for hypoglycemia in a domestic ferret (*Mustela putorius furo*). *J Am Vet Med Assoc*. 2015;246:451-454.
9. Burgess M, Garner M. Clinical aspects of inflammatory bowel disease in ferrets. *Exot DVM*. 2002;4(2):29-34.
10. Carpenter JW. *Personal observation*; 2017.
11. Chen S, Michels D, Culpepper E. Nonsurgical management of hyperadrenocorticism in ferrets. *Vet Clin Exot Anim*. 2014;17:35-49.
12. Coburn DR, Morris JA. The treatment of *Salmonella typhimurium* infection in ferrets. *Cornell Vet*. 1949;39:198.
13. Couturier J, Huynh M, Boussarie D, et al. Autoimmune myasthenia gravis in a ferret. *J Am Vet Med Assoc*. 2009;235:1462-1466.
14. Fisher M, Beck W, Hutchinson MJ. Efficacy and safety of selamectin (Stronghold®/Revolution™) used off-label in exotic pets. *Intern J Appl Res Vet Med*. 2007;5:87-96.
15. Fox JG, Bell JA. Diseases of the genitourinary system. In: Fox JG, Marini RP, eds. *Biology and Diseases of the Ferret*. 3rd ed. Ames: Wiley Blackwell; 2014:335-361.
16. Fox JG, Lee A. The role of *Helicobacter* species in newly recognized gastrointestinal diseases of animals. *Lab Anim Sci*. 1997;47:222-227.
17. Fox JG, Marini RP. *Helicobacter mustelae* infection in ferrets: pathogenesis, epizootiology, diagnosis, and treatment. *Semin Avian Exot Pet Med*. 2001;10:36-44.
18. Giral M, Garcia-Olma DC, Gomez-Juarez M, et al. Anaesthetic effect in the ferret of alfaxalone alone and in combination with medetomidine or tramadol: a pilot study. *Lab Anim*. 2014;48:313-320.
19. Greenacre CB. Incidence of adverse events in ferrets vaccinated with distemper or rabies vaccine: 143 cases (1995-2001). *J Am Vet Med Assoc*. 2003;223:663-665.
20. Greenacre CB, Dowling M, Nobrega-Lee M. Histoplasmosis in a group of domestic ferrets (*Mustela putorius furo*). *ExoticsCon*. 2015;363.
21. Hawkins MG. Advances in exotic mammal clinical therapeutics. *Vet Clin N Am Exot Anim Pract*. 2015;18:323-327.
22. Hein J, Spreyer F, Sauter-Louis C, et al. Reference ranges for laboratory parameters in ferrets. *Vet Rec*. 2012;171:218.
23. Hess L. Insulin glargine treatment of a ferret with diabetes mellitus. *J Am Vet Med Assoc*. 2012;241:1490-1494.
24. Hoppes SM. The senior ferret. *Vet Clin North Am Exot Anim Pract*. 2010;13:107-121.
25. Jepson L. Ferrets. In: Jepson L, ed. *Exotic Animal Medicine: A Quick Reference Guide*. 2nd ed. St. Louis: Elsevier; 2016:1-42.

26. Johnson D. Current therapies for ferret adrenal disease. *Proc Atlantic Coast Vet Conf.* 2006;1-7.
27. Johnson-Delaney C. Ferrets: anaesthesia and analgesia. In: Keeble E, Meredith A, eds. *BSAVA Manual of Rodents and Ferrets*. Gloucester, UK: British Small Animal Veterinary Association; 2009:245-253.
28. Johnson-Delaney CA. *Ferret Medicine and Surgery*. Boca Raton: CRC Press; 2017:457-467.
29. Katzenbach JE, Wittenburg LA, Allweiler SI, et al. Pharmacokinetics of single-dose buprenorphine, butorphanol, and hydromorphone in the domestic ferret (Mustela putorius furo). J Exot Pet Med. In press.
30. Keeble E. Endocrine diseases in small mammals. *In Pract.* 2001;23:570-585.
31. Kiupel M, Perpinan D. Viral diseases of ferrets. In: Fox JG, Marini RP, eds. *Biology and Diseases of the Ferret*. 3rd ed. Ames: Wiley Blackwell; 2014:439-517.
32. Ko JC, Marini RP. Anesthesia. In: Fox JG, Marini RP, eds. *Biology and Diseases of the Ferret*. 3rd ed. Ames: Wiley Blackwell; 2014:259-283.
33. Ko JC, Heaton-Jones TG, Nicklin CF, et al. Comparison of sedative and cardiorespiratory effects of diazepam, acepromazine, and xylazine in ferrets. *J Am Anim Hosp Assoc.* 1998;34:234-241.
34. Ko JC, Nicklin CF, Montgomery T, et al. Comparison of anesthetic and cardiorespiratory effects of tiletamine-zolazepam-xylazine and tiletamine-zolazepam-xylazine-butorphanol in ferrets. *J Am Anim Hosp Assoc.* 1998;34:164-174.
35. Kraus MS, Morrisey JK. Cardiovascular and other diseases. In: Quesenberry KE, Carpenter JW, eds. *Ferrets, Rabbits, and Rodents: Clinical Medicine and Surgery*. 3rd ed. St. Louis: Saunders/Elsevier; 2012:62-77.
36. Larsen KS, Siggurdsson H, Mencke N. Efficacy of imidacloprid, imidacloprid/permethrin and phoxim for flea control in the Mustelidae (ferrets, mink). *Parasitol Res.* 2005;97:S107-S112.
37. Lennox A. GI disease in ferrets. Available at: https://www.cliniciansbrief.com/article/gi-disease-ferrets. Published Sept 2013. Accessed May 25, 2017.
38. Lennox A. Alternative surgical options for elective altering in exotic companion mammals. *ExoticsCon.* 2015;435-444.
39. Lewington JH. Appendix. In: Lewington JH, ed. *Ferret Husbandry, Medicine and Surgery*. Oxford: Butterworth Heinemann; 2000:273-282.
40. Longley L. Ferret anaesthesia. In: Longley L, ed. *Anaesthesia of Exotic Pets*. Philadelphia: Saunders/Elsevier; 2008:85-95.
41. Malik R, Martin P, McGill J, et al. Successful treatment of invasive nasal cryptococcosis in a ferret. *Aust Vet J.* 2000;78:158-159.
42. Malka S, Hawkins MG, Zabolotzky SM, et al. Immune-mediated pure red cell aplasia in a domestic ferret. *J Am Vet Med Assoc.* 2010;237:695-700.
43. Marini RP. Physical examination, preventive medicine, and diagnosis in the ferret. In: Fox JG, Marini RP, eds. *Biology and Diseases of the Ferret*. 3rd ed. Ames: Wiley Blackwell; 2014:235-258.
44. Marini RP, Fox JG, Taylor NS, et al. Ranitidine bismuth citrate and clarithromycin, alone or in combination, for eradication of *Helicobacter mustelae* infection in ferrets. *Am J Vet Res.* 1999;60:1280-1286.
45. Marini RP, Ryden EB, Rosenblad WD, et al. Functional islet cell tumor in six ferrets. *J Am Vet Med Assoc.* 1993;202:430-433.
46. Maurer KJ, Fox JG. Diseases of the gastrointestinal system. In: Fox JG, Marini RP, eds. *Biology and Diseases of the Ferret*. 3rd ed. Ames: Wiley Blackwell; 2014:363-375.
47. Mayer J, Erdman SE, Fox JG. Diseases of the hematopoietic system. In: Fox JG, Marini RP, eds. *Biology and Diseases of the Ferret*. 3rd ed. Ames: Wiley Blackwell; 2014:311-334.
48. Melillo A. Applications of serum protein electrophoresis in exotic mammals. *Vet Clin North Am Exot Anim Pract.* 2013;16:211-225.
49. Meredith A. *Small Animal Formulary—Part B: Exotic Pets*. 9th ed. British Small Animal Veterinary Association: Gloucester; 2015.

50. Miller DS, Eagle RP, Zabel S, et al. Efficacy and safety of selamectin in the treatment of *Otodectes cynotis* infestation in domestic ferrets. *Vet Rec.* 2006;159:748.
51. Morrisey JK. Ferrets: therapeutics. In: Keeble E, Meredith A, eds. *BSAVA Manual of Rodents and Ferrets*. Gloucester, UK: British Small Animal Veterinary Association; 2009:237-244.
52. Morrisey JK. Ferrets. In: Carpenter JW, ed. *Exotic Animal Formulary*. 4th ed. St. Louis: Elsevier Saunders; 2013:560-594.
53. Morrisey JK, Carpenter JW. Formulary. In: Quesenberry KE, Carpenter JW, eds. *Ferrets, Rabbits, and Rodents: Clinical Medicine and Surgery*. 3rd ed. St. Louis: Saunders/Elsevier; 2012:566-575.
54. Neuwirth L, Isaza R, Bellah J, et al. Adrenal neoplasia in seven ferrets. *Vet Radiol Ultrasound.* 1993;34:340-346.
55. Patterson MM, Kirchain SM. Comparison of three treatments for control of ear mites in ferrets. *Lab Anim Sci.* 1999;49:655-657.
56. Patterson MM, Fox JC, Eberhard ML. Parasitic diseases. In: Fox JG, Marini RP, eds. *Biology and Diseases of the Ferret*. 3rd ed. Ames: Wiley Blackwell; 2014:553-572.
57. Perpinan D, Ramis A, Tomas A, et al. Outbreak of canine distemper in domestic ferrets (*Mustela putorius furo*). *Vet Rec.* 2008;163:246-250.
58. Pinon C, Huynh M. Flexible gastrointestinal endoscopy in ferrets. *ExoticsCon.* 2015;459-463.
59. Pollock CG. Disorders of the urinary and reproductive systems. In: Quesenberry KE, Carpenter JW, eds. *Ferrets, Rabbits, and Rodents: Clinical Medicine and Surgery*. 3rd ed. St. Louis: Saunders/Elsevier; 2012:46-61.
60. Powers LV. Bacterial and parasitic diseases of ferrets. *Vet Clin North Am Exot Anim Pract.* 2009;12:531-561.
61. Ramer JC, Benson KG, Morrisey JK, et al. Effects of melatonin administration on the clinical course of adrenocortical disease in domestic ferrets. *J Am Vet Med Assoc.* 2006;229:1743-1748.
62. Rodeheffer C, von Messling V, Milot S, et al. Disease manifestations of canine distemper virus infection in ferrets are modulated by vitamin A status. *J Nutr.* 2007;137:1916-1922.
63. Rosenthal KR, Wyre NR. Endocrine diseases. In: Quesenberry KE, Carpenter JW, eds. *Ferrets, Rabbits, and Rodents: Clinical Medicine and Surgery*. 3rd ed. St. Louis: Saunders/Elsevier; 2012:86-102.
64. Sapienza JS, Porcher D, Collins BR, et al. Tonometry in clinically normal ferrets (*Mustela putorius furo*). *Prog Vet Comp Ophthalmol.* 1991;1:291-294.
65. Schwarz LA, Solano M, Manning A, et al. The normal upper gastrointestinal examination in the ferret. *Vet Radiol Ultrasound.* 2003;44:165-172.
66. Silverman S, Tell LA. *Radiology of Rodents, Rabbits, and Ferrets: an Atlas of Normal Anatomy and Positioning*. St. Louis: Elsevier Saunders; 2005.
67. Vella D. Cryptococcosis. In: Mayer J, Donnelly TM, eds. *Clinical Veterinary Advisor: Birds and Exotic Pets*. St. Louis: Elsevier Saunders; 2013:439.
68. Wagner RA. Ferret cardiology. *Vet Clin North Am Exot Anim Pract.* 2009;12:115-134.
69. Wagner RA. Diseases of the cardiovascular system. In: Fox JG, Marini RP, eds. *Biology and Diseases of the Ferret*. 3rd ed. Ames: Wiley Blackwell; 2014:401-419.
70. Wagner RA, Bailey EM, Schneider JF, et al. Leuprolide acetate treatment of adrenocortical disease in ferrets. *J Am Vet Med Assoc.* 2001;218:1272-1274.
71. Wagner RA, Piche CA, Jöchle W, et al. Clinical and endocrine responses to treatment with deslorelin acetate implants in ferrets with adrenocortical disease. *Am J Vet Res.* 2005;66:910-914.
72. Wyre NR, Michels D, Chen S. Selected emerging diseases in ferrets. *Vet Clin North Am Exot Anim Pract.* 2013;16:469-493.

Chapter 12 Miniature Pigs

Valarie V. Tynes | Kristie Mozzachio

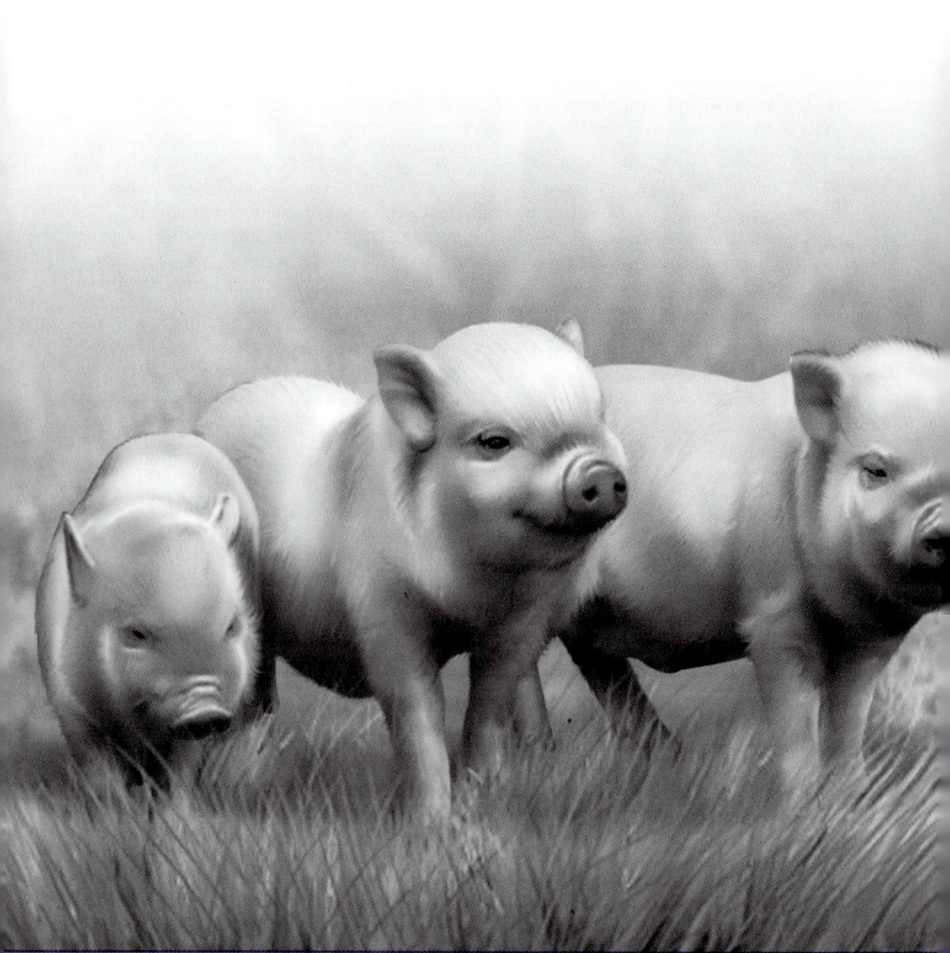

TABLE 12-1 Antimicrobial Agents Used in Miniature Pigs.[a]

Agent	Dosage	Comments
Amoxicillin	10-22 mg/kg PO q12-24h[14]	
	11-13 mg/kg PO q24h[3]	
Amoxicillin/clavulanate (Clavamox, Pfizer)	11-13 mg/kg PO q12[21]-24h[10]	
	12.5-25 mg/kg PO q12h[25,b]	
Ampicillin	20 mg/kg SC, IM q8h[3]	
	6.5 mg/kg IM q24h[10]	
• Sodium	10-20 mg/kg SC, IM, IV q6-8h[14,25,b]	
	20-40 mg/kg PO q8h[25,b]	
• Trihydrate	4.4-22 mg/kg IM q8-24h[14]	
	10-50 mg/kg SC, IM q12-24h[25,b]	
Apramycin (Apralan, Elanco)	10-20 mg/kg PO q12-24h[10]	
Ceftiofur	3-10 mg/kg IM q24h[10]	
• Hydrochloride (Excenel, Zoetis)	3-5 mg/kg IM q24h[14] × 3 days[25]	
• Sodium (Naxcel, Zoetis)	3-5 mg/kg IM q24h[14] × 3 days[25]	No more than 2 mL/injection site[c]
• Long acting (Excede, Zoetis)	5 mg/kg IM[c] q3-5d[21]	
Ceftriaxone	50-75 mg/kg IM, IV q24h[28]	
Cephalexin	10-30 mg/kg PO q6-12h[21,25,b]	
Cephradine (Velosef, Bristol-Myers Squibb)	25-50 mg/kg PO q12h[28]	
Clindamycin	11-33 mg/kg q12h PO[21,25,b]	Tusk abscesses
Doxycycline	3-5 mg/kg PO q12h[21,25,b]	Tick-associated illness
	10 mg/kg PO q24h[25,b]	
Enrofloxacin (Baytril, Bayer)	2.5-5 mg/kg IM q24h[25,30]	Extra-label use prohibited in food-producing animals; oral form extremely unpalatable to pigs making PO administration nearly impossible, even with compounded flavoring[21]
	7.5 mg/kg SC, IM[c]	
Florfenicol (Nuflor, Intervet)	15 mg/kg IM q48h[25]	
	20 mg/kg IM q48h[14]	
	20 mg/kg PO, IM, IV q48h[17]	
Nuflor 2.3% concentrate solution	400 mg/gal drinking water × 5 days[25]	

Continued

TABLE 12-1 Antimicrobial Agents Used in Miniature Pigs. (cont'd)

Agent	Dosage	Comments
Gentamicin	5 mg/kg PO q24h[10]	
	10-15 mg/kg SC, IM q24h[25]	
	1.1-2.2 mg/kg × 3 days in drinking water[25]	Colibacillosis and swine dysentery
Lincomycin	10 mg/kg IM q24h[10]	Mycoplasma
	11 mg/kg IM q24h[14,25]	
	8.4 mg/kg q24h in drinking water[14] × 5-10 days[25]	Swine dysentery
Metronidazole	Anaerobes: 15 mg/kg PO q12h[25,b]	Prohibited in food-producing animals
	Giardia: 12-15 mg/kg PO q12h for 8 days[25,b]	
	15-20 mg/kg PO q12h[15]	
Neomycin	10 mg/kg PO q6h[10]	
	11 mg/kg PO q24h[2]	
Oxytetracycline	44-55 mg/kg PO q24h[3]	
	7-11 mg/kg IM q24h[3]	
• Long acting (Liquamycin LA-200, Zoetis)	1.4-2.3 mg/kg q24h IM × maximum 4 days[c]	
Penicillin G, procaine	15,000-25,000 U/kg IM q24h[25]	
	20,000-45,000 U/kg IM q24h[10]	
	20,000-60,000 U/kg IM q24h[14]	
Spectinomycin (Spectam, Merial)	6.6-22 mg/kg IM q12-24h[25]	
	50-100 mg/pig PO[25]	
Tetracycline	10-20 mg/kg IM q24h[10]	Enteritis and pneumonia
	11 mg/kg q12h in water or as a bolus[25]	
• Long acting	20 mg/kg IM q48h[10]	
Trimethoprim/ sulfadiazine	15 mg/kg PO q12h[25,b]	
	30 mg/kg PO q12-24h[25,b]	
	30 mg/kg PO q24h[14]	
Tulathromycin (Draxxin, Zoetis)	2.5 mg/kg IM as a single injection[25]	Draxxin 25 formulation available for small pigs
Tylosin (Tylan, Elanco)	9 mg/kg IM q12-24h[10]	

[a]Not to be used in animals for human consumption.
[b]Authors note: In the past, in the absence of published dosages specific to swine, the authors have often found it necessary to rely upon canine dosages published by Papich (2016) when treating pet pigs. This has generally been found to be safe and effective.
[c]From product insert.

TABLE 12-2 Antiparasitic Agents Used in Miniature Pigs.[a]

Agent	Dosage	Comments
Dichlorvos	11.2-21.6 mg/kg PO once[25] 20 mg/kg PO[2]	
Doramectin (Dectomax, Zoetis)	0.3 mg/kg IM[16,25]	Use same as ivermectin; may cause less discomfort than ivermectin when injected[21]
Fenbendazole (Safe-Guard, Intervet)	3 mg/kg PO q24h × 3 days[16] 9 mg/kg PO in divided doses × 3-12 days[b]	Whipworms
Ivermectin	0.3 mg/kg PO, SC, IM[4,5,25]	Repeat in 10-14 days for sarcoptic mange; PO dosing ineffective for treating sarcoptic mange; may cause pain on injection[21]
Levamisole	10 mg/kg PO[2] 8 mg/kg in drinking water[25]	
Piperazine	200 mg/kg PO[2] 110 mg/kg in drinking water[25]	
Pyrantel pamoate	6.6 mg/kg PO, repeat prn[4,5] 22 mg/kg in feed, once[21,25]	Can give ½ of this dose initially if suspect high parasite burden; in 7-10 days, repeat with full dose[21]
Sulfadimethoxine (Albon, Zoetis)	25 mg/kg PO[2] 55 mg/kg PO as loading dose followed by 27.5 mg/kg PO q12h[25,c]	Coccidia

[a]Not to be used in animals for human consumption.
[b]From product insert.
[c]Authors note: In the past, in the absence of published dosages specific to swine, the authors have often found it necessary to rely upon canine dosages published by Papich (2016) when treating pet pigs. This has generally been found to be safe and effective.

TABLE 12-3 Chemical Restraint/Anesthetic Agents Used in Miniature Pigs.[a]

Agent	Dosage	Comments
Acepromazine	0.1-0.45 mg/kg IM[3]	Tranquilization; slow onset of action; inconsistent results
	0.2-1.1 mg/kg IM[5]	Higher doses reportedly produce more profound tranquilization
Acepromazine (A)/ ketamine (K)	(A) 0.5-1.1 mg/kg IM, followed in 15 min by (K) 15-33 mg/kg IM[3] (A) 1.1 mg/kg + (K) 33 mg/kg IM, SC[29]	
Atipamezole	For IM dose, see comments	Reverses detomidine and dexmedetomidine, and potentially other α_2-adrenergic agonists; actual volume is same as volume used for detomidine (1 mg/mL) or dexmedetomidine (0.5 mg/mL)

Continued

TABLE 12-3 Chemical Restraint/Anesthetic Agents Used in Miniature Pigs. (cont'd)

Agent	Dosage	Comments
Atropine	0.02-0.05 mg/kg SC, IM, IV[29]	Anesthesia adjunct; increases heart rate, decreases GI and respiratory secretions
Azaperone (Stresnil, Schering-Plough)	— 0.25-0.5 mg/kg IM[4] 0.25-2 mg/kg IM[24] 2 mg/kg IM[4] 2-8 mg/kg IM, SC[9,24,29] 5-8 mg/kg IM[3]	See also ketamine for combinations Relaxation, sedation, without ataxia up to 0.5 mg/kg dose Moderate sedation; doses exceeding 2 mg/kg likely to produce negative side effects such as hypotension, bradycardia, and decreased cardiac output and contractility[24]
Azaperone (Az)/midazolam (Mi)/± atropine (At)	(Az) 4 mg/kg + (Mi) 0.5 mg/kg ± (At) 0.04 mg/kg IM[3]	Moderate to deep sedation; no analgesia
Butorphanol	—	See detomidine, dexmedetomidine, ketamine, tiletamine/zolazepam, xylazine for combinations; see Table 12-4 for analgesic doses
Detomidine (Dormosedan, Zoetis)	—	Detomidine combinations follow
Detomidine (De)/butorphanol (B)/Midazolam (Mz)	(De) 0.06-0.125 mg/kg + (B) 0.3-0.4 mg/kg + 0.3-0.4 (Mz) IM[24]	Rapid, smooth induction with excellent relaxation
Dexmedetomidine (Dexdomitor, Zoetis)	—	See dexmedetomidine/midazolam/butorphanol for combination
Dexmedetomidine (De)/midazolam (Mi)/butorphanol (B)	(De) 0.01-0.04 mg/kg + (Mi) 0.1-0.3 mg/kg + (B) 0.2-0.4 mg/kg IM[20,21]	Can substitute xylazine 1 mg/kg (for dexmedetomidine)
Diazepam	— 0.1-0.5 mg/kg PO[24,33] 0.5-1.5 mg/kg IV[30] 0.5-2 mg/kg IM[3] 5.5-8.5 mg/kg IM[7]	See ketamine for combination Calming for car trip or veterinary examination Sedation; rarely used in conscious pigs since venous access is extremely difficult Effective muscle relaxation Sedation
Fentanyl	0.02-0.04 mg/kg SC, IM, IV q2h[25,b] 0.02-0.05 mg/kg, IM, IV[18]	
Fentanyl/droperidol (Innovar-Vet, Schering-Plough)	1 mL/10-14 kg IM[35] 1 mL/9-25 kg IM[5,18]	Sedation; maximum effect in 20 min; analgesia with some mild sedation Tranquilization; minor procedures

TABLE 12-3 Chemical Restraint/Anesthetic Agents Used in Miniature Pigs. (cont'd)

Agent	Dosage	Comments
Flumazenil	0.02 mg/kg IV[25]	Benzodiazepine (midazolam, diazepam) reversal; use with caution if ketamine is only other agent being used
	1 mg/10-15 mg midazolam IM[7]	
Glycopyrrolate	0.004-0.01 mg/kg SC, IM, IV[29]	Anesthesia adjunct; increases heart rate, decreases GI and respiratory secretions; use with caution as heart may be overtaxed; atropine preferred[20]
Guaifenesin(G)/ketamine (K)/xylazine (X)	0.5-1 mg/kg IV to induce unpremedicated pig; decrease dose by 50% if sedative or tranquilizer given prior to induction[35]	Administer atropine IM prior to induction. Combination prepared using (G) (50 mg/mL), (K) (2 mg/mL), and (X) (1 mg/mL); induction; maintain at 2 mL/kg/h; rarely used since IV access is impractical in conscious pigs
Isoflurane (or sevoflurane)	4%-5% induction or to effect[21,33]	Especially recommended for sick or debilitated pigs and for those <8 weeks of age
	1%-3% maintenance[20,21,33]	
Ketamine	Use only in combination	Ketamine combinations follow; see guaifenesin, tiletamine/zolazepam for additional combinations
		Used alone results in poor muscle relaxation, poor visceral analgesia, and rough recovery (hyperkinesia, severe and prolonged ataxia, distress vocalizations),[24] especially IM; use with other agents
Ketamine (K)/azaperone (Az)	(K) 15 mg/kg + (Az) 2 mg/kg IM, SC[9,29]	
Ketamine (K)/diazepam (D)	(K) 8-10 mg/kg + (D) 1-2 mg/kg IM[3]	
	(K) 15-20 mg/kg + (D) 2 mg/kg IM, SC[9,29]	
	(D) 1-2 mg/kg IM, followed by (K) 12-20 mg/kg IM[5]	Short-term anesthesia; prolong with (K) 2-4 mg/kg IV prn; minimal analgesia; smoother recovery than ketamine alone[5]
Ketamine(K)/midazolam (Mi)	(K) 10 mg/kg + (Mi) 1 mg/kg IM[3]	This drug combination can cause profound hypothermia[29]
Ketamine (K)/xylazine (X)	(K) 15-20 mg/kg + (X) 2 mg/kg IM, SC[3,9,29]	Anesthesia; rough recovery
	(K) 10 mg/kg + (X) 1 mg/kg IM[20]	
	(X) 2.2 mg/kg IM, followed by (K) 12-20 mg/kg IM[5]	Short-term anesthesia; prolong with (K) 2-4 mg/kg IV prn

Continued

TABLE 12-3 Chemical Restraint/Anesthetic Agents Used in Miniature Pigs. (cont'd)

Agent	Dosage	Comments
Ketamine (K)/xylazine (X)/butorphanol (B)	(K) 5 mg/kg + (X) 2 mg/kg + (B) 0.22 mg/kg IM[3]	Anesthesia; butorphanol enhances analgesia
	(K) 11 mg/kg + (X) 2 mg/kg + (B) 0.22 mg/kg IM[7]	
Ketamine (K)/xylazine (X)/midazolam (Mi)	(K) 5-10 mg/kg + (X) 1 mg/kg + (Mi) 0.2 mg/kg IM[20]	Can substitute dexmedetomidine (for xylazine) at 10-40 mcg/kg
Ketamine (K)/xylazine (X)/oxymorphone (O)	(K) 2 mg/kg + (X) 2 mg/kg + (O) 0.075 mg/kg IV[29]	
Lidocaine 2%	Topical[18]	Spray onto larynx 2 min before intubation to prevent laryngospasm
Lidocaine/prilocaine (EMLA cream, AstraZeneca)	Topical[18]	Apply to skin at time of premedication to ease intravenous access; may take 20-30 min to take effect
Midazolam	—	See azaperone, dexmedetomidine, ketamine, xylazine for combinations
	0.1-0.5 mg/kg IM, IV[9,29]	Sedation
Naloxone (P/M Naloxone, Schering-Plough)	0.5-2 mg/kg IV[29]	Narcotic reversal; given to effect prn
Nitrous oxide	—	Nitrous oxide and oxygen at equal levels (1-2 L/min) before isoflurane induction; may help calm animal during mask induction[33]
Pentobarbital	20-40 mg/kg IV[9,29]	Anesthesia with some analgesia
Promazine hydrochloride	0.4-1 mg/kg IV[13]	Tranquilization
	0.5-2 mg/kg IM[13]	Tranquilization
Sevoflurane	—	See isoflurane
Thiamylal	6.6-30 mg/kg IV[9,29]	Induction
Tiletamine/zolazepam (Telazol, Fort Dodge)	—	Tiletamine/zolazepam combinations follow
		Poor muscle relaxation; may cause rough recovery;[24,33] avoid using as sole agent
		Anesthesia with good analgesia
Tiletamine/zolazepam (T)/ketamine (K)/xylazine (X)	—	Reconstitute (T) (500 mg) with 2.5 mL (K) (100 mg/mL) and 2.5 mL (X) (100 mg/mL), instead of sterile water; mixture has 50 mg/mL each of tiletamine, zolazepam, ketamine, xylazine; rough recovery
	2.2-4.4 mg/kg IM[5]	Induction; maintain with 2.2 mg/kg IV prn
	0.03 mL/kg IM[21]	Heavy sedation; useful prior to euthanasia

TABLE 12-3 Chemical Restraint/Anesthetic Agents Used in Miniature Pigs. (cont'd)

Agent	Dosage	Comments
Tiletamine/zolazepam (T)/xylazine (X)	(T) 2 mg/kg + (X) 2 mg/kg IV[4]	Not routinely recommended; difficult venous access in a conscious pig makes this impractical
	(T) 4-6 mg/kg + (X) 2.2 mg/kg IM[4,9]	Anesthesia; rapid induction; poor muscle relaxation; may have rough recovery
	(T) 4.4 mg/kg + (X) 4.4 mg/kg IM, SC[29]	
	(T) 4.4 mg/kg + (X) 2.2-4.4 mg/kg IM[3]	
	(T) 4.4-6 mg/kg + (X) 1.1-4.4 mg/kg IM[7]	
	(X) 2.2 mg/kg, then (T) 2-4 mg/kg IM[13]	Anesthesia duration of 30-40 min; the use of two separate injections makes this an impractical choice
Tiletamine/zolazepam (T)/xylazine (X)/butorphanol (B)	(T) 0.6 mg/kg + (X) 2-3 mg/kg + (B) 0.3-0.4 mg/kg IM[24]	
	(T) 4.4 mg/kg + (X) 2.2 mg/kg + (B) 0.22 mg/kg IM, SC[29]	
Xylazine	—	See also guaifenesin, ketamine, tiletamine/zolazepam for combinations
	0.5-3 mg/kg IM[5]	Sedation; tranquilization; some analgesia; deep sedation seldom encountered
Xylazine (X)/butorphanol (B)/midazolam (Mi)	(X) 2-3 mg/kg + (B) 0.3-0.4 mg/kg + (Mi) 0.3-0.4 mg/kg IM[24]	Antagonize xylazine with atipamezole or yohimbine and butorphanol with naltrexone; xylazine or midazolam can be administered as a premedicant or concurrently[24]
Yohimbine	0.25-0.5 mg/kg SC, IM[25,b]	α_2-antagonist (xylazine, dexmedetomidine, detomidine reversal)
	0.11 mg/kg IV[25,b]	
	0.3 mg/kg SC, IM, IV[7]	

[a]Not to be used in animals for human consumption.
[b]Authors note: In the past, in the absence of published dosages specific to swine, the authors have often found it necessary to rely upon canine dosages published by Papich (2016) when treating pet pigs. This has generally been found to be safe and effective.

TABLE 12-4 Analgesic Agents Used in Miniature Pigs.[a]

Agent	Dosage	Comments
Aspirin	10-20 mg/kg PO q6-8h[22,25,29]	Also antiinflammatory and antipyretic; use enteric coated tablets
Bupivicaine (multi-vesicular liposomal)	Infiltrate surgical site with 100-200 mg/site[25,b]	Local anesthetic
Buprenorphine	0.005-0.01 mg/kg IM q12h[11] 0.005-0.01 mg/kg IM, IV q8-12h[18] 0.005-0.02 mg/kg IM q6-12h[3] 0.01-0.05 mg/kg SC, IM, IV q6-12h[22] 0.01-0.05 mg/kg SC, IM q8-12h[29] 0.05-0.1 mg/kg IM q8-12h[9]	
Butorphanol	0.05-0.2 mg/kg SC, IV q3-4h[11] 0.1-0.3 mg/kg SC, IM q8-12h[29] 0.1-0.3 mg/kg SC, IM q4-6h[3,9] 0.2-0.4 mg/kg SC, IM, IV q2-6h[22]	
Carprofen[c]	1-4 mg/kg SC q24h[3] 2 mg/kg SC q24h[29] 2.2 mg/kg SC q12h[22] 2-3 mg/kg PO q12h[9,29] 2-4 mg/kg SC, IV q24h[17] 4.4 mg/kg SC q24h[22]	
Dexamethasone	0.01-0.04 mg/kg IM[21]	Antiinflammatory used in treating arthritis; administer once then switch to oral medications
Etodolac[c]	10-15 mg/kg PO q24h[22]	
Fentanyl	0.03-0.1 mg/kg/h IV (CRI)[3] 0.005-0.01 mg/kg SC, IM, IV q2h[25,b] 0.02-0.05 mg/kg IM, IV prn[22] 0.02-0.05 mg/kg IM q2h[9] 0.02-0.1 mg/kg/h IV CRI[22]	Analgesia
Fentanyl, transdermal patch	12.5 or 25 µg/h/27-82 kg[22]	Intense or prolonged pain or when oral or injectable analgesics are not an option; apply 12 h before surgery[22]; may last up to 72 h
Flunixin meglumine (Banamine, Schering Plough)	0.5-1 mg/kg SC, IV q12-24h[11] 1.1 mg/kg SC, IM, IV q12-24h[22] 1-2 mg/kg SC q24h[3] 2.2 mg/kg IM once[25]	
Gabapentin	5-15 mg/kg PO q12h, then increase gradually to as high as 40 mg/kg PO q8-12h prn[21,25,b]	

TABLE 12-4 Analgesic Agents Used in Miniature Pigs. (cont'd)

Agent	Dosage	Comments
Hydromorphone	0.1-0.2 mg/kg IV q2h[22]	
	0.2 mg/kg SC, IM q4-6h[22]	
Ibuprofen[c]	10 mg/kg PO q6-8h[22]	
Ketoprofen[c]	1 mg/kg PO q24h up to 5 d[22,25,b]	
	1-3 mg/kg PO, SC, IM q24h[29]	
	3 mg/kg PO, SC, IM, IV q24h[3,22,25]	
Meloxicam[c]	0.1-0.4 mg/kg PO q24h[21,22]	
	0.4 mg/kg SC, IM q24h[22,29]	
Meperidine (Demerol, Winthrop Breon)	2-10 mg/kg IM q4h[9,11]	
	10 mg/kg SC q8h[29]	
Morphine	0.2 mg/kg (max total dose 20 mg) IM q4h or prn[11]	
	0.2 mg/kg SC, IM q4h[22]	
	0.2-0.5 mg/kg IM q4h[20]	
	0.2-1 mg/kg IM q4h[3]	
Oxymorphone	0.1-0.2 mg/kg SC, IM, IV, re-dose at 0.05-0.1 mg/kg q1-2h[22]	
	0.15 mg/kg IM, SC q8-12h[29]	
	0.15 mg/kg IM q4h[9]	
Pentazocine (Talwin-V, Pharmacia & Upjohn)	1.5-3 mg/kg IM, SC q4h[9,29]	
	2-5 mg/kg SC, IM, IV q4h[22]	
Phenylbutazone	4 mg/kg IV q24h[22,25]	Also antiinflammatory and antipyretic
	4-8 mg/kg PO q12h[22]	
	5-20 mg/kg PO q12h[29]	
	10-20 mg/kg PO q12h[9]	
Prednisone	0.5-1 mg/kg PO q12-24h initially, then taper to q48h[22]	Antiinflammatory used in treating arthritis
Tramadol	2-4 mg/kg PO q6h-24h[22]	

[a]Not to be used in animals for human consumption.
[b]Authors note: In the past, in the absence of published dosages specific to swine, the authors have often found it necessary to rely upon canine dosages published by Papich (2016) when treating pet pigs. This has generally been found to be safe and effective.
[c]Potential exists for gastrointestinal upset and gastric ulcers, although these are uncommon in the pet pig; should be given with food and gastrointestinal protectants.

TABLE 12-5 Miscellaneous Agents Used in Miniature Pigs.[a]

Agent	Dosage	Comments
Dantrolene sodium (Dantrium, Procter & Gamble)	1-3 mg/kg IV[25]	Malignant hyperthermia
	5 mg/kg PO ($\pm$) 8h[8]	For treatment
	2-5 mg/kg IV q8h[8]	For treatment and prevention
	3.5-5 mg/kg IV[3]	
	5 mg/kg PO,[8,25] IV[9]	Malignant hyperthermia; treatment and prevention
Dexamethasone	0.1 mg/kg IM, IV[23]	Shock; laryngeal edema
Dextrose	10 mL/kg of 10% solution IP[4]	Hypoglycemic neonate
	20 mL/kg of 5% solution IP[4]	
Famotidine	0.1-0.2 mg/kg PO, SC, IM, IV q12h[21,24,b]	Reduce gastric acid secretion
Glucosamine (G)/chondroitin sulfate (C)	(G) 12 mg/kg + (C) 3.8 mg/kg PO q12h × 4 wk[22]	Loading dose
	(G) 4 mg/kg + (C) 1.3 mg/kg q12h[22]	Maintenance dose
Hydrogen peroxide	1 mL/5 kg PO[30]	Induces vomiting; some animals may require larger dose
Ipecac syrup	7-15 mL/animal PO[30]	Induces vomiting
Iron dextran	25 mg/animal IM in first few days of life; may repeat in 2-3 wk[26]	Iron deficiency in baby pigs; uncommon in miniature pigs so rarely used as a part of routine management practices
Kaolin/pectin	1-2 mL/kg PO q2-6h[25,b]	Antidiarrheal
Metoclopramide	0.2-0.5 mg/kg q6-8h PO, IM, IV[21,25,b]	Prevent postoperative ileus; start with the lower end of the dose to prevent cramping
Oxytocin	5-10 U/animal IM[25]	Dystocia, if not obstructed
	10-20 U/animal IM[4]	Dystocia, if not obstructed
Pentobarbital	1 mL/4.5 kg (1 mL/10 lb) IV[21,25,b]	Euthanasia
	>150 mg/kg IV[9,29]	
	100-150 mg/kg IV[3]	
Polysulfated glycosaminoglycan (Adequan, Novartis)	4.4 mg/kg IM once, then 3.3 mg/kg q4d × 7 treatments[15]	May not see results until after 3-4 treatments; if good clinical results after first 8 treatments, then decrease frequency to weekly for 1 month, then 2 ×/month, then monthly as needed for maintenance
Prostaglandin F$_2$-α (Lutalyse, Pharmacia & Upjohn)	5 mg/animal IM[4]	Induces parturition in 24-30 h when given within 3 days of expected parturition; causes abortion after 12 days of gestation
	8 mg and 5 mg (in a 25-kg pig) 12 h apart[16]	For inducing estrus; estrus should occur 3-7 days later

[a]Not to be used in animals for human consumption.
[b]Authors note: In the past, in the absence of published dosages specific to swine, the authors have often found it necessary to rely upon canine dosages published by Papich (2016) when treating pet pigs. This has generally been found to be safe and effective.

TABLE 12-6 Hematologic and Serum Biochemical Values of Miniature Pigs.

Measurement	Mean (Reference Range)[6,a]	Mean (Reference Range)[3,b]	Mean (Reference Range)[12,c]
Hematology			
PCV (%)	36 (22-50)	—	—
Hematocrit (%)	—	32-61	35-56
RBC ($10^6/\mu L$)	5.7 (3.6-7.8)	5.30-9.25	5.6-9.3
Hgb (g/dL)	12 (7.8-16.2)	9-17	10.9-17.0
MCV (fL)	63 (55-71)	40-73	46.0-72.5
MCH (pg)	21 (18-24)	15.2-26.4	13.7-24.3
MCHC (g/dL)	33.5 (31-36)	29.4-37.9	29.6-34.5
Platelets ($10^3/\mu L$)	310 (204-518)	148-898	152-845
WBC ($10^3/\mu L$)	11.5 (5.2-17.9)	4.4-26.4	6.9-32.4
Neutrophils ($10^3/\mu L$)	5.7 (0-11.4)	—	1.8-6.4
Band cells ($10^3/\mu L$)	0.03 (0-0.19)	—	0.0-24.6
Lymphocytes ($10^3/\mu L$)	5.3 (0.8-9.8)	—	2.1-17.3
Monocytes ($10^3/\mu L$)	0.2 (0-0.67)	—	0.2-1.3
Eosinophils ($10^3/\mu L$)	0.14 (0-0.73)	—	0-1.5
Basophils ($10^3/\mu L$)	0.15 (0-0.61)	—	0-0.5
Fibrinogen (g/L)	2 (1-4)	—	—
Chemistries			
ALP (U/L)	65 (27-160)	—	166-576
ALT (U/L)	53 (11-95)	20-106	—
AST (U/L)	32 (16-64)	13-53	15-90
Bilirubin, total (mg/dL)	0.25 (0.2-0.45)	0.0-0.3	0.1-0.41
BUN (mg/dL)	9.7 (4.2-15.1)	—	5.7-29
Chloride (mEq/L)	110 (106-113)	94-140	95-114
Creatine kinase (U/L)	701 (213-2852)	37-6000	—
Creatinine (mg/dL)	1.7 (1-2.3)	0.5-2.0	0.5-1.1
GGT (U/L)	35 (15-56)	25-86	20.4-96.4
Glucose (mg/dL)	105 (60-175)	43-153	56-123
Potassium (mEq/L)	4.3 (3.7-5)	3.5-7.4	3.9-7.7
Protein, total (g/dL)	7.7 (6.6-8.9)	6.0-9.4	4.9-9.4
Albumin (g/dL)	4.3 (3.6-5)	2.9-5.6	2.9-5.6
Globulin (g/dL)	—	1.4-5.2	1.4-3.7
Sodium (mEq/L)	144 (139-149)	132-153	139-153
TCO_2 (mEq/L)	24 (8-31)	—	20-29
Calcium (mg/dL)	—	8.6-12.6	9.3-11.7
Phosphorus (mg/dL)	—	4.9-9.8	5.0-10.7

[a] $n=100$, 2- to 10-year-old healthy, Vietnamese potbellied pigs.
[b] Combined ranges for adult Yucatan micropig, Gottingen, Sinclair, Yucatan, and Hanford minipigs weighing 35-70 kg and 70-90 kg.
[c] Combined ranges for male and female Hanford, Yucatan micropig, and male and female Gottingen minipigs.

TABLE 12-7 Urinalysis Reference Values for Miniature Pigs.[1,16,21,34]

Parameter	Reference Value
Specific gravity	1.010-1.050
pH	6.9 (range 5-8)
Color	Yellow-dark amber; may be slightly cloudy
Protein	Negative to trace
Red blood cells (per HPF)	0-5
White blood cells (per HPF)	0-5
Crystals	Common, occasionally pathologic;[21] calcium oxalate or triple phosphate crystals
Bacteria	Numerous in voided samples; only significant if numerous WBCs also present

TABLE 12-8 Biological and Physiological Data of Miniature Pigs.[3,5,12,16,19,22]

Parameter	Value
Life expectancy	14-21 yr (avg 15-18)
Respiratory rate (breaths/min)	
Newborn	50-60
Weaned pigs	25-40
10-15 wk	30-40
15-26 wk	25-35
Adult	12-18
Heart rate (beats/min)	
Newborn	200-250
Weaned pigs	90-100
10-15 wk	80-90
15-26 wk	75-85
Adult	70-80
Rectal temperature	37.6-39°C (99.7-102.2°F); diurnal variation in body temperature exists; temperature decreases as age increases
Weight	
Birth	250-450 g
Adult	34-91 kg (avg 55)
Reproduction	
Puberty	
• Boars	3 mo of age
• Gilts	3.5-4 mo of age
Estrous cycle	17-25 days (avg 21)
Standing heat duration	1-3 days
Ovulation	
• Gilts	24-36 h after onset of estrus
• Sows	30-44 h after onset of estrus
Gestation length	112-116 days (avg 114)
Litter size	2-15 piglets (avg 6-8)

TABLE 12-9 Preventive Medicine Recommendations for Miniature Pigs.[5,12,16,21,32]

Recommended Vaccinations

Pet pigs	
• Erysipelas	8-12 wk of age; repeat in 3-4 wk; revaccinate semiannually or annually
• Leptospirosis	8-12 wk of age; repeat in 3-4 wk; revaccinate semiannually or annually; substantial risk of high fever after use[16]
• Pneumonia (*Actinobacillus pleuropneumoniae*)	8-12 wk of age; repeat in 3-4 wk; revaccinate semiannually or annually
• Rabies	Off-label use but recommended if at risk of exposure; 14-16 wk of age; revaccinate annually
Breeder pigs	
• Erysipelas	8-12 wk of age; repeat in 3-4 wk; revaccinate 3 wk before breeding
• Leptospirosis	8-12 wk of age; repeat in 3-4 wk; revaccinate 3 wk before breeding; substantial risk of high fever after use[16]
• Parvovirus	5-6 mo of age; repeat in 3-4 wk; revaccinate 3-8 wk before breeding; boars should be revaccinated semiannually
• Pneumonia (*Actinobacillus pleuropneumoniae*)	Sows: 5 and 2 wk before farrowing Piglets: 3-8 wk of age; repeat in 3 wk

Selected Disease Vaccinations for Higher Risk Pigs

Colibacillosis (baby pig scours) (*E. coli*)	Sows: 5 and 2 wk before first farrowing, and 2 wk before each subsequent farrowing
Other enteritides (rotavirus, TGE virus, *Clostridium, Salmonella*)	Sows: 5 and 2 wk before farrowing
Atrophic rhinitis (*Bordetella bronchiseptica, Pasteurella multocida* [types A and D])	Sows: 7 and 3 wk before first farrowing, and 3 wk before each subsequent farrowing
	Piglets: 1 wk of age; repeat in 3 wk
	Boars: semiannually or annually
Pneumonia (*Mycoplasma hyopneumoniae*)	Sows: 5 and 2 wk before first farrowing, and 2 wk before each subsequent farrowing
	Piglets: 1 wk of age; repeat in 2-3 wk
	Boars: semiannually or annually
Tetanus toxoid	Vaccinate after surgery or trauma or annually when exposure is likely
Tetanus antitoxin	Administer 500-1500 U (depending on body weight) after surgery, dental procedure, or trauma; if not current on tetanus vaccine and where exposure is likely

Continued

TABLE 12-9 Preventive Medicine Recommendations for Miniature Pigs. (cont'd)

Neonatal Care

Preferred environmental temperature at 1-7 days of age	33-35°C (91-95°F); may be lowered 1.7-2.8°C (3-5°F) each wk for 4-6 wk until weaned
Colostrum	15-20 mL in 2-3 feedings within first 12 h of life
Castration	<3 mo of age and older
Ovariohysterectomy or ovariectomy	3-4 mo of age and older, but may be performed as early as 6 wk of age
Tusk (canine) removal	Not recommended
Tusk (canine) trimming	As needed

Fecal Examination

Young (6 wk to 6 mo of age)	Bimonthly
Adults	Semiannually if potential for exposure

TABLE 12-10 Blood Collection Sites in Miniature Pigs.[21,24,27,30,34]

Venipuncture Site	Comments
Cranial vena cava/right brachiocephalic vein	Anesthesia required for safety
Right external jugular vein	Short, fat neck of most pet pigs makes this challenging; best if pig is anesthetized; advance a ≥1.5-inch needle cranially in the jugular furrow, angled slightly medially while applying slight negative pressure
Cephalic vein	Thick skin makes this difficult; cut down may be required; reasonable choice for catheterization for fluid or medication administration if pig is sedated or moribund
Radial vein	Can be easily sampled in a properly restrained, awake patient; vein runs along medial aspect of front leg and landmarks are readily palpable
Lateral auricular vein	Easiest in debilitated or very cooperative pigs; good for obtaining very small blood samples; recommended for most routine catheterization
Subcutaneous abdominal vein	Easy to visualize and access in most large, cooperative pigs

TABLE 12-11 Recommendations for Feeding Miniature Pigs.[21,31]

- Miniature pet pigs should be offered feeds made specifically for the miniature pig.
- A rate of 1%-2% of the pig's body weight daily, depending upon life stage, is usually appropriate, *or*
  - Piglet: ½ cup per 15-20 lb per day
  - Adult: 1 cup per 50-80 lb per day
- The pig's current body condition should be the most important consideration when determining how much to feed.
- Divide daily ration into 2-3 meals daily when possible; ideally broadcast food on a grassy area, or place in food-dispensing toys or in rooting boxes.
- Some manufacturers of feeds for miniature pigs:

  Heartland Animal Health, Inc;
  www.healthypigs.com

  Mazuri Exotic Animal Nutrition;
  www.mazuri.com

  Ross Mill Farm's
  Champion Pet Pig Feed;
  www.rossmillfarm.com

TABLE 12-12   Tips for Oral Dosing of Miniature Pigs.[21,33]

- Choose flavored pediatric liquid formulations whenever possible.
- Mix medications with food items known to be favored by the individual; most pigs prefer sweets, including:
  - Jams or jelly, placed on a small piece of bread
  - Fruit flavored gelatin
  - Peanut butter
  - Bread, cookies, pastry, etc.
  - Fruit juice
- If a medication is known to be bitter, a few spoonfuls of peanut butter and jelly smeared on a piece of bread is recommended; if the pig tastes the medication, it will likely refuse this offering on the second dose; be prepared to change the food item for each dose.
- Small tablets can be placed inside a grape and will be consumed readily by most individuals.
- Medications can be mixed with fruit juice and frozen into cubes.

REFERENCES

1. Almond GW, Stevens JB. Urinalysis techniques for swine practitioners. *Compend Contin Educ Vet* 1995;17:121-129.
2. Boldrick L. *Veterinary Care of Pot-Bellied Pet Pigs.* Orange, CA: All Publishing Co; 1993:122-123.
3. Bollen PJA, Hansen AK, Alstrup AKO. *The Laboratory Swine.* 2nd ed. Boca Raton: CRC Press; 2010:11-13, 45-71.
4. Braun WF, Jr. Casteel SW. Potbellied pigs – miniature porcine pets. *Vet Clin N Am: Small Anim Pract* 1993;23:1149-1177.
5. Braun WF, Jr. Potbellied pigs: general medical care. In: Bonagura JD, ed. *Kirk's Current Veterinary Therapy XII—Small Animal Practice.* Philadelphia: WB Saunders Co; 1995:1388-1392.
6. Brockus CW, Mahaffey EA, Bush S, et al. Hematologic and serum biochemical reference intervals for Vietnamese potbellied pigs (*Sus scrofa*). *Comp Clin Path* 2005;13:162-165.
7. Calle PP, Morris PJ. Anesthesia for nondomestic suids. In: Fowler ME, Miller RE, eds. *Zoo and Wild Animal Medicine: Current Therapy 4.* Philadelphia: WB Saunders Co; 1999:639-646.
8. Claxton-Gill MS, Cornick-Seahorn JL, Gamboa JC, et al. Suspected malignant hyperthermia syndrome in a miniature pot-bellied pig anesthetized with isoflurane. *J Am Vet Med Assoc* 1993;203:1434-1436.
9. Flecknell P, Lofgren JLS, Dyson MC, et al. Preanesthesia, anesthesia, analgesia, and euthanasia. In: Fox JG, Anderson LC, Otto G, et al., eds. *Laboratory Animal Medicine.* 3rd ed. St. Louis: Elsevier; 2015:1162-1168.
10. Friendship RM. Antimicrobial drug use in swine. In: Giguère S, Prescott JF, Baggot JD, et al., eds. *Antimicrobial Therapy in Veterinary Medicine.* 4th ed. Ames: Blackwell Publishing; 2006:535-543.
11. Heard DJ. Principles and techniques of anesthesia and analgesia for exotic practice. *Vet Clin North Am Small Anim Pract* 1993;23:1301-1327.
12. Helke KL, Ezell PC, Duran-Struuck R, Swindle MM. Biology and diseases of swine. In: Fox JG, Anderson LC, Otto G, et al., eds. *Laboratory Animal Medicine.* 3rd ed. St. Louis: Elsevier; 2015:695-769.
13. Johnson L. Physical and chemical restraint of miniature pet pigs. In: Reeves DE, ed. *Care and Management of Miniature Pet Pigs.* Santa Barbara: Veterinary Practice Publishing Co; 1993:59-66.
14. Langston VC. Antimicrobial use in food animals (Table 5). In: Howard JL, Smith RA, eds. *Current Veterinary Therapy 4—Food Animal Practice.* Philadelphia: WB Saunders Co; 1999:26.
15. Lawhorn B. Personal communication. 2016.
16. Lawhorn B. Potbellied pigs. In: Aiello SE, ed. *The Merck Veterinary Manual.* 11th ed. Kenilworth, NJ: Merck & Co; 2016:1929-1937.
17. Liu J, Fung K, Chen Z, et al. Pharmacokinetics of florfenicol in healthy pigs and in pigs experimentally infected with *Actinobacillus pleuropneumoniae*. *Antimicrob Agents Chemother* 2003;47:820-823.

18. Longley L. Fancy pigs anaesthesia. In: Longley L, ed. *Anaesthesia of Exotic Pets*. New York: Elsevier Saunders; 2008:112-126.
19. Lord LK, Wittum TE, Anderson DE, et al. Resting rectal temperature of Vietnamese potbellied pigs. *J Am Vet Med Assoc* 1999;215:342-344.
20. Messenger K. Personal communication. 2016.
21. Mozzachio K. Personal observation. 2016.
22. Mozzachio K, Tynes VV. Recognition and treatment of pain in pet pigs. In: Eggers CM, Love L, Doherty T, eds. *Pain Management in Veterinary Practice*. Ames: Wiley Blackwell; 2014:383-389.
23. Murison PJ. Delayed dyspnoea in pigs possibly associated with endotracheal intubation. *Vet Anaesth Analg* 2001;28:226.
24. Padilla LR, Ko JC. Nondomestic suids. In: West G, Heard D, Caulkett N, eds. *Zoo Animal and Wildlife Immobilization and Anesthesia*. 2nd ed. Ames: Wiley Blackwell; 2014:773-785.
25. Papich MG. *Saunders Handbook of Veterinary Drugs*. 4th ed. St. Louis: Elsevier; 2016.
26. Reeves DE. Neonatal care of miniature pet pigs. In: Reeves DE, ed. *Care and Management of Miniature Pet Pigs*. Santa Barbara: Veterinary Practice Publishing Co; 1993:41-45.
27. Snook CS. Use of the subcutaneous abdominal vein for blood sampling and intravenous catheterization in potbellied pigs. *J Am Vet Med Assoc* 2001;219:809-810.
28. Swindle MM. Minipigs as pets. *Proc North Am Vet Conf* 1993;648-649.
29. Swindle MM, Sistino JJ. Anesthesia, analgesia, and perioperative care. In: Swindle MM, Smith AC, eds. *Swine in the Laboratory*. 3rd ed. Boca Raton: CRC Press; 2016:39-87.
30. Tynes VV. Emergency care for potbellied pigs. *Vet Clin North Am Exot Anim Pract* 1998;1:177-189.
31. Tynes VV. Potbellied pig husbandry and nutrition. *Vet Clin North Am Exot Anim Pract* 1999;2:193-207.
32. Tynes VV. Vaccinating the pet potbellied pig. *Exot DVM* 2000;2.1:11-13.
33. Tynes VV. Personal observation. 2016.
34. Van Metre DC, Angelos SM. Miniature pigs. *Vet Clin North Am Exot Anim Pract* 1999;2:519-537.
35. Wertz EM, Wagner AE. Anesthesia in potbellied pigs. *Compend Contin Educ Vet* 1995;17:369-383.

Chapter 13 Primates

Kathryn C. Gamble

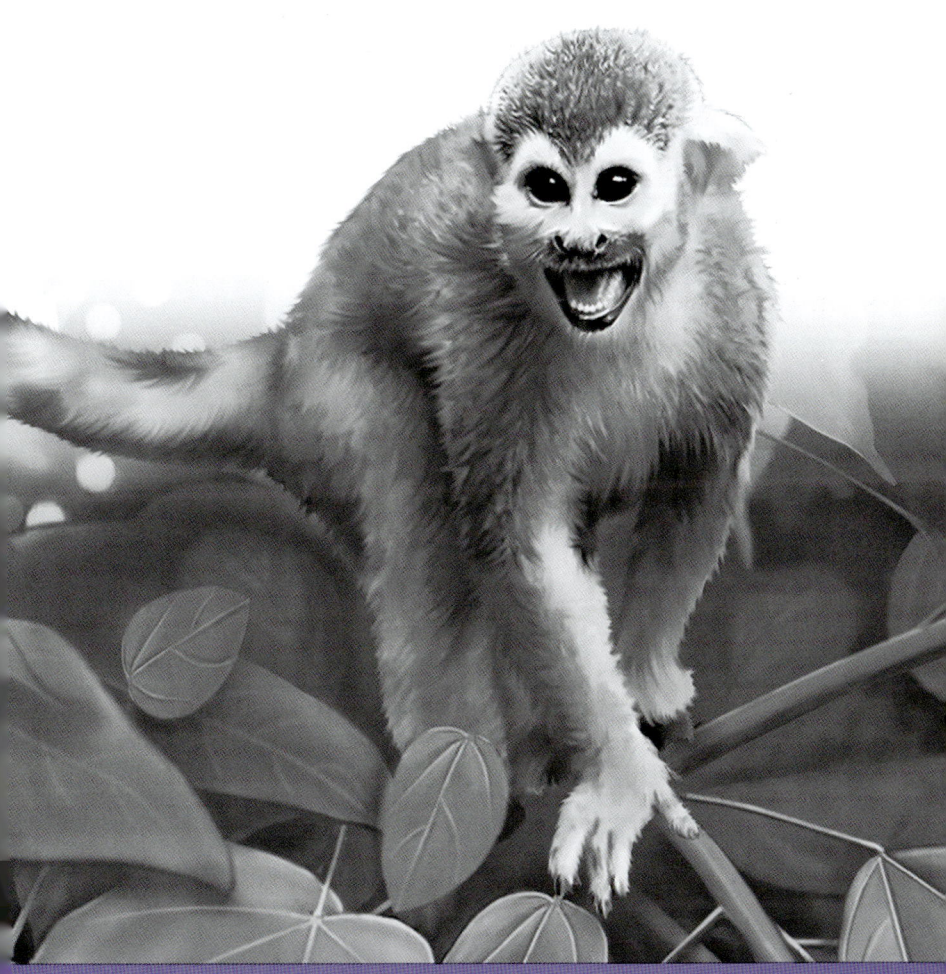

TABLE 13-1 Antimicrobial and Antifungal Agents Used in Primates.

Agent	Dosage	Species/Comments
Amikacin	2-3 mg/kg IM q24h[59]	
	2.3 mg/kg IM q24h[3]	Chimpanzees
	5 mg/kg IM q8h[3]	Monkeys
Amoxicillin	6.7-13.3 mg/kg PO, IM q8h[3]	Monkeys
	7 mg/kg PO q8h[86]	Macaques/quadruple treatment for *Helicobacter pylori* with clarithromycin, omeprazole, bismuth subsalicylate
	10-15 mg/kg PO q12h[7]	Eulemurs
	10-20 mg/kg PO q12h[90]	Prosimians
	11 mg/kg PO q12h or SC, IM q24h[44,59]	
	500 mg/animal PO, IM, IV q8h[3]	Chimpanzees
Amoxicillin trihydrate, clavulanic potassium	6.7-13.3 mg/kg PO q8h[3]	Monkeys
	13.75 mg/kg PO q12h[3]	Chimpanzees
	15 mg/kg PO q12h[59]	
Amphotericin B	0.5 mg/kg IV 3 ×/wk suspended in 30 mL of 5% dextrose, increased to 1.7 mg/kg[86]	Swamp monkey ($n=1$)/*Cryptococcus*; discontinued due to nephrotoxicity
	150 µg/kg IV 3 ×/wk × 2-4 mo[41]	Common marmosets
Ampicillin	10-30 mg/kg SC, IM, IV q6-8h[7,90]	Prosimians, *Eulemur*
	20 mg/kg PO, IM, IV q8h[3]	Chimpanzees
	25-50 mg/kg/day IM, IV divided q6-8h[3]	Monkeys
	150-200 mg/kg/day IM, IV divided q3-4h[3]	Monkeys/meningitis, septicemia
Azithromycin	—	In humans, associated with increased cardiac arrhythmogenicity;[75] use with caution in older great apes
	5-10 mg/kg PO q24h[3,7,90]	Chimpanzees,[3] prosimians[7,90]
	25 mg/kg PO q24h × 7 days, or 40 mg/kg PO q24h × 7 days, or 70 mg/kg PO q24h × 4 days[73]	Macaques/antimalarial
	30-50 mg/kg IM q12h × 7-14 days[41] 40 mg/kg PO q24h[44]	*Campylobacter*-associated diarrhea
	40 mg/kg PO once, then 20 mg/kg PO q24h × 4 days[3]	Monkeys
Cefadroxil	20 mg/kg PO q12h[86]	Prosimians
Cefazolin sodium	8-16 mg/kg IM q8h[5]	*Eulemur*
	10-30 mg/kg IM, IV q8h[90]	Prosimians
	20 mg/kg IM, IV q8h[3]	Monkeys
	25 mg/kg IM, IV q12h[3,44] × 7 days[81]	Chimpanzees,[3] rhesus macaques[81]

TABLE 13-1 Antimicrobial and Antifungal Agents Used in Primates. (cont'd)

Agent	Dosage	Species/Comments
Cefovecin (Convenia, Zoetis)	8 mg/kg SC[9,68,74]	In studies of both New World primates[68] and Old World primates,[9,68,74] pharmacokinetics were not consistent with those of dogs and cats; not considered effective in nonhuman primates[9,68,74]
Ceftazidime	1 g IM, IV q6-12h[3]	Chimpanzees
	50 mg/kg IM, IV q8h[3,59]	Monkeys
Ceftiofur	1.1-2.2 mg/kg IM q24h[7,90]	Prosimians, *Eulemur*
	2 mg/kg IM q24h[3]	Chimpanzees
	2.2 mg/kg IM q24h[44]	Monkeys
Ceftiofur CFA (Excede, Zoetis)	5 mg/kg SC once[81]	Rhesus macaques/PK; with plasma concentrations >0.2 μg/mL for at least 2 days
	20 mg/kg SC once[53]	Lion-tailed macaques; *Streptococcus* toxic shock
	20 mg/kg SC once[81]	Rhesus macaques/PK; with plasma concentrations >0.2 μg/mL for at least 7 days
Ceftriaxone	10 mg/kg IV[85]	Macaques, chimpanzees/PK
	25 mg/kg IM, IV q24h[44]	
	50 mg/kg IM q24h[3]	Monkeys
	50-100 mg/kg IM q12-24h[3]	Chimpanzees
Cephalexin	1-4 g q8-12h[3]	Chimpanzees
	10 mg/kg IM q12h[29]	
	20 mg/kg PO q12h[7,59]	*Eulemur*[7]
	30 mg/kg PO q12h[3]	Monkeys
Cephalothin	25 mg/kg IM q12h[86]	Macaques
Chloramphenicol palmitate	20 mg/kg IM q12h[29]	
	25 mg/kg PO q8h[3]	Monkeys (infants)
Chloramphenicol sodium succinate	20 mg/kg IM q12h[3]	Chimpanzees
	33.3 mg/kg IM q8h[3]	Monkeys
	50 mg/kg SC q8h[3]	Chimpanzees
Ciprofloxacin	10 mg/kg PO q12h[3]	Monkeys
	16-20 mg/kg PO q12h[3]	Chimpanzees
	20 mg/kg PO q12h[59]	
Clarithromycin	10 mg/kg PO q12h × 10 days[86]	Macaques/quadruple treatment of *Helicobacter pylori*; see amoxicillin
	20 mg/kg PO q24h[8]	Macaques/PK
	250-500 mg/animal PO q12h × 7-14 days[3]	Chimpanzees

Continued

TABLE 13-1 Antimicrobial and Antifungal Agents Used in Primates. (cont'd)

Agent	Dosage	Species/Comments
Clindamycin	10 mg/kg PO q12h[59]	
	12.5 mg/kg IM q8h[3]	Monkeys
	150-300 mg/animal PO q6h[3]	Chimpanzees
	300-600 mg/animal IM q8-12h[3]	Chimpanzees
Doxycycline	2-5 mg/kg PO q12h[3]	Chimpanzees
	2.5 mg/kg PO q12h × 1 day, then 2.5 mg/kg PO q24h[3]	Monkeys
	3-4 mg/kg PO q12h[59]	
	5-10 mg/kg PO q12h[90]	Prosimians
Enrofloxacin	5 mg/kg SC q12h[29]	
	5 mg/kg IM q24h[44]	
	5 mg/kg PO, SC, IM q24h[59,90]	Prosimians[90]/hallucinations in humans[59]
	5 mg/kg PO, IM q24h[7] × 6 days[50]	Rhesus macaques/PK; *Shigella flexneri*
	5 mg/kg PO, IM q12-24h[3]	Chimpanzees, monkeys
Erythromycin	15-20 mg/kg/day IM q12h[3]	Monkeys
	30-50 mg/kg IM q12h[44]	
	35 mg/kg PO q8h[3]	Monkeys
	75 mg/kg PO q12h × 10 days[59]	*Campylobacter*-associated diarrhea
Ethambutol	Start 15 mg/kg, then 25 mg/kg PO q24h[3]	Chimpanzees/antituberculosis drug
Florfenicol	50 mg/kg IM q48h[21]	
Fluconazole	2-3 mg/kg PO q24h × 30 days[86]	Macaques/coccidioidomycosis; prolonged treatment; relapses may occur
	18 mg/kg PO q12-24h[59,86]	Swamp monkey (*n*=1)/*Cryptococcus*; treated concurrently with flucytosine
Flucytosine	50-150 mg/kg/day PO divided q6h[3]	Chimpanzees
	143 mg/kg PO q24h[86]	Swamp monkey (*n*=1)/see fluconazole
Flurofamide	25 mg/animal PO q12h × 3 doses[41]	Common marmosets/*Ureaplasma*; bacterial urease inhibitor
Furazolidone	10 mg/kg PO q12h[3]	Monkeys
	10-15 mg/kg PO q24h[86]	
	100 mg/animal PO q6h[3]	Chimpanzees
Gentamicin	2-4 mg/kg IM, IV q12h[3]	Monkeys, chimpanzees
	3 mg/kg IM q6-8h[89]	Baboons/PK
	3-5 mg/kg SC, IM q24h[44]	
Griseofulvin	20 mg/kg PO q24h[3,59]	Monkeys
	25 mg/kg PO q24h for 30-60 days[69]	Common marmosets/dermatophytosis
	200 mg/kg PO once every 10 days[3,59]	Monkeys[3]
	500 mg/day PO divided q6-24h[3]	Chimpanzees

TABLE 13-1 Antimicrobial and Antifungal Agents Used in Primates. (cont'd)

Agent	Dosage	Species/Comments
Isoniazid	5 mg/kg PO q24h[3]	Monkeys
	30-50 mg/kg PO q24h × 9 mo[3]	Chimpanzees/active tuberculosis
	300 mg PO q24h[3]	Chimpanzee/prophylaxis; treat concurrently with rifampin
Itraconazole	5-10 mg/kg PO q12h[41]	Common marmosets/dermatophytosis
	10 mg/kg PO q24h[59]	Fungal (yeast) gastroenteritis
Ketoconazole	5-10 mg/kg PO q12h[3] × 30 days[69]	Monkeys
	10-30 mg/kg PO q24h × 60 days[41]	Common marmosets
	200-400 mg/day PO[3]	Chimpanzees
Levofloxacin	—	In humans, associated with increased cardiac arrhythmogenicity;[75] use with caution in older great apes
	500 mg PO q24h[3]	Chimpanzees
Metronidazole	25 mg/kg PO q24h[90]	Prosimians
	25 mg/kg PO q12h[3,59]	Chimpanzees
	25-30 mg/kg PO divided q12h[86]	*Clostridium;* treat concurrently with tylosin
	50 mg/kg PO q12h[3]	Monkeys
Minocycline	4 mg/kg PO[3]	Monkeys
	200 mg, then 100 mg, IV (slow)[3]	Chimpanzees
	200 mg PO q12h[3]	Chimpanzees
Neomycin	10 mg/kg PO q12h[29]	
	50 mg/kg PO q12h[3]	Monkeys
Nystatin	100,000 U/animal PO q8h[3]	Monkeys
	100,000 U/kg PO q24h × 10 days[41]	Common marmosets/*Candida*
	200,000 U/animal PO q6h[44,59]	Gastrointestinal candidiasis; continue 48 hr after clinical recovery
	500,000-1,000,000 U/animal PO q8h[3]	Chimpanzees
Ofloxacin	200-400 mg PO, IV constant rate infusion[3]	Chimpanzees
Oxacillin	16.7 mg/kg IM q8h[3]	Monkeys
Oxytetracycline	10 mg/kg SC, IM q24h[3,59]	Monkeys
	25-50 mg/kg PO[3]	Monkeys
	250-300 mg/day PO, IM divided q8-24h[3]	Chimpanzees
Penicillin G, benzathine	20,000-60,000 U/kg IM q12-24h[3,44]	Monkeys[3]
Penicillin G, procaine	20,000 U/kg IM q12h[59]	
	20,000-40,000 U/kg SC, IM q12h[3]	Monkeys
	22,000 U/kg IM q24h[3]	Chimpanzees
Penicillin VK	11 mg/kg PO q6h[3]	Chimpanzees

Continued

TABLE 13-1 Antimicrobial and Antifungal Agents Used in Primates. (cont'd)

Agent	Dosage	Species/Comments
Pentamidine isethionate	4 mg/kg IM, IV q24h × 14 days[86]	Great apes/*Pneumocystis*; slow IV infusion; associated with profound hypotension, cardiac arrhythmias
Rifampin	600 mg PO, IV q24h[3]	Chimpanzees/tuberculosis; treat concurrently with or without isoniazid
Streptomycin	1-2 g/day divided q6-24h[3]	Chimpanzees
	2.5-5 mg/kg IM q12h[3]	Monkeys
Sulfadimethoxine	50 mg/kg first day, then 25 mg/kg IM q24h[3]	Monkeys
Tetracycline	20 mg/kg PO q8h[3]	Monkeys
	20-25 mg/kg PO q8-12h[3]	Chimpanzees
Ticarcillin/clavulanate	65-100 mg/kg IV q8h[3]	Monkeys
	200-300 mg/kg/day divided evenly q4-6h[3]	Chimpanzees
Tilmicosin	—	Shown to be fatal in humans and nonhuman primates when injected[71]
Trimethoprim/sulfa	30 mg/kg PO, IM q24h[7]	Prosimians
Trimethoprim/sulfadiazine	15 mg/kg PO q12h[59]	
	30 mg/kg SC, IM q24h[59]	
Trimethoprim (T)/sulfamethoxazole (S)	4 mg/kg PO, SC q8h[3]	Monkeys
	(T) 4 mg/kg + (S) 20 mg/kg PO q12h[44]	Useful to treat shigellosis[69]
	(T) 5 mg/kg + (S) 25 mg/kg PO q6h[86]	Great apes/*Pneumocystis carini*
	15-20 mg/kg/day IV divided q6-12h[2] or 800 mg/animal PO q12h[3]	Chimpanzees
	25 mg/kg PO, IM q12h[90]	Prosimians
Tylosin	2 mg/kg IM q24h[3]	Monkeys
	5 mg/kg PO q12h[86]	*Clostridium*; treat concurrently with metronidazole
	20 mg/kg IM q24h × 10 days[13]	Rhesus macaques/chronic diarrhea
Vancomycin	20 mg/kg IM, IV q12h[3]	Monkeys
	500 mg/animal PO q6h × 7-10 days; can give IV slow[3]	Chimpanzees

TABLE 13-2 Antiparasitic Agents Used in Primates.

Agent	Dosage	Species/Comments
Albendazole	10 mg/kg PO[7]	*Eulemur*[7]
	10 mg/kg PO q24h × 6 wk[41]	Common marmosets/*Encephalitozoon cuniculi*
	20 mg/kg PO q12h × 5 days[51]	Geoffroy's tamarins ($n=3$)/*Angiostrongylus*; treat concurrently with prednisolone

TABLE 13-2 Antiparasitic Agents Used in Primates. (cont'd)

Agent	Dosage	Species/Comments
Albendazole (cont'd)	25 mg/kg PO q12h × 5 days[19,59]	New World primates, Old World primates/*Filaroides, Giardia*,[19] gastrointestinal nematodes[59]
	28.5 mg/animal PO q12h × 10 days × 3 at 10 day intervals[94]	Red ruffed lemur (*n* = 1)/cysticercosis; administer with praziquantel (SC)
	50 mg/kg PO q12h × 16 days[33,41]	Common marmosets, cotton-topped tamarins/*Acanthocephalus* sp.
	100 mg/kg PO q12h × 3 days, then repeat 2 × weekly × 4 treatments[33,41]	Common marmosets, cotton-topped tamarins/*Acanthocephalus* sp.
Amitraz	250 ppm dip for 2-5 min duration q14d × 4 treatments or until resolution of skin lesions[19,40,59]	Red-handed tamarins (*n* = 2)/demodectic mange; no hair clipping or bathing; not rinsed after treatment; dried by hot-air; ataxia (transient)
Bunamidine	25-100 mg/kg PO once[19]	New World primates, Old World primates/cestodes
Chloroquine	2.5-5 mg/kg IM q24h × 4-7 days[19]	New World primates, Old World primates/*Plasmodium;* follow with primaquine; give drugs separately to prevent toxicity
	5 mg/kg PO, IM q24h × 14 days[19]	New World primates, Old World primates/*Entamoeba histolytica*
	10 mg/kg IM q24h × 2 days, then 5 mg/kg IM q24h on day 3[86]	*Plasmodium* sp.; treat concurrently with primaquine
	10 mg/kg via nasogastric tube day 1 AM; 5 mg/kg via nasogastric tube day 1 PM, days 2 and 3 q24h[3]	Monkeys
	10 mg/kg PO, IM once, then 5 mg/kg 6 hr later, then 5 mg/kg q24h × 2 days[19,86]	New World primates, Old World primates/*Plasmodium* sp.; treat concurrently with primaquine
Clindamycin	12.5 mg/kg PO, IM q12h × 28 days[19]	New World primates, Old World primates/toxoplasmosis
	12.5-25 mg/kg PO q12h × 28 days[59]	*Toxoplasma* infection
Diethylcarbamazine	50 mg/kg PO q24h × 10 days[86]	Squirrel monkeys/filariasis; effective against microfilaria and adults
Diiodohydroxyquinoline (iodoquinol)	12 mg/kg PO q8h × 10-20 days[3]	Monkeys
	12-16 mg/kg PO q8h[86]	Great apes (infants, juveniles)/*Balantidium coli*
	30-40 mg/kg PO q24h × 3-21 days; 14-21 days for *Balantidium coli;* 21 days for *Entamoeba histolytica*[86]	Great apes/minimal absorption; use with other agents for invasive disease
	35-50 mg/kg PO q24h × 21 days[86]	Great apes (juvenile)
	630 mg PO q8h × 20 days[3]	Chimpanzees
Dithiazanine	10-20 mg/kg PO q24h × 3-10 days[19]	New World primates, Old World primates/*Strongyloides;* low margin of safety

Continued

TABLE 13-2 Antiparasitic Agents Used in Primates. (cont'd)

Agent	Dosage	Species/Comments
Doxycycline	2.5 mg/kg PO q12h × 1 day, q24h × 10 days[19]	New World primates, Old World primates/*Balantidium*
Fenbendazole	10-20 mg/kg PO q24h × 30 days[41]	Common marmosets/*Encephalitozoon cuniculi*
	10-25 mg/kg PO q24h × 3-10 days[19]	New World primates, Old World primates/*Anatrichosoma cynomolgi*
	20 mg/kg PO q24h × 7 days[19]	New World primates, Old World primates/*Prosthenorchis*
	20 mg/kg PO q24h × 14 days[19,59]	New World primates, Old World primates/*Strongyloides, Filaroides,*[19] gastrointestinal nematodes[59]
	25 mg/kg PO once, repeat in 7 days[19]	New World primates, Old World primates/*Ancylostoma*
	50 mg/kg PO q24h × 3 days,[22,59,77] repeat in 2 wk[44]	Baboons/[77] gastrointestinal nematodes, *Filaroides,*[59] *Trichuris trichura;*[77] New World primates/*Capillaria hepatica*[22]
	50 mg/kg PO q24h × 3-14 days[19]	New World primates, Old World primates
	50 mg/kg PO q24h × 5 days[41]	Common marmosets/*Baylisascaris*
	50 mg/kg PO q24h × 14 days[19,41]	Common marmosets/*Filaroides* sp., *Trichospiura leptostoma*
	50 mg/kg PO q24h × 3 days, repeat in 3 wk[3]	Chimpanzees/for monkeys repeat in 3 mo
	50 mg/kg PO every 2 wk until infection resolved[41]	Common marmosets/*Capillaria hepatica*
Fipronil (9.8% soln)	0.2 mL/kg topically every 6 wk[19]	Prosimians/*Cuterebra* sp., ticks
Furazolidone	5 mg/kg PO q6h × 7 days[86]	Great apes (juveniles)/*Giardia* sp.
	100 mg/animal PO q6h × 7 days[86]	Great apes (adults)/*Giardia* sp.; more palatable, but less effective than other agents
Ivermectin	0.2 mg/kg PO[27]	Lemurs
	0.2 mg/kg PO,[3,7] SC,[3,12,44] IM[7,44]	Chimpanzees, monkeys, *Eulemur*[7]
	0.2 mg/kg PO, SC, IM, repeat in 10-14 days[19,59]	
	0.2 mg/kg SC or topically, repeat after 4 wk[41]	Common marmosets/*Anatrichosoma, Sarcoptes, Demodex, Dipetalonema,* pentastomids
	0.3 mg/kg PO every 7 days × 4 treatments[42]	Callitrichids/*Gongylonema* sp.
Levamisole	2.5 mg/kg PO q24h × 14 days[86]	Prosimians/*Physaloptera*
	5 mg/kg PO, repeat in 21 days[19,59]	*Strongyloides, Trichuris, Spiruroides*[59]
	7.5 mg/kg SC, repeat in 14 days[19]	New World primates, Old World primates/*Trichuris, Ancylostoma*

TABLE 13-2 Antiparasitic Agents Used in Primates. (cont'd)

Agent	Dosage	Species/Comments
Mebendazole	3 mg/kg PO q24h × 10 days[19]	New World primates, Old World primates/*Ancylostoma*
	10-20 mg/kg PO[7] q12h × 3 days, repeat in 14 days[86]	*Eulemur*,[7] prosimians/gastrointestinal nematodes
	15 mg/kg PO q24h × 3 days[19]	*Strongyloides, Necator, Pterygodermatites, Trichuris*
	22 mg/kg PO q24h × 3 days, repeat in 14 days[19,44] or repeat in 3 wk[41]	Common marmosets[41]/*Giardia* sp.[44]
	22 mg/kg PO q24h × 3 days, repeat in 10-14 days[86]	Gastrointestinal nematodes
	40 mg/kg PO q24h × 3 days, repeat 3-4 times per year for prevention[19]	New World primates, Old World primates/*Pterygodermatites*
	40 mg/kg PO q24h × 30 days[59]	*Strongyloides, Trichuris, Pterygodermatites*
	50 mg/kg PO q12h × 3 days[3]	Monkeys
	70 mg/kg PO q24h × 3 days[19]	New World primates/oral spiruridiasis
	100 mg/animal PO q12h × 3 days[3]	Chimpanzees, monkeys
	100 mg/kg PO q12h × 3 days, repeat in 3 wk[3]	Monkeys/*Trichurus*
Mefloquine	25 mg/kg PO once via nasogastric tube[3]	Monkeys
	Active infection: 1250 mg PO once; preventive: 250 mg PO q7d[19]	Chimpanzees
Metronidazole	10-16.7 mg/kg PO q8h × 5-10 days[19]	New World primates, Old World primates/*Giardia*
	17.5-25 mg/kg PO q12h × 10 days[19]	Enteric flagellates and amoebas
	20 mg/kg PO q12h[41]	Common marmosets/*Entamoeba*
	25 mg/kg PO q12h × 5 days[19]	New World primates, Old World primates/*Giardia*
	25 mg/kg PO q12h × 10 days[59]	Enteric protozoans
	25 mg/kg PO q24h[90]	Prosimians
	30-50 mg/kg q24h × 5-10 days[41]	Common marmosets/*Giardia*
	30-50 mg/kg PO q12h × 5-10 days[86]	*Balantidium coli*
	30-50 mg/kg PO q24h × 5-10 days[19,41,44]	Common marmosets/*Giardia*[41]
	35 mg/kg PO q24h × 3 days[70]	Macaques/*Trichomonas vaginalis*
Milbemycin oxime	1 mg/kg PO q24h every 30 days for 3 mo[77]	Baboons/*Trichuris trichiura*
Moxidectin	0.5 mg/kg PO, IM once[19]	New World primates, Old World primates/*Strongyloides*
Niclosamide	37.5 mg PO q24h × 5 days[3]	Monkeys
	100 mg/kg once[19]	New World primates, Old World primates/intestinal cestodiasis
Nifurtimox	15-20 mg/kg PO q8h × 90 days[41]	Common marmosets/*Trypanosoma cruzi*

Continued

TABLE 13-2 Antiparasitic Agents Used in Primates. (cont'd)

Agent	Dosage	Species/Comments
Nitazoxanide	5 mg/kg PO q24h[41]	Common marmosets/*Cryptosporidium*
	25 mg/kg PO q24h × 5-7 days[90]	Prosimians/protozoa
Oxytetracycline	1500 mg/animal q24h IV constant rate infusion[86]	Gorillas (n=2)/*Balantidium coli*
Paromomycin	10 mg/kg PO q8h × 5-10 days[86]	Great apes/*Entamoeba*
	10-20 mg/kg PO q12h × 5-10 days[19]	New World primates, Old World primates/*Balantidium coli*
	12.5-15 mg/kg PO q12h × 5-10 days[19]	New World primates/amoebae; minimal enteric absorption
	15 mg/kg PO q12h × 28 days[34,41]	Common marmosets (n=2)/*Cryptosporidium*
	100 mg/kg PO q24h × 10 days[19]	Cercopithecids
Praziquantel	5 mg/kg IM[44]	Cestodes
	5 mg/kg PO, SC, IM once[3,44]	Monkeys
	15-20 mg/kg PO, IM[19,44,86]	New World primates, Old World primates/trematodes[86]
	20 mg/kg PO, IM once[59]	Cestodes
	20 mg/kg PO q8h × 1 day[3]	Chimpanzees
	23 mg/animal PO at 10 day intervals × 3 treatments[94]	Red ruffed lemur (n=1)/subcutaneous cysticercosis; treat concurrently with albendazole
	40 mg/kg PO, IM[19,59]	Trematodes,[19,59] cestodes[19]
Primaquine	0.3 mg/kg PO via nasogastric tube q24h × 14 days[3,86]	Monkeys/[3]*Plasmodium*; treat concurrently with chloroquine[86]
	0.3 mg/kg PO q24h × 14 days[19]	New World primates, Old World primates/treat with chloroquine; give drugs separately to prevent toxicity
Pyrantel pamoate	5-10 mg/kg PO,[7] repeat in 2 wk[90]	*Eulemur*,[7] prosimians/nematodes[90]
	6 mg/kg PO[27]	Lemurs
	10 mg/kg PO, repeat in 3 wk[3]	Chimpanzees
Pyrimethamine	0.5 mg/kg PO q12h[41]	Common marmosets/*Encephalitozoon cuniculi*; treat concurrently with trimethoprim/sulfamethoxazole and folic acid for encephalitozoonosis or toxoplasmosis
	2 mg/kg PO q24h × 3 days, then 1 mg/kg PO q24h × 28 days[86]	Great apes/*toxoplasmosis*; maximum dose of 100 mg/animal q24h for days 1-3 and 25 mg/animal q24h for 28 days; treat concurrently with sulfadiazine
	10 mg/kg PO q24h[19]	*Plasmodium*; folic acid antagonist so monitor for deficiency
Pyrvinium	5 mg/kg PO once, repeat every 6 mo[19]	New World primates, Old World primates/pinworms

TABLE 13-2 Antiparasitic Agents Used in Primates. (cont'd)

Agent	Dosage	Species/Comments
Quinacrine	2 mg/kg PO q8h × 7 days[19,86]	New World primates, Old World primates/may cause gastrointestinal upset in squirrel monkeys;[19] great apes/*Giardia;* maximum dose of 300 mg/day[86]
	10 mg/kg PO q8h × 5 days[19]	New World primates, Old World primates/*Giardia*
Ronnel	55 mg/kg PO or topically q72h × 4 treatments, then every 7 days for 3 mo[19]	Lung mites
Sulfadiazine	25-50 mg/kg PO q6h[86]	Great apes/toxoplasmosis, maximum dose of 6 g/animal/day; treat concurrently with pyrimethamine
	100 mg/kg PO q24h[19]	Toxoplasmosis; treat concurrently with pyrimethamine
Sulfadimethoxine	50 mg/kg PO once, then 25 mg/kg q24h[19]	Coccidiosis
Tetracycline	15 mg/kg PO q8h × 10-14 days[86]	Great apes (infants, juveniles)/*Balantidium coli*
	25-50 mg/kg PO q24h × 5-10 days[86]	Great apes/*Entamoeba, Balantidium*
	500-1000 mg/animal PO q8h × 10-14 days[86]	Great apes (adults)/*Balantidium coli*
Thiabendazole	50 mg/kg PO[7] q24h × 2 days[3,19]	*Eulemur,*[7] infant monkeys[3]/*Necator*[19]
	50 mg/kg PO × 3-5 days[90]	Prosimians/nematodes
	75-100 mg/kg PO q24h once, repeat in 21 days[19]	New World primates, Old World primates
	100 mg/kg PO q24h[3]	Monkeys (adult)
	100 mg/kg PO once, repeat in 3 wk[44]	*Strongyloides*
	750-1500 mg/animal PO q24h × 2 days or 7 days[3,19]	Chimpanzees/visceral larval migrans
Tinidazole	40-45 mg/kg PO q24h × 6 days[90]	Prosimians/protozoa
	150 mg/kg PO q24h once, then 77 mg/kg PO q24h on day 4[19,41,52]	Marmosets/*Giardia*
Toltrazuril	7 mg/kg PO q24h × 2 days[41]	Common marmosets/toxoplasmosis; treat concurrently with trimethoprim/sulfamethoxazole
Trimethoprim/sulfa	15 mg/kg PO q12h[59]	Toxoplasmosis
Trimethoprim/sulfamethoxazole	30 mg/kg PO q12h for at least 3 wk[41]	Common marmosets/*Encephalitozoon cuniculi;* treat concurrently with folic acid and pyrimethamine for encephalitozoonosis or toxoplasmosis

TABLE 13-3 Chemical Restraint/Anesthetic/Analgesic Agents Used in Primates.

Agent	Dosage	Species/Comments
Acepromazine	—	See butorphanol and ketamine for combinations
	0.1-0.5 mg/kg IM, IV[3]	Monkeys
	0.5-1 mg/kg PO,[59] SC, IM[3]	Chimpanzees
Acetaminophen	5-10 mg/kg PO q6h[41,59,72]	New World primates, juvenile macaques, common marmosets/pyrexia, mild pain
	6 mg/kg PO q8h[3]	Monkeys
	10-15 mg/kg PO q8-12h[91]	Prosimians
	15-20 mg/kg rectal[72]	
	500-1000 mg/animal PO q8h[3]	Chimpanzees
Acetaminophen/codeine suspension (120 mg/12 mg per 5 mL)	10-15 mL PO q6h[3]	Chimpanzees
Acetylsalicylic acid (aspirin)	—	NSAID; analgesic; antipyretic;[59] avoid aspirin based products during viral infections due to concerns of Reyes syndrome[65]
	5-10 mg/kg PO q4-6h[3,41,59,86]	Monkeys, common marmosets, chimpanzees use q6h
	10-20 mg/kg PO q8-12h[91]	Prosimians
	20 mg/kg PO q8-12h[3]	Monkeys
	20 mg/kg PO q12h[2]	Rhesus macaques/platelet aggregation was significantly decreased
Alphaxalone	—	Injectable steroid anesthetic; available in the United States as Alfaxan but not yet reported as sole agent for doses
	18 mg/kg IM, IV[86]	Marmosets, small primates/Saffan (9 mg/mL alphaxalone in 12 mg/mL); therefore 13.5 mg of reported dose was calculated as alphaxalone
Atipamezole (Antisedan, Zoetis)	IM use only per label	Specific α_2-adrenergic antagonist; more specific for medetomidine and dexmedetomidine than for xylazine; as a general rule, atipamezole is dosed at the same volume of medetomidine or dexmedetomidine;[38] atipamezole dose is 5 × dose of medetomidine or 10 × dose of dexmedetomidine on mg basis[20]
	0.15-0.3 mg/kg IM, IV[3,72]	Chimpanzees;[3] use lower dose in monkeys[3] and baboons[72]
	0.2 mg/kg IV[72]	Squirrel monkeys
	0.25 mg/kg IM, IV[72]	Macaques
Bupivacaine (0.5%)	1.2 mg/kg epidural as two 0.6 mg/kg doses at 2 min, then 20 min[86]	Rhesus macaques/epidural analgesia
	2 mg/kg maximum perineurally[25]	Macaques/local anesthetic

TABLE 13-3 Chemical Restraint/Anesthetic/Analgesic Agents Used in Primates. (cont'd)

Agent	Dosage	Species/Comments
Buprenorphine	—	Opioid agonist-antagonist; analgesia[35]
	0.005-0.01 mg/kg SC,[38] IM, IV q6-12h[29]	Rhesus macaques, marmosets
	0.005-0.01 mg/kg SC, IM, IV q6-12h[35]	
	0.005-0.03 mg/kg IM, IV q6-12h[41]	Common marmosets
	0.01 mg/kg IM, IV q6-8h[66,72]	Macaques/PK; not to exceed 0.3 mg/animal IM q8h in chimpanzees[72]
	0.01 mg/kg IM q12h[16]	Rhesus macaques/postoperative analgesia
	0.01-0.02 mg/kg SC, IM, IV q8-12h[91]	Prosimians
	0.01-0.02 mg/kg IM q12h[59]	
	0.01-0.05 mg/kg IM, SC q8-12h[44]	
	0.03 mg/kg IM q12h[46,66] or IV bolus[46]	Macaques/PK
	Sustained-release: 0.2 mg/kg SC once[66]	Macaques/single injection; plasma concentrations 0.1 ng/mL
Butorphanol	—	In primates, butorphanol behaves more as an agonist with intermediate efficacy; may cause profound respiratory depression—reverse with naloxone[41,59,67]
	0.01-0.02 mg/kg SC, IM, IV q6-12h[41]	Common marmosets
	0.013 mg/kg IM q8h[16]	Rhesus macaques
	0.02 mg/kg IM q3-4h[59]	
	0.02 mg/kg SC, IV q8h[3,72]	New World primates
	0.05 mg/kg IM q8h[3,72]	Monkeys,[3] macaques[72]
	0.1-0.15 mg/kg SC q6h[44]	
	0.1-0.2 mg/kg IM q12-48h[86]	
	0.1-0.4 mg/kg IM[7]	Eulemurs
	0.1-0.4 mg/kg SC, IM, IV q3-4h[91]	Prosimians
Butorphanol (B)/ acepromazine (A)	(B) 0.013 mg/kg + (A) 0.02 mg/kg IM[86]	Macaques/premedication for general anesthesia; butorphanol could be substituted with buprenorphine (0.01 mg/kg) and ketamine (10 mg/kg)
Butorphanol (B)/ dexmedetomidine (D)/ ketamine (K)	(B) 0.3-0.4 mg/kg + (D) 0.02 mg/kg + (K) 3-5 mg/kg IM[90,91]	Prosimians/can exchange ketamine with 0.2-0.3 mg/kg IM midazolam
Carfentanil	—	This product is no longer available commercially in the United States; prior publications suggest substantial concern with use of this product, both alone and in combinations, for use in nonhuman primates[20,45,86]
Carprofen	2 mg/kg PO q12h[3]	Chimpanzees, monkeys
	2-4 mg/kg PO, SC, IV q12-24h[38,41,59,72,86]	NSAID; analgesia; antipyretic; half-life varies with species; COX-1 selectivity[59]
	3-4 mg/kg IV, SC once[28]	Macaques/preoperatively

Continued

TABLE 13-3 Chemical Restraint/Anesthetic/Analgesic Agents Used in Primates. (cont'd)

Agent	Dosage	Species/Comments
Celecoxib	200 mg/animal PO q12-24h[3]	Chimpanzees/COX-2 NSAID
Deracoxib (Deramaxx, Eli Lilly)	2 mg/kg PO q24h[3]	Chimpanzees/COX-2 NSAID; chronic use
	4 mg/kg PO q24h[3]	Chimpanzees
Diazepam	—	Used often as an adjuvant with ketamine
	0.25-0.5 mg/kg PO, IV[7,90]	Prosimians, lemurs
	0.25-0.5 mg/kg IM, IV[3]	Chimpanzees
	0.5-1 mg/kg PO[3,59,86]	Chimpanzees[3]
	0.5-1 mg/kg IM, IV[3]	Monkeys/seizures
	0.5-2.5 mg/kg IV[91]	Prosimians
	1 mg/kg IM[29]	Marmosets
	5 mg/animal PO[20]	Gorillas (juvenile)
Droperidol	2.5-10 mg/animal IM[3]	Chimpanzees/given 30-60 min prior to procedure
Etomidate	0.1 mg/kg/min IV constant rate infusion[26]	Rhesus macaques/maintenance
	1 mg/kg IV[26]	Rhesus macaques/induction
Fentanyl	—	Produced respiratory depression and analgesia at dosages as low as 2 μg/kg IV, and apnea was seen consistently at 60 μg/kg[67]
	0.001-0.03 mg/kg/h IV constant rate infusion[90,91]	Prosimians
	0.05-0.15 μg/kg IM as needed[3]	Monkeys
	1-2 μg/kg as an adjunct to general anesthesia; 50-150 μg/kg as sole anesthetic[18]	Great apes
	5-10 μg/kg IV bolus[72] or IV constant rate infusion[3,25] or 10-25 μg/kg/h IV constant rate infusion[72]	Rhesus macaques, baboons,[72] chimpanzees[3]
	8 μg/kg IV[87]	Rhesus macaques ($n=6$)/PK; published with error in dose
	10-15 μg/kg PO as lollipops[20]	Orangutans, gorillas/adequate sedation in 30-45 min; chimpanzees suboptimal effects
	25 μg/kg/h (5-10 kg); 50 μg/kg/h (10 kg) q48-72h[3]	Monkeys/transdermal patch
Fentanyl/droperidol (Innovar-Vet, Janssen)	0.05 mL/kg IM[3]	New World primates
	0.1-0.3 mL/kg IM[3]	Chimpanzees, monkeys
Flumazenil	0.02 mg/kg IV[72,91]	Patas monkeys, prosimians
	0.025 mg/kg IV[20,86]	Chimpanzees, gorillas/did not significantly enhance speed or quality of recovery

TABLE 13-3 Chemical Restraint/Anesthetic/Analgesic Agents Used in Primates. (cont'd)

Agent	Dosage	Species/Comments
Flunixin meglumine	0.25-0.5 mg/kg SC, IM, IV q24h[91]	Prosimians
	0.3-1 mg/kg SC, IV q12-24h[59,86]	NSAID; analgesia; antipyretic
	1 mg/kg IM q12h[25]	Rhesus macaques
	2 mg/kg IM q12h[3]	Monkeys
Hydrocodone bitartrate	5 mg/animal PO q4-6h prn[3]	Chimpanzees
Hydromorphone	0.2 mg/kg IM, IV bolus q4h[47]	Rhesus macaques/PK; whole-body pruritus, sedation, and decreased appetite
Ibuprofen	7 mg/kg PO q12h[3,72]	Old World primates, New World primates/NSAID; mild analgesia[72]
	10 mg/kg PO q8-12h[91]	Prosimians
	20 mg/kg PO q24h[41,59]	Common marmosets
	200-400 mg/animal PO q8h[3]	Chimpanzees
Isoflurane	1%-3% maintenance[59,72]	Marmosets, chimpanzees
Ketamine	—	Tranquilization; anesthesia; mg/kg dose increases as size of animal decreases; causes seizures in lemurs when used as sole agent so not recommended for use alone in prosimians[90]
	5 mg/kg IM[86]	Great apes/follow with inhalant anesthetic; ketamine provides a shorter recovery time than tiletamine-zolazepam
	5 mg/kg IV[3]	Monkeys
	5-12 mg/kg IM[67]	Monkeys
	5-15 mg/kg IM, IV[59,91]	Prosimians[91]
	5-15 mg/kg PO, IM, IV or rectally[18]	Great apes/in general 6-10 mg/kg should allow safe initial immobilization
	5-40 mg/kg IM[3]	Chimpanzees
	10 mg/kg IM[3]	Monkeys
	10-15 mg/kg IM[3]	New World primates
Ketamine (K)/acepromazine (A)	(K) 4 mg/kg + (A) 0.4 mg/kg IM[27]	Lemurs
Ketamine (K)/detomidine (Det)	(K) 9.6 mg/kg + (Det) 0.32 mg/kg PO[20]	Gorillas
	(K) 10 mg/kg + (Det) 0.5 mg/kg PO[60]	Gorillas ($n=6$), mandrill baboons ($n=7$)/reduced the reaction to darting
Ketamine (K)/dexmedetomidine (De)	(K) 2-4 mg/kg + (De) 0.02-0.03 mg/kg IM[19]	Medium to large primates
Ketamine (K)/medetomidine[a] (Me)	—	Medetomidine is no longer commercially available; can be compounded;[a] replaced with dexmedetomidine; recoveries can be quite sudden even without reversal[20]

Continued

TABLE 13-3 Chemical Restraint/Anesthetic/Analgesic Agents Used in Primates. (cont'd)

Agent	Dosage	Species/Comments
Ketamine (K)/ medetomidinea (Me) (cont'd)	(K) 2 mg/kg + (Me) 0.03-0.04 mg/kg[18]	Chimpanzees
	(K) 2-4 mg/kg + (Me) 0.04-0.06 mg/kg IM[19]	Medium to large primates
	(K) 2-6 mg/kg + (Me) 0.03-0.06 mg/kg IM[3,86]	Chimpanzees
	(K) 3 mg/kg + (Me) 0.02-0.03 mg/kg IM[20]	Orangutans
	(K) 3-4 mg/kg + (Me) 0.15 mg/kg IM[56,67,72,84]	Macaques, capuchins
	(K) 5 mg/kg + (Me) 0.01 mg/kg IM[41]	Common marmosets
	(K) 5 mg/kg + (Me) 0.05 mg/kg IM[67]	Japanese macaques
	(K) 5-7.5 mg/kg IM + (Me) 0.05-0.1 mg/kg IM, IV[59,67]	Use higher dosages for smaller primates
Ketamine (K)/ medetomidine[a] (Me)/ butorphanol (B)	—	Medetomidine is no longer commercially available; can be compounded;[a] replaced with dexmedetomidine
	(K) 2-3 mg/kg + (Me) 0.02-0.03 mg/kg + (B) 0.2-0.4 mg/kg[20]	Great apes
	(K) 3 mg/kg + (Me) 0.04 mg/kg + (B) 0.4 mg/kg IM[86,92]	Ring-tailed lemurs/anesthesia; long duration of action
Ketamine (K)/midazolam (Mi)	(K) 1-2 mg/kg + (Mi) 0.03 mg/kg IM[20]	Orangutans
	(K) 2.5 mg/kg + (Mi) 0.25 mg/kg IM[20]	Chimpanzees
	(K) 4-20 mg/kg IM + (Mi) 0.05-0.2 mg SC, IM[38]	
	(K) 5 mg/kg + (Mi) 0.1 mg/kg IM[72]	Baboons
	(K) 8 mg/kg + (Mi) 0.2 mg/kg IM[6,72]	Macaques/up to 1 mg/kg IM of midazolam[44,56]
	(K) 9 mg/kg + (Mi) 0.05 mg/kg IM[20]	Gorillas
	(K) 10 mg/kg + (Mi) 1 mg/kg IM[32,67]	Marmosets
	(K) 15 mg/kg + (Mi) 0.05-0.09 mg (lower body weight)[35] or 0.05-0.15 mg (higher body weight) IV[72]	
Ketamine (K)/ tiletamine-zolazepam (T)	(K) 1-3 mg/kg + (T) 2-4 mg/kg IM[18]	Great apes/combination reduces amount of ketamine needed for induction
Ketamine (K)/xylazine (X)	(K) 5 mg/kg + (X) 0.5-1 mg/kg[67]	Monkeys
	(K) 5-7 mg/kg + (X) 1-1.4 mg/kg IM[20]	Orangutans
	(K) 5-10 mg/kg + (X) 0.25-0.3 mg/kg SC, IM[38]	
	(K) 7 mg/kg + (X) 0.6 mg/kg IM[3,72]	Monkeys, macaques
	(K) 10 mg/kg + (X) 0.25 mg/kg for 45 min, or (X) 2 mg/kg for 138 min sedation[72]	Macaques
	(K) 10-20 mg/kg IM + (X) 3 mg/kg IM[3]	New World primates
	(K) 15-20 mg/kg IM + (X) 1 mg/kg IM[2,20,72]	Chimpanzees[20]

TABLE 13-3 Chemical Restraint/Anesthetic/Analgesic Agents Used in Primates. (cont'd)

Agent	Dosage	Species/Comments
Ketoprofen	2 mg/kg IM q24h[20]	Gorilla ($n=1$)
	2 mg/kg IM, IV q24h[3,44]	Chimpanzees, monkeys[3]
	2 mg/kg PO, SC, IM, IV[91]	Prosimians/NSAID; reduce prosimians to 1 mg/kg q24h after first dose
	5 mg/kg IM q6-8h[86]	Macaques
	5 mg/kg IM q24h[25]	
Ketorolac	0.5-1 mg/kg[67] SC, IM q8-12h × 4 days[38]	NSAID
	15-30 mg/animal IM[72]	Baboons
	30 mg/animal PO q6h[3,72]	Chimpanzees
	60 mg/animal PO once[3]	Chimpanzees
Lidocaine	2-4 mg/kg[18]	Great apes/preferred to bupivacaine for dental procedures
	6 mg/kg maximum perineurally[25]	Macaques/local anesthetic
Medetomidine[a]	—	Medetomidine is a more selective, potent and specific α_2-agonist than xylazine; can be compounded; replaced with dexmedetomidine
	0.01-0.035 mg/kg IM[3,44]	Monkeys[3]
	0.1 mg/kg PO[20]	Great apes
	0.1 mg/kg SC, IM[72]	Squirrel monkeys, baboons
	0.15 mg/kg[72]	Macaques
Medetomidine (Me)[a]/ midazolam (Mi)	(Me) 0.03-0.06 mg/kg + (Mi) 0.3 mg/kg IM[67]	Japanese macaques
Meloxicam	0.1 mg/kg PO q24h[11]	Cynomolgus macaques/PK; sustained-release formation (0.6 mg/kg SC) achieved adequate steady-state plasma concentration for 2-3 days; PO formulation limited use
	0.1-0.2 mg/kg SC q24h[29] up to 3 days[72]	Marmosets, rhesus macaques/NSAID
	0.2 mg/kg IM q24h[11]	Cynomolgus macaques/PK; see above dose for cynomolgus macaques; IM provided adequate plasma concentrations for 12-24 hr
	0.2-0.3 mg/kg PO, SC, IM q24h × 4 days[38]	Lower dose—common marmosets,[41] macaques[72]
	0.3 mg/kg PO, SC q24h[2]	Rhesus macaques/platelet aggregation was not affected
Meperidine	2 mg/kg IM[72]	Macaques
	2-4 mg/kg IM,[72] IV q30-60 min[3]	Baboons, monkeys/analgesia
	50-150 mg/animal PO[72] q3-4h prn[3]	Chimpanzees

Continued

TABLE 13-3 Chemical Restraint/Anesthetic/Analgesic Agents Used in Primates. (cont'd)

Agent	Dosage	Species/Comments
Midazolam	—	See ketamine and medetomidine for combinations
	0.05-0.1 mg/kg IM, slow IV[3,44]	Monkeys[3]
	0.1-0.3 mg/kg IM,[7,91] IV[91]	Eulemurs, prosimians
	0.5 mg/kg PO[59]	More applicable in larger species
	0.7-1.2 mg/kg PO[20]	Gorillas, chimpanzees, orangutans
	1-2.5 mg/animal IV, or 5 mg/animal IV[3]	Chimpanzees
Morphine	—	Opioid analgesia; dose dependent respiratory depression[59]
	0.01-0.1 mg/kg IV[3,72]	Chimpanzees
	0.15 mg/kg epidurally[72]	Baboons
	1 mg/kg PO, SC, IM, IV q4h[59]	
	1-2 mg/kg SC,[72,86] IM, IV q4h[3,72]	Monkeys, macaques, baboons, squirrel monkeys
	1-2 mg/kg SC, IM q6h[41]	Common marmosets
Nalbuphine	0.5 mg/kg IM, IV q3-4h[86]	Agonist-antagonist opioid
	2.5-5 mg/kg IM q3-4h[3]	Monkeys
	10 mg SC, IM, IV q3-6h as needed[3]	Chimpanzees
Naloxone	—	Opioid antagonist/reversal;[59] short acting; a second dose may be necessary to avoid the return of respiratory depression[72]
	0.015 mg/kg SC, IM, IV[3,72]	Chimpanzees
	0.01-0.05 mg/kg IM, IV[41,59]	Common marmosets[41]
	0.02 mg/kg IM[91]	Prosimians
	0.1 mg/kg SC, IM, IV as needed[3]	Monkeys
	0.1-0.2 mg as needed[72]	Macaques, baboons, squirrel monkeys, common marmosets
Naproxen	5 mg/kg PO q24h[3]	Chimpanzees
	10 mg/kg PO q12h[86]	Lemurs
Nitrous oxide (N$_2$O)	Up to 60% with O$_2$[38]	Not acceptable as sole agent
Oxymorphone	—	Opioid analgesia
	0.025 mg/kg SC, IM, IV q4-6h[3]	New World primates
	0.075 mg/kg IV bolus[49]	New World primates, rhesus macaques ($n=4$), titi monkeys ($n=4$)/PK
	0.075 mg/kg IM, IV q4-6h[72]	Squirrel monkeys, marmosets
	0.15 mg/kg SC, IM, IV q4-6h[3,44,49,72]	Old World primates,[49] macaques, baboons,[72] monkeys[3]
	1-1.5 mg/animal SC, IM q4-6h[3,72]	Chimpanzees
Pentobarbital (pentobarbitone sodium)	—	The product has considerable variation between species; severe respiratory depression; inability to modulate depth of anesthesia;[38] should be used for euthanasia only, not for sedation

TABLE 13-3 Chemical Restraint/Anesthetic/Analgesic Agents Used in Primates. (cont'd)

Agent	Dosage	Species/Comments
Propofol	—	Dose to maintain anesthesia in great apes 5-10 × less than human dose;[18] use sterile technique due to vehicle
	0.3-0.5 mg/kg/min constant rate infusion[44]	
	1 mg/kg IV[44]	Induction
	1-2 mg/kg IV bolus, followed by constant rate infusion to effect[3,72]	Chimpanzees
	2 mg/kg IV bolus[58]	Neonatal rhesus macaques ($n=4$)/induction
	2-4 mg/kg/min IV constant rate infusion[72]	Baboons
	2-5 mg/kg IV bolus;[41] maintenance with 0.3-0.4 mg/kg/min IV constant rate infusion[72]	Common marmosets, macaques
	2.5-5 mg/kg IV bolus; maintenance with 0.3-0.4 mg/kg/min constant rate infusion[3]	Monkeys
	3-6 mg/kg IV[91]	Prosimians
	5 mg/kg IV bolus at 0.6 mg/kg/min[61]	Japanese macaques ($n=5$)/step down started at 0.6 mg/kg/min, then 0.3 mg/kg/min for 10 min, then 0.2 mg/kg/min for 100 min
	5-10 mg/kg IV, then 0.3-0.6 mg/kg IV constant rate infusion[29]	Marmosets
Sevoflurane	1 MAC = 2%[72]	Macaques
Thiamylal sodium	15-25 mg/kg IV to effect[3]	Monkeys/barbiturate anesthesia
Thiopental	—	Barbiturate anesthesia
	5-7 mg/kg IV if combined with ketamine[72]	Macaques
	15-17 mg/kg/h IV constant rate infusion[72]	Baboons
	25 mg/kg IV to effect[3]	Monkeys
Tiletamine-zolazepam (Telazol, Fort Dodge; Zoletil, Virbac)	—	Can concentrate in vial; see ketamine for combination
	1-2.5 mg/kg IM[3]	New World primates
	1.5-3 mg/kg IM[86]	
	2-5 mg/kg IM[19]	New World primates, Old World primates
	2-6 mg/kg IM[20,72]	Chimpanzees, gorillas, orangutans (up to 6.9 mg/kg)
	3-5 mg/kg IM[3,44,72,91]	Prosimians/for restraint only[44]
	4-6 mg/kg IM[72,86]	Macaques, baboons
	5-8 mg/kg IM[3]	Chimpanzees, monkeys
	10 mg/kg[67,72,78]	Squirrel monkeys,[72] chimpanzees[78]

Continued

TABLE 13-3 Chemical Restraint/Anesthetic/Analgesic Agents Used in Primates. (cont'd)

Agent	Dosage	Species/Comments
Tiletamine-zolazepam (T)/medetomidine (Me)[a]	(T) 0.8-2.3 mg/kg + (Me) 0.02-0.06 mg/kg IM[20,67]	Orangutans, monkeys, gibbons, macaques
	(T) 1-3 mg/kg + (Me) 0.02-0.06 mg/kg[67]	Monkeys, macaques, gibbons
	(T) 1.25 mg/kg + (Me) 0.03 mg/kg IM[72]	Chimpanzees
	(T) 2 mg/kg + (Me) 0.03 mg/kg IM[78]	Chimpanzees
	(T) 3 mg/kg + (Me) 0.05 mg/kg IM[63]	Chimpanzees
	(T) 3 mg/kg IM + (Me) 0.1 mg/kg PO[63]	Chimpanzees
Tramadol	1-4 mg/kg PO q12h[91]	Prosimians
	1.5 mg/kg IV q24h[48]	Rhesus macaques/PK; sedation, pruritus
	3 mg/kg PO[48]	Rhesus macaques/PK; PO bioavailability poor; oral dosages of 4-20 × this dose may be required for analgesia
Xylazine	—	See ketamine for combination
	0.5-6 mg/kg IM[3]	Monkeys
	1.1 mg/kg IV[3]	Chimpanzees
	2.2 mg/kg IM[3]	Chimpanzees
Yohimbine	0.1 mg/kg IM, IV[3]	Monkeys, chimpanzees (0.11 mg/kg)
	0.125-0.25 mg/kg IM[20]	Chimpanzees
	0.5 mg/kg IV or 1 mg/kg IM[72,86]	Macaques/xylazine reversal
Zuclopenthixol (Clopixol, Lundbeck)	0.1-0.36 mg/kg PO q12h[20]	Gorillas/antipsychotic drug; not approved for use in the United States

[a]Medetomidine is no longer commercially available although it can be obtained from select compounding services (i.e., Wildlife Pharmaceuticals, www.zoopharm.net); limited data on the efficacy and safety of dexmedetomidine in primates; the effects of the v/v use of the two drugs may not be equivalent, so the dose of dexmedetomidine may need to be adjusted based on clinical response.

TABLE 13-4 Miscellaneous Agents Used in Primates.

Agent	Dosage	Species/Comments
Allopurinol	200-600 mg PO q24h[3]	Chimpanzees
Aminophylline	10 mg/kg IV[3,27]	Chimpanzees,[3] lemurs
	25-100 mg/animal PO q24h[3]	Monkeys
Amlodipine	0.1 mg/kg PO q24h[3]	Chimpanzees/antihypertensive agent
Atropine	0.02-0.04 mg/kg SC, IM, IV[72]	Chimpanzees; for marmosets use higher dose
	0.02-0.05 mg/kg SC,[41] IM[72]	Macaques, baboons, common marmosets

TABLE 13-4 Miscellaneous Agents Used in Primates. (cont'd)

Agent	Dosage	Species/Comments
Atropine sulfate	0.01 mg/kg IM[20]	Orangutan ($n=1$)
	0.02-0.04 mg/kg SC, IM, IV[3]	Monkeys
	0.02-0.05 mg/kg SC, IM, IV[3]	Chimpanzees
	0.04 mg/kg IM[20]	Gorillas
	2-5 mg/animal IM[20]	Chimpanzees (juvenile)
Azathioprine	1-2 mg/kg PO q24h[3]	Monkeys/immunosuppressive agent; purine antagonist
	1-2.5 mg/kg PO q24h[3]	Chimpanzees
Benazepril	0.25-0.5 mg/kg PO q24h[41]	Common marmosets/less nephrotoxicity than enalapril
Bisacodyl	10-15 mg PO as needed[3]	Chimpanzees
Bismuth subsalicylate	10 mg/kg PO q12h[86]	Macaques/quadruple treatment for *Helicobacter pylori*; see amoxicillin (Table 13.1)
	30 mL PO as needed[3]	Chimpanzees
	40 mg/kg PO q8-12h[3]	Monkeys
Budesonide	0.5 mg/animal PO q24h × 8 wk, then 0.75 mg PO q24h × 8 wk[41]	Common marmosets/marmoset wasting syndrome
Calcitonin	10 U/kg q48h × 3 wk[41]	Common marmosets/must be normocalcemic
Calcitriol	0.03 mg/kg PO q24h[3]	Chimpanzees
Calcium glubionate	1 mL/kg PO q12h[41]	Common marmosets/metabolic bone disease
Calcium gluconate	200 mg/kg SC, IM, IV[3,86]	Chimpanzees/hypocalcemia; hyperkalemia; prophylaxis and therapy of nutritional secondary hyperparathyroidism
Captopril	1 mg/kg PO[86]	ACE inhibitor and vasodilator
Carvedilol	3.125 mg PO q12h × 2 wk, then 6.25 mg PO q12h, increase as needed[3]	Chimpanzees
Cimetidine	5-10 mg/kg PO[41]	Common marmosets/*Helicobacter*
	10 mg/kg PO, IM q8h[3]	Monkeys/gastrointestinal ulceration
	300 mg/animal PO, IM, slow IV q6-8h[3]	Chimpanzees
Cisapride	0.2 mg/kg PO q12h × 3 wk[86]	Macaques/promotes gastrointestinal motility; compounded in United States
Dapsone	50 mg/animal PO q24h; 100 mg/animal PO q24h[3]	Chimpanzees/use higher dose with leprosy
Depoprovera	2.5-5 mg/kg IM[80]	Old World primates/contraception for 45-90 days; higher doses for smaller species
	5 mg/kg IM[7,80]	Prosimians/contraception for 30-45 days, during breeding season (Nov-March)
	20 mg/kg IM[80]	New World primates/contraception for 30 days

Continued

TABLE 13-4 Miscellaneous Agents Used in Primates. (cont'd)

Agent	Dosage	Species/Comments
Deslorelin (Suprelorin, Virbac)	4.7 mg SC implant effective for 6 mo; 9.4 mg SC implant effective for 12 mo[41,59,80]	GnRH antagonist implant; need secondary contraception of megesterol acetate (not depoprovera) for 7 days prior to and postimplantation
Dexamethasone	0.25-1 mg/kg PO, IM q24h[3]	Monkeys
Digoxin	0.005-0.01 mg/kg PO q12h or IV as needed[3]	Chimpanzees
	0.01 mg/kg PO q24h[41]	Common marmosets/congestive heart failure
	2-12 µg/kg PO, IM, IV divided q12-24h[3]	Monkeys/maintenance dose
Diphenhydramine	5 mg/kg/day PO, IM,[27] IV, daily total may be divided q6-8h[3]	Monkeys,[3] lemurs[27]
	25-50 mg/animal PO, IM, IV q6-8h[3]	Chimpanzees
Dobutamine	2.5-10 µg/kg/min IV constant rate infusion[3]	Chimpanzees, monkeys/adrenergic β_1 agonist; increases cardiac output
Docusate sodium (DSS)	10-40 mg/animal PO[3]	Monkeys
	50-200 mg/animal PO[3]	Chimpanzees
Dopamine	2-5 µg/kg/min IV constant rate infusion[3]	Chimpanzees, monkeys/low to moderate doses; positive inotropic effects and renal vasodilation
	2-10 µg/kg/min IV constant rate infusion[18]	Great apes/stimulates dopaminergic, α and β adrenergic receptors; positive inotrope which significantly can improve blood pressures intraoperatively
	5-15 µg/kg/min IV constant rate infusion[3]	Monkeys
Doxapram	2 mg/kg IV[3]	Chimpanzees/respiratory stimulant
Duloxetine	30-60 mg/kg PO q12h[54]	Drill ($n=1$)/serotonin-norepinephrine reuptake inhibitor
Enalapril	0.015-0.125 mg/kg PO q12-24h[86]	Gorillas/antihypertensive
	0.3 mg/kg PO, IV[3]	Chimpanzees/ACE inhibitor; balanced vasodilator
	0.5 mg/kg PO q48h[41]	Common marmosets
Enoxaparin sodium	20 mg SC q24h × 10 days, repeat in 2 mo[68]	Rhesus macaque ($n=1$)/deep vein thrombosis; low-molecular weight heparin
Ephedrine	0.1-0.5 mg/animal SC, IM, IV, IC[3]	Monkeys
	1.25-2.5 mg/kg IV[72]	Macaques, baboons/vasopressor; safest during maternal hypotension
	2.5 mg/kg IV bolus[72]	Use when hypotension is accompanied by bradycardia
Epinephrine	0.1-0.5 mg/animal SC, IV, IM, IC[3]	Monkeys
	0.2-0.4 mg/kg diluted in 5 mL sterile water,[41] IT if ≥3 kg or 1:10,000 dilution[31]	Common marmosets/cardiac arrest
	0.2-1 mg/animal SC, IM; 0.5-10 mg IV, IC[3]	Chimpanzees

TABLE 13-4 Miscellaneous Agents Used in Primates. (cont'd)

Agent	Dosage	Species/Comments
Fluoxetine	0.45 mg/kg PO q24h[86]	Bonobo ($n=1$)[86]/antianxiety; serotonin reuptake inhibitor; antidepressant used to moderate abnormal behaviors[76]
	0.5-1 mg/kg PO q24h[3]	Chimpanzees
	2 mg/kg PO q24h[55] × 1-4 wk[30]	Rhesus macaques ($n=6$)/reduction of self-biting behavior, but not self-directed stereotypes; venlafaxine ineffective
Folic acid	15 μg/kg PO q24h[3]	Monkeys
	500 μg/kg PO[3]	Chimpanzees
Furosemide	1-2 mg/kg PO, IM, IV[3]	Chimpanzees/diuresis; congestive heart failure; pulmonary edema
	1-4 mg/kg PO, SC q12h[41]	Common marmosets/congestive heart failure
	1-4 mg/kg IV[3]	Monkeys
	2-4 mg/kg IM q8h[3]	Monkeys
Glipizide	1.25 mg/kg PO q24h[86]	Titi monkey ($n=1$)/sulfonylurea; gestational diabetes
Glycopyrrolate	0.004 mg/kg IM, IV[3]	Chimpanzees
	0.004-0.008 mg/kg IM[3]	Monkeys
	0.005-0.01 mg/kg IM[20,72]	Macaques, baboons, chimpanzees[72]
	0.01 mg/kg IM[16,20]	Rhesus macaques,[16] orangutan[20]
	1 mg/animal PO q8h[3]	Chimpanzees
GnRH immunocontraceptive vaccine (GonaCon, USDA Wildlife Services)	500 μg dose IM[24]	Vervet monkeys/1 of 3 monkeys (adjuvant 1) cycled at 33 wk; 3 of 3 monkeys (adjuvant 2) cycled 25 wk; both had localized swelling at injection site
Guaifenesin	10-20 mL PO q4-6h[3]	Chimpanzees
Guanfacine	—	Self-injurious behavior; decreased agitation without profound sedation
	0.3 mg/kg PO, IM q12h × 5-10 days, followed by gradual reduction to 0.15 mg/kg q24h over 30 days[57]	Baboon ($n=1$)/recurrence controlled by returning to 0.3 mg/kg q12h
	0.5 mg/kg PO, IM q12h × 5-10 days, followed by gradual reduction to 0.25 mg/kg q24h over 30 days[57]	Macaques ($n=2$)/recurrence controlled by returning to 0.5 mg/kg q12h
Haloperidol	0.03-0.05 mg/kg IM q12h[3]	Monkeys
	0.5-5 mg PO q8-12h[3]	Chimpanzees
	60 mg PO q24h[76]	Gorilla ($n=1$)/antipsychotic; treat concurrently with sulpiride; extrapyramidal symptoms; neuroleptic malignant syndrome is a rare but potential side effect

Continued

TABLE 13-4 Miscellaneous Agents Used in Primates. (cont'd)

Agent	Dosage	Species/Comments
Heparin	5000-10,000 units IV q6h; 10,000-20,000 units SC q12h[3]	Chimpanzees
Human chorionic gonadotropin (hCG)	5000-10,000 U IM[3]	Chimpanzees
Hydrochlorothiazide	1 mg/kg PO q24h[3]	Chimpanzees
Hydrocortisone sodium succinate	5 mg/kg IM, IV q12h[3]	Chimpanzees
Insulin, NPH	0.1 U/animal SC q12h[41]	Common marmosets/glucose monitoring
	0.25-0.5 U/kg SC q24h[3]	Chimpanzees/starting dose; diabetes mellitus; diabetic ketoacidosis
	0.5 U/kg q24h[86]	Advisable to start with this dose and reevaluate with blood glucose
	2.5 U/kg divided into 2 doses IM[86]	Cynomolgus macaques/use combination of short-acting and longer-acting insulin (70:30); dose is highly variable
Iron dextran	10 mg/kg IM q7d[3]	Monkeys
	11-22 mg/kg IM[3]	Chimpanzees
Isoproterenol	0.05-2 µg/kg/min IV constant rate infusion[3]	Monkeys/nonselective β-adrenergic agonist
	0.1-1 µg/kg/min IV constant rate infusion or 0.02-0.06 mg IV bolus[3]	Chimpanzees
Lactulose	0.25-1.1 mL/kg PO q8-12h[41]	Common marmosets
Leuprolide acetate (Lupron)	Effective contraception for 1-6 mo	New World primates/GnRH antagonist implant; need secondary contraception of megesterol acetate (*not* depoprovera) for 7 days prior to and postimplant placement[80]
	0.3 mg/kg IM every 4 wk[3]	
	3.75 mg suspension once/mo for 6 mo[39]	Allen's swamp monkey ($n=1$)/uterine fibroids and ovarian cysts
Levothyroxine	0.05 mg/animal PO q24h; incremental changes of 0.025 mg q24h at 30 day intervals up to 0.1 mg q24h[86]	Gorilla ($n=1$)/hypothyroidism; monitor TSH and T_4 q6-8wk
Lidocaine	0.7-1.4 mg/kg IV as needed[3]	Monkeys, chimpanzees at 1-1.5 mg/kg IV and max of 3 mg/kg
	1-2 mg/kg IV bolus[41,72]	Common marmosets[41]
	20-50 µg/kg/min IV constant rate infusion[72]	Ventricular arrhythmia
Lisinopril	0.25-0.5 mg/kg PO q24h[3]	Chimpanzees
Loperamide	0.04 mg/kg PO q8h[3]	Monkeys
	4 mg/animal PO prn[3]	Chimpanzees
Mannitol (25%)	0.25-0.5 g/kg IV over 5-10 min[3]	Monkeys/diuretic
	0.5-1 g/kg IV constant rate infusion[3]	Chimpanzees
	1.65-2.2 g/kg IV over 20 min[3]	Monkeys/cerebral edema

TABLE 13-4 Miscellaneous Agents Used in Primates. (cont'd)

Agent	Dosage	Species/Comments
Medroxyprogesterone acetate	5 mg/kg IM q6wk[59]	Lemurs/seasonal contraceptive
	5-10 mg/animal PO q24h × 5-10 days[3]	Monkeys/contraceptive
	150 mg/animal IM once q3mo[3] or q30d[23]	Chimpanzees, monkeys/contraceptive;[3] rhesus macaques/endometriosis[23]
Megestrol acetate	800 mg/animal PO q24h[3]	Chimpanzees
Melengestrol acetate implant (MGA, WildPharm)	—	Implant must be ethylene oxide sterilized then degassed for 2 wk before surgical placement; available only in United States
	0.06 g/kg[80]	Great apes, gibbons
	0.1 g/kg[80]	Old World primates, except colobinae (0.15 g/kg)
	0.25 g/kg[80]	Lemurs
	0.4 g/kg[80]	Howler monkeys
	0.5 g/kg[80]	Spider monkeys, saki monkeys, cebids
	0.7 g/kg[80]	New World primates other than howler, spider, saki, capuchin, and squirrel monkeys; not recommended in *Callimico*[41,80]
	1 g/kg[80]	Squirrel monkeys
Metformin	5-10 mg/kg PO q12h[41]	Common marmosets/oral hypoglycemic
Metoclopramide	0.2-0.5 mg/kg IM q8-24h[3]	Monkeys/antiemetic; stimulates motility of upper gastrointestinal tract
	0.4 mg/kg PO,[20] IM, slow IV q8-24h[3]	Chimpanzees
Milk thistle (silymarin)	4-15 mg/kg PO q8-12h[41]	Common marmosets
Mirtazapine	15 mg PO q24h[15]	Mandrill ($n=1$)/antianxiety
Misoprostol	5 μg/kg PO q6h; 1-3 μg/kg intravaginal[3]	Chimpanzees
Nitroglycerin (2% ointment)	3 mm topically q12-24h[41]	Common marmosets/congestive heart failure
	7.5 mg topically q8h[3]	Chimpanzees
Nitroprusside	0.3-10 μg/kg/min IV constant rate infusion[3]	Chimpanzees
Norepinephrine	0.05-0.1 μg/kg/min IV constant rate infusion[72]	Hypotension
	0.2-0.4 μg/kg/min IV constant rate infusion[3]	Chimpanzees
Omeprazole	0.4 mg/kg PO q12h × 10 days[86]	Macaques/quadruple treatment of *Helicobacter pylori*; see amoxicillin (Table 13.1)
Ondansetron	1-2 mg/kg PO × 2 doses[86]	Macaques/antiemetic
Oxytocin	0.5-1 U/min IV constant rate infusion[3]	Chimpanzees
	1-2 U IM every 20 min × 4 doses[41]	Common marmosets
	2 U/dose as needed[3]	Monkeys
	5-30 U/animal SC, IV as needed[3]	Chimpanzees

Continued

TABLE 13-4 Miscellaneous Agents Used in Primates. (cont'd)

Agent	Dosage	Species/Comments
Paroxetine	0.3 mg/kg PO q12-24h[86]	Bonobo ($n=1$)/antianxiety
PGF_2 alpha	1 mg/kg IM q24h[3]	Monkeys
Phenobarbital	1-6 mg/kg PO, or 2 mg/kg IV[3]	Monkeys/seizures
Phentolamine mesylate	5-10 mg SC, IV[3]	Chimpanzees/antihypertensive
Phenylephrine	1-2 µg/kg IV bolus, followed by 0.5-1 µg/kg/min IV constant rate infusion[72]	Drug of choice to treat isoflurane-induced hypotension
Phenytoin	2.5 mg/kg PO q12h, increase as needed[3]	Monkeys
	125 mg PO q8h, increase as needed[3]	Chimpanzees
Pimobendan	0.2 mg/kg PO q24h[41]	Common marmosets/congestive heart failure
Polysulfated glycosaminoglycan (Adequan, Luitpold Pharmaceuticals)	2 mg/kg IM q3-5d × 2-3 mo[3]	Monkeys
	2-3 mg/kg IM q4d × 2 mo[3]	Chimpanzees
Potassium chloride	0.5-1 mEq/kg/h IV[3]	Chimpanzees, monkeys
	20-100 mEq PO q24h[3]	Chimpanzees, monkeys
Prednisolone sodium succinate	1 mg/kg PO q24h[41]	Common marmosets/myelofibrosis
	10 mg/kg IM, IV[3,27]	Chimpanzees, monkeys,[3] lemurs/shock[27]
Prednisone	0.5-2 mg/kg PO[3]	Monkeys
	0.5-2.2 mg/kg PO[3]	Chimpanzees
Probencid	1 g/animal PO q12h × 7 days[3]	Chimpanzees
Procainamide	50 mg/kg/day PO divided q6h[3]	Chimpanzees
Prochlorperazine	0.12 mg/kg IM, IV[3]	Monkeys/antiemetic
	5-10 mg PO, IM, IV q8-24h[3]	Chimpanzees
Propanolol	0.25-1 mg/kg PO q8-12h[3]	Chimpanzees
Quinidine	100-200 mg/animal PO q8-12h[3]	Chimpanzees
Ranitidine	0.5 mg/kg PO q12h[3]	Monkeys
	150 mg/animal PO q8-12h[3]	Chimpanzees
Ribavirin	150 mg/kg IM q24h × 6 days[33]	Callitrichid hepatitis virus
S-Adenosylmethionine (SAM-e) (Denosyl, Nutramax)	18 mg/kg PO q24h[3]	Chimpanzees
Spironolactone	20-300 mg/day divided q8-24h[3]	Chimpanzees
Stanozolol	2 mg/animal PO q6-8h[3]	Chimpanzees
	5-10 mg/kg IM q4-7d[3]	Monkeys
Sucralfate	0.5 g/animal PO; maintenance q12h, active ulcer q6h × 4-6 wk[3]	Monkeys/prevent or treat gastric ulcers
	1 g/animal PO q12h[3]	Chimpanzees
Sulpiride	400-800 mg/animal PO q24h[76]	Gorilla ($n=1$)/antipsychotic; treat concurrently with haloperidol; extrapyramidal symptoms; neuroleptic malignant syndrome is rare but potential side effect

TABLE 13-4 Miscellaneous Agents Used in Primates. (cont'd)

Agent	Dosage	Species/Comments
Telmisartan	1 mg/kg PO[41]	Common marmosets/protein losing nephropathy
Terbutaline	0.05 mg/kg IM, IV[18]	Great apes/bronchodilator
	5 mg/animal PO q24h[3]	Chimpanzees
Theophylline	5 mg/kg, then 2-4 mg/kg PO q6-8h[3]	Chimpanzees
Tolbutamine	250 mg/animal PO q24h, then 100 mg/animal PO q48h[86]	Capuchin monkey ($n=1$)/non–insulin-dependent diabetes mellitus
Triamcinolone	0.2-2 mg/kg IM prn[3] or q3d[86]	Monkeys
Vitamin B_{12}	3-5 mL PO, IM, IV[3]	Chimpanzees
Vitamin C (ascorbic acid)	—	Vitamin C is an essential nutrient for nonhuman primates[59,64,71]
	1-4 mg/kg PO q24h[41]	Common marmosets/maintenance; up to 25 mg/kg/day[59]
	3-6 mg/kg PO q24h to prevent scurvy[69]	
	4-25 mg/kg PO q24h[3]	Chimpanzees
	25 mg/kg PO, IM[86] q12h × 5 days[41]	Macaques,[86] common marmosets[41]/deficiency situation
	30 mg/kg IM q24h[3]	Monkeys
Vitamin D_3	—	Vitamin D is an essential nutrient for nonhuman primates;[10] elevated concentration that is not D_2 is required for New World primates[64]
	20 U/kg PO q24h[3]	Chimpanzees
	110 U/100 g[59]	New World primates/UVB light
	2000 U/kg[41]	Common marmosets
	5000 U ergocalciferol depot (sesame oil) IM once at age 4 mo and ergocalciferol 400 U PO q24h from age 4 mo until weaning[43]	Infant chimpanzees/prevention of rickets
Vitamin E	3.75 U/kg PO q24h[3]	Chimpanzees
Vitamin K_1	1 mg/kg PO, IM q8h[3]	Chimpanzees
	1-5 mg/animal IM q24h[3]	Monkeys
Winstrol	2-4 mg PO q24h[3]	Chimpanzees
Zinc	2.5 µg/animal PO q24h × 3 days[3]	Monkeys
	75 mg PO q12h as needed[3]	Chimpanzees
Zuclopenthixol	10-25 mg PO q8h[76]	Gorilla ($n=1$)/aggression; tapered with a decrease of 5 mg/wk; antipsychotic; extrapyramidal symptoms; neuroleptic malignant syndrome is a rare but potentially side effect

TABLE 13-5 Hematologic and Serum Biochemical Values of Primates.[19,37,41,59,62,90,93]

Measurement	Baboon (Papio spp.)	Capuchin Monkey (Cebus sp.)	Chimpanzee (Pan troglodytes)	Common Marmoset (Callithrix jacchus)[b]	Ring-Tailed Lemur (Lemur catta)
Hematology					
PCV (%)	45	45-53	38-51	45-48	44-57
RBC ($10^6/\mu L$)	4.5-4.8	6	4.7-6.4	2.5-10.4	6.7-8.6
Hgb (g/dL)	13	14-17	7.6-10.7	15.1-15.5	13.8-17.2
WBC ($10^3/\mu L$)	14.1	5-24	7.3-15.7	3-15	4.8-12.5
Neutrophils (%)	60.5	55	3.0-10.7[a]	28-55	1.2-7.5[a]
Lymphocytes (%)	36	41	2.0-7.3[a]	43-67	1.7-5.7[a]
Monocytes (%)	1.5	1.8	64.8-572.2[a]	0.4-2.1	0-0.8[a]
Eosinophils (%)	1.5	1.6	68.8-629.6[a]	0.5-0.6	0-0.7[a]
Basophils (%)	0.4	<1	0-23.6[a]	0.3-1.3	0-0.1[a]
Platelets ($10^3/\mu L$)	406	108-187	130-379	390-490	161-379
Chemistries					
ALT (U/L)	12-20	13-43	20.5-62.1	9.5-10.2	36-154
AST (U/L)	22-28	21-57	12.1-56.6	160-182	12-80
Bilirubin (mg/dL)	0.3-0.4	0-4	0.2-0.6	0.5-0.6	0.2-1
BUN (mg/dL)	8-14	24-44	8.3-17.8	13.0-38.5	13-29
Calcium (mg/dL)	8-10	10	7.8-10.5	9.5-10.2	8.8-10.4
Cholesterol (mg/dL)	60-134	170-254	166.8-295.8	89-292	1.6-3.0
Glucose (mg/dL)	80-95	44-94	66-118	95-257	66-222
Phosphorus (mg/dL)	5.5-8.5	7	1.5-4.9	1.6-10.4	3.3-6.7
Protein, total (g/dL)	6-7	7.5-8.7	6.7-8.4	4.1-8.9	6.5-8.1

Measurement	Rhesus Macaque (Macaca mulatta)	Spider Monkey (Ateles spp.)	Squirrel Monkey (Saimiri sciureus)	Tamarin (Saguinus spp.)
Hematology				
PCV (%)	39-43	35-40	43-56	45
RBC ($10^6/\mu L$)	4.5-6	5.5	7.1-10.9	6.6
Hgb (g/dL)	12.7	16	12.9-17	15.5
WBC ($10^3/\mu L$)	11.5-12.4	10-12	5.1-10.9	12.6-14.4
Neutrophils (%)	20-56	52	36-66	43-64
Lymphocytes (%)	40-76	40	27-55	34-49
Monocytes (%)	0-2	3	0-6	2-5
Eosinophils (%)	1-3	5	0-11	1-1.2
Basophils (%)	0-1	0-1	<1	0.1
Platelets ($10^3/\mu L$)	130-144	239-343	112	331-650

TABLE 13-5 Hematologic and Serum Biochemical Values of Primates. (cont'd)

Measurement	Rhesus Macaque (*Macaca mulatta*)	Spider Monkey (*Ateles* spp.)	Squirrel Monkey (*Saimiri sciureus*)	Tamarin (*Saguinus* spp.)
Chemistries				
ALT (U/L)	145-171	8-78	59-99	7-14
AST (U/L)	20-34	42-210	56-118	49-59
Bilirubin (mg/dL)	0.10-0.66	0.1-1.0	0.1-0.53	0.14-0.26
BUN (mg/dL)	14.2-19.6	25.9	23-39	6-12
Calcium (mg/dL)	8.1-11.3	12.8	8.3-9.7	10
Cholesterol (mg/dL)	94-162	76-278	127-207	69
Glucose (mg/dL)	53-87	82.3	52-108	125-189
LDH (U/L)	201-665	—	271-490	0-1578
Phosphorus (mg/dL)	4-6	2.1-8.5	3.3-7.7	3-6
Protein, total (g/dL)	6.1-7.1	10.2	6.9-8.1	6.2-8.6

[a]These values are reported as absolute differential as $10^3/\mu L$ for more accuracy when they were available.
[b]Chemistry values for this species were not obtained from standard deviation but direct high and low values for $n=21$ animals as reported in the cited study.[93]

TABLE 13-6 Biologic and Physiologic Data of Primates.[4,19,20,31,59,62,79,90]

Species	Temperature °C (°F)	Respiratory (breaths/min)	Heart Rate (beats/min)	Avg Adult Wt (kg) M/F	Estrus Length (days)	Gestation (days)	Weaning Age (days)	Median Life Expectancy (yrs)
Baboon (*Papio* sp.)	37-39 (98.6-103.1)	22-35	85-90	14-41; males 50% larger	32-36	154-193	180-450	30-45
Capuchin monkey (*Cebus* sp.)	37-38.5 (98.6-101.3)	30-50	165-225	3.5-3.9/2.5-3	18-23	180	270	50
Chimpanzee (*Pan troglodytes*)	34.6-38.7 (94.3-101.7)	20-60	60-200	45-90/40-80	28-53	215-239	1440	31.7-37.4
Common marmoset (*Callithrix jacchus*)	38.4-39.1 (101.1-102.4)	36-44	204-399	0.34-0.35	16-30	141-145	40-120	8-12
Ring-tailed lemur (*Lemur catta*)	37.9-38.1 (100.2-100.6)	30-60	168-210	2-3	39	130-136	90-120	16.5
Rhesus macaque (*Macaca mulatta*)	37-39 (98.6-103.1)	35-50	98-122	6-11/4-9	24-40	144-210	210-420	18-23.8
Spider monkey (*Ateles* sp.)	—	—	—	6-10/6-8	26	225-232	365	24.4
Squirrel monkey (*Saimiri sciureus*)	37-38.5 (98.6-101.3)	20-50	200-350	0.75-1.1	7-16	140-180	180	14.6
Tamarin (*Saguinus* sp.)	—	—	—	0.225-0.9	15	140	60-90	11.5

TABLE 13-7 Identifying Characteristics of Small Nonhuman Primates by their Taxonomic Classification.[19,31,79,90]

Characteristic	Prosimians	New World Monkeys (Platyrrhini)	Old World Monkeys (Catarrhini)
Tapetum	Yes	—	—
Moist rhinarium	Yes	—	—
Specialized scent glands	Yes	—	—
Uterus	Bicornuate	Simplex	Simplex
Placenta	Epitheliochorial	Hemochorial	Hemochorial
Closed orbits	—	Yes	Yes
Incisor comb	Yes	—	—
Dental formula	2.1.3.3./2.1.3.3. (36)	2.1.3.3./2.1.3.3. (36)	2.1.2.3./2.1.2.3. (32)
Grooming claw	Yes	—	—
Prehensile tail	—	Yes	—
Nostrils	At end of rhinarium	Round, directed laterally	Narrowed, directed ventrally
Claws or nails	Claws	Claws	Nails
Ischial callosities	—	—	Yes

TABLE 13-8 ECG Intervals and Durations.[5,41,82]

Species	P Wave duration (sec)	PR Interval (sec)	QT Interval (sec)	QRS Duration (sec)
Baboon (*Papio* sp.)	0.02-0.06	0.05-0.09	0.13-0.19	0.01-0.05
Capuchin monkey (*Cebus* sp.)	0.02-0.04	0.07-0.09	0.14-0.16	0.01-0.03
Chimpanzee (*Pan troglodytes*)	<0.12	0.104-0.242	0.327-0.445	0.059-0.103
Common marmoset (*Callithrix jacchus*)	0.021-0.029	0.052-0.062	0.088-0.156	—
Rhesus macaque (*Macaca mulatta*)	0.03-0.05	0.08-0.1	0.18-0.22	0.02-0.04
Squirrel monkey (*Saimiri sciureus*)	0.02-0.04	0.05-0.07	0.14-0.16	0.01-0.03

TABLE 13-9 Preventive Medicine Recommendations for Primates.[19,35,36,41,59,62]

Procedure	Schedule	Comments
Routine examination	Annually for small or medium nonhuman primates; q2-3yr great apes	Routine: physical examination, hemogram, serum biochemical analysis, serum banking, rectal culture, mycobacterial screening, radiographs, ultrasound By institution history: viral serology, vaccination
Tuberculin skin testing (Intradermal Mammalian Old Tuberculin, Synbiotics)	0.1 mL ID via 27 g needle; test at routine examination intervals	Typically, the test is placed intrapalpebrally so test site can be examined without restraint; an alternative site, or used for subsequent screening, is the areolar area; following test placement, test is evaluated visually at 24, 48, and 72 hr; a positive reaction is erythema, edema, induration, or combination of these signs persisting for >48 hr; false positives (especially in orangutans) and false negatives (anergic animals) can occur; comparative testing with evaluation of hemogram, comparative antigens (e.g., avian purified protein derivative), thoracic radiographs, mycobacterial culture of tracheal or gastric lavage assists interpretation; imported primates to the United States have testing dictated by Centers for Disease Control and Prevention with three negative intradermal tests required over a 30-day interval; for all caretakers, tuberculin screening for in-contact staff is recommended annually; comparative testing could include serologic testing for gamma interferon, but often this methodology is not available reliably as a commercial test for nonhuman primates; although it is available for humans, these products were not validated for nonhuman primates.
	0.05 mL ID via 27 g needle; test annually[37]	Commonly used dose reduction for callitrichids and similar sized New World primates; see previous comments
Fecal parasite examination	q3-12mo based on collection history or when abnormal fecal quality is present	Direct wet mount of fresh feces for protozoa; flotation and/or sedimentation procedures for parasite ova; trichrome stains can be used to identify protozoal cysts; direct staining of fecal smears for cell populations
Fecal culture	At collection entry; at routine examination schedule; based on collection history or when abnormal fecal quality is present	Culture for *Salmonella, Shigella, Campylobacter, Yersinia*; may take multiple samples to identify asymptomatic carriers of *Salmonella* or *Shigella*

CHAPTER 13 Primates 607

TABLE 13-10 Immunization Recommendations for Primates.[a]

Species	Immunization	Dose/Schedule	Comments
Prosimians	Rabies		There are no specific recommendations for prosimians[91]
			Killed vaccine only; consider with elevated exposure risk situations[91]
	Tetanus	Tetanus toxoid	Used in some institutions;[91] of note, current preparations are combined with *Diphtheria* prophylaxis
New World primates	Measles		Measles in New World primates is a severe disease that may be associated with epizootics of high morbidity and mortality; in callitrichids, the virus targets the gastrointestinal tract;[59] in the United States, only an attenuated measles/mumps/rubella vaccine is available; however, it is rarely recommended due to declined human incidence of this disease and extensive vaccination of humans[19,59]
	Rabies	Volume of vaccine adjusted by body size:[19] callitrichids, 0.05-0.1 mL; medium-sized primates, 0.25 mL;[69] larger primates, 0.5 mL	Used by some institutions in rabies-endemic areas; use only killed virus preparation[69]
		1 mL dose of killed vaccine IM (quadriceps muscle) days 2,7,12,19,33 postexposure and single dose of human rabies immunoglobulin IM 5 days postexposure[86]	Capuchin monkeys/postexposure prophylaxis in monkeys that had direct contact with rabid bats; animals developed and maintained levels of rabies virus neutralizing antibody >0.05 U/mL by 67 days postexposure[86]
	Tetanus	Volume of tetanus toxoid adjusted by body size:[19] callitrichids, 0.05-0.1 mL; medium-sized primates, 0.25 mL; larger primates, 0.5 mL	New World monkeys are susceptible to *Clostridium tetani*;[19] of note, current preparations are combined with *Diphtheria* prophylaxis
Old World primates	Measles		In the United States, only an attenuated measles/mumps/rubella vaccine is available; however, it is rarely recommended due to declined human incidence of this disease and extensive vaccination of humans[19]
	Rabies	Volume of vaccine adjusted by body size:[19] medium-sized primates, 0.25 mL; larger primates, 0.5 mL	Used by some institutions in rabies-endemic areas; use only killed virus preparation
	Tetanus	Volume of tetanus toxoid adjusted by body size:[19] medium-sized primates, 0.25 mL; larger primates, 0.5 mL	Old World monkeys are susceptible to tetanus;[19,83] of note, current preparations are combined with *Diphtheria* prophylaxis

Continued

TABLE 13-10 Immunization Recommendations for Primates. (cont'd)

Species	Immunization	Dose/Schedule	Comments
Great apes	Measles	MMR II (live-attenuated product; Merck) – 12-15 mo; 4-6 yr of age[62]	Optional;[62] risk of shedding live virus and susceptibility of pregnant females and fetus is unquantified but rubella component has fetal concerns labeled in pregnant humans; from Attenuvax (Merck) product vaccine, seroconversion occurred in Western lowland gorillas and persisted for at least 11 yr following 1, 2, or 3 vaccinations on 12 mo, 15 mo, and 10 yr of age or 2 doses separated by 2-4 wk for unvaccinated, seronegative adults[14]
	Polio	Inactivated poliovirus – 2, 4, 6-18 mo; 4-6 yr[62]	Although human adult vaccination in the United States is no longer considered necessary, catch-up protocols exist for pediatric patients
	Rabies		Used by some institutions in rabies-endemic areas; use only killed virus preparation[62]
	Tetanus	Diphtheria, tetanus, pertussis (DTaP) – 2, 4, 6, 15-18 mo; 11-12 yr; q10yr[62]	Based on human schedule; of note, current products are combined with Diphtheria prophylaxis

[a]Vaccination protocols are highly individualized to institutional risk with considerations of potential exposure, age of animals, outdoor housing, access to humans, and community health profiles of the in-access human population.[62] Additionally, killed vaccine products are strongly encouraged whenever possible with caution of live or attenuated products for monitoring for vaccine-induced disease. It also should be noted that immunoprophylaxis products vary with availability to the medical community and human health issues and, therefore, absolute recommendations are not possible. Sources to consider for planning a program-specific approach include: www.cdc.gov, American Academy of Pediatrics publications,[1] Conn's Current Therapy (published annually),[17] AAZV's Infectious Diseases of Concern to Captive and Free-Ranging Animals in North America,[33] and species care guidelines available on www.aza.org.

TABLE 13-11　Nonhuman Primate Laboratories.

Antech Diagnostics
17672-B Cowan Avenue, Irvine, CA 92614, USA
ANTECH West: 1-800-745-4725; ANTECH East: 1-800-872-1001; ANTECH Test Express: 1-888-397-8378
http://www.antechdiagnostics.com/Main/TestGuide.aspx

Arbovirus Diagnostic Laboratory
3156 Rampart Road, Fort Collins, CO 80521, USA
970-221-6400
http://www.cdc.gov/ncezid/dvbd/specimensub/arboviral-shipping.html

B Virus Research and Resource Laboratory
Dr. Julia Hilliard
Georgia State University, Viral Immunology Center, 161 Jesse Hill Jr Dr., Atlanta, GA 30303, USA
For emergency: 404-358-8168
http://www2.gsu.edu/~wwwvir/

BioReliance, Serology/PCR Laboratories
14920 Broschart Rd., Rockville, MD 20850, USA
301-610-2227
http://www.bioreliance.com/us/services

Centers for Disease Control and Prevention
1600 Clifton Rd. Atlanta, GA 30329, USA
800-232-4636
http://www.cdc.gov/

Clinical Parasitology Diagnostic Service Laboratory
University of Tennessee College of Veterinary Medicine, 2407 River Drive, Knoxville, TN 37996, USA
865-974-5645
https://vetmed.tennessee.edu/vmc/dls/Pages/default.aspx

Colorado State University Veterinary Diagnostic Laboratory
300 West Drake Road, Ft. Collins, CO 80526
970-297-1281
http://csu-cvmbs.colostate.edu/vdl/Pages/default.aspx

Comparative Pathology Laboratory
University of Miami, Clinical Research Building, 1120 NW 14th Street, 14th Floor, Suite 1409, Miami, FL 33136, USA
305-243-7284
http://www.pathology.med.miami.edu/clinical-pathology

Diagnostic Center for Population and Animal Health (DCPAH)
Clinical Pathology Laboratory, A215 Veterinary Medical Center, Michigan State University, East Lansing, MI 48824, USA
517-355-1774
https://www.dcpah.msu.edu/Sections/

IDEXX Laboratories, Inc.
One IDEXX Drive, Westbrook, ME 04092, USA
1-207-556-0300
1-800-548-6733
https://www.idexx.com/small-animal-health/products-and-services/products-and-services.html

Infectious Diseases Laboratory
University of Georgia College of Veterinary Medicine
110 Riverbend Rd., Riverbend North, Room 150, University of Georgia, Athens, GA 30602, USA
Lab: 706-542-5812
http://www.vet.uga.edu/idl/

Infectious Disease Pathology Activity
CDC (MS-G32), 1600 Clifton Rd, NE, Atlanta, GA 30333, USA
1-800-232-4636

Continued

TABLE 13-11 Nonhuman Primate Laboratories. (cont'd)

Kansas State University Diagnostic Laboratory
Kansas State University, 1800 Denison Avenue, Manhattan, KS 66506, USA
785-532-5650
http://www.ksvdl.org/

Louisiana Animal Disease Diagnostic Laboratory
School of Veterinary Medicine, 1909 Skip Bertman Drive, Room 1519, Baton Rouge, LA 70803, USA
225-578-9777
http://www.lsu.edu/vetmed/laddl/index.php

MiraVista Diagnostics
4705 Decatur Blvd., Indianapolis, IN 46241, USA
317-856-2681
http://miravistalabs.com/veterinary-fungal-infections/

New York State Veterinary Diagnostic Laboratory
Cornell University, 240 Farrier Rd, Ithaca, NY 14852, USA
607-253-3900
https://ahdc.vet.cornell.edu/test/list.aspx?Species=16&Test_Name=&TstTyp=&WebDisc=

North Carolina State University College of Veterinary Medicine Vector Borne Disease Diagnostic Laboratory
1060 William Moore Drive, Room 462A Raleigh, NC 27607, USA
919-513-8279
https://cvm.ncsu.edu/research/labs/diagnostic-testing-labs/

Northwest ZooPath
654 W Main St., Monroe, WA 98272, USA
360-794-0630
http://www.zoopath.com/

Pathogen Detection Laboratory
California National Primate Research Center, University of California, Road 98 & Hutchison
Davis, CA 95616, USA
530-752-8242
http://www.cnprc.ucdavis.edu/our-services/core-services/pathogen-detection-laboratory-core-2/services/

Primate Diagnostic Services Laboratory (PDSL)
Washington National Primate Research Center
University of Washington, 3000 Western Ave, B-411, Seattle, WA 98195, USA
206-543-0440
https://www.wanprc.org/

Texas A&M Veterinary Medical Diagnostic Laboratory
PO Box Drawer 3040, College Station, TX 77841, USA
979-845-3414
888-646-5623
https://tvmdl.tamu.edu/

The Fungus Testing Laboratory
Department of Pathology, Room 329E, Mail Code 7750, The University of Texas Health Science Center at San Antonio, San Antonio, TX 78229, USA
210-567-4131
http://pathology.uthscsa.edu/strl/fungus/index.shtml

UC Davis Coccidioidomycosis Serology Laboratory, 3416 One Shields Avenue, Davis, CA 95616, USA530-752-9402
http://www.ucdmc.ucdavis.edu/medmicro/cocci-lab.html

USDA-APHIS-VS-NVSL
1920 Dayton Ave. (packages), Ames, IA 50010, USA
515-337-7266
https://www.aphis.usda.gov/aphis/ourfocus/animalhealth/lab-info-services/ct_laboratory_information_services

TABLE 13-11	Nonhuman Primate Laboratories. (cont'd)

Veterinary Molecular Diagnostics, Inc.
5989 Meijer Dr., Suite 5, Milford, OH 45150, USA
513-576-1808
http://www.vmdlabs.com/

Virus Reference Laboratories, Inc. (VRL)
P.O. Box 40100, 7540 Louis Pasteur Road, San Antonio, TX 78229, USA
877-615-7275
http://www.vrlsat.com/nhp

Zoological Pathology Program
3300 Golf Road, Brookfield, IL 60513, USA
312-585-9050
http://vetmed.illinois.edu/vet-resources/veterinary-diagnostic-laboratory/zoological-pathology-program/

Zoologix Inc.
9811 Owensmouth Avenue, Suite 4, Chatsworth, CA 91311, USA
818-717-8880
http://zoologix.com/primate/index.htm

REFERENCES

1. American Academy of Pediatrics. Available at: https://www.aap.org/; 18 December 2016.
2. Anderson KE, Austin J, Escobar EP, et al. Platelet aggregation in rhesus macaques (*Macaca mulatta*) in response to short-term meloxicam administration. *J Am Assoc Lab Anim Sci* 2013;52:590-594.
3. Association of Primate Veterinarians. Nonhuman Primate Formulary. https://www.primatevets.org/education; 18 December 2016.
4. Association of Zoos and Aquariums. *Species Survival Statistics*. Available at: https://www.aza.org/assets/2332/survival_statistics_library_-_expires_1_dec_2016.pdf; 18 December 2016.
5. Atencia R, Revuelta L, Somauroo JD, et al. Electrocardiogram reference intervals for clinically normal wild-born chimpanzees (*Pan troglodytes*). *Am J Vet Res* 2015;76:688-693.
6. Authier S, Chaurand F, Legaspi M, et al. Comparison of three anesthetic protocols for intraduodenal drug administration using endoscopy in rhesus monkeys (*Macaca mulatta*). *J Am Assoc Lab Anim Sci* 2006;45:73-79.
7. AZA Prosimian Taxon Advisory Group. *Eulemur Care Manual*. Silver Spring: Association of Zoos and Aquariums; 2013.
8. Badyal DK, Garg SK. Effect of clarithromycin on the pharmacokinetics of carbamazepine in rhesus monkeys. *Methods Find Exp Clin Pharmacol* 2000;22:581-584.
9. Bakker J, Thuesen LR, Braskamp G, et al. Single subcutaneous dosing of cefovecin in rhesus monkeys (*Macaca mulatta*): a pharmacokinetic study. *J Vet Pharmacol Therap* 2011;34:464-468.
10. Bartlett SL, Chen TC, Murphy H, et al. Assessment of serum 25-hydroxy vitamin D concentrations in two collections of captive gorillas (*Gorilla gorilla gorilla*). *J Zoo Wildl Med* 2017;48:144-151.
11. Bauer C, Frost P, Kirschner S. Pharmacokinetics of 3 formulations of meloxicam in cynomolgus macaques (*Macaca fascicularis*). *J Am Assoc Lab Anim Sci* 2014;53:502-511.
12. Bentzel DE, Bacon DJ. Comparison of various anthelmintic therapies for the treatment of *Trypanoxyuris microon* infection in owl monkeys (*Aotus nancymae*). *Comp Med* 2007;57:206-209.
13. Blackwood RS, Tarara RP, Christe KL, et al. Effects of the macrolide drug tylosin on chronic diarrhea in rhesus macaques (*Macaca mulatta*). *Comp Med* 2008;58:81-87.
14. Blasier MW, Travis DA, Barbiers R. Retrospective evaluation of measles antibody titers in vaccinated captive gorillas (*Gorilla gorilla gorilla*). *J Zoo Wildl Med* 2005;36:198-203.

15. Bodley K, Ley J. Management of behavioral disorders in zoo primates: two cases at Melbourne Zoo. *Proc Annu Conf Am Assoc Zoo Vet* 2014;73.
16. Bohm RP, Rockar RA, Ratterree MS, et al. A method of video-assisted thorascopic surgery for collection of thymic biopsies in rhesus monkeys (*Macaca mulatta*). *Contemp Top Lab Anim Sci* 2000;39:24-26.
17. Bope ET, Kellerman RD, eds. *Conn's Current Therapy 2016*. Philadelphia: Elsevier; 2016.
18. Brainard B, Darrow EJ. Sedation and anesthesia in the great apes—an overview. *Proc Annu Conf Am Assoc Zoo Vet* 2013;26-35.
19. Calle PP, Joslin JO. New World and Old World monkeys. In: Miller RE, Fowler RE, eds. *Zoo and Wild Animal Medicine*. Vol 8. St. Louis: Elsevier; 2015:301-335.
20. Cerveny S, Sleeman J. Great apes. In: West G, Heard D, Caulkett N, eds. *Zoo Animal and Wildlife Immobilization and Anesthesia*. 2nd ed. Ames: John Wiley & Sons; 2014:573-584.
21. Cook AL, St Claire M, Sams R. Use of florfenicol in non-human primates. *J Med Primatol* 2004;33:127-133.
22. Correia J, Noiva R, Pissarra H, et al. Four cases of *Calodium hepaticum* infection in non-human primates from the Lisbon Zoological Garden, Portugal. *Proc Int Conf Dis Zoo Wild Anim* 2011;13-22.
23. Cruzen CL, Baum ST, Colman RJ. Glucoregulatory function in adult rhesus macaques (*Macaca mulatta*) undergoing treatment with medroxyprogesterone acetate for endometriosis. *J Am Assoc Lab Anim Sci* 2011;50:921-925.
24. Dascanio JJ, Hegler A, Hall E, et al. Efficacy of gonadotropin-releasing hormone (GnRH) vaccine (GonaCon™) on reproduction function in female vervet monkeys (*Chlorocebus aethiops*). *Proc Annu Conf Am Assoc Zoo Vet* 2014;180.
25. DiVincenti L. Analgesic use in nonhuman primates undergoing neurosurgical procedures. *J Am Assoc Lab Anim Sci* 2013;52:10-16.
26. Fanton JW, Zar SR, Ewert DL, et al. Cardiovascular responses to propofol and etomidate in long-term instrumented rhesus monkeys (*Macaca mulatta*). *Comp Med* 2000;5:303-308.
27. Feeser P, White F. Medical management of *Lemur catta*, *Varecia variegata*, and *Propithecus verreauxi* in natural habitat enclosures. *Proc Annu Conf Am Assoc Zoo Vet/Am Assoc Wildl Vet* 1992;320-323.
28. Flecknell PA. Clinical experience with NSAIDs in macaques. *Lab Primate Newsl* 2004;44:4.
29. Flecknell PA. *Laboratory Animal Anaesthesia*. 4th ed. Waltham: Elsevier/Academic Press; 2016.
30. Fontenot MB, Musso MW, McFatter RM, et al. Dose-finding study of fluoxetine and venlafaxine for the treatment of self-injurious and stereotypic behavior in rhesus macaques (*Macaca mulatta*). *J Am Assoc Lab Anim Sci* 2009;48:176-184.
31. Fortman JD, Hewett TA, Bennett BT, eds. *The Laboratory Nonhuman Primate*. Boca Raton: CRC Press; 2002.
32. Furtado MM, Nunes AL, Intelizano TR, et al. Comparison of racemic ketamine versus (S+) ketamine when combined with midazolam for anesthesia of *Callithrix jacchus* and *Callithrix penicillata*. *J Zoo Wildl Med* 2010;41:389-394.
33. Gamble KC, Clancy MM, eds. *Infectious Diseases of Concern to Captive and Free-Ranging Animals in North America*. 2nd ed. Yulee: Infectious Disease Committee, American Association of Zoo Veterinarians; 2013.
34. Hahn NE, Capuano SV. Successful treatment of cryptosporidiosis in 2 common marmosets (*Callithrix jacchus*) by using paromycin. *J Am Assoc Lab Anim Sci* 2010;49:873-875.
35. Hellebrekers LJ, Hedenqvist P. Laboratory animal analgesia, anesthesia, and euthanasia. In: Hau J, Schapiro SJ, eds. *Handbook of Laboratory Animal Science*. Vol 1. 3rd ed. Boca Raton: CRC Press; 2011:485-534.
36. Hrapkiewicz K, Medina L. *Nonhuman primates*. *Clinical Laboratory Animal Medicine*. 3rd ed. Ames: Blackwell Publishing; 2007:280-329.
37. Ihrig M, Tassinary LG, Bernacky B, et al. Hematologic and serum biochemical reference intervals for the chimpanzee (*Pan troglodytes*) categorized by age and sex. *Comp Med* 2001;51:30-37.

38. Institutional Animal Care and Use Committee of the University of California San Francisco. *Nonhuman Primate Formulary. Anesthesia and Analgesia in Laboratory Animals at UCSF.* Available at: http://www.iacuc.ucsf.edu/Proc/awNHPFrm.asp; 18 December 2016.
39. Jafarey Y, Hanley C, Berlinski R, et al. Management of uterine fibroids and ovarian cysts with leuprolide acetate in an Allen's swamp monkey (*Allenopithecus nigroviridus*). *Proc Annu Conf Am Assoc Zoo Vet* 2012;236.
40. James SB, Raphael BL. Demodicosis in red-handed tamarins (*Saguinus midas*). *J Zoo Wildl Med* 2000;31:251-254.
41. Jepson L. *Exotic Animal Medicine: A Quick Reference Guide.* 2nd ed. St. Louis: Elsevier; 2016.
42. Johnson-Delaney CA. Parasites of captive nonhuman primates. *Vet Clin North Am Exot Anim Pract* 2009;12:563-581.
43. Junge RE, Gannon FH, Porton I, et al. Management and prevention of vitamin D deficiency rickets in captive-born juvenile chimpanzees (*Pan troglodytes*). *J Zoo Wildl Med* 2000;31:361-369.
44. Kahn CM, ed. Nonhuman primates. In: *The Merck Veterinary Manual.* 10th ed. Whitehouse Station: Merck & Co; 2010:1681-1687.
45. Kearns KS, Swenson B, Ramsay EC. Oral induction of anesthesia with droperidol and transmucosal carfentanil citrate in chimpanzees (*Pan troglodytes*). *J Zoo Wildl Med* 2000;31:185-189.
46. Kelly KR, Pypendop BH, Christe KL. Pharmacokinetics of buprenorphine following intravenous and intramuscular administration in male rhesus macaques (*Macaca mulatta*). *J Vet Pharmacol Ther* 2014;37:480-485.
47. Kelly KR, Pypendop BH, Christe KL. Pharmacokinetics of hydromorphone after intravenous and intramuscular administration in male rhesus macaques (*Macaca mulatta*). *J Am Assoc Lab Anim Sci* 2014;53:512-516.
48. Kelly KR, Pypendop BH, Christe KL. Pharmacokinetics of tramadol following intravenous and oral administration in male rhesus macaques (*Macaca mulatta*). *J Vet Pharmacol Ther* 2015;38:375-382.
49. Kelly KR, Pypendop BH, Grayson JK, et al. Pharmacokinetics of oxymorphone in titi monkeys (*Callicebus* spp.) and rhesus macaques (*Macaca mulatta*). *J Am Assoc Lab Anim Sci* 2011;50:212-220.
50. Klein H, Hasselschwert D, Handt L, et al. A pharmacokinetics study of enrofloxacin and its active metabolite ciprofloxacin after oral and intramuscular dosing of enrofloxacin in rhesus monkeys (*Macaca mulatta*). *J Med Primatol* 2008;37:177-183.
51. Kottwitz JJ, Perry KK, Rose HH, et al. Angiostrongylus cantonensis infection in captive Geoffroy's tamarins (*Saguinus geoffroyi*). *J Am Vet Med Assoc* 2014;245:821-827.
52. Kramer JA, Hachey AM, Wachtman LM, et al. Treatment of giardiasis in common marmosets (*Callithrix jacchus*) with tinidazole. *Comp Med* 2009;59:174-179.
53. Kummrow MS, Mätz-Rensing K. High mortality due to streptococcal toxic shock syndrome in a captive colony of lion-tailed macaques (*Macaca silenus*). *Proc Joint Conf Am Assoc Zoo Vet/Euro Assoc Zoo Wildl Vet/Intnl Zoo Wildl* 2016;159-160.
54. Kummrow MS, Schwittlick U, Wohlsein P, et al. Treatment of suspected diabetes type I induced polyneuropathy in a drill (*Mandrillus leucophaeus*). *Proc Int Conf Dis Zoo Wild Anim* 2011;23.
55. Laudenslager ML, Clarke AS. Antidepressant treatment during social challenge prior to 1 year of age affects immune and endocrine responses in adult macaques. *Psychiatry Res* 2000;95: 25-34.
56. Lee VK, Flynt KS, Haag LM, et al. Comparison of the effects of ketamine, ketamine-medetomidine, and ketamine-midazolam on physiologic parameters and anesthesia-induced stress in rhesus (*Macaca mulatta*) and cynomolgus (*Macaca fascicularis*) macaques. *J Am Assoc Lab Anim Sci* 2010;49:57-63.
57. Macy JD, Beattie TA, Morgenstern SE, et al. Use of guanfacine to control self-injurious behavior in two rhesus macaques (*Macaca mulatta*) and one baboon (*Papio anubis*). *Comp Med* 2000; 50:419-425.

58. Martin LD, Dissen GA, McPike MJ, et al. Effects of anesthesia with isoflurane, ketamine, or propofol on physiologic parameters in neonatal rhesus macaques (*Macaca mulatta*). *J Am Assoc Lab Anim Sci* 2014;53:290-300.
59. Masters N. Primates. In: Meredith A, Johnson-Delaney C, eds. *BSAVA Manual of Exotic Pets*. 5th ed. Quedgeley: British Small Animal Veterinary Association; 2010:148-166.
60. Miller M, Weber M, Mangold B, et al. Use of oral detomidine and ketamine for anesthetic induction in nonhuman primates. *Proc Annu Conf Am Assoc Zoo Vet* 2000;179-180.
61. Miyabe-Nishiwaki T, Masui K, Kaneko A, et al. Evaluation of the predictive performance of a pharmokinetic model for propofol in Japanese macaques (*Macaca fuscata fuscata*). *J Vet Pharmacol Ther* 2013;36:169-173.
62. Murphy HW. Great apes. In: Miller RE, Fowler ME, eds. *Zoo and Wild Animal Medicine*. 8th ed. St. Louis: Elsevier; 2015:336-354.
63. Naples LM, Langan JN, Kearns KS. Comparison of the anesthetic effects of oral transmucosal versus injectable medetomidine in combination with tiletamine-zolazepam for immobilization of chimpanzees (*Pan troglodytes*). *J Zoo Wildl Med* 2010;41:50-62.
64. National Research Council of the Academies. *Vitamins. Nutrient Requirements of Nonhuman Primates*. 2nd ed Washington DC: The National Academic Press; 2003:113-149.
65. National Reye's Syndrome Foundation. Aspirin Lists. Available at: http://reyessyndrome.org/aspirinlists.html; 18 December 2016.
66. Nunamaker EA, Halliday LC, Moody DE, et al. Pharmacokinetics of 2 formulations of buprenorphine in macaques (*Macaca mulatta* and *Macaca fascicularis*). *J Am Assoc Lab Anim Sci* 2013;52:48-56.
67. Ølberg RA, Sinclair M. Monkeys and gibbons. In: West G, Heard D, Caulkett N, eds. *Zoo Animal and Wildlife Immobilization and Anesthesia*. Ames: John Wiley & Sons; 2014:561-571.
68. Papp R, Popovic A, Kelly N, et al. Pharmokinetics of cefovecin in squirrel monkey (*Saimiri sciureus*), rhesus macaques (*Macaca mulatta*), and cynomolgus macaques (*Macaca fascicularis*). *J Am Assoc Lab Anim Sci* 2010;49:805-808.
69. Parrott T. *Nonhuman primates*. Available at: *The Merck Veterinary Manual*. 11th ed. Whitehouse Station: Merck & Co; 2016. www.merckvetmanual.com/exotic-and-laboratory-animals/nonhuman-primates/overview-of-nonhuman-primates. Accessed December 18.
70. Patton DL, Cosgrove YT, Agnew KJ, et al. Development of a nonhuman primate model Trichomonas vaginalis infection. *Sex Transm Dis* 2006;33:743-746.
71. Plumb DC. *Plumb's Veterinary Drug Handbook*. 7th ed. PharmaVet Inc: Stockholm; 2011.
72. Popilskis SJ, Lee DR, Elmore DB. Anesthesia and analgesia in nonhuman primates. In: Fish RE, Brown MJ, Danneman PJ, et al. *Anesthesia and Analgesia in Laboratory Animals*. 2nd ed. New York: Academic Press; 2008:336-363.
73. Puri SK, Singh N. Azithromycin: antimalarial profile against blood- and sporozoite-induced infections in mice and monkeys. *Exp Parasitol* 2000;94:8-14.
74. Raabe BM, Lovaglio J, Grover GS, et al. Pharmokinetics of cefovecin in cynomolgus macaques (*Macaca fascicularis*), olive baboons (*Papio anubis*), and rhesus macaques (*Macaca mulatta*). *J Am Assoc Lab Anim Sci* 2011;50:389-395.
75. Rao GA, Mann JR, Shoaibi A, et al. Azithromycin and levofloxacin use and increased risk of cardiac arrhythmia and death. *Ann Fam Med* 2014;12:121-127.
76. Redrobe SP. Neuroleptics in great apes, with specific reference to modification of aggressive behavior in a male gorilla. In: Fowler ME, Miller RE, eds. *Zoo and Wild Animal Medicine*. 6th ed. St. Louis: Saunders Elsevier; 2008:243-250.
77. Reichard MV, Wolf RF, Carey DW, et al. Efficacy of fenbendazole and milbemycin oxime for treating baboons (*Papio cynocephalus anubis*) infected with *Trichuris trichiura*. *J Am Assoc Lab Anim Sci* 2007;46:42-45.
78. Rodriguez P Rio Lopez del, Sanchez C, Stembridge M, et al. Comparison of indirect blood pressure values in chimpanzees (*Pan troglodytes*) anesthetized with two anesthetic protocols: tiletamine-zolazepam and tiletamine-zolazepam-medetomidine. *Proc Annu Conf Am Assoc Zoo Vet* 2014;31.

79. Rowe N. *The Pictorial Guide to the Living Primates.* New York: Pogonias Press; 1996.
80. Saint Louis Zoo. Contraception Methods, Rodriguez P, Rio Lopez del, Sanchez C, Stembridge M. https://www.stlzoo.org/animals/scienceresearch/reproductivemanagementcenter/contraception recommendatio/contraceptionmethods; 18 December 2016.
81. Salyards GW, Knych HK, Hill AE, et al. Pharmacokinetics of ceftiofur crystalline free acid in male rhesus macaques (*Macaca mulatta*) after subcutaneous administration. *J Am Assoc Lab Anim Sci* 2015;54:557-563.
82. Sasseville VG, Hotchkiss CE, Levesque PC, et al. Hematopoietic, cardiovascular, lymphoid and mononuclear phagocyte systems of nonhuman primates. In: Abee C, Mansfield K, Tardif SD, et al. *Nonhuman Primates in Biomedical Research: Diseases.* 2nd ed. London: Elsevier; 2012:357-384.
83. Springer DA, Phillippi-Falkenstein K, Smith G. Retrospective analysis of wound characteristics and tetanus development in captive macaques. *J Zoo Wildl Med* 2009;40:95-102.
84. Sun FJ, Wright DE, Pinson DM. Comparison of ketamine versus combination of ketamine and medetomidine in injectable anesthetic protocols: chemical immobilization in macaques and tissue reaction in rats. *Contemp Top Lab Anim Sci* 2003;42:32-37.
85. Sundelof JG, Hajdu R, Gill CJ, et al. Pharmacokinetics of L-749,345, a long-acting carbapenem antibiotic, in primates. *Antimicrob Agents Chemother* 1997;41:1743-1748.
86. Valverde CR, Lemoy MJ. Primates. In: Carpenter JW, ed. *Exotic Animal Formulary.* 4th ed. St. Louis: Elsevier; 2013:614-661.
87. Valverde CR, Mama KR, Kollias-Baker C, et al. Pharmacokinetics and cardiopulmonary effects of fentanyl in isoflurane-anesthetized rhesus monkeys (*Macaca mulatta*). *Am J Vet Res* 2000;61:931-934.
88. Wathen AB, Myers DD, Zajkowski P, et al. Enoxaparin treatment of spontaneous deep vein thrombosis in a chronically catheterized rhesus macaque (*Macaca mulatta*). *J Am Assoc Lab Anim Sci* 2009;48:521-526.
89. Watson JR, Stoskopf MK, Rozmiarek H, et al. Kinetic study of serum gentamicin concentrations in baboons after single dose administration. *Am J Vet Res* 1991;52:1285-1287.
90. Williams CV. Prosimians. In: Miller RE, Fowler ME, eds. *Zoo and Wild Animal Medicine.* 8th ed. St. Louis: Elsevier; 2015:291-301.
91. Williams CV, Junge RE. Prosimians. In: West G, Heard D, Caulkett N, eds. *Zoo Animal and Wildlife Immobilization and Anesthesia.* 2nd ed. Ames: John Wiley & Sons; 2014:551-559.
92. Williams CV, Glenn KM, Levine JF, et al. Comparison of the efficacy and cardiorespiratory effects of medetomidine-based anesthetic protocols in ring-tailed lemurs (*Lemur catta*). *J Zoo Wildl Med* 2003;34:163-170.
93. Yamada N, Sato J, Kanno T, et al. Morphological study of progressive glomerulonephropathy in common marmosets (*Callithrix jacchus*). *Toxicol Pathol* 2013;41:1106-1115.
94. Young LA, Morris PJ, Keener L, et al. Subcutaneous *Taenia crassiceps* cysticercosis in a red-ruffed lemur (*Varecia variegata rubra*). *Proc Annu Conf Am Assoc Zoo Vet* 2000;251-252.

Chapter 14 **Wildlife**

David L. McRuer | *Heather Barron*

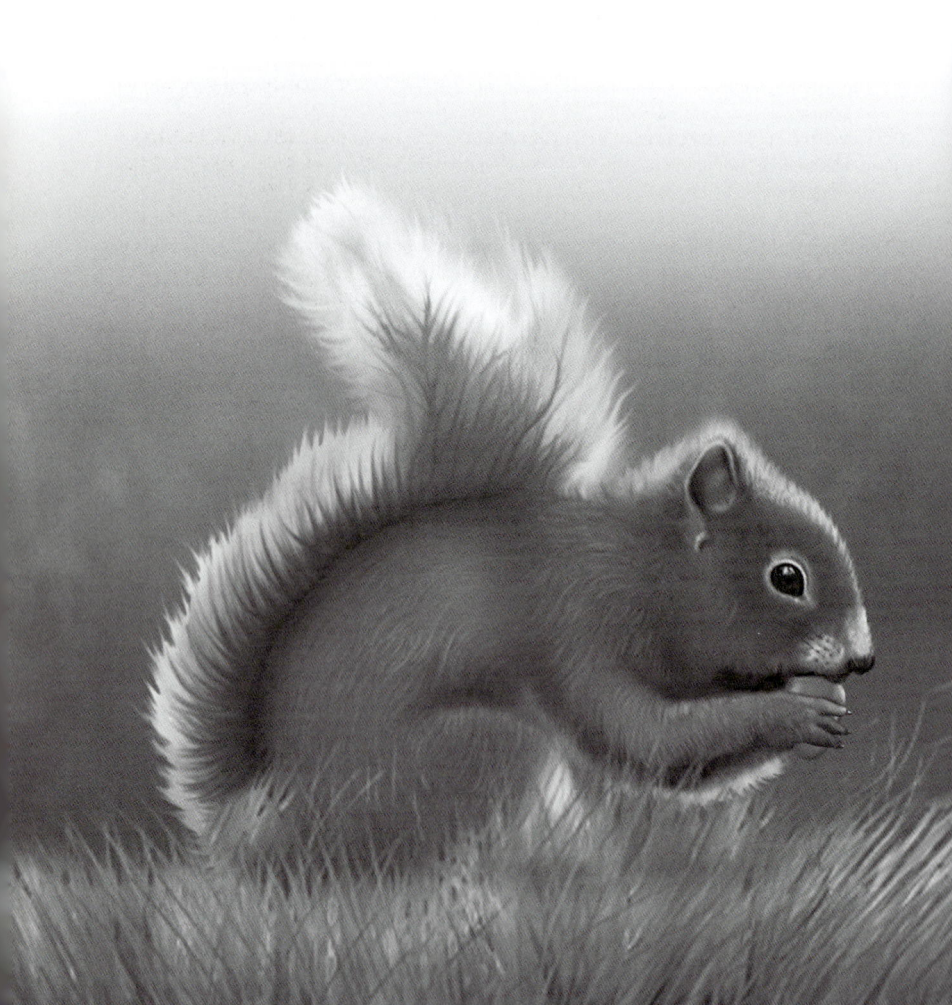

TABLE 14-1 Checklist for the Care of Sick, Injured, or Orphaned Wildlife.[a-c]

The information contained within this section is designed to help a veterinarian triage and provide basic stabilizing care to injured or orphaned wildlife. The veterinarian is strongly encouraged to transfer these animals to or consult with experienced wildlife veterinarians or wildlife rehabilitators as soon as possible. In addition, any individual working with wildlife should check with state and federal officials on permit requirements. In the event of bites inflicted by rabies vector species or wild mammals showing neurologic signs to persons or domestic pets, the local health department should be contacted regarding appropriate rabies prevention procedures.

A. Regulations and reporting
   a. Permits: check with state and federal officials on laws and permit requirements for hospitalizing wildlife; if you do not have permits, stabilize the animal and transport it to a permitted facility as soon as possible.
   b. Species reporting: check with state wildlife officials for a list of reportable endangered, threatened, or listed species; these may vary from state to state.
   c. Illegal activity: report injuries caused by illegal activities such as gunshot wounds to nongame species to local, state, or federal wildlife authorities.
   d. Reportable diseases: reportable or foreign animal diseases diagnosed in wildlife should be reported to the USDA-APHIS Area veterinarian-in-charge (https://www.aphis.usda.gov/aphis/ourfocus/animalhealth/contact-us).
   e. Banded birds: band numbers on federally banded birds should be reported to the US Geological Survey Bird Banding Laboratory (http://www.pwrc.usgs.gov/bbl/).
   f. Advise the public not to approach rabies vector species and to contact local authorities instead. In addition, bats should never be handled bare handed. If a rescuer has handled a rabies vector species, report any potential rabies exposure (bite or contact with saliva through broken skin or mucous membranes) to the local health department.

B. Patient background
   a. Is the "orphan" truly an orphan? If not, return to nest or site found because natural parents provide the best care. Human scent will not cause rejection of the young by the mother.
      i. Fledgling birds normally spend time on the ground before gaining full flight ability. The parents will continue to feed and guard the fledgling.
      ii. Adult rabbits and deer normally leave their young unattended for much of the day. Parents will return to the site where offspring were left to reunite, often hours later. Check for a "milk line" in young rabbits to determine if they were recently fed.
   b. Get precise information. When was animal found? Exact location? Circumstances? Has any medical or supportive care been provided?
   c. The rescue location of many turtle species is particularly important as they have high site fidelity.
   d. Obtain rescuer's name, address, and phone number in case further details are required.

C. Initial patient triage
   a. What is medically wrong with the animal? Can it be treated, survive the rehabilitation period (sometimes months), and be released or placed into an education program? Check with experienced wildlife veterinarians if unsure. Unfortunately, euthanasia is often required.
   b. Address life-threatening problems first. ABC: Check that the *airway* is clear, the animal is *breathing,* and *cardiac beat and pulse* are present. Provide cardiopulmonary resuscitation if needed.
   c. Control hemorrhage. Total blood loss of more than 1% of body weight is considered an emergency. Remove broken blood feathers by pulling the feather shaft out of the follicle with straight, steady pressure. Apply direct pressure to hemorrhage sites. Use topical epinephrine, cautery, and ligation if needed.
   d. Assess for shock. Evaluate neonates for hypoglycemia and hypothermia. Clinical signs include cold extremities, pale and tacky mucous membranes, and rapid heart rate. Treat with fluids and supplemental heat if needed, and treat hypoglycemia with intravenous or oral dextrose. Treat hyperthermia with fluids, placing the patient in a cool place and spraying limbs with cool water.
   e. Perform full examination once the patient is stable. Examination may need to be delayed, limited to a cursory exam, or done in stages to minimize patient stress.
      i. If possible, determine the species, gender, life stage, body condition, and weight.
      ii. Is zoonotic disease or infectious disease a concern? Isolate the patient if necessary.

Continued

TABLE 14-1	Checklist for the Care of Sick, Injured, or Orphaned Wildlife. (cont'd)

D. Develop treatment and supportive care plan
   a. Assume most wildlife patients are 10% dehydrated on admission. Provide hydrating solutions and electrolyte support for the first 24 to 48 hours parenterally (Normosol, 2.5% dextrose, LRS, 0.9% saline) or orally with a multispecies electrolyte solution (e.g., Pedialyte [Abbott], Gatorade [Gatorade], or Bounce Back [Manna Pro]). Continue to treat if ongoing fluid losses occur. Most birds, reptiles, and mammals can be triaged with fluids based on an assumed maintenance rate of 40-60 mL/kg/day, 10-25 mL/kg/day, and 60 mL/kg/day, respectively.
   b. Provide supplemental heat to neonates at 80-90°F (27-32°C). Keep heating pads on low to prevent thermal burns. Use wrapped hot water bottles and warmed air.
   c. Treat and prevent infection. Most open wounds will require antimicrobial therapy.
   d. Provide analgesia and antiinflammatory medications if needed. Nonsteroidal antiinflammatory drugs are useful for soft-tissue injury, head trauma, and spinal trauma. Although steroids are used by some clinicians to treat acute spinal trauma and shock, their use in shock, especially in birds, may be controversial and is generally not recommended. Opioids are useful for severe soft-tissue injury and fractures.
   e. Develop a nutritional plan. Attempt to calculate the calories needed for each day's feeding. Except for neonates, do not provide food for the first 24 hours while the animal is being rehydrated. Emaciated animals may need special diets (Emerald Nutritional Care System [Lafeber]; Carnivore and Critical Care [Oxbow]) to avoid refeeding syndrome.
   f. Neonatal mammals must be stimulated to urinate and defecate by gently brushing anal and genital areas with moist cotton or clean tissue after each feeding.
   g. Determine appropriate housing. The main goals are safety and to reduce stress on the animal by preventing noise and visual stimulation. In general, minimize contact to people and domestic animals. Wildlife should not be kept in close proximity to domestic animals while being housed for veterinary care.

E. Rehabilitation
   a. Contact the International Wildlife Rehabilitation Council (866-871-1869; https://theiwrc.org/), the National Wildlife Rehabilitators Association (320-230-9920; www.nwrawildlife.org), or State Rehabilitation Associations to find a rehabilitator near you.
   b. Transfer the animal to a qualified rehabilitator for continued therapy and to prepare the animal for release.
   c. Rehabilitators are often familiar with animal nutrition and natural history and can provide initial supportive care recommendations as well.

F. Release criteria
   a. Animals must meet the following criteria in order to be released to the wild:
      i. Initial illness or injury is resolved with no risk of recurrence. Animals must have normal laboratory values if tested.
      ii. All secondary problems have been resolved.
      iii. The animal does not pose an unnatural risk to the wild population, humans, or the environment. It is not likely to spread pathogens or contribute to disease processes in other ways. The animal does not pose a zoonotic risk.
      iv. The animal can effectively avoid predators.
      v. The animal is able to find food by foraging or hunting in the wild. This requires adequate vision and locomotive skills.
      vi. The animal can function reasonably within the population and can reproduce.
      vii. The animal displays proper species behavior (not improperly imprinted) and the fight or flight behavioral response.
      viii. The animal must be the correct age and weight for independent survival.
      ix. The animal must possess pelage or plumage that is adequate for that species to survive. The animal must exhibit waterproof pelage/plumage sufficient for that species.

TABLE 14-1 Checklist for the Care of Sick, Injured, or Orphaned Wildlife. (cont'd)

b. Animals should be released at the original site of capture unless conservation efforts or safety considerations dictate otherwise. Animals should be released in their natural environment and habitat suitable for species survival but in areas away from traffic, people, and pets. The habitat must be within carrying capacity for the species. Release diurnal species in the morning and nocturnal species at dusk. Check local and state laws regarding release of rabies vector species and deer.
c. Animals that cannot be returned to the wild for any reason should be euthanized unless they can be legally placed in educational, breeding, or research programs.

[a]See references in appendices.
[b]For information on nutritional management of captive wildlife, see Carpenter JW, ed. *Exotic Animal Formulary*. 3rd ed. St. Louis: Saunders/Elsevier; 2005.
[c]*Web resources:*
National Wildlife Rehabilitation Association—http://www.nwrawildlife.org
International Wildlife Rehabilitation Council—http://theiwrc.org/
Wildlife Center of Virginia—www.wildlifecenter.org
USGS National Wildlife Health Center—http://www.nwhc.usgs.gov/
U.S. Fish and Wildlife Service—http://www.fws.gov/
Southeastern Cooperative Wildlife Disease Study—http://vet.uga.edu/scwds
Birds of North America Online—https://birdsna.org/Species-Account/bna/home
World Organization for Animal Health—http://www.oie.int/
National Association of State Public Health Veterinarians—http://www.nasphv.org/

TABLE 14-2 Considerations for Developing a Wildlife Policy in Private Practice.[2,4,15,34,56,76,78,79,83,84]

Topic		Notes
General Considerations		
		Whether your practice admits wildlife or not, all veterinary clinics should have a wildlife policy to ensure injured and orphaned wildlife receive timely care, regulatory and public health guidelines are followed, and a consistent message is presented to the public regarding the practice's willingness to see wildlife. Wildlife policies do not need to be complicated and are often built on lessons learned from prior wildlife patients and experiences.
Treating injured and orphaned wildlife		Although practitioners should not feel obligated to treat wildlife, referral information should be on-hand to expedite appropriate treatment and/or supportive care. The referral list should contain contact information for veterinarians that treat wildlife, permitted wildlife rehabilitators, referral wildlife hospitals, game wardens, wildlife biologists, animal control officers, and state and federal wildlife agencies. It may be advantageous to build a network of volunteer transporters able to quickly move the wild animal to an appropriate location for initial or additional treatment. Depending on the comfort level and expertise of the veterinarians and staff, the clinic may decide to see only certain types of wildlife, may treat to stabilize and transfer, or admit only severely injured animals for humane euthanasia.
Legalities		Practitioners need to be aware of local, state, and federal laws pertaining to wildlife. Endangered, threatened, and listed species need to be reported immediately to the appropriate authorities. Practitioners should also check with local wildlife agencies and veterinary licensing boards for guidance on how long wildlife may be in a practitioner's possession without rehabilitation permits. The state veterinarian and local APHIS Veterinary Services need to be contacted if you suspect or confirm a notifiable animal disease. The state public health agency needs to be contacted if you suspect or confirm a notifiable disease of public health concern.

Continued

TABLE 14-2 Considerations for Developing a Wildlife Policy in Private Practice. (cont'd)

Topic	Notes
Preparedness and safety	Does the practice have the necessary restraint devices, enclosures, food, and experienced veterinarians and staff to provide treatment and supportive care to wildlife? Is there a space to house wildlife away from domestic animals? Are biosecurity measurements in place to prevent the spread of potential infectious diseases or parasites? Appropriate personal protective equipment should be onsite and appropriate for the species. Additional considerations include reservoir or vector status of the animal, rabies immunization and titers of staff, and general safety for staff, clients, domestic patients, and the public.
Euthanasia	Injured wildlife may require humane euthanasia to alleviate pain and suffering due to injuries that are either severe or nonconducive to release or placement in an education program. Euthanasia of wild animals should be conducted according to the AVMA Guidelines on Euthanasia or the AAZV Guidelines for the Euthanasia of Nondomestic Animals. Wildlife authorities should be contacted if a wild animal is fitted with a band, transmitter, tag, or other identification device. Consideration of carcass disposal is necessary, the usual means being incineration, burial/landfill, composting, or newer evolving technologies. Animals euthanized with pentobarbital should never be disposed in a manner that makes the carcass accessible to scavenging and subsequent secondary pentobarbital toxicosis. All carcasses, parts, and feathers from bald eagles and golden eagles must be sent to the National Eagle Repository. According to the Migratory Bird Treaty Act, it is illegal to keep carcasses, parts and feathers from any migratory bird without an appropriate federal permit.

TABLE 14-3 Recommendations for Safe Restraint of Native Wildlife.[5,9,11,12,19,28,47,49,54,57,58,70,72,75]

Topic	Notes[a]
	Wild animals may carry a variety of infectious and parasitic diseases that may present a health risk to veterinary staff, clients, the public, and domestic patients. It is strongly advised to wear a primary barrier (latex gloves) when handling wild animals.
Badgers, coyotes, foxes, bobcats, and lynx	Young kits/cubs weighing less than 1 kg can be handled by wearing latex gloves under long leather gloves and caught up by wrapping in a thick towel or blanket. For long procedures or fractious adults, anesthetize by injectable/inhalant combinations. Inject larger animals (over 3 kg) using squeeze cage, netting, or syringe pole. Do not scruff animals for restraint because they can still turn and bite. Restrain by grasping the head around the back of the neck and holding the dorsal pelvis with the legs aimed away from your abdomen to avoid personal injury. Use muzzles to prevent biting.
Raccoons	Infants/juveniles may be restrained by the scruff of the neck or by holding the shoulder area of the forelegs with one leg in each hand. Animals tend to scream, grasp, or bite at the gloves and may urinate with handling. Restrain older juveniles and adults with chemical or a combination of chemical and gas anesthesia.
Skunk	Limit handling in this species to avoid being sprayed from the musk glands. Wear eye protection when handling. For young animals, attempt to drape a towel or plastic sheet and tuck the tail between the hind legs to decrease the possibility of being sprayed. Restrain older juveniles and adults with chemical and/or gas anesthesia.

TABLE 14-3 Recommendations for Safe Restraint of Native Wildlife. (cont'd)

Topic	Notes
River otters	Natural defense is to bite, grasp, and twist which may cause significant tissue trauma. Appropriate protective gear includes elbow-length leather gloves for protection against teeth and nails. Adult animals may need to be anesthetized for restraint.
Opossums	Appropriate protective gear includes elbow-length leather gloves for protection against teeth and nails. Anesthesia may be required for examination of adults.
Rabbits and hares	Appropriate protective gear includes a towel or light gloves for adults. Cover with a towel before picking up to reduce stress. Restrain so that the patient cannot kick its hind legs and injure its back. Avoid overhandling and anesthetize for prolonged restraint.
Wild rodents	Adults of these species can deliver hard bites. Appropriate protective wear includes leather gloves to the elbow. Use nets for initial restraint of larger rodents. A noose-style catch pole may be appropriate for initial restraint of large beavers.
Birds of prey	Appropriate protective gear includes leather gloves (garden gloves for small species and up to the elbows or higher for larger hawks and eagles) and protective eyewear. A leather welder's jacket may be used for large raptors such as eagles. Raptors will use talons for primary defense but may also use their beak. Restrain feet first and head second. A body grab should be used if the bird has a known leg injury. A towel may be placed over the body before restraint to reduce wing flapping. Vulture defense includes regurgitation. Keeping the patient's neck extended will reduce regurgitation efforts. Keep the patient's eyes covered with a hood or light cloth during handling to reduce patient stress.
Passerines, woodpeckers, doves, etc.	Appropriate protective gear includes light leather gloves. Patients may become stressed or overheat with handling. Watch the patient closely and perform procedures in stages if needed. Secure smaller birds using fore and middle fingers around the base of the head and the bird's back pressed against your palm. Do not compress the body by grasping too tightly as this may compromise breathing. Cup doves, pigeons, and similar species in a light towel.
Waterfowl, pelagic, and wading birds	Appropriate protective gear includes vinyl or light leather gloves. Powdered latex gloves and bare hands are inappropriate for waterfowl, pelagic birds, and other species that require waterproofing of the feathers. Handle passerine-sized precocial birds the same as altricial birds. Waterfowl and large wading birds should be restrained by securing the legs with one hand, tucking the bird's body between your side and the arm restraining the legs, and securing the head and neck with the opposite hand. Long-billed birds such as herons and loons require the handler to wear goggles and/or face shields to protect the eyes.
Insectivorous bats	Appropriate protective gear includes latex gloves under leather garden gloves. Place the bat gently in a soft cloth and cover. Expose portions of the bat to perform a physical exam. Cotton tip applicators are useful to examine wing membranes, head and oral cavity, integument, etc.
Snakes	Nonvenomous snakes may be restrained by grasping the head just behind the mandibles and securing the body with the other hand. An additional handler is needed for every 3-4 feet of snake to support the spine. Venomous snakes should be restrained only by experts using snake hooks and tongs to handle and clear plastic tubes for restraint.

Continued

TABLE 14-3 Recommendations for Safe Restraint of Native Wildlife. (cont'd)

Topic	Notes
Chelonians	Chelonians may scratch with claws or bite. Appropriate handling gear includes latex gloves. Nonaggressive species may be restrained by grasping the sides of the shell between the front and back legs. Larger turtles, especially snapping turtles, require a hand under the caudal third of the plastron and the other hand grasping the tail or the caudal carapace. Snapping turtles can extend the head and neck two-thirds their body length caudally. Consider using a toilet plunger over a snapping turtle's head to reduce the risk of biting.
Lizards	Place the index finger and thumb around the base of the mandibles to secure the head and prevent biting. Use the free hand to restrain the hind legs and tail. Never grab lizards by the tail, especially in species with tail autonomy. To calm lizards, a vagal response can be created by placing cotton balls over the eyes and securing with bandage material.

[a]Although this outline is intended to provide general guidelines for the care of injured wildlife, the veterinarian is strongly encouraged to transfer these animals to experienced rehabilitators as soon as possible and/or to contact rehabilitators if questions arise. In addition, any individual working with wildlife should check with state and federal officials on permit requirements.

TABLE 14-4 Recommendations for Venipuncture Sites in Native Wildlife.[19,22,28,31,35,57,62,65,68,72,75]

Topic	Notes
Badgers, river otters, skunks, coyotes, foxes, raccoons, bobcats, lynx	Medial saphenous vein, lateral saphenous vein, jugular vein, cephalic vein, ventral coccygeal vein, femoral vein, cranial vena cava (in otters)
Opossums	Lateral coccygeal and ventral tail vein/artery, cephalic vein, saphenous vein, pouch vein in females
Rabbits and hares	Jugular vein, cephalic vein, femoral vein, lateral saphenous vein
Wild rodents	Small rodents often require cranial vena cava venipuncture under anesthesia; larger species have accessible jugular veins, cephalic veins, and medial and lateral saphenous veins; beavers have accessible tail vein
Birds of prey	Jugular vein (right is larger), basilic vein in either wing, medial metatarsal vein (use caution when working near talons)
Passerines, woodpeckers, doves, etc.	Right jugular vein; basilic vein in larger birds is an alternative site
Waterfowl, pelagic, and wading birds	Medial metatarsal vein is preferred; jugular vein and basilic veins are secondary sources
Insectivorous bats	Need 24 μL for a manual complete blood cell count; venipuncture sites include heart, infraorbital sinus, jugular, peripheral vessels (median vein, cephalic vein, uropatagial vein)
Snakes	Heart (snakes >200 g; dorsal recumbency; insertion of needle under central abdominal scale at 45° angle caudal to heart; pericardial fluid contamination can occur), jugular vein (needle is inserted parallel or perpendicular to the ribs and 9 ventral scales cranial to the heart), or ventral coccygeal vein; venomous snakes should only be handled by professionals using appropriate equipment (tongs, hooks, clear snake-handling tubes)
Chelonians	Jugular, dorsal venous sinus/dorsal coccygeal vein, subcarapacial venous sinus; less commonly used vessels include brachial venous plexus, femoral venous plexus, and femoral vein; all sites except the jugular vein may be subject to lymph contamination
Lizards	Ventral coccygeal vein (accessed laterally or ventrally), jugular, ventral abdominal/coelomic vein

CHAPTER 14 Wildlife

TABLE 14-5 Recommendations for Meat Withdrawal Times in Game Species for Select Medications.[3,14,27,82,89]

Drug use in wild animals is considered extra-label and as such is regulated by the Food and Drug Administration (FDA) through the Animal Medicinal Drug Use Clarification Act (AMDUCA). This act is divided into food-producing animals and non–food-producing animals. Drug residues in game animals are a potential public health risk to those who consume the meat. Game animals are defined by the FDA as "an animal, the products of which are food, that is not classified as livestock, sheep, swine, goat, horse, mule or other equine, or as poultry or fish." Game animals include mammals such as deer, antelope, rabbit, squirrel, opossum, raccoon, nutria, or muskrat, and nonaquatic reptiles such as land snakes. The FDA classifies wild game birds as "poultry" and includes "migratory waterfowl or game birds, pheasant, partridge, quail, grouse, or pigeon."

Practitioners need to be aware of potential meat withdrawal times (defined as the time between drug administration and when the meat can safely be consumed by a human) when administering drugs to game species during or just before established hunting and trapping seasons. There are very few established withdrawal times for wildlife, and practitioners should check the Food Animal Residue Avoidance Database (FARAD) for guidance on drug administration in game species that could be consumed. If a game animal cannot be held until the meat withdrawal time has passed, it should be identified with a unique number and warning that the meat should not be consumed. Permission to tag wildlife may also require permission from state or federal authorities.

Some drugs may never be used in food-producing animals throughout the year. These include: chloramphenicol, clenbuterol, diethylstilbestrol, dimetridazole, ipronidazole, metronidazole, other nitromidazoles, furazolidone, nitrofurazone, glycopeptides, and fluoroquinolones. Adamantane and neuraminidase inhibitors are prohibited in wild game birds. The following is a list of recommended withdrawal times for select drugs used in wildlife.

Agent	Meat Withdrawal Time (days)	Agent	Meat Withdrawal Time (days)
Acepromazine	14	Naloxone	30
Atipamezole	14	Naltrexone	30
Diazepam	14	Penicillin (long-acting)	21
Diprenorphine	30	Tolazoline	30
Etorphine	30	Xylazine	30
Ivermectin	49	Yohimbine	30
Ketamine	3	Zolazepam and tiletamine (1:1)	14
Medetomidine	14		

TABLE 14-6 Antimicrobial Agents Used in Wild Mammals.[a-c]

Agent	Dosage	Species/Comments
Amikacin	10-15 mg/kg SC, IM, IV q12h[90]	Rodents
	20 mg/kg SC q24h[7]	Bats
	1.25 g/20 g methylmethacrylate[85]	To make antibiotic impregnated polymethylmethacrylate beads
Amoxicillin	10-20 mg/kg PO q8h[67]	Rats, mice, squirrels, bats, raccoons, opossums, wild felids, canids; do not use in rabbits and certain species of rodents
Amoxicillin/ clavulanic acid (Clavamox, Zoetis)	—	Do not use in rabbits and certain species of rodents
	13-22 mg/kg PO q8-12h[67,74]	Rats, mice, squirrels, bats, raccoons, opossums, wild felids, canids

Continued

TABLE 14-6 Antimicrobial Agents Used in Wild Mammals. (cont'd)

Agent	Dosage	Species/Comments
Ampicillin sodium/ sulbactam (Unasyn, Pfizer)	—	Stable for 3 days refrigerated and 3 mo frozen
	10-20 mg/kg IM, IV q8h[67]	For infections susceptible to amoxicillin/clavulanate in patients unable to receive oral doses
Ampicillin trihydrate	—	Do not use in rabbits and certain species of rodents
	6.6 mg/kg SC, IM q12h[67]	Canids, felids
	20-30 mg/kg SC, IM, IV q8h[67,74]	Rats, mice, squirrels, raccoons, opossums
Azithromycin (Zithromax, Pfizer)	5-10 mg/kg PO q24h × 3-5 days[67]	Carnivores
	20 mg/kg PO q24h[7]	Bats
Cefazolin sodium	—	Do not use in rabbits and rodents
	10-30 mg/kg SC, IM, IV q8h[67]	Carnivores
	2 g/20 g methylmethacrylate[85]	To make antibiotic impregnated polymethylmethacrylate beads
Cefovecin (Convenia, Zoetis)	8 mg/kg SC once, repeat in 10 days if indicated	Carnivores; based on authors' experience in raccoons, foxes, otters[8,54]
Ceftazidime	25-30 mg/kg IM, IV q8-12h[67]	Carnivores
Ceftiofur crystalline-free acid (Excede, Zoetis)	7 mg/kg SC[45,81]	Carnivores
Cephalexin	—	Do not use in rabbits and certain species of rodents
	22-60 mg/kg PO q6-12h[7,67]	Rats, mice, bats, squirrels, raccoons, opossums, wild felids, canids
Clindamycin	—	Do not use in rabbits, rodents, and ruminants[58,69]
	11-33 mg/kg PO q24h[67]	Felids
	15-30 mg/kg PO q12h[67]	Carnivores
Doxycycline	2.5-5 mg/kg PO q12h[68]	Rabbits, rodents
	5-10 mg/kg PO q12h[67]	Carnivores
Enrofloxacin	—	Injectable may cause tissue necrosis; in general, more than one IM injection not advised; appears stable when compounded; dilute 1:10 to reduce irritation
	5 mg/kg PO q24h[67]	Felids/contraindicated in young, growing animals
	5-10 mg/kg PO, IM q12h[21]	Rabbits, rodents
	5-20 mg/kg PO, IM, IV q24h[67]	Canids/contraindicated in young, growing animals
Metronidazole	10-15 mg/kg PO q12h[67]	Felids
Penicillin G procaine	—	Do not use in rabbits or rodents
	20,000-40,000 IU/kg IV q6h or SC, IM q12h[67]	Carnivores
Piperacillin/ tazobactam (Zosyn, Wyeth)	50 mg/kg IV q8h[67]	Canids

TABLE 14-6 Antimicrobial Agents Used in Wild Mammals. (cont'd)

Agent	Dosage	Species/Comments
Trimethoprim/ sulfadiazine (Tribrissen, Schering-Plough)	15 mg/kg PO q12h[67] 15-30 mg/kg PO q12h[7,67]	Felids Canids, bats
Tylosin (Tylan, Elanco)	— 10-40 mg/kg PO q12h[67]	Not recommended for use in rodents; injectable may cause tissue necrosis Carnivores

[a]Additional drug doses for other classes of wild animals may be found in other chapters of this formulary.
[b]"Carnivores" may include wild North American felids, canids, procyonids, ursids, and mustelids.
[c]Many species of wildlife are hunted for human consumption. Drugs prohibited for use in food animals should not be administered to these species if they will be released to the wild and/or consumed by humans. See www.farad.org for list of drugs.

TABLE 14-7 Antiparasitic Agents Used in Wild Mammals.[a-c]

Agent	Dosage	Species/Comments
Fenbendazole (Panacur, Intervet)	—	Toxicosis reported in porcupines and rabbits[32,88]
	10-25 mg/kg PO q24h × 5 days[51]	Prairie dogs, other rodents
	25 mg/kg PO q24h × 5 days[6]	Marsupials/*Capillaria*
	25-50 mg/kg PO q12h × 10-14 days[67]	Canids, felids/*Paragonimus*
	50 mg/kg PO q24h × 3-5 days[67]	Canids, felids/ascarids, hookworms, whipworms, *Taenia*
	50 mg/kg PO q24h × 3-7 days[67]	Canids, felids/*Giardia*
Fipronil	—	Most species/do *not* use in rabbits[68]
	Mix 1 mL fipronil with 4 mL 70% isopropyl alcohol; apply 0.5 mL to 15 g bat; 0.7 mL to 20 g bat; 1 mL to 25 g bat[7]	Bats
Imidacloprid/ moxidectin (Advantage Multi, Bayer)	0.2 mg/kg topically prn[87] Mix 0.1 mL imidacloprid with 0.9 mL water[7]	Most species Bats/imidacloprid only; apply 1 drop of solution to back of head
Ivermectin	—	Intravenous lipid emulsion has been successfully used to treat ivermectin toxicosis in mammals[49]
	0.2-0.4 mg/kg PO, SC q7d[1,68]	Most species/many endoparasites and ectoparasites; continue 2 wk past negative skin scrape for mites
	100 μg/kg PO once[7]	Bats/toxicosis possible; higher doses not recommended[18]
Metronidazole	15-25 mg/kg PO q12h × 5-7 days[67]	Carnivores/*Giardia*
	10-40 mg/kg PO q24h[10]	Rodents
Moxidectin	0.2-0.4 mg/kg PO q7-10d × 3-6 doses[87]	Carnivores, rabbits

Continued

TABLE 14-7 Antiparasitic Agents Used in Wild Mammals. (cont'd)

Agent	Dosage	Species/Comments
Nitenpyram (Capstar, Novartis)	—	Capstar wound flush: one 11.4 mg tablet crushed and mixed with 30 mL sterile 0.9% NaCl or water[55]
	11.4 mg (1 tablet) PO for animals weighing 0.9-11.36 kg[67]	Carnivores/fleas, myiasis
Praziquantel (Droncit, Bayer)	5-10 mg/kg PO, SC[67]	Carnivores/cestodes
	20-25 mg/kg PO q24h × 3-10 days[67]	Carnivores/trematodes
Pyrantel pamoate	5-10 mg/kg PO after meal q2-3wk[44,67]	Carnivores
Sulfadimethoxine (Albon, Zoetis)	25-50 mg/kg PO q24h[1,51,71]	Most species

[a]Additional drug doses for other classes of wild animals may be found in other chapters of this formulary.
[b]"Carnivores" may include wild North American felids, canids, procyonids, ursids, and mustelids.
[c]Many species of wildlife are hunted for human consumption. Drugs prohibited for use in food animals should not be administered to these species if they will be released to the wild and/or consumed by humans. See www.farad.org for list of drugs.

TABLE 14-8 Antifungal Agents Used in Wild Mammals.[a-c]

Agent	Dosage	Species/Comments
Amphotericin B	0.25 mg/kg IV 3×/wk; maximum dose 8 mg/kg; 4 mg/kg if used with an azole[60]	Carnivores/efficacy against aspergillosis may be low; MIC indicated[77]
Griseofulvin	1 mg/kg IV q24h[73]	Rabbits, rodents
		Administer with fatty meal; may cause bone marrow depression; monitor CBC during treatment
	25 mg/kg PO q12h or 50 mg/kg PO q24h[60]	Carnivores/dermatophytosis; continue therapy 2 wk beyond clinical resolution
	25 mg/kg PO q24h × 28 days[1,39]	Rabbits, rodents, Virginia opossums, eastern grey squirrels/dermatophytosis
Itraconazole (Itrafungol, Elanco)	—	Give with meal for most effective absorption; monitor liver function
	5-10 mg/kg PO q24h[38,67]	Carnivores, rabbits
Nystatin 100,000 IU/mL suspension	—	Apply topically to oral lesions
	5,000 IU/kg PO q8-12h[59]	Opossums
	50,000-150,000 IU topically q6-8h[67]	Carnivores/oral candidiasis
Terbinafine	8-20 mg/kg PO q24h[38]	Rabbits
	10-20 mg/kg PO q24h[67]	Carnivores/dermatophytosis; can do pulse therapy (7 days on, 21 days off)
Voriconazole	—	Not recommended in felids due to significant side effects
	4 mg/kg PO q12h[67]	Canids

[a]Additional drug doses for other classes of wild animals may be found in other chapters of this formulary.
[b]"Carnivores" may include wild North American felids, canids, procyonids, ursids, and mustelids.
[c]Many species of wildlife are hunted for human consumption. Drugs prohibited for use in food animals should not be administered to these species if they will be released to the wild and/or consumed by humans. See www.farad.org for list of drugs.

TABLE 14-9 Chemical Restraint/Anesthetic Agents Used in Wild Mammals.[a-c]

Agent	Dosage	Species/Comments
Acepromazine	0.5-2.5 mg/kg IM[37]	Prairie dogs
	0.1 mg/kg IM[37]	Beavers, porcupines
Alfaxalone (Alfaxan, Jurox)	5-10 mg/kg IM or 1.5 mg/kg IV[74]	Most species
Atipamezole (Antisedan, Zoetis)	—	Dexmedetomidine and medetomidine reversal; give same volume SC, IV, IP as medetomidine and dexmedetomidine (dexmedetomidine is used at one-half the dose of medetomidine but the same volume due to higher concentration); medetomidine is no longer commercially available, but can be compounded
Atropine sulfate	0.03-0.05 mg/kg SC[67]	Most species/preanesthetic dose; may not be effective in lagomorphs and some rodents
Dexmedetomi-dine (Dexdomitor, Zoetis)	0.05-1 µg/kg IM, IV (use lower end of range if giving IV)[36]	Most species/generally insufficient alone to produce sedation in most wild mammals; combine with opioids and/or benzodiazepines; see ketamine for combinations
Diazepam (available as a 1 mg/mL oral solution)	0.1-1 mg/kg IM, PO[37]	Beavers, porcupines
	0.5-2 mg/kg IM, SC, PO[7]	Bats
	1-2.5 mg/kg PO, IM, IP[37]	Prairie dogs
Flumazenil	0.01-0.05 mg/kg IM, IV, IO; repeat q1h prn[67]	If using 5 mg/mL midazolam and 0.1 mg/mL flumazenil, use 2 × the volume of midazolam given
Glycopyrolate	0.01 mg/kg SC, IM[37]	Beavers, porcupines
	0.01-0.02 mg/kg SC, IM[37]	Prairie dogs
Ketamine	—	Combinations frequently used by the authors; most can be followed by intubation and inhalant anesthetic drugs if general anesthesia is required; concentrated formulations of ketamine (200 mg/mL), butorphanol (30-50 mg/mL), and medetomidine (10 or 20 mg/mL) are available from compounding pharmacies and are advised for larger mammals; sustained release (SR) products available from compounding pharmacies; can also be combined with benzodiazepines
	30-100 mg/kg SC[7]	Bats
Ketamine (K)/ medetomidine (M)	(K) 2-5 mg/kg + (M) 0.04-0.1 mg/kg IM[26]	Carnivores
Ketamine (K)/medetomidine (M)/dexmede-tomidine (D)/butorphanol (B)	(K) 2-4 mg/kg + (M) 0.02 mg/kg + (B) 0.04-0.2 mg/kg or 0.01 mL/lb IM each of (K) 100 mg/mL, (D) 0.5 mg/mL, and (B) 10 mg/mL[26]	Carnivores/deepen anesthesia with isoflurane for invasive procedures; reverse dexmedetomidine with equal volume of atipamezole IM (wait at least 30 min after ketamine is administered)

Continued

TABLE 14-9 Chemical Restraint/Anesthetic Agents Used in Wild Mammals. (cont'd)

Agent	Dosage	Species/Comments
Midazolam	0.1-0.5 mg/kg IM[37]	Beavers, porcupines
	0.2-0.5 mg/kg IM, IV[26]	Carnivores/preanesthetic or sedative
	1-2 mg/kg IM, IP[37]	Prairie dogs
Propofol	—	Reduce dose with hypoproteinemia; supplemental oxygen recommended; induces profound respiratory depression; be prepared to ventilate
	3-7 mg/kg IV slowly to effect[67]	Carnivores
	0.1-0.6 mg/kg/min constant rate infusion[36]	Carnivores/sedation at lower doses; light anesthesia at higher doses

[a]Additional drug doses for other classes of wild animals may be found in other chapters of this formulary.
[b]"Carnivores" may include wild North American felids, canids, procyonids, ursids, and mustelids.
[c]Many species of wildlife are hunted for human consumption. Drugs prohibited for use in food animals should not be administered to these species if they will be released to the wild and/or consumed by humans. See www.farad.org for list of drugs.

TABLE 14-10 Analgesic and Nonsteroidal Antiinflammatory Agents Used in Wild Mammals.[a-c]

Agent	Dosage	Species/Comments
Buprenorphine	0.01-0.02 mg/kg SC, IM q12h; may be administered via transmucosal route at higher dosage of 0.02-0.03 mg/kg q12h[68]	Felids
	0.01-0.05 mg/kg SC, IM, IV, IP, oral transmucosal q6-12h[23,29]	Most species
	0.1 mg/kg SC q24h[7]	Bats
Buprenorphine-SR (Buprenorphine SR-LAB, ZooPharm)	—	Acquired from compounding pharmacy; sustained release; shelf life 1 yr; refrigerate
	0.06-0.12 mg/kg SC q72h[13]	Carnivores
Butorphanol	1-2 mg/kg SC q48-72h[25,46]	Rodents
	—	Can be compounded at 30-50 mg/mL by compounding pharmacy
	0.1-0.5 mg/kg SC, IM, IV q2-4h[67]	Carnivores
	2 mg/kg SC, IM q4h[90]	Prairie dogs
Carprofen	2-5 mg/kg SC, PO q12h[24]	Rodents
	2.2 mg/kg PO q12h[67]	Canids/not recommended for felids
Fentanyl	Transdermal patch 1-5 µg/kg/h[67]	Most species/dysphoria more prevalent at higher end of dose range
Gabapentin	5-10 mg/kg PO q12h[67]	Carnivores/anecdotal dosage
	100 mg/kg PO q24h[33]	Rodents
Ketoprofen	2-5 mg/kg SC q24h[7]	Bats

TABLE 14-10 Analgesic and Nonsteroidal Antiinflammatory Agents Used in Wild Mammals. (cont'd)

Agent	Dosage	Species/Comments
Meloxicam	0.1 mg/kg PO q24h[7]	Bats
	0.2 mg/kg PO, SC, IV, then 0.1 mg/kg PO q24h[67]	Canids
	Label dosage: 0.3 mg/kg SC once for 3-4-day effect;[67] Extra-label dosage: 0.2 mg/kg PO once, then 0.1 mg/kg PO q24h in food for 3-4 days[8]	Felids, raccoons, Virginia opossums, skunks
Morphine	1 mg/kg PO q24h × 29 days[17]	Rabbits
	1-2 mg/kg PO, SC q24[8]	Rodents
	0.1-0.5 mg/kg SC, IM q4-6h[67]	Felids/not recommended to use alone
	0.5-2 mg/kg SC, IM q4-6h[67]	Canids
Tramadol	—	Compounded suspension has a shelf life of 90 days at 5°C/41°F[86]
	0.5-2 mg/kg PO q12h[67]	Felids
	3-5 mg/kg PO q8-12h[67]	Canids
Lidocaine	—	Toxic dose varies with species; use lowest dose possible
	<3 mg/kg[90]	Felids
	<4 mg/kg[90]	Canids
Bupivicaine	—	Toxic dose varies with species; use lowest dose possible
	2 mg/kg[90]	Carnivores

[a]Additional drug doses for other classes of wild animals may be found in other chapters of this formulary.
[b]"Carnivores" may include wild North American felids, canids, procyonids, ursids, and mustelids.
[c]Many species of wildlife are hunted for human consumption. Drugs prohibited for use in food animals should not be administered to these species if they will be released to the wild and/or consumed by humans. See www.farad.org for list of drugs.

TABLE 14-11 Agents Used in Wild Mammal Emergencies.[a-c]

Agent	Dosage	Species/Comments
Activated charcoal	1-4 g/kg with 5-10 mL of water per g of charcoal PO q4-6h[67]	Carnivores
Atropine (0.54 mg/mL)	2-3 g/kg PO[43]	Rabbits, rodents
	0.02-0.04 mg/kg IM, IV[67]	Carnivores; bradycardia
	0.04 mg/kg IV, IO; repeat q3-5min prn for maximum of 3 doses or 0.08-0.1 mg/kg intra-tracheal; dilute with 5-10 mL sterile water before administration[67]	Carnivores; cardiopulmonary resuscitation
	0.04-0.05 mg/kg SC, IM[36,37]	Most species/preanesthetic
	0.2-0.5 mg/kg; give ¼ dose IV and remainder SC, IM[67]	Organophosphate toxicity

Continued

TABLE 14-11 Agents Used in Wild Mammal Emergencies. (cont'd)

Agent	Dosage	Species/Comments
Crystalloid fluids (isotonic) bolus volume for shock	0.8-1 mg/kg SC, IM[61]	Rabbits/many have serum atropinase and need higher doses
	90 mL/kg 1st hr[40]	Most species/administer one quarter of total dose over 15 min, then reassess heart rate, blood pressure, mucous membranes
Crystalloid fluids (maintenance)	40-60 mL/kg/day[80]	Carnivores
Diazepam	0.5-1 mg/kg IV, intranasally, rectally; repeat 2 × prn[67]	Carnivores/status epilepticus or cluster seizures
Dexamethasone sodium phosphate; methylprednisolone sodium succinate	—	High dose (e.g., 30 mg/kg IV), fast-acting corticosteroids are no longer recommended for use in shock or CNS trauma (still controversial); recent studies have not demonstrated significant benefit and it actually may cause increased deleterious effects[67]
Dextrose 50%	0.5 mL/kg IV bolus (dilute by half to make a 25% solution), follow up with constant rate infusion of 5% dextrose in a balanced electrolyte solution[67]	Most species/hypoglycemia
	0.25 mL/kg of 50% dextrose diluted 50% w/saline[50]	Small mammal CPR
Edetate calcium disodium (CaEDTA)	—	Nephrotoxic; consider administration of fluids during treatment to maintain hydration
	25 mg/kg SC q6-12h × 5 days[16,51,67]	Most species/recheck lead levels after 5 days of treatment; if still elevated, allow 5-7 day rest period before restarting treatment
Epinephrine 1:1000 (1 mg/mL)	—	Most species
	0.01 mg/kg IV/IO epinephrine administered every 3-5 min[50,67,69]	Low-dose; early in CPR is recommended
	0.1 mg/kg IV, IO[50,67,69]	High-dose; consider after prolonged CPR
	0.1-0.2 mg/kg IV, IO, intratracheal[50,67,69]	Dilute in 5-10 mL sterile water or saline for intratracheal administration
Furosemide	1-4 mg/kg IM, IV q4-12h[42]	Rabbits/pulmonary edema
	2-4 mg/kg IM, IV q1-2h until respiration improves[67]	Carnivores/pulmonary edema, ascites
Hetastarch	1-2 mL/kg/h IV constant rate infusion[67]	Canids/do not exceed 25 mL/kg/day
	1-2 mL/kg/h IV constant rate infusion[67]	Felids/do not exceed 10 mL/kg/day
	5-10 mL/kg IV bolus over 15-30 min[40]	Felids
	10-20 mL/kg IV bolus 15-30 min[40]	Carnivores
Mannitol	0.5-1.5 g/kg IV over 10-20 min[67]	Most species/traumatic brain injury; repeat q6-8h prn for maximum of 3 boluses and only if patient is showing response

TABLE 14-11 Agents Used in Wild Mammal Emergencies. (cont'd)

Agent	Dosage	Species/Comments
Pralidoxime (2-PAM)	20 mg/kg SC, IM, IV (slowly) q6-12h until nicotinic signs are present[67]	Carnivores
Saline (NaCl; hypertonic; 7.5%)	4-6 mL/kg slow bolus[67]	Most species/head trauma, pulmonary contusions; consider using with a colloid to prolong effect

[a]Additional drug doses for other classes of wild animals may be found in other chapters of this formulary.
[b]"Carnivores" may include wild North American felids, canids, procyonids, ursids, and mustelids.
[c]Many species of wildlife are hunted for human consumption. Drugs prohibited for use in food animals should not be administered to these species if they will be released to the wild and/or consumed by humans. See www.farad.org for list of drugs.

TABLE 14-12 Miscellaneous Agents Used in Wild Mammals.[a-c]

Agent	Dosage	Species/Comments
Acetylcysteine	Nebulize 50 mg as a 2% solution diluted with saline[60,67]	Most species/can be stored in refrigerator for 6 mo; do not freeze
Calcium gluconate	—	Dilute the 23% solution 1:1 with saline or sterile water for IM or IV administration
	50-100 mg/kg IV for 10-20 min[67]	Most species/hyperkalemic cardiotoxicity (serum K >8 mEq/L); monitor ECG
	94-140 mg/kg IV slowly to effect[67]	Most species/hypocalcemia; monitor respiration and cardiac rhythm during administration; halt administration if arrhythmias occur
Cimetidine	5-10 mg/kg PO, SC, IM, IV q6-12h[44,67,71]	Most species
Diphenhydramine	2 mg/kg PO, SC[7,67]	Most species
Famotidine	0.5 mg/kg PO, SC, IM, IV q6-12h[60,67]	Most species
Iron dextran	10-20 mg/kg IM followed by oral therapy[67]	Carnivores
Isoxuprine	1 mg/kg PO q24h[67]	Canids
Lactulose	0.25-0.5 mL/kg PO q6-8h until stools are loose[67]	Carnivores
Loperamide	0.1 mg/kg PO q8h × 3 days, then q24h × 2 days (give in 1 mL water)[44,60]	Most species
Maropitant (Cerenia, Zoetis)	0.5-1 mg/kg SC, IV slow q24h	Carnivores
	2-4 mg/kg PO q24h up to 5 consecutive days[60,67]	Carnivores
Meclizine	2-12 mg/kg PO q12-24h[44,60,67]	Most species
Metoclopramide	0.2-0.5 mg/kg PO, SC q6-8h[51,60,67]	Carnivores, rodents, rabbits
Omeprazole	0.5-1 mg/kg PO q24h[67]	Carnivores
Oxytocin	0.2-3 IU/kg SC, IM, IV[53,64]	Most species
Simethicone (66 mg/mL)	60 mg/kg PO q8-12h or at every feeding for infants[60]	Most species (adult or infant)/also consider burping nursing neonates after every feeding

Continued

TABLE 14-12   Miscellaneous Agents Used in Wild Mammals. (cont'd)

Agent	Dosage	Species/Comments
Sucralfate	25-125 mg/kg PO q8h[41,71]	Most species/give 30-60 min after histamine-2 blockers
Vitamin B complex	10-20 mg/kg SC, IM q8-12h prn[67]	Carnivores/dose based on thiamine (B_1)

[a]Additional drug doses for other classes of wild animals may be found in other chapters of this formulary.
[b]"Carnivores" may include wild North American felids, canids, procyonids, ursids, and mustelids.
[c]Many species of wildlife are hunted for human consumption. Drugs prohibited for use in food animals should not be administered to these species if they will be released to the wild and/or consumed by humans. See www.farad.org for list of drugs.

REFERENCES

1. Adamcak A, Otten B. Rodent therapeutics. In: Fronefield SA, ed. *Vet Clin North Am Exot Anim Pract* 3:2000:221-240.
2. American Veterinary Medical Association. *Guidelines for the Euthanasia of Animals.* Available at: https://www.avma.org/KB/Policies/Documents/euthanasia.pdf. Accessed Dec 15, 2016.
3. American Veterinary Medical Association. *Guidelines for Veterinary Prescription Drugs.* Available at: https://www.avma.org/KB/Policies/Pages/Guidelines-for-Veterinary-Prescription-Drugs.aspx. Accessed Dec 15, 2016.
4. American Veterinary Medical Association. *Wildlife Decision Tree.* Available at: https://www.avma.org/KB/Resources/Reference/wildlife/Pages/default.aspx. Accessed Dec 15, 2016.
5. Arent LR. *Raptors in Captivity.* Blaine, WA: Hancock House Publishers; 2007.
6. Baker DG, Cook LF, Johnson EM, Lamberski N. Prevalence, acquisition, and treatment of *Didelphostrongylus hayesi* (Nematoda: Metastrongyloidea) infection in opossums (*Didelphis virginiana*). *J Zoo Wildl Med* 1995;26:403-408.
7. Barnard SM, ed. *Bats in Captivity Volume 1—Biological and Medical Aspects.* Washington, DC: Logos Press; 2009:493-558.
8. Barron H. *Personal observation;* 2016.
9. Beckwith S. Rehabilitation of orphan river otters. *Proc Nat Wildl Rehab Symp* 2003;21:51-60.
10. Brown C, Donnelly TM. Disease problems of small rodents. In: Quesenberry KE, Carpenter JW, eds. *Ferrets, Rabbits, and Rodents: Clinical Medicine and Surgery.* 3rd ed. St. Louis: Elsevier/Saunders; 2012:354-372.
11. Carpenter JW, ed. *Exotic Animal Formulary.* 3rd ed. St. Louis: Saunders/Elsevier; 2005.
12. Carpenter JW, ed. *Exotic Animal Formulary.* 4th ed. St. Louis: Elsevier; 2013.
13. Catbagan DL, Quimby JM, Mama KR, et al. Comparison of the efficacy and adverse effects of sustained-release buprenorphine hydrochloride following subcutaneous administration and buprenorphine hydrochloride following oral transmucosal administration in cats undergoing ovariohysterectomy. *Am J Vet Res* 2011;72:461-466.
14. Cattet M. A CCWHC technical bulletin: drug residues in wild meat—addressing a public health concern. *Canadian Cooperative Wildlife Health Centre: Newsletter & Publications.* Paper 46. 2003.
15. Cornell Waste Management Institute. US Mortality and Butcher Waste Disposal Laws. Available at: http://compost.css.cornell.edu/mapsdisposal.html. Published 2014. Accessed Dec 15, 2016.
16. Deeb BJ, Carpenter JW. Neurologic and musculoskeletal diseases. In: Quesenberry KE, Carpenter JW, eds. *Ferrets, Rabbits, and Rodents: Clinical Medicine and Surgery.* 2nd ed. St. Louis: WB Saunders Co; 2004:209.
17. Delk KW, Carpenter JW, Kukanich B, et al. Pharmacokinetics of meloxicam administered orally to rabbits (*Oryctolagus cuniculus*) for 29 days. *Am J Vet Res* 2014;75:195-199.
18. DeMarco JH, Heard DJ, Fleming GJ, et al. Ivermectin toxicosis after topical administration in dog-faced fruit bats (*Cynopterus brachyotis*). *J Zoo Wildl Med* 2002;33:147-150.

19. Derrell CJ, Olfert ED. Rodents. In: Fowler ME, ed. *Zoo and Wild Animal Medicine*. 2nd ed. Philadelphia: WB Saunders Co; 1986:727-747.
20. Desmarchelier M, Troncy E, Fitzgerald G, et al. Analgesic effects of meloxicam administration on postoperative orthopedic pain in domestic pigeons (*Columba livia*). *Am J Vet Res* 2012;73:361-367.
21. Donnelly TM. Disease problems of small rodents. In: Quesenberry KE, Carpenter JW, eds. *Ferrets, Rabbits, and Rodents: Clinical Medicine and Surgery*. 2nd ed. St. Louis: WB Saunders Co; 2004:305-306.
22. Duerr R. *Personal communication*; 2016.
23. Flecknell PA. Analgesia of small mammals. In: Heard DJ, ed. *Vet Clin North Am Exot Anim Pract*. 4:2001:47-56.
24. Flecknell PA, Orr HE, Roughan JV, et al. Comparison of the effects of oral or subcutaneous carprofen or ketoprofen in rats undergoing laparotomy. *Vet Rec* 1999;144:65-67.
25. Foley PL, Liang H, Crichlow AR. Evaluation of a sustained-release formulation of buprenorphine for analgesia in rats. *J Am Assoc Lab Anim Sci* 2011;50:198-204.
26. Fontenot DK. Exotic carnivore restraint, anesthesia and analgesia. *Proc Am Assoc Zoo Vet Annu Pre-Conf* 2009;1-7.
27. Food Animal Residue Avoidance Databank (Farad). Available at: http://www.farad.org/. Accessed Dec 15, 2016.
28. Fowler ME, Miller RE, eds. *Zoo and Wild Animal Medicine*. 5th ed. St. Louis: WB Saunders Co; 2003.
29. Gades NM, Danneman PJ, Wixson SK, et al. The magnitude and duration of the analgesic effect of morphine, butorphanol, and buprenorphine in rats and mice. *Contemp Top Lab Anim Sci* 2000;39:8-13.
30. Gentz EJ, Harrenstein LA, Carpenter JW. Dealing with gastrointestinal, genitourinary, and musculoskeletal problems in rabbits. *Vet Med* 1995;90:365-372.
31. Graham JE, Heatley JJ. Emergency care of raptors. *Vet Clin North Am Exot Anim Pract* 2007;10:395-418.
32. Graham J, Garner MM, Reavill DR. Benzimidazole toxicosis in rabbits: 13 cases (2003 to 2011). *J Exot Pet Med* 2014;23:188-195.
33. Griggs RB, Bardo MT, Taylor BK. Gabapentin alleviates affective pain after traumatic nerve injury. *Neuroreport* 2015;26:522-527.
34. Guidelines for the Euthanasia of Nondomestic Animals. American Association of Zoo Veterinarians. 2006. Available at: http://www.aazv.org/?441. Accessed July 2, 2017.
35. Harrison GJ, Lightfoot TL, eds. *Clinical Avian Medicine*. Palm Beach: Spix Publishing; 2006.
36. Hawkins MG, Pascoe PJ. Anesthesia, analgesia, and sedation of small mammals. In: Quesenberry KE, Carpenter JW, eds. *Ferrets, Rabbits, and Rodents: Clinical Medicine and Surgery*. 3rd ed. St. Louis: Elsevier Saunders; 2012:429-451.
37. Heard DJ. Rodents. In: West G, Heard D, Caulkett N, eds. *Zoo Animal & Wildlife Immobilization and Anesthesia*. 2nd ed. Ames: Wiley Blackwell Publishing; 2014:893-903.
38. Hess L. Dermatologic diseases. In: Quesenberry KE, Carpenter JW, eds. *Ferrets, Rabbits, and Rodents: Clinical Medicine and Surgery*. 2nd ed St. Louis: WB Saunders Co; 2004:199.
39. Hillyer EV. Dermatologic diseases. In: Hillyer EV, Quesenberry KE, eds. *Ferrets, Rabbits, and Rodents: Clinical Medicine and Surgery*. St. Louis: WB Saunders Co; 1997:212-219.
40. Hoareau G. *Shock Proc Pac Vet Conf* 2015;17-18.
41. Hoefer HL, Fox JG, Bell JA. Gastrointestinal diseases. In: Quesenberry KE, Carpenter JW, eds. *Ferrets, Rabbits, and Rodents: Clinical Medicine and Surgery*. 3rd ed. St. Louis: Elsevier Saunders; 2012:27-45.
42. Huston SH. Cardiovascular diseases. In: Quesenberry KE, Carpenter JW, eds. *Ferrets, Rabbits, and Rodents: Clinical Medicine and Surgery*. 2nd ed. St. Louis: WB Saunders Co; 2004:213.
43. Idid SZ, Lee CY. Effects of Fuller's earth and activated charcoal on oral absorption of paraquat in rabbits. *Clin Exp Pharmacol Physiol* 1996;23:679-681.

44. Ivey ES, Morrisey JK. Therapeutics for rabbits. In: Fronefield SA, ed. *Vet Clin North Am Exot Anim Pract* 3:2000:183-220.
45. Jankowski G, Adkesson MJ, Langan JN, et al. Cystic endometrial hyperplasia and pyometra in three captive African hunting dogs (*Lycaeon pictus*). *J Zoo Wildl Med* 2012;43:99-100.
46. Jirkof P, Tourvieille A, Cinelli P, et al. Buprenorphine for pain relief in mice: repeated injections vs sustained-release depot formulation. *Lab Anim* 2015;49:177-187.
47. Johnson-Delaney CA. What every veterinarian needs to know about Virginia opossums. *Exot DVM* 2005;6:38-43.
48. Kidwell JH, Buckley GJ, Allen AE, et al. Use of IV lipid emulsion for treatment of ivermectin toxicosis in a cat. *J Am Anim Hosp Assoc* 2014;50:59-61.
49. Lafeber Company (Cornell, IL). Available at: http://www.lafebervet.com. Accessed Dec 15, 2016.
50. Lichtenberger M. Emergency and critical care of small mammals. In: Quesenberry KE, Carpenter JW, eds. *Ferrets, Rabbits, and Rodents: Clinical Medicine and Surgery*. 3rd ed. St. Louis: Elsevier Saunders; 2012:532-544.
51. Lightfoot TL. Therapeutics of African pygmy hedgehogs and prairie dogs. *Vet Clin North Am Exot Anim Pract* 2000;3:155-172.
52. Luther E. *Answering the Call of the Wild*. Toronto: Toronto Wildlife Center; 2010.
53. Mans C, Donnelly TM. Disease problems of chinchillas. In: Quesenberry KE, Carpenter JW, eds. *Ferrets, Rabbits, and Rodents: Clinical Medicine and Surgery*. 3rd ed. St. Louis: Elsevier Saunders; 2012:311-325.
54. McRuer DL, Barron HW. *Personal observation;* 2016.
55. Miller EA. Parasite identification. *Proc Fl Wildl Rehab Assoc Symp* 2014;1-49.
56. Miller EA, ed. *Minimum Standards of Wildlife Rehabilitation*. 4th ed. St. Cloud: National Wildlife Rehabilitation Association; 2012.
57. Mitchell M, Tully T, eds. *Manual of Exotic Pet Practice*. St. Louis: Saunders/Elsevier; 2009.
58. Moore AT, Joosten S. *Principles of Wildlife Rehabilitation*. National Wildlife Rehabilitation Association: St. Cloud; 1997.
59. Ness RD, Johnson-Delaney CA. Sugar gliders. In: Quesenberry KE, Carpenter JW, eds. *Ferrets, Rabbits, and Rodents: Clinical Medicine and Surgery*. 3rd ed. St. Louis: Elsevier/Saunders; 2012:393-410.
60. Oglesbee BL. Guinea pigs. In: Oglesbee BL, ed. *Blackwell's Five Minute Veterinary Consult: Small Mammal*. 2nd ed. Ames: Wiley Blackwell; 2011:226-341.
61. Olson ME, Vizzutti D, Marck DW, et al. The parasympatholytic effects of atropine sulfate and glycopyrrolate in rats and rabbits. *Can J Vet Res* 1994;58:254-258.
62. Olsson A. Blood collection and hematological values. In: Barnard SM, ed. *Bats in Captivity Vol 1. Biological and Medical Aspects*. Washington DC: Logos Press; 2009:339-380.
63. Oxbow Animal Health (Murdock, NE). Available at: http://www.oxbowanimalhealth.com. Accessed Dec 15, 2016.
64. Pare JA, Paul-Murphy J. Disorders of the reproductive and urinary systems. In: Quesenberry KE, Carpenter JW, eds. *Ferrets, Rabbits, and Rodents: Clinical Medicine and Surgery*. 2nd ed. St. Louis: WB Saunders Co; 2004:183-193.
65. Paul-Murphy J. Critical care of the rabbit. *Vet Clin North Am Exot Anim Pract* 2007;10:437-461.
66. Plumb DC. *Plumb's Veterinary Drug Handbook*. 7th ed. Wiley-Blackwell: Ames; 2011.
67. Plumb DC. *Plumb's Veterinary Drug Handbook*. 8th ed. Wiley-Blackwell: Ames; 2015.
68. Quesenberry KE, Carpenter JW, eds. *Ferrets, Rabbits, and Rodents: Clinical Medicine and Surgery*. 2nd ed. St. Louis: WB Saunders Co; 2004.
69. Ramer JC, Paul-Murphy J, Benson KG. Evaluating and stabilizing critically ill rabbits—Part I. *Comp Cont Educ Pract* 1999;21:30-40.
70. Reed-Smith J, Ball J. *North American River Otter Husbandry Notebook*. 2nd ed. John Ball Zoological Garden: Grand Rapids; 2001.
71. Riggs SM, Mitchell MA. Chinchillas. In: Mitchell MA, Tully TN, eds. *Manual of Exotic Pet Practice*. St. Louis: Saunders/Elsevier; 2009:474-492.

72. Samour JH, ed. *Avian Medicine.* 3rd ed. St. Louis: Elsevier; 2016.
73. Sanati H, Ramos CF, Bayer AS, et al. Combination therapy with amphotericin B and fluconazole against invasive candidiasis in neutropenic-mouse and infective-endocarditis rabbit models. *Antimicrob Agents Chemother* 1997;41:1345-1348.
74. Schott R. Triaging the wildlife patient. *Proc Student Chap Am Vet Med Assoc Symp* 2015.
75. Scott D. *Raptor Rehabilitation.* Lulu: Raleigh; 2010.
76. *Secondary Pentobarbital Poisoning in Wildlife.* Fact Sheet. Available at: https://www.fws.gov/mountain-prairie/poison.pdf. Accessed Dec 15, 2016.
77. Silvanose C, Bailry T, Di Somma A. In vitro sensitivity of *Aspergillus* species isolated from respiratory tract of falcons. *Vet Scan Online Vet J* 2011;6(95):1-6.
78. State and Territorial Fish and Wildlife Offices. Available at: https://www.fws.gov/offices/statelinks.html. Accessed Dec 15, 2016.
79. State and Territorial Public Health Offices. Available at: https://www.cdc.gov/mmwr/international/relres.html. Accessed Dec 15, 2016.
80. Thomovsky E. Basics of fluid therapy: crystalloids and colloids. *Proc Atl Coast Vet Conf* 2015;33-37.
81. Travis E, Duncan M, Weber M, et al. Ileocecocolic strictures in two captive cheetahs (*Acinonyx jubatus jubatus*). *J Zoo Wildl Med* 2007;38:574-578.
82. United States Department of Health and Human Services. *Food Code.* College Park; 2013.
83. United States Fish and Wildlife Service. *Migratory Bird Treaty Act.* Available at: https://www.fws.gov/birds/policies-and-regulations/laws-legislations/migratory-bird-treaty-act.php. Accessed Dec 15, 2016.
84. United States Fish and Wildlife Service. *National Eagle Repository.* Available at: https://www.fws.gov/eaglerepository/. Accessed Dec 15, 2016.
85. Vennen KM, Mitchell MA. Rabbits. In: Mitchell MA, Tully TN, eds. *Manual of Exotic Pet Practice.* St. Louis: Saunders Elsevier; 2009:375-405.
86. Wagner DS, Johnson CE. Stability of oral liquid preparations of tramadol in strawberry syrup and a sugar free vehicle. *Am J Health-Syst Pharm* 2003;60:1268-1270.
87. Wagner R, Wendlberger U. Field efficacy of moxidectin in dogs and rabbits naturally infested with *Sarcoptes* spp., *Demodex* spp. and *Psoroptes* spp. mites. *Vet Parasitol* 2000;93:149-158.
88. Weber MA, Miller MA, Neiffer DL, et al. Presumptive fenbendazole toxicosis in North American porcupines. *J Am Vet Med Assoc* 2006;228:1240-1242.
89. Western Association of Fish and Wildlife Agencies. *A model protocol for purchase, distribution and use of pharmaceuticals in wildlife.* Available at: www.dfw.state.or.us/wildlife/docs/WWHC_DRUG_PROTOCOL2009.pdf. Accessed Dec 15, 2016.
90. Yarto-Jaramillo E. Rodentia. In: Miller RE, Fowler ME, eds. *Fowler's Zoo and Wild Animal Medicine.* Vol. 8:St. Louis: Elsevier/Saunders; 2015:384-422.

Chapter 15 Select Topics for the Exotic Animal Veterinarian

Julie Swenson | James W. Carpenter

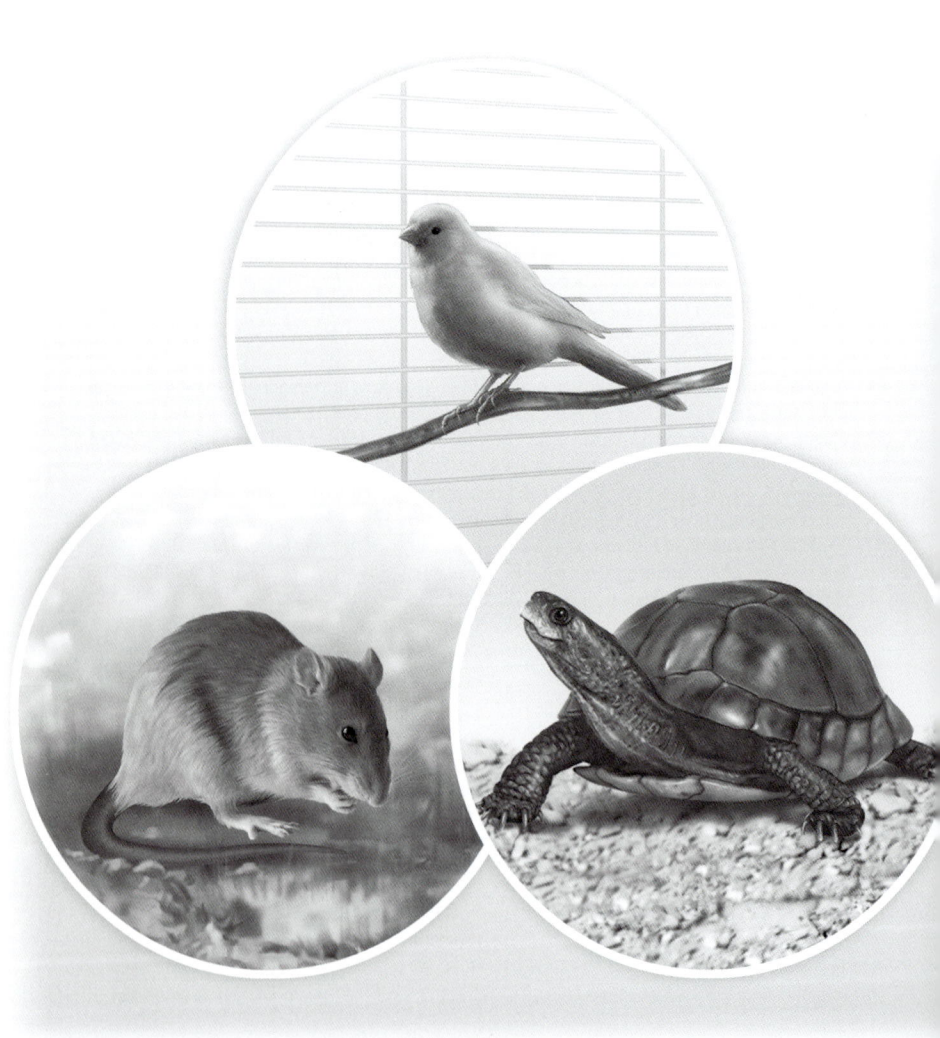

CHAPTER 15 Select Topics for the Exotic Animal Veterinarian

TABLE 15-1 Classification of Select Antimicrobials Used in Exotic Animal Medicine.

Class	Antimicrobial Agent
Benzyl penicillins[a]	Benzathine penicillin G
	Procaine penicillin G
Extended-spectrum penicillins[a]	
Aminopenicillins	Amoxicillin
	Ampicillin
Antipseudomonal penicillins	
Carboxypenicillins	Carbenicillin
	Ticarcillin
Piperazine penicillins	Piperacillin
Carbapenems[b]	Imipenem
	Meropenem
β-lactamase inhibitors	Ampicillin[a]/sulbactam
	Piperacillin[a]/tazobactam
Clavulanic acid	Amoxicillin[a]/clavulanate
	Ticarcillin[a]/clavulanate
First-generation cephalosporins[a]	Cefadroxil
	Cefazolin
	Cefovecin
	Cefpodoxime
	Cephalexin
Third-generation cephalosporins[a]	Cefixime
	Cefotaxime
	Ceftazidime
	Ceftiofur
Fourth-generation cephalosporins[a]	Cefepime
	Cefpirome
Macrolides[b]	Clarithromycin
	Erythromycin
	Tilmicosin
	Tylosin
Azalides[b]	Azithromycin
Ketolides[b]	Telithromycin
Tetracyclines[b]	Chlortetracycline
	Doxycycline
	Oxytetracycline
	Tetracycline
Chloramphenicol (or its derivative)[b]	Chloramphenicol
	Florfenicol
Lincosamides[c]	Clindamycin
	Lincomycin
	Pirlimycin

Continued

TABLE 15-1 Classification of Select Antimicrobials Used in Exotic Animal Medicine. (cont'd)

Class	Antimicrobial Agent
Aminoglycosides[a]	Amikacin
	Gentamicin
	Kanamycin
	Neomycin
	Streptomycin
	Tobramycin
Aminocyclitols[b]	Spectinomycin
Nitroimidazole[d]	Metronidazole
	Ronidazole
Sulfonamides[b]	Sulfachlorpyridazine
	Sulfadiazine
	Sulfadimethoxine
	Sulfamethazine
	Sulfamethoxazole
	Sulfaquinoxaline
	Sulfathiazole
	Sulfisoxazole
Trimethoprim[a]	Trimethoprim
Trimethoprim/sulfas[a]	Trimethoprim/sulfadiazine
	Trimethoprim/sulfamethoxazole
Quinolones[b]	Nalidixic acid
Fluoroquinolones[a]	Ciprofloxacin
	Danofloxacin
	Difloxacin
	Enrofloxacin
	Marbofloxacin
	Orbifloxacin

[a]Bactericidal.
[b]Bacteriostatic.
[c]Bacteriostatic or bactericidal.
[d]Cidal vs. amoebae, *Giardia*, *Trichomonas*, and most obligate anaerobes; inactive vs. most aerobic bacteria or facultative anaerobes.

CHAPTER 15 Select Topics for the Exotic Animal Veterinarian

TABLE 15-2 General Efficacy of Select Antimicrobial Agents Used in Exotic Animals.

Infectious Agent	Antimicrobial Agent
Gram-positive bacteria	
Gram-positive bacteria (in general)	• Aminoglycosides (select) (amikacin, gentamicin) • Azalides (i.e., azithromycin) • Cephalosporins • Chloramphenicol • Erythromycin • Florfenicol • Fluoroquinolones • Lincosamides • Macrolides • Penicillins • Tetracyclines
Staphylococcus spp.	• Aminoglycosides (select) (amikacin, gentamicin) • Azithromycin • β-lactams (early-generation) • Cephalosporins (cefovecin, cefpodoxime) • Chloramphenicol • Clindamycin • Fluoroquinolones • Lincosamides • Macrolides • Penicillin/β-lactamase inhibitor (amoxicillin/clavulanate, ampicillin/sulbactam, piperacillin/tazobactam, ticarcillin/clavulanate) • Trimethoprim/sulfas
Streptococcus spp.	• Azithromycin • β-lactams (early-generation) • Cephalosporins • Chloramphenicol • Clindamycin • Lincosamides • Macrolides • Penicillins • Tetracyclines • Trimethoprim/sulfas
Clostridium spp. and other anaerobes	• Azithromycin • Cephalosporins (cefotetan, cefoxitin) • Chloramphenicol • Clindamycin • Erythromycin • Florfenicol • Lincomycin • Metronidazole[a] • Penicillins (amoxicillin/clavulanate) • Tetracyclines
Gram-negative bacteria	
Enterobacteriaceae (in general)	• Aminoglycosides (amikacin, gentamicin) • Azalides • Carbapenems • Cephalosporins (third/fourth-generation) • Fluoroquinolones • Penicillins (extended-spectrum) • Trimethoprim/sulfas

Continued

TABLE 15-2 General Efficacy of Select Antimicrobial Agents Used in Exotic Animals. (cont'd)

Infectious Agent	Antimicrobial Agent
Campylobacter spp.	• Amoxicillin • Azithromycin • Ceftriazone • Chloramphenicol • Clindamycin • Doxycycline • Erythromycin • Fluoroquinolones • Furazolidone • Gentamicin • Neomycin
Pasteurella spp. (resistance may occur)	• Aminoglycosides (amikacin, gentamicin) • Chloramphenicols (chloramphenicol, florfenicol) • Erythromycin • Fluoroquinolones • Penicillins • Sulfonamides • Tetracyclines • Trimethoprim/sulfas
Pseudomonas spp. (often resistant)	• Aminoglycosides (frequently in combination with an advanced-generation β-lactam) • Carbapenems • Ceftazidime and fourth-generation cephalosporins (frequently in combination with an aminoglycoside) • Chloramphenicol • Fluoroquinolones • Penicillins (advanced-generation) (carbenicillin, ticarcillin; frequently in combination with an aminoglycoside)
Salmonella spp.	• Aminoglycosides • Chloramphenicol • Fluoroquinolones • Penicillins (advanced-generation) • Trimethoprim/sulfas
Chlamydia	• Azithromycin • Enrofloxacin (vs. some species) • Erythromycin • Tetracyclines (doxycyline)
***Mycoplasma* spp**.	• Azithromycin • Chloramphenicol • Clindamycin • Enrofloxacin • Lincosamides • Macrolides • Tetracyclines

[a]Effective vs. most obligate anaerobes; inactive vs. most aerobic bacteria or facultative anaerobes.

CHAPTER 15 Select Topics for the Exotic Animal Veterinarian

TABLE 15-3 Antimicrobial Therapy Used in Exotic Animals According to Site of Infection.[a,b]

Site of Infection	Antimicrobial Agent
Bacteremia, septicemia	
Aerobic bacteria	Aminoglycoside with a penicillin or cephalosporin
	Cephalosporins (third-generation)
	Fluoroquinolone with amoxicillin
	Penicillins (penicillin, amoxicillin, amoxicillin/clavulanate, ampicillin/sulbactam)
Anaerobic bacteria	Azithromycin
	Cefoxitin, cefotetan
	Chloramphenicol
	Clindamycin
	Florfenicol
	Metronidazole
	Penicillin
Soft-tissue infection	Azithromycin
	Cephalosporins
	Clindamycin or metronidazole (vs. anaerobes)
	Fluoroquinolones
	Fluoroquinolone with metronidazole (vs. polymicrobial aerobic and anaerobic infections)
	Penicillin/β-lactamase inhibitor (amoxicillin/clavulanate)
	Tetracyclines
	Trimethoprim/sulfas
Respiratory tract	Azithromycin
	Cephalosporins
	Chloramphenicol
	Clindamycin (includes anaerobes)
	Enrofloxacin (vs. *Mycoplasma*, etc.)
	Florfenicol
	Macrolides (vs. *Mycoplasma*)
	Metronidazole (vs. anaerobes)
	Penicillins
	Tetracyclines (vs. *Mycoplasma* and *Chlamydia*)
	Trimethoprim/sulfas
Alimentary tract	Amoxicillin
	Cephalosporins
	Fluoroquinolones
	Metronidazole (vs. anaerobes)
	Neomycin
	Tetracyclines
	Trimethoprim/sulfas

Continued

TABLE 15-3 Antimicrobial Therapy Used in Exotic Animals According to Site of Infection. (cont'd)

Site of Infection	Antimicrobial Agent
Skin	Amoxicillin/clavulanate
	Azithromycin
	Cephalosporins
	Clindamycin
	Erythromycin
	Fluoroquinolones
	Lincomycin
	Trimethoprim/sulfas
Bone and/or joint	Aminoglycosides
	Azithromycin
	Cephalosporins
	Cephalosporins (third-generation) with clindamycin (vs. anaerobes)
	Clindamycin
	Fluoroquinolones
	Lincosamides
	Penicillins (extended-spectrum)
	Penicillins with clindamycin (vs. anaerobes)
Urinary tract	Cephalosporins (cefadroxil, cefazolin, cephalexin)
	Fluoroquinolones
	Penicillins (amoxicillin, amoxicillin/clavulanate, ampicillin)
	Sulfisoxazole
	Tetracyclines
	Trimethoprim/sulfas
Central nervous system	Azithromycin
	Cephalosporins (third-generation) (excluding cefovecin, cefpodoxime)
	Chloramphenicol (encephalitis)
	Florfenicol
	Fluoroquinolones (meningitis)
	Metronidazole (vs. anaerobes)
	Penicillins (in cases of inflammation)
	Trimethoprim/sulfas
Reproductive tract	Amoxicillin/clavulanate
	Chloramphenicol
	Clindamycin (vs. anaerobes)
	Fluoroquinolones
	Florfenicol
	Trimethoprim/sulfas

[a]Definitive therapy should be based on bacterial culture and sensitivity and host species involved.
[b]Modified from: Carpenter JW, ed. *Exotic Animal Formulary.* 4th ed. St. Louis: Elsevier-Saunders; 2013; Papich MG. *Saunders Handbook of Veterinary Drugs. Small and Large Animal.* 4th ed. St. Louis: Elsevier; 2016; Plumb DC, ed. *Plumb's Veterinary Drug Handbook.* 8th ed. Ames: Wiley Blackwell; 2015.

TABLE 15-4 Antimicrobial Combination Therapies Commonly Used in Exotic Animals.[a]

Antimicrobial Agent	Synergistic or Combination Agent
Aminoglycosides[b] (amikacin, gentamicin)	Cephalosporins, clindamycin, fluoroquinolones, lincomycin, metronidazole, penicillins (amoxicillin, ampicillin, carbenicillin, piperacillin, ticarcillin), trimethoprim/sulfas
Amoxicillin	Clavulanate
Ampicillin	Sulbactam
Cephalosporin	Aminoglycosides,[b] clindamycin, fluoroquinolones, metronidazole, semi-synthetic penicillins
Clindamycin	Aminoglycosides, cephalosporins (third-generation), enrofloxacin, penicillins
Fluoroquinolones (enrofloxacin, ciprofloxacin, marbofloxacin)	Aminoglycosides,[b] cephalosporins (third-generation), clindamycin, metronidazole, penicillins (extended-spectrum)
Lincomycin	Aminoglycosides,[b] spectinomycin
Metronidazole	Amikacin, azithromycin, carbenicillin, cefazolin, cefotaxime, chloramphenicol, enrofloxacin, gentamicin, marbofloxacin, others as indicated
Ormetoprim	Sulfadimethoxine
Penicillins (ampicillin, carbenicillin, piperacillin)	Aminoglycosides,[b] fluoroquinolones
Penicillins, early generation	Aminoglycosides,[b] third-generation cephalosporins, fluoroquinolones
Ticarcillin	Clavulanate
Trimethoprim	Sulfadiazine, sulfamethoxazole
Tylosin	Oxytetracycline

[a]Indicated when synergy is advantageous in definitive therapy, to treat polymicrobial infections, to broaden empiric coverage, or to attempt to prevent the development of antimicrobial resistance.
[b]Generally amikacin, occasionally gentamicin.

TABLE 15-5 Select Laboratories Conducting Exotic Animal Diagnostic Procedures.

Laboratory	Select Tests/Procedures
Animal Health Diagnostic Center College of Veterinary Medicine Cornell University PO Box 5786 Ithaca, NY 14852 USA (607) 253-3900 ahdc.vet.cornell.edu	General: Chemistry, hematology, clotting panels, histopathology, microbiology, necropsy, parasitology, virology Avian: *Chlamydia, Cryptosporidium, Giardia, Mycobacterium, Mycoplasma*, infectious bronchitis virus, infectious bursal disease, influenza virus, paramyxovirus, West Nile virus, viral isolation, blood lead/zinc Mammal: Ferret enteric coronavirus, ferret influenza virus, mink enteric coronavirus, ferret adrenal testing Reptile: *Cryptosporidium, Salmonella*
Antech Diagnostics 10 Executive Boulevard Farmingdale, NY 11735 USA (800) 745-4725 (West) (800) 872-1001 (East)	General: Chemistry, electrophoresis, hematology, microbiology, virology Avian: *Mycoplasma, Chlamydia, Aspergillus*, polyomavirus, psittacine beak and feather disease virus, West Nile virus, sex determination, blood lead/zinc

Continued

TABLE 15-5 Select Laboratories Conducting Exotic Animal Diagnostic Procedures. (cont'd)

Laboratory	Select Tests/Procedures
(800) 341-3440 (Canada) antechdiagnostics.com	Mammal: *Pasteurella, Encephalitozoon, Treponema, Toxoplasma,* ferret adrenal panel, distemper virus, Aleutian disease virus Reptile: *Mycoplasma*
Avian Biotech International Animal Genetics, Inc. 1336 Timberlane Road Tallahassee, FL 32312 USA (800) 514-9672 (850) 386-1145 avianbiotech.com	Avian: *Bordetella, Chlamydia, Mycobacterium, Salmonella, Aspergillus, Candida, Cryptosporidium, Giardia,* paramyxovirus, pigeon circovirus, polyomavirus, psittacine beak and feather disease virus, herpes virus, influenza virus, West Nile virus, Pacheco's disease, sex determination
Avian & Exotic Animal Clin Path Labs 2712 North Highway 68 Wilmington, OH 45177 USA (937) 383-3347 (800) 350-1122 avianexoticlab.com	General: Chemistry, electrophoresis, hematology, histopathology, microbiology, parasitology, toxicology, virology Avian: *Chlamydia, Salmonella, Aspergillus, Histoplasma, Cryptosporidium, Giardia, Sarcocystis,* adenovirus, influenza virus, Pacheco's disease, paramyxovirus, polyomavirus, West Nile virus, blood iron/lead/zinc Mammal: Heartworm testing, *Toxoplasma,* distemper virus Herps: *Cryptosporidium, Giardia,* chytrid, inclusion body disease, ophidian paramyxovirus
Avian and Wildlife Laboratory Division of Comparative Pathology University of Miami School of Medicine 1611 NW 12th Avenue Miami, FL 33136 USA (305) 585-6303 cpl.med.miami.edu	General: Chemistry, electrophoresis, hematology Avian: *Aspergillus, Chlamydia, Cryptosporidium,* Pacheco's virus, polyomavirus, psittacine beak and feather disease virus, sex determination Mammal: CAR bacillus, *Clostridium piliforme, Mycoplasma, Pasteurella, E. cuniculi,* guinea pig adenovirus, coronavirus, Kilham's rat virus, lymphocytic choriomeningitis virus, mouse hepatitis virus, minute virus of mice, pneumonia virus of mice, parainfluenza virus 3, parvovirus, rotavirus, Sendai virus, Theiler's murine encephalomyelitis virus
Diagnostic Center for Population and Animal Health Michigan State University 4125 Beaumont Road Lansing, MI 48910 USA (517) 353-1683 animalhealth.msu.edu	General: Chemistry, hematology, histopathology, microbiology, necropsy, protein electrophoresis, toxicology, virology Avian: *Chlamydia, Mycobacterium, Mycoplasma, Aspergillus, Cryptosporidium, Salmonella,* Newcastle disease virus, infectious bronchitis virus, infectious laryngotracheitis virus, influenza virus, West Nile virus, blood lead Mammal: *Cryptosporidium, Giardia, Salmonella,* Aleutian disease virus, ferret enteric coronavirus, ferret rotavirus Herps: *Mycoplasma, Salmonella, Cryptosporidium*
Diagnostic Laboratory Service College of Veterinary Medicine University of Tennessee 2407 River Drive Knoxville, TN 37996 USA (865) 974-8387 vetmed.tennessee.edu/vmc/dls	General: Chemistry, endocrinology, hematology, histopathology, microbiology, necropsy, parasitology, toxicology, virology Avian: *Chlamydia, Mycobacterium, Mycoplasma, Aspergillus, Cryptosporidium,* sex determination Mammal: *Giardia,* influenza A virus, ferret adrenal panel, rabbit adrenal panel Herps: *Mycoplasma, Cryptosporidium,* herpesvirus, ophidian paramyxovirus, ranavirus

CHAPTER 15 Select Topics for the Exotic Animal Veterinarian

TABLE 15-5 Select Laboratories Conducting Exotic Animal Diagnostic Procedures. (cont'd)

Laboratory	Select Tests/Procedures
Georgia Veterinary Diagnostic Laboratories College of Veterinary Medicine University of Georgia 501 DW Brooks Drive Athens, GA 30602 USA (706) 542-5568 vet.uga.edu/dlab/	General: Chemistry, hematology, histopathology, microbiology, necropsy, parasitology, toxicology, virology Avian: *Chlamydia, Mycobacterium, Mycoplasma, Salmonella, Aspergillus, Cryptosporidium, Plasmodium,* herpesvirus, influenza virus, Newcastle disease virus, West Nile virus, Pacheco's disease Mammal: *Bordetella, Clostridium* (toxin panel), *Francisella tularensis, Helicobacter, Lawsonia, Mycobacteria, Mycoplasma, Pasteurella, Salmonella, Treponema, Encephalitozoon,* herpesvirus, influenza A virus, lymphocytic choriomeningitis virus, morbiliviruses, mouse hepatitis virus, mouse reoviruses, murine norovirus, paramyxovirus, pneumonia virus of mice, rabies virus, rodent parvoviruses, Sendai virus, simian virus 5, Tyzzer's disease Herps: *Cryptosporidium, Mycoplasma, Salmonella,* adenovirus, herpesvirus, ranavirus Aquatic: Aquatic bacterial and fungal cultures (including *Mycobacterium* and *Mycoplasma*)
Kansas State Veterinary Diagnostic Laboratory College of Veterinary Medicine Kansas State University 1800 Denison Avenue Manhattan, KS 66506 USA (866) 512-5650 vet.k-state.edu/depts/dmp/service	General: Chemistry, hematology, histopathology, microbiology, necropsy, parasitology, protein electrophoresis, toxicology, virology Avian: *Bordetella, Chlamydia, Salmonella, Aspergillus, Cryptosporidium,* influenza virus, Newcastle disease virus, West Nile virus, blood lead Mammal: *Francisella tularensis, Lawsonia, Giardia, Cryptosporidium,* influenza virus, rabies virus Herps: *Salmonella*
National Veterinary Services Laboratory USDA-APHIS-VS-NVSL PO Box 844 Ames, IA 50010 USA (515) 337-7266 aphis.usda.gov/aphis/ourfocus/ animalhealth/lab-info-services	General: Microbiology, virology Avian: *Avibacterium paragallinarum, Bordetella, Chlamydia, Mycoplasma, Mycoplasma, Ornithobacterium rhinotracheale, Pasteurella, Salmonella,* adenoviruses, avian pox virus, chicken anemia virus, duck viral enteritis virus, encephalomyelitis virus, goose parvovirus, herpesviruses, infectious bronchitis virus, infectious bursal disease, infectious laryngotracheitis, influenza virus, Marek's disease, metapneumovirus, nephritis virus, paramyxoviruses, reoviruses, rotavirus, West Nile virus Mammal: *Francisella tularensis* Aquatic: Various bacterial and viral testing options for aquaculture (contact lab for arrangements)
Northwest ZooPath 654 West Main Street Monroe, WA 98272 USA (360) 794-0630 zoopath.com	General: Pathology
Research Associates Laboratory 14556 Midway Road Dallas, TX 75224 USA (972) 960-2221 vetdna.com	General: Microbiology, virology Avian: *Bartonella, Bordetella, Chlamydia, Cryptosporidium, Helicobacter, Mycobacterium, Mycoplasma, Salmonella, Aspergillus, Candida,* avian gastric yeast, *Giardia,* plasmodium, adenoviruses, circoviruses, duck enteritis virus, herpesviruses, Marek's disease, polyomavirus, poxvirus, psittacine beak and feather disease virus, sex determination

Continued

TABLE 15-5 Select Laboratories Conducting Exotic Animal Diagnostic Procedures. (cont'd)

Laboratory	Select Tests/Procedures
	Mammal: *Anaplasma, Babesia, Bartonella, Bordetella, Brucella, Campylobacter, Chlamydia, Clostridium, Coxiella, E. coli, Ehrlichia, Francisella tularensis, Helicobacter, Lawsonia intracellularis, Pasteurella, Mycobacterium, Mycoplasma, Candida, Cryptosporidium, Encephalitozoon, Entamoeba, Enterocytozoon, Giardia, Hepatozoon, Plasmodium, Sarcocystis, Spironucleus, Toxoplasma,* Aleutian disease, astrovirus, distemper virus, ferret epizootic catarrhal enteritis, hantavirus, hepatitis E virus, lymphocytic choriomeningitis virus, myxomavirus, orthopoxvirus, rabies virus, West Nile virus
	Herps: *Campylobacter, Clostridium, Mycobacterium, Mycoplasma, Pasteurella, Salmonella, Aspergillus, Candida,* CANV, chytrid, *Cryptosporidium, Entamoeba, Giardia, Plasmodium, Spironucleus,* arenavirus, atadenovirus, herpesviruses, iridovirus, fibropapillomatosis, ophidian paramyxovirus, ranavirus, sunshine virus, West Nile virus
	Aquatic: Bacterial, viral, and parasitic testing (see Web site for extensive list)
Texas Veterinary Medical Diagnostic Laboratory Texas A&M University 1 Sippel Road College Station, TX 77843 USA (979) 845-3414 (888) 646-5623 tvmdl.tamu.edu	General: Chemistry, hematology, histopathology, microbiology, necropsy, protein electrophoresis, toxicology, virology Avian: *Chlamydia, Mycobacterium, Mycoplasma, Salmonella, Aspergillus, Cryptosporidium,* avian encephalomyelitis virus, duck enteritis virus, infectious bronchitis virus, infectious bursal disease virus, infectious laryngotracheitis virus, influenza virus, paramyxoviruses, reovirus, reticuloendotheliosis virus, West Nile virus, blood lead/zinc/iron Mammal: *Bordetella, E. coli, Mycoplasma, Salmonella, Cryptosporidium, Giardia,* distemper virus, rabies virus Herps: *Mycoplasma, Salmonella, Cryptosporidium*
Veterinary Medical Diagnostic Lab College of Veterinary Medicine University of Missouri PO Box 6023 Columbia, MO 65205 USA (573) 882-6811 vmdl.missouri.edu	General: Histopathology, microbiology, necropsy, toxicology, virology Avian: *Bordetella, Chlamydia, Mycoplasma, Ornithobacterium rhinotracheale, Salmonella, Cryptosporidium,* avian encephalitis virus, hemorrhagic enteritis virus, infectious bronchitis virus, influenza virus, Newcastle disease virus, rotavirus, blood lead/zinc
Veterinary Molecular Diagnostics, Inc. 5989 Meijer Drive, Suite 5 Milford, OH 45150 USA (513) 576-1808 vmdlabs.com	General: Molecular diagnostics Avian: *Bordetella, Chlamydia, Mycobacterium, Mycoplasma, Aspergillus,* avian gastric yeast, adenovirus, bornavirus, circoviruses, coronavirus, polyomavirus, psittacine beak and feather disease virus, psittacine herpes virus, West Nile virus, sex determination Mammal: *Campylobacter, Helicobacter, Lawsonia, Encephalitozoon,* Aleutian disease virus, epizootic catarrhal enteritis virus Herps: *Cryptosporidium, Mycoplasma,* bearded dragon atadenovirus
Wisconsin Veterinary Diagnostic Laboratory University of Wisconsin 455 Easterday Lane	General: Histopathology, microbiology, necropsy, virology Avian: *Bordetella, Chlamydia, Mycoplasma, Salmonella, Cryptosporidium,* avian encephalitis virus, duck viral enteritis virus, infectious bronchitis virus, infectious bursal disease virus,

TABLE 15-5 Select Laboratories Conducting Exotic Animal Diagnostic Procedures. (cont'd)

Laboratory	Select Tests/Procedures
Madison, WI 53706 USA (608) 262-5432 (800) 608-8387 wvdl.wisc.edu	infectious laryngotracheitis virus, influenza virus, paramyxovirus, pneumovirus, polyomavirus, poxvirus, psittacine herpes virus, turkey hemorrhagic enteritis virus, West Nile virus Herps: *Mycoplasma, Salmonella*
Zoo/Exotic Pathology Service 2825 Kovr Drive West Sacramento, CA 95605 USA (916) 725-5100 zooexotic.com	General: Pathology
Zoologix, Inc 9811 Owensmouth Avenue Suite 4 Chatsworth, CA 91311 USA (818) 717-8880 zoologix.com	General: Molecular diagnostics Avian: *Avibacterium paragallinarum, Bordetella, Chlamydia, Mycobacterium, Mycoplasma, Ornithobacterium rhinotracheale, Salmonella, Aspergillus, Candida, Atoxoplasma, Cryptosporidium, Plasmodium,* adenovirus, bornavirus, circovirus, herpesvirus, infectious bronchitis virus, infectious bursal disease virus, infectious laryngotracheitis virus, influenza virus, Newcastle disease virus, Pacheco's disease, polyomavirus, poxvirus, psittacine beak and feather disease virus, reovirus, West Nile virus Mammal: *Bordetella, Campylobacter, E. coli, Francisella tularensis, Helicobacter, Lawsonia intracellularis, Mycobacterium, Mycoplasma, Pasteurella, Salmonella, Giardia, Treponema,* Aleutian disease virus, hantavirus, lymphocytic choriomeningitis virus, mink enteritis virus, monkeypox, mouse adenovirus, mouse cytomegaloviruses, mouse hepatitis virus, mouse minute virus, mouse norovirus, mouse parvovirus, mouse polyoma virus, mouse pox virus, mouse rotavirus, pneumonia virus of mice, rabbit fibroma virus, rabies virus, rat coronavirus, reovirus, rotavirus, Sendai virus, sialodacryoadenitis virus, Tyzzer's disease Herps: *Mycobacterium, Mycoplasma, Salmonella,* chytrid fungus, *Cryptosporidium,* ranavirus
Zoo Medicine Service College of Veterinary Medicine University of Florida PO Box 100126 Gainesville, FL 32610 USA (352) 392-4700 (ext. 5700) http://labs.vetmed.ufl.edu/sample-requirements/zoo-med-infections/	General: Consensus polymerase chain reaction (PCR) and sequencing Herps: *Chlamydiales, Mycobacterium, Mycoplasma,* coccidia, *Cryptosporidium,* microsporidians, pentastomids, adenoviruses, arenaviruses, astroviruses, erythrocytic iridoviruses, ferlaviruses, herpesviruses, orthoreoviruses, papillomaviruses, paramyxoviruses, poxviruses, ranaviruses, rhabdoviruses

TABLE 15-6 Professional Associations for Veterinarians Interested in Exotics.[a]

Organization	Web Site
American Association of Wildlife Veterinarians	aawv.net
American Association of Zoo Veterinarians	aazv.org
American Board of Veterinary Practitioners	abvp.com
American College of Zoological Medicine	aczm.org
American Society of Laboratory Animal Practitioners	aslap.org
Association of Amphibian and Reptilian Veterinarians	arav.org
Association of Avian Veterinarians	aav.org
Association of Exotic Mammal Veterinarians	aemv.org
Association of Primate Veterinarians	primatevets.org
Association of Sugar Glider Veterinarians	asgv.org
Association of Zoo Veterinary Technicians	azvt.org
British Veterinary Zoological Society	bvzs.org
Canadian Association of Zoo and Wildlife Veterinarians	cazwv.org
European Association of Zoo and Wildlife Veterinarians	eazwv.org
International Association for Aquatic Animal Medicine	iaaam.org
National Wildlife Rehabilitators Association	nwrawildlife.org

[a]Web sites accessed on August 2, 2016.

TABLE 15-7 Exotic Animal Online Resources for Practitioners.[a]

Site Name	Web Site	Description
American Society for the Prevention of Cruelty to Animals	aspca.org	Contains an Animal Poison Control Center and general pet care guidelines
Amphibian Diseases Home Page	arwh.org/amphibian-dz-homepage	Australian page focusing on current information on amphibian diseases
Animal Diversity Web	animaldiversity.org	Taxonomic site from the University of Michigan Museum of Zoology
Avibase	avibase.bsc-eoc.org	Searchable database with taxonomic information and photographs of the world's bird species
Biodidac	biodidac.bio.uottawa.ca	Bank of digital resources for teaching biology; includes anatomy line drawings
BioOne	bioone.org	Resource database collection of bioscience research journals; contains multiple peer-reviewed exotic journals

TABLE 15-7   Exotic Animal Online Resources for Practitioners. (cont'd)

Site Name	Web Site	Description
Center for Agricultural Bioscience International	cabi.org	Resource database collection of agricultural and bioscience journals; contains multiple peer-reviewed exotic journals
Convention on International Trade in Endangered Species	cites.org	International agreement between governments concerning the international trade of wild animals and plants
The Colyer Institute	colyerinstitute.org	Center for the study of oral disease and nutrition in exotic animals
Dental Anatomy	arbl.cvmbs.colostate.edu/hbooks/pathphys/digestion/pregastric/dentalanat.html	Includes information and images of dental anatomy of rabbits and rodents (from Colorado State University)
Diseases of Research Animals (DORA)	dora.missouri.edu	Teaching resources from the University of Missouri regarding diseases seen in species commonly kept for research purposes
Exotic DVM	exoticdvm.com	Web site for the *Exotic DVM* magazine
Exotic Pet Vet Net	exoticpetvet.net	Web site of veterinary articles from exotic veterinarians
The Humane Society	humanesociety.org	Includes care sheets for many exotic species
International Species Information System (recently renamed: Species 360)	species360.org (previous Web site: isis.org)	Global network of animal management professionals
International Union for the Conservation of Nature	iucn.org	Organization dedicated to finding pragmatic solutions to environment and development challenges; produces the IUCN Red List of Threatened Species
International Veterinary Information System	ivis.org	Online veterinary book publisher with free access to multiple online books
An Introduction to Ratite Ranching and Medicine	instruction.cvhs.okstate.edu/kocan/ostrich/ostbk2a1.htm	Online book of ratite medicine from Oklahoma State University
Medirabbit	medirabbit.com	Rabbit medicine articles and video demonstrations
The Merck Veterinary Manual	merckvetmanual.com	*Merck Veterinary Manual* online including exotic animals with normal physiological parameters
PubMed	ncbi.nlm.nih.gov/pubmed	Digital Archive of the US National Library of Medicine; contains multiple peer-reviewed exotic journals
Species 360 (formerly International Species Information System)	species360.org	Global network of animal management professionals
Tufts University Open Courseware, Zoological Medicine Course	ocw.tufts.edu/Course/60	Open access course notes from the Tufts University College of Veterinary Medicine Zoological Medicine Course

Continued

TABLE 15-7 Exotic Animal Online Resources for Practitioners. (cont'd)

Site Name	Web Site	Description
University of Pennsylvania Computer Aided Learning	research.vet.upenn.edu/Home/tabid/5849/Default.aspx	Computer Aided Learning Program from the University of Pennsylvania School of Veterinary Medicine; includes Special Species Clinical Pathology and Special Species Radiology Sections
USDA APHIS	aphis.usda.gov	United States Department of Agriculture, Animal Plant Health Inspection Service
Veterinary Information Network	vin.com	Member-based network of veterinary consultants; large bank of information on zoo and exotic animals
Veterinary Partner	veterinarypartner.com	Partner to the Veterinary Information Network, contains information and handouts for clients concerning medical diseases
World Organization for Animal Health (OIE)	oie.int	Intergovernmental organization responsible for improving animal health worldwide

[a]Web sites accessed on August 1, 2016. Please note that Elsevier Inc. and the editor of the *Exotic Animal Formulary*, 5th ed. have not reviewed all of the content of these sites and, therefore, cannot confirm the accuracy of the information presented.

TABLE 15-8 Captive Husbandry Web Sites for Owners of Exotic Animals.[a]

Category	Site Name	Web Site	Description
Aquatics	Fish Channel	fishchannel.com	Web site with information on tropical and saltwater aquariums including a large variety of species-specific information
	Fish Lore	fishlore.com	Tropical fish, freshwater aquarium, and saltwater aquarium information Web site
	Fish Tank Guide	fish-tank-guide.com	Web site including information on basic tank care, fish care, and medical information. Also contains some species-specific information on common aquarium fish
	Goldfish Society of America	goldfishsociety.org	Association for goldfish enthusiasts; includes husbandry and care information
	International Fancy Guppy Association	ifga.org	Association dedicated to the Fancy Show Guppy; contains general starter information and medical information on guppies
Herptile	Bearded Dragon Care	beardeddragoncare.net	Web site dedicated to provide bearded dragon care information to pet lizard owners
	Boa Tips	boatips.com	Web site for pet snakes; includes husbandry and care articles as well as species-specific information and photographs

CHAPTER 15　Select Topics for the Exotic Animal Veterinarian　651

TABLE 15-8　Captive Husbandry Web Sites for Owners of Exotic Animals. (cont'd)

Category	Site Name	Web Site	Description
	Box Turtle Care and Conservation	boxturtlesite.info	Web site for natural history and captive care of North American box turtles
	Chameleon Care and Information Center	chameleoninfo.com	Web site devoted to chameleons; includes husbandry and care articles
	Frog World	frogworld.net	Web site concerning natural history, husbandry, and care of multiple frog species
	Green Iguana Society	greenigsociety.org	Society dedicated to providing quality information on iguana care; contains husbandry and care articles as well as some medical information
	Lizard Landscapes	lizard-landscapes.com	Web site with husbandry and care information for multiple species of reptiles; also contains information on building cage landscapes
	The Lizard Lounge	the-lizard-lounge.com	Web site containing husbandry and care information as well as taxonomy, photographs, natural history, and medical information on multiple species of lizards
	Melissa Kaplan's Herp Care Collection	anapsid.org	Web site containing husbandry and care articles on amphibians, reptiles, and invertebrates
	Pet Snakes	pet-snakes.com	Web site containing husbandry and care information as well as listings of some exotic animal vet clinics by states
	Poison Dart Frogs	poisondartfrog.co.uk	Web site containing husbandry and care information on *Dendrobates* species
	Reptile Web	reptilesweb.com	A world reptile amphibian information center; contains husbandry and care information for reptiles, amphibians, and invertebrates
	Tortoise Trust	tortoisetrust.org	Web site with information on turtles and tortoises including species care sheets and husbandry articles
	World Chelonian Trust	chelonia.org	Web site with information on turtles and tortoises including species care sheets and chelonian taxonomy.
Avian	African Love Bird Society	africanlovebirdsociety.org	Association dedicated to keeping, breeding, and showing of love birds; contains husbandry and care information along with information on the nine species
	American Budgerigar Society	abs1.org	Society for information about keeping, breeding, and exhibiting budgerigars

Continued

TABLE 15-8 Captive Husbandry Web Sites for Owners of Exotic Animals. (cont'd)

Category	Site Name	Web Site	Description
	American Dove Association	americandoveassociation.com	Association for dove enthusiasts; contains husbandry and care information along with information on the different species
	American Federation of Aviculture	afabirds.org	Nonprofit organization whose purpose is to represent all aspects of aviculture and to educate the public about keeping and breeding birds in captivity
	American Ostrich Association	ostrich.org	Association to establish the standards for the highest quality American ostrich products to ensure the long-term viability of the industry
	Foraging For Parrots	foragingforparrots.com	Web site on how to make foraging toys for psittacine birds
	International Cockatiel Society	cockatiels.org	Society dedicated to providing information on the proper care, handling, maintenance, and breeding of cockatiels
	National Finch and Softbill Society	nfss.org	Society dedicated to promoting the enjoyment of keeping and breeding finches and softbills
	Parrot A.L.E.R.T.	parrotalert.org	Web site for reporting lost and found parrots; also includes husbandry articles
	Parrot Outreach Society	parrotoutreachsociety.org	Society dedicated to helping birds find homes; includes basic bird care articles
	World Parrot Trust	parrots.org	Organization to promote survival of all parrot species in the wild and to advocate for the welfare of individual birds in our homes
Mammal	American Fancy Rat and Mouse Association	afrma.org	Association to promote and encourage the breeding and exhibition of fancy rats and mice for show and pets
	American Ferret Association	ferret.org	Association to promote the domestic ferret as a companion animal through public education via shows, newsletters, legislative education, and other venues
	American Gerbil Society	agsgerbils.org	Society providing support and education to breeders, caregivers, and gerbil enthusiasts
	American Rabbit Breeders Association	arba.net	Association dedicated to the promotion, development, and improvement of the domestic rabbit and cavy
	Cheeky Chinchilla	cheekychinchillas.com	Husbandry and care information for chinchillas
	Ferret Universe	ferretuniverse.com	Husbandry and care information for ferrets

CHAPTER 15 Select Topics for the Exotic Animal Veterinarian

TABLE 15-8 Captive Husbandry Web Sites for Owners of Exotic Animals. (cont'd)

Category	Site Name	Web Site	Description
	Ferret Village	ferretvillage.org	Message boards concerning ferrets
	Gerbil Care	gerbilcare.org	Husbandry and care information for gerbils
	Guinea Lynx	guinealynx.info	Husbandry and care information for guinea pigs
	Hamster Hideout	hamsterhideout.com	Husbandry and care information for hamsters
	Hamsterific	hamsterific.com	Husbandry and care information for hamsters
	House Rabbit Society	rabbit.org	Society that rescues rabbits from animal shelters and educates the public on rabbit care and behavior
	International Ferret Congress	ferretcongress.org	Organization to enhance the welfare of the domestic ferret as a companion animal
	International Hedgehog Association	hedgehogclub.com	Association to educate the public in the care and betterment of hedgehogs
	My House Rabbit	myhouserabbit.com	Web site celebrating house rabbits and educating the public about rabbit care and behavior
	North American Sugar Glider Association	mynasga.org	Association to provide information to persons considering getting a sugar glider for a family pet
	Pet Hamster Care	pethamstercare.com	Husbandry and care information for hamsters
	Rat Guide	ratguide.com	A layman's guide to health, medication use, breeding, and responsible care of pet rats
	Sugarglider	sugarglider.com	Husbandry and care information for sugar gliders
	Weasel Words	weaselwords.com	Husbandry and care information for ferrets

[a]Web sites accessed on August 1, 2016. Please note that Elsevier Inc. and the editor of the *Exotic Animal Formulary*, 5th ed. have not reviewed all of the content of these sites and therefore cannot confirm the accuracy of the information presented.

TABLE 15-9 Emergency Drug Doses (in mL) Commonly Used in Exotic Animals.[a]

Emergency Drug			Gerbils, Hamsters, Mice, Rats							Guinea Pigs, Chinchillas		
Drug	Conc	Route	25 g	50 g	75 g	100 g	125 g	150 g	250 g	500 g	0.5 kg	1 kg	1.5 kg
Epinephrine	0.01 mg/mL	IV, IM, IO	0.01	0.02	0.02	0.03	0.04	0.05	0.08	0.15	0.15	0.3	0.45
Atropine	0.54 mg/mL	IM, SC	0.03	0.04	0.06	0.07	0.09	0.11	0.19	0.37	0.37	0.74	1.11
Glycopyrrolate	0.2 mg/mL	IM, SC	0.01	0.01	0.01	0.01	0.02	0.02	0.03	0.05	0.05	0.1	0.15
Dex SP	4 mg/mL	IV, IM	0.03	0.06	0.09	0.13	0.16	0.19	0.32	0.63	0.63	1.25	1.87
Doxapram	20 mg/mL	IV, SC	0.02	0.03	0.04	0.05	0.07	0.08	0.13	0.25	0.25	0.5	0.75
Diazepam	5 mg/mL	IV, IM, IO	0.01	0.03	0.05	0.06	0.08	0.09	0.15	0.3	0.3	0.6	0.9
Furosemide	5 mg/mL	IV, IM, SC	0.02	0.04	0.06	0.08	0.1	0.12	0.2	0.4	0.4	0.8	0.12

Emergency Drug			Rabbits							Ferrets		
Drug	Conc	Route	0.5 kg	1 kg	1.5 kg	2 kg	3 kg	4 kg	5 kg	0.5 kg	1 kg	1.5 kg	2 kg
Epinephrine	1 mg/mL	IV, IM, IO	0.5	1.0	1.5	2.0	3.0	4.0	5.0	0.1	0.2	0.3	0.4
Atropine	0.54 mg/mL	IM, SC	0.5	0.9	1.4	1.9	2.8	3.7	4.6	0.05	0.1	0.15	0.2
Glycopyrrolate	0.2 mg/mL	IM, SC	0.05	0.1	0.15	0.2	0.3	0.4	0.5	0.03	0.05	0.08	0.1
Dex SP	4 mg/mL	IV, IM	0.25	0.5	0.75	1.0	1.5	2.0	2.5	1.0	2.0	3.0	4.0
Doxapram	20 mg/mL	IV, SC	0.13	0.25	0.38	0.5	0.75	1.0	1.3	0.05	0.1	0.15	0.2
Diazepam	55 mg/mL	IV, IM, IO	0.3	0.6	0.9	1.2	1.8	2.4	3.0	0.2	0.4	0.6	0.8
Furosemide	50 mg/mL	IV, IM, SC	0.04	0.08	0.12	0.16	0.24	0.32	0.4	0.04	0.08	0.12	0.16
Diphenhydramine	50 mg/mL	IV, IM	—	—	—	—	—	—	—	0.02	0.04	0.06	0.08

CHAPTER 15 Select Topics for the Exotic Animal Veterinarian

TABLE 15-9 Emergency Drug Doses (in mL) Commonly Used in Exotic Animals. (cont'd)

Emergency Drug			Avian (Psittacine Birds)										
Drug	Conc	Route	0.05 kg	0.1 kg	0.2 kg	0.3 kg	0.4 kg	0.5 kg	0.6 kg	0.7 kg	0.8 kg	0.9 kg	1.0 kg
Epinephrine	1 mg/mL	IV, IM, IO	0.05	0.1	0.2	0.3	0.4	0.5	0.6	0.7	0.8	0.9	1.0
Atropine	0.54 mg/mL	IM, SC	0.05	0.09	0.19	0.28	0.37	0.46	0.56	0.65	0.74	0.83	0.93
Doxapram	20 mg/mL	IV, IM, IO	0.05	0.1	0.2	0.3	0.4	0.5	0.6	0.7	0.8	0.9	1.0
Dex SP	4 mg/mL	IV, IM	0.05	0.1	0.2	0.3	0.4	0.5	0.6	0.7	0.8	0.9	1.0
Ca gluconate	100 mg/mL	IV, IM	0.05	0.1	0.2	0.3	0.4	0.5	0.6	0.7	0.8	0.9	1.0
Diazepam	5 mg/mL	IV, IM, IO	0.01	0.02	0.04	0.06	0.08	0.1	0.12	0.14	0.16	0.18	0.2

Emergency Drug			Reptiles							
Drug	Conc	Route	0.1 kg	0.25 kg	0.5 kg	0.75 kg	1 kg	2 kg	3 kg	4 kg	5 kg	6 kg	7 kg
Atropine	0.54 mg/mL	IV, IM, SC	0.01	0.02	0.04	0.06	0.07	0.15	0.22	0.3	0.37	0.44	0.52
Glycopyrrolate	0.2 mg/mL	IV, IM	0.01	0.02	0.03	0.04	0.05	0.1	0.15	0.2	0.25	0.3	0.35
Dex SP	4 mg/mL	IV, IM	0.01	0.02	0.03	0.05	0.06	0.13	0.19	0.25	0.31	0.38	0.44
Diazepam	5 mg/mL	IV, IM, ICe	0.05	0.12	0.25	0.38	0.5	1.0	1.5	2.0	2.5	3.0	3.5
Ca gluconate	100 mg/mL	IV, IO, SC	0.1	0.3	0.5	0.75	1.0	2.0	3.0	4.0	5.0	6.0	7.0

[a]Modified from Kottwitz J, Kelleher S. Emergency drugs: Quick reference chart for exotic animals. *Exotic DVM* 2003;5.5:23-25.

TABLE 15-10 Fluid Solutions Used in Exotic Animal Medicine.

Solution Type	Solution	Na+ (mEq/L)	K+ (mEq/L)	Cl− (mEq/L)	Ca++ (mEq/L)	Mg++ (mEq/L)	Buffer (mEq/L)	Osmolality (mOsm/L)	pH
Crystalloids	Ringer's solution	147	4	156	4	0	0	310	5-7.5
	Lactated Ringer's solution	130	4	109	3	0	28 (lactate)	275	6-7.5
	0.9% NaCl	154	0	154	0	0	0	308	4.5
	5% Dextrose	0	0	0	0	0	0	252	4-6.5
	2.5% Dextrose/0.45% NaCl	77	0	77	0	0	0	280	4.5
	Plasma-Lyte	140	5	98	0	3	27 (acetate) 23 (gluconate)	294	4-6.5
	Normosol-R	140	5	98	0	3	27 (acetate) 23 (gluconate)	294	6.6
Colloids	Dextran 6% and 0.9% NaCl	154	0	154	0	0	0	310	3-7.0
	Hetastarch	154	0	154	0	0	0	309	5.5
	Pentastarch	154	0	154	0	0	0	326	5.0

TABLE 15-11 Common Abbreviations Used in Prescription Writing.

a.c.	before meals	o.d.	right eye
a.d.	right ear	o.s.	left eye
ad lib	at pleasure	o.u.	both eyes
adm	administer	oz	ounce
aq	water	p.c.	after meals
a.s.	left ear	PO (p.o.)	per os
a.u.	both ears	prn (p.r.n.)	as needed
b.i.d.	twice a day	q. (q)	every
c.	with	q.d.	every day
cap(s)	capsule(s)	q4h	every 4 hours, etc.
cc	cubic centimeter	q24h	once a day
disp	dispense	q.i.d.	four times a day
fl oz	fluid ounce	q.o.d.	every other day
g (gm)	gram	q.s.	a sufficient quantity
gr	grain	®	trademarked name
gtt(s)	drop(s)	SC (SQ)	subcutaneously
h (hr)	hour	Sig:	instructions to patient
h.s.	at bedtime	sol'n	solution
IM	intramuscularly	stat	immediately
inj	inject	susp	suspension
IP	intraperitoneally	tab(s)	tablet(s)
IV	intravenously	Tbs	tablespoon
kg	kilogram	t.i.d.	three times a day
lb	pound	tsp	teaspoon
mg	milligram	ut dict.	as directed
mL	milliliter		

TABLE 15-12 Common Weight, Liquid Measure, Length, Percentage, and Milliequivalent Conversions.

Weights

1 milligram (mg) = 1000 micrograms (mcg orig) = 0.015 grain
1 grain (gr) = 64.8 mg (≈65 mg)
1 gram (g) = 15.43 grains (≈15 grains) = 1000 mg
1 kilogram (kg) = 1000 g = 2.2 lb
1 ounce (oz) = 28.35 g
1 pound (lb) = 454 g = 16 oz = 0.45 kg
2.2 pound = 1 kg

Liquid Measures

1 drop = 0.05 (1/20) milliliter (mL)
1 cubic centimeter (cc) = 1 mL
1 liter (L) = 1000 mL
1 teaspoon (tsp) = 5 mL
1 tablespoon (Tbs) = 15 mL
1 fluid ounce (fl oz) = 29.57 mL (≈30 mL)
1 pint = 473.2 mL (≈473 mL)
1 quart = 2 pints = 32 fl oz = 0.946 L
1 gallon = 4 quarts = 3.785 L
1 cup = 8 fl oz = 237 mL = 16 Tbs

Linear Measures

1 millimeter (mm) = 0.039 inches (in)
1 centimeter (cm) = 0.39 in
1 meter (m) = 39.37 in
1 inch (in) = 2.54 cm
1 foot (ft) = 30.48 cm
1 yard (yd) = 91.44 cm

Percentage Equivalents

0.1% solution = 1 mg per mL
1% solution = 10 mg per mL
10% solution = 100 mg per mL

Milliequivalents

1 mEq Na = 23 mg Na = 58.5 mg NaCl
1 g Na = 2.54 g NaCl = 43 mEq Na
1 g NaCl = 0.39 g Na = 17 mEq Na
1 mEq K = 39 mg K = 74.5 mg KCl
1 g K = 1.91 g KCl = 26 mEq K
1 g KCl = 0.52 g K = 13 mEq K
1 mEq Ca = 20 mg Ca
1 g Ca = 50 mEq Ca
1 mEq Mg = 0.12 g $MgSO_4 \times 7H_2O$
1 g Mg = 10.2 g $MgSO_4 \times 7H_2O$ = 82 mEq Mg

CHAPTER 15 Select Topics for the Exotic Animal Veterinarian   659

TABLE 15-13 Equivalents of Celsius (Centigrade) and Fahrenheit Temperature Scales.[a]

°C	°F	°C	°F	°C	°F
0	32.0	17	62.6	34	93.2
1	33.8	18	64.4	35	95.0
2	35.6	19	66.2	36	96.8
3	37.4	20	68.0	37	98.6
4	39.2	21	69.8	38	100.4
5	41.0	22	71.6	39	102.2
6	42.8	23	73.4	40	104.0
7	44.6	24	75.2	41	105.8
8	46.4	25	77.0	42	107.6
9	48.2	26	78.8	43	109.4
10	50.0	27	80.6	44	111.2
11	51.8	28	82.4	45	113.0
12	53.6	29	84.2	46	114.8
13	55.4	30	86.0	47	116.6
14	57.2	31	87.8	48	118.4
15	59.0	32	89.6	49	120.2
16	60.8	33	91.4	50	122.0

[a]Conversions: °C = 5/9 × (°F − 32); °F = 9/5 × (°C) + 32.

TABLE 15-14 System of International (SI) Units Conversion Factors of Hematology Commonly Used in Exotic Animal Medicine.[a]

Component	Conventional (USA) Units	SI Unit
Hemoglobin (Hgb)	g/dL	g/L
Red blood cells (RBC)	× 10^6/μL	× 10^{12}/L
Reticulocytes	%	%
Mean corpuscular volume (MCV)	fL	fL
Mean corpuscular Hgb (MCH)	pg	pg
Mean corpuscular Hgb concentration (MCHC)	g/dL	g/L
Platelets	× 10^3/μL	× 10^9/L
White blood cells (WBC)	× 10^3/μL	× 10^9/L
Neutrophils (segmented)	× 10^3/μL	× 10^9/L
Neutrophils (bands)	× 10^3/μL	× 10^9/L
Lymphocytes	× 10^3/μL	× 10^9/L
Monocytes	× 10^3/μL	× 10^9/L
Eosinophils	× 10^3/μL	× 10^9/L
Basophils	× 10^3/μL	× 10^9/L

[a]Adapted from *Veterinary Laboratory Medicine: Interpretation and Diagnosis,* Meyer DH, Harvey JW, 3rd ed., Copyright, 2004, with permission from Elsevier.

TABLE 15-15 System of International (SI) Units Conversion Factors of Clinical Chemistries Commonly Used in Exotic Animal Medicine.[a]

Component	Conventional (USA) Units	Conversion Factor (x)	SI Unit
Albumin	g/dL	10	g/L
Alkaline phosphatase	U/L	1.0	IU/L
ALT (SGPT)	U/L	1.0	IU/L
Ammonia (NH_3)	μg/dL	0.5871	μmol/L
Amylase	U/L	1.0	IU/L
AST (SGOT)	U/L	1.0	IU/L
Bilirubin	mg/dL	17.10	μmol/L
Calcium	mg/dL	0.2495	mmol/L
Carbon dioxide	mEq/L	1.0	mmol/L
Chloride	mEq/L	1.0	mmol/L
Cholesterol	mg/dL	0.02586	mmol/L
Copper	μg/dL	0.16	μmol/L
Cortisol	μg/dL	27.59	nmol/L
Creatine kinase	U/L	1.0	IU/L
Creatinine	mg/dL	88.40	μmol/L
Fibrinogen	mg/dL	0.01	g/L
Glucose	mg/dL	0.05551	mmol/L
Iron	μg/dL	0.1791	μmol/L
Lipase			
Sigma Tietz	U/dL	280	IU/L
Cherry-Crandall	U/L	1.0	IU/L
Lipid, total	mg/dL	0.01	g/L
Magnesium	mEq/L	0.5	mmol/L
Osmolality	mOsm/kg	1.0	mmol/kg
Phosphate (as inorganic P)	mg/dL	0.3229	mmol/L
Potassium	mEq/L	1.0	mmol/L
Protein (total)	g/dL	10	g/L
Sodium	mEq/L	1.0	mmol/L
Thyroxine (T_4)	μg/dL	12.87	nmol/L
Triglycerides	mg/dL	0.011	mmol/L
Tri-iodothyronine (T_3)	μg/dL	15.6	nmol/L
Urea nitrogen	mg/dL	0.3570	mmol/L[b]
Uric acid	mg/dL	59.48	umol/L

[a]Adapted from *Veterinary Laboratory Medicine: Interpretation and Diagnosis*, Meyer DH, Harvey JW, 3rd ed., Copyright, 2004, with permission from Elsevier.
[b]Urea.

CHAPTER 15 Select Topics for the Exotic Animal Veterinarian

TABLE 15-16 Select Compounding Pharmacies.[a,b]

State	City	Name	Web Site	Phone
AR	Conway	US Compounding Pharmacy[b]	uscompounding.com	800-718-3588
AZ	Scottsdale	Diamondback Drugs	diamondbackdrugs.com	866-646-2223
AZ	Phoenix	Roadrunner Pharmacy	roadrunnerpharmacy.com	877-518-4589
CA	Bakersfield	Precision Pharmacy	myprecisionpharmacy.com/vet	877-734-3338
	Bellflower	B&B Pharmacy and Health Care Center[b]	bbpharmacy.com	800-231-8905
	Encino	Valley Drug and Compounding	valleydrug.net	818-788-0635
	La Habra	Central Drugs Compounding Pharmacy	centraldrugsrx.com	877-447-7077
	Los Angeles	American Health Solutions Pharmacy	ahsrx.com	800-337-2844
	Merced	Valley Prescription and Compounding Pharmacy[b]	valleyrxandcompounding.com	209-722-5765
	North Hollywood	E-Compounding Pharmacy	ecompounding.com/pharmacy	800-366-4961
	Placerville	Grandpa's Compounding Pharmacy	grandpas-rx.com	530-622-2323
	Rancho Cucamonga	Parkview Compounding Pharmacy[b]	parkviewrx.com	800-605-0166
	San Jose	Leiter's Pharmacy	leiters.com	800-292-6773
	San Rafael	Golden Gate Veterinary Pharmacy[b]	ggvetrx.com	415-455-5590
CO	Monument	Monument Pharmacy	monumentpharmacy.com	800-595-7565
CT	Southington	Beacon Compounding Pharmacy	beaconcompounding.com	860-628-3972
DE	Newark	Save Way Pharmacy	savewaypharmacy.com	302-369-5520
FL	Gainesville	Westlab Pharmacy[b]	westlabpharmacy.com	352-373-8111
IL	Chicago	Braun PharmaCare	braunrx.com	773-549-0634
	Naperville	Martin Avenue Pharmacy[b]	martinavenue.com	630-355-6400
IN	Fort Wayne	Fort Wayne Custom Rx[b]	fwcustomrx.com	260-490-3447
KS	Arkansas City	Taylor Drug	taylordrug.net	800-567-3733
	Lenexa	Midwest Compounders Pharmacy	mwcpharmacy.com	888-245-3012
	Overland Park	Stark Pharmacy[b]	starkpharmacy.com	913-345-3800
MA	Scituate	Animal Pharm, LLC	animalpharmllc.com	866-544-3010
MI	Imlay	Creative Compounding Center	ccc-rx.com	800-672-2177
	Saginaw	Healthway Compounding Pharmacy[b]	healthwayrx.com	866-883-8868
MN	Saint Peter	Soderlund Village Drug	villagedrug.com	800-603-8196
MO	Jackson	Horst Pharmacy	horstpharmacy.com	800-640-5940
NE	Ord	Good Life Pharmacy	goodliferx.com	800-752-5694

Continued

TABLE 15-16 Select Compounding Pharmacies. (cont'd)

State	City	Name	Web Site	Phone
NH	Littleton	Eastern States Compounding Pharmacy[b]	easternstatescompounding.com	603-444-0094
NJ	Swedesboro	Wedgewood Pharmacy	wedgewoodpharmacy.com	800-331-8272
NY	Canandaigua	Animal Pharmacy	animalpharmacy.net	800-663-5261
	Cross River	Cross River Pharmacy and Compounding Center	crossriverpharmacy.com	914-763-3152
	Jamestown	Pharmacy Innovations	pharmacyinnovations.net	716-720-5121
OH	Cincinnati	Tri-State Compounding Pharmacy[b]	tristaterx.com	513-624-7333
	Fairview Park	Nature's Pharmacy	naturescompound.com	440-331-8509
OR	Tualatin	Northwest Compounders	northwestcompounders.com	800-968-0742
PA	Hatboro	Philadelphia Professional Compounding Agency	ppcpharmacy.com	215-672-8552
	Pitcairn	Yakim's Compounding Pharmacy	yakims.com	800-368-3112
RI	South Kingstown	Bayview Pharmacy	bayviewrx.com	401-284-4505
TN	Cordova	Regel PharmaLab	regelpharmalab.com	866-907-3435
TX	Houston	BCP Veterinary Pharmacy	bcpvetpharm.com	800-481-1729
UT	Sandy	Meds for Vets	medsforvets.com	866-633-4838
VA	Alexandria	Alexandria Medical Arts Pharmacy & Compounding Lab[b]	amapharmacy.com	703-549-4350
WA	Bellevue	Custom Prescriptions[b]	custom-prescriptions.com	425-289-0347
	Puyallup	Bealls Compounding Pharmacy	beallspharmacy.com	253-858-8444
	Seattle	Ballard Plaza Pharmacy	ballardplazapharmacy.com	888-782-6354
WI	Milwaukee	Pet Apothecary	petapothecary.com	414-247-8633

[a]Web sites accessed on September 1, 2016.
[b]Accredited by the Pharmacy Compounding Accreditation Board (PCAB). Accessed November 15, 2016.

TABLE 15-17 Additional Compounding Resources.[a]

Name	Contact	Description
AVMA Compounding FAQs	Web site: Avma.org/KB/Resources/FAQs/Pages/Compounding-FAQs.aspx	FAQ regarding veterinary compounding
Compounding Today	Web site: compoundingtoday.com	Several databases including flavoring recommendations by species, requires a login but does offer a 14-day free trial
Fagron	Web site: us.fagron.com	Compounding bases and flavorings
FDA Compounding Resources	Web site: fda.gov/AnimalVeterinary/ResourcesforYou/ucm268128.htm#Compounding_of_Animal_Drugs	Information regarding legal requirements for compounding
Flavorx	Web site: flavorx.com	In house compounding kits
Humco	Web site: humcocompounding.com	Compounding bases and flavorings
Medisca	Web site: medisca.com	Compounding flavors and recipes
Perrigo	Web site: perrigo.com	Compounding bases and flavorings
Trissel's Stability of Compounded Formulations, 5th ed[b]	Publisher: American Pharmacists Association	Monographs on various commonly compounded drugs
U.S. Pharmacopeial Convention	Web site: usp.org/usp-healthcare-professionals/compounding	Compounding standards and resources

[a]Web sites accessed on September 1, 2016.
[b]Trissel LA, American Pharmacists Association. *Trissel's Stability of Compounded Formulations/Lawrence A Trissel.* 3rd ed. Washington, DC: American Pharmacists Association, 2005.

Index

Note: Page numbers followed by *t* indicate tables.

A
Abbreviations, used in prescription writing, 657*t*
Abnormalities
  of standard avian biochemical profile, 312–313*t*
  of standard avian hematology profile, 311*t*
Acemannan, for birds, 267–270*t*
Acepromazine
  for birds, 218–236*t*
  for ferrets, 536–539*t*
  for hedgehogs, 447–448*t*
  for miniature pigs, 561–565*t*
  for primates, 586–594*t*
  for rabbits, 503–511*t*
  for reptiles, 93–103*t*
  for rodents, 467–470*t*
  for sugar gliders, 434–435*t*
  for wild mammals, 627–628*t*
Acepromazine/ketamine, for miniature pigs, 561–565*t*
Acepromazine/propofol, for reptiles, 93–103*t*
Acetaminophen
  for backyard poultry and waterfowl, 404–405*t*
  for birds, 236–239*t*
  for primates, 586–594*t*
  for rabbits, 503–511*t*
  for rodents, 470–473*t*
Acetaminophen/codeine suspension, for primates, 586–594*t*
Acetic acid
  for birds, 189–195*t*, 275–283*t*
  glacial
    for fish, 25–30*t*
    for invertebrates, 5–6*t*
N-Acetyl-L-cysteine, for birds, 246–248*t*
Acetylcysteine
  for rodents, 476–479*t*
  for wild mammals, 631–632*t*
Acetylsalicylic acid
  for birds, 236–239*t*, 275–283*t*
  for ferrets, 539–540*t*
  for primates, 586–594*t*
  for rabbits, 503–511*t*
  for rodents, 470–473*t*
Acriflavine
  for amphibians, 58–60*t*
  for fish, 17–24*t*
Activated charcoal
  for birds, 248–252*t*, 272*t*
  for ferrets, 543–549*t*
  for rabbits, 513–517*t*
  for wild mammals, 629–631*t*
Activated charcoal-kaolin suspension, for reptiles, 113–116*t*
Acyclovir
  for backyard poultry and waterfowl, 391*t*
  for birds, 189–197*t*

Acyclovir (*Continued*)
  for hedgehogs, 449–450*t*
  for reptiles, 86–87*t*
Adrenal gland disease agents, for ferrets, 542–543*t*
Adrenocorticotropic hormone (ACTH), for birds, 240–245*t*
Aerobic bacteria, antimicrobial therapy for, 641–642*t*
African grey parrot (*Psittacus* spp.)
  biologic and physiologic values of, 307–308*t*
  hematologic and biochemical values of, 284–292*t*
  lipoprotein panel of, 314*t*
  T_4 values of, 315*t*
African Love Bird Society, websites for owners of exotic animals, 650–653*t*
African spurred tortoise (*Centrochelys sulcata*), hematologic and serum biochemical values of, 117–136*t*
Aglepristone, for rodents, 476–479*t*
Albaconazole, for rabbits, 498–499*t*
Albendazole
  for backyard poultry and waterfowl, 391–398*t*
  for birds, 197–217*t*
  for fish, 25–30*t*
  for primates, 580–585*t*
  for rabbits, 500–502*t*
  for reptiles, 89–93*t*
  for rodents, 464–466*t*
Aldabra tortoise (*Aldabrachelys gigantea*), hematologic and serum biochemical values of, 117–136*t*
Alexandria Medical Arts Pharmacy & Compounding Lab, 661–662*t*
Alfalfa pellets, for anorectic or debilitated reptiles, 139–140*t*
Alfaxalone
  for amphibians, 60–64*t*
  for birds, 218–236*t*
  for ferrets, 536–539*t*
  for fish, 31–33*t*
  for invertebrates, 6–9*t*
  for rabbits, 503–511*t*
  for rodents, 467–470*t*
  for wild mammals, 627–628*t*
Alfaxalone/fentanyl, for birds, 218–236*t*
Alfaxalone/fentanyl/midazolam, for birds, 218–236*t*
Alfaxalone/midazolam, for birds, 218–236*t*
Alimentary tract infection, antimicrobial therapy for, 641–642*t*
Allopurinol
  for birds, 275–283*t*
  for primates, 594–601*t*
  for reptiles, 113–116*t*
Aloe vera, for birds, 275–283*t*
Alpha chloralose, for birds, 218–236*t*
Alpha-tocopherol, for amphibians, 65–67*t*

INDEX

Alphachloralose for backyard poultry and waterfowl, 399–403t
Alphadolone, for backyard poultry and waterfowl, 399–403t
Alphaxalone
 for backyard poultry and waterfowl, 399–403t
 for primates, 586–594t
 for reptiles, 93–103t
Alphaxalone/medetomidine, for reptiles, 93–103t
Aluminum hydroxide
 for birds, 275–283t
 for hedgehogs, 449–450t
 for rabbits, 513–517t
 for reptiles, 113–116t
 for rodents, 476–479t
Amantadine
 for birds, 189–197t
 for ferrets, 539–540t, 543–549t
Amazon parrot (*Amazona* spp.)
 biologic and physiologic values of, 307–308t
 hematologic and biochemical values of, 284–292t
 lipoprotein panel of, 314t
 T_4 values of, 315t
American alligator (*Alligator mississippiensis*)
 environmental, dietary, and reproductive characteristics of, 137–138t
 hematologic and serum biochemical values of, 117–136t
American Association of Wildlife Veterinarians, 648t
American Association of Zoo Veterinarians, 648t
American Board of Veterinary Practitioners, 648t
American Budgerigar Society, websites for owners of exotic animals, 650–653t
American College of Zoological Medicine, 648t
American Dove Association, websites for owners of exotic animals, 650–653t
American Fancy Rat and Mouse Association, websites for owners of exotic animals, 650–653t
American Federation of Aviculture, websites for owners of exotic animals, 650–653t
American Ferret Association, websites for owners of exotic animals, 650–653t
American Gerbil Society, websites for owners of exotic animals, 650–653t
American Health Solutions Pharmacy, 661–662t
American kestrel (*Falco sparverius*)
 biologic and physiologic values of, 309–310t
 hematologic and biochemical values of, 298–306t
American Ostrich Association, websites for owners of exotic animals, 650–653t
American Rabbit Breeders Association, websites for owners of exotic animals, 650–653t
American Society for the Prevention of Cruelty to Animals, 648–650t
American Society of Laboratory Animal Practitioners, 648t
Amidotrizoate, for reptiles, 113–116t
Amikacin
 for amphibians, 54–55t
 for backyard poultry and waterfowl, 377–389t
 for birds, 168–189t, 246–248t, 270–271t
 for ferrets, 533–534t
 for fish, 17–24t
 for hedgehogs, 444–445t
 for primates, 576–580t

Amikacin (*Continued*)
 for rabbits, 495–498t
 for reptiles, 82–86t
 for rodents, 460–463t
 for wild mammals, 623–625t
Amikacin sulfate, for sugar gliders, 433t
Aminocyclitols, 637–638t
Aminoglycosides, 637–638t
Aminoloid, for birds, 275–283t
Aminopentamide hydrogen sulfate, for birds, 275–283t
Aminophylline
 for birds, 246–248t, 272–283t
 for ferrets, 540–541t
 for primates, 594–601t
 for reptiles, 113–116t
 for rodents, 476–479t
Amitraz
 for ferrets, 535–536t
 for hedgehogs, 446t
 for invertebrates, 5–6t
 for primates, 580–585t
 for rodents, 464–466t
Amitriptyline
 for birds, 253–257t
 for rodents, 476–479t
Amlodipine
 for ferrets, 540–541t
 for primates, 594–601t
Ammonium solution, for birds, 275–283t
Amoxicillin
 for backyard poultry and waterfowl, 377–389t
 for ferrets, 533–534t
 for fish, 17–24t
 for hedgehogs, 444–445t
 for miniature pigs, 559–560t
 for primates, 576–580t
 for reptiles, 82–86t
 for rodents, 460–463t
 for sugar gliders, 433t
Amoxicillin/clavulanic acid
 for birds, 168–189t
 for ferrets, 533–534t
 for hedgehogs, 444–445t
 for miniature pigs, 559–560t
Amoxicillin sodium, for birds, 168–189t
Amoxicillin trihydrate
 for backyard poultry and waterfowl, 377–389t
 for birds, 168–189t
 for primates, 576–580t
Amphibian Diseases Home Page, 648–650t
Amphibians, 53–80
 analgesic agents for, 60–64t
 anesthetic agents for, 60–64t
 antifungal agents for, 56–57t
 antimicrobial agents for, 54–55t
 antiparasitic agents for, 58–60t
 blood collection sites in, 71t
 chemical restraint agents for, 60–64t
 differential diagnoses by predominant signs in, 71–74t
 hormones used in, 65t
 miscellaneous agents for, 65–67t
 nematode parasites in, 75t
 physiologic and hematologic values of, 68–70t

Amphibians (*Continued*)
quarantine protocols for, 75–77t
selected disinfectants for, 74t
Amphotericin B
for amphibians, 56–57t
for backyard poultry and waterfowl, 409t
for birds, 189–195t, 246–248t, 263–267t
for ferrets, 533–534t
for primates, 576–580t
for rabbits, 498–499t, 511–513t
for reptiles, 87–89t
for rodents, 460–463t
for wild mammals, 626t
Amphotericin B liposome, for birds, 246–248t
Ampicillin
for ferrets, 533–534t
for fish, 17–24t
for hedgehogs, 444–445t
for invertebrates, 2–4t
for miniature pigs, 559–560t
for primates, 576–580t
for reptiles, 82–86t
for rodents, 460–463t
Ampicillin sodium, for birds, 168–189t
Ampicillin sodium/sulbactam, for wild mammals, 623–625t
Ampicillin trihydrate
for backyard poultry and waterfowl, 377–389t
for birds, 168–189t
for wild mammals, 623–625t
Amprolium
for backyard poultry and waterfowl, 391–398t
for birds, 197–217t
for ferrets, 535–536t
for rabbits, 500–502t
An Introduction to Ratite Ranching and Medicine, 648–650t
Anaerobic bacteria, antimicrobial therapy for, 641–642t
Analgesic agents
for amphibians, 60–64t
for backyard poultry and waterfowl, 399–403t
for birds, 218–236t
for ferrets, 539–540t
for fish, 31–33t
for hedgehogs, 448–449t
for invertebrates, 6–9t
for miniature pigs, 566–567t
for primates, 586–594t
for rabbits, 503–511t
for reptiles, 104–106t
for rodents, 470–473t
for sugar gliders, 435t
for wild mammals, 628–629t
Anastrozole, for ferrets, 542–543t
Anesthetic agents
for amphibians, 60–64t
for backyard poultry and waterfowl, 399–403t
for birds, 218–236t
for ferrets, 536–539t
for fish, 31–33t
for hedgehogs, 447–448t
for invertebrates, 6–9t
for miniature pigs, 561–565t
for primates, 586–594t

Anesthetic agents (*Continued*)
for rabbits, 503–511t
for reptiles, 93–103t
for rodents, 467–470t
for sugar gliders, 434–435t
for wild mammals, 627–628t
Animal Diversity Web, 648–650t
Animal Health Diagnostic Center, 643–647t
Animal Medicinal Drug Use Clarification Act (AMDUCA), 623t
Animal Pharm, LLC, 661–662t
Animal Pharmacy, 661–662t
Anorectic animals
birds as, gavage feeding in, 319t
reptiles as, 139–140t
Anseriformes
biologic and physiologic values of, 415t
hematologic and serum biochemical values of, 413t
Antech Diagnostics, 643–647t
9, 10 Anthraquinone, for backyard poultry and waterfowl, 411t
Antiepileptic agents, for birds, 253–257t
Antifungal agents
for amphibians, 56–57t
for backyard poultry and waterfowl, 390t
for birds, 189–195t
for ferrets, 533–534t
for fish, 17–24t
for hedgehogs, 445t
for invertebrates, 2–4t
for primates, 576–580t
for rabbits, 498–499t
for reptiles, 87–89t
for rodents, 460–463t
for sugar gliders, 433t
for wild mammals, 626t
Antimicrobials
according to site of infection, 641–642t
for amphibians, 54–55t
for backyard poultry and waterfowl, 377–389t
for birds, 168–189t
classification of, 637–638t
combination therapies, 643t
for ferrets, 533–534t
for fish, 17–24t
general efficacy of, 639–640t
for hedgehogs, 444–445t
-impregnated polymethylmethacrylate (PMMA) agents, for birds, 270–271t
for invertebrates, 2–4t
for miniature pigs, 559–560t
partial list of, 416t
for primates, 576–580t
for rabbits, 495–498t
for reptiles, 82–86t
for rodents, 460–463t
for sugar gliders, 433t
for wild mammals, 623–625t
Antiparasitic agents
for amphibians, 58–60t
for backyard poultry and waterfowl, 391–398t
for birds, 197–217t
for ferrets, 535–536t
for fish, 25–30t
for hedgehogs, 446t

Antiparasitic agents (*Continued*)
  for invertebrates, 5–6t
  for miniature pigs, 561t
  for primates, 580–585t
  for rabbits, 500–502t
  for reptiles, 89–93t
  for rodents, 464–466t
  for sugar gliders, 433–434t
  for wild mammals, 625–626t
Antipseudomonal penicillins, 637–638t
Antiviral agents
  for backyard poultry and waterfowl, 391t
  for birds, 196–197t
  for reptiles, 86–87t
Apomorphine, for ferrets, 543–549t
Apple cider, for birds, 275–283t
Apramycin
  for backyard poultry and waterfowl, 377–389t
  for miniature pigs, 559–560t
Aquatic birds, nutritional recommendations for rehabilitation of, 322t
Arginine vasopressin, for birds, 275–283t
Arginine vasotocin
  for birds, 275–283t
  for reptiles, 106–108t
  with dystocia, 142–143t
Argon, for backyard poultry and waterfowl, 410–411t
Armor All Protectant, for birds, 275–283t
Arrhythmias, in birds, 331t
Arthropods, as common captive invertebrate taxa, 11t
Artificial sea salts, for fish, 25–30t
Ascorbic acid, 258–263t
  for primates, 594–601t
Asparaginase
  for birds, 267–270t
  for rodents, 476–479t
L-asparaginase
  for ferrets, 543–549t
  for reptiles, 113–116t
Aspirin
  for backyard poultry and waterfowl, 404–405t
  for birds, 236–239t, 275–283t
  for miniature pigs, 566–567t
Association of Amphibian and Reptilian Veterinarians, 648t
Association of Avian Veterinarians, 648t
Association of Exotic Mammal Veterinarians, 648t
Association of Primate Veterinarians, 648t
Association of Sugar Glider Veterinarians, 648t
Association of Zoo Veterinary Technicians, 648t
Atenolol
  for birds, 275–283t
  for ferrets, 540–541t
  for rodents, 470–474t
Atipamezole
  for amphibians, 60–64t
  for backyard poultry and waterfowl, 399–403t
  for birds, 218–236t
  for ferrets, 536–539t
  for fish, 31–33t
  for hedgehogs, 447–448t
  for miniature pigs, 561–565t
  for primates, 586–594t
  for rabbits, 503–511t

Atipamezole (*Continued*)
  for reptiles, 93–103t
  for rodents, 467–470t
  for wild mammals, 627–628t
Atorvastatin, for birds, 275–283t
Atracurium
  for birds, 263–267t
  for rabbits, 503–511t
Atropine
  for amphibians, 65–67t
  for birds, 263–267t
  doses of, 654–655t
  for ferrets, 536–541t, 543–549t
  for fish, 34–36t
  for hedgehogs, 447–450t
  for miniature pigs, 561–565t
  for primates, 594–601t
  for rabbits, 503–513t
  for reptiles, 93–103t
  for rodents, 467–470t, 473–479t
  for sugar gliders, 434–435t
  for wild mammals, 629–631t
Atropine sulfate
  for backyard poultry and waterfowl, 399–403t
    toxicologic conditions of, 407–408t
  for birds, 218–236t, 248–252t, 272–274t
  for primates, 594–601t
  for wild mammals, 627–628t
Avian & Exotic Animal Clin Path Labs, 643–647t
Avian and Wildlife Laboratory Division of Comparative Pathology, 643–647t
Avian Biotech International Animal Genetics, Inc., 643–647t
Avian encephalomyelitis, vaccine for, 421–422t
Avian species. *See* Birds
Avibase, 648–650t
AVMA Compounding FAQs, 663t
Azalides, 637–638t
Azaperone
  for birds, 218–236t
  for miniature pigs, 561–565t
Azathioprine
  for ferrets, 543–549t
  for primates, 594–601t
Azithromycin (A)
  for birds, 168–189t
  for ferrets, 533–534t
  for fish, 17–24t
  for primates, 576–580t
  for rabbits, 495–498t, 511–513t
  for reptiles, 82–86t
  for rodents, 460–463t
  for wild mammals, 623–625t
Aztreonam, for fish, 17–24t

B

Baby foods, for anorectic or debilitated reptiles, 139–140t
Bacitracin
  for amphibians, 56–57t
  for rabbits, 511–513t
Bacitracin methylene disalicylate
  for backyard poultry and waterfowl, 377–389t
  for birds, 168–189t

INDEX   669

Bacitracin/neomycin/polymyxin B sulfate, for birds, 263–267t
Bacitracin ophthalmic ointment, for hedgehogs, 444–445t
Bacitracin zinc ointment
  for backyard poultry and waterfowl, 377–389t
  for reptiles, 82–86t
Backyard poultry and waterfowl, 376–431
  antifungal agents for, 390t
  antimicrobial agents for, 377–389t
  antiparasitic agents for, 391–398t
  antiviral and immunomodulating agents for, 391t
  chemical restraint/anesthetic/analgesic agents for, 399–403t
  euthanasia agents for, 410–411t
  hormones and steroids for, 406t
  meat and egg withdrawal for, sources of information on, 420t
  miscellaneous agents for, 411t
  nebulization agents for, 406–407t
  nonsteroidal antiinflammatory agents for, 404–405t
  nutritional/mineral support for, 408–409t
  oncologic agents for, 410t
  ophthalmologic agents for, 409t
  serological tests for, 417–418t
  toxicologic conditions of, agents for, 407–408t
  vaccines for, 421–422t
  water and feed consumption rates for, 420t
Bacteremia, antimicrobial therapy for, 641–642t
Bacteria, nitrifying
  for fish, 34–36t
  for invertebrates, 9–10t
Bald eagle (*Haliaeetus leucocephalus*)
  biologic and physiologic values of, 309–310t
  hematologic and biochemical values of, 298–306t
Ball python (*Python regius*)
  environmental, dietary, and reproductive characteristics of, 137–138t
  hematologic and serum biochemical values of, 117–136t
Ballard Plaza Pharmacy, 661–662t
Barium
  for ferrets, 543–549t
  for rabbits, 513–517t
Barium sulfate
  for birds, 275–283t
  for invertebrates, 9–10t
  for reptiles, 113–116t
  for rodents, 476–479t
Barn owl (*Tyto alba*)
  biologic and physiologic values of, 309–310t
  hematologic and biochemical values of, 298–306t
Barred owl (*Strix varia*)
  biologic and physiologic values of, 309–310t
  hematologic and biochemical values of, 298–306t
Batrachochytrium dendrobatidis, disinfectants for, 74t
Bayview Pharmacy, 661–662t
B&B Pharmacy and Health Care Center, 661–662t
BCP Veterinary Pharmacy, 661–662t
Beacon Compounding Pharmacy, 661–662t
Bealls Compounding Pharmacy, 661–662t
Bearded Dragon Care, websites for owners of exotic animals, 650–653t
Bearded dragon (*Pogona vitticeps*)

Bearded dragon (*Pogona vitticeps*) (*Continued*)
  environmental, dietary, and reproductive characteristics of, 137–138t
  hematologic and serum biochemical values of, 117–136t
Becaplermin, for fish, 34–36t
Benazepril
  for birds, 275–283t
  for ferrets, 540–541t
  for primates, 594–601t
  for rabbits, 513–517t
  for rodents, 473–474t
Benzalkonium chloride
  for amphibians, 56–60t
  for fish, 17–24t
  for inverte brates, 2–4t
Benzathine penicillin
  for rabbits, 495–498t
  for reptiles, 82–86t
Benzocaine
  for amphibians, 60–64t
  for birds, 218–236t
  for fish, 31–33t, 36–37t
  for invertebrates, 6–10t
Benzylpenicillin, 637–638t
  for rabbits, 495–498t
Besifloxacin, for rabbits, 511–513t
Betaxolol, for rabbits, 511–513t
Bicalutamide, for ferrets, 542–543t
Biochemical values
  abnormalities of standard avian, 312–313t
  of Passeriformes, 295t
  of Piciformes and Columbiformes, 297–298t
  of Psittaciformes, 284–292t
    juvenile, 293–294t
  of raptors, 298–306t
  of ratites, 296t
Biodidac, 648–650t
Biologic values
  of birds, 307–308t
  of ferrets, 550–551t
  of hedgehogs, 452t
  of miniature pigs, 570t
  of primates, 604t
  of rabbits, 519t
  of rodents, 482t
  of sugar gliders, 438t
BioOne, 648–650t
Biotin
  for backyard poultry and waterfowl, 408–409t
  for birds, 258–263t
Birds, 167–375
  abnormalities of standard biochemical profile of, 312–313t
  abnormalities of standard hematology profile of, 311t
  analgesic agents for, 218–236t
  anesthetic agents for, 218–236t
  anorectic, gavage feeding in, 319t
  antifungal agents for, 189–195t
  antimicrobial agents for, 168–189t
  antimicrobial-impregnated polymethylmethacrylate (PMMA) agents for, 270–271t
  antiparasitic agents for, 197–217t

Birds (*Continued*)
  antiviral and immunomodulating agents for, 196–197t
  approximate resting respiratory rates of, 316t
  arrhythmias in, 331t
  biologic and physiologic values of, 307–308t
  blood gases of, 314t
  blood pressure values of, 330t
  calculation of enteral feeding requirements for, 320t
  cardiopulmonary resuscitation for, 326–327t
  chemical restraint agents for, 218–236t
  chemotherapeutic protocols used in, 325t
  dystocia or egg binding in, management of, 323t
  ECG measurements in, 332t
  echocardiographic reference intervals in, 333t
  emergencies in, agents for, 272–274t
  euthanasia agents for, 274t
  fluid therapy for, 318t
  hematologic and biochemical values of
    Passeriformes, 295t
    Piciformes and Columbiformes, 297–298t
    Psittaciformes, 284–294t
    raptors, 298–306t
    ratites, 296t
  hormones and steroids for, 240–245t
  lipoprotein panel of, 314t
  miscellaneous agents for, 275–283t
  mycobacteriosis in, 324t
  nebulization agents for, 246–248t
  nonsteroidal antiinflammatory agents for, 236–239t
  nutritional/mineral support and supplementation for, 258–263t
  oncologic agents and radiation therapy for, 267–270t
  ophthalmic diagnostic tests for, 317t
  ophthalmologic agents for, 263–267t
  psychotherapeutic agents for, 334–336t
  psychotropic and antiepileptic agents for, 253–257t
  raptors, 309–310t, 317t, 322t
  ratites, 307–308t
  routes of administration and maximum suggested volumes of fluid therapy for, 319t
  sources of formulated and medicated diets for, 321t
  spectral Doppler echocardiographic reference intervals in, 333t
  supportive care procedures used in companion medicine, 318t
  T_4 values of, 315t
  toxicologic conditions of, agents for, 248–252t
  treatment of oiled, 272t
  urinalysis values of, 316t
  vaccines for, 328–329t
  wild, nutritional recommendations for rehabilitation of, 322t
Bisacodyl, for primates, 594–601t
Bismuth subcitrate, for ferrets, 543–549t
Bismuth subsalicylate
  for birds, 272t, 275–283t
  for ferrets, 543–549t
  for primates, 594–601t
Bismuth sulfate, for birds, 248–252t
Bleomycin
  for ferrets, 543–549t
  for reptiles, 113–116t
Blood
  collection sites, in amphibians, 71t.
    see also Venipuncture sites
  gases, of birds, 314t
  pressure values in birds, 330t
  volumes of rodents with safe-bleeding volume recommendations, 483t
Blood python (*Python curtus*), hematologic and serum biochemical values of, 117–136t
Blood transfusion
  homologous, for birds, 272–274t
  for rabbits, 513–517t
Blue and gold macaw (*Ara ararauna*)
  hematologic and biochemical values of, 293–294t
  T_4 values of, 315t
Blue-tongued skink (*Tiliqua scincoides*), hematologic and serum biochemical values of, 117–136t
Boa constrictor (*Boa constrictor*)
  environmental, dietary, and reproductive characteristics of, 137–138t
  hematologic and serum biochemical values of, 117–136t
Boa Tips, websites for owners of exotic animals, 650–653t
Body weight, conversion to body surface area, in ferrets, 554t
Boldenone undecylenate, for birds, 240–245t
Bone cement, for birds, 270–271t
Bone infection, antimicrobial therapy for, 641–642t
Botulinum antitoxin
  for birds, 248–252t
  type C
    for birds, 248–252t
    for toxicologic conditions, of backyard poultry and waterfowl, 407–408t
Box Turtle Care and Conservation, websites for owners of exotic animals, 650–653t
Braun PharmaCare, 661–662t
Brewer's yeast
  for birds, 258–263t
  for ferrets, 543–549t
British Veterinary Zoological Society, 648t
Bromhexine, for rodents, 476–479t
Bromhexine HCl, for birds, 275–283t
Bronchoalveolar lavage (BAL), in rabbits, 523t
Bronopol, for fish, 17–24t
Budesonide
  for ferrets, 543–549t
  for primates, 594–601t
Budgerigar parakeet (*Melopsittacus undulatus*)
  biologic and physiologic values of, 307–308t
  hematologic and biochemical values of, 284–292t
Bunamidine, for primates, 580–585t
Bupivacaine
  for ferrets, 536–540t
  for hedgehogs, 449–450t
  for miniature pigs, 566–567t
  for primates, 586–594t
  for rabbits, 503–511t
  for reptiles, 93–106t
  for rodents, 467–470t
  for sugar gliders, 434–435t
  for wild mammals, 628–629t

Bupivacaine HCl
 for backyard poultry and waterfowl, 399–403t
 for birds, 218–236t
Buprenorphine
 for amphibians, 60–64t
 for ferrets, 539–540t
 for hedgehogs, 447–449t
 for miniature pigs, 566–567t
 for primates, 586–594t
 for rabbits, 503–511t
 for reptiles, 104–106t
 for RGIS, 522–523t
 for rodents, 470–473t
 for sugar gliders, 434–435t
 sustained release, for birds, 218–236t
 for wild mammals, 628–629t
Buprenorphine HCl
 for backyard poultry and waterfowl, 399–403t
 for birds, 218–236t
Buprenorphine-SR, for wild mammals, 628–629t
Buprenorphine SR-LAB, for rabbits, 503–511t
Burmese python (*Python bivittatus*), hematologic and serum biochemical values of, 117–136t
Buserelin acetate depot, for birds, 240–245t
Buspirone HCl, for birds, 253–257t
Butorphanol (B)
 for amphibians, 60–64t
 for backyard poultry and waterfowl, 399–403t
 for ferrets, 536–540t
 for fish, 31–33t
 for hedgehogs, 447–449t
 for invertebrates, 6–9t
 for miniature pigs, 561–567t
 for primates, 586–594t
 for rabbits, 503–511t
 for reptiles, 93–106t
 for RGIS, 522–523t
 for rodents, 470–473t
 for sugar gliders, 434–435t
 for wild mammals, 628–629t
Butorphanol (B)/acepromazine (A), for primates, 586–594t
Butorphanol (B)/dexmedetomidine (D)/ketamine (K), for primates, 586–594t
Butorphanol/medetomidine, for reptiles, 93–103t
Butorphanol/midazolam
 for birds, 218–236t
 for reptiles, 93–103t
Butorphanol tartrate
 for backyard poultry and waterfowl, 399–403t
 for birds, 218–236t

C

Cabergoline
 for birds, 240–245t
 for ferrets, 543–549t
 for rodents, 476–479t
Caffeine, for amphibians, 65–67t
Caique (*Pionites* spp.), hematologic and biochemical values of, 284–292t
Calcitonin
 for birds, 240–245t
 for primates, 594–601t
 for reptiles, 106–108t
  with metabolic bone diseases, 144–145t

Calcitonin (*Continued*)
 for sugar gliders, 436t
Calcitriol, for primates, 594–601t
Calcium
 for backyard poultry and waterfowl, 408–409t
 for birds, 258–263t
 for reptiles
  with dystocia, 142–143t
  with metabolic bone diseases, 144–145t
  as nutritional/mineral/fluid support, 108–113t
Calcium borogluconate, for birds, 258–263t
Calcium carbonate, for reptiles, 108–113t
Calcium chloride, for birds, 258–263t
Calcium EDTA (edetate calcium disodium)
 for birds, 248–252t
 for ferrets, 543–549t
 for rabbits, 513–517t
 for reptiles, 113–116t
 for rodents, 476–479t
 for toxicologic conditions, of backyard poultry and waterfowl, 407–408t
Calcium glubionate
 for amphibians, 65–67t
 for birds, 258–263t
 for primates, 594–601t
 for reptiles, 108–113t
 for sugar gliders, 436t
Calcium gluconate
 for amphibians, 65–67t
 for birds, 258–263t, 272–274t
 doses of, 654–655t
 for hedgehogs, 449–450t
 for primates, 594–601t
 for reptiles, 108–113t
 for rodents, 474–475t
 for sugar gliders, 436t
 for wild mammals, 631–632t
Calcium gluconate/borogluconate, for reptiles, 108–113t
Calcium glycerophosphate/calcium lactate, for reptiles, 108–113t
Calcium lactate/calcium glycerophosphate, for birds, 258–263t
Calcium levulinate, for birds, 258–263t
Cambendazole, for birds, 197–217t
Campylobacter spp., antimicrobial agents for, 639–640t
Canadian Association of Zoo and Wildlife Veterinarians, 648t
Canary (*Serinus canaria*)
 biologic and physiologic values of, 307–308t
 hematologic and biochemical values of, 295t
 T_4 values of, 315t
Captan powder, for rodents, 460–463t
Captive husbandry web sites, websites for owners of exotic animals, 650–653t
Captopril
 for ferrets, 540–541t
 for primates, 594–601t
Carbamazepine, for birds, 253–257t
Carbapenems, 637–638t
Carbaryl 5%
 for backyard poultry and waterfowl, 391–398t
 for birds, 197–217t
Carbaryl powder
 for ferrets, 535–536t

Carbaryl powder (*Continued*)
  for rabbits, 500–502t
  for reptiles, 89–93t
  for rodents, 464–466t
  for sugar gliders, 433–434t
Carbenicillin
  for amphibians, 54–55t
  for birds, 168–189t, 246–248t
  for reptiles, 82–86t
Carbimazole, for rodents, 476–479t
Carbon, activated
  for fish, 34–36t
  for invertebrates, 9–10t
Carbon dioxide (CO_2)
  for backyard poultry and waterfowl, 410–411t
  for birds, 274t
  for fish, 31–33t, 36–37t
  for invertebrates, 6–9t
Carbon monoxide (CO)
  for backyard poultry and waterfowl, 410–411t
  for birds, 274t
Carboplatin
  for birds, 267–270t
  for reptiles, 113–116t
Cardiac measurements, for hedgehogs, 455t
Cardiopulmonary agents, for ferrets, 540–541t
Cardiopulmonary resuscitation, for birds, 326–327t
Cardiovascular agents, for rodents, 473–474t
Carfentanil
  for birds, 218–236t
  for primates, 586–594t
Carnidazole, for birds, 197–217t
L-Carnitine
  for birds, 258–263t, 267–270t
  for sugar gliders, 436t
Carnivore Care
  for hedgehogs, 449–450t
  for reptiles, 108–113t
Carnivore Critical Care, for amphibians, 65–67t
Carp pituitary extract, for fish, 34–36t
Carpet python (*Morelia spilota* ssp.), hematologic and serum biochemical values of, 117–136t
Carprofen
  for backyard poultry and waterfowl, 404–405t
  for birds, 236–239t
  for ferrets, 539–540t
  for hedgehogs, 448–449t
  for miniature pigs, 566–567t
  for primates, 586–594t
  for rabbits, 503–511t
  for reptiles, 104–106t
  for rodents, 470–473t
  for wild mammals, 628–629t
Carvedilol
  for primates, 594–601t
  for rodents, 470–474t
Cefadroxil
  for birds, 168–189t
  for ferrets, 533–534t
  for primates, 576–580t
Cefazolin
  for backyard poultry and waterfowl, 377–389t
  for birds, 168–189t, 270–271t
  for rabbits, 495–498t

Cefazolin (*Continued*)
  for reptiles, 82–86t
Cefazolin sodium
  for primates, 576–580t
  for wild mammals, 623–625t
Cefoperazone, for reptiles, 82–86t
Cefotaxime
  for birds, 168–189t, 246–248t, 270–271t
  for rabbits, 495–498t
  for reptiles, 82–86t
Cefovecin
  for backyard poultry and waterfowl, 377–389t
  for birds, 168–189t
  for ferrets, 533–534t
  for fish, 17–24t
  for primates, 576–580t
  for reptiles, 82–86t
  for wild mammals, 623–625t
Cefovecin sodium, for sugar gliders, 433t
Cefoxitin, for birds, 168–189t
Cefquinome, for backyard poultry and waterfowl, 377–389t
Ceftazidime
  for amphibians, 54–55t
  for birds, 168–189t, 270–271t
  for fish, 17–24t
  for invertebrates, 2–4t
  for primates, 576–580t
  for rabbits, 495–498t
  for reptiles, 82–86t
  for wild mammals, 623–625t
Ceftiofur
  for backyard poultry and waterfowl, 377–389t
  for birds, 168–189t, 270–271t
  extended release formulation, 168–189t
  for miniature pigs, 559–560t
  for primates, 576–580t
  for rabbits, 495–498t
  for reptiles, 82–86t
Ceftiofur crystalline-free acid
  for primates, 576–580t
  for wild mammals, 623–625t
Ceftiofur sodium, for hedgehogs, 444–445t
Ceftriaxone
  for backyard poultry and waterfowl, 377–389t, 406–407t
  for birds, 168–189t
  for miniature pigs, 559–560t
  for primates, 576–580t
  for rabbits, 495–498t
Cefuroxime, for reptiles, 82–86t
Celecoxib
  for birds, 236–239t
  for rodents, 470–473t
Cellulose powder, for rabbits, 513–517t
Celsius temperature scales, equivalents of, 659t
Center for Agricultural Bioscience International, 648–650t
Central Drugs Compounding Pharmacy, 661–662t
Central nervous system infection, antimicrobial therapy for, 641–642t
Cephalexin
  for backyard poultry and waterfowl, 377–389t
  for birds, 168–189t
  for hedgehogs, 444–445t

Cephalexin (*Continued*)
  for miniature pigs, 559–560t
  for primates, 576–580t
  for rabbits, 495–498t
  for reptiles, 82–86t
  for rodents, 460–463t
  for sugar gliders, 433t
  for wild mammals, 623–625t
Cephaloridine, for ferrets, 533–534t
Cephalosporins
  first-generation, 637–638t
  fourth-generation, 637–638t
  third-generation, 637–638t
Cephalothin
  for backyard poultry and waterfowl, 377–389t
  for birds, 168–189t
  for primates, 576–580t
  for rabbits, 495–498t
  for reptiles, 82–86t
Cephradine
  for birds, 168–189t
  for miniature pigs, 559–560t
Cerebrospinal fluid values, in rabbits, 520t
Chameleon Care and Information Center, websites for owners of exotic animals, 650–653t
Charcoal, for rodents, 474–479t
Cheeky Chinchilla, websites for owners of exotic animals, 650–653t
Chelonians
  environmental, dietary, and reproductive characteristics of, 137–138t
  tracheal/pulmonary and colonic lavage for, 141t
  urinalysis values of, 139t
  venipuncture sites in, 141–142t
Chemical restraint agents
  for amphibians, 60–64t
  for backyard poultry and waterfowl, 399–403t
  for birds, 218–236t
  for ferrets, 536–539t
  for fish, 31–33t
  for hedgehogs, 447–448t
  for invertebrates, 6–9t
  for miniature pigs, 561–565t
  for primates, 586–594t
  for rabbits, 503–511t
  for reptiles, 93–103t
  for rodents, 467–470t
  for sugar gliders, 434–435t
  for wild mammals, 627–628t
Chemotherapy
  for birds, 325t
  for ferrets, 552–554t
Chinese (Asian) water dragon (*Physignathus cocincinus*), hematologic and serum biochemical values of, 117–136t
Chitosan, for ferrets, 543–549t
Chlamydia, antimicrobial agents for, 639–640t
Chlorambucil
  for backyard poultry and waterfowl, 410t
  for birds, 267–270t
  for ferrets, 543–549t
  for reptiles, 113–116t
Chloramine-T, for fish, 17–30t
Chloramphenicol, 637–638t

Chloramphenicol (*Continued*)
  for amphibians, 54–57t
  for birds, 246–248t
  for ferrets, 533–534t
  for fish, 17–24t
  for hedgehogs, 444–445t
  for invertebrates, 2–4t
  for rabbits, 495–498t
  for reptiles, 82–86t
  for rodents, 460–463t
  for sugar gliders, 433t
Chloramphenicol ophthalmic drops, for birds, 263–267t
Chloramphenicol palmitate
  for birds, 168–189t
  for primates, 576–580t
Chloramphenicol sodium succinate, for primates, 576–580t
Chloramphenicol succinate
  for backyard poultry and waterfowl, 377–389t
  for birds, 168–189t
Chlorhexidine
  for birds, 168–189t
  for hedgehogs, 444–445t
  for reptiles, 82–89t
Chlorhexidine shampoo
  for hedgehogs, 444–445t
  for rabbits, 498–499t
Chlorine, for birds, 168–189t
Chlorine/chloramine neutralizer
  for fish, 34–36t
  for invertebrates, 9–10t
Chloroquine
  for primates, 580–585t
  for reptiles, 89–93t
Chloroquine diphosphate, for fish, 25–30t
Chloroquine phosphate
  for backyard poultry and waterfowl, 391–398t
  for birds, 197–217t
Chlorpheniramine, for ferrets, 543–549t
Chlorpheniramine maleate
  for rabbits, 513–517t
  for rodents, 476–479t
Chlorpromazine, for birds, 253–257t
Chlortetracycline
  for backyard poultry and waterfowl, 377–389t
  for birds, 168–189t
  for hedgehogs, 444–445t
  for rabbits, 495–498t
  for reptiles, 82–86t
  for rodents, 460–463t
Chlortetracycline bisulfate, for backyard poultry and waterfowl, 377–389t
Cholestyramine
  for rabbits, 513–517t
  for rodents, 476–479t
Chondroitin sulfate, for rabbits, 513–517t
CHOP therapy, for reptiles, 113–116t
Cimetidine
  for birds, 275–283t
  for ferrets, 543–549t
  for hedgehogs, 449–450t
  for primates, 594–601t
  for rabbits, 513–517t
  for reptiles, 113–116t

INDEX

Cimetidine (*Continued*)
  for rodents, 476–479t
  for wild mammals, 631–632t
Ciprofloxacin
  for amphibians, 54–55t
  for backyard poultry and waterfowl, 377–389t
  for birds, 168–189t, 270–271t
  for ferrets, 533–534t
  for fish, 17–24t
  for hedgehogs, 444–445t
  for primates, 576–580t
  for rabbits, 495–498t, 511–513t
  for reptiles, 82–86t
  for rodents, 460–463t
  for sugar gliders, 433t
Ciprofloxacin HCl, for birds, 263–267t
Ciprofloxacin ophthalmic ointment, for reptiles, 82–86t
Cisapride
  for birds, 275–283t
  for ferrets, 543–549t
  for primates, 594–601t
  for rabbits, 513–517t
  for reptiles, 113–116t
  for RGIS, 522–523t
  for rodents, 476–479t
  for sugar gliders, 436t
Cisplatin
  for birds, 267–270t
  for reptiles, 113–116t
Citrate phosphate dextrose adenine solution (CPDA), for birds, 275–283t
Citric acid, for birds, 275–283t
Clarithromycin, 495–498t
  for birds, 168–189t
  for ferrets, 533–534t
  for hedgehogs, 444–445t
  for primates, 576–580t
  for reptiles, 82–86t
  for rodents, 460–463t
Clavulanic acid, 637–638t
  for backyard poultry and waterfowl, 377–389t
  for sugar gliders, 433t
Clavulanic potassium, for primates, 576–580t
Clazuril
  for backyard poultry and waterfowl, 391–398t
  for birds, 197–217t
Clindamycin
  for birds, 168–189t, 270–271t
  for ferrets, 533–534t
  for hedgehogs, 444–445t
  for miniature pigs, 559–560t
  for primates, 576–585t
  for reptiles, 82–86t
  for rodents, 460–463t
  for sugar gliders, 433t
  for wild mammals, 623–625t
Clinicare, for reptiles, 108–113t
Clofazimine, for birds, 168–189t
Clomipramine
  for birds, 253–257t
  for rodents, 476–479t
Clonazepam, for birds, 253–257t
Clonidine, for rodents, 470–473t
Clopidol, for backyard poultry and waterfowl, 391–398t

Clorsulon
  for backyard poultry and waterfowl, 391–398t
  for birds, 197–217t
Closantel, for fish, 25–30t
Clostridium spp., antimicrobial agents for, 639–640t
Clotrimazole
  for birds, 189–195t, 246–248t
  for rabbits, 498–499t
  for reptiles, 87–89t
Clove oil (eugenol)
  for amphibians, 60–64t
  for fish, 31–33t
  for invertebrates, 6–9t
Cloxacillin
  for birds, 168–189t
  for ferrets, 533–534t
Cobalamin, for ferrets, 543–549t
Coccidiosis, vaccine for, 421–422t
Cockatiel (*Nymphicus hollandicus*)
  biologic and physiologic values of, 307–308t
  hematologic and biochemical values of, 284–292t
  T_4 values of, 315t
Cockatoos (Cacatuidae)
  biologic and physiologic values of, 307–308t
  hematologic and biochemical values of, 284–294t
  T_4 values of, 315t
Codeine
  for amphibians, 60–64t
  for rabbits, 503–511t
  for rodents, 470–473t
Coelenterates, 11t
Colchicine, for birds, 275–283t
Colloids, 656t
Colonic lavage, for reptiles, 141t
Columbiformes
  biologic and physiologic values of, 307–308t
  hematologic and biochemical values of, 297–298t
Combination therapies, antimicrobials, 643t
Commercial dry or moist diets, for anorectic or debilitated reptiles, 139–140t
Common captive invertebrate taxa, 11t
Compounding pharmacies, 661–662t
Compounding resources, 663t
Compounding Today, 663t
Constant rate infusion (CRI) protocols, for rabbits, 511t
Conures (*Aratinga* and *Pyrrhura* spp.)
  biologic and physiologic values of, 307–308t
  hematologic and biochemical values of, 284–292t
  T_4 values of, 315t
Convention on International Trade in Endangered Species, 648–650t
Copper sulfate ("bluestone")
  for backyard poultry and waterfowl, 390t
  for birds, 275–283t
  for fish, 25–30t
Corn snake (*Pantherophis guttata*), hematologic and serum biochemical values of, 117–136t
Coumaphos, for birds, 197–217t
Creative Compounding Center, 661–662t
Crested gecko (*Rhacodactylus ciliatus*)
  environmental, dietary, and reproductive characteristics of, 137–138t
  hematologic and serum biochemical values of, 117–136t
Critical Care for Herbivores, for reptiles, 108–113t

INDEX 675

Crocodilians
　environmental, dietary, and reproductive
　　characteristics of, 137–138t
　venipuncture sites in, 141–142t
Cross River Pharmacy and Compounding Center,
　　661–662t
Crotamiton, for birds, 197–217t
Crystalloids, 656t
　for wild mammals, 629–631t
Custom Prescriptions, 661–662t
Cyanoacrylate surgical adhesive, for amphibians,
　　65–67t
Cyclizine, for rabbits, 513–517t
Cyclophosphamide
　for birds, 267–270t
　for ferrets, 543–549t
　for reptiles, 113–116t
　for rodents, 476–479t
Cycloserine, for birds, 168–189t
Cyclosporine
　for birds, 189–197t, 275–283t
　for ferrets, 543–549t
　for rabbits, 511–513t
　for rodents, 476–479t
Cypermethrin
　for backyard poultry and waterfowl, 391–398t
　for birds, 197–217t
Cyproheptadine
　for ferrets, 543–549t
　for rabbits, 513–517t
　for rodents, 476–479t
Cyproheptadine HCl, for RGIS, 522–523t
Cyromazine, for rabbits, 500–502t
Cytarabine, for ferrets, 543–549t

D

Danofloxacin, for reptiles, 82–86t
Danofloxacin mesylate
　for backyard poultry and waterfowl, 377–389t
　for birds, 168–189t
Dantrolene sodium, for miniature pigs, 568t
Dapsone, for primates, 594–601t
Debilitated reptiles, force-feeding, 139–140t
Decoquinate
　for backyard poultry and waterfowl, 391–398t
　for ferrets, 535–536t
　for rabbits, 500–502t
Deferiprone
　for birds, 248–252t
　for toxicologic conditions, of backyard poultry and
　　waterfowl, 407–408t
Deferoxamine mesylate, for birds, 248–252t
Delmadinone, for birds, 240–245t, 253–257t
Deltamethrin, for birds, 197–217t
Demecarium bromide, for birds, 263–267t
Dental Anatomy, 648–650t
2-deoxy-2-fluoro-d-glucose, for birds, 275–283t
Deoxycorticosterone, for ferrets, 542–543t
Depoprovera, for primates, 594–601t
Deracoxib, for primates, 586–594t
Desert tortoise (Gopherus agassizii)
　environmental, dietary, and reproductive
　　characteristics of, 137–138t
　hematologic and serum biochemical values of,
　　117–136t

Desflurane, for birds, 218–236t
Deslorelin
　for birds, 240–245t, 253–257t
　for ferrets, 542–543t
　for primates, 594–601t
Deslorelin acetate
　for reptiles, 106–108t
　for rodents, 476–479t
Deslorelin implant, for birds, 267–270t
Desmopressin, for birds, 240–245t
Desoxycholate form, for rabbits, 498–499t
Detergent, for birds, 272t
Detomidine
　for backyard poultry and waterfowl, 399–403t
　for birds, 218–236t
Detomidine/butorphanol/midazolam, for miniature
　　pigs, 561–565t
Dex SP, emergency drug doses of, 654–655t
Dexamethasone
　for amphibians, 65–67t
　for birds, 240–245t, 263–267t
　for ferrets, 535–536t
　for fish, 34–36t
　for hedgehogs, 444–445t, 448–449t
　for miniature pigs, 566–568t
　for primates, 594–601t
　for rabbits, 500–502t, 513–517t
　for reptiles, 106–108t
　for rodents, 474–479t
　for sugar gliders, 436t
Dexamethasone sodium phosphate
　for birds, 240–248t, 272–274t
　for ferrets, 543–549t
　for reptiles, 106–108t
　for wild mammals, 629–631t
Dexmedetomidine
　for amphibians, 60–64t
　for birds, 218–236t
　for ferrets, 536–539t
　for fish, 31–33t
　for hedgehogs, 447–448t
　for miniature pigs, 561–565t
　for rabbits, 503–511t
　for reptiles, 93–103t
　for rodents, 467–470t
　for sugar gliders, 434–435t
　for wild mammals, 627–628t
Dexmedetomidine/alfaxalone, for
　　birds, 218–236t
Dexmedetomidine/butorphanol, for
　　ferrets, 536–539t
Dexmedetomidine HCl, for birds, 218–236t
Dexmedetomidine/ketamine, for reptiles, 93–103t
Dexmedetomidine/ketamine/butorphanol, for birds,
　　218–236t
Dexmedetomidine/ketamine/morphine, for reptiles,
　　93–103t
Dexmedetomidine/midazolam, for birds, 218–236t
Dexmedetomidine/midazolam/butorphanol, for
　　miniature pigs, 561–565t
Dexmedetomidine/midazolam/ketamine, for reptiles,
　　93–103t
Dexmedetomidine/thiafentanil oxalate/
　　tiletamine-zolazepam, for birds, 218–236t
Dextran 70, for birds, 272–274t

Dextroketamine, for reptiles, 93–103*t*
Dextroketamine/midazolam, for reptiles, 93–103*t*
Dextrose
  for amphibians, 65–67*t*
  for birds, 258–263*t*, 272–274*t*
  for ferrets, 543–549*t*
  for miniature pigs, 568*t*
  in water, for reptiles, 108–113*t*
Dextrose 50%, for wild mammals, 629–631*t*
Diagnoses. *See* Differential diagnoses
Diagnostic Center for Population and Animal Health, 643–647*t*
Diagnostic Laboratory Service, 643–647*t*
Diagnostic procedures, laboratories conducting, 643–647*t*
Diamondback Drugs, 661–662*t*
Diatomaceous earth, for backyard poultry and waterfowl, 391–398*t*
Diatrizoate meglumine, for invertebrates, 9–10*t*
Diatrizoate meglumine sodium, for birds, 258–263*t*
Diatrizoate sodium, for invertebrates, 9–10*t*
Diazepam
  for amphibians, 60–64*t*
  for backyard poultry and waterfowl, 399–403*t*
  for birds, 218–236*t*, 253–257*t*
  doses of, 654–655*t*
  for ferrets, 536–539*t*
  for hedgehogs, 447–448*t*
  for miniature pigs, 561–565*t*
  for primates, 586–594*t*
  for rabbits, 503–511*t*
  for reptiles, 93–103*t*
  for rodents, 467–470*t*, 474–475*t*
  for sugar gliders, 434–435*t*
  for wild mammals, 627–631*t*
Diazepam/ketamine, for hedgehogs, 447–448*t*
Diazoxide
  for ferrets, 543–549*t*
  for rodents, 476–479*t*
Dichlorophenamide, for rabbits, 511–513*t*
Dichlorophene, for birds, 197–217*t*
Dichlorvos
  for miniature pigs, 561*t*
  for reptiles, 89–93*t*
Diclazuril
  for backyard poultry and waterfowl, 391–398*t*
  for birds, 197–217*t*
  for rabbits, 500–502*t*
Diclofenac
  for backyard poultry and waterfowl, 404–405*t*
  for birds, 236–239*t*, 263–267*t*
  for rodents, 470–473*t*
Diclofenac sodium, for rabbits, 511–513*t*
Dietary characteristics
  of hedgehogs, 452–453*t*
  of reptiles, 137–138*t*
  of sugar gliders, 439–440*t*
Diethylcarbamazine, for primates, 580–585*t*
Diethylstilbestrol diphosphate, for birds, 240–245*t*
Diets and commercial products
  for birds, 321*t*
  for reptiles, 145–149*t*
Differential diagnoses, for amphibians, 71–74*t*
Difloxacin

Difloxacin (*Continued*)
  for fish, 17–24*t*
  for rabbits, 495–498*t*
Diflubenzuron
  for fish, 25–30*t*
  for invertebrates, 5–6*t*
Digoxin
  for backyard poultry and waterfowl, 411*t*
  for birds, 275–283*t*
  for ferrets, 540–541*t*
  for primates, 594–601*t*
  for rabbits, 513–517*t*
  for rodents, 470–474*t*
Dihydrostreptomycin, for reptiles, 82–86*t*
Diiodohydroxyquinoline, for primates, 580–585*t*
Diltiazem
  for ferrets, 540–541*t*
  for rabbits, 513–517*t*
  for rodents, 470–474*t*
Dimercaprol, for birds, 248–252*t*
Dimercaptosuccinic acid, for birds, 248–252*t*
Dimethyl phosphonate, for fish, 25–30*t*
Dimethylsulfoxide (DMSO), for birds, 236–239*t*, 275–283*t*
Dimetridazole
  for backyard poultry and waterfowl, 391–398*t*
  for birds, 197–217*t*
  for fish, 25–30*t*
  for reptiles, 89–93*t*
  for rodents, 464–466*t*
Dinitolmide, for backyard poultry and waterfowl, 391–398*t*
Dinoprost tromethamine, for birds, 240–245*t*
Dinoprostone, for birds, 240–245*t*
Dinoprostone gel, for reptiles, with dystocia, 142–143*t*
Dioctyl sodium sulfosuccinate
  for birds, 275–283*t*
  for reptiles, 113–116*t*
Diphenhydramine
  for birds, 248–257*t*, 267–270*t*, 275–283*t*
  emergency drug doses of, 654–655*t*
  for ferrets, 543–549*t*
  for primates, 594–601*t*
  for rabbits, 513–517*t*
  for reptiles, 113–116*t*
  for rodents, 474–479*t*
  for wild mammals, 631–632*t*
Diphenoxylate, with atropine, for birds, 275–283*t*
Diphenylhydantoin, for rodents, 476–479*t*
Diprenorphine, for birds, 218–236*t*
Dipyrone
  for birds, 236–239*t*
  for rodents, 470–473*t*
Diquat dibromide, for fish, 17–24*t*
Disease testing, in rodents, 486–487*t*
Diseases, zoonotic
  in hedgehogs, 454*t*
  in rodents, 485–486*t*
Diseases of Research Animals (DORA), 648–650*t*
Disinfectants, for amphibians, 74*t*
Disoprofol, for reptiles, 93–103*t*
Distilled water, for amphibians, 58–60*t*
Dithiazanine, for primates, 580–585*t*
Dobutamine
  for birds, 218–236*t*, 272–274*t*

Dobutamine (*Continued*)
  for ferrets, 540–541*t*
  for primates, 594–601*t*
Docusate sodium (DSS), for primates, 594–601*t*
Dog/cat food, for anorectic or debilitated reptiles, 139–140*t*
Dopamine
  for birds, 272–274*t*
  for primates, 594–601*t*
  for rodents, 470–475*t*
Dopamine HCl, for birds, 218–236*t*
Doramectin
  for birds, 197–217*t*
  for fish, 25–30*t*
  for miniature pigs, 561*t*
  for rabbits, 500–502*t*
  for rodents, 464–466*t*
Dorzolamide
  for rabbits, 511–513*t*
  for rodents, 476–479*t*
Dosing
  of emergency drug, 654–655*t*
  of miniature pigs, 573*t*
Doxapram
  for backyard poultry and waterfowl, 411*t*
  for birds, 272–274*t*
  doses of, 654–655*t*
  for ferrets, 540–541*t*, 543–549*t*
  for fish, 34–36*t*
  for hedgehogs, 449–450*t*
  for primates, 594–601*t*
  for rabbits, 513–517*t*
  for reptiles, 93–103*t*
  for rodents, 474–475*t*
  for sugar gliders, 436*t*
Doxepin, for birds, 253–257*t*
Doxorubicin
  for birds, 267–270*t*
  for ferrets, 543–549*t*
  for reptiles, 113–116*t*
Doxycycline
  for amphibians, 54–55*t*, 65–67*t*
  for backyard poultry and waterfowl, 377–389*t*
  for birds, 168–189*t*, 197–217*t*
  for ferrets, 533–534*t*
  for fish, 17–24*t*
  for hedgehogs, 444–445*t*
  for miniature pigs, 559–560*t*
  for primates, 576–585*t*
  for rabbits, 495–498*t*
  for reptiles, 82–86*t*
  for rodents, 460–463*t*
  for wild mammals, 623–625*t*
Doxycycline hyclate, for birds, 168–189*t*, 246–248*t*
Doxycycline monohydrate, for rabbits, 511–513*t*
Doxycycline recipes, used in Psittacines, 321*t*
Droperidol, for primates, 586–594*t*
Duloxetine
  for primates, 594–601*t*
  for rodents, 470–473*t*
Dwarf caiman (*Paleosuchus palpebrosus*), hematologic and serum biochemical values of, 117–136*t*
Dystocia
  in birds, management of, 323*t*
  in reptiles, 142–143*t*

E

E-Compounding Pharmacy, 661–662*t*
Eastern box turtle (*Terrapene carolina*)
  environmental, dietary, and reproductive characteristics of, 137–138*t*
  hematologic and serum biochemical values of, 117–136*t*
Eastern screech owl (*Megascops asio*)
  biologic and physiologic values of, 309–310*t*
  hematologic and biochemical values of, 298–306*t*
Eastern States Compounding Pharmacy, 661–662*t*
Echinacea, 189–197*t*
Echinoderms, 11*t*
Echocardiographic measurements, in rodents, 488*t*
Eclectus parrot (*Eclectus roratus*)
  biologic and physiologic values of, 307–308*t*
  hematologic and biochemical values of, 284–292*t*
  T_4 values of, 315*t*
Edetate calcium disodium (CaEDTA), for wild mammals, 629–631*t*
Edetate disodium, for birds, 263–267*t*
EDTA-Tris, with atropine, for birds, 275–283*t*
EDTA-tromethamine, for birds, 275–283*t*
Egg binding, in birds, management of, 323*t*
Egg withdrawal, in backyard poultry and waterfowl, 420*t*
Electrocardiographic values, in rabbits, 520–521*t*
Electrolyte solutions
  for anorectic or debilitated reptiles, 139–140*t*
  for reptiles, 108–113*t*
Emamectin, for fish, 25–30*t*
Emeraid Carnivore
  for amphibians, 65–67*t*
  for hedgehogs, 449–450*t*
Emeraid Exotic Carnivore
  for anorectic or debilitated reptiles, 139–140*t*
  for reptiles, 108–113*t*
Emeraid Herbivore
  for anorectic or debilitated reptiles, 139–140*t*
  for reptiles, 108–113*t*
Emeraid Omnivore
  for anorectic or debilitated reptiles, 139–140*t*
  for reptiles, 108–113*t*
Emerald tree boa (*Corallus caninus*), hematologic and serum biochemical values of, 117–136*t*
Emergencies, agents used in, for wild mammals, 629–631*t*
Emergency drugs
  for birds, 272–274*t*
  doses, for exotic animals, 654–655*t*
  for rodents, 474–475*t*
Emodepside
  for rabbits, 500–502*t*
  for reptiles, 89–93*t*
  for rodents, 464–466*t*
Emu (*Dromaius novaehollandiae*)
  biologic and physiologic values of, 307–308*t*
  hematologic and biochemical values of, 296*t*
Enalapril
  for birds, 275–283*t*
  for ferrets, 540–541*t*
  for hedgehogs, 449–450*t*
  for primates, 594–601*t*
  for rabbits, 513–517*t*
  for rodents, 470–474*t*
  for sugar gliders, 436*t*

Endocrine values, in rodents, 487t
Enflurane
 for ferrets, 536–539t
 for hedgehogs, 447–448t
Enilconazole
 for birds, 246–248t
 for hedgehogs, 445t
 for rodents, 460–463t
Enilconazole emulsion, for birds, 189–195t
Enoxaparin sodium, for primates, 594–601t
Enrofloxacin
 for amphibians, 54–55t
 for backyard poultry and waterfowl, 377–389t
 for birds, 168–189t, 246–248t, 270–271t
 for ferrets, 533–534t
 for fish, 17–24t
 for hedgehogs, 444–445t
 for invertebrates, 2–4t
 for miniature pigs, 559–560t
 for primates, 576–580t
 for rabbits, 495–498t
 for reptiles, 82–86t
 for RGIS, 522–523t
 for rodents, 460–463t
 and silver sulfadiazine solution, for amphibians, 54–55t
 for sugar gliders, 433t
 for wild mammals, 623–625t
Enteral feeding, for birds, 320t
Enterobacteriaceae, antimicrobial agents for, 639–640t
Environmental characteristics, of reptiles, 137–138t
Ephedrine
 for primates, 594–601t
 for rodents, 474–479t
Epinephrine
 for birds, 272–274t
 emergency drug doses of, 654–655t
 for ferrets, 540–541t, 543–549t
 for fish, 34–36t
 for hedgehogs, 449–450t
 for primates, 594–601t
 for rabbits, 513–517t
 for reptiles, 93–103t
 for rodents, 470–475t
 for sugar gliders, 436t
 for wild mammals, 629–631t
Epoetin alfa
 for ferrets, 543–549t
 for rabbits, 513–517t
Eprinomectin, for rabbits, 500–502t
Epsom salts, for backyard poultry and waterfowl, 390t
Erythromycin
 for backyard poultry and waterfowl, 377–389t
 for birds, 168–189t, 246–248t
 for ferrets, 533–534t
 for fish, 17–24t
 for hedgehogs, 444–445t
 for primates, 576–580t
 for rodents, 460–463t
Erythromycin phosphate, for backyard poultry and waterfowl, 377–389t
Erythromycin thiocyanate, for backyard poultry and waterfowl, 377–389t
Erythropoietin, for hedgehogs, 449–450t
Essential fatty acids, for birds, 258–263t

Estradiol benzoate
 for backyard poultry and waterfowl, 406t
 for birds, 240–245t
Ethambutol
 for birds, 168–189t
 for primates, 576–580t
Ethanol
 for fish, 31–33t, 36–37t
 for invertebrates, 6–9t
Ethanol/menthol, for invertebrates, 6–9t
Etilefrine, for rodents, 470–474t
Etodolac
 for miniature pigs, 566–567t
 for reptiles, 104–106t
Etomidate
 for ferrets, 536–539t
 for fish, 31–33t
 for primates, 586–594t
 for rabbits, 503–511t
Etorphine
 for birds, 218–236t
 for reptiles, 93–103t
Etorphine/acepromazine, for birds, 218–236t
Etorphine/acepromazine/xylazine, for birds, 218–236t
Etorphine HCl, for birds, 218–236t
Etorphine/ketamine, for birds, 218–236t
Eugenol (clove oil)
 for amphibians, 60–64t
 for fish, 31–33t, 36–37t
 for invertebrates, 6–9t
Eurasian eagle owl (*Bubo bubo*)
 biologic and physiologic values of, 309–310t
 hematologic and biochemical values of, 298–306t
European Association of Zoo and Wildlife Veterinarians, 648t
Euthanasia agents
 for backyard poultry and waterfowl, 399–403t
 for birds, 274t
 for fish, 36–37t
Exotic animal online resources, for practitioners, 648–650t
 captive husbandry web sites, 650–653t
Exotic DVM, 648–650t
Exotic Pet Vet Net, 648–650t

F
F10, for birds, 246–248t
F10 super concentrate disinfectant, for reptiles, 87–89t
Fagron, 663t
Fahrenheit temperature scales, equivalents of, 659t
Famciclovir
 for backyard poultry and waterfowl, 391t
 for reptiles, 86–87t
Famotidine
 for ferrets, 543–549t
 for hedgehogs, 449–450t
 for miniature pigs, 568t
 for rabbits, 513–517t
 for reptiles, 113–116t
 for rodents, 476–479t
 for wild mammals, 631–632t
Fatty acids, for birds, 258–263t
FDA Compounding Resources, 663t

Febantel
  for amphibians, 58–60t
  for birds, 197–217t
  for rabbits, 500–502t
Fecal transfaunation, for rabbits, 513–517t
Feed consumption rate, for backyard poultry and waterfowl, 420t
Feed estimates, for hand-rearing sugar gliders, 441t
Feline Clinical Care Liquid, for amphibians, 65–67t
Fenbendazole
  for amphibians, 58–60t
  for backyard poultry and waterfowl, 391–398t
  for birds, 197–217t
  for ferrets, 535–536t
  for fish, 25–30t
  for hedgehogs, 446t
  for miniature pigs, 561t
  for primates, 580–585t
  for rabbits, 500–502t
  for reptiles, 89–93t
  for rodents, 464–466t
  for sugar gliders, 433–434t
  for wild mammals, 625–626t
Fentanyl
  for amphibians, 60–64t
  for hedgehogs, 447–448t
  for miniature pigs, 561–567t
  for primates, 586–594t
  for rabbits, 503–511t
  for reptiles, 104–106t
  for rodents, 467–473t
  for wild mammals, 628–629t
Fentanyl citrate
  for backyard poultry and waterfowl, 399–403t
  for birds, 218–236t
  for ferrets, 536–540t
Fentanyl/droperidol
  for ferrets, 536–539t
  for miniature pigs, 561–565t
  for primates, 586–594t
Fentanyl/midazolam, for birds, 218–236t
Fentanyl patch, for rabbits, 503–511t
Ferret Universe, websites for owners of exotic animals, 650–653t
Ferret Village, websites for owners of exotic animals, 650–653t
Ferrets, 532–557
  adrenal gland disease agents for, 542–543t
  analgesic agents for, 539–540t
  anesthetic agents for, 536–539t
  antifungal agents for, 533–534t
  antimicrobial agents for, 533–534t
  antiparasitic agents for, 535–536t
  biochemical values of, 549–550t
  biologic data of, 550–551t
  cardiopulmonary agents for, 540–541t
  chemical restraint agents for, 536–539t
  chemotherapy protocols for lymphoma in, 552–554t
  hematologic values of, 549–550t
  miscellaneous agents for, 543–549t
  physiologic data of, 550–551t
  protein electrophoresis values for, 550t

Ferrets (Continued)
  schedule of vaccinations and routine prophylactic care for, 552t
  urinalysis values of, 551t
Ferric subsulfate, for birds, 275–283t
Ferrous sulfate, for rabbits, 513–517t
Finasteride, for ferrets, 542–543t
Fipronil
  for birds, 197–217t
  for ferrets, 535–536t
  for primates, 580–585t
  for rabbits, 500–502t
  for reptiles, 89–93t
  for rodents, 464–466t
  for wild mammals, 625–626t
Fipronil spray, for hedgehogs, 446t
Fish, 16–52
  analgesic agents for, 31–33t
  anesthetic agents for, 31–33t
  antifungal agents for, 17–24t
  antimicrobial agents for, 17–24t
  antiparasitic agents for, 25–30t
  chemical restraint agents for, 31–33t
  euthanasia agents for, 36–37t
  hematologic values of, 37–44t
  miscellaneous agents for, 34–36t
  serum biochemical values of, 37–44t
Fish Channel, websites for owners of exotic animals, 650–653t
Fish Lore, websites for owners of exotic animals, 650–653t
Fish Tank Guide, websites for owners of exotic animals, 650–653t
Flavorx, 663t
Flea products (feline), for hedgehogs, 446t
Florfenicol
  for amphibians, 56–57t
  for fish, 17–24t
  for miniature pigs, 559–560t
  for primates, 576–580t
  for rabbits, 495–498t
Fluanisone
  for ferrets, 536–539t
  for rabbits, 503–511t
  for rodents, 467–470t
Flubendazole
  for backyard poultry and waterfowl, 391–398t
  for birds, 197–217t
Fluconazole
  for amphibians, 56–57t
  for backyard poultry and waterfowl, 390t
  for birds, 189–195t
  for ferrets, 533–534t
  for invertebrates, 2–4t
  for primates, 576–580t
  for rabbits, 498–499t, 511–513t
  for reptiles, 87–89t
Flucytosine
  for backyard poultry and waterfowl, 390t
  for birds, 189–195t
  for primates, 576–580t
Fludrocortisone, for ferrets, 543–549t
Fluid support
  for reptiles, 108–113t
  solutions used in exotic animal medicine, 656t

Fluid therapy
  for amphibians, 75–77t
  for birds, 272t
    routes of administration and maximum
      suggested volumes of, 319t
  for RGIS, 522–523t
Flumazenil
  for backyard poultry and waterfowl,
    399–403t
  for birds, 218–236t
  for miniature pigs, 561–565t
  for primates, 586–594t
  for rabbits, 503–511t
  for reptiles, 93–103t
  for rodents, 467–470t
  for wild mammals, 627–628t
Flumequine
  for birds, 168–189t
  for fish, 17–24t
Flumethasone, for birds, 240–245t
Flunixin meglumine
  for amphibians, 60–64t
  for backyard poultry and waterfowl, 404–405t
  for birds, 236–239t
  for ferrets, 539–540t, 543–549t
  for hedgehogs, 448–449t
  for miniature pigs, 566–567t
  for primates, 586–594t
  for rabbits, 503–511t
  for reptiles, 104–106t
  for rodents, 470–473t
Fluoroquinolones, 637–638t
Fluoxetine
  for birds, 253–257t
  for primates, 594–601t
  for rodents, 476–479t
  for sugar gliders, 436t
Flurbiprofen sodium
  for ferrets, 543–549t
  for rabbits, 511–513t
Flurofamide, for primates, 576–580t
Flutamide, for ferrets, 542–543t
Folic acid
  for backyard poultry and waterfowl, 408–409t
  for primates, 594–601t
Food Animal Residue Avoidance Database (FARAD),
  623t
Food-producing animals, various designations of
  drugs in, definition of, 419t
Foraging For Parrots, websites for owners of exotic
  animals, 650–653t
Force-feeding reptiles, 139–140t
Formalin
  for amphibians, 58–60t
  for fish, 17–30t
  for invertebrates, 2–6t
Formic acid, for invertebrates, 5–6t
Fort Wayne Custom Rx, 661–662t
Fospropofol, for reptiles, 93–103t
Fowl cholera, vaccine for, 421–422t
Fowl cholera bacterin, vaccine for, 421–422t
Fowl pox, vaccine for, 421–422t
Freshwater
  for fish, 25–30t
  for invertebrates, 5–6t

Frog World, websites for owners of exotic animals,
  650–653t
Fumagillin
  for birds, 263–267t
  for invertebrates, 5–6t
Furazolidone
  for backyard poultry and waterfowl, 377–389t
  for birds, 168–189t
  for fish, 17–24t
  for invertebrates, 2–4t
  for primates, 576–585t
  for rabbits, 495–498t
Furosemide
  for birds, 275–283t
  doses of, 654–655t
  for ferrets, 540–541t
  for fish, 34–36t
  for hedgehogs, 449–450t
  for primates, 594–601t
  for rabbits, 513–517t
  for reptiles, 113–116t
  for rodents, 470–479t
  for sugar gliders, 436t
  for wild mammals, 629–631t
Fusidic acid, for rabbits, 511–513t

G
Gabapentin
  for birds, 218–236t, 253–257t
  for ferrets, 539–540t
  for miniature pigs, 566–567t
  for rabbits, 503–511t
  for rodents, 470–473t
  for wild mammals, 628–629t
Gadolinium-diethylenetriamine pentaacetic acid, for
  ferrets, 543–549t
Gadopentate dimeglumine, for birds, 275–283t
Galapagos tortoise (*Chelonoidis nigra*), hematologic
  and serum biochemical values of, 117–136t
Gallamine, for reptiles, 93–103t
Galliformes
  biologic and physiologic values of, 414t
  hematologic and serum biochemical values of, 412t
Gallium-67 citrate, for birds, 275–283t
Game animals, 623t
Garter snake (*Thamnophis sirtalis*), environmental,
  dietary, and reproductive characteristics of,
  137–138t
Gatifloxacin, for rabbits, 511–513t
Gavage feeding, of anorectic birds, 319t
Gemfibrozil, for birds, 275–283t
Gentamicin
  for amphibians, 54–55t
  for birds, 168–189t, 246–248t, 270–271t
  for ferrets, 533–534t
  for fish, 17–24t
  for hedgehogs, 444–445t
  for miniature pigs, 559–560t
  for primates, 576–580t
  for rabbits, 495–498t, 511–513t
  for reptiles, 82–86t
  for rodents, 460–463t
  for sugar gliders, 433t
Gentamicin/betamethasone ophthalmic drops, for
  reptiles, 82–86t

INDEX 681

Gentamicin ophthalmic drops, for hedgehogs, 444–445t
Gentamicin ophthalmic ointment, for reptiles, 82–86t
Gentamicin sulfate
  for backyard poultry and waterfowl, 377–389t
  for birds, 263–267t
Gentian violet, for birds, 275–283t
Georgia Veterinary Diagnostic Laboratories, 643–647t
Gerbil Care, websites for owners of exotic animals, 650–653t
Gila monster (*Heloderma suspectum*), hematologic and serum biochemical values of, 117–136t
Glauber's salt, for birds, 248–252t
Glipizide
  for birds, 240–245t, 275–283t
  for primates, 594–601t
Glucagon, for ferrets, 543–549t
Glucans, for fish, 34–36t
Glucosamine (G)/chondroitin sulfate (C), for miniature pigs, 568t
Glutamine, for ferrets, 543–549t
Glyceryl trinitrate, for rodents, 470–474t
Glycopyrrolate
  for birds, 218–236t
  emergency drug doses of, 654–655t
  for ferrets, 536–539t
  for hedgehogs, 449–450t
  for miniature pigs, 561–565t
  for primates, 594–601t
  for rabbits, 503–511t
  for reptiles, 93–103t
  for rodents, 467–470t, 473–475t
  for sugar gliders, 434–435t
  for wild mammals, 627–628t
Glycosaminoglycan, for birds, 275–283t
GnRH immunocontraceptive vaccine, for primates, 594–601t
sGnRHa + domperidone, for fish, 34–36t
Golden eagle (*Aquila chrysaetos*)
  biologic and physiologic values of, 309–310t
  hematologic and biochemical values of, 298–306t
Golden Gate Veterinary Pharmacy, 661–662t
Goldfish Society of America, websites for owners of exotic animals, 650–653t
Gonadotropin-releasing hormone (GnRH)
  for amphibians, 65t
  for ferrets, 543–549t
  for rodents, 476–479t
Good Life Pharmacy, 661–662t
Gopher snake (*Pituophis catenifer*), hematologic and serum biochemical values of, 117–136t
Gopher tortoise (*Gopherus polyphemus*), hematologic and serum biochemical values of, 117–136t
Gram-negative bacteria, antimicrobial agents for, 639–640t
Gram-positive bacteria, antimicrobial agents for, 639–640t
Grandpa's Compounding Pharmacy, 661–662t
Great gray owl (*Strix nebulosa*), hematologic and biochemical values of, 298–306t
Great-horned owl (*Bubo virginianus*), hematologic and biochemical values of, 298–306t
Greek tortoise (*Testudo graeca*), environmental, dietary, and reproductive characteristics of, 137–138t

Green iguana (*Iguana iguana*), hematologic and serum biochemical values of, 117–136t
Green Iguana Society, websites for owners of exotic animals, 650–653t
Green sea turtle (*Chelonia mydas*), hematologic and serum biochemical values of, 117–136t
Green tree python (*Morelia viridis*), hematologic and serum biochemical values of, 117–136t
Grey-cheeked parakeet (*Brotogeris pyrrhoptera*), hematologic and biochemical values of, 284–292t
Griseofulvin
  for birds, 189–195t
  for ferrets, 533–534t
  for hedgehogs, 445t
  for primates, 576–580t
  for rabbits, 498–499t
  for reptiles, 87–89t
  for rodents, 460–463t
  for sugar gliders, 433t
  for wild mammals, 626t
Grit, for birds, 248–252t
Growth and development, of sugar gliders, 439t
Guaifenesin
  for birds, 275–283t
  for primates, 594–601t
Guaifenesin (G)/ketamine (K)/xylazine (X), for miniature pigs, 561–565t
Guanfacine, for primates, 594–601t
Guinea Lynx, websites for owners of exotic animals, 650–653t
Gyrfalcon (*Falco rusticolus*)
  biologic and physiologic values of, 309–310t
  hematologic and biochemical values of, 298–306t

H

Hairball laxative, for ferrets, 543–549t
Halofuginone, for backyard poultry and waterfowl, 391–398t
Haloperidol
  for birds, 253–257t
  for fish, 34–36t
  for primates, 594–601t
  for reptiles, 93–103t
Hamster Hideout, websites for owners of exotic animals, 650–653t
Hamsterific, websites for owners of exotic animals, 650–653t
Hand-rearing feed estimates
  for orphaned hedgehogs, 453t
  for sugar gliders, 441t
Harris hawk (*Parabuteo unicinctus*)
  biologic and physiologic values of, 309–310t
  hematologic and biochemical values of, 298–306t
Hawksbill sea turtle (*Eretmochelys imbricata*), hematologic and serum biochemical values of, 117–136t
Healthway Compounding Pharmacy, 661–662t
Hedgehogs, 443–458
  analgesic agents for, 448–449t
  anesthetic agents for, 447–448t
  antifungal agents for, 445t
  antimicrobial agents for, 444–445t
  antiparasitic agents for, 446t
  biologic and physiologic values of, 452t

Hedgehogs (*Continued*)
  cardiac measurements in, 455t
  chemical restraint agents for, 447–448t
  differential diagnoses based on physical examination findings in, 454t
  hand-rearing orphaned, 453t
  hematologic and serum biochemical values of, 451t
  injection and venipuncture sites in, 453–454t
  miscellaneous agents for, 449–450t
  preventive medicine for, 454t
  suggested diets for, 452–453t
  vocalizations in, 454t
  zoonotic diseases carried by, 454t
Hematologic values
  abnormalities of standard avian, 311t
  of amphibians, 68–70t
  of Anseriformes, 413t
  of ferrets, 549–550t
  of fish, 37–44t
  of Galliformes, 412t
  of hedgehogs, 451t
  of miniature pigs, 569t
  of Passeriformes, 295t
  of Piciformes and Columbiformes, 297–298t
  of primates, 602–603t
  of Psittaciformes, 284–292t
    juvenile, 293–294t
  of rabbits, 517–518t
  of raptors, 298–306t
  of ratites, 296t
  of reptiles, 117–136t
  of rodents, 481t
  of sugar gliders, 437t
Hemicellulose, for birds, 258–263t
Hemoglobin glutamer-200
  for backyard poultry and waterfowl, 411t
  for birds, 272–274t
Hemorrhagic enteritis, vaccine for, 421–422t
Heparin
  for birds, 275–283t
  for ferrets, 543–549t
  for primates, 594–601t
  for rodents, 476–479t
Heparin/aloe vera, for birds, 275–283t
Herbivore critical care diet, for RGIS, 522–523t
Hetastarch
  for amphibians, 65–67t
  for birds, 272–274t
  for hedgehogs, 449–450t
  for rabbits, 513–517t
  for rodents, 474–475t
  for wild mammals, 629–631t
Hexyl ether pyropheophorbide-a, for birds, 267–270t
High protein powders, for anorectic or debilitated reptiles, 139–140t
Hill's Feline, for amphibians, 65–67t
Hormones
  for amphibians, 65t
  for backyard poultry and waterfowl, 399–403t
  for birds, 240–245t
  for reptiles, 106–108t
Horst Pharmacy, 661–662t
House Rabbit Society, websites for owners of exotic animals, 650–653t

Human chorionic gonadotropin (hCG)
  for amphibians, 65t
  for birds, 240–245t
  for ferrets, 543–549t
  for fish, 34–36t
  for primates, 594–601t
  for rabbits, 513–517t
  for rodents, 476–479t
Humco, 663t
Hummingbirds, nutritional recommendations for rehabilitation of, 322t
Husbandry, captive, 650–653t
Hyaluronidase
  for birds, 275–283t
  for hedgehogs, 449–450t
  for reptiles, 93–103t
Hydrochlorothiazide
  for primates, 594–601t
  for reptiles, 113–116t
Hydrocodone, for rodents, 470–473t
Hydrocodone bitartrate, for primates, 586–594t
Hydrocortisone
  for birds, 240–245t
  for fish, 34–36t
Hydrocortisone sodium succinate
  for ferrets, 543–549t
  for primates, 594–601t
Hydrogen peroxide
  for ferrets, 543–549t
  for fish, 17–30t, 34–36t
  for invertebrates, 9–10t
  for miniature pigs, 568t
Hydromorphone
  for birds, 218–236t
  for ferrets, 539–540t
  for hedgehogs, 448–449t
  for miniature pigs, 566–567t
  for primates, 586–594t
  for rabbits, 503–511t
  for reptiles, 104–106t
  for RGIS, 522–523t
  for rodents, 470–473t
Hydroxyapatite cement, for birds, 270–271t
Hydroxychloroquine sulfate, for birds, 197–217t
Hydroxyethyl starch, for reptiles, 108–113t
Hydroxyzine
  for birds, 253–257t, 275–283t
  for ferrets, 543–549t
  for rabbits, 513–517t
Hygromycin B
  for backyard poultry and waterfowl, 391–398t
  for birds, 197–217t
Hyperimmune serum, for ferrets, 540–541t
Hypertonic saline, for amphibians, 65–67t

I
Ibuprofen
  for birds, 236–239t
  for ferrets, 539–540t
  for miniature pigs, 566–567t
  for primates, 586–594t
  for rabbits, 503–511t
  for rodents, 470–473t
Imidacloprid
  for ferrets, 535–536t

Imidacloprid (*Continued*)
  for hedgehogs, 446t
  for rabbits, 500–502t
  for reptiles, 89–93t
  for rodents, 464–466t
Imidacloprid 10% + moxidectin 1%, for hedgehogs, 446t
Imidacloprid/moxidectin, for wild mammals, 625–626t
Imidapril hydrochloride, for rodents, 470–474t
Imidocarb dipropionate, for birds, 197–217t
Imiquimod cream, for birds, 189–197t
Immunizations. *See* Vaccinations
Immunomodulating agents
  for backyard poultry and waterfowl, 391t
  for birds, 196–197t
Indian star tortoise (*Geochelone elegans*), hematologic and serum biochemical values of, 117–136t
Indigo snake (*Drymarchon corais*), hematologic and serum biochemical values of, 117–136t
Indomethacin, for rodents, 470–473t
Infection site, antimicrobials and, 641–642t
Infectious bronchitis, Newcastle disease combination and, vaccine for, 421–422t
Infectious laryngotracheitis, vaccine for, 421–422t
Inhalant anesthetics, for backyard poultry and waterfowl, 410–411t
Injection sites, for hedgehogs, 453–454t
Injured wildlife, care of, 617–619t
Inositol, for birds, 258–263t
Insulin
  for birds, 240–245t
  glargine, for ferrets, 543–549t
  NPH
    for ferrets, 543–549t
    for primates, 594–601t
  for reptiles, 106–108t
  for rodents, 476–479t
  ultralente, for ferrets, 543–549t
Insulin/dextrose 50%, for birds, 272–274t
Interferon-α, for ferrets, 543–549t
Interferon α_2, for birds, 189–197t
International Association for Aquatic Animal Medicine, 648t
International Cockatiel Society, websites for owners of exotic animals, 650–653t
International Fancy Guppy Association, websites for owners of exotic animals, 650–653t
International Ferret Congress, websites for owners of exotic animals, 650–653t
International Hedgehog Association, websites for owners of exotic animals, 650–653t
International Species Information System, 648–650t
International Union for the Conservation of Nature, 648–650t
International Veterinary Information System, 648–650t
Invertebrates, 1–15
  analgesic agents for, 6–9t
  anesthetic agents for, 6–9t
  antifungal agents for, 2–4t
  antimicrobial agents for, 2–4t
  antiparasitic agents for, 5–6t
  chemical restraint agents for, 6–9t
  common captive taxa of, 11t
  miscellaneous agents for, 9–10t

Iodine
  for birds, 258–263t
  tincture, 275–283t
  for invertebrates, 2–4t
  1% solution, for birds, 189–195t
  potentiated, for fish, 17–24t
  for reptiles, 108–113t
  for rodents, 476–479t
Iodine compound, for reptiles, 113–116t
Iohexol
  for birds, 275–283t
  for ferrets, 543–549t
  for invertebrates, 9–10t
  for reptiles, 113–116t
Ipecac
  for ferrets, 543–549t
  for miniature pigs, 568t
Ipronidazole, for birds, 197–217t
Iron, for birds, 258–263t
Iron dextran
  for birds, 258–263t, 272t
  for ferrets, 543–549t
  for hedgehogs, 449–450t
  for primates, 594–601t
  for rabbits, 513–517t
  for reptiles, 108–113t
  for wild mammals, 631–632t
Isoeugenol, for amphibians, 60–64t
Isoflurane
  for amphibians, 60–64t
  for backyard poultry and waterfowl, 399–403t
  for birds, 218–236t, 263–267t, 274t
  for ferrets, 536–539t
  for fish, 31–33t
  for hedgehogs, 447–448t
  for invertebrates, 6–9t
  for miniature pigs, 561–565t
  for primates, 586–594t
  for rabbits, 503–511t
  for reptiles, 93–103t
  for rodents, 467–470t
  for sugar gliders, 434–435t
Isoflurane/sevoflurane, for fish, 36–37t
Isoniazid
  for birds, 168–189t
  for primates, 576–580t
Isoproterenol
  for ferrets, 540–541t
  for primates, 594–601t
Isotretinoin, for ferrets, 543–549t
Isoxsuprine
  for birds, 275–283t
Isoxuprine
  for wild mammals, 631–632t
Itraconazole
  for amphibians, 56–57t
  for backyard poultry and waterfowl, 390t
  for birds, 189–195t, 246–248t, 270–271t
  for ferrets, 533–534t
  for fish, 17–24t
  for hedgehogs, 445t
  for invertebrates, 2–4t
  for primates, 576–580t
  for rabbits, 498–499t
  for reptiles, 87–89t
  for rodents, 460–463t

Itraconazole (*Continued*)
  for sugar gliders, 433*t*
  for wild mammals, 626*t*
Ivermectin
  for amphibians, 58–60*t*
  for backyard poultry and waterfowl, 391–398*t*, 409*t*
  for birds, 197–217*t*
  for ferrets, 535–536*t*
  for fish, 25–30*t*
  for hedgehogs, 446*t*
  for invertebrates, 5–6*t*
  for miniature pigs, 561*t*
  for primates, 580–585*t*
  for rabbits, 500–502*t*
  for reptiles, 89–93*t*
  for rodents, 464–466*t*
  for sugar gliders, 433–434*t*
  for wild mammals, 625–626*t*

J
Jardine's parrot (*Poicephalus gulielmi*)
  hematologic and biochemical values of, 284–292*t*
  T_4 values of, 315*t*
Joint infection, antimicrobial therapy for, 641–642*t*
Juvenile Psittaciformes, hematologic and biochemical values of, 293–294*t*

K
K-Y jelly, for reptiles, 113–116*t*
Kanamycin
  for birds, 168–189*t*
  for reptiles, 82–86*t*
Kanamycin sulfate, for fish, 17–24*t*
Kansas State Veterinary Diagnostic Laboratory, 643–647*t*
Kaolin/pectin
  for birds, 275–283*t*
  for ferrets, 543–549*t*
  for miniature pigs, 568*t*
  for rodents, 476–479*t*
Ketamine
  for amphibians, 60–64*t*
  for backyard poultry and waterfowl, 399–403*t*
  for ferrets, 536–540*t*
  for fish, 31–33*t*, 36–37*t*
  for hedgehogs, 447–448*t*
  for invertebrates, 6–9*t*
  for miniature pigs, 561–565*t*
  for primates, 586–594*t*
  for rabbits, 503–511*t*
  for reptiles, 93–103*t*
  for rodents, 467–470*t*
  for sugar gliders, 434–435*t*
  for wild mammals, 627–628*t*
Ketamine/acepromazine
  for birds, 218–236*t*
  for ferrets, 536–539*t*
  for primates, 586–594*t*
Ketamine/azaperone, for miniature pigs, 561–565*t*
Ketamine/butorphanol, for reptiles, 93–103*t*
Ketamine/butorphanol/medetomidine, for birds, 218–236*t*
Ketamine/detomidine, for primates, 586–594*t*
Ketamine/dexmedetomidine
  for ferrets, 536–539*t*

Ketamine/dexmedetomidine (*Continued*)
  for fish, 36–37*t*
  for primates, 586–594*t*
  for reptiles, 93–103*t*
Ketamine/diazepam
  for birds, 218–236*t*
  for ferrets, 536–539*t*
  for miniature pigs, 561–565*t*
  for reptiles, 93–103*t*
Ketamine HCl
  for backyard poultry and waterfowl, 399–403*t*
  for birds, 218–236*t*
Ketamine/medetomidine
  for birds, 218–236*t*
  for ferrets, 536–539*t*
  for fish, 31–33*t*
  for hedgehogs, 447–448*t*
  for primates, 586–594*t*
  for reptiles, 93–103*t*
  for wild mammals, 627–628*t*
Ketamine/medetomidine/butorphanol, for primates, 586–594*t*
Ketamine/medetomidine/dexmedetomidine/butorphanol, for wild mammals, 627–628*t*
Ketamine/medetomidine/midazolam, for reptiles, 93–103*t*
Ketamine/medetomidine/morphine, for reptiles, 93–103*t*
Ketamine/midazolam
  for birds, 218–236*t*
  for ferrets, 536–539*t*
  for hedgehogs, 447–448*t*
  for miniature pigs, 561–565*t*
  for primates, 586–594*t*
  for reptiles, 93–103*t*
Ketamine/midazolam/butorphanol, for birds, 218–236*t*
Ketamine/propofol, for reptiles, 93–103*t*
Ketamine/tiletamine/zolazepam
  for birds, 218–236*t*
  for primates, 586–594*t*
Ketamine/xylazine
  for birds, 218–236*t*
  for ferrets, 536–539*t*
  for miniature pigs, 561–565*t*
  for primates, 586–594*t*
  for reptiles, 93–103*t*
Ketamine/xylazine/acepromazine, for birds, 218–236*t*
Ketamine/xylazine/butorphanol, for miniature pigs, 561–565*t*
Ketamine/xylazine/midazolam, for miniature pigs, 561–565*t*
Ketamine/xylazine/oxymorphone, for miniature pigs, 561–565*t*
Ketoconazole
  for amphibians, 56–57*t*
  for backyard poultry and waterfowl, 390*t*
  for birds, 189–195*t*
  for ferrets, 533–534*t*
  for fish, 17–24*t*
  for hedgehogs, 445*t*
  for primates, 576–580*t*
  for rabbits, 498–499*t*
  for reptiles, 87–89*t*
  for rodents, 460–463*t*

Ketolides, 637–638t
Ketoprofen
  for backyard poultry and waterfowl, 404–405t
  for birds, 236–239t
  for fish, 31–33t
  for miniature pigs, 566–567t
  for primates, 586–594t
  for rabbits, 503–511t
  for rodents, 470–473t
  for wild mammals, 628–629t
Ketorolac, for primates, 586–594t
Ketorolac tromethamine, for rabbits, 511–513t
Kingsnake (*Lampropeltis getula*)
  environmental, dietary, and reproductive characteristics of, 137–138t
  hematologic and serum biochemical values of, 117–136t

L
Laboratories, non-human primate, 609–611t
β-lactamase inhibitors, 637–638t
Lactated Ringer's solution (LRS)
  for hedgehogs, 449–450t
  for rabbits, 513–517t
  for reptiles, 108–113t
  for rodents, 474–475t
Lactobacilli
  for birds, 258–263t
  for hedgehogs, 449–450t
  for rabbits, 513–517t
Lactobacillus acidophilus, for birds, 258–263t
Lactulose
  for birds, 272t, 275–283t
  for hedgehogs, 449–450t
  for primates, 594–601t
  for reptiles, 113–116t
  for rodents, 476–479t
  for wild mammals, 631–632t
Lactulose syrup, for ferrets, 543–549t
Lasalocid
  for backyard poultry and waterfowl, 391–398t
  for rabbits, 500–502t
Laxative, for amphibians, 65–67t
Lecirelin, for birds, 240–245t
Leiter's Pharmacy, 661–662t
Length conversions, 658t
Leopard gecko (*Eublepharis macularius*),
  environmental, dietary, and reproductive characteristics of, 137–138t
Leopard tortoise (*Stigmochelys pardalis*), hematologic and serum biochemical values of, 117–136t
Leuprolide acetate
  for birds, 240–245t, 253–257t, 267–270t
  for ferrets, 542–543t
  for primates, 594–601t
  for reptiles, 106–108t
  for rodents, 476–479t
Levamisole
  for amphibians, 58–60t
  for backyard poultry and waterfowl, 391–398t
  for birds, 197–217t
  for fish, 25–30t
  for hedgehogs, 446t
  for invertebrates, 5–6t
  for miniature pigs, 561t

Levamisole (*Continued*)
  for primates, 580–585t
  for reptiles, 89–93t
  for rodents, 464–466t
  for sugar gliders, 433–434t
Levetiracetam
  for birds, 253–257t
  for rabbits, 513–517t
  for rodents, 476–479t
Levofloxacin, for primates, 576–580t
Levonorgestrel depot form, for backyard poultry and waterfowl, 406t
Levothyroxine
  for backyard poultry and waterfowl, 406t
  for birds, 240–245t
  for ferrets, 543–549t
  for primates, 594–601t
  for reptiles, 106–108t
  for rodents, 476–479t
Lidocaine
  for amphibians, 60–64t
  for backyard poultry and waterfowl, 399–403t
  for birds, 218–236t
  for ferrets, 536–539t
  for fish, 31–33t
  for invertebrates, 6–9t
  for miniature pigs, 561–565t
  for primates, 586–601t
  for rabbits, 503–511t, 513–517t
  for reptiles, 93–106t
  for RGIS, 522–523t
  for rodents, 470–474t
  for sugar gliders, 434–435t
  for wild mammals, 628–629t
Lidocaine/morphine, for reptiles, 104–106t
Lidocaine/prilocaine, for miniature pigs, 561–565t
Lime sulfur
  for ferrets, 533–536t
  for hedgehogs, 445t
  for rabbits, 498–502t
Lime sulfur dip, for rodents, 460–466t
Lincomycin
  for backyard poultry and waterfowl, 377–389t, 406–407t
  for birds, 168–189t, 246–248t
  for ferrets, 533–534t
  for miniature pigs, 559–560t
  for reptiles, 82–86t
  for sugar gliders, 433t
Lincomycin HCl, for backyard poultry and waterfowl, 377–389t
Lincomycin hydrochloride monohydrate, for backyard poultry and waterfowl, 377–389t
Lincomycin/spectinomycin, for birds, 168–189t
Lincosamides, 637–638t
Linear measures, 658t
Linoleic acid, for backyard poultry and waterfowl, 408–409t
γ-Linolenic acid, for backyard poultry and waterfowl, 408–409t
Lipoprotein panel, of birds, 314t
Liposomal form, for rabbits, 498–499t
Liquid measures, 658t
Lisinopril, for primates, 594–601t
Lizards

Lizards (*Continued*)
  environmental, dietary, and reproductive characteristics of, 137–138*t*
  tracheal/pulmonary and colonic lavage for, 141*t*
  venipuncture sites in, 141–142*t*
Loggerhead sea turtle (*Caretta caretta*), hematologic and serum biochemical values of, 117–136*t*
Loperamide
  for ferrets, 543–549*t*
  for primates, 594–601*t*
  for rabbits, 513–517*t*
  for rodents, 476–479*t*
  for wild mammals, 631–632*t*
Lorazepam, for birds, 253–257*t*
Lories
  biologic and physiologic values of, 307–308*t*
  hematologic and biochemical values of, 284–292*t*
  T_4 values of, 315*t*
Lorikeets
  biologic and physiologic values of, 307–308*t*
  hematologic and biochemical values of, 284–292*t*
Lovebirds (*Agapornis* spp.)
  biologic and physiologic values of, 307–308*t*
  hematologic and biochemical values of, 284–292*t*
  T_4 values of, 315*t*
Lufenuron
  for ferrets, 535–536*t*
  for fish, 25–30*t*
  for hedgehogs, 446*t*
  for rabbits, 500–502*t*
Lugol's 5% solution, for invertebrates, 2–4*t*
Lugol's iodine, for birds, 258–263*t*
Lupron, for ferrets, 542–543*t*
Luteinizing hormone, for amphibians, 65*t*
Luteinizing releasing hormone analog (LRH-A), for fish, 34–36*t*
Lymphoma, in ferrets, 552–554*t*
Lysine, for hedgehogs, 449–450*t*

M

Macaws (*Ara* and *Anodorhynchus* spp.)
  biologic and physiologic values of, 307–308*t*
  hematologic and biochemical values of, 284–294*t*
Macrolides, 637–638*t*
Maduramicin ammonium, for backyard poultry and waterfowl, 391–398*t*
Magnesium chloride, for invertebrates, 6–9*t*
Magnesium hydroxide, for rodents, 476–479*t*
Magnesium hydroxide/activated charcoal, for birds, 248–252*t*, 275–283*t*
Magnesium sulfate
  for birds, 248–252*t*, 258–263*t*, 275–283*t*
  for invertebrates, 6–9*t*
  for toxicologic conditions, of backyard poultry and waterfowl, 407–408*t*
Maintenance crystalloid solution, for reptiles, 108–113*t*
Malachite green
  for fish, 25–30*t*
  for reptiles, 87–89*t*
  zinc-free, for fish, 17–24*t*
Mannitol
  for birds, 272–283*t*
  for ferrets, 543–549*t*
  for primates, 594–601*t*

Mannitol (*Continued*)
  for rodents, 474–475*t*
  for wild mammals, 629–631*t*
Marbofloxacin
  for backyard poultry and waterfowl, 377–389*t*
  for birds, 168–189*t*
  for rabbits, 495–498*t*, 511–513*t*
  for reptiles, 82–86*t*
  for rodents, 460–463*t*
  for sugar gliders, 433*t*
Marek's disease, vaccine for, 421–422*t*
Maropitant
  for birds, 275–283*t*
  for wild mammals, 631–632*t*
Maropitant citrate
  for rabbits, 503–511*t*, 513–517*t*
  for reptiles, 113–116*t*
  for RGIS, 522–523*t*
  for sugar gliders, 436*t*
Martin Avenue Pharmacy, 661–662*t*
Maximum suggested volumes of fluid therapy, for birds, 319*t*
Meat withdrawal, in backyard poultry and waterfowl, 420*t*
Mebendazole
  for backyard poultry and waterfowl, 391–398*t*
  for birds, 197–217*t*
  for ferrets, 535–536*t*
  for fish, 25–30*t*
  for hedgehogs, 446*t*
  for primates, 580–585*t*
  for reptiles, 89–93*t*
  for rodents, 464–466*t*
Meclizine
  for rabbits, 513–517*t*
  for wild mammals, 631–632*t*
Medetomidine
  for backyard poultry and waterfowl, 399–403*t*
  for birds, 218–236*t*
  for fish, 31–33*t*
  for hedgehogs, 447–448*t*
  for primates, 586–594*t*
  for rabbits, 503–511*t*
  for reptiles, 93–103*t*
  for rodents, 467–470*t*
  for sugar gliders, 434–435*t*
Medetomidine/ketamine/fentanyl, for hedgehogs, 447–448*t*
Medetomidine/midazolam, for primates, 586–594*t*
Medirabbit, 648–650*t*
Medisca, 663*t*
Medroxyprogesterone acetate
  for birds, 240–245*t*
  for primates, 594–601*t*
Meds for Vets, 661–662*t*
Mefloquine, for primates, 580–585*t*
Mefloquine HCl, for birds, 197–217*t*
Megestrol acetate
  for birds, 240–245*t*, 253–257*t*
  for primates, 594–601*t*
Melarsomine dihydrochloride
  for birds, 197–217*t*
  for ferrets, 535–536*t*
Melatonin
  for ferrets, 542–543*t*

Melatonin (*Continued*)
  for toxicologic conditions, of backyard poultry and waterfowl, 407–408t
Melengestrol acetate implant, for primates, 594–601t
Melissa Kaplan's Herp Care Collection, websites for owners of exotic animals, 650–653t
Meloxicam
  for amphibians, 60–67t
  for backyard poultry and waterfowl, 404–405t
  for birds, 236–239t
  for ferrets, 539–540t
  for hedgehogs, 448–449t
  for miniature pigs, 566–567t
  for primates, 586–594t
  for rabbits, 503–511t
  for reptiles, 104–106t
  for RGIS, 522–523t
  for rodents, 470–473t
  for sugar gliders, 435t
  for wild mammals, 628–629t
Melphalan, for reptiles, 113–116t
Menthol, for invertebrates, 5–6t
Mepacrine HCl, for birds, 197–217t
Meperidine
  for birds, 218–236t
  for ferrets, 539–540t
  for miniature pigs, 566–567t
  for primates, 586–594t
  for reptiles, 104–106t
  for rodents, 470–473t
Meperidine/midazolam, for reptiles, 93–103t
Meropenem, for birds, 168–189t, 270–271t
Metabolic bone diseases, in reptiles, 144–145t
Metamizole, for rodents, 470–473t
Metaproterenol, for ferrets, 540–541t
Metformin, for primates, 594–601t
Methadone
  for reptiles, 104–106t
  for rodents, 470–473t
Methimazole
  for reptiles, 113–116t
  for rodents, 476–479t
Methocarbamol
  for backyard poultry and waterfowl, 411t
  for birds, 275–283t
Methohexital, for reptiles, 93–103t
Methohexital sodium, for backyard poultry and waterfowl, 399–403t
Methotrexate
  for ferrets, 543–549t
  for reptiles, 113–116t
Methoxyflurane, for birds, 274t
Methylene blue
  for amphibians, 56–57t, 65–67t
  for fish, 17–30t
Methylmethacrylate, for invertebrates, 9–10t
Methylprednisolone
  for birds, 267–270t
  for hedgehogs, 448–449t
  for reptiles, 106–108t
Methylprednisolone acetate, for birds, 240–245t
Methylprednisolone sodium succinate, for wild mammals, 629–631t
Methylsulfonylmethane (MSM), for rabbits, 511–513t
Methyltestosterone, for fish, 34–36t

Metildigoxin, for rodents, 470–474t
Metipranolol, for rabbits, 511–513t
Metoclopramide
  for backyard poultry and waterfowl, 411t
  for birds, 275–283t
  for ferrets, 543–549t
  for hedgehogs, 449–450t
  for miniature pigs, 568t
  for primates, 594–601t
  for rabbits, 513–517t
  for reptiles, 113–116t
  for RGIS, 522–523t
  for rodents, 476–479t
  for sugar gliders, 436t
  for wild mammals, 631–632t
Metomidate
  for fish, 31–33t
  for reptiles, 93–103t
Metomidate HCl
  for amphibians, 60–64t
  for backyard poultry and waterfowl, 399–403t
Metronidazole
  for amphibians, 54–55t, 58–60t
  for backyard poultry and waterfowl, 377–389t, 391–398t
  for birds, 168–189t, 197–217t, 270–271t
  for ferrets, 533–536t
  for fish, 25–30t
  for hedgehogs, 446t
  for invertebrates, 5–6t
  for miniature pigs, 559–560t
  for primates, 576–585t
  for rabbits, 495–498t, 500–502t
  for reptiles, 82–86t, 89–93t, 108–113t
  for RGIS, 522–523t
  for rodents, 460–466t
  for sugar gliders, 433–434t
  for wild mammals, 623–626t
Metyrapone, for rodents, 476–479t
Mexiletine, for birds, 275–283t
Micafungin, for rabbits, 498–499t, 511–513t
Miconazole
  for amphibians, 56–57t
  for birds, 189–195t, 246–248t, 263–267t
  for fish, 17–24t
  for rabbits, 498–499t
  for reptiles, 87–89t
Midazolam
  for backyard poultry and waterfowl, 399–403t
  for ferrets, 536–539t
  for hedgehogs, 447–448t
  for miniature pigs, 561–565t
  for primates, 586–594t
  for rabbits, 503–511t
  for reptiles, 93–103t
  for RGIS, 522–523t
  for rodents, 467–470t
  for sugar gliders, 434–435t
  for wild mammals, 627–628t
Midazolam/buprenorphine, for hedgehogs, 447–448t
Midazolam/butorphanol
  for ferrets, 536–539t
  for hedgehogs, 447–448t
Midazolam HCl
  for backyard poultry and waterfowl, 399–403t

Midazolam HCl (*Continued*)
   for birds, 218–236t
Midwest Compounders Pharmacy, 661–662t
Milbemycin, for reptiles, 89–93t
Milbemycin oxime
   for backyard poultry and waterfowl, 391–398t
   for birds, 197–217t
   for ferrets, 535–536t
   for invertebrates, 5–6t
   for primates, 580–585t
Milk snake (*Lampropeltis triangulum*), hematologic and serum biochemical values of, 117–136t
Milk thistle (*Silybum marianum*)
   for birds, 196–197t, 267–270t, 275–283t
   for ferrets, 543–549t
   for hedgehogs, 449–450t
   for primates, 594–601t
   for reptiles, 113–116t
   for rodents, 476–479t
Milliequivalent conversions, 658t
Mineral oil
   for birds, 275–283t
   for invertebrates, 9–10t
Mineral support
   for backyard poultry and waterfowl, 408–409t
   for birds, 258–263t
   for reptiles, 108–113t
Miniature pigs, 558–574
   analgesic agents for, 566–567t
   anesthetic agents for, 561–565t
   antimicrobial agents for, 559–560t
   antiparasitic agents for, 561t
   biologic and physiologic data of, 570t
   blood collection sites in, 572t
   chemical restraint agents for, 561–565t
   feeding recommendations for, 572t
   hematologic and serum biochemical values for, 569t
   miscellaneous agents for, 568t
   oral dosing of, 573t
   preventive medicine recommendations for, 571–572t
   urinalysis reference values for, 570t
Minocycline
   for birds, 168–189t
   for primates, 576–580t
   for rabbits, 495–498t
Miporamicin, for backyard poultry and waterfowl, 377–389t
Mirtazapine
   for primates, 594–601t
   for rabbits, 513–517t
Miscellaneous agents
   for amphibians, 65–67t
   for birds, 275–283t
   for ferrets, 543–549t
   for fish, 34–36t
   for hedgehogs, 449–450t
   for invertebrates, 9–10t
   for miniature pigs, 568t
   for primates, 594–601t
   for rabbits, 513–517t
   for reptiles, 113–116t
   for rodents, 476–479t
   for sugar gliders, 436t

Misoprostol
   for ferrets, 543–549t
   for primates, 594–601t
Mitotane
   for ferrets, 542–543t
   for rodents, 476–479t
Mollusks, as common captive invertebrate taxa, 11t
Monensin
   for backyard poultry and waterfowl, 391–398t
   for birds, 197–217t
   for rabbits, 500–502t
Monument Pharmacy, 661–662t
Morphine
   for amphibians, 60–64t
   for ferrets, 536–540t
   for fish, 31–33t
   for invertebrates, 6–9t
   for miniature pigs, 566–567t
   for primates, 586–594t
   for rabbits, 503–511t
   for reptiles, 104–106t
   for rodents, 470–473t
   for wild mammals, 628–629t
Morphine sulfate
   for backyard poultry and waterfowl, 399–403t
   for birds, 218–236t
Moxidectin
   for amphibians, 58–60t
   for birds, 197–217t
   for ferrets, 535–536t
   for hedgehogs, 446t
   for primates, 580–585t
   for rabbits, 500–502t
   for reptiles, 89–93t
   for rodents, 464–466t
   for wild mammals, 625–626t
Moxifloxacin, for rabbits, 495–498t, 511–513t
MS-222
   for fish, 31–33t
   for invertebrates, 6–9t
Multivitamin products, for reptiles, 108–113t
Mupirocin, for hedgehogs, 444–445t
My House Rabbit, websites for owners of exotic animals, 650–653t
Mycobacteriosis, in birds, 312–313t
Mycoplasma spp., antimicrobial agents for, 639–640t
Mynah (*Gracula religiosa*)
   biologic and physiologic values of, 307–308t
   hematologic and biochemical values of, 295t

N
Nalbuphine
   for ferrets, 539–540t
   for primates, 586–594t
   for rodents, 470–473t
Nalbuphine HCl, for birds, 218–236t
Nalidixic acid, for fish, 17–24t
Nalorphine, for amphibians, 60–64t
Naloxone
   for amphibians, 60–64t
   for ferrets, 536–539t
   for hedgehogs, 447–449t
   for miniature pigs, 561–565t
   for primates, 586–594t
   for rabbits, 503–511t

INDEX 689

Naloxone (*Continued*)
  for reptiles, 93–106*t*
  for rodents, 467–470*t*
Naloxone HCl, for birds, 218–236*t*, 253–257*t*
Naltrexone, for amphibians, 60–64*t*
Naltrexone HCl, for birds, 218–236*t*, 253–257*t*
Nandrolone
  for rabbits, 513–517*t*
  for reptiles, 106–108*t*
Nandrolone decanoate, for ferrets, 543–549*t*
Nandrolone laurate, for birds, 240–245*t*
Naproxen, for primates, 586–594*t*
Narasin, for backyard poultry and waterfowl, 391–398*t*
Natamycin, for birds, 263–267*t*
National Finch and Softbill Society, websites for owners of exotic animals, 650–653*t*
National Veterinary Services Laboratory, 643–647*t*
National Wildlife Rehabilitators Association, 648*t*
Nature's Pharmacy, 661–662*t*
Nebulization agents
  for backyard poultry and waterfowl, 406–407*t*
  for birds, 246–248*t*
Nematode parasites, amphibians with, 75*t*
Neomycin
  for amphibians, 56–57*t*
  for backyard poultry and waterfowl, 377–389*t*
  for birds, 168–189*t*
  for ferrets, 533–534*t*
  for fish, 17–24*t*
  for hedgehogs, 444–445*t*
  for invertebrates, 2–4*t*
  for miniature pigs, 559–560*t*
  for primates, 576–580*t*
  for rabbits, 500–502*t*, 511–513*t*
  for rodents, 460–463*t*
Neomycin/polymyxin B/dexamethasone, for birds, 263–267*t*
Neomycin/polymyxin B/gramicidin, for birds, 263–267*t*
Neomycin sulfate
  for backyard poultry and waterfowl, 377–389*t*
  for reptiles, 82–86*t*
Neostigmine, for reptiles, 93–103*t*
Netilmicin
  for ferrets, 533–534*t*
  for rabbits, 495–498*t*
Newcastle's disease, vaccine for, 421–422*t*
Niacin
  for backyard poultry and waterfowl, 408–409*t*
  for birds, 258–263*t*
Nicarbazin
  for backyard poultry and waterfowl, 391–398*t*, 411*t*
  for birds, 275–283*t*
Niclosamide
  for birds, 197–217*t*
  for fish, 25–30*t*
  for primates, 580–585*t*
  for rodents, 464–466*t*
Nicotinic acid, for birds, 258–263*t*
Nifurpirinol, for fish, 17–24*t*
Nifurtimox, for primates, 580–585*t*
Nitazoxanide
  for ferrets, 533–534*t*
  for primates, 580–585*t*

Nitenpyram
  for rodents, 464–466*t*
  for wild mammals, 625–626*t*
Nitrifying bacteria
  for fish, 34–36*t*
  for invertebrates, 9–10*t*
Nitrofuran, for backyard poultry and waterfowl, 377–389*t*
Nitrofurazone
  for backyard poultry and waterfowl, 377–389*t*
  for birds, 168–189*t*
  for fish, 17–24*t*
  for invertebrates, 2–4*t*
  for reptiles, 89–93*t*
Nitrogen, for backyard poultry and waterfowl, 410–411*t*
Nitroglycerin
  for ferrets, 540–541*t*
  for primates, 594–601*t*
Nitroimidazole, 637–638*t*
Nitroprusside, for primates, 594–601*t*
Nitrous oxide/isoflurane/vecuronium, for birds, 218–236*t*
Nitrous oxide (N_2O)
  for birds, 218–236*t*
  for miniature pigs, 561–565*t*
  for primates, 586–594*t*
Nonhuman primate laboratories, 609–611*t*
Nonsteroidal antiinflammatory agents
  for backyard poultry and waterfowl, 404–405*t*
  for birds, 236–239*t*
  for wild mammals, 628–629*t*
Norepinephrine, for primates, 594–601*t*
Norfloxacin
  for backyard poultry and waterfowl, 377–389*t*
  for birds, 168–189*t*
North American Sugar Glider Association, websites for owners of exotic animals, 650–653*t*
Northern saw-whet owl (*Aegolius acadicus*), hematologic and biochemical values of, 298–306*t*
Northwest Compounders, 661–662*t*
Northwest ZooPath, 643–647*t*
Nortriptyline, for birds, 253–257*t*
Novobiocin, for backyard poultry and waterfowl, 377–389*t*
Novobiocin sodium, for backyard poultry and waterfowl, 377–389*t*
Nucleotide, for fish, 34–36*t*
Nuflor, for miniature pigs, 559–560*t*
Nutri-Cal, for ferrets, 543–549*t*
Nutritional support and data
  for backyard poultry and waterfowl, 408–409*t*
  for birds, 258–263*t*
  for reptiles, 108–113*t*
  for rodents, 485*t*
Nystatin
  for amphibians, 1% cream, 56–57*t*
  for backyard poultry and waterfowl, 390*t*
  for birds, 189–195*t*
  for hedgehogs, 444–445*t*
  for primates, 576–580*t*
  for rabbits, 498–499*t*
  for reptiles, 87–89*t*
  for rodents, 460–463*t*

Nystatin (*Continued*)
  for sugar gliders, 433t
  for wild mammals, 626t

O

Octreotide, for ferrets, 543–549t
Ofloxacin
  for amphibians, 54–55t
  for primates, 576–580t
  for rabbits, 495–498t
Oiled birds, treatment of, 272t
Oleandomycin
  for backyard poultry and waterfowl, 377–389t
  for birds, 168–189t
Olive oil, for reptiles, 89–93t
Omega-3, for birds, 258–263t
Omega-6, for birds, 258–263t
Omeprazole
  for ferrets, 543–549t
  for primates, 594–601t
  for rabbits, 513–517t
  for wild mammals, 631–632t
Oncologic agents
  for backyard poultry and waterfowl, 410t
  for birds, 267–270t
Ondansetron
  for ferrets, 543–549t
  for primates, 594–601t
Ophthalmic diagnostic tests
  in avian species, 420t
  in birds, 317t
Ophthalmologic agents
  for backyard poultry and waterfowl, 409t
  for birds, 263–267t
  for rabbits, 511–513t
Oral dosing, of miniature pigs, 573t
Oral electrolyte solutions, for birds, 272t
Orange-winged Amazon parrot (*Amazona amazonica*), hematologic and biochemical values of, 284–292t
Orbifloxacin
  for backyard poultry and waterfowl, 377–389t
  for hedgehogs, 444–445t
  for rabbits, 495–498t
Oregano essential oil, for backyard poultry and waterfowl, 391–398t
Ormetoprim
  for backyard poultry and waterfowl, 391–398t
  for rabbits, 500–502t
Ormetoprim-sulfadimethoxine
  for backyard poultry and waterfowl, 377–389t
  for birds, 168–189t, 197–217t
Ornate box turtle (*Terrapene ornata*), hematologic and serum biochemical values of, 117–136t
Orphaned wildlife, care of, 617–619t
Oseltamivir phosphate, for ferrets, 543–549t
Ostrich (*Struthio camelus*)
  biologic and physiological values of, 307–308t
  hematologic and biochemical values of, 296t
Oxacillin, for primates, 576–580t
Oxfendazole
  for amphibians, 58–60t
  for birds, 197–217t
  for reptiles, 89–93t

Oxibendazole, for rabbits, 500–502t
Oxolinic acid
  for fish, 17–24t
  for invertebrates, 2–4t
Oxybuprocaine, for birds, 263–267t
Oxycodone, for rodents, 470–473t
Oxygen
  for amphibians, 65–67t
  for fish, 34–36t
  for invertebrates, 9–10t
Oxyglobin, for birds, 272–274t
Oxymorphone
  for ferrets, 539–540t
  for miniature pigs, 566–567t
  for primates, 586–594t
  for rabbits, 503–511t
  for reptiles, 104–106t
  for rodents, 470–473t
Oxytetracycline
  for amphibians, 54–55t, 58–60t
  for backyard poultry and waterfowl, 377–389t, 406–407t
  for birds, 168–189t, 246–248t, 270–271t
  for ferrets, 533–534t
  for fish, 17–24t
  for hedgehogs, 444–445t
  for invertebrates, 2–4t
  for miniature pigs, 559–560t
  for primates, 576–585t
  for rabbits, 495–498t
  for reptiles, 82–86t
  for rodents, 460–463t
Oxytetracycline ophthalmic ointment, for hedgehogs, 444–445t
Oxytetracycline/polymyxin B, for birds, 263–267t
Oxytocin
  for backyard poultry and waterfowl, 406t
  for birds, 240–245t
  for ferrets, 543–549t
  for miniature pigs, 568t
  for primates, 594–601t
  for rabbits, 513–517t
  for reptiles, 106–108t
    with dystocia, 142–143t
  for rodents, 476–479t
  for wild mammals, 631–632t

P

Pacific pond turtle (*Actinemys marmorata*), hematologic and serum biochemical values of, 117–136t
Painted turtle (*Chrysemys picta*)
  environmental, dietary, and reproductive characteristics of, 137–138t
  hematologic and serum biochemical values of, 117–136t
Pancreatic enzyme powder, for birds, 258–263t
Panther chameleon (*Furcifur pardalis*), hematologic and serum biochemical values of, 117–136t
Pantothenic acid, for backyard poultry and waterfowl, 408–409t
Papaya enzyme, for birds, 272t
Parakeets, hematologic and biochemical values of, 284–292t
Parasites, nematode, amphibians with, 75t

INDEX 691

Parconazole, for backyard poultry and waterfowl, 390t
Parkview Compounding Pharmacy, 661–662t
Paromomycin
 for amphibians, 58–60t
 for birds, 197–217t
 for ferrets, 535–536t
 for invertebrates, 2–4t
 for primates, 580–585t
 for reptiles, 89–93t
Paroxetine
 for birds, 253–257t
 for primates, 594–601t
Parrot A.L.E.R.T., websites for owners of exotic animals, 650–653t
Parrot Outreach Society, websites for owners of exotic animals, 650–653t
Parrotlets (*Forpus* spp.), hematologic and biochemical values of, 284–292t
Parrots, hematologic and biochemical values of, 284–292t
Passeriformes
 biologic and physiologic values of, 307–308t
 hematologic and biochemical values of, 295t
Pasteurella spp., antimicrobial agents for, 639–640t
Peanut butter, for birds, 248–252t, 275–283t
Penciclovir, for backyard poultry and waterfowl, 391t
Penicillamine
 for birds, 248–252t
 for ferrets, 543–549t
 for toxicologic conditions, of backyard poultry and waterfowl, 407–408t
Penicillin
 for backyard poultry and waterfowl, 377–389t
 extended-spectrum, 637–638t
 for reptiles, 82–86t
 for sugar gliders, 433t
Penicillin benzathine/procaine, for birds, 168–189t
Penicillin G
 for backyard poultry and waterfowl, 377–389t
 benzathine, for primates, 576–580t
 for birds, 168–189t
 for ferrets, 533–534t
 for hedgehogs, 444–445t
 for miniature pigs, 559–560t
 procaine
  for primates, 576–580t
  for wild mammals, 623–625t
 for rabbits, 495–498t, 511–513t
 for reptiles, 82–86t
 for rodents, 460–463t
Penicillin procaine
 for backyard poultry and waterfowl, 377–389t
 for birds, 168–189t
Penicillin VK, for primates, 576–580t
Pentamidine isethionate
 for ferrets, 533–534t
 for primates, 576–580t
Pentastarch, for birds, 272–274t
Pentazocine
 for ferrets, 539–540t
 for miniature pigs, 566–567t
 for rabbits, 503–511t
 for rodents, 470–473t
Pentobarbital
 for fish, 31–33t

Pentobarbital (*Continued*)
 for miniature pigs, 561–565t, 568t
 for primates, 586–594t
 for rabbits, 503–511t
 for reptiles, 93–103t, 113–116t
 for rodents, 467–470t
Pentobarbital sodium
 for amphibians, 60–64t
 for backyard poultry and waterfowl, 410–411t
 for birds, 218–236t, 274t
 for primates, 586–594t
Pentobarbital sodium + sodium phenytoin, for amphibians, 60–64t
Pentosan polysulphate, for rodents, 476–479t
Pentoxifylline
 for birds, 275–283t
 for ferrets, 543–549t
Percentage conversions, 658t
Peregrine falcon (*Falco peregrinus*)
 biologic and physiologic values of, 309–310t
 hematologic and biochemical values of, 298–306t
Perflutren lipid microspheres, for birds, 275–283t
Permethrin
 for birds, 197–217t
  high-cis, 197–217t
 for hedgehogs, 446t
 for rabbits, 500–502t
 for reptiles, 89–93t
 for rodents, 464–466t
Perrigo, 663t
Pet Apothecary, 661–662t
Pet Hamster Care, websites for owners of exotic animals, 650–653t
Pet Snakes, websites for owners of exotic animals, 650–653t
Pet-Tinic, for ferrets, 543–549t
Pethidine
 for reptiles, 104–106t
 for rodents, 470–473t
PGF$_2$ alpha, for primates, 594–601t
Pharmacy Innovations, 661–662t
Phenobarbital
 for primates, 594–601t
 for rodents, 476–479t
Phenobarbital sodium, for birds, 253–257t
Phenoxybenzamine
 for ferrets, 543–549t
 for rodents, 476–479t
2-phenoxyethanol
 for fish, 31–33t, 36–37t
 for invertebrates, 6–9t
Phentolamine mesylate, for primates, 594–601t
Phenylarsonic acid, for backyard poultry and waterfowl, 391–398t
Phenylbutazone
 for birds, 236–239t
 for miniature pigs, 566–567t
Phenylephrine
 for birds, 263–267t
 for primates, 594–601t
 for rabbits, 511–513t
 for rodents, 476–479t
Phenytoin, for primates, 594–601t
Philadelphia Professional Compounding Agency, 661–662t

Physiologic values
  of amphibians, 68–70t
  of birds, 307–308t
  of ferrets, 550–551t
  of hedgehogs, 452t
  of miniature pigs, 570t
  of primates, 604t
  of rabbits, 519t
  of rodents, 482t
  of sugar gliders, 438t
Physostigmine, for amphibians, 65–67t
Phytonadione, for birds, 248–252t, 258–263t
Piciformes, hematologic and biochemical values of, 297–298t
Pigeon (*Columba livia*)
  biologic and physiologic values of, 307–308t
  hematologic and biochemical values of, 297–298t
  T_4 values of, 315t
Pigs. *See* Miniature pigs
Pilocarpine, for rabbits, 511–513t
Pimaricin, for birds, 263–267t
Pimobendan
  for birds, 275–283t
  for ferrets, 540–541t
  for hedgehogs, 449–450t
  for primates, 594–601t
  for rabbits, 513–517t
  for reptiles, 113–116t
  for rodents, 470–474t
  for sugar gliders, 436t
Pionus parrots (*Pionus* spp.)
  hematologic and biochemical values of, 284–292t
  lipoprotein panel of, 314t
  T_4 values of, 315t
Piperacillin
  for amphibians, 54–55t
  for birds, 168–189t, 246–248t
  for hedgehogs, 444–445t
  for reptiles, 82–86t
Piperacillin/tazobactam
  for birds, 168–189t
  for wild mammals, 623–625t
Piperazine
  for amphibians, 58–60t
  for backyard poultry and waterfowl, 391–398t
  for birds, 197–217t
  for fish, 25–30t
  for miniature pigs, 561t
  for rabbits, 500–502t
  for reptiles, 89–93t
  for sugar gliders, 433–434t
Piperazine adipate, for rodents, 464–466t
Piperazine citrate
  for ferrets, 535–536t
  for rodents, 464–466t
Piperazine penicillins, 637–638t
Piperonyl butoxide/pyrethrin, for birds, 197–217t
Piperonyl butoxide/pyrethrin/methoprene, for birds, 197–217t
Piroxicam
  for birds, 236–239t
  for rabbits, 503–511t
  for rodents, 470–473t
Poison Dart Frogs, websites for owners of exotic animals, 650–653t

Policosanol, for birds, 275–283t
Polymerized bovine hemoglobin, for reptiles, 108–113t
Polymyxin B
  for amphibians, 56–57t
  for birds, 168–189t
  for hedgehogs, 444–445t
  for rabbits, 511–513t
Polymyxin B sulfate
  for birds, 246–248t
  for reptiles, 82–86t
Polymyxin B sulfate/bacitracin/neomycin sulfate, for fish, 17–24t
Polyprenol, for ferrets, 543–549t
Polysulfated glycosaminoglycan (PSGAG)
  for backyard poultry and waterfowl, 411t
  for birds, 275–283t
  for miniature pigs, 568t
  for primates, 594–601t
  for rabbits, 513–517t
Ponazuril
  for amphibians, 58–60t
  for birds, 197–217t
  for reptiles, 89–93t
  for rodents, 464–466t
Porfimer sodium, for birds, 267–270t
Posaconazole, for rabbits, 498–499t
Potassium bromide
  for birds, 253–257t
  for ferrets, 543–549t
Potassium chloride
  for backyard poultry and waterfowl, 410–411t
  for birds, 258–263t, 272–274t
  for invertebrates, 6–9t
  for primates, 594–601t
  for reptiles, 113–116t
Potassium citrate
  for rabbits, 513–517t
  for rodents, 476–479t
Potassium permanganate
  for amphibians, 56–60t
  for fish, 17–30t
  for invertebrates, 5–6t
Povidone-iodine
  for birds, 168–195t, 275–283t
  for invertebrates, 5–6t
  for reptiles, 82–86t
Pralidoxime (2-PAM)
  for birds, 248–252t
  for wild mammals, 629–631t
Pralidoxime mesylate, for toxicologic conditions, of backyard poultry and waterfowl, 407–408t
Praziquantel
  for amphibians, 58–60t
  for backyard poultry and waterfowl, 391–398t
  for birds, 197–217t, 246–248t
  for ferrets, 535–536t
  for fish, 25–30t
  for hedgehogs, 446t
  for primates, 580–585t
  for rabbits, 500–502t
  for reptiles, 89–93t
  for rodents, 464–466t
  for sugar gliders, 433–434t
  for wild mammals, 625–626t

Prazosin, for ferrets, 543–549t
Precision Pharmacy, 661–662t
Prednisolone
   for birds, 240–245t
   for hedgehogs, 448–449t
   for rabbits, 513–517t
   for reptiles, 104–108t
   for rodents, 474–479t
   for sugar gliders, 436t
Prednisolone acetate
   for birds, 263–267t
   for rabbits, 511–513t
Prednisolone sodium succinate
   for amphibians, 65–67t
   for birds, 240–245t, 272–274t
   for primates, 594–601t
   for reptiles, 106–108t
Prednisone
   for backyard poultry and waterfowl, 410t
   for birds, 240–245t, 267–270t
   for ferrets, 543–549t
   for miniature pigs, 566–567t
   for primates, 594–601t
   for rabbits, 513–517t
   for reptiles, 106–108t
   for rodents, 476–479t
Pregnant mare serum gonadotropin (PMSG), for amphibians, 65t
Prehensile-tailed skink (*Corucia zebrata*), hematologic and serum biochemical values of, 117–136t
Prescription writing, common abbreviations used in, 657t
Preventive medicine
   for hedgehogs, 454t
   for miniature pigs, 571–572t
   for primates, 606t
Prilocaine, for rabbits, 503–511t
Primaquine
   for backyard poultry and waterfowl, 391–398t
   for birds, 197–217t
   for primates, 580–585t
Primates, 575–615
   analgesic agents for, 586–594t
   anesthetic agents for, 586–594t
   antifungal agents for, 576–580t
   antimicrobial agents for, 576–580t
   antiparasitic agents for, 580–585t
   biologic data of, 604t
   chemical restraint agents for, 586–594t
   ECG intervals and durations in, 605t
   hematologic values of, 602–603t
   immunization recommendations for, 607–608t
   miscellaneous agents for, 594–601t
   nonhuman primate laboratories for, 609–611t
   physiologic data of, 604t
   preventive medicine recommendations for, 606t
   serum biochemical values of, 602–603t
   taxonomic classification of, 605t
Probenecid
   for birds, 275–283t
   for primates, 594–601t
   for reptiles, 113–116t
Probucol, for birds, 275–283t
Procainamide, for primates, 594–601t
Procaine
   for invertebrates, 6–9t
   for miniature pigs, 559–560t
   for rabbits, 495–498t
Procarbazine, for ferrets, 543–549t
Prochlorperazine
   for primates, 594–601t
   for rabbits, 513–517t
Professional associations, for veterinarians, 648t
Progesterone, for amphibians, 65t
Proligestone, for ferrets, 543–549t
Promazine hydrochloride, for miniature pigs, 561–565t
Proparacaine, for reptiles, 104–106t
Propentofylline
   for birds, 275–283t
   for rodents, 470–474t
Propionibacterium acnes, for birds, 196–197t
Propofol
   for amphibians, 60–64t
   for backyard poultry and waterfowl, 399–403t
   for birds, 218–236t
   for ferrets, 536–539t
   for fish, 31–33t, 36–37t
   for primates, 586–594t
   for rabbits, 503–511t
   for reptiles, 93–103t
   for rodents, 467–470t
   for wild mammals, 627–628t
Propranolol
   for birds, 275–283t
   for ferrets, 540–541t
   for primates, 594–601t
   for reptiles, with dystocia, 142–143t
Propylene phenoxetol, for invertebrates, 6–9t
Prostaglandin E_2
   for backyard poultry and waterfowl, 406t
   for birds, 240–245t
Prostaglandin $F_{2\alpha}$
   for backyard poultry and waterfowl, 406t
   for birds, 240–245t
   for ferrets, 543–549t
   for miniature pigs, 568t
   for reptiles, with dystocia, 142–143t
Proxymetacaine, for birds, 263–267t
Pseudoephedrine, for rodents, 476–479t
Pseudomonas spp., antimicrobial agents for, 639–640t
Pseudoephedrine, for ferrets, 540–541t
Psittaciformes
   biologic and physiologic values of, 307–308t
   doxycycline recipes for, 321t
   hematologic and biochemical values of, 284–292t
   juvenile, 293–294t
   ophthalmic diagnostic tests in, 317t
   routes of administration and maximum suggested volumes of fluids for, 319t
Psittacines, doxycycline recipes used in, 321t
Psychotherapeutic agents, for birds, 334–336t
Psychotropic agents, for birds, 253–257t
Psyllium, for birds, 248–252t, 275–283t
PubMed, 648–650t
Pulmonary lavage, for reptiles, 141t
Pyrantel pamoate
   for amphibians, 58–60t
   for birds, 197–217t

Pyrantel pamoate (*Continued*)
  for ferrets, 535–536*t*
  for fish, 25–30*t*
  for miniature pigs, 561*t*
  for primates, 580–585*t*
  for rabbits, 500–502*t*
  for reptiles, 89–93*t*
  for rodents, 464–466*t*
  for wild mammals, 625–626*t*
Pyremethamine, for ferrets, 533–534*t*
Pyrethrin powder, for sugar gliders, 433–434*t*
Pyrethrin spray, for reptiles, 89–93*t*
Pyrethrins
  for birds, 197–217*t*
  for ferrets, 535–536*t*
  for rabbits, 500–502*t*
  for rodents, 464–466*t*
Pyridostigmine, for ferrets, 543–549*t*
Pyrimethamine
  for backyard poultry and waterfowl, 391–398*t*
  for birds, 197–217*t*
  for ferrets, 535–536*t*
  for primates, 580–585*t*
Pyrvinium, for primates, 580–585*t*

Q

Quaker parakeet (*Myopsitta monachus*), hematologic and biochemical values of, 284–292*t*
Quarantine protocols, for amphibians, 75–77*t*
Quinacrine
  for primates, 580–585*t*
  for reptiles, 89–93*t*
Quinacrine HCl, for birds, 197–217*t*
Quinaldine sulfate, for fish, 31–33*t*, 36–37*t*
Quinidine, for primates, 594–601*t*
Quinine sulfate, for reptiles, 89–93*t*
Quinolones, 637–638*t*

R

Rabbit gastrointestinal syndrome (RGIS), treatment for, 522–523*t*
Rabbits, 494–531
  analgesic agents for, 503–511*t*
  anesthetic agents for, 503–511*t*
  antifungal agents for, 498–499*t*
  antimicrobial agents for, 495–498*t*
  antiparasitic agents for, 500–502*t*
  biologic data of, 519*t*
  blood glucose and sodium levels as prognostic indicators, 518*t*
  bronchoalveolar lavage in, 523*t*
  cerebrospinal fluid values in, 520*t*
  chemical restraint agents for, 503–511*t*
  clinical signs and behavioral changes used in assessment of pain in, 523–524*t*
  constant rate infusion (CRI) protocols for, 511*t*
  determining sex of mature, 521*t*
  drugs reported to be toxic in, 521–522*t*
  echocardiographic values in, 520–521*t*
  electrocardiographic values in, 520–521*t*
  hematologic values of, 517–518*t*
  miscellaneous agents for, 513–517*t*
  ophthalmologic agents for, 511–513*t*
  physiologic data of, 519*t*

Rabbits (*Continued*)
  sedative agents for, 503–511*t*
  serum biochemical values of, 517–518*t*
  with signs of upper respiratory disease, 524*t*
  suspected *Encephalitozoon cuniculi* infections in, 524*t*
  urinalysis values in, 519*t*
Radiated tortoise (*Astrochelys radiata*), hematologic and serum biochemical values of, 117–136*t*
Radiation therapy, for birds, 267–270*t*
Rafoxanide, for birds, 197–217*t*
Rainbow boa (*Epicrates cenchria*), hematologic and serum biochemical values of, 117–136*t*
Ranavirus, disinfectants for, 74*t*
Ranitidine
  for primates, 594–601*t*
  for rabbits, 513–517*t*
  for RGIS, 522–523*t*
  for rodents, 476–479*t*
Ranitidine bismuth citrate, for ferrets, 543–549*t*
Ranitidine HCl, for ferrets, 543–549*t*
Raptors
  biologic and physiologic values of, 309–310*t*
  hematologic and biochemical values of, 298–306*t*
  nutritional recommendations for rehabilitation of, 322*t*
  ophthalmic diagnostic tests in, 317*t*
Rat Guide, websites for owners of exotic animals, 650–653*t*
Rat snake (*Elaphe obsoleta*), hematologic and serum biochemical values of, 117–136*t*
Ratites
  biologic and physiologic values of, 307–308*t*
  hematologic and biochemical values of, 296*t*
Red-eared slider (*Trachemys scripta elegans*), environmental, dietary, and reproductive characteristics of, 137–138*t*
Red-footed tortoise (*Chelonoidis carbonaria*), hematologic and serum biochemical values of, 117–136*t*
Red-tailed hawk (*Buteo jamaicensis*), hematologic and biochemical values of, 298–306*t*
Regel PharmaLab, 661–662*t*
Rehabilitation, of wild birds, nutritional recommendations for, 322*t*
Releasing hormone, for amphibians, 65*t*
Replacement crystalloid solutions, for reptiles, 108–113*t*
Reproductive characteristics
  of reptiles, 137–138*t*
  of rodents, 484*t*
Reproductive tract infection, antimicrobial therapy for, 641–642*t*
Reptile Web, websites for owners of exotic animals, 650–653*t*
Reptiles, 81–166
  analgesic agents for, 104–106*t*
  anesthetic agents for, 93–103*t*
  antifungal agents for, 87–89*t*
  antimicrobial agents for, 82–86*t*
  antiparasitic agents for, 89–93*t*
  antiviral agents for, 86–87*t*
  chemical restraint agents for, 93–103*t*
  dystocia in, 142–143*t*

Reptiles (*Continued*)
 environmental, dietary, and reproductive characteristics of, 137–138t
 force-feeding anorectic or debilitated, 139–140t
 hematologic values of, 117–136t
 hormones and steroids for, 106–108t
 metabolic bone diseases in, 144–145t
 miscellaneous agents for, 113–116t
 nutritional/mineral/fluid support for, 108–113t
 serum biochemical values of, 117–136t
 source of diets and other commercial products for, 145–149t
 tracheal/pulmonary and colonic lavage for, 141t
 urinalysis values of, 139t
 venipuncture sites in, 141–142t
Research Associates Laboratory, 643–647t
Reserpine, for fish, 34–36t
Resorantel, for birds, 197–217t
Respiratory tract infection, antimicrobial therapy for, 641–642t
Resting respiratory rates, of birds, 316t
Reticulated python (*Python reticulatus*), hematologic and serum biochemical values of, 117–136t
Rhea (*Rhea* spp.)
 biologic and physiologic values of, 307–308t
 hematologic and biochemical values of, 296t
Ribavirin, for primates, 594–601t
Riboflavin, for backyard poultry and waterfowl, 408–409t
Rifabutin, for birds, 168–189t
Rifampicin, for birds, 168–189t
Rifampin
 for birds, 168–189t
 for primates, 576–580t
 for rabbits, 495–498t
Rifampin/pefloxacin, for birds, 270–271t
Rifampin/piperacillin, for birds, 270–271t
Ringer's solution
 amphibian, 65–67t
 for reptiles, 108–113t
Roadrunner Pharmacy, 661–662t
Robenidine HCl, for backyard poultry and waterfowl, 391–398t
Rocuronium, for reptiles, 93–103t
Rocuronium bromide, for birds, 263–267t
Rodents, 459–493
 analgesic agents for, 470–473t
 anesthetic agents for, 467–470t
 antifungal agents for, 460–463t
 antimicrobial agents for, 460–463t
 antiparasitic agents for, 464–466t
 biologic data of, 482t
 blood volumes with safe-bleeding volume recommendations in, 483t
 cardiovascular agents for, 473–474t
 chemical restraint agents for, 467–470t
 common and scientific names of, 480t
 disease testing in, 486–487t
 echocardiographic measurements in, 488t
 electrocardiographic measurements in, 488t
 emergency drugs for, 474–475t
 endocrine values in, 487t
 hematologic values of, 481t
 miscellaneous agents for, 476–479t
 nutritional data for, 485t

Rodents (*Continued*)
 physiologic data of, 482t
 reproductive data for, 484t
 serum biochemical values of, 481t
 sex determination of, 485t
 urinalysis reference values of, 483t
 zoonotic diseases in, 485–486t
Romark, for ferrets, 533–534t
Ronidazole
 for amphibians, 58–60t
 for birds, 197–217t
 for rodents, 464–466t
Ronnel, for primates, 580–585t
Ropivacaine, for backyard poultry and waterfowl, 399–403t
Rosuvastatin, for birds, 275–283t
Rosy boa (*Lichanura trivirgata*), hematologic and serum biochemical values of, 117–136t
Routes of administration, of birds, 319t
Routine prophylactic care, for ferrets, 552t
Russian tortoise (*Testudo horsfieldii*)
 environmental, dietary, and reproductive characteristics of, 137–138t
 hematologic and serum biochemical values of, 117–136t

S

S-Adenosylmethionine (SAM-e)
 for ferrets, 543–549t
 for primates, 594–601t
 for reptiles, 113–116t
 for rodents, 476–479t
Safe-bleeding volume recommendations, in rodents, 483t
Saline
 hypertonic, for rodents, 474–475t
 for wild mammals, 629–631t
Salmonella spp., antimicrobial agents for, 639–640t
Salt
 for amphibians, 58–60t
 for fish, 25–30t, 34–36t
Sand boa (*Eryx* sp.), environmental, dietary, and reproductive characteristics of, 137–138t
Sarafloxacin
 for backyard poultry and waterfowl, 377–389t
 for fish, 17–24t
Satureja montana (winter savory extract), for invertebrates, 2–4t
Savannah monitor (*Varanus exanthematicus*), hematologic and serum biochemical values of, 117–136t
Save Way Pharmacy, 661–662t
Saw palmetto, for ferrets, 543–549t
Seawater, for fish, 25–30t
Sedative agents, for rabbits, 503–511t
Selamectin
 for amphibians, 58–60t
 for birds, 197–217t
 for ferrets, 535–536t
 for hedgehogs, 446t
 for rabbits, 500–502t
 for rodents, 464–466t
 for sugar gliders, 433–434t

Selenium
  for birds, 258–263t
  for reptiles, 108–113t
Senegal parrot (*Poicephalus senegalus*)
  hematologic and biochemical values of, 284–292t
  T_4 values of, 315t
Septicemia, antimicrobial therapy for, 641–642t
Serological tests, for backyard poultry and waterfowl, 417–418t
Serum biochemical values
  of Anseriformes, 413t
  of Columbiformes, 297–298t
  of ferrets, 549–550t
  of fish, 37–44t
  of Galliformes, 412t
  of hedgehogs, 451t
  of miniature pigs, 569t
  of Passeriformes, 295t
  of primates, 602–603t
  of Psittaciformes, 284–292t
  of rabbits, 517–518t
  of raptors, 298–306t
  of ratites, 296t
  of reptiles, 117–136t
  of rodents, 481t
  of sugar gliders, 437t
Sevelamer, for rabbits, 513–517t
Sevoflurane
  for amphibians, 60–64t
  for backyard poultry and waterfowl, 399–403t
  for birds, 218–236t
  for ferrets, 536–539t
  for hedgehogs, 447–448t
  for invertebrates, 6–9t
  for miniature pigs, 561–565t
  for primates, 586–594t
  for rabbits, 503–511t
  for reptiles, 93–103t
  for rodents, 467–470t
  for sugar gliders, 434–435t
Sex determination, of rodents, 485t
Sharp-shinned hawk (*Accipiter striatus*)
  biologic and physiologic values of, 309–310t
  hematologic and biochemical values of, 298–306t
Short-eared owl (*Asio flammeus*), hematologic and biochemical values of, 298–306t
Sick wildlife, care of, 617–619t
Sildenafil, for birds, 275–283t
Sildenafil citrate, for rodents, 476–479t
Silver sulfadiazine cream
  for birds, 168–195t
  for fish, 17–24t
  for invertebrates, 2–4t
  for rabbits, 495–498t
  for reptiles, 82–86t
Silymarin
  for birds, 196–197t, 267–270t, 275–283t
  for rabbits, 513–517t
  for rodents, 476–479t
Simethicone
  for rabbits, 513–517t
  for RGIS, 522–523t
  for wild mammals, 631–632t
Skin infection, antimicrobial therapy for, 641–642t
Skin-So-Soft (Avon), for birds, 275–283t

Sliders (*Trachemys scripta* spp.), hematologic and serum biochemical values of, 117–136t
Snakes
  environmental, dietary, and reproductive characteristics of, 137–138t
  tracheal/pulmonary and colonic lavage for, 141t
  venipuncture sites in, 141–142t
Snowy owl (*Bubo scandiaca*)
  biologic and physiologic values of, 309–310t
  hematologic and biochemical values of, 298–306t
Soderlund Village Drug, 661–662t
Sodium benzoate, for birds, 189–195t, 275–283t
Sodium bicarbonate
  for birds, 272–274t
  for fish, 31–33t
  for rabbits, 513–517t
  for reptiles, 113–116t
Sodium bicarbonate tablets
  for fish, 31–33t
  for invertebrates, 6–9t
Sodium chloride
  for amphibians, 56–60t
  for birds, 246–248t, 258–263t
  for fish, 25–30t, 34–36t
  for reptiles, 108–113t
Sodium pentobarbital, for invertebrates, 6–9t
Sodium sulfate, for birds, 248–252t
Sodium tetradecyl sulfate, for birds, 275–283t
Sodium thiosulfate
  for amphibians, 65–67t
  for fish, 34–36t
  for invertebrates, 9–10t
Soft-tissue infection, antimicrobial therapy for, 641–642t
Somatostatin, for birds, 240–245t
Songbirds, nutritional recommendations for rehabilitation of, 322t
Species 360, 648–650t
Spectinomycin
  for backyard poultry and waterfowl, 377–389t
  for birds, 168–189t, 246–248t
  for miniature pigs, 559–560t
  for rabbits, 495–498t
Spectinomycin sulfate tetrahydrate, for backyard poultry and waterfowl, 377–389t
Spectral Doppler echocardiographic reference intervals, in birds, 333t
Spiny-tailed lizard (*Uromastyx* spp.), hematologic and serum biochemical values of, 117–136t
Spiramycin
  for birds, 168–189t
  for hedgehogs, 444–445t
  for reptiles, 89–93t
Spironolactone
  for birds, 275–283t
  for primates, 594–601t
STA solution, for birds, 189–195t
Stanozolol
  for primates, 594–601t
  for rabbits, 513–517t
  for reptiles, 106–108t
Staphylococcus spp., antimicrobial agents for, 639–640t
Stark Pharmacy, 661–662t
Sterile water, for birds, 246–248t
Steroids

INDEX 697

Steroids (Continued)
  for backyard poultry and waterfowl, 399–403t
  for birds, 240–245t
  for reptiles, 106–108t
Streptococcus spp., antimicrobial agents for, 639–640t
Streptomycin
  for backyard poultry and waterfowl, 377–389t
  for birds, 168–189t
  for primates, 576–580t
  for reptiles, 82–86t
Strontium (Sr-90), for birds, 267–270t
Succimer (DMSA)
  for birds, 248–252t
  for rabbits, 513–517t
Succinylcholine, for reptiles, 93–103t
Sucralfate
  for birds, 275–283t
  for ferrets, 543–549t
  for hedgehogs, 449–450t
  for primates, 594–601t
  for rabbits, 513–517t
  for reptiles, 113–116t
  for rodents, 476–479t
  for wild mammals, 631–632t
Sugar gliders, 432–442
  analgesic agents for, 435t
  anesthetic agents for, 434–435t
  antifungal agents for, 433t
  antimicrobial agents for, 433t
  antiparasitic agents for, 433–434t
  biologic values of, 438t
  chemical restraint agents for, 434–435t
  dietary components for, 439–440t
  feed estimates for hand-rearing, 441t
  growth and development of, 439t
  hematologic values of, 437t
  miscellaneous agents for, 436t
  physiologic values of, 438t
  serum biochemical values of, 437t
  suggested diets for, 440t
  urinalysis values of, 438t
Sugarglider web site, 650–653t
Sulfachlorpyrazine, for birds, 197–217t
Sulfachlorpyridazine
  for backyard poultry and waterfowl, 391–398t
  for birds, 168–189t, 197–217t
Sulfachlorpyridazine/trimethoprim, for backyard poultry and waterfowl, 377–389t
Sulfadiazine
  for amphibians, 54–55t, 58–60t
  for backyard poultry and waterfowl, 377–389t, 391–398t
  for primates, 580–585t
  for reptiles, 82–86t, 89–93t
Sulfadimethoxine
  for backyard poultry and waterfowl, 377–389t, 391–398t
  for birds, 168–189t, 197–217t, 246–248t
  for ferrets, 533–536t
  for hedgehogs, 444–446t
  for invertebrates, 2–4t
  for miniature pigs, 561t
  for primates, 576–585t
  for rabbits, 495–498t, 500–502t
  for reptiles, 82–86t, 89–93t

Sulfadimethoxine (Continued)
  for rodents, 464–466t
  for wild mammals, 625–626t
Sulfadimethoxine/ormetoprim
  for fish, 17–24t
  for invertebrates, 2–4t
Sulfadimidine
  for hedgehogs, 446t
  for reptiles, 89–93t
Sulfadimidine sodium, for birds, 197–217t
Sulfamerazine
  for rabbits, 500–502t
  for reptiles, 89–93t
  for rodents, 464–466t
Sulfamethazine
  for amphibians, 54–55t, 58–60t
  for backyard poultry and waterfowl, 377–389t, 391–398t
  for birds, 197–217t
  for ferrets, 533–534t
  for rabbits, 495–498t, 500–502t
  for reptiles, 89–93t
  for rodents, 464–466t
Sulfamethoxazole
  for backyard poultry and waterfowl, 377–389t, 391–398t
  for reptiles, 82–86t
  for sugar gliders, 433t
Sulfamethoxazole/trimethoprim, for invertebrates, 2–4t
Sulfamethoxine, for rabbits, 500–502t
Sulfamethoxypyrazine, for rodents, 464–466t
Sulfaquinoxaline
  for backyard poultry and waterfowl, 377–389t, 391–398t
  for birds, 197–217t
  for rabbits, 495–498t, 500–502t
  for reptiles, 89–93t
  for rodents, 464–466t
Sulfasalazine, for rabbits, 513–517t
Sulfasoxazole, for ferrets, 533–534t
Sulfathalidine, for ferrets, 533–534t
Sulfonamides
  for birds, 197–217t
  for exotic animal medicine, 637–638t
  for rodents, 460–463t
Sulpiride, for primates, 594–601t
Supportive care procedures, in companion bird medicine
System of International (SI) units conversion factors
  of clinical chemistries, 660t
  of hematology, 659t

T

T_4 values, of birds, 315t
Tamoxifen, for reptiles, 113–116t
Tamoxifen citrate
  for backyard poultry and waterfowl, 406t
  for birds, 240–245t
Tannic acid, for birds, 258–263t
Tapentadol, for reptiles, 104–106t
Taurine, for rodents, 470–474t
Taylor Drug, 661–662t
Tea, for birds, 248–252t, 258–263t
^{99m}Technetium-diethylenetriaminepenta-acetic acid, for birds, 275–283t

^{99m}Technetium-disofenin, for birds, 275–283t
^{99m}Technetium-mebrofenin, for birds, 275–283t
Tegu lizard (*Tupinambis* spp.), hematologic and serum biochemical values of, 117–136t
Telmisartan, for primates, 594–601t
Temperature elevation, for amphibians, 56–57t
Tepoxalin, for backyard poultry and waterfowl, 404–405t
Terbinafine
    for birds, 189–195t, 246–248t
    for hedgehogs, 445t
    for rabbits, 498–499t, 511–513t
    for reptiles, 87–89t
    for rodents, 460–463t
    for wild mammals, 626t
Terbinafine hydrochloride, for amphibians, 56–57t
Terbutaline
    for birds, 246–248t, 272–283t
    for ferrets, 540–541t
    for primates, 594–601t
    for reptiles, 113–116t
    for rodents, 476–479t
Testosterone, for birds, 240–245t
Tetanus antitoxin, for birds, 248–252t
Tetracaine, for birds, 263–267t
Tetracycline
    for amphibians, 54–55t, 58–60t
    for backyard poultry and waterfowl, 377–389t
    for birds, 168–189t
    for exotic animal medicine, 637–638t
    for ferrets, 533–534t
    for invertebrates, 2–4t
    for miniature pigs, 559–560t
    for primates, 576–585t
    for rabbits, 495–498t
    for rodents, 460–463t
Tetracycline/furaltadone, for birds, 197–217t
Texas Veterinary Medical Diagnostic Laboratory, 643–647t
The Colyer Institute, 648–650t
The Humane Society, 648–650t
The Lizard Lounge, websites for owners of exotic animals, 650–653t
The Merck Veterinary Manual, 648–650t
Theophylline
    for birds, 275–283t
    for ferrets, 540–541t
    for hedgehogs, 449–450t
    for primates, 594–601t
    for rodents, 476–479t
Theophylline elixir, for ferrets, 543–549t
Therapeutic agent, for fish, 34–36t
Thermal support, for RGIS, 522–523t
Thiabendazole
    for amphibians, 58–60t
    for backyard poultry and waterfowl, 391–398t
    for birds, 197–217t
    for ferrets, 535–536t
    for fish, 25–30t
    for hedgehogs, 444–445t
    for primates, 580–585t
    for rabbits, 500–502t
    for reptiles, 89–93t
    for rodents, 464–466t
Thiafentanil oxalate/medetomidine, for birds, 218–236t

Thiamazole, for rodents, 476–479t
Thiamine
    for backyard poultry and waterfowl, 408–409t
    for birds, 258–263t, 272t
    for rodents, 476–479t
Thiamphenicol, for fish, 17–24t
Thiamylal
    for miniature pigs, 561–565t
    for rabbits, 503–511t
Thiamylal sodium, for primates, 586–594t
Thiopental
    for primates, 586–594t
    for rabbits, 503–511t
    for reptiles, 93–103t
Thiostrepton, for hedgehogs, 444–445t
Thymol, for invertebrates, 5–6t
Thyroid releasing hormone, for birds, 240–245t
Thyroid-stimulating hormone (TSH)
    for birds, 240–245t
    for ferrets, 543–549t
    for rodents, 476–479t
Thyroxine, for ferrets, 543–549t
Tiamulin
    for backyard poultry and waterfowl, 377–389t
    for birds, 168–189t
Tiamulin/chlortetracycline, 377–389t
Ticarcillin
    for birds, 168–189t
    for reptiles, 82–86t
Ticarcillin/clavulanate
    for birds, 168–189t
    for primates, 576–580t
Tiletamine
    for backyard poultry and waterfowl, 399–403t
    for rabbits, 503–511t
    for rodents, 467–470t
    for sugar gliders, 434–435t
Tiletamine/zolazepam
    for amphibians, 60–64t
    for birds, 218–236t
    for ferrets, 536–539t
    for hedgehogs, 447–448t
    for miniature pigs, 561–565t
    for primates, 586–594t
    for reptiles, 93–103t
Tiletamine/zolazepam/dexmedetomidine/butorphanol, for ferrets, 536–539t
Tiletamine/zolazepam/ketamine/xylazine, for miniature pigs, 561–565t
Tiletamine-zolazepam/medetomidine, for primates, 586–594t
Tiletamine/zolazepam/xylazine
    for ferrets, 536–539t
    for miniature pigs, 561–565t
Tiletamine/zolazepam/xylazine/butorphanol
    for ferrets, 536–539t
    for miniature pigs, 561–565t
Tilmicosin
    for backyard poultry and waterfowl, 377–389t
    for birds, 168–189t
    for primates, 576–580t
    for rabbits, 495–498t
Timolol, for rabbits, 511–513t
Tincture of iodine, for birds, 275–283t
Tinidazole

Tinidazole (*Continued*)
    for backyard poultry and waterfowl, 391–398*t*
    for primates, 580–585*t*
    for rodents, 464–466*t*
Tissue plasminogen activator (rTPA), for birds, 263–267*t*
Tobramycin
    for backyard poultry and waterfowl, 377–389*t*
    for birds, 168–189*t*, 263–267*t*, 270–271*t*
    for fish, 17–24*t*
    for rabbits, 495–498*t*, 511–513*t*
    for reptiles, 82–86*t*
Toco toucan (*Ramphastos toco*), hematologic and biochemical values of, 297–298*t*
Tolazoline HCl, for birds, 218–236*t*
Tolbutamine, for primates, 594–601*t*
Tolfenamic acid, for rodents, 470–473*t*
Tolnaftate, for reptiles, 87–89*t*
Toltrazuril
    for backyard poultry and waterfowl, 391–398*t*
    for birds, 197–217*t*
    for hedgehogs, 446*t*
    for primates, 580–585*t*
    for rabbits, 500–502*t*
    for reptiles, 89–93*t*
    for rodents, 464–466*t*
Toremifene, for rodents, 476–479*t*
Tortoise Trust, websites for owners of exotic animals, 650–653*t*
Toxic drugs, in rabbits, 521–522*t*
Toxicologic conditions, of birds, agents for, 248–252*t*
Tracheal lavage, for reptiles, 141*t*
Tramadol
    for ferrets, 539–540*t*
    for hedgehogs, 448–449*t*
    for miniature pigs, 566–567*t*
    for primates, 586–594*t*
    for rabbits, 503–511*t*
    for reptiles, 104–106*t*
    for rodents, 470–473*t*
    for wild mammals, 628–629*t*
Tramadol HCl
    for backyard poultry and waterfowl, 399–403*t*
    for birds, 218–236*t*
Tri-State Compounding Pharmacy, 661–662*t*
Triamcinolone
    for birds, 263–267*t*
    for hedgehogs, 444–445*t*, 448–449*t*
    for primates, 594–601*t*
Tricaine methanesulfonate
    for amphibians, 60–64*t*
    for fish, 31–33*t*, 36–37*t*
    for invertebrates, 6–9*t*
    for reptiles, 113–116*t*
Trichlorfon (dimethyl phosphonate), for fish, 25–30*t*
Trientine, for ferrets, 543–549*t*
Trifluralin, for invertebrates, 2–4*t*
Trilostane
    for birds, 275–283*t*
    for ferrets, 542–543*t*
    for hedgehogs, 449–450*t*
    for rodents, 476–479*t*
Trimebutine, for RGIS, 522–523*t*

Trimethoprim
    for backyard poultry and waterfowl, 377–389*t*, 391–398*t*
    for birds, 168–189*t*
    for exotic animal medicine, 637–638*t*
    for ferrets, 533–534*t*
    for rodents, 460–463*t*
    for sugar gliders, 433*t*
Trimethoprim/sulfadiazine
    for amphibians, 54–55*t*
    for birds, 168–189*t*, 197–217*t*
    for miniature pigs, 559–560*t*
    for primates, 576–580*t*
    for reptiles, 82–86*t*
    for wild mammals, 623–625*t*
Trimethoprim/sulfamethoxazole
    for amphibians, 54–55*t*, 58–60*t*
    for birds, 168–189*t*, 197–217*t*
    for fish, 17–24*t*
    for hedgehogs, 444–445*t*
    for primates, 576–585*t*
    for rabbits, 495–498*t*
    for reptiles, 89–93*t*
Triple antibiotic ointment, for fish, 17–24*t*
Tris EDTA (Tricide-Neo, Molecular Therapeutics), for invertebrates, 2–4*t*
Trissel's Stability of Compounded Formulations, 5th ed, 663*t*
Tropicamide, for rabbits, 511–513*t*
Trovafloxacin, for rabbits, 511–513*t*
Trypsin-balsam of Peru castor oil, for birds, 275–283*t*
d-Tubocurarine, for birds, 263–267*t*
Tufts University Open Courseware, Zoological Medicine Course, 648–650*t*
Tulathromycin, for miniature pigs, 559–560*t*
Turkey vulture (*Cathartes aura*)
    biologic and physiologic values of, 309–310*t*
    hematologic and biochemical values of, 298–306*t*
Tylosin
    for backyard poultry and waterfowl, 377–389*t*, 406–407*t*
    for birds, 168–189*t*, 246–248*t*, 263–267*t*
    for ferrets, 533–534*t*
    for hedgehogs, 444–445*t*
    for invertebrates, 2–4*t*
    for miniature pigs, 559–560*t*
    for primates, 576–580*t*
    for rabbits, 495–498*t*
    for reptiles, 82–86*t*
    for rodents, 460–463*t*
    for wild mammals, 623–625*t*
Tyrode's solution, for birds, 275–283*t*

U

Umbrella cockatoo (*Cacatua alba*), hematologic and biochemical values of, 293–294*t*
University of Pennsylvania Computer Aided Learning, 648–650*t*
Urate oxidase, for birds, 275–283*t*
Urinalysis values
    of birds, 316*t*
    of ferrets, 551*t*
    of miniature pigs, 570*t*
    of rabbits, 519*t*

Urinalysis values (*Continued*)
  of reptiles, 139*t*
  of rodents, 483*t*
  of sugar gliders, 438*t*
Urinary tract infection, antimicrobial therapy for, 641–642*t*
Uromastyx species, environmental, dietary, and reproductive characteristics of, 137–138*t*
Ursodeoxycholic acid, for birds, 275–283*t*
Ursodiol, for ferrets, 543–549*t*
U.S. Pharmacopeial Convention, 663*t*
US Compounding Pharmacy, 661–662*t*
USDA APHIS, 648–650*t*
UVA/UVB, for reptiles, with metabolic bone diseases, 144–145*t*

V

Vaccinations
  for backyard poultry and waterfowl, 421–422*t*
  for birds, 328–329*t*
  for ferrets, 552*t*
  for miniature pigs, 571–572*t*
Valacyclovir, for reptiles, 86–87*t*
Valley Drug and Compounding Pharmacy, 661–662*t*
Valley Prescription and Compounding Pharmacy, 661–662*t*
Vancomycin
  for primates, 576–580*t*
  for rabbits, 495–498*t*, 511–513*t*
  for rodents, 460–463*t*
Vasopressin, for birds, 272–274*t*
Vecuronium bromide, for birds, 263–267*t*
Vecuronium/nitrous oxide/isoflurane, for birds, 263–267*t*
Vegetable oil, for birds, 275–283*t*
Veiled chameleon (*Chameleo calyptratus*)
  environmental, dietary, and reproductive characteristics of, 137–138*t*
  hematologic and serum biochemical values of, 117–136*t*
Venipuncture sites
  in hedgehogs, 453–454*t*
  in reptiles, 141–142*t*
Verapamil
  for rabbits, 513–517*t*
  for rodents, 470–474*t*
Vetark Professional Critical Care Formula (CCF) powder, for anorectic or debilitated reptiles, 139–140*t*
Veterinarians
  exotic animal online resources for, 648–650*t*
  professional associations for, 648*t*
Veterinary Feed Directive (VFD) Order Information, 416*t*
Veterinary Information Network, 648–650*t*
Veterinary Medical Diagnostic Lab College of Veterinary Medicine, 643–647*t*
Veterinary Molecular Diagnostics, Inc., 643–647*t*
Veterinary Partner, 648–650*t*
Vincristine
  for ferrets, 543–549*t*
  for reptiles, 113–116*t*
Vincristine sulfate
  for backyard poultry and waterfowl, 410*t*
  for birds, 267–270*t*

Vinegar, for birds, 189–195*t*, 275–283*t*
Virginiamycin, for backyard poultry and waterfowl, 377–389*t*
Vitamin A
  for amphibians, 65–67*t*
  for birds, 258–263*t*
  for ferrets, 543–549*t*
  for hedgehogs, 449–450*t*
  for rabbits, 513–517*t*
  for reptiles, 108–113*t*
  for rodents, 476–479*t*
  for sugar gliders, 436*t*
Vitamin B complex
  for birds, 258–263*t*
  for ferrets, 543–549*t*
  for hedgehogs, 449–450*t*
  for rabbits, 513–517*t*
  for reptiles, 108–113*t*
  for RGIS, 522–523*t*
  for rodents, 476–479*t*
  for sugar gliders, 436*t*
  for wild mammals, 631–632*t*
Vitamin B_1
  for amphibians, 65–67*t*
  for birds, 258–263*t*, 272*t*
  for reptiles, 108–113*t*
Vitamin B_{12}
  for backyard poultry and waterfowl, 408–409*t*
  for birds, 258–263*t*
  for primates, 594–601*t*
  for reptiles, 108–113*t*
Vitamin C
  for backyard poultry and waterfowl, 408–409*t*
  for birds, 258–263*t*
  for ferrets, 543–549*t*
  for hedgehogs, 449–450*t*
  for primates, 594–601*t*
  for rabbits, 513–517*t*
  for reptiles, 108–113*t*
  for rodents, 476–479*t*
Vitamin D, for rodents, 476–479*t*
Vitamin D_3
  for amphibians, 65–67*t*
  for backyard poultry and waterfowl, 408–409*t*
  for birds, 258–263*t*
  for primates, 594–601*t*
  for reptiles, 108–113*t*
  with metabolic bone diseases, 144–145*t*
Vitamin E
  for amphibians, 65–67*t*
  for backyard poultry and waterfowl, 408–409*t*
  for birds, 258–263*t*
  for primates, 594–601*t*
  for reptiles, 108–113*t*
  for rodents, 476–479*t*
  for sugar gliders, 436*t*
Vitamin E/γ-linolenic acid, for birds, 258–263*t*
Vitamin K
  for ferrets, 543–549*t*
  for rabbits, 513–517*t*
  for sugar gliders, 436*t*
Vitamin K_1
  for backyard poultry and waterfowl, 408–409*t*
  for birds, 248–252*t*, 258–263*t*
  for primates, 594–601*t*

Vitamin K₁ (*Continued*)
  for reptiles, 108–113t
  for rodents, 476–479t
Vocalizations, in hedgehogs, 454t
Voriconazole
  for amphibians, 56–57t
  for backyard poultry and waterfowl, 390t
  for birds, 189–195t, 246–248t
  for rabbits, 498–499t, 511–513t
  for reptiles, 87–89t
  for wild mammals, 626t
Voriconazole/F10 super concentrate disinfectant, for reptiles, 87–89t

W
Water
  consumption rate, for backyard poultry and waterfowl, 420t
  for reptiles, 89–93t
Water dragon (*Physignathus cocincinus*), environmental, dietary, and reproductive characteristics of, 137–138t
Water monitor (*Varanus salvator*), hematologic and serum biochemical values of, 117–136t
Weasel Words, websites for owners of exotic animals, 650–653t
Wedgewood Pharmacy, 661–662t
Weight conversions, 658t
Westlab Pharmacy, 661–662t
Wild bird rehabilitation, selected nutritional recommendations for, 416t
Wild rodents. *See* Rodents
Wildlife, 616–635
  mammals in
    analgesic and nonsteroidal antiinflammatory agents for, 628–629t
    antifungal agents for, 626t
    antimicrobial agents for, 623–625t
    antiparasitic agents for, 625–626t
    chemical restraint/anesthetic agents for, 627–628t
    emergencies in, agents for, 629–631t
    miscellaneous agents for, 631–632t
    meat withdrawal times and, 623t
    policy in private practice, considerations for, 619–620t
    safe restraint of, recommendations for, 620–622t
    sick, injured, or orphaned, checklist for care of, 617–619t
    venipuncture sites in, recommendations for, 622t
Winstrol, for primates, 594–601t
Winter savory extract (*Satureja montana*), for invertebrates, 2–4t
Wisconsin Veterinary Diagnostic Laboratory, 643–647t
Wood turtle (*Glyptemys insculpta*), hematologic and serum biochemical values of, 117–136t
World Chelonian Trust, websites for owners of exotic animals, 650–653t
World Organization for Animal Health (OIE), 648–650t
World Parrot Trust, websites for owners of exotic animals, 650–653t

X
Xylazine
  for backyard poultry and waterfowl, 399–403t
  for birds, 218–236t
  for ferrets, 536–539t
  for hedgehogs, 447–448t
  for invertebrates, 6–9t
  for miniature pigs, 561–565t
  for primates, 586–594t
  for rabbits, 503–511t
  for reptiles, 93–103t
  for rodents, 467–470t
  for sugar gliders, 434–435t
Xylazine/butorphanol, for birds, 218–236t
Xylazine/butorphanol/midazolam, for miniature pigs, 561–565t

Y
Yakim's Compounding Pharmacy, 661–662t
Yeast, for ferrets, 543–549t
Yeast cell derivatives, for birds, 275–283t
Yohimbine
  for ferrets, 536–539t
  for hedgehogs, 447–448t
  for miniature pigs, 561–565t
  for primates, 586–594t
  for rabbits, 503–511t
  for reptiles, 93–103t
  for rodents, 467–470t
  for sugar gliders, 434–435t
Yohimbine HCl
  for backyard poultry and waterfowl, 399–403t
  for birds, 218–236t

Z
Zanamivir, for ferrets, 543–549t
Zeolite
  for fish, 34–36t
  for invertebrates, 9–10t
Zinc, for primates, 594–601t
Zolazepam
  for backyard poultry and waterfowl, 399–403t
  for rabbits, 503–511t
  for rodents, 467–470t
  for sugar gliders, 434–435t
Zonisamide, for birds, 253–257t
Zoo/Exotic Pathology Service, 643–647t
Zoo Medicine Service, 643–647t
Zoologix, Inc, 643–647t
Zoonotic diseases
  carried by hedgehogs, 454t
  in rodents, 485–486t
Zuclopenthixol, for primates, 586–601t